Respiratory Care Equipment

Respiratory Care Equipment

Richard D. Branson, RRT
Assistant Professor of Surgery
Division of Trauma and Critical Care
Department of Surgery
University of Cincinnati Medical Center
Cincinnati, Ohio

Dean R. Hess, PhD, RRT
Instructor in Anesthesia
Harvard Medical School
Assistant Director of Respiratory Care
Massachusetts General Hospital
Boston, Massachusetts

Robert L. Chatburn, RRT
Director of Pediatric Respiratory Care
Rainbow Babies and Children's Hospital
Clinical Instructor in Pediatrics
Case Western Reserve University
Cleveland, Ohio

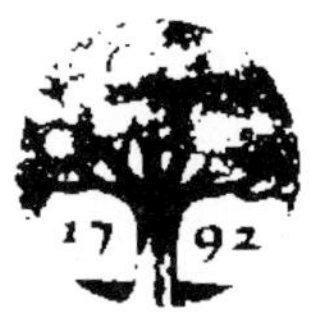

J.B. LIPPINCOTT COMPANY
Philadelphia

Sponsoring Editor: Andrew M. Allen
Coordinating Editorial Assistant: Laura W. Dover
Project Editor: Karen S. Huffman
Indexer: Katherine Pitcoff
Design Coordinator: Doug Smock
Interior Designer: Holly Reid McLaughlin
Cover Designer: Louis Fuiano
Production Manager: Helen Ewan
Production Coordinator: Nannette Winski
Compositor: Graphic Sciences Corporation
Printer/Binder: Courier Book Company, Westford
Cover Printer: Lehigh Press

6 5 4 3 2

∞This paper meets the requirements of ANSI/NISO Z39,48–1992 (Permanence of paper).

Library of Congress Cataloging in Publications Data
Respiratory care equipment / [edited by] Richard D. Branson, Dean R. Hess, Robert L. Chatburn.
p. cm.
Includes bibliographical references and index.
ISBN 0-397-54995-4
1. Respiratory therapy—Equipment and supplies. 2. Respiratory intensive care—Equipment and supplies. I. Branson, Richard D. II. Hess, Dean R. III. Chatburn, Robert L.
[DNLM: 1. Respiratory Therapy—instrumentation. WF 26 R4322 1995]
RC735.I5R4728 1995
681′.761—dc20
DNLM/DLC
for Library of Congress 94-22641
CIP

Any procedure or practice described in this book should be applied by the healthcare practitioner under appropriate supervision in accordance with professional standards of care used with regard to the unique circumstances that apply in each practice situation. Care has been taken to confirm the accuracy of information presented and to describe generally accepted practices. However, the authors, editors, and publisher cannot accept any responsibility for errors or omissions or for any consequences from application of the information in this book and make no warranty express or implied, with respect to the contents of the book.

Every effort has been made to ensure drug selections and dosages are in accordance with current recommendations and practice. Because of ongoing research, changes in government regulations and the constant flow of information on drug therapy, reactions and interactions, the reader is cautioned to check the package insert for each drug for indications, dosages, warnings and precautions, particularly if the drug is new or infrequently used.

To Captain S.K. Branson, USMC (ret) and Lois Lee Branson, RN,
for their love, example, and sacrifice,
all of which become clearer with the passage of time.
RICHARD D. BRANSON

For Susan, Terri, and Lauren—
thanks for your support; and for all of the instructors,
students, patients, therapists, physicians, and nurses
who have influenced my career for the past twenty years.
DEAN HESS

To my daughters, Maya and Kendra,
and to those rare individuals who know that knowledge
is no substitute for wisdom.
ROBERT L. CHATBURN

CONTRIBUTORS

Michael J. Banner, PHD, RRT
Associate Professor of Anesthesiology and Physiology
Director, Anesthesiology Research Laboratories
University of Florida College of Medicine
Gainesville, Florida

Richard D. Branson, RRT
Assistant Professor of Surgery
Division of Trauma and Critical Care
Department of Surgery
University of Cincinnati Medical Center
Cincinnati, Ohio

Robert L. Chatburn, RRT
Director of Pediatric Respiratory Care
Rainbow Babies and Children's Hospital
Clinical Instructor in Pediatrics
Case Western Reserve University
Cleveland, Ohio

David A. Desautels, MPA, RRT
Administrative Director
Wound and Hyperbaric Center
St. Joseph's Hospital
Tampa, Florida

Vijay M. Deshpande, MS, RRT
Assistant Professor
Department of Cardiopulmonary Care Services
Georgia State University
Atlanta, Georgia

F. Herbert Douce, MS, RRT, RPFT
Assistant Professor and Director
Respiratory Therapy Division
School of Allied Medical Professions
The Ohio State University
Columbus, Ohio

Robert R. Fluck, Jr., MS, RRT
Associate Professor and Clinical Coordinator
Department of Respiratory Care and Cardiorespiratory Sciences
SUNY, Health Science Center
Syracuse, New York

Ann Grahm, CRNA
Formerly Nurse Consultant
Food and Drug Administration
Silver Springs, Maryland

John M. Graybeal, CRTT
Research Assistant in Neuroanesthesia
Department of Anesthesia
Penn State University
Hershey, Pennsylvania

Dean R. Hess, PHD, RRT
Instructor in Anesthesia, Harvard Medical School
Assistant Director of Respiratory Care, Massachusetts General Hospital
Boston, Massachusetts

Robert M. Kacmarek, PHD, RRT
Assistant Professor of Anesthesia, Harvard Medical School
Director of Respiratory Care, Massachusetts General Hospital
Boston, Massachusetts

Samsun Lampotang, PHD
Assistant Professor of Anesthesiology and Mechanical Engineering
University of Florida College of Medicine
Gainesville, Florida

Robert Langenderfer, MED, RRT
Assistant Professor of Respiratory Care Program
Northern Kentucky University
Highland Heights, Kentucky

Christopher Maxwell, BA, MGA, RRT
Vice President, Ancillary Services
Community General Osteopathic Hospital
Harrisburg, Pennsylvania

Robert F. Moran, MS, PHD, FCCM, FAIC
Senior Technical Liaison
Ciba-Corning Diagnostics Corporation
Medfield, Massachusetts

Dennis A. Silage, PHD
Professor of Electrical Engineering
Department of Electrical Engineering
College of Engineering and Architecture
Temple University
Philadelphia, Pennsylvania

Mark L. Simmons, MSED, RRT, RPFT
Program Director
School of Respiratory Therapy
York Hospital
York, Pennsylvania

FOREWORD

All heath care givers recognize the importance of understanding human anatomy, physiology, and pathology. The importance of thoroughly understanding medical equipment and supplies, however, is less recognized. Often it is assumed that knowledge about equipment is much less important than knowledge about patients.

But, wait a minute! A medical device also has its anatomy, physiology, and potential pathologies. Furthermore, many devices are extensions of patients and must not be considered separately from them. A mechanical ventilator is an excellent example. In essence, it is an extension of the patient's own lung. Like the patient's lung, the ventilator can be looked at from the viewpoints of anatomy (structure), physiology (function), and pathology (operational problems). The more dependent a patient is on mechanical ventilation, the more important it is that the ventilator's "anatomy" be correct (eg, it has the right size tubing to ventilate an infant), that its "physiology" be appropriate (eg, it can support an apneic patient), and that its potential "pathologies" (eg, disconnections in the gas-delivery system) be anticipated, recognized, and treated if they occur.

Some medical devices, then, are clearly extensions of patients. Others are extensions of caregivers. The stethoscope is an obvious example, serving to augment the clinician's ears. Some devices are extensions of both the patient and the caregiver. The mechanical ventilator, referred to above as an extension of the patient's lung, is also an extension of the clinician, who uses his mind and hands to regulate it to affect the lung.

To use another analogy, think of the old adage that a chain is only as strong as its weakest link. What that really says is that every link must be adequately strong. When it comes to the medical equipment in the chains of therapy or diagnosis, two possible weak links must be kept in mind. One weak link is equipment or supplies that are not adequate for the job; the other is a caregiver who either lacks knowledge about the equipment or fails to use his or her knowledge.

The value of this book is that it can prepare the willing reader to be a strong link in respiratory care that involves equipment and supplies; this includes nearly every respiratory care procedure. The aspects of pulmonary care that do not require equipment—such as some forms of chest physiotherapy—are rare.

The anatomy of human beings does not visibly change in a clinician's lifetime, whereas several generations of ventilators, oximeters, resuscitators, and the like are almost certain to appear in any 10-year, or even 5-year, era of medical care. With this *changing* "anatomy" comes new or altered aspects of the "physiology" of the devices in question. And, despite new vigilance, advancing technology does not come without its own "pathology." Therefore, in a sense, the respiratory care practitioner has one of the most challenging situations in all of health care—keeping up with frequent changes, even revolutions, in medical devices and supplies.

This book's editors, Rich Branson, Dean Hess, and Rob Chatburn are researchers and equipment evaluators of the first rank. Through their many publications, they have been educators in the best sense of the term. Their strong backgrounds encompass medicine, surgery, neonatology/pediatrics, formal teaching, and clinical and bench research. I have known these three men for many years, working with them as authors and as members of the Editorial Board of the science journal in our profession. Rich Branson, Dean Hess and Rob Chatburn are consummate professionals who have often shared their knowledge with their colleagues everywhere. This book is the latest example of that.

It has been said that the sense of perfection at the Rolls-Royce automobile factory is such that even the doorman won't let a bad product out the gate. I believe that we can trust Branson, Hess, and Chatburn to have acted as equally concerned "doormen" here, making sure that this is the Rolls-Royce of respiratory care equipment textbooks.

PHILIP KITTREDGE, RRT
Editor of *Respiratory Care*, 1968–1989

PREFACE

The relationship between equipment and the respiratory care profession is time honored and intimate. Technological advancements and the evolving role of the respiratory care practitioner have traveled parallel paths. This text is intended to provide practitioners with the principles of operation, appropriate use, and intricacies of the myriad of devices used in respiratory care.

We have written this text using the principles applied to peer-reviewed publications. We have gathered information from the literature, used the most recent references, avoided speculation, and hopefully, dispelled many of the "myths" perpetuated by historic texts. We have tried to concentrate on principles of operation, appropriate application, and limitations of types of devices rather than specific brands. The ventilator chapters are the exception to this, of course.

Research for this text demonstrated a paucity of information on monitoring in previous publications. In an effort to highlight the expanding role of respiratory care practitioners in diagnostics and non-invasive monitoring, we have dedicated four chapters to these topics. These chapters include the basics related to measurement of blood gases and pH, the noninvasive monitoring of oxygenation and ventilation, the principles of flow, volume and pressure monitoring, and the application of monitoring devices in the care of patients from the home to the intensive care unit.

Mechanical ventilation represents the ultimate technical challenge for the practitioner. This text introduces the complete classification system developed by Chatburn, followed by descriptions of intensive care unit ventilators, transport ventilators, home care ventilators, and high frequency ventilators according to the classification system. This consistent format allows ventilators to be compared in a way not available in any other text. Only commercially available ventilators, or those with a second life being used in extended care facilities, are discussed. This text also includes chapters on disinfection and sterilization, hyperbaric oxygen therapy, the role of computers in respiratory care equipment, and the federal regulations related to the development, testing, and use of equipment. These topics have never been treated in such detail before.

Understanding the appropriate clinical application of respiratory care devices is as essential to the practitioner as understanding their operating principles. In an effort to facilitate this process, we have included an extract of each of the relevant American Association for Respiratory Care Clinical Practice Guidelines at the end of appropriate chapters. We believe these guidelines, coupled with the wealth of practical information within each chapter, will provide readers the best of both worlds.

We believe this text will be useful to anyone involved in the delivery of respiratory care. Respiratory care students as well as advanced practitioners should find the information practical and enlightening. Physicians, nurses, and other health care professionals involved in treating patients with respiratory diseases should also find this text helpful.

In an attempt to make the text more user friendly, we have included key words, an outline, and objectives for each chapter. A glossary is also provided.

Authors for the text were selected for their leadership role in the profession and their publication records. Four of the authors are among the five most published authors from the professional journal *Respiratory Care*, over the past decade. Each of the authors has used their own unique style and experience to bring the principles and topics to life.

We hope this text meets the approval of the respiratory care community, and we welcome comments and critiques that will make future editions more useful.

ACKNOWLEDGMENTS

As senior editor, I have reserved the right to acknowledge those people who have been instrumental in the long and arduous task of bringing this book to fruition. I do this for selfish reasons as well as to fully acknowledge the contributions of my co-editors, Dean Hess and Rob Chatburn.

First and foremost, I would like to thank my family, without whom any accomplishment would be meaningless. My wife, Patty; children, Carolynn, Christopher, Lauren, and Richard, provide the foundation from which my life grows. Words fail to express my love and appreciation for each of you.

Many people tolerated my frequent absences of body and mind to allow this book to be completed. I would like to thank my best friend, Bob Campbell, RRT, whose zest for life and work were both an inspiration and a diversion; Ken Davis, MD, my boss and friend, who constantly reminds me of the qualities men and fathers should have; and Jacqui Roberts, who encouraged, cajoled, and threatened as well as typed, edited, and proofread. I also want to thank Josef Fischer, MD, Chairman of the Department of Surgery at the University of Cincinnati, for his support of a Respiratory Therapist in his Department.

Dean Hess, PhD, RRT, revived the text at the half-way point. His knowledge of equipment theory, appropriate clinical application, and his practical writing style form the basis for the first ten chapters of the book. Beside his many honors and awards, Dean is a role model for other practitioners. He has been chair of the AARC Clinical Practice Guidelines Committee, Chair of the Editorial Board of Respiratory Care, and is the most published author in the history of the Journal. He is also a man of conviction, admirable honesty, and modesty. I am honored to be his co-author, co-editor, and friend.

Rob Chatburn, RRT, created the template for discussion of ventilators in the text and wrote the classification chapter specifically for this text. The "Chatburn Classification System" has been used extensively by others and represents the future of understanding mechanical ventilators. At present, this contribution, which has taken nearly 5 years to finalize, is greatly unappreciated. In 20 years, when the Chatburn Classification is the standard system taught in every school, the true importance of this work will finally be realized. I am proud to have had a small part in the development of the classification system and am always humbled by Rob's ability to analyze and clarify the most difficult subjects.

Finally, I would like to thank those people who have guided my career down the appropriate paths: Jim Hurst, MD, who taught me about critical care and not to live within the boundaries constructed by others; Forrest M. Bird, MD, PhD, ScD, who has been a good friend, untiring teacher, and inspiration; Pat Brougher, RRT, who has excused my tirades and taught me to be a better writer by example; Phil Kittredge, RRT, who encouraged my early writing, broadened my horizons through his communications, and has been a good friend and mentor; and Ray Masferrer, RRT, who reminds me what it means to be a friend and what it means to be a man.

RICHARD D. BRANSON, RRT
Assistant Professor of Surgery
University of Cincinnati

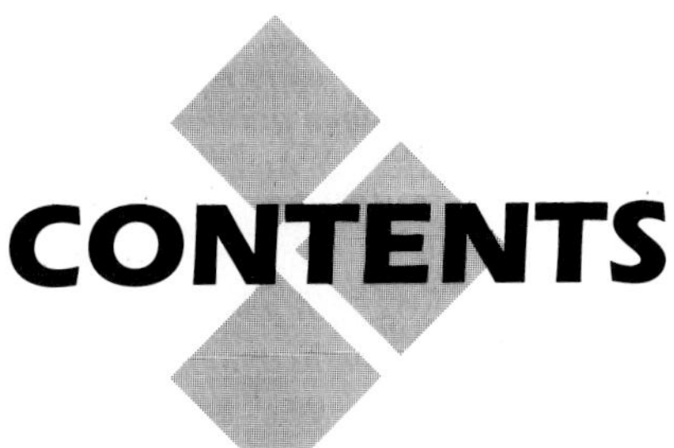

CONTENTS

AARC CLINICAL PRACTICE GUIDELINES

Extracts from the American Association for Respiratory Care's Clinical Practice Guidelines are included in relevant chapters. Indications, Contraindications, Hazards and Complications from each Clinical Practice Guideline are included.

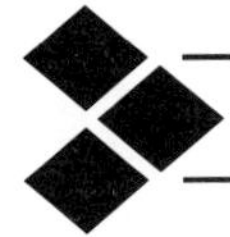

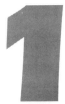

Physical Properties of Gases and Principles of Gas Movement

Vijay M. Deshpande
Dean R. Hess
Richard D. Branson

OBJECTIVES

1. Compare solids, liquids, and gases.
2. Compare the Celsius, Fahrenheit, and Kelvin scales of temperature measurement.
3. Define absolute zero temperature.
4. Calculate temperature conversions between Celsius, Fahrenheit, and Kelvin scales.
5. Distinguish between gauge pressure and absolute pressure.
6. Define Avogadro's law, Boyle's law, Charles' law, Gay-Lussac's law, and Dalton's law of partial pressures.
7. Use Henry's law and Graham's law to describe diffusion.
8. Define the law of continuity.
9. Distinguish between laminar and turbulent flow.
10. Explain Poiseuille's law.
11. Use the Reynold's number to predict laminar or turbulent flow.
12. Explain the use of Bernoulli's principle, Venturi's principle, and constant-pressure jet mixing to produce acceleration of gas flow.

KEY TERMS

absolute pressure
absolute scale
atom
Avogadro's law
Bernoulli's principle
Boyle's law
Celsius
Charles' law
combined gas law
constant-pressure jet mixing
Dalton's law of partial pressures
diffusion
Fahrenheit
Fick's law
fluid
gas
gauge pressure
Gay-Lussac's law
Graham's law
Henry's law
Kelvin
kinetic theory
laminar flow
law of continuity
liquid
molecule
Ohm's law
pressure
resistance
Reynold's number
solid
standard atmospheric pressure
temperature
turbulent flow
Venturi's principle
viscosity
volume

Introduction

Respiratory care practitioners commonly use technology in the treatment of patients with lung disease. They are expected to be familiar with the physical properties of gases and to use the principles of basic physics to understand the operation of respiratory care equipment. In this chapter the basic principles of gas physics are discussed as to how they relate to respiratory care equipment.

Basic Principles

The atom is the smallest unit of matter, whereas a molecule is the smallest stable unit of any substance. Most atoms can combine with other atoms to produce compounds that are different from those of the reacting atoms. Molecular reactions to create various compounds form the basis of chemistry. An atom of oxygen, O, is less stable than a molecule of oxygen, O_2. When two atoms of hydrogen react with one atom of oxygen, they form the compound water (H_2O), a molecule more stable than the atoms oxygen and hydrogen.

States of Matter

All matter exists in three states: solids, liquids, and gases. The state of matter depends on the molecular activity of the substance. A solid is a substance that has a fixed shape and volume. The molecules of a solid are relatively fixed in relation to one another. Their motion is limited to vibration around a fixed point. This molecular characteristic gives solids a crystalline structure, and thus a fixed volume and shape (Fig. 1-1*A*). As the intermolecular distances increase, the cohesive forces decrease and allow the molecular mobility observed in liquids (see Fig. 1-1*B*). In gases, the intermolecular forces are the weakest, allowing molecules to move freely at random (see Fig. 1-1*C*). This phenomenon allows gas molecules to assume the volume of their container.

The cohesive intermolecular forces can be reduced by applying energy, usually in the form of heat. A typical change in the state of matter can be observed when ice melts and when water boils. When changing to a higher state (solid→liquid→gas), energy must be added to matter. On the other hand, changing to a lower state (gas→liquid→solid) results in the release of energy. An unheated humidifier, such as those used in respiratory therapy, will be cooler than the ambient temperature due to evaporative cooling.

Physical Characteristics of Gases

Gas Movement

According to the kinetic theory, gas molecules are widely separated and move at high velocities. Their motion is random, allowing them to expand indefi-

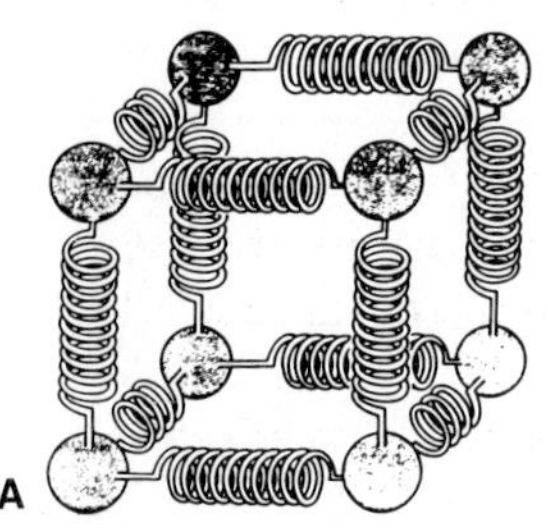

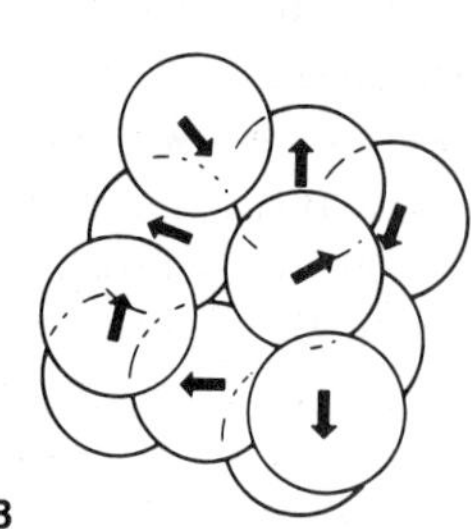

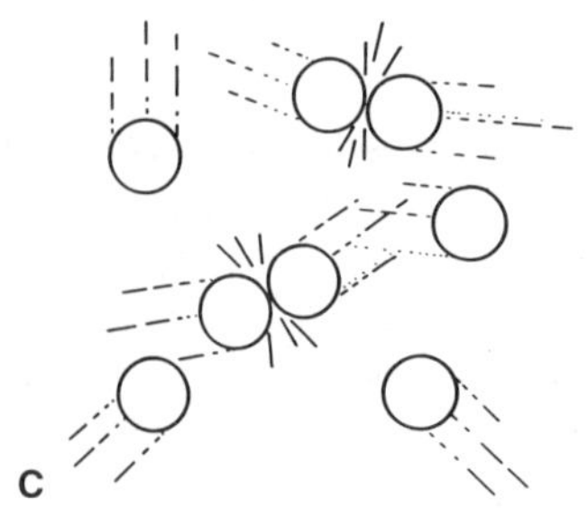

Figure 1-1. Molecular behavior in solids, liquids, and gases. (A.) Molecules in solids oscillate around a fixed point. (B.) Liquid molecules are relatively free and move over each other. (C.) Gas molecules are far apart from each other, freely move in a random motion, and collide frequently.

nitely unless they are confined in a container. Confined gas molecules, moving at high speeds, collide with one another and with the walls of the container. The gas molecules are elastic and bounce away from each other and the container walls.

Temperature

The kinetic theory of gases uses temperature as a measure of the average velocity of gas molecules. When a gas is heated, the kinetic energy of the molecules increases, promoting increased movement (velocity) of the molecules. On the other hand, removing heat from gas molecules slows their random motion. This effect of changes in the kinetic energy (motion energy) is responsible for changing the average velocity of gas molecules. If the kinetic activity of a molecule is stopped completely, the molecule will be stationary. This represents absolute zero temperature.

Temperature Scales

To measure the velocity of molecules (temperature), at least two reference points must be determined for calibration of a thermometer. Since water is an abundant liquid, the two reference points selected were the freezing point and the boiling point of water at standard atmospheric pressure (760 mm Hg). Temperature scales commonly used in medicine are the Celsius (centigrade), the Kelvin (absolute), and the Fahrenheit scales. The Celsius scale assigns the freezing point of water to 0°C and the boiling point to 100°C. All the temperatures within these points were scaled conveniently into 100 parts (Fig. 1-2). The Kelvin, or absolute, scale utilizes the same degree size as the Celsius scale; however, the zero point of this scale represents the theoretical absolute zero. This temperature (0°K) is approximately −273°C. Thus, 0°C corresponds to 273°K, water boils at 373°K (100°C), and any Celsius temperature can be expressed in Kelvin scale by adding 273°. See Equation Box 1-1.

The Fahrenheit temperature scale is based on the coldest temperature that can be achieved by mixing salt, ice, and water. This temperature was arbitrarily assigned 0°F. The acceptable standard calibration points on this scale make the freezing point of water 32°F, body temperature 98.6°F, and the boiling point of water 212°F.

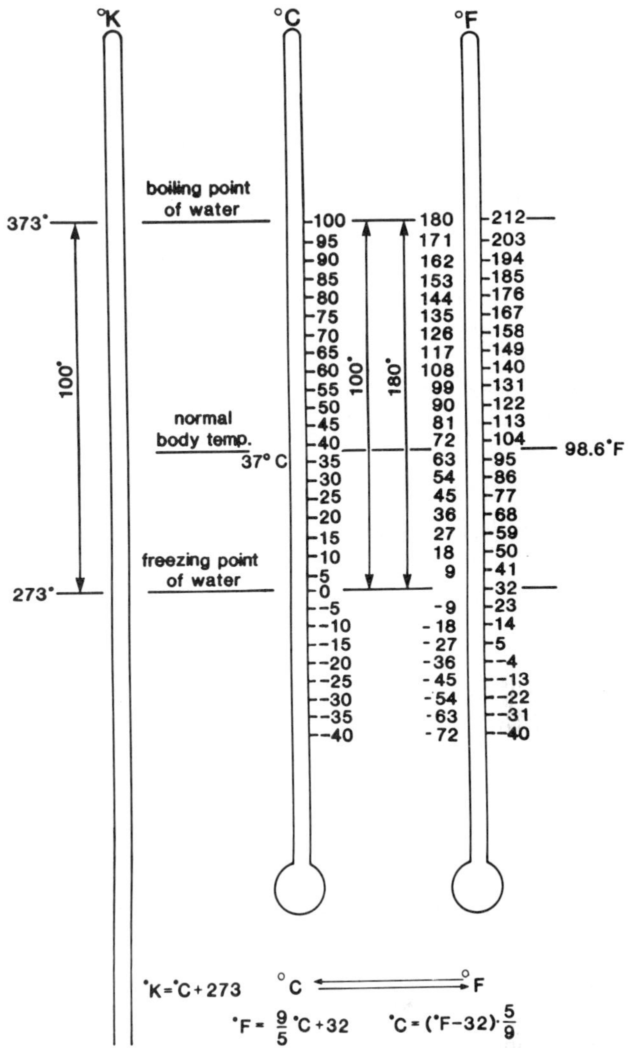

Figure 1-2. Three commonly used temperature scales: Kelvin, Celsius, and Fahrenheit. The two reference calibration scales are the freezing point of water (0°C, 32°F, and 273°K) and the boiling point of water (100°C, 212°F, and 373°K). Note that 5 degrees of the Celsius scale is equivalent to 9 degrees on the Fahrenheit scale. Thus, temperature conversions from the Celsius to the Fahrenheit scale are performed using the equation $°F = \frac{9}{5}°C + 32$, whereas the reverse conversion requires the same starting point by subtracting 32 from the Fahrenheit scale before using the ratio: $°C = (°F - 32) \cdot \frac{5}{9}$. The Kelvin scale is simply 273 greater than the Celsius scale.

Temperature Conversions

Figure 1-2 indicates the relative differences in the three temperature scales. The Celsius is the most logical and commonly used scientific temperature scale. The Kelvin temperature ideally indicates the change in the velocity of molecules, since 0°K represents no molecular movement. The Kelvin temperature is commonly used in quantifying changes in temperature, pressure, and volume, in accordance with gas laws. The Fahrenheit scale is seldom used scientifically. Mathematical operations to convert temperatures from one scale to another are based on the difference in degree size and their respective zero points.

Figure 1-2 indicates that the temperature differences between the freezing and boiling points of water are 180°F and 100°C. Thus, a Celsius degree is 180/100 or 9/5 times greater than a Fahrenheit degree. However, the zero points for these two scales are different. The Fahrenheit zero is 32° below the Celsius zero.

Equation Box 1-1: Temperature Conversions

$$°K = °C + 273°$$

$$°C = \frac{5}{9}(°F - 32)$$

$$°F = \frac{9}{5}°C + 32$$

Equation Box 1-2: Pressure

$$P = \frac{F}{A}$$

where P = pressure, F = force, and A = area.

$$P = H \cdot D$$

where H = height and D = density.

Thus, conversion of Celsius to Fahrenheit involves multiplying the Celsius temperature by a factor of 9/5 and adding 32°. See Equation Box 1-1. The conversion of Fahrenheit to Celsius can be accomplished by subtracting 32° from the Fahrenheit temperature and then multiplying by 5/9. See Equation Box 1-1.

Pressure

Pressure is the result of the molecular collisions of gas molecules with each other and the walls of their container. The greater the number of gas molecules, the higher will be the pressure. If gas temperature is increased, the average velocity of the gas molecules increases, resulting in an increased frequency of the molecular bombardment with the walls of the container, and pressure rises. The smaller the volume of the container, the higher the frequency of the collisions of gas molecules with the container, resulting in an increased pressure. Thus, the factors affecting pressure are the number of molecules, the gas temperature, and the volume of the container.

Pressure is defined as force per unit surface area. See Equation Box 1-2. If the force applied increases, there is an increase in pressure. Force is determined primarily by mass. For example, a larger person (greater mass) will exert a greater force (and pressure) on dependent skin and its vasculature and thus be at greater risk for pressure sores (decubitus ulcers). Likewise, a gas with a greater pressure (eg, 50 psi) will exert a greater force than a gas with a lower pressure (eg, 20 psi).

Pressure represents an important parameter in studying behavior of gases. Factors affecting pressure are similar for all gases. For example, pressure is increased when gases are compressed, and increased temperature increases pressure. Atmospheric pressure is measured by a barometer, and the pressure of any gas mixture is measured by a manometer.

For a fluid (liquids and gases), pressure is also determined by the height and density of the fluid. See Equation Box 1-2. A greater height or density produces a greater pressure. Due to this relationship, a column of mercury will exert more pressure than an equal column of water and a 100-cm column will exert more pressure than a 50-cm column.

Pressure can be expressed as gauge pressure or absolute pressure. The pressure measured on a manometer is the pressure above atmospheric pressure and is called gauge pressure. Absolute pressure is the sum of gauge pressure and atmospheric pressure. In practice, pressure is often stated as the height of the column and density is ignored. For example, if the pressure of a gas is stated as 50 cm H_2O, this means that the pressure of the gas is sufficient to raise a column of H_2O 50 cm against atmospheric pressure. A pressure of 50 mm Hg would mean that the pressure is great enough to raise a column of Hg 50 mm against atmospheric pressure.

Various units of pressure are used and include atmospheres (atm), inches of mercury (in Hg), millimeters of mercury (mm Hg), centimeters of water (cm H_2O), kilopascal (kPa), and pounds per square inch (psi). In respiratory care, pressure is commonly measured in atmospheres, millimeters of mercury, centimeters of water, and pounds per square inch. Torr is also used and is equivalent to millimeters of mercury.

The atmospheric pressure at sea level is relatively stable and provides a baseline pressure to facilitate conversions to other units. One atmosphere is equivalent to 760 mm Hg, 760 torr, 29.9 in Hg, 1034 cm H_2O, 33.9 ft fresh H_2O, 14.7 psi, 101.3 kPa, and 1.014×10^6 dynes/cm^2. See Equation Box 1-3 for derivations of pressure conversions. Table 1-1 lists some useful conversion units.

Volume

One of the major predicaments in dealing with gases relates to its quantitative unit of weight (grams) or volume (liters). Chemists and physicists have established a uniform quantitative unit, the mole. A mole, or gram-molecular weight, corresponds to the molecular weight expressed in grams. One mole of O_2 weighs 32 g, whereas one mole of CO_2 weighs 44 g.

One mole of any gas contains 6.02×10^{23} molecules (Avogadro's number). Avogadro's law states that equal volumes of all gases, at the same temperature and pressure, occupy the same volume. According to Avogadro's law, 1 mole of dry gas at 0°C and 1 atm occupies a volume of 22.4 L. This can be used to calcu-

Equation Box 1-3: Pressure Conversions

$$1 \text{ atmosphere} = 14.7 \text{ psi} = 760 \text{ mm Hg}$$

$$\therefore 14.7 \text{ psi} = 760 \text{ mm Hg } \textit{or}$$

$$1 \text{ psi} = \frac{760 \text{ mm Hg}}{14.7} \textit{ or}$$

$$1 \text{ psi} = 51.7 \text{ mm Hg}$$

$$1 \text{ atmosphere} = 760 \text{ mm Hg} = 1034 \text{ cm } H_2O$$

$$\therefore 760 \text{ mm Hg} = 1034 \text{ cm } H_2O \textit{ or}$$

$$1 \text{ mm Hg} = \frac{1034 \text{ cm } H_2O}{760} \textit{ or}$$

$$1 \text{ mm Hg} = 1.36 \text{ cm } H_2O$$

$$1 \text{ atmosphere} = 14.7 \text{ psi} = 1034 \text{ cm } H_2O$$

$$\therefore 14.7 \text{ psi} = 1034 \text{ cm } H_2O \textit{ or}$$

$$1 \text{ psi} = \frac{1034 \text{ cm } H_2O}{14.7} \textit{ or}$$

$$1 \text{ psi} = 70.34 \text{ cm } H_2O$$

late gas density. A mole of any gas will have a mass equal to its molecular weight, and the corresponding molar volume will be 22.4 L. Thus, the density of any gas can be calculated by dividing its gram molecular weight by 22.4. See Equation Box 1-4. Note that gases with lower molecular weights have lower densities. He/O_2 (heliox) gas mixtures are sometimes used in respiratory care because of the low density of these gas mixtures.

Gas Laws

The effects of changes in temperature, pressure, volume, and mass on the physical behavior of gases can be predicted on the basis of the gas laws. These describe the behavior of gases under ideal conditions, which assumes that the intermolecular forces between gas molecules are negligible and that the volume of gas molecules can be ignored. The gases used in respiratory care are considered to be ideal gases when applying the following gas laws. The following discussion is presented for dry conditions (ie, absolute humidity = zero).

Boyle's Law

Boyle's law explains the relationship between gas volume (V) and absolute pressure (P) at a constant temperature and mass of gas. Boyle's law states that the volume of a gas decreases as the absolute pressure exerted by the gas increases, and vice versa. See Equation Box 1-5. For example, a volume of 1000 mL of an ideal gas at 1 atm will reduce to 500 mL when the absolute pressure is doubled.

TABLE 1-1. Pressure Conversions

From (Units)	To (Units)	Conversion Factor
psi	mm Hg	51.7 mm Hg/psi
psi	cm H_2O	70 cm H_2O/psi
mm Hg	cm H_2O	1.36 cm H_2O/mm Hg
kPa	mm Hg	7.5 mm Hg/kPa
kPa	cm H_2O	10 cm H_2O/kPa
mm Hg	dynes/cm^2	1335 dynes/cm^2/mm Hg
cm H_2O	mm Hg	0.735 mm Hg/cm H_2O
cm H_2O	psi	0.0142 psi/cm H_2O

A common physiologic application of Boyle's law is observed in the mechanics of breathing. Figure 1-3 illustrates that during inspiration, when the diaphragm and the respiratory muscles contract, intrathoracic volume increases. Since the temperature is maintained at a constant value (37°C), according to Boyle's law the intrathoracic pressure decreases (−2 cm H_2O to −6 cm H_2O). This decrease in intrapleural pressure results in flow of gas into the lungs.

Clinically, the principle of Boyle's law is used to calculate the compressible volume in ventilator circuits. During positive-pressure breathing, the increase in pressure decreases the volume in ventilator circuit. During volume ventilation, this results in decreased volume delivered to the patient (see Chapter 13). Boyle's law is also employed in the body plethysmograph for measurement of thoracic gas volumes (see Chapter 10).

Equation Box 1-4: Gas Density

$$D = \frac{\text{mass}}{\text{volume}}$$

$$D_{gas} = \frac{\text{molecular weight}}{22.4 \text{ L}}$$

$$D_{N_2} = \frac{28 \text{ g}}{22.4 \text{ L}} = 1.25 \text{ g/L}$$

$$D_{He} = \frac{4 \text{ g}}{22.4 \text{ L}} = 0.1785 \text{ g/L}$$

$$D_{CO_2} = \frac{44 \text{ g}}{22.4 \text{ L}} = 1.965 \text{ g/L}$$

$$D_{O_2} = \frac{32 \text{ g}}{22.4 \text{ L}} = 1.43 \text{ g/L}$$

Equation Box 1-5:
Boyle's Law

$$P \cdot V = \text{constant}$$

where P is absolute pressure and V is volume.

$$P_1 \cdot V_1 = P_2 \cdot V_2$$

where P_1 is the initial absolute pressure, V_1 is the initial volume, P_2 is the final absolute pressure, and V_2 is the final volume.

For example, what happens to a 100-mL volume of gas if pressure increases from 0 mm Hg to 50 mm Hg?

$P_1 = 0$ mm Hg + 760 mm Hg = 760 mm Hg absolute

$V_1 = 100$ mL

$P_2 = 50$ mm Hg + 760 mm Hg = 810 mm Hg absolute

$$V_2 = \frac{P_1 \cdot V_1}{P_2} = \frac{760 \text{ mm Hg} \cdot 100 \text{ mL}}{810 \text{ mm Hg}} = 93.8 \text{ mL}$$

In other words, the volume decreases from 100 mL to 93.8 mL.

Charles' Law

According to Charles' law, for a given mass and pressure of a gas, the volume varies directly with the absolute temperature. See Equation Box 1-6. Figure 1-4 illustrates the effect of increased temperature on gas volume at a constant applied pressure. As the gas temperature is increased by 1°C, the volume increases by 1/273 of the original volume. The reverse is also true. As gas temperature is decreased, there is a decrease in the original volume. Theoretically, if the gas is cooled to −273°C (absolute zero), the volume will decrease to zero.

Inspired air at room temperature expands in the lungs, which are at body temperature (37°C). Thus, if a 500-mL volume of air is inspired at 25°C (298°K), the volume of the gas in the lungs (37°C or 310°K) will be 520 mL (ambient temperature and pressure to body temperature and pressure under dry conditions). A similar increase in gas volume occurs when gas is warmed before delivery to the patient, as during mechanical ventilation.

Gay-Lussac's Law

The relationship between absolute pressure and temperature at a constant mass and volume is described by Gay-Lussac's law, which states that absolute pressure varies directly with temperature. See Equation Box 1-7. An increase in temperature results in an increase in pressure, and vice versa.

In respiratory care, gas cylinders are commonly used to deliver therapeutic gases. These cylinders have a fixed volume. An increase in temperature increases the gas pressure in the cylinder. A safety relief system prevents excessive pressure inside the cylinder as a result of increased gas temperature. An example of the cooling that occurs with a decrease in pressure is that of gas leaving a medical gas cylinder. As gas leaves the cylinder, its pressure decreases to atmospheric pressure. This decrease in pressure is associated with a drop in temperature, and thus the regulator attached to the cylinder feels cold.

Combined Gas Law

All three gas laws (Boyle's, Charles', and Gay-Lussac's) can be combined to describe a predictable relationship between pressure, volume, and temperature. This is known as the combined gas law. The combined gas law indicates that for a given mass of gas, the original conditions of pressure, volume, and temperature are equal to the final conditions of pressure, volume, and temperature. See Equation Box 1-8.

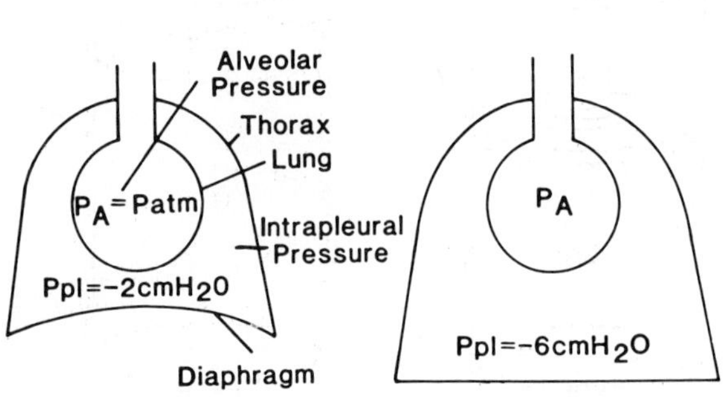

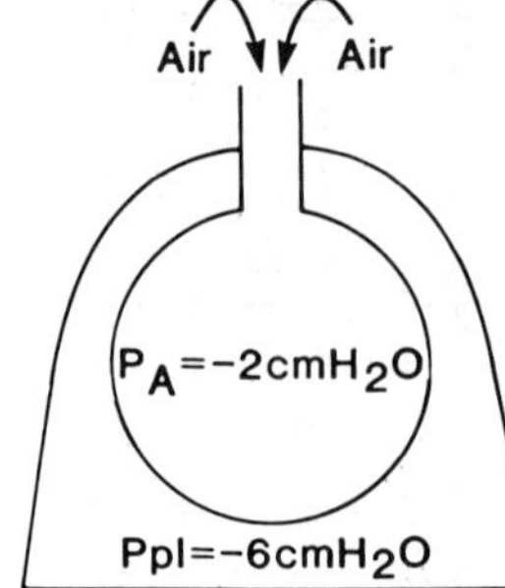

End Exhalation   Beginning of Inspiration   Inspiration

Figure 1-3. Application of Boyle's law in the normal mechanics of breathing. Intrathoracic expansion at constant body temperature promotes a decrease in the intrathoracic pressure from −2 to −6 cm H_2O, resulting in expansion of the lung. Consequently, intrapulmonic pressure decreases, creating a pressure gradient from atmosphere to the lungs and inspiration occurs.

Equation Box 1-6:
Charles' Law

$$\frac{V}{T} = \text{constant}$$

where V is volume and T is absolute temperature.

$$\frac{V_1}{T_1} = \frac{V_2}{T_2}$$

where V_1 is the initial volume, T_1 is the initial temperature, V_2 is the final volume, and T_2 is the final temperature.

For example, what happens to a 273-mL volume of gas if temperature increases from 0°C to 1°C?

$T_1 = 0 + 273 = 273$ absolute degrees

$T_2 = 1 + 273 = 274$ absolute degrees

$V_1 = 273$ mL

$$V_2 = \frac{V_1}{T_1} \cdot T_2 = \frac{273}{273} \cdot 274 \text{ mL} = 274 \text{ mL}$$

In other words, the volume increases by 1 mL.

Equation Box 1-7:
Gay-Lussac's Law

$$\frac{P}{T} = \text{constant}$$

where P is absolute pressure and T is absolute temperature.

$$\frac{P_1}{T_1} = \frac{P_2}{T_2}$$

where P_1 is the initial absolute pressure, T_1 is the initial absolute temperature, P_2 is the final absolute pressure, and T_2 is the final absolute temperature.

For example, what happens to a pressure of 10 mm Hg if the temperature increases from 25°C to 30°C?

$P_1 = 10$ mm Hg + 760 mm Hg = 770 mm Hg absolute

$T_1 = 25 + 273 = 298$ absolute degrees

$T_2 = 30 + 273 = 303$ absolute degrees

$$P_2 = \frac{P_1}{T_1} \cdot T_2 = \frac{770}{298} \cdot 303 = 783 \text{ mm Hg absolute}$$

In other words, the pressure increases by 13 mm Hg, or from 10 mm Hg to 23 mm Hg gauge pressure.

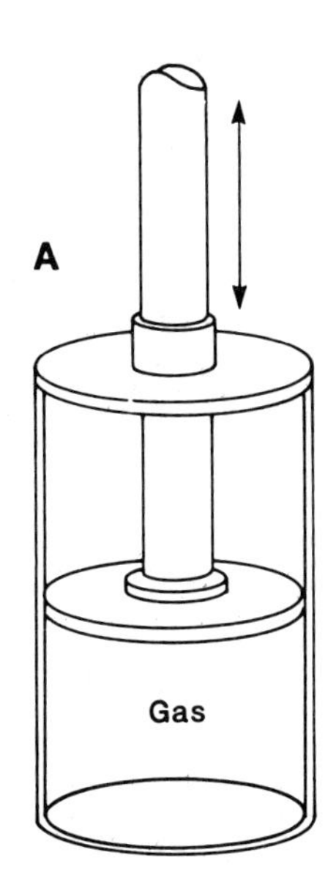

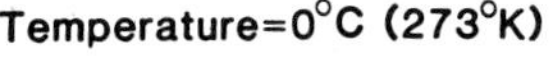

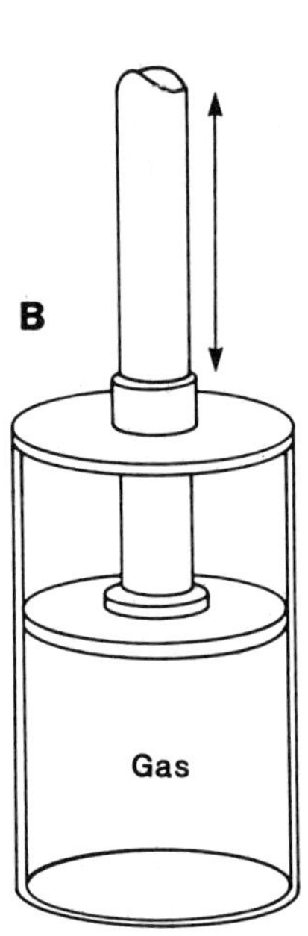

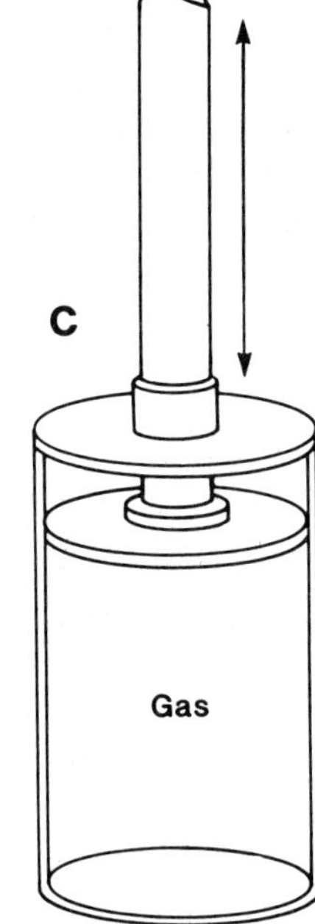

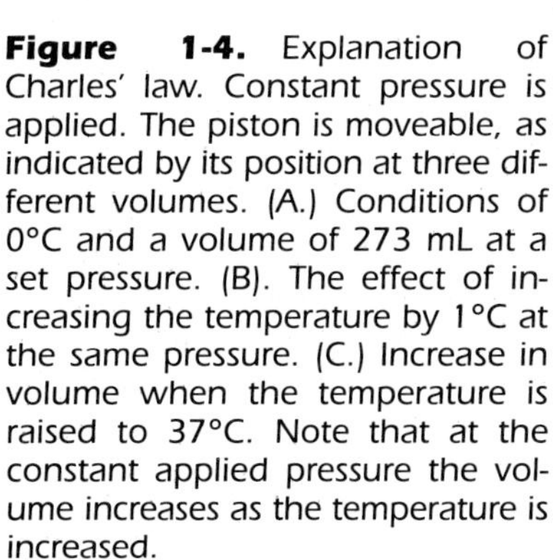

Figure 1-4. Explanation of Charles' law. Constant pressure is applied. The piston is moveable, as indicated by its position at three different volumes. (A.) Conditions of 0°C and a volume of 273 mL at a set pressure. (B). The effect of increasing the temperature by 1°C at the same pressure. (C.) Increase in volume when the temperature is raised to 37°C. Note that at the constant applied pressure the volume increases as the temperature is increased.

Equation Box 1-8:
Combined Gas Laws

$$\frac{P \cdot V}{T} = \text{constant}$$

where P is absolute pressure, V is volume, and T is absolute temperature.

$$\frac{P_1 \cdot V_1}{T_1} = \frac{P_2 \cdot V_2}{T_2}$$

where P_1 is the initial pressure, V_1 is the initial volume, T_1 is the initial temperature, P_2 is the final pressure, V_2 is the final volume, and T_2 is the final temperature.

For example, what happens to the volume of gas if its initial volume is 500 mL, pressure is 25 mm Hg, and temperature is 25°C and the pressure increases to 40 mm Hg and the temperature drops to 15°C?

$P_1 = 25 + 760 = 785$ mm Hg absolute

$V_1 = 500$ mL

$T_1 = 25 + 273 = 298$ absolute degrees

$P_2 = 40 + 760 = 800$ mm Hg absolute

$T_2 = 15 + 273 = 288$ mm Hg

$$V_2 = \frac{P_1 \cdot V_1 \cdot T_2}{P_2 \cdot T_1} = \frac{785 \cdot 500 \cdot 288}{800 \cdot 298} = 474 \text{ mL}$$

Equation Box 1-9:
Dalton's Law

$$P_{total} = P_A + P_B + P_C + \ldots P_i$$

where P_A, P_B, P_C, and Pi represent the partial pressures of gases A, B, C, and i in the mixture.

For example, atmospheric air is composed of 20.9% oxygen, 79% nitrogen, and 0.1% trace gases. Thus, at sea level

$$P_{atm} = P_{O_2} + P_{N_2} + P_{trace}$$

$$760 \text{ mm Hg} = (760 \cdot 0.209) + (760 \cdot 0.79) + (760 \cdot 0.001)$$

$$760 \text{ mm Hg} = 159 \text{ mm Hg } (P_{O_2}) + 600 \text{ mm Hg } (P_{N_2}) + 1 \text{ mm Hg } (P_{trace})$$

As another example, if barometric pressure is 750 mm Hg and the oxygen concentration is 50%, then the P_{O_2} is 375 mm Hg.

Equation Box 1-10:
Fick's Law

$$V_{gas} \propto \frac{A}{T} \cdot D_{gas} \cdot (P_1 - P_2)$$

where V_{gas} is the volume of gas that diffuses across a membrane, A is the surface area for diffusion, T is the thickness of the membrane, D_{gas} is the diffusibility of the gas (solubility coefficient ÷ density), and $P_1 - P_2$ is the partial pressure gradient.

The diffusibility of a gas is determined by its solubility coefficient and density.

$$D_{O_2} = \frac{0.023}{\left(\frac{32}{22.4}\right)} = 0.0192$$

$$D_{CO_2} = \frac{0.51}{\left(\frac{44}{22.4}\right)} = 0.364$$

Thus, the diffusibility of CO_2 is 19 times greater than that of O_2 (0.364 ÷ 0.0192 = 19).

Dalton's Law of Partial Pressures

Dalton's law of partial pressures states that the total pressure of a mixture of gases is equal to the sum of partial pressures of each constituent gas. Furthermore, the partial pressure exerted by each constituent gas is proportional to its concentration in the mixture. See Equation Box 1-9.

There are several implications of Dalton's Law. If the atmospheric pressure decreases, the partial pressures of all gases, including oxygen, will decrease. Thus, the inspired P_{O_2} will decrease at a high altitude. If the oxygen concentration increases, then the inspired P_{O_2} will increase, and vice versa. The P_{O_2} can be raised to very high levels if 100% oxygen is combined with hyperbaric conditions (see Chapter 4).

Gas Movement

Diffusion

Diffusion is the passive molecular movement of molecules from a region of high concentration to a region of low concentration. For gases, a higher concentration implies a higher partial pressure. Thus, the driving force in gaseous diffusion is the partial pressure gradient.

Fick's Law

Fick's law describes the relationship between factors influencing diffusion. See Equation Box 1-10. Diffusion through tissues or membranes depends on surface area of the membrane, the concentration gradient across the membrane, a diffusion rate constant based on Henry's law and Graham's law, and the thickness of the membrane. In pulmonary diseases such as pulmonary emphysema and pulmonary fibrosis, a diffusion defect is expected since the area of the diffusing surface is reduced in emphysema and the thickness of the diffusing surface is increased in fibrosis.

Henry's Law

Henry's law states that the amount of gas that dissolves in a liquid depends on two factors, the partial pressure of the gas and the solubility coefficient of the gas. The solubility coefficient is the amount of gas that can be dissolved in 1 mL of a liquid and varies inversely with temperature. The solubility coefficient of O_2 in plasma at 37°C and 760 mm Hg pressure is 0.023 mL and that of CO_2 in plasma is 0.510 mL. For commonly performed clinical calculation, the solubility coefficient of 0.003 mL is used for oxygen. This is based on 100 mL of plasma and 1 mm Hg pressure at 37°C.

Graham's Law

Graham's law describes the diffusion of gases through liquids. According to Graham's law, the rate of diffusion is inversely proportional to the square root of the gas density. This means that lighter gas molecules will diffuse faster than heavier molecules if only gas density is considered. In a liquid medium, both Henry's and Graham's laws influence diffusion rate. A physiologic application of Henry's law and Graham's law is observed in the gas exchange of O_2 and CO_2 across the alveolar-capillary membrane of the lungs. See Equation Box 1-10. Quantitatively, CO_2 diffuses approximately 20 times faster than oxygen across the alveolar-capillary membrane.

Gas Flow

Bulk gas flow occurs as the result of a pressure gradient. Fluid physics describes gas flow as a phenomenon of gas movement from a region of higher kinetic activity (higher pressure) to a region of lesser kinetic activity (lower pressure). Since gases demonstrate the ability to flow, they are included with liquids in the general term "fluids."

Law of Continuity

The law of continuity quantifies the flow of a fluid moving through a tube. Flow varies directly with cross-sectional area and velocity. If cross-sectional area increases, flow will increase or velocity will decrease. See Equation Box 1-11. Due to the law of continuity, the velocity of gas flow will be less through small airways of the lungs where the total cross-sectional area is greater. The law of continuity also indicates that the blood flow through capillaries is slower than in the aorta or pulmonary artery. Physiologically, this serves the purpose of allowing more time for gas exchange between the capillary blood and the lungs or tissues.

Equation Box 1-11:
Law of Continuity

$$\text{flow} \propto \text{cross-sectional area} \cdot \text{velocity}$$

For example, the left ventricle pumps blood through the aorta to the systemic circulation and the right ventricle pumps blood through the pulmonary circulation (Fig. 1-5). In both cases, the same amount of blood flow (cardiac output) is flowing through the blood vessels. According to the law of continuity:

$$\text{cardiac output (blood flow)} \propto A_1 \cdot V_1 = A_2 \cdot V_2$$

where A_1 is the cross-sectional area of the aorta or pulmonary artery, V_1 is the velocity of blood flow through the aorta or pulmonary artery, A_2 is the cross-sectional area of the systemic or pulmonary capillaries, and V_2 is the velocity of blood flow through the capillaries. Knowing that the cross-sectional areas of the capillaries (A_2) is greater than that of the aorta or pulmonary artery (A_1), the velocity of blood flow is less in the capillaries ($V_1 > V_2$).

Laminar Flow

Laminar flow is a smooth, streamlined flow with few directional changes. This type of flow exists in concentric cylindrical layers. As the molecules move along the wall of the a rigid tube, the frictional resistance with the wall decreases the forward motion of the molecules closest to the wall. Thus, the layer closest to the wall is almost stationary. The next layer experiences less frictional resistance and thus advances further. The forward velocity of each layer increases from the wall of the tube to the center of the tube. The overall velocity pattern resembles a parabola (Fig. 1-6*A*). The molecules at the center of the tube advance at a greater velocity than those at the sides of the tube.

Laminar flow implies movement of smoothly sliding layers, or lamina, in one direction and parallel to each other. During this type of flow, molecular friction develops between adjacent layers. Slower-moving molecular layers reduce the overall velocity of the faster-moving layers. This phenomenon is called viscosity. Laminar flow is observed in tube systems that are rigid, smooth, and unobstructed. The diameter of these tubes is relatively uniform. The pressure gradi-

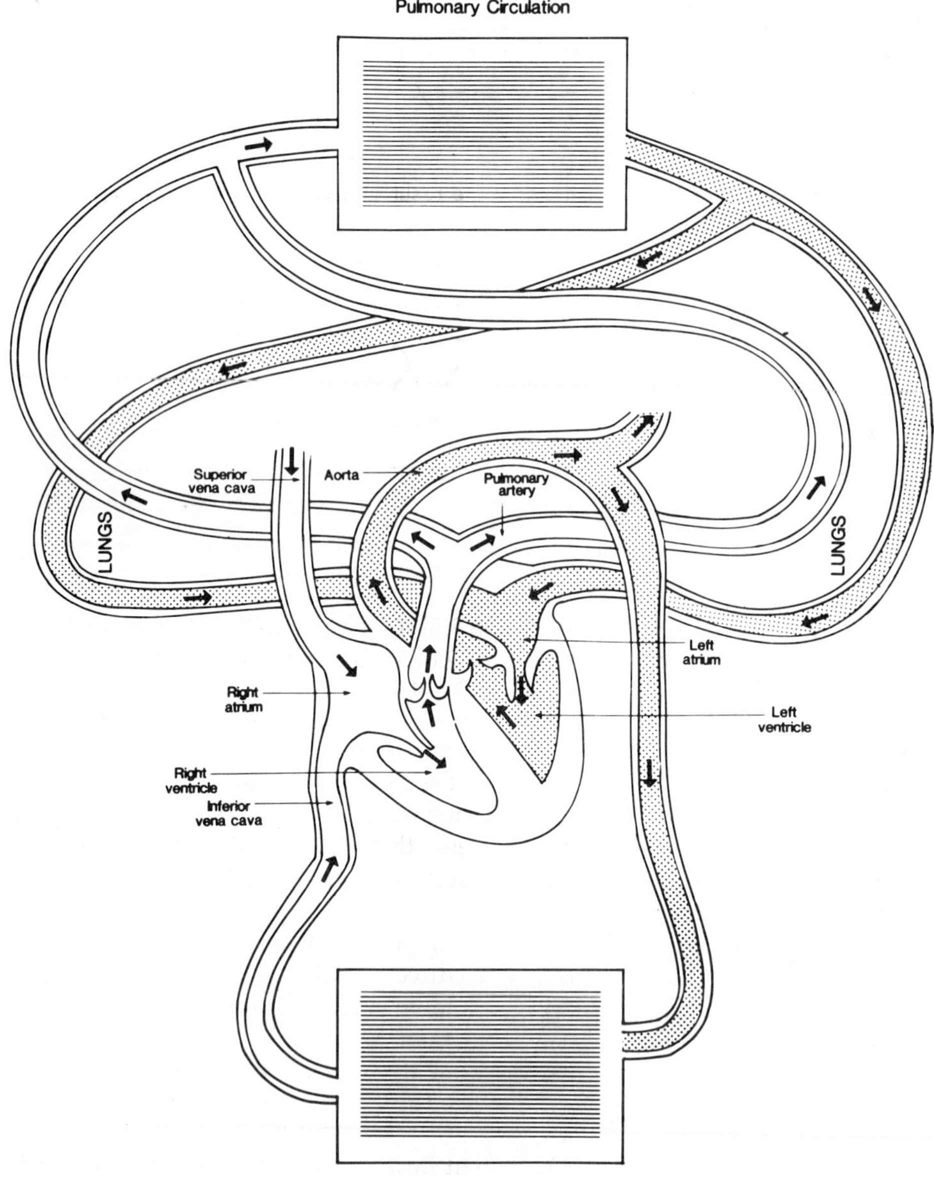

Figure 1-5. Schematic of the cardiopulmonary system. The large increase in the surface area of the pulmonary capillaries and the systemic capillaries profoundly decreases the velocity of the blood flow, facilitating gas exchange.

ent required to produce and maintain laminar flow is proportional to the flow and the resistance (Ohm's law). If resistance increases, flow decreases. If the pressure gradient increases, flow increases. See Equation Box 1-12.

Various factors influence flow characteristics and resistance. The relationship of these factors during laminar flow in a rigid cylindrical tube is expressed by Poiseuille's law. Poiseuille's law states that resistance to flow varies directly with the length of the tube and inversely with the radius of the tube. However, radius is quantitatively more important because resistance varies with the fourth power of the radius. See Equation Box 1-13.

The viscosity of the gas also affects resistance during laminar flow. However, in clinical respiratory care, changes in viscosity are insignificant because the composition of the gas is not changed. Thus, the primary factor that determines airway resistance during laminar flow is the radius of the airways. The radius of the airway remains relatively unchanged unless obstruction occurs, such as with increased sputum, tumor, or foreign body.

Equation Box 1-12:
Ohm's Law for Laminar Flow

$$\Delta P = \dot{V} \cdot R$$

where ΔP is the pressure gradient, $\dot{V}$ is the gas flow, and R is the resistance to gas flow.

P1→ →P2

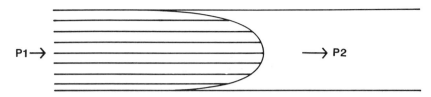

A. Laminar Flow in a smooth rigid tube resulting from a pressure gradient of P1–P2

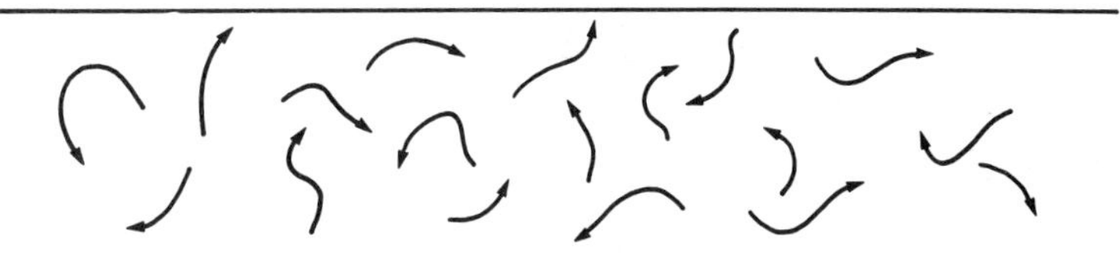

B. Turbulent flow

Figure 1-6. (A.) Laminar flow through a rigid tube. Note the advancement of the fluid molecules in a parabolic pattern. (B.) In turbulent flow, the molecules move in any direction. The pressure required to maintain laminar flow is lower than that required to maintain turbulent flow of the same magnitude.

A common clinical example is the asthmatic patient in acute bronchospasm. In this case, the radius of the airway is significantly decreased, increasing the airway resistance. In the case of a spontaneously breathing patient, this increase in resistance will increase the work of breathing. During mechanical ventilation, the increase in airway resistance will increase the pressure required by the ventilator to deliver the tidal volume.

In respiratory physiology, the length of the airway is constant. With respiratory equipment applications, it is important to recognize that the length of the conducting tube may not remain constant. If the length of the tube is increased, resistance will increase and flow will decrease unless the pressure gradient is increased. The opposite effect will occur if the length of the tube decreases.

Turbulent Flow

Turbulent flow (see Fig. 1-6*B*) is characterized by disorderly flowing vortices known as eddy currents. The flow moves at a uniform velocity. Molecular movement is more random and rapid. The change from laminar flow to turbulent flow is prompted by an increase in velocity, an increase in gas density, an increase in diameter of the tube, or a decrease in the viscosity of the gas. This relationship is known as Reynold's number. See Equation Box 1-14. A Reynold's number less than 2000 indicates laminar flow, whereas a number exceeding 2000 is considered turbulent flow.

The driving pressure required to produce turbulent flow varies directly with resistance and the square of flow. Thus, more pressure is required to produce turbulent flow than laminar flow. See Equation Box 1-15. For turbulent flow, resistance is determined by the length of the tube, radius of the tube, and density of the gas.

Turbulent flow is affected by gas density (and not viscosity), whereas laminar flow is affected by gas viscosity (but not density). Turbulent flow is sometimes said to be density dependent, whereas laminar flow is density independent. In the tracheobronchial tree, a laminar flow normally exists in airways less than 2 mm in diameter. Turbulent flow is observed in the upper respiratory tract and large central airways. Thus, overall tracheobronchial flow is a combination

Equation Box 1-13: Poiseuille's Law

$$R \propto \frac{8 \cdot n \cdot \ell}{\pi \cdot r^4}$$

Because:

$$\Delta P = \dot{V} \cdot R$$

Then:

$$\dot{V} \propto \frac{\pi \cdot r^4 \cdot \Delta P}{8 \cdot n \cdot \ell}$$

where π is 3.14, r is the radius of the tube, ΔP is the pressure gradient, n is the viscosity of the gas, and l is the length of the tube.

Equation Box 1-14: Reynold's Number

$$R_N \propto \frac{V \cdot D \cdot d}{n}$$

where V is velocity, D is the diameter of the tube, d is gas density, and n is gas viscosity.

Equation Box 1-15:
Ohm's Law and Poiseuille's Law for Turbulent Flow

$$\Delta P = \dot{V}^2 \cdot R$$

and

$$R \propto \frac{d \cdot \ell}{4 \cdot \pi \cdot r^5}$$

then

$$\dot{V}^2 \propto \frac{4 \cdot \pi \cdot r^5 \cdot \Delta P}{d \cdot \ell}$$

where ΔP is the pressure gradient, $\dot{V}$ is the gas flow, R is the resistance to gas flow, d is density of the gas, ℓ is the length of the tube, and r is the radius of the tube.

Equation Box 1-16:
Bernoulli's Principle

The kinetic energies at points A and B in Figure 1-7 are $\frac{1}{2}(mv_1^2)$ and $\frac{1}{2}(mv_2^2)$, respectively, m is the mass of the fluid and v_1 and v_2 represent the linear velocities at points A and B. According to the law of conservation of energy

Energy at point A = Energy at point B

$$P_1 + \tfrac{1}{2}(mv_1^2) = P_2 + \tfrac{1}{2}(mv_2^2)$$

or

$$P_1 - P_2 = \tfrac{1}{2} \cdot m \cdot (v_2^2 - v_1^2)$$

In other words, the gradient $P_1 - P_2$ is proportional to the gradient $v_2^2 - v_1^2$.

of laminar and turbulent flow (turbulent flow in larger airways and laminar flow in smaller airways).

Acceleration of Gas Flow

An increased pressure gradient enhances gas flow from a higher pressure to a lower pressure. Thus, driving pressure can be increased to accelerate gas flow. Normally, if one wishes to accelerate gas flow, the driving pressure must be increased. Clinically, increasing driving pressure is not always feasible. Acceleration of gas flow can also be achieved by employing other methods. Bernoulli's and Venturi's principles provide a means for accelerating gas flows. These principles not only accelerate delivery of gas but also permit delivery of a precise and predictable flow. Another method of gas flow acceleration uses the jet mixing principle based on viscous shearing forces.

Bernoulli's Principle

Fluid flow through a tube can be explained by the first law of thermodynamics, which states that energy cannot be created or destroyed using ordinary conditions, energy is conserved when transformed from one form to another, and the sum of all energy is constant. Applied to fluid flow, this can be restated in relation to fluid mechanics. Pressure energy and velocity energy at any given point are the same as that at another point along the fluid flow in a tube. If a tube is tapered, the fluid velocity increases with a resultant decrease in pressure distal to the constriction.

Bernoulli's principle (Fig. 1-7) states that the sum of the pressure and the kinetic energy has the same value at all points along a streamline. See Equation Box 1-16. As a result of tapering or constriction to a gas flow, velocity increases. To conserve the total fluid energy, this acceleration in velocity energy is balanced by a decrease in pressure energy. If the driving pressure is kept constant, the smaller the orifice size of the tubing constriction, the higher the velocity of the fluid, and the greater the pressure drop past the orifice (Fig. 1-8).

A physiologic application of Bernoulli's principle is observed in advanced arteriosclerosis (Fig. 1-9). The constricted coronary artery, due to accumulation of plaque on its inner walls, decreases blood flow to the heart muscle. To maintain adequate blood flow through the constricted artery, the driving pressure is increased by increased contraction of the heart. If the delivered velocity is sufficiently high, the lateral wall pressure decreases, collapsing the artery, owing to

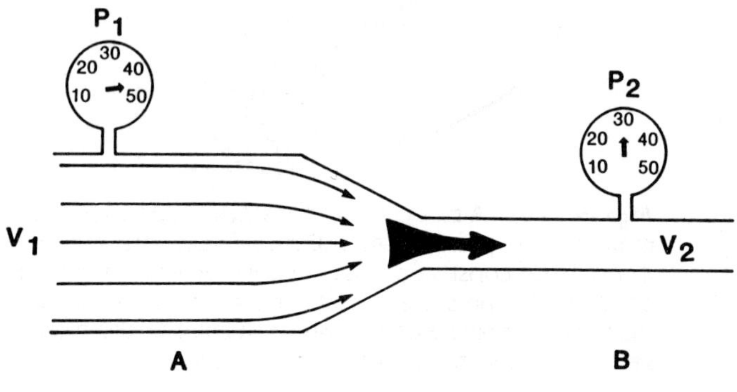

Figure 1-7. Bernoulli's principle. A and B are two sections of a tube through which a fluid (gas) flow is generated. The tubing is constricted, and V_1 and V_2 indicate the linear velocities. According to Bernoulli's principle, the fluid velocity increases as it travels through a constriction, resulting in a pressure drop: $V_2 > V_1$ and $P_2 < P_1$.

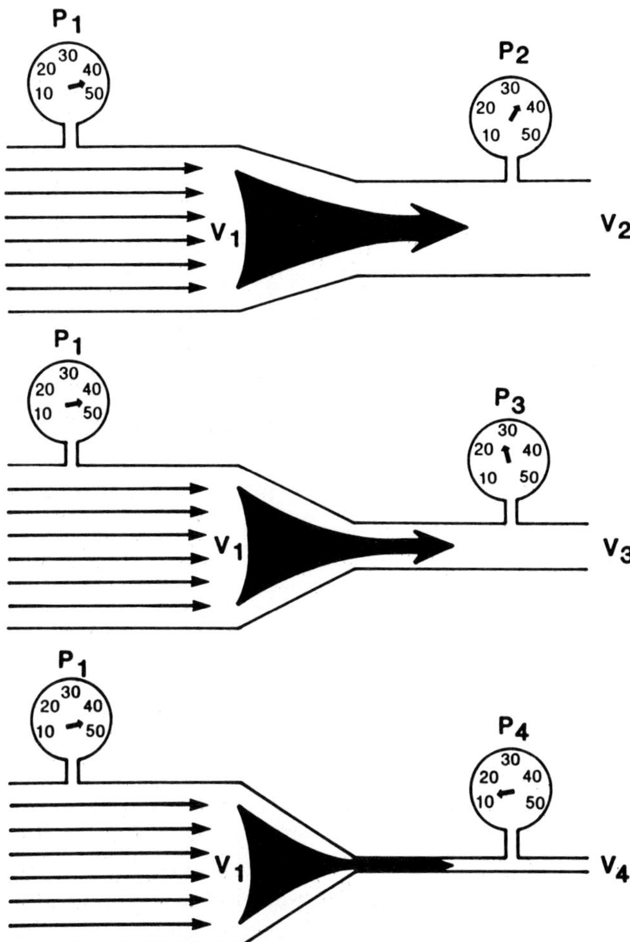

Figure 1-8. As the orifice size of the constriction is decreased, the velocity of the fluid exiting the orifice increases and a greater pressure drop results: $V_4 > V_3 > V_2 > V_1$ and $P_1 > P_2 > P_3 > P_4$.

higher external pressure. The flow is momentarily interrupted and the Bernoulli effect is eliminated. The blood vessel then reopens owing to arterial pressure. As blood flows through the constricted artery, the internal pressure decreases and the artery closes again. This periodic closure and opening of the blood vessel is known as vascular flutter.

In respiratory therapy equipment, gases often flow through a restriction, or orifice. This results in an increase in the velocity of the gas and a corresponding decrease in its pressure.

Venturi's Principle

If flow occurs through constricted tubing, the pressure drop distal to the constriction can be used to entrain a second fluid to mix with the main flow. The Venturi principle states that the pressure drop distal to the restriction can be restored to the driving pressure by funneling the passage immediately distal to the constriction at an angle of divergence less than 15 degrees.

Figure 1-10 depicts the construction of a Venturi tube. The pressure drop across an obstruction is restored provided the angle of divergence is less than 15 degrees. Furthermore, the flow increases owing to entrainment of the second fluid.

Clinically, venturi devices are used to increase gas flows. Since a second gas can be entrained using the Venturi principle, this can be used to deliver a precise oxygen concentration to patients by mixing air with oxygen. Aerosol delivery for humidification and nebulization of medications is also accomplished by using the Venturi principle (see Chapter 5).

Constant-Pressure Jet Mixing

In respiratory care, an oxygen delivery system known as a Venturi mask or an air-entrainment mask is commonly used to provide the patient with a precise, predictable oxygen concentration. Although it is called an air-entrainment mask, the principle of operation for this device is constant-pressure jet mixing and not venturi entrainment.[1] The mixing of air with the driving gas (O_2) occurs at the constant ambient pressure. Unlike venturi entrainment, which is based on a pressure drop, the entrainment of the ambient air results from viscous interaction between the driving gas flow and the stationary ambient air.

The theory of viscous shearing interaction can be compared with the theory describing laminar flow, discussed previously (see Fig. 1-6*A*). A concentric cylindrical forward velocity pattern (parabolic pat-

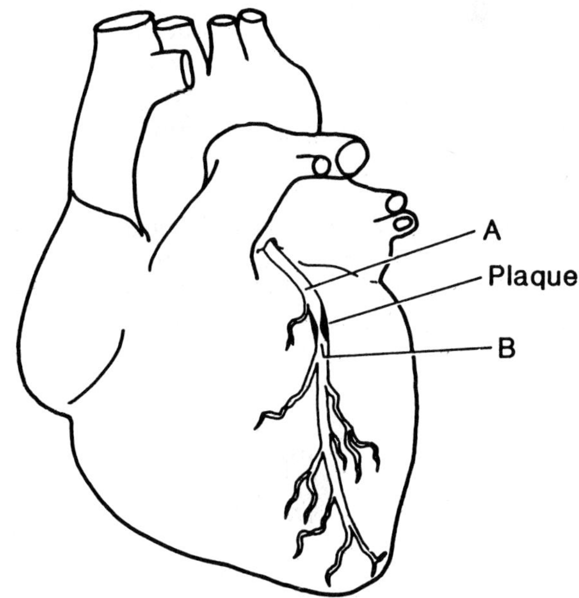

Figure 1-9. A blood vessel constricted due to plaque formation. The pressure at point A forces the blood flow through the constriction, resulting in decrease in pressure at point B. The pressure outside the blood vessel is greater than that at point B and causes a collapse of the blood vessel. This demonstrates Bernoulli's principle.

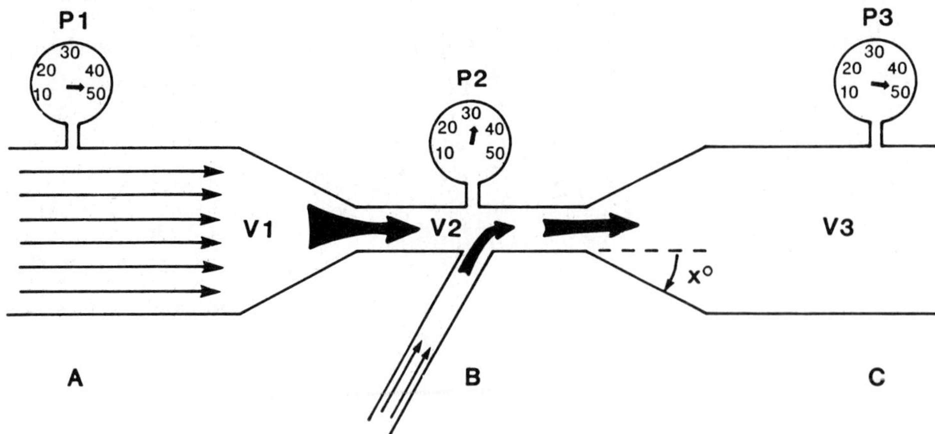

Figure 1-10. Venturi's Principle. A, B, and C represent three sections of a tube in which section A has a higher cross-sectional area than section B. Gas flow through section A enters section B at a higher velocity owing to constriction of the tubing. According to Bernoulli's principle, pressure decreases ($P_1 > P_2$). This pressure drop facilitates entrainment of a second fluid into the main flow. The original pressure, P_1, can be restored if the angle of divergence of the tubing (angle X) is less than 15 degrees.

tern) develops as a result of frictional resistance offered by the cylindrical wall of the tubing. In this case, the molecules closest to the wall have the slowest forward velocity and the molecules in the center of the tube have the highest forward velocity. Each layer of molecules is decelerated by the frictional viscous resistance in proportion to their distance from the wall. When this principle is applied to two fluids, one moving and the other stationary, the stationary fluid decelerates the moving fluid whereas the moving fluid attempts to accelerate the stationary fluid. The net result is the development of a viscous shearing layer. Since fluids can be deformed relatively easily, the viscous shearing force promotes movement of layers of the stationary fluid into the path of the moving fluid.

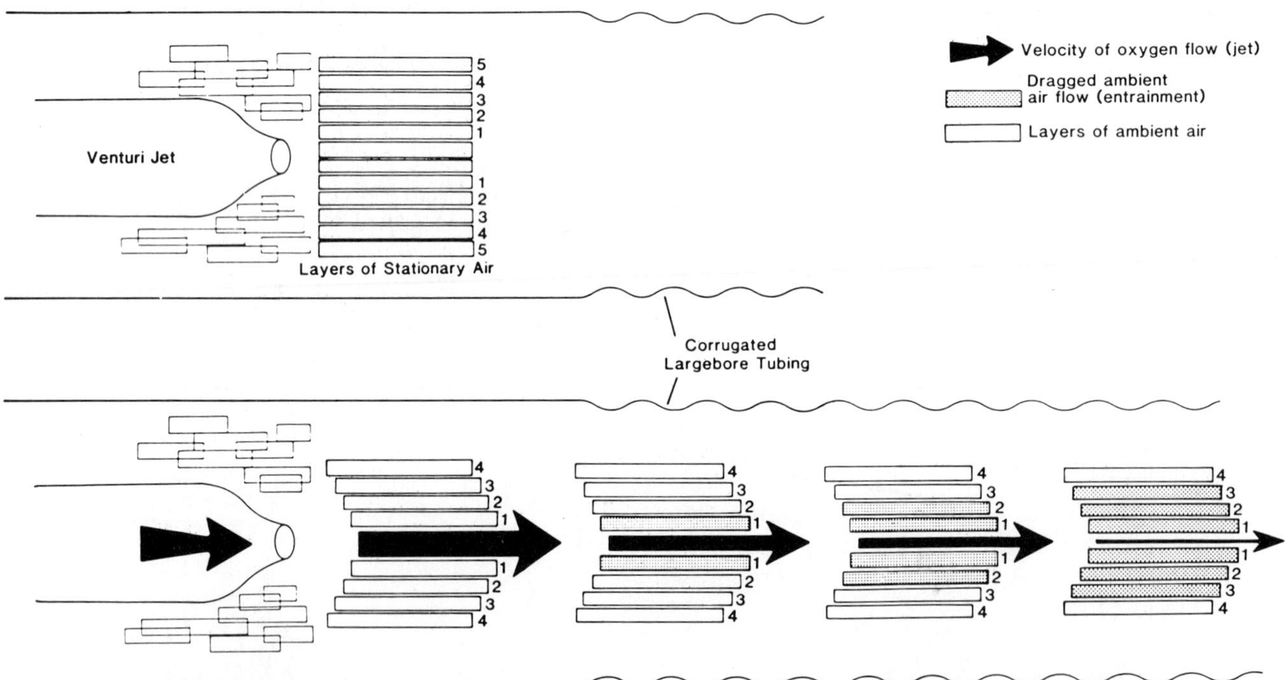

Figure 1-11. Operation of a Venturi mask by jet mixing principle. Numbers 1, 2, 3, 4, and 5 represent imaginary stationary layers of ambient air at the exit port of the Venturi jet. As the gas flow (oxygen in this case) is initiated, a high-velocity oxygen jet advances through the nozzle, attempting to accelerate adjacent air layers. The stationary layers of air attempt to decelerate the advancing oxygen jet. As the stationary layers of air are deformed, a "staircase" effect develops in the proximity of the main jet flow. Thus, layer 1 advances farther than layer 2, which in turn, advances farther than layer 3, and so on. Subsequently, these layers are drawn into the main flow of gas produced by the jet, increasing the total flow and oxygen flow is diluted by incoming layers of air. The jet mixing is a function of the jet orifice size (jet velocity) and is independent of the jet flow.

Operation of a Venturi Mask Powered by Oxygen

As shown in Figure 1-11, layers of ambient air are in a stationary condition outside the jet orifice before initiating any oxygen flow. Velocity refers to the forward, linear movement of the gas molecules per unit time whereas flow indicates the volume of gas leaving the orifice or nozzle per unit time. On initiating the flow of oxygen, the velocity of the gas increases as it exits the constricted port. The high-velocity oxygen flow imparts some of its kinetic energy to the stationary ambient air, distorting adjacent layers of the air. As the forward velocity of oxygen is decelerated by the stationary layers of air, it accelerates the stationary layers, and viscous shearing results in a "staircase" effect on the adjacent layers of the ambient air. This gas dilution is the result of jet mixing due to viscous shearing force and not due to the Venturi entrainment based on a pressure drop phenomenon.

Reference

1. Scacci R. Air entrainment masks: Jet mixing is how they work. Respir Care 1979;24:928.

Additional Reading

Adriani J. The Chemistry and Physics of Anesthesia, 2nd ed. Springfield, IL: Charles C Thomas, 1972.

Brooks S. Integrated Basic Sciences, 4th ed. St. Louis: CV Mosby, 1979.

Ewen D, et al. Physics for Career Education. Englewood Cliffs, NJ: Prentice-Hall, 1974.

Kimball WR. Fluid mechanics. In: Kacmarek RM, Hess D, Stoller JK, eds. Monitoring in Respiratory Care. St. Louis: Mosby–Year Book, 1993.

Nave C, Nave B. Physics for the Health Sciences, 3rd ed. Philadelphia: WB Saunders, 1985.

Serway RA, Faughn JS. College Physics. Philadelphia: WB Saunders, 1985.

Wojciechowski W. Respiratory Care Sciences—An Integrated Approach. New York: John Wiley & Sons, 1985.

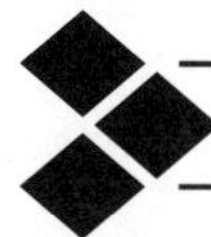

2

Compressed Gases: Manufacture, Storage, and Piping Systems

Robert Langenderfer
Richard D. Branson

OBJECTIVES

1. Define a medical gas.
2. Describe the components of a medical gas distribution system.
3. Explain the advantages and disadvantages of using a bulk liquid oxygen system.
4. State the role of gas distribution system alarms and the appropriate response to an alarm.
5. Describe the safety systems used in a medical gas distribution system to prevent accidental delivery of the wrong gas.

(continued)

OBJECTIVES, (continued)

6. Explain the methods and reasons for testing a medical gas distribution system.
7. Describe the most common problems associated with a medical gas distribution system.
8. Define a medical gas cylinder.
9. Describe the function of a cylinder valve and explain the difference between the two kinds.
10. Describe the safety systems used with medical gas cylinders, including the pin index safety system, cylinder markings, cylinder color, and cylinder labels.
11. Describe the safe handling and storage of medical gas cylinders.
12. Calculate the duration of cylinder gas flow given the gauge pressure, cylinder size, and flow rate.
13. Describe the advantages, disadvantages, uses, and hazards of portable liquid oxygen systems.
14. Describe the two types of oxygen concentrators.

KEY TERMS

bulk oxygen system
compressed gas
liquefied compressed gas
medical gas
medical gas container
medical gas cylinder
nonliquefied compressed gas
oxygen concentrator
oxygen enricher
psi
psia
psig
station outlet

Introduction

The delivery of medical gas therapy is one of the foundations of the respiratory care profession. Early respiratory care practitioners were often referred to as "oxygen orderlies" since their primary responsibility was the delivery and set-up of oxygen tanks. This was before oxygen and air were routinely piped into the patient's room. Today the respiratory care practitioner should not only be familiar with tanks and other containers but also with the characteristics of medical gases, their source, and appropriate handling.

Much of the information in this chapter is obtained from publications of the National Fire Protection Agency (NFPA)[1] and the Compressed Gas Association (CGA).[2] Although the material in this chapter provides an overview of important systems, theory of operation, and potential problems, we encourage readers to refer to these publications for pertinent regulations and detailed procedure descriptions.

Medical Gases

Medical gases are gases that have been refined and purified according to specifications contained in the *United States Pharmacopeia* (USP) (Table 2-1). They are intended for human use in the diagnosis and treatment of disease. Medical gases can be subdivided into three groups: therapeutic gases, laboratory gases, and anesthetic gases. Therapeutic gases include air, oxygen, and mixtures of helium and oxygen or carbon dioxide and oxygen. Laboratory gases are often used during diagnostic tests or in the calibration of equipment and include helium, nitrogen, and carbon monoxide. Anesthetic gases include cyclopropane, ethylene, and nitrous oxide and are used in conjunction with oxygen to provide the appropriate anesthetic effect during an operative procedure.

Oxygen

Oxygen (O_2) is an elemental gas that possesses several unique physical and chemical characteristics, the most important being its ability to support life. At normal atmospheric pressure and temperature, O_2 exists as an odorless, tasteless, colorless gas. It represents one fifth of the earth's atmosphere by volume (22.99%) and nearly one fourth by weight (23.2%). Although the percentage of O_2 in the atmosphere is constant, the partial pressure varies as barometric pressure (P_B) changes. See Chapter 1, Equation Box 2-1, and Table 2-2.

TABLE 2-1. Physical Properties of Some Commonly Used Medical Gases

Property	Air	Carbon Dioxide	Helium	Nitrogen	Nitrous Oxide	Oxygen
Symbol	Air	CO_2	He	N	N_2O	O_2
Color	Colorless	Colorless	Colorless	Colorless	Colorless	Colorless
Odor	Odorless	Odorless	Odorless	Odorless	Odorless	Odorless
Taste	Tasteless	Tasteless/slight acid taste	Tasteless	Tasteless	Tasteless	Tasteless
Life support compatibility	Supports life	Will not support life	Will not support life	Will not support life	Will not support life	Supports life
Flammability	Nonflammable	Nonflammable	Nonflammable	Nonflammable	Nonflammable, supports combustion	Nonflammable, supports combustion
Molecular weight	28.975	44.01	4.003	28.013	44.013	31.999
Percent by mole	—	0.0335	0.000524	78.084	—	20.946
Percent by weight	—	0.045	—	75.5	—	23.2
Partial pressure (ATPD)	—	0.25 mm Hg	—	01.75 mm Hg	—	158 mm Hg
Viscosity*	182.7×10^{-6}	148×10^{-6}	194.1×10^{-6}	—	—	201.8×10^{-6}
Density*	1.2 kg/m^3	1.833 kg/m^3	0.1656 kg/m^3	1.1605 kg/m^3	1.9703 $kg/m^{3\dagger}$	1.326 kg/m^3
Specific gravity	1.0	1.524	0.138	0.967	1.529	1.1049
Boiling point	−194.3°C	−29°C	−268.9°C	−195.8°C	−88.47°C	−183°C
Critical temperature	−140.7°C	31.1°C	−267.9°C	−147.0°C	36.5°C	−118.6°C
Critical pressure	547 psia	1070.6 psia	33 psia	493 psia	1054 psia	731.4 psia
Triple point	—	−56.6°C at 75.1 psia	—	−210°C at 1.82 psia	−90.83°C at 12.74 psia	218.8°C at 0.220 psia
Solubility H_2O at 0°C	0.0292	0.90	0.0086	0.023	1.3	0.0489

*All values referenced to 21.1°C and 1 atmosphere.

†Values for H_2O are at 0°C and 1 atmosphere.

D at 1 atmosphere.

Equation Box 2-1: Effects of Barometric Pressure on Partial Pressure of Oxygen

At one atmosphere (760 mm Hg), the partial pressure of oxygen (PO_2) is 159 mm Hg. The partial pressure for any barometric pressure (PB) can be calculated using the following formula:

$$PO_2 = (PB) \cdot FIO_2$$

Changes in PO_2 are most often encountered during ascent to a higher altitude. At an altitude of 30,000 feet (PB = 266), PO_2 decreases by 70%.

$$PO_2 = (226) \cdot 0.21$$

$$PO_2 = 47.5 \text{ mm Hg}$$

These changes in PO_2 account for the need to pressurize aircraft during high-altitude flight and explain why the normal partial pressure of oxygen in arterial blood (PaO_2) is variable according to geography. Table 2-2 compares PB and PO_2 at different altitudes.

Another important physical characteristic of O_2 is its ability to support combustion. Materials that will burn in room air will burn vigorously and at a higher temperature in the presence of oxygen. Petroleum products (eg, oil, grease) will ignite easily, occasionally from a simple spark caused by friction or from the energy created by impact, and will burn violently. Oxygen itself, however, is nonflammable.

The molecular bonding characteristics of oxygen are also unique. To form the molecule O_2, two oxygen atoms combine by sharing two electrons in the outer shell orbital. This "sharing" of electrons gives O_2 a paramagnetic quality. A paramagnetic oxygen analyzer (see Chapter 9) exploits this unique characteristic of oxygen to measure the PO_2 of a gas sample.

Oxygen Used in Respiratory Care

Oxygen for medical use is often stored as a liquid to reduce the size of the container required to house it.

TABLE 2-2. Effects of Altitude on Barometric Pressure and Partial Pressure of Oxygen

Altitude (ft)	Barometric Pressure (mm Hg)	PO_2 (mm Hg)
Sea level	760	159
5,000	623	132
10,000	523	109
20,000	349	73
30,000	226	47

Oxygen becomes a liquid at temperatures below its boiling point, −183°C. As a liquid, O_2 is a pale blue color and is 1.14 times heavier than water. When the temperature of liquid O_2 is greater than −118.6°C, it will return to the gaseous state regardless of the pressure exerted. This is known as the critical temperature. At the critical temperature, O_2 will return to the liquid state if compressed by 731.4 psia. This is known as the critical pressure.

At normal atmospheric conditions, the density of O_2 (1.329 kg/m^3) is greater than air but less than carbon dioxide. The density of a gas is important in measurement and control of flow and volume. This is why each gas has a separate flowmeter to accurately regulate gas delivery.

Manufacture of Oxygen

The most significant method for manufacturing O_2 is accomplished by the fractional distillation of liquefied air. This method is also known as the Joule-Kelvin method because it is based on the Joule-Kelvin principle. This principle states that when gases under pressure are released into a vacuum, the gas molecules will tend to lose their kinetic energy. In the vacuum, the reduction in kinetic energy causes a decrease in temperature as well as a reduction in the cohesive forces between molecules. This is an essential part of the liquefaction of air.

The process of fractional distillation (shown in Fig. 2-1) can be divided into three stages: (1) purification, (2) liquefaction, and (3) distillation.

1. *Purification.* Using a large compressor, room air is first compressed to 1500 psig. This increase in pressure results in a rise in temperature (according to Gay-Lussac's law) that is dissipated by use of a water-cooled heat exchanger. The air is then further compressed to 2000 psig, passed through an aftercooler, and delivered to a countercurrent heat exchanger at room temperature. By using waste nitrogen as a coolant, the air is cooled to −50°F. This process causes water vapor to freeze and be removed from the system.
2. *Liquefaction.* In a second heat exchanger, gas is cooled to −40°F by the evaporation of liquid ammonia, eliminating any remaining water vapor. A third heat exchanger cools the air to −265°F, with the pressure remaining at 200 psig. At this point, no liquefaction has taken place, since the critical pressure of air is 532 psig. For liquefaction to take place, the air is released into a separator and expanded to 90 psig. Releasing the pressure causes a further reduction in temperature and partial liquefaction.
3. *Distillation.* In the separator, gas and liquid are pumped through separate streams into the distillation column. The liquid portion enters the top of

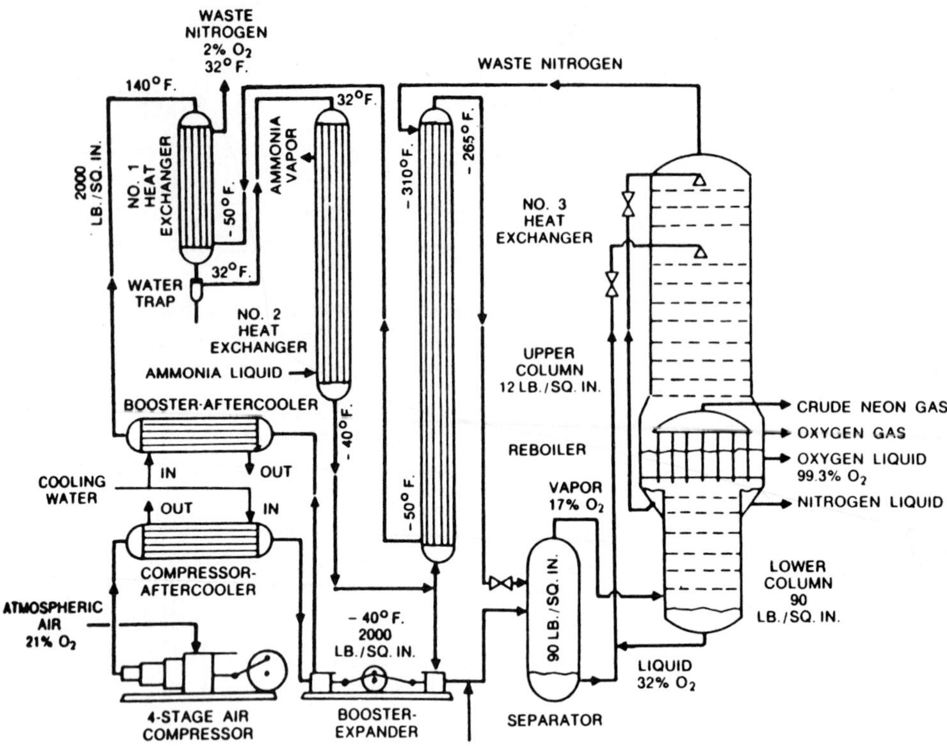

Figure 2-1. Fractional distillation plant for the production of liquid oxygen from air (Joule-Kelvin method). (Courtesy of Union Carbide Corp, Indianapolis, IN)

the distillation column and passes over a series of cylindrical shells that contain metal trays. As the liquid passes down over the trays, vapor from the separator passes through them. The falling liquid becomes richer in oxygen (as nitrogen boils off) and the rising vapor becomes richer in nitrogen. At the bottom of the column, liquid oxygen forms but contains a few impurities. These include the gases argon and krypton. The oxygen is reboiled with precise control of temperature and pressure. These gases evaporate (their boiling points are lower), leaving 99.9% pure O_2.[2]

Other methods for preparing large amounts of oxygen are mainly historical and include electrolysis of water and heating metallic oxides (barium oxide, mercuric oxide).[2] Oxygen concentrators are discussed later in this chapter.

Compressed Air

The earth's natural atmosphere consists of the colorless, odorless, tasteless gas we call air. Air is actually a mixture of other gases, the major constituents being oxygen and nitrogen. Several other trace gases are present in small to insignificant amounts. Table 2-3 lists the typical concentration of air at 1 atmosphere (ATA). Air is considered nonflammable and, by virtue of its second most abundant constituent (oxygen), can support life. The density of air is 1.2 kg/m^3, slightly less than that of oxygen. Air can be stored as a transparent liquid, which has a slight bluish tint, and if carbon dioxide is present in sufficient quantities, it takes on a milky appearance. The boiling point of air is −194.3°C.

Manufacture of Compressed Air

The abundant uses of compressed air outside the medical field have resulted in the CGA specifying grades of air.[2] In gaseous form, these are A through J, with J being the medical form. Compressed medical air is 19.5% to 23.5% oxygen, is anhydrous, and contains a minimum level of impurities (eg, dioxides, hydrocarbons).

There are three methods by which medical-grade air can be obtained. The first, and least common, is by the combination of oxygen and nitrogen in the appro-

TABLE 2-3. Typical Concentration of Air at One Atmosphere

Gas	Percentage by Mole	Percentage by Weight
Nitrogen	78.084	75.5
Oxygen	20.946	23.2
Argon	0.934	1.33
Carbon dioxide	0.0335	0.045
Hydrogen	0.00005	—
Neon	0.001818	—
Helium	0.000524	—
Krypton	0.000114	—
Xenon	0.0000087	—

priate concentrations. This is expensive compared with other methods and is only done in unusual circumstances. Large quantities of liquid air can be manufactured by either the Linde or the Claude process. Both methods use the compression and reexpansion of the air to cool the gas, finally resulting in liquefaction. Of the two, the Claude process is more efficient, only requiring pressure to be increased to 30 atm. The Linde process requires pressures in excess of 200 atm to produce liquefaction.

Most air is supplied on site from bedside compressors or large compressors, which supply gas to multiple bedsides through a piping system. Compressors are discussed later in this chapter.

Carbon Dioxide

Carbon dioxide (CO_2) is a naturally occurring compound that represents approximately 0.03% of the earth's atmosphere by volume. CO_2 is a by-product of human respiration, the combustion of fossil fuels, and fermentation, and is released during the decay of animal and vegetable remains. At normal atmospheric conditions, CO_2 is an odorless, tasteless, colorless gas that is nontoxic in the presence of sufficient oxygen and relatively nonreactive. Since CO_2 is an acid gas, some individuals believe it has a "pungent"' odor and a slight acid taste.[2] CO_2 is heavier and more dense than either air or oxygen, is nonflammable, and is incapable of supporting life. At its triple point (−56.6°C and 60.43 psig) CO_2 can exist simultaneously in all three phases. At even lower temperatures and normal atmospheric pressure CO_2 will go directly from a solid to a gas (sublimation), bypassing the liquid state. This is commonly observed when solid CO_2 (dry ice) appears to be "smoking" when left out in normal atmospheric conditions. The critical temperature of CO_2 is 28.05°C, making it easily liquefied under pressure. In a compressed medical gas cylinder, CO_2 will exist as both a liquid and a gas. In these instances, determining the volume remaining in the cylinder requires that the cylinder be weighed.

The medical applications of CO_2 usually dictate that it be delivered in conjunction with O_2 in 95%/5% or 90%/10% mixtures. In these instances, none of the CO_2 will remain in liquid form. Tanks of 100% CO_2 are often used for calibration of blood gas analyzers.

Manufacture of Carbon Dioxide

Unrefined CO_2 is obtained from the combustion of carbonaceous fuels (coal, coke, natural gas, and oil), as a by-product from the fermentation of sugar during alcohol production, and from natural wells and springs. Before use, this CO_2 is refined and purified to 99.5% or higher, depending on its application. Aside from its medical use, CO_2 is widely used to carbonate beverages, as a food preservative, and as a shielding gas during welding.[2]

In its liquid form, CO_2 is used in fire extinguishers and in cooling systems as a refrigerant. Solid CO_2 is frequently used for shipping items that would perish at normal temperatures.

Helium

Helium (He) is a rare, naturally occurring gas that occupies a very small portion of the earth's atmosphere (5 ppm). It is nonflammable, odorless, tasteless, colorless, and chemically inert. Helium is the second lightest atmospheric element (only hydrogen is lighter) and has an extremely low density (0.1656 kg/m^3) approximately one-sixth that of air. The medical use of He includes diagnostic applications (in the determination of lung volumes and in the assessment of airway obstruction) and as a therapeutic mixture with O_2 to treat patients with severe airway obstruction. The latter uses the low density properties of He as a method to increase flow through narrowed orifices. Commercially, He is used for lifting lighter-than-air airships, as a gas shield during arc welding, as a coolant in nuclear reactors, as a protective atmosphere during the manufacture of germanium and silicon crystals for transistors, and in the production of highly reactive metals (titanium and zirconium).[2]

Manufacture of Helium

Most He is recovered from natural gas wells containing as much a 2% He. The largest of these wells are located in Saskatchewan (Canada), near the Black Sea, and in the southwestern United States. Like CO_2, raw He is refined through a process of liquefaction and purification, resulting in a product 99.9% pure. Helium can also be obtained in small amounts from the atmosphere by fractionation.

Nitrous Oxide

Nitrous oxide (N_2O) is an analgesic gas often referred to as "laughing gas." At normal atmospheric conditions, nitrous oxide is an odorless, colorless, tasteless gas. Nitrous oxide is nonflammable but will support combustion to a degree less than O_2 but more than room air. It is slightly heavier and more dense than CO_2. The principle medical use of nitrous oxide is as a general anesthetic during surgical procedures. Although nitrous oxide is nontoxic, its use without sufficient O_2 (minimum 20%) will result in death by asphyxia.

Commercially, nitrous oxide is used as a propellant for aerosol products and as a refrigeration fluid during the immersion freezing of food products.

Manufacture of Nitrous Oxide

The majority of nitrous oxide is manufactured by the thermal decomposition of ammonium nitrate. This reaction produces large amounts of nitrous oxide and water as well as small amounts of highly toxic oxides. These are removed by a series of scrubbing towers, and the water is removed by condensation and finally by passing the refined nitrous oxide through a desiccant material.[2]

Nitrogen

Nitrogen (N_2) is the most abundant gas in the earth's atmosphere (78.03%). At normal atmospheric conditions, it is a colorless, odorless, tasteless, inert gas. Nitrogen is less dense than both air and O_2 and has a lower boiling point. It will not support life or combustion and is nonflammable. Nitrogen is used medically as a calibration gas for many types of gas analyzers, usually providing the zero reference point, and in the pulmonary function laboratory, as a diagnostic gas. Commercially, nitrogen has a tremendous variety of uses including as a refrigerant for numerous food products, for the preservation of live tissues (eg, blood, livestock sperm), and as an important part of numerous classified projects in the United States missile and space programs.[2]

Manufacture of Nitrogen

Nitrogen is produced in large quantities during the liquefaction of air, as described previously in the discussion of O_2 manufacturing. Table 2-1 compares characteristics of medical gases.

Medical Gas Distribution Systems

Respiratory care practitioners work every day with oxygen, medical compressed air, and other medical gases and seldom think about where these gases come from or how they travel to the patient's bedside. It is only when equipment malfunctions or new construction is being done that the therapist needs to know about hospital gas supply and piping systems. On the other hand, when the oxygen supply system for an entire hospital fails suddenly, the magnitude of the threat is indeed terrifying. Ventilated patients in the intensive care unit, oxygen-dependent patients on the floors, newborns in the nursery, and surgery patients in the operating room may all be in mortal danger if the oxygen system fails. Because the potential magnitude of the disaster is so great, it is imperative that the respiratory care practitioner understand the oxygen supply system and know what to do if an oxygen supply failure occurs.

When new construction dictates the need for additions to the current piping system or installation of a new one, respiratory care practitioners should be included when planning and testing the system. Appropriate decisions regarding the number and locations of outlets can prevent future expense and inconvenience. Care should be taken not to overlook remote hospital locations where patients may be taken for therapeutic or diagnostic procedures.

Standards

Several nongovernmental agencies have published standards for hospital piping systems. These include the CGA, the NFPA, the International Standards Organization (ISO), the Canadian Standards Association (CSA), and the American Society of Mechanical Engineers (ASME).[1–5] And although these agencies have no regulatory authority, these standards are often written into state and local laws.

Compliance with standards is often left to individual hospitals and suppliers, although more recently compliance with these standards is required by the Joint Commission on the Accreditation of Healthcare Organizations (JCAHO).

The respiratory care department and physical plant personnel are frequently jointly responsible for the medical gas distribution system and should be familiar with these standards. Feeley and Hedley-Whyte found that in 1976 compliance with NFPA standards was uncommon.[6]

Bulk Gas Delivery Systems

A bulk gas delivery system consists of the central supply with monitoring and alarm systems, the piping that delivers gas to patient care areas, and the terminal units at each point of use. A bulk oxygen system is any assembly of equipment and interconnecting piping that has a storage capacity of more than 20,000 cubic feet of oxygen, including unconnected reserves on hand at the site.[1] Bulk delivery systems for nitrous oxide, air, and carbon dioxide may also be part of a hospital's gas distribution system.

The supply of bulk gas for any gas distribution system is known as the central supply. The central supply may be located outside (the control panel must be protected from the elements), in an enclosure used specifically for this purpose, or in a room used specifically for this purpose that is enclosed within a building used for other purposes.[1] Access to the central supply should be limited to individuals responsible for the care and safety of the system.

The central oxygen supply system varies in construction and components depending on the demand for oxygen and site of use. Three typical supply systems are the (1) cylinder supply system without a reserve supply, also known as an alternating supply system; (2) cylinder supply system with a reserve supply; and (3) bulk supply system with reserve supply.

The alternating supply system is shown in Figure 2-2. Two banks of cylinders each with its own pressure regulator and each containing a minimum of an average day's supply of oxygen are used. Each bank must have a least two cylinders, and more than a day's supply may be necessary if the hospital is located in a remote area. Cylinders from each bank are connected to a high-pressure header that combines them into a single continuous supply. Check valves are placed between each cylinder and the header to prevent loss of gas due to a leak in a single cylinder. These check valves operate as one-way valves, allowing flow from the cylinder to the header but not from the header back toward the cylinder. With this system, the bank in use is considered the primary supply and the secondary bank the stand-by supply. When the primary supply can no longer meet system demands, the secondary supply automatically switches on and becomes the primary supply. This is accomplished at the changeover or activating switch. The activating switch is sensitive to differences in supply pressure and closes gas flow from the primary supply when it falls below a predetermined pressure. Together, the primary and secondary supplies are known as the operating supply. After the switch-over from the primary to secondary supplies, full cylinders should be placed in the primary supply bank. Alternating supply systems are typically used to supply nitrous oxide and carbon dioxide in large facilities or oxygen in small facilities.

A cylinder system with a reserve supply is shown in Figure 2-3. In this system, the operating supplies consist of the primary and secondary supply (usually liquid oxygen). The reserve supply consists of a minimum of three cylinders and must either have a check valve between each cylinder and the header or an activating switch that signals when less than a day's supply remains in the reserve.

The primary and secondary supplies typically have check valves prior to the header but are not required if a check valve is present between the primary supply line and the point where the reserve system intersects the main line.

In this system, the reserve is only used in emergency situations when neither the primary nor secondary systems can supply system demands. When this occurs, a signal alerting the switch-over should warn the appropriate personnel. Reserve systems can also be used when maintenance or repair of the operating supply is required.

A pressure regulator and pressure relief valve are placed at the end of the central supply system prior to piping that leads to the hospital. In some instances two pressure regulators are used in series in case one should fail. All final pressure regulators must be installed in tandem with a bypass system between them. This allows the regulator to be serviced without interrupting gas delivery.

Most bulk oxygen supply systems at large facilities use a stationary liquid system as the operating supply. A typical bulk supply system is shown in Figure 2-4.

The bulk supply system consists of the liquid operating supply and a reserve supply consisting of a bank of cylinders or smaller liquid system. In many in-

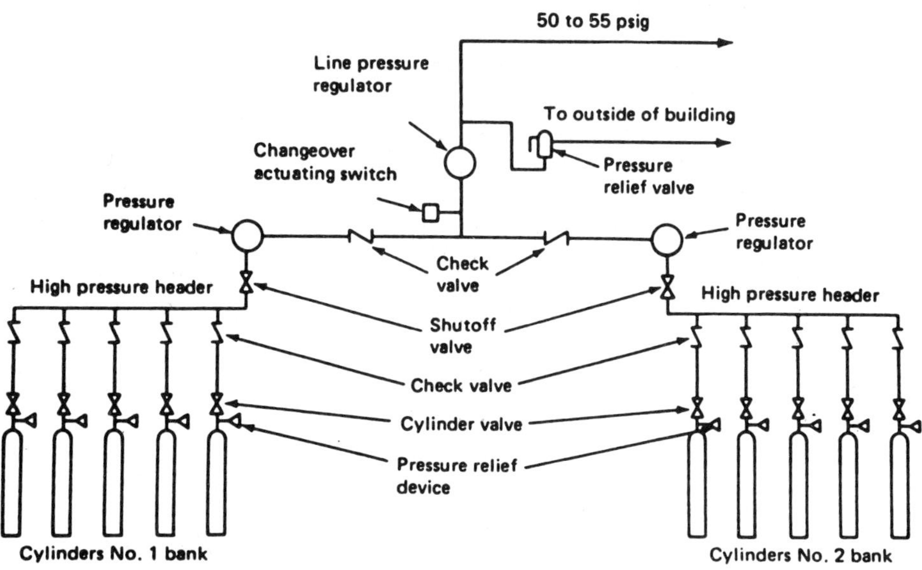

Figure 2-2. A typical cylinder supply system without a reserve supply or alternating supply system. (From Klein PE. Health Care Facilities Handbook. 4th Ed. National Fire Protection Association. Quincy, MA 1993)

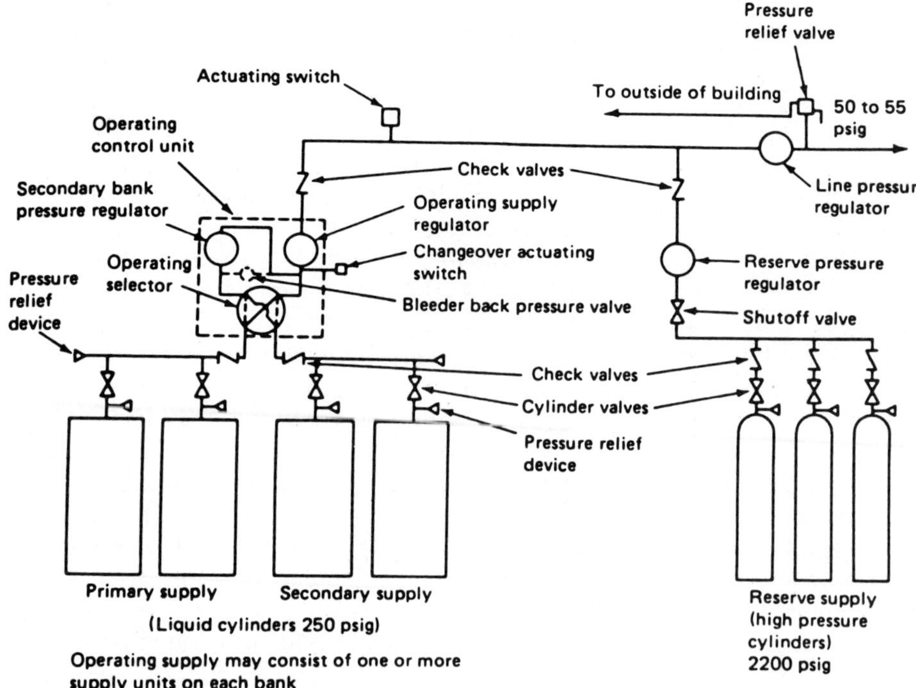

Figure 2-3. A typical cylinder supply system with a reserve supply. (From Klein PE. Health Care Facilities Handbook. 4th Ed. National Fire Protection Association. Quincy, MA 1993)

stances, demand is too great to be met economically and efficiently with cylinders. As with the other systems we have described, the bulk system requires a pressure regulator and check valve between each gas supply and the main gas supply line. A check valve is also required in the main gas supply line upstream from the point of intersection with the secondary or reserve supply.

Manually operated shutoff valves must be installed upstream of each pressure regulator. Pressure relief valves are placed in the main supply line and set to vent gas to the atmosphere at a pressure 50% greater than normal line pressure.

All bulk oxygen systems must also have an emergency oxygen supply connection incorporated into the piping system outside the building served. This

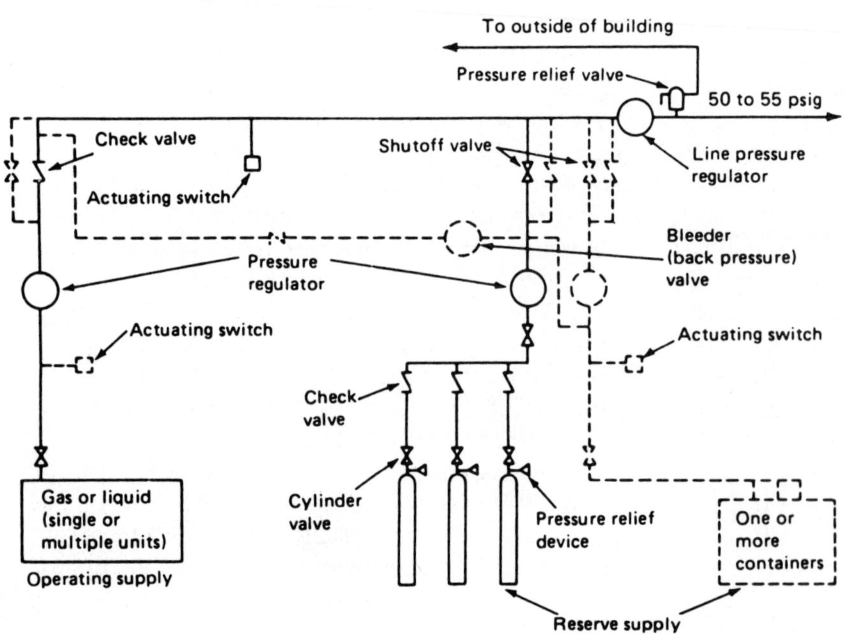

Figure 2-4. A typical bulk supply system. (From Klein PE. Health Care Facilities Handbook. 4th Ed. National Fire Protection Association. Quincy, MA 1993)

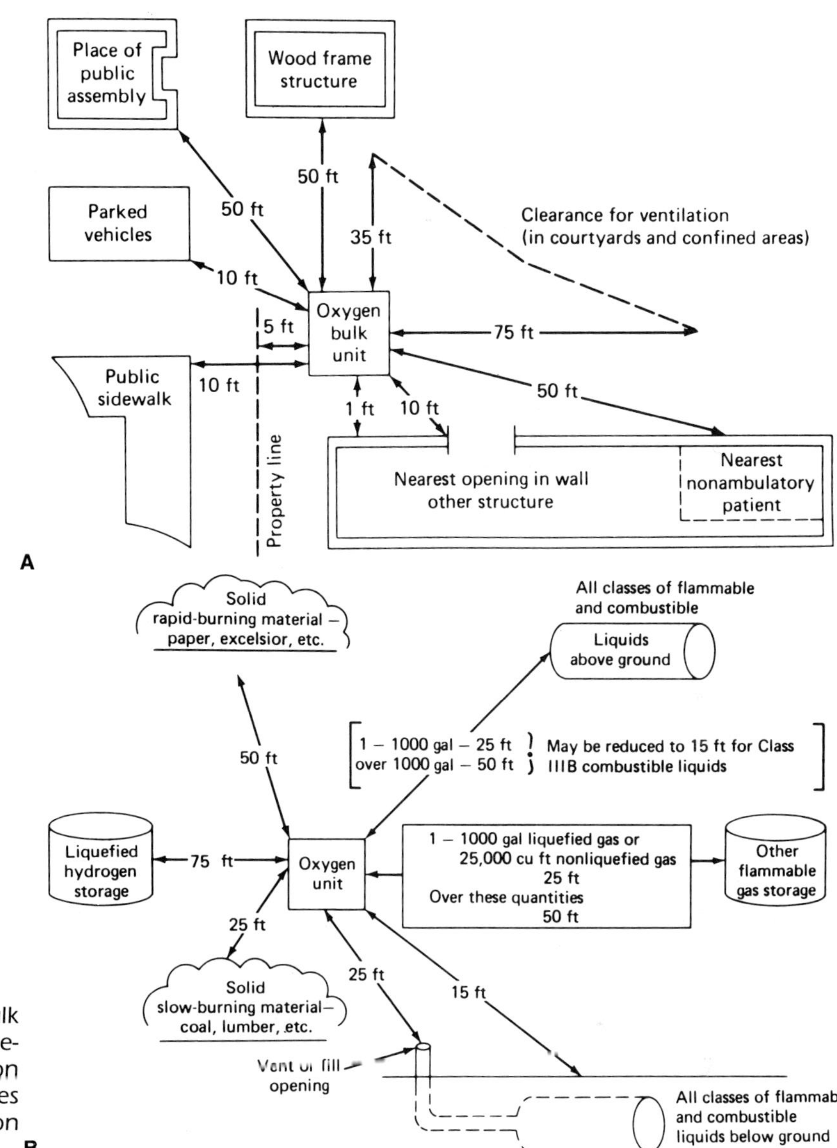

Figure 2-5. (A) Distance between the bulk oxygen unit and exposures. (B) Distance between the bulk oxygen unit and ignition sources. (From Klein PE. Health Care Facilities Handbook. 4th Ed. National Fire Protection Association. Quincy, MA 1993)

connection allows a temporary auxiliary source of gas to be connected in emergencies. This inlet must be labeled "Emergency low pressure gaseous oxygen inlet," be downstream of the main supply shutoff valve, and be physically protected to prevent tampering or unauthorized access. This T-shaped connection must have a check valve and pressure relief valve installed prior to the main supply line. These emergency connections are typically serviced by trailer units. Trailer units are large cylinders of liquid oxygen that can be towed to the distribution area. Trailer units may also be used when maintenance or repair of the central supply is needed.

Bulk Liquid Oxygen

Liquid oxygen is both less expensive and more convenient to store than oxygen in cylinders, making it the preferable method when large quantities of oxygen are required. A cubic foot of liquid oxygen at a temperature of −300°F produces 860 cubic feet of gaseous oxygen at 70°F. Compared with cylinder supply systems, liquid oxygen requires less storage space and less frequent deliveries from suppliers. Additionally, the expense and problems associated with handling large numbers of cylinders are eliminated.

Liquid oxygen systems are typically refilled from supply trucks without interrupting service. Hoses from these supply trucks are indexed to prevent misfilling. Smaller liquid systems may be exchanged on trailers from the supplier to the hospital and back again.

Liquid oxygen systems are installed near ground level to allow easy filling. The NFPA regulates the site requirements for liquid systems, dictating the proximity of potential ignition sources. Figure 2-5 shows the position of bulk oxygen systems and exposures.

Liquid oxygen is stored in a large, double-walled, stainless steel tank constructed like a giant thermos bottle (Fig. 2-6). The space between two steel shells is filled with an insulating material, and then a vacuum is drawn on the insulating space to further reduce heat transfer. As oxygen is needed in the hospital, liquid oxygen goes from the storage tank through a vaporizer coil where heat is absorbed from the environment. As the temperature of the liquid oxygen rises above −297°F, the liquid vaporizes into gaseous oxygen and increases tremendously in volume (by a factor of 860). So much heat is required for vaporization that ambient air is suddenly cooled, and water vapor from the ambient air condenses and freezes on the vaporizer coils. These coils will be caked with layers of ice on even the hottest days. Figure 2-7 is a picture of the bulk liquid oxygen system at the University of Cincinnati.

Compressed Air

Compressed air can be provided to the hospital in a manner similar to oxygen by banks of cylinders, but it is more frequently supplied by motor-driven compressors. In general, air from cylinders is cleaner and drier than air delivered by compressors, but the use of air compressors is considerably less expensive.

Like oxygen supply systems, compressed air delivery systems are regulated by the NFPA. Typically, a compressed air system uses two compressors. These compressors are usually equivalent in size and function and can operate simultaneously or alternately, depending on system demands. In the event of failure, each compressor must be capable of delivering 100% of the calculated peak demand. In larger systems using more than two compressors the peak demand must be met when the largest compressor is out of service.

A typical two-compressor system is shown in Figure 2-8. Each compressor must have its own pressure relief valve, check valves between the compressor and header, and isolation valves to prevent backflow through the off-cycle compressor. The compressors take in ambient air and compress it to above working pressure. Air for an entire hospital is usually supplied by a liquid-sealed rotary compressor. Compressed air is delivered to an aftercooler where moisture is eliminated by decreasing the temperature of the gas such that water vapor is condensed. Gas then travels to a receiver or reservoir tank from which air can be drawn as required. The receiver must be equipped with a pressure gauge, pressure relief valve, automatic drain (to eliminate water), and a visual sight to inspect patency of the drain. The receiver helps maintain a steady air stream to the pressure regulator, helps further condense water vapor, and reduces wear on the compressor. A dryer located between the receiver and regulator removes any remaining moisture. The importance of delivering dry air to the station outlet is discussed later. Recently, the NFPA has made recommendations for monitoring air downstream from the dryer. This includes monitoring dew point and humidity to ensure adequate function of the aftercooler and dryer as well as monitoring contaminants (carbon dioxide, carbon monoxide, hydrocarbons, and particulate matter).[1]

Location of the compressor ambient air intake is particularly important in eliminating contaminants. The intakes should be located outside the hospital where air is free from dirt, smoke, fumes, and odors. Attention should be paid to potential sources of contaminants, such as automobile exhaust and exhaust from other hospital areas (eg, anesthetic scavenging

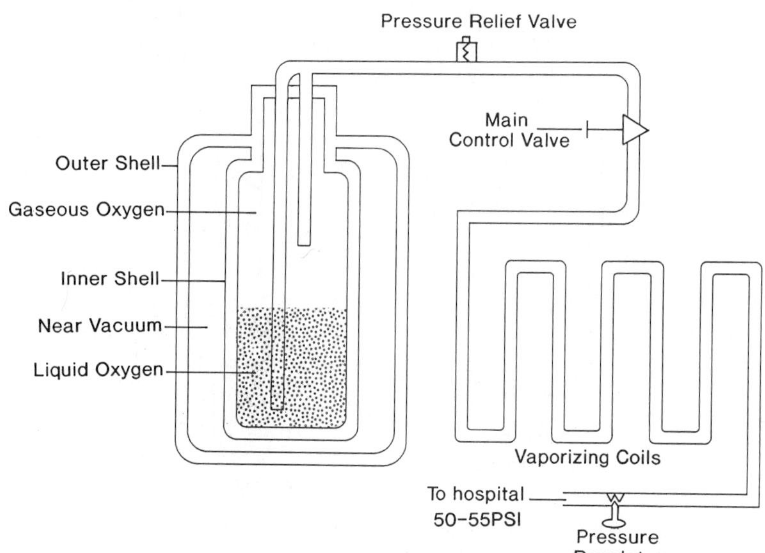

Figure 2-6. A fixed station for bulk liquid oxygen storage.

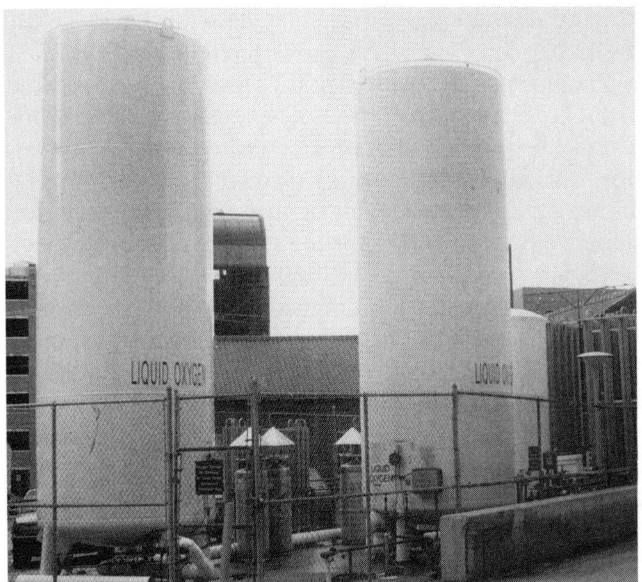

Figure 2-7. The bulk liquid oxygen system at the University of Cincinnati.

systems). In areas where local air conditions may exceed USP levels for contaminants, filtering systems should be used. Filters are typically placed between each intake and compressor and between each compressor and the aftercooler. When filters are used, they must be installed in duplex to allow maintenance and repair without interrupting service.

Medical-grade air delivered by compressors should be clean and dry, but it is not sterile. Many respiratory care devices are equipped with filters to prevent damage to equipment caused by contaminated air.

Piping Distribution Systems

Piping systems deliver gas through a system of seamless type K or L copper or brass pipe. These pipes must be identified by labeling at least every 20 feet and at least once in each room and building floor. Labeling is essential to prevent improper cross-connections and alert maintenance personnel to the contents of individual pipes. Oxygen is typically installed in 0.5-inch outside diameter pipe and other gases in 0.375-inch outside diameter as additional protection from cross connections.

Considerable variation exists in the actual distribution of piping through the hospital. A typical gas distribution system is shown in Figure 2-9. Piping systems include the pipes, pressure relief valves, zone valves, alarms, and terminal units. Three classes of pipes are usually identified as described below:

- *Main lines.* Pipes that connect the operating supply to risers, branch lines, or both.
- *Risers.* Pipes installed vertically that connect the main line with branch lines on each floor of the building.

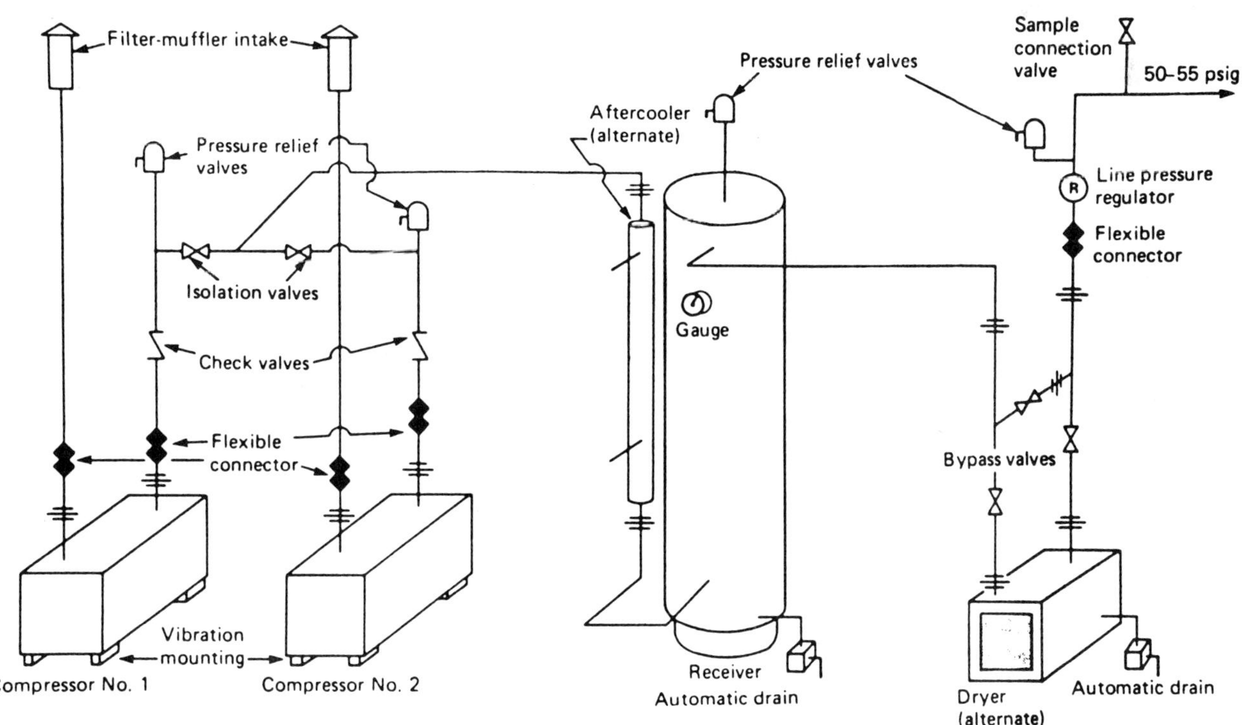

Figure 2-8. A duplex medical air compressor system. (From Klein PE. Health Care Facilities Handbook. 4th Ed. National Fire Protection Association. Quincy, MA 1993)

- *Branch (lateral) lines.* Pipes that travel from the risers to individual rooms or group of rooms on the same floor of the building.

Pressure Relief Valves

Pressure relief valves are required in the bulk liquid oxygen container, above each air compressor, and downstream of the main line pressure regulator. Additionally, a pressure relief valve should be installed upstream of any zone valve to prevent overpressurization of a part of the system when the zone valve is closed. Pressure relief valves are usually set at 50% greater than working pressure.

Zone Valves

Zone valves are typically located in branch and riser lines and allow isolation of a room or rooms during emergencies or maintenance and repair without shutting off the entire system. Zone valves are also known as shutoff valves, isolation valves, or section valves.

Zone valves should be located in easily accessible areas where caregivers can access them in emergencies. Respiratory care practitioners should know the location of all zone valves in their area of responsibility. Zone valves are usually installed in boxes with easily removable windows (Fig. 2-10). These valves are quarter-turn valves (Fig. 2-11) and allow service downstream from the zone valve to be discontinued by moving the handle from the 3 o'clock to the 6 o'clock position.

A zone valve is required at the outlet of the operating supply, upstream from the main line zone valve. This allows the operating supply to be completely separated from the piping network in case of operating supply failure and a secondary system (trailer unit) to be installed. The zone valve for the operating supply must be located near the operating supply. Another zone valve must be installed at the point where the main line enters the building. This zone valve allows isolation of the entire hospital and should be in a readily accessible location but protected from possible tampering.

Zone valves are also required in each riser supplied from the main line adjacent to the riser connection and in each branch line serving non–"life-support" patient rooms. A zone valve is required outside each "life-support" or "critical care" area and installed in a position to be operated from a standing position in an emergency. Separate zone valves are also required outside each anesthetizing location in the operating room. Zone valves in the operating room must be located outside the individual room.

Medical Gas Distribution System Alarms

All gas distribution systems require alarms to monitor the operating supply, reserve supply, and pressure in the main and local supply lines.

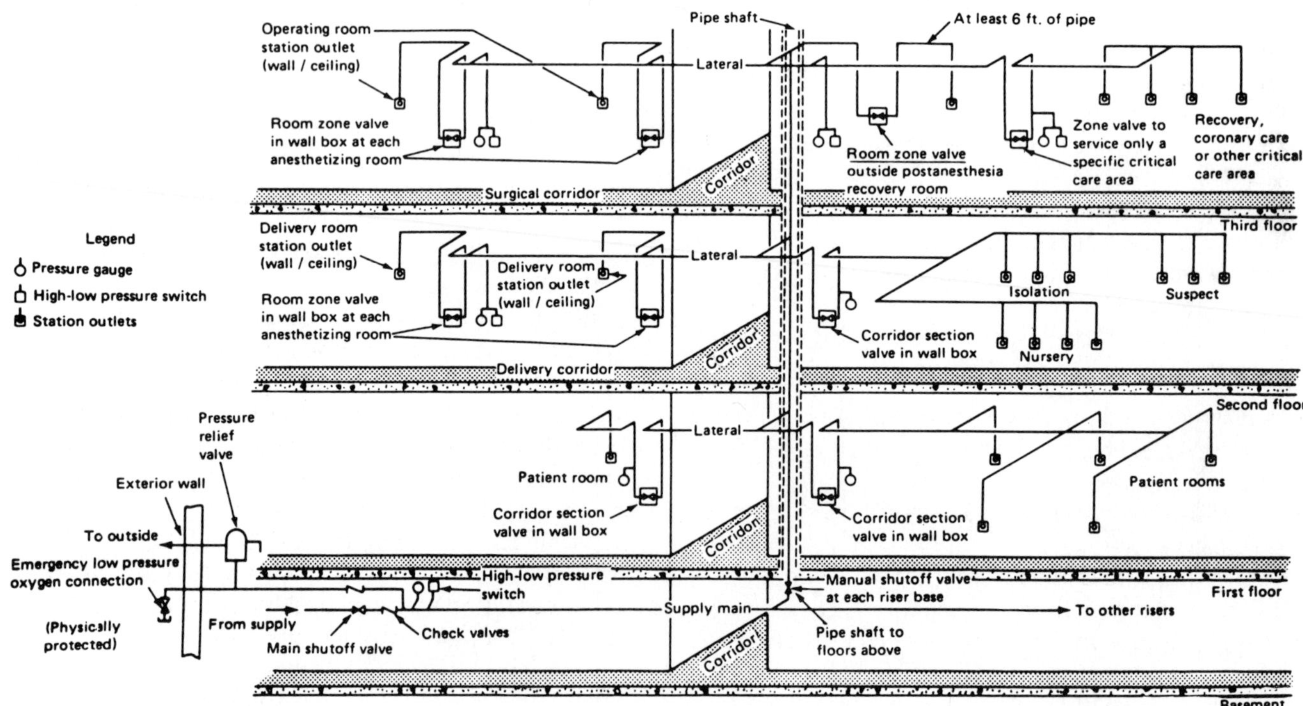

Figure 2-9. Location of valves, pressure switches, and piping for a medical gas distribution system. (From Klein PE. Health Care Facilities Handbook. 4th Ed. National Fire Protection Association. Quincy, MA 1993)

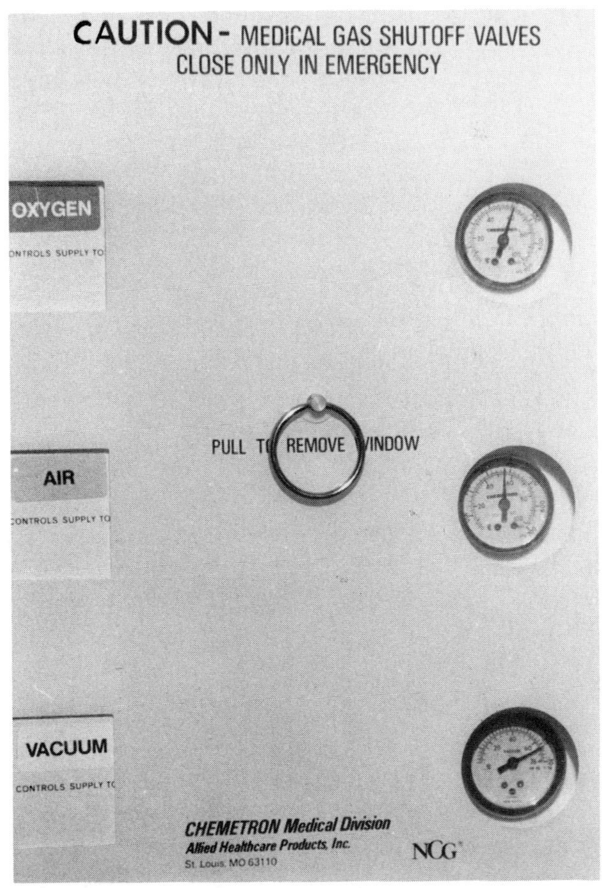

Figure 2-10. Zone valve covered by a removable window.

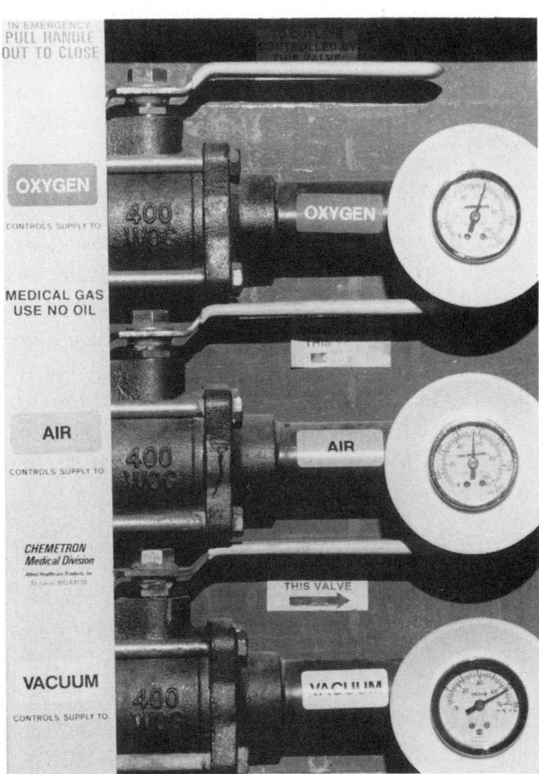

Figure 2-11. Zone valves for air, oxygen, and vacuum. These are manually operated quarter-turn valves. Each valve should be clearly labeled as to the gas within.

Master Alarm Systems

A master alarm system consisting of two signal panels in separate locations monitors the operating supply and main line pressure. Separate monitoring locations are required to ensure continuous surveillance. Ideally these alarms are placed in the office of the individual responsible for gas system maintenance and in either the security office or telephone operator's area. Master alarms should be audible and signals should be visual and noncancellable.

The following conditions should result in an audible or noncancellable visual alarm:

- A changeover from the primary to secondary bank occurs, or just before the reserve supply goes into operation.
- When the reserve supply is reduced to one average day's supply.
- When pressure in the reserve supply is too low to allow proper function.
- When pressure in the main line increases or decreases from normal operating pressure.
- When the level of liquid in the bulk liquid oxygen supply reaches a predetermined level.
- When dew point in the compressed air system exceeds a threshold.

Area Alarm Systems

Area alarm systems are required in vital care areas, including critical care units, operating rooms, and recovery rooms. These alarms must provide an audible and noncancellable visual alarm if operating pressure changes 20% from normal operating pressure.[1] In critical care units the area alarm should be installed in the specific line serving that area downstream of the zone valve (Fig. 2-12). Area alarms should be labeled appropriately and installed near the point of use to ensure responsible surveillance.

Employees responsible for monitoring area alarms should be trained to respond appropriately. Responses vary according to area and hospital policy but should include notification of respiratory care personnel and individuals responsible for maintenance of the piping system. Appropriate response to an alarm should be documented in the hospital's policy and procedure manual, and new employees should be trained accordingly. Feeley and Hedley-Whyte[6] have reported instances when area alarms have sounded and hospital employees did not know what to do.

Pressure Gauges

Pressure gauges are important in monitoring line pressures, allowing the cause of alarms to be easily identified. Pressure gauges must be installed in the main line adjacent to the actuating switch and in each area alarm panel. Gauges should be labeled appropriately, color coded, and readable from a standing position.

Station Outlets

Station outlets or terminal units are the final component of the piping system. The station outlet is the point where equipment (eg, ventilators, flowmeters) is connected and disconnected from the gas distribution system.

Station outlets are made up of the base block, face plate, primary valve, secondary valve, and the connection point. The base block is the portion of the station outlet connected to the piping system. A base block is similar in function to an electric outlet at the end of an electric wiring system. The face plate covers the base block and must be permanently marked with the name and/or symbol of the delivered gas. Face plates are also color coded for easy identification.

The primary and secondary valves are safety or check valves that open to allow gas flow when the male probe is inserted and automatically closes when the probe is disengaged (Fig. 2-13). These valves prevent loss of gas when equipment is disconnected from the station outlet. Two valves are used to allow maintenance of the station outlet without excessive loss of gases. It is important to remember that these check valves will allow gas to flow in either direction. In general, if equipment is turned off, it should be disconnected from the gas source.

Diameter Index Safety System and Quick Connecters

To prevent misconnection of gases each station outlet will accept only a gas-specific connecter. This is accomplished by using a threaded Diameter Index Safety System connector or a nonthreaded quick connecter. The Diameter Index Safety System was developed by the CGA for medical gases at 200 psig or less. This connection consists of a body, nipple, and nut assembly. The body contains two specifically sized "bores," the nipple, and two specifically sized "shoulders" (Fig. 2-14). The small bore (BB) mates with the small shoulder (MM), and the large bore (CC) mates with the large shoulder (NN). Inappropriate connections are prevented by changing bore sizes in opposite directions. As BB gets larger, CC gets smaller. In this manner, only properly mated parts are allowed to achieve a threaded connecter.

Quick connecters allow the noninterchangeability of the Diameter Index Safety System but speed up connection by using a single action rater than a threaded connection. Essentially, quick connecters are "plugged in" to the station outlet like plugging in an electric device.

There are a variety of quick connect devices, each different in size and shape. Two of the most common are the national compressed gas (NCG) and Ohio quick connecters (Fig. 2-15). All quick connecters consist of a pair of nonthreaded, gas-specific male and female connecters. Noninterchangeability is ensured by different sizes, shapes, and configurations of the mating portions (Fig. 2-16). There are no standards for quick connecters, and individual manufacturers are responsible for ensuring noninterchangeability. Quick connecters are more convenient than Diameter Index Safety System fittings but are more prone to leaks.

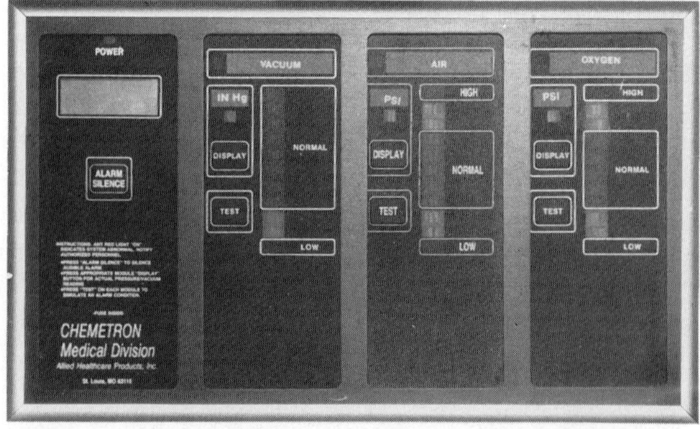

Figure 2-12. Area alarm system for an intensive care unit. Gas pressures for air, oxygen, and vacuum are displayed, and an alarm is activated if pressure deviates ±20% from normal operating pressure. Push buttons allow the alarm system to be tested for proper operation.

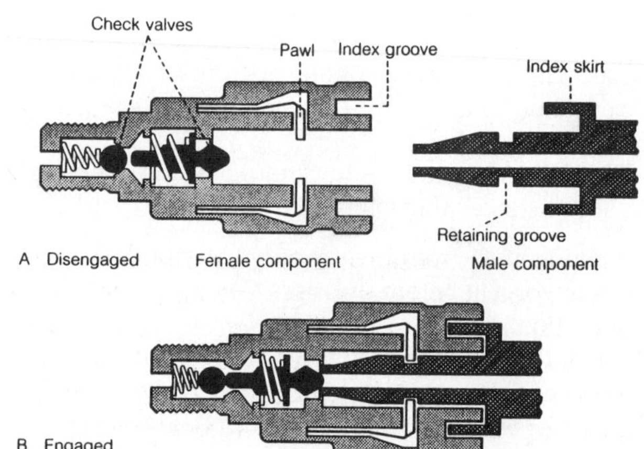

Figure 2-13. Quick disconnect system for a medical gas station outlet. The check valves represent primary and secondary valves. (A.) The male connector is disengaged, and the check valves prevent leakage of gas. (B.) The male connector is engaged, allowing gas to flow to the appropriate device. (From Barnes TA. Core Textbook of Respiratory Care Practice, 2nd ed. St. Louis: CV Mosby, 1994)

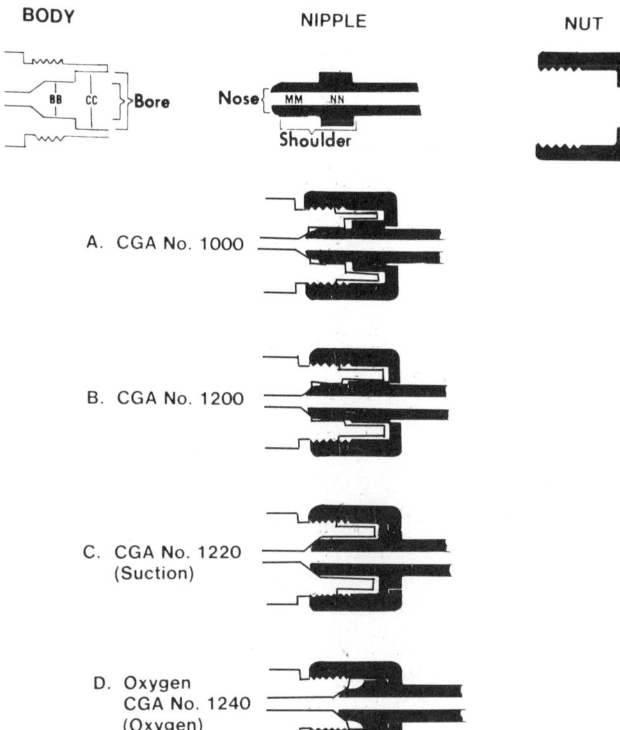

Figure 2-14. Diameter index safety system. A through D. As the CGA number increases the small shoulder becomes larger and the large diameter becomes smaller. If improper assembly is attempted, either MM will be too large for BB or NN will be too large for CC. (From Dorsch JA, Dorsch SE. Understanding Anesthesia Equipment. Baltimore: Williams & Wilkins, 1994)

Testing and Verification of Medical Gas Distribution Systems

After installation of a new piping system, or an addition to an existing one, testing to identify leaks and ensure that there are no cross-connections to other piping systems should be accomplished. Problems with piping systems occur most frequently after additional piping is connected to the existing system.

Pressure Testing

Pressure testing is used to detect leaks in the system. Leaks represent lost gases and lost money. Leaks in oxygen pipelines are particularly dangerous since they create a fire hazard. Before installation of the alarm systems and pressure gauges, the piping system should be pressure tested. This is accomplished by exposing the piping system to a pressure of 150 psig with oil-free air or nitrogen. Each joint in the system is tested for leaks using a leak detection solution. All leaks should be repaired and the test repeated.

After installation of alarms and pressure gauges the entire system should be exposed to a pressure 20% greater than operating pressure for 24 hours. Leak detection should be undertaken and repairs made as necessary.

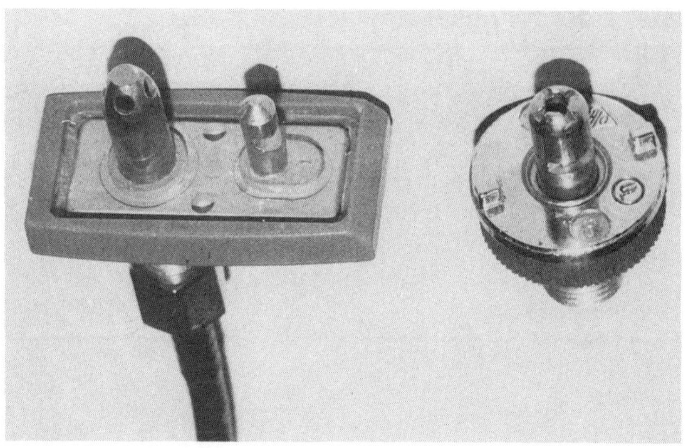

Figure 2-15. Examples of NCG and Ohio quick connectors for oxygen.

Testing for cross-connections is accomplished to verify that each station outlet delivers the gas shown on the outlet label and that proper connecting fittings are present. Cross-connection testing requires that gases be tested one at a time. All gases except the one to be tested are turned off. Each individual station outlet is then tested to determine that the test gas is being dispensed only from outlets of the gas system being tested.

Alternatively, all gas systems can be reduced to atmospheric pressure and then increased to the pressures shown in Table 2-4.

Once pressure in each system is adjusted, each station outlet is tested using a pressure gauge and the appropriate gas-specific connecter. Pressure on the test gauge for a given gas supply should match the pressure shown above.

Additional testing is accomplished by testing the percentage of oxygen coming from each station outlet with an oxygen analyzer. Compressed air should contain 21% oxygen, nitrous oxide should contain 0%

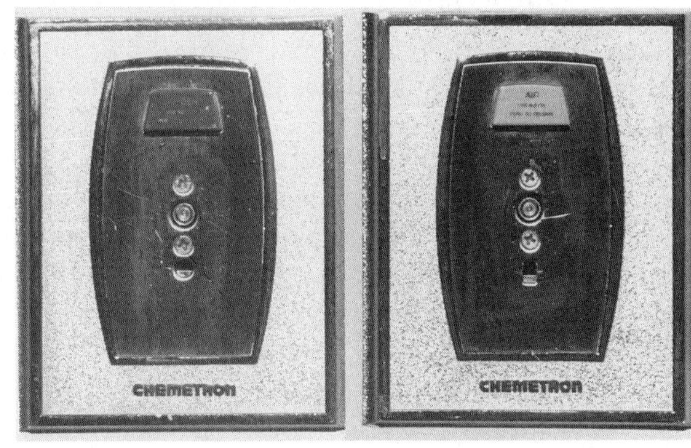

Figure 2-16. Station outlet for NCG connectors of air and oxygen.

TABLE 2-4. Pressures of Medical Gases

	Pressure	
Medical Gas	Psig	kPa Gauge
Gas mixtures	20	140
Nitrogen	30	210
Nitrous oxide	40	280
Oxygen	50	350
Compressed air	60	420

oxygen, and the oxygen system should supply 100% oxygen. If a mass spectrometer is available, the actual concentrations of other gases should also be verified.

Component Testing

The central supply system should be checked to verify that the changeover from primary to secondary supplies and from primary to reserve supplies function properly and the appropriate signals are activated. The reserve supply should be checked to ensure that the reserve in-use signal and reserve low supply alarm work as required. Pressure relief valves should vent excessive pressure to atmosphere at a pressure 50% above normal line pressure and reseat when pressure returns to normal. The low liquid level alarm in the bulk oxygen supply should be tested for proper function. Alarms in the compressed air system should be tested and function of the safety valve and automatic drain verified.

Zone valves should be tested to ensure they control only that area they are intended to control and that labeling is appropriate. Zone valves should also be tested for tightness. This is done by closing the zone valve, releasing pressure through a station outlet, and monitoring downstream pressure for 30 minutes. If pressure increases during the 30 minute time interval, the valve is not tight.

Cleaning, Purging, and Purity

After installation of the piping, but before installation of station outlets and other components, the line must be blown clear using oil-free, dry air, or nitrogen. Once this is complete, each gas is connected to its system and all outlets are opened in progressive order, starting at the source and ending at the farthest outlet from the source. This is known as purging and continues until particulate contamination is eliminated. Testing for particulates is accomplished by allowing the purge gas to flow through a white cloth material at 100 L/min. When no evidence of discoloration is present, particulates are considered negligible.

It is important to remember that the purge gas must be eliminated from the piping system before use. There are reports of patient deaths caused by failure to purge nitrogen gas from the oxygen pipeline.[7]

Periodic Testing

Periodic testing and inspection of piping systems should be done on a regular basis and the results recorded. Zone valves should be tested to verify proper function and tightness. Area alarms should be tested monthly to verify appropriate operation of audible and visual signals. Supply system alarms should be tested annually. Pressure relief valves should be checked to determine appropriate venting of excess pressure and reseating of the valve.

Air intakes for the compressed air system should be inspected quarterly for evidence of contamination. Pressure gauges and water level alarms in the receivers should be checked annually. Function of the automatic drain and water (from condensation) in the receiver should be checked daily.

Station outlets should be inspected annually for ease of insertion, locking and unlocking of the connecter, gas leakage, wear, and damage.

Problems and Troubleshooting

Most problems associated with piping systems are the result of poor communication between maintenance and clinical departments, lack of understanding by hospital personnel, and unfamiliarity with emergency measures.

By far the most often reported problem is low or inadequate pressure.[8] If pressure falls too low, ventilators will cease to operate and air–oxygen mixtures may change drastically. Causes of low line pressure include the following:

- Inadvertent interruption of gas during construction
- Fire[9,10]
- Motor vehicle accidents (typically involving the operating supply)[6]
- Environmental forces (eg, earthquake, hurricane)[11]
- Damage or depletion of the operating supply[12,13]
- Human error (inadvertent closure of a zone valve[14] and improper adjustment of a main line regulator[7])
- Equipment failure: zone valve leaks,[15–17] reserve supply failure,[18] regulator malfunction,[19,20] failure of switchover systems[19]
- Obstruction of the pipeline (by debris left behind during installation)[21,22]
- Quick connect failures: improper fit,[23–25] breaking,[26,27] obstruction of the connector,[27,28] disconnection of the station outlet[29]

In the event of an oxygen or air source failure, a disaster plan should be in place. Anderson and Brock-Utne[30] have developed a strategy to deal with oxygen pipeline supply failure. In the operating room and intensive care unit, complete loss of oxygen can be disastrous. In some instances, an emergency supply of cylinders may be used. The bank of cylinders can be connected into a station outlet downstream of the zone valve. If failure occurs, the zone valve is closed and the oxygen supply turned on. This allows the emergency supply to provide oxygen to all station outlets downstream of the zone valve.

High pressure is also commonly reported,[6] but it does not pose the threat that low-pressure situations do. Pressure relief valves are installed to prevent high-pressure problems, but these only operate at a pressure 50% greater than normal line pressure. Additionally, these devices may fail. Consequences of high pressure include damage to regulators, flowmeters, and other equipment. High-pressure situations typically result from regulator failure.

Alarm failure or disconnection is not uncommon[5,31] but can be prevented by a regular maintenance program. Alarms may also sound erroneously owing to uncalibrated pressure sensors. This creates a situation in which caregivers ignore the alarms due to frequent false alarms. Appropriate personnel should be trained to respond to gas distribution alarms. Failure to respond to an alarm, failure to understand the procedure following an alarm signal, or failing to follow the procedure are human errors that can result in dire consequences.[5,32]

Cross-connection of gases can occur at the operating supply, in the distribution system, at station outlets, and in ancillary devices. Cross-connection is uncommon, but the results are often devastating. Practitioners should remember that the alarm system only detects pressure, not gas type or concentration. Several cases have been reported in which the liquid oxygen operating supply was accidentally filled with nitrogen or argon.[31,33,34] Likewise, the wrong cylinders have been connected to the distribution system.[35] In the latter case, two patients died when nitrous oxide cylinders were connected to the oxygen system.

Actual cross-connection of pipelines has been reported during new construction and after additions to the existing system.[36–46] This underscores the importance of testing procedures described earlier in this chapter. Improperly labeled station outlets result in a situation similar to that of cross-connections and have been reported.[47–49] Improperly installed station outlets may also allow the wrong quick connecter to be installed.[50–53] This can allow air to be delivered instead of oxygen, with the possibility of a hypoxic gas mixture being delivered to the patient. At least one case has been described in which carbon dioxide was delivered instead of oxygen during anesthesia, with resultant hypercarbia.[54]

Several reports have described a cross connection of air and oxygen pipelines through the air—oxygen blender of a mechanical ventilator.[54–63] In each of these reports, the ventilator was turned off but remained connected to the air and oxygen systems. Depending on the differences in air and oxygen pipeline pressures, this either allowed air to flow into the oxygen pipeline or oxygen to flow into the air pipeline. When ventilators and other air–oxygen blending systems are not in use, they should be disconnected from both gas sources.

Gas Contamination

Particulate matter in the gas distribution system in the form of oil, metal fillings, solder flux, and other hydrocarbons can seriously damage equipment and is hazardous if inhaled by the patient. The presence of particulate matter is common after new construction and addition to existing pipelines. Proper cleaning and purging of the lines as previously described can help eliminate this problem.

Oil has been isolated in air systems due to inappropriate lubrication and care of air compressors.[64] Contamination by cleaning solvents has also been reported,[65] even though use of organic solvents to clean fittings or other components is prohibited.

Compressed air can be contaminated by improper installation of air intakes and failure to eliminate water vapor. Lackore and Perkins[66] reported a case in which an air intake filter was soaked in cleaning fluid and replaced before being allowed to dry. Another report found that the air intake was located next to the ambulance entrance. Exhaust from waiting ambulances was entrained into the air system.[67]

Humidity is a common problem in compressed air systems and can result in major damage to ventilators and great expense.[68,69,70] The presence of water also allows the growth and passage of bacteria in the air system.[71,72] Compressed air is not sterile, and appropriate filters should be used.

Medical Gas Cylinders

A medical gas cylinder is a tank containing a high-pressure gas or gas mixture at a pressure in excess of 2000 psig.[1] Cylinders are frequently used to supply oxygen during transport or to remote locations of the hospital.

Medical gas cylinders are made of steel, aluminum, or chrome-molybdenum. Steel and chrome-molybdenum are most frequently used and are the most durable. Aluminum cylinders are useful during air transport and at home where weight is a major concern. Use of aluminum cylinders is particularly useful during magnetic resonance imaging.

Cylinders are constructed using a variety of methods. A cylinder can be made by forcing a hardened steel press through a softer mass of cylinder material called a billet, shaping the billet into a steel tube. The bottom and top of the steel tube are heated, shaped, and closed, with the neck at the top threaded for a valve stem. Alternately, steel bands can be spun or wrapped around a mold and then sealed together under extreme heat. After the mold is removed, the bottom is welded closed and the top is threaded for the valve stem. The bottom of a cylinder is flat so it can stand up on one end.

Cylinder Valves

Cylinders are filled and emptied by means of a valve threaded into the neck of the cylinder. This valve is turned counterclockwise to open the cylinder and use its contents or clockwise to close the cylinder and stop the discharge of contents. Small cylinders, sizes A through E, require the use of a small hand wrench or handle to open the cylinder. Large cylinders have a permanently attached hand wheel to open and close the valve. If the valve is open, turning the valve stem clockwise will lower the end of the valve stem against the seat and shut off gas flow. Turning the handle counterclockwise raises the valve stem and opens a channel from the valve seat to the exit port through which the gas passes. On an E cylinder, the exit port is surrounded by a plastic washer that prevents the high pressure gas from leaking between the valve port and the regulator yoke.

Direct-Acting

Cylinder valves are typically known as direct-acting (packed) or indirect-acting (diaphragm) valves. Packed or direct-acting valves use a resilient packing to prevent leaks around the threads (Fig. 2-17). The term *direct-acting* refers to the fact that as the stem turns, so does the seat. Large direct-acting cylinder valves use a driver square to transmit force to the seat. Direct-acting valves are capable of withstanding high pressures.

Indirect-Acting

Diaphragm, or indirect-acting, cylinder valves get their name from a diaphragm positioned between the stem and the seat (Fig. 2-18). Turning the stem raises or lowers the diaphragm, opening or closing the valve. A spring around the seat opposes the pressure applied by the diaphragm. Diaphragm cylinder valves are more expensive than packed valves but are less prone to leakage and can be fully opened with a one-half to three-quarter turn. Packed valves usually require two to three turns.

Pressure Relief Devices

Pressure relief or safety relief devices are part of every cylinder valve. The pressure relief device allows gas to vent to atmosphere when pressure in the cylinder rises above a critical pressure. High pressure in a cylinder is usually the result of overfilling or high temperature.

Pressure relief devices fit into three types: frangible disks, fusible plugs, and spring-loaded devices. A frangible disk is a metal disk constructed to burst when a specified dangerous pressure is reached. When the disk ruptures, the gas escapes safely through discharge vents (Fig. 2-19*B*). A fusible plug is made of metal alloy with a low melting point. As described by Gay-Lussac's law, excessive gas pressure will generate high temperatures, melting the fusible plug and allowing gas to escape and pressure to fall. These are typically used with small cylinders. A spring-loaded device uses a vented cap to hold a spring against a metal disk over a port in the gas container. These are typically used with large cylinders. If pressure becomes excessive, the disk is pushed back, compressing the spring and opening an escape channel (see Fig. 2-19*A*).

Indexed Safety Connections

Cylinder valves are built with indexed safety connections so that only the proper regulators for the gas contained can be used. Small cylinders, sizes A through E, use the Pin Index Safety System, and large cylinders use the American Standard System. The Pin Index Safety System consists of two holes bored in assigned places in the valve with two corresponding pins on the regulator yoke (Fig. 2-20). The pin and hole positions are specified for each gas by the CGA (Table 2-5). Large cylinders use a size configuration and thread indexed safety connection system called the American Standard System of the CGA (CGA-ASS). The shape of the gas outlet nipple, the diameter, and the size of the threads is specified for each gas. The proper regulator has a nipple receptacle and hex-nut with corresponding configuration and threading (Fig. 2-21).

Specifications for large cylinder connections are shown in the following example for oxygen: 0.903-14-RH-EXT. The first number (0.903) is the diameter (in inches) of the cylinder outlet, the second number (14) is the number of threads per inch, and the letters (RH-EXT) indicate whether the threads are right or left handed and external (EXT) or internal (INT).

Cylinders

Cylinder Sizes

Cylinders are identified by letter codes to indicate size and gas capacity (Table 2-6). Cylinders most frequently used in respiratory care are E and H cylinders. Sizes AA through E are known as small cylinders and are used for portable oxygen supplies

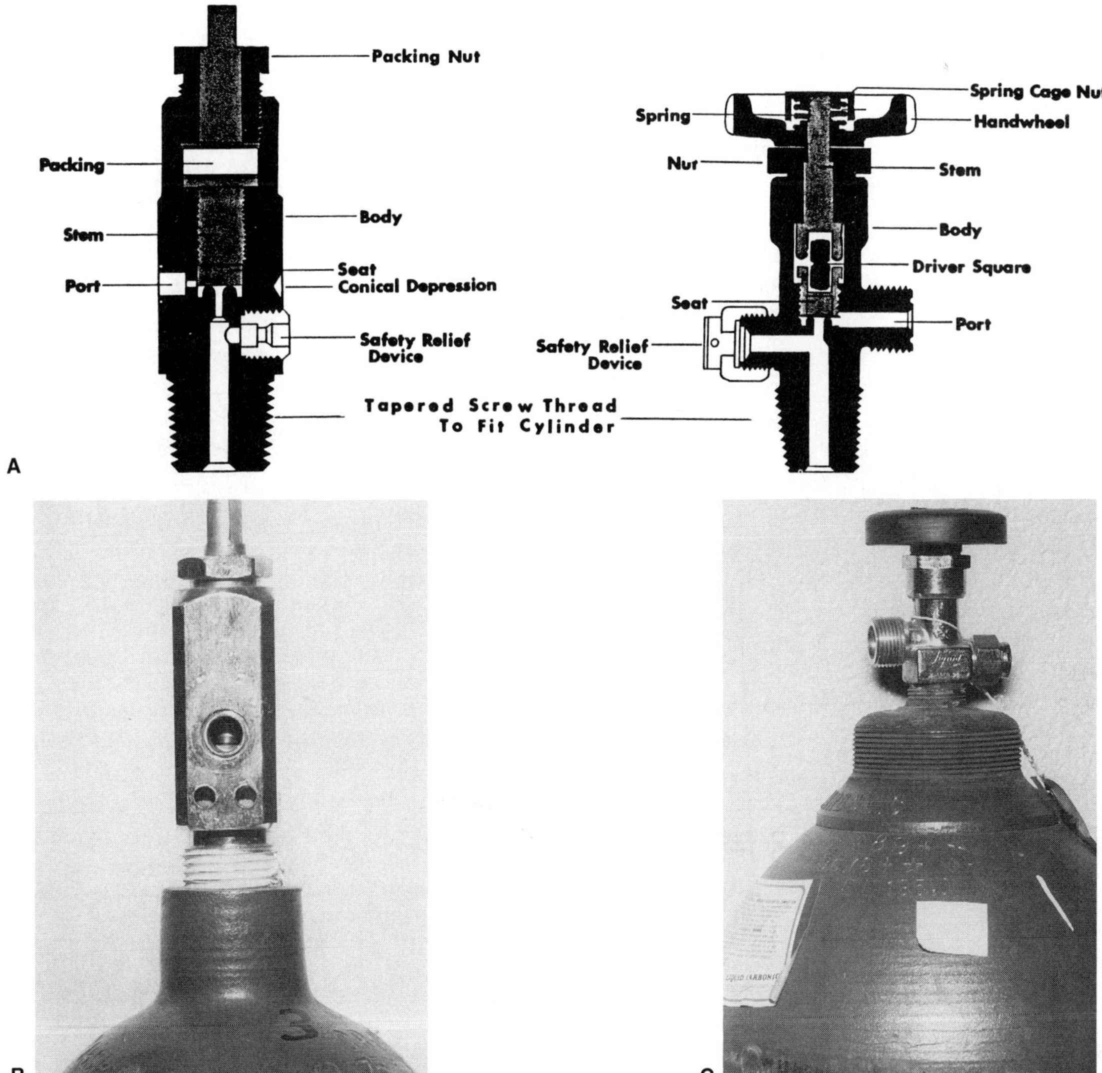

Figure 2-17. (A.) Small cylinder (left) and large (right) packed valves. The packing seals the stem and prevents leaks. Turning the stem on the large cylinder valve counterclockwise causes the stem to turn in its thread, opening the valve. (A. from Dorsch JA, Dorsch SE. Understanding Anesthesia Equipment. Baltimore: Williams & Wilkins, 1991) used with permission.) (B) and (C) are pictures of a small and large cylinder valve, respectively.

and anesthetic gases. Small cylinders use a connector known as a yoke, which contains the gas-specific Pin Index Safety System to access cylinder contents. Sizes F through K are known as large cylinders. These cylinders use the CGA-ASS threaded connectors to access cylinder contents.

Cylinder Color and Markings

Color is used to help identify cylinder contents and avoid confusion. The United States color code is shown in Table 2-7. Cylinders containing a single gas are of a uniform color. Cylinders containing a gas mixture use both colors to indicate the contents. For example, a 5% CO_2, 95% O_2 tank is green with gray shoulders (the part sloping up to the cylinder valve). Color coding should be used as a guide. Practitioners should always check the label to identify cylinder contents before use.

The Department of Transportation (DOT) requires specific, permanent markings on every cylinder. These markings are stamped on the shoulder at the front and rear of the tank (Fig. 2-22). The front of a cylinder corresponds to the gas outlet.

Labels and Tags

Each cylinder must bear a label on its shoulder that uses the CGA marking system (Fig. 2-23). This label names the cylinder contents on the left and denotes the hazard class of the gas in a color-coded diamond figure. The diamond indicates whether the gas is non-

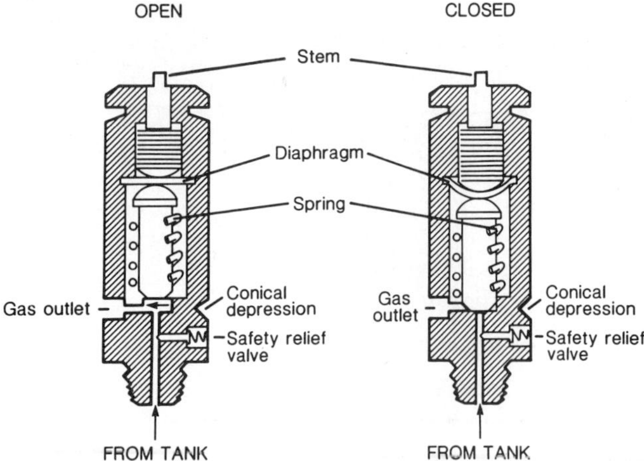

Figure 2-18. Small diaphragm (indirect-acting) cylinder valve in the open (left) and closed (right) position.

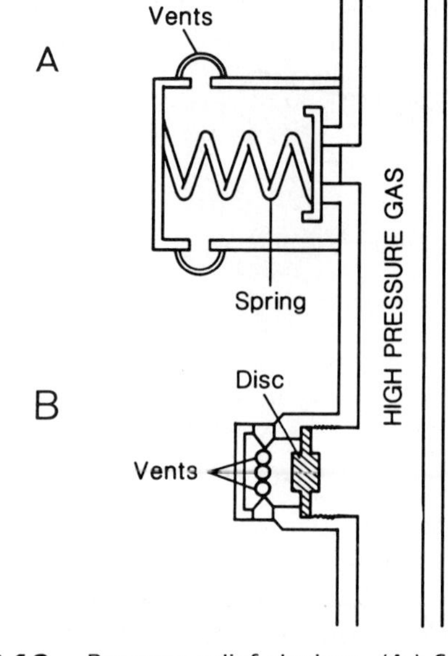

Figure 2-19. Pressure relief devices. (A.) Spring-loaded device. When gas pressure is excessive, the spring is compressed to the left, allowing gas to escape. When pressure returns to normal, the spring reseats and prevents gas from escaping. (B.) Frangible disk. When gas pressure is excessive, the disk ruptures, allowing gas to escape to atmosphere through a series of vents.

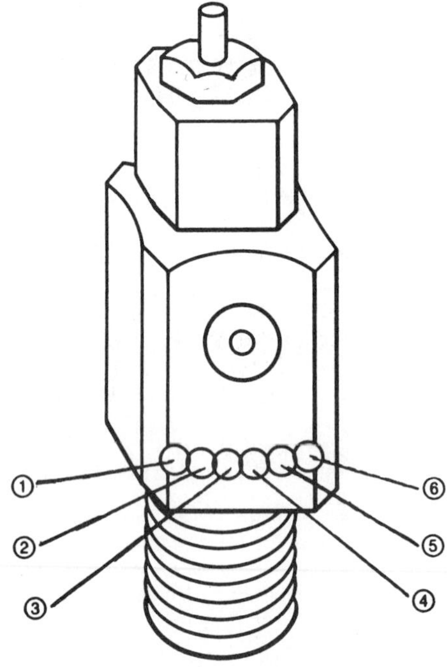

Figure 2-20. Pin Index Safety System pin positions.

TABLE 2-5. Pin Index Safety System Pin and Hole Positions for Medical Gases

Gas	Index Pins
Air	1, 5
Carbon dioxide	1, 6
Cyclopropane	3, 6
Helium	4, 6
Nitrogen	1, 4
Nitrous oxide	3, 5
Oxygen	2, 5
Oxygen/carbon dioxide (> 7% CO_2)	1, 6
Oxygen/carbon dioxide (< 7% CO_2)	2, 6
Oxygen/helium (He > 80.5%)	4, 6
Oxygen/helium (He < 80.5%)	2, 4

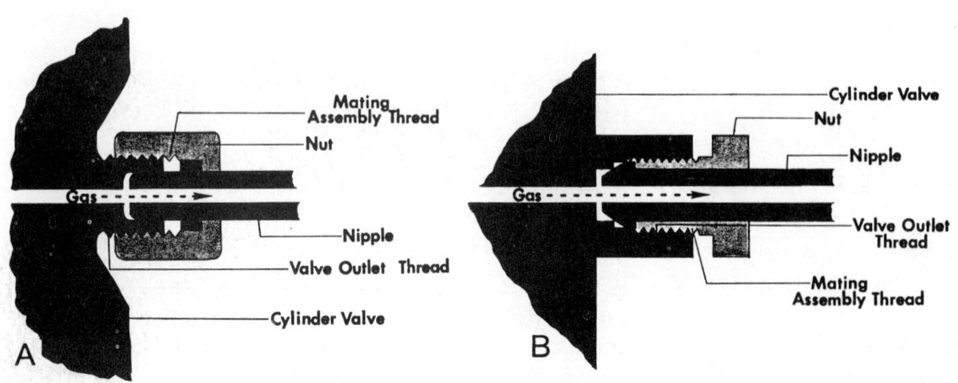

Figure 2-21. Valve outlet connections for large cylinders. (A.) Threads are on the outside of the cylinder valve outlet, and the nut screws are over the valve outlet. (B.) The valve outlet thread is internal, so the nut screws into the outlet. (From Dorsch JA, Dorsch SE. Understanding Anesthesia Equipment. Baltimore: Williams & Wilkins, 1991)

TABLE 2-6. Medical Gas Cylinder Letter Codes, Size, and Weight, Pressure, and Volume at 70°F

Cylinder Size	Empty Weight (lb)	Dimensions: OD × Length (in)	Volume and Pressure	Air	CO_2	He	N_2O	O_2
D	11	4.5 × 17	Liters	375	940	300	940	360
			psig	1,900	838	1,600	745	2,200
E	14	4.25 × 26	Liters	625	1,590	500	1,590	620
			psig	1,900	838	1,600	745	2,200
G	97	8.5 × 51	Liters	4,040	12,300	4,000	13,800	5,300
			psig	1,900	838	1,600	745	2,200
H	119	9.25 × 51	Liters	6,550	—	6,000	15,800	6,900
			psig	2,200	—	2,200	745	2,200

flammable (green), flammable (red), or an oxidizer (yellow). A signal word (Danger, Warning, Caution) is also provided if release of the gas would cause an immediate, less than immediate, or no immediate hazard. A second diamond may be added if the contents are poisonous (as in the case of chlorine). After the signal word is a statement of hazards describing the danger and a precautionary statement on avoiding injury. The label also lists the name and address of the cylinder's manufacturer or distributor.

Tags are attached around the cylinder valve and identify its contents. A tag has three perforated sections labeled full, in use, and empty. When the cylinder is first set up, the full portion should be removed. When the cylinder is empty, the "in use" portion should be removed. Following this simple procedure can help prevent depletion of the cylinder during use and the associated consequences.

Inspection and Testing

All cylinders must be inspected and tested every 5 or 10 years. The date (month and year) of every test is stamped on the rear of the cylinder. Cylinders are inspected visually both internally and externally. External inspection includes looking for dents, rust, damage to paint, and corrosion. The hammer or dead ring test is performed at each refilling. This test requires lightly striking the cylinder on the side and listening to the tone created. A good cylinder will produce a clean, ringing tone lasting 2 to 3 seconds. If the tone is flat or fades immediately, damage should be suspected. Possible causes of damage include fire, corrosion, and oil or water contamination.

TABLE 2-7. Color Coding and Labeling of Gas Cylinders

Gas	Color
Oxygen	Green (international color—white)
Carbon dioxide	Gray
Cyclopropane	Orange
Ethylene	Red
Helium	Brown
Nitrogen	Black
Air	Yellow (international color—black and white)
CO_2–O_2 mixture	Gray shoulder/green body
He–O_2 mixture	Brown shoulder/green body

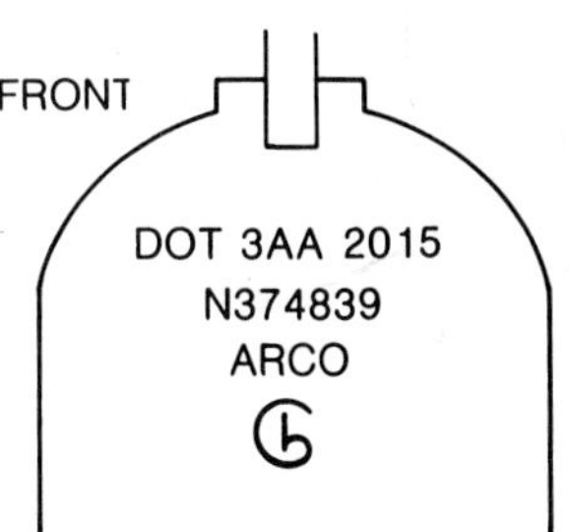

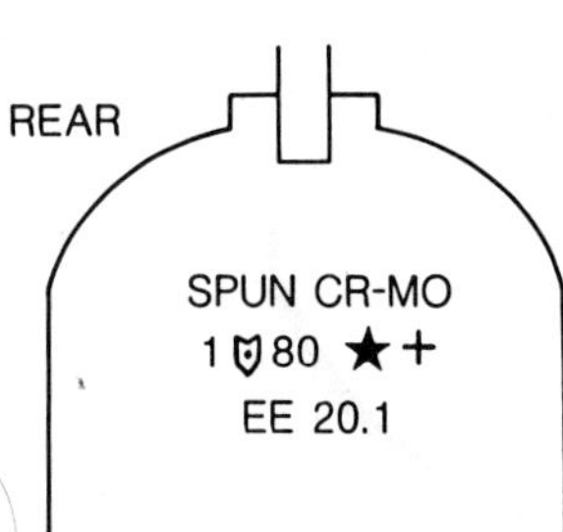

Figure 2-22. Front and rear cylinder markings. Front: DOT 3AA indicates the material used in construction. 2015 is the filling pressure of the cylinder (2015 psig). The second line contains a letter (N) identifying the cylinder size and its serial number (374839). The third line identifies the owner (ARCO) and is followed by a manufacturer's or inspector's mark. Rear: Spun CR-MO is the method of manufacture, in this case spun chrome-molybdenum. The second line contains the original safety test (1/80) by month and year. The star indicates testing must be performed every 10 years, and the + indicates the cylinder may be filled to 110% of its service pressure. EE 20.1 represents the elastic expansion in cubic centimeters used during testing.

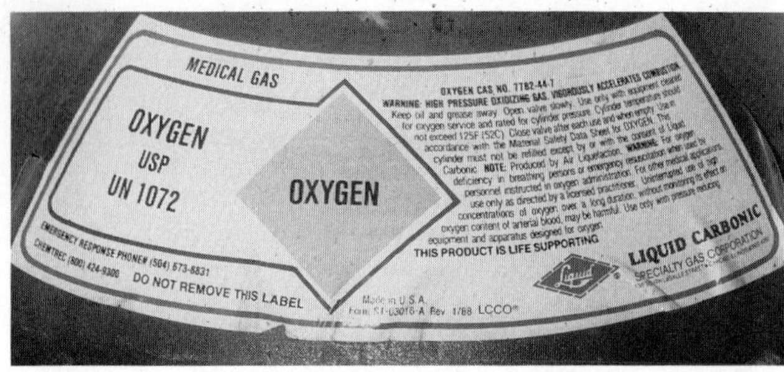

Figure 2-23. Cylinder label using the CGA marking system.

Internal visual inspection requires dropping a light into the neck of the cylinder and rotating the cylinder to visualize the entire inner surface. Corrosion and rust should be identified, and scale (usually caused by moisture) should be removed. Suspicious findings on internal inspection should lead to formal testing.

Formal testing of cylinders is accomplished under CGA guidelines using hydrostatic testing (Fig. 2-24). Hydrostatic testing involves immersing the cylinder into a water jacket container. Both the cylinder and the jacket are filled with water. With water in the cylinder at atmospheric pressure, the water level in the water jacket is recorded. Water pressure in the cylinder is increased to 3000 psig and the water level in the jacket monitored. When the cylinder is under pressure, some of the water in the jacket is displaced due to cylinder expansion. When cylinder pressure is released, some water returns to the water jacket. The volume of water initially displaced is known as total expansion of the cylinder. The final displaced volume represents permanent expansion. Total expansion minus permanent expansion equals wall thickness of the cylinder. A calculation of cylinder suitability is then accomplished by determining the percentage of permanent expansion. This value is obtained by dividing 100 times the permanent expansion by the total expansion. If a cylinder fails to meet DOT specifications, it is rejected. Rejected cylinders may be scrapped or used to contain a gas (such as helium) that has a lower maximum pressure when the cylinder is full.

The CGA permits substitutes for hydrostatic testing in some instances. These include the proof pressure method and the direct expansion method. Both tests have methodologic problems that make them inferior to hydrostatic testing.

Cylinder Safety

Rules and regulations for cylinder safety are often quoted verbatim from the CGA's *Handbook of Compressed Gases*.[2] We encourage all respiratory care departments to use this book as a reference. The list of safety rules runs some 20 pages. In the interest of space and economy, the important safety and storage rules are listed below.

Storage

- A definite area should be designated for cylinder storage.
- The cylinder storage area should be constructed of fire-resistant materials.
- The cylinder storage area should be cool, dry, and well ventilated. Proper ventilation prevents gas from accumulating if leaks are present.
- Full and empty cylinders should be stored in separate areas to prevent confusion.
- Flammable gases should not be stored with oxidizing gases (eg, oxygen, air).
- Large cylinders should be stored upright, with the protective cap on, and restrained from being knocked over by a chain or other restraint.
- Cylinders should be protected from the elements to prevent rusting and from possible tampering.
- The cylinder storage area should have signs outside the door such as "Gas Cylinders. Remove to a safe place in case of fire" and "Authorized Personnel Only."
- Inside the cylinder storage area warning signs such as, "No Smoking, No Open Flames or Sparks, No Oil or Grease, and No Combustible Material" should be posted.

Transport

Safe handling of cylinders includes the following:

- During transportation cylinder valve caps should be kept in place.
- Cylinders should be transported on suitable carts equipped with a restraining chain. Cylinders should not be dragged, slid, or rolled to their destination.
- Petroleum-based lubricants *should never be* in contact with cylinder valves, regulators, high-pressure hoses, or fittings.
- Always use the appropriate CGA connector to access cylinder contents. Do not attempt to interchange regulators.
- Cylinder valves should be opened slowly to allow dissipation of heat. When in use, the valve should be fully opened.
- Cylinders should not be exposed to temperatures greater than 54°C, sparks, or open flame.
- Unlabeled cylinders should be returned to the vendor.
- When not in use, the cylinder valve should be in the closed position.

Transfilling

Transfilling is the process of filling one cylinder (usually smaller) from another cylinder (usually larger). Transfilling is frequently done by manufacturers and distributors but is generally best avoided by users. The process of transfilling can be hazardous. High

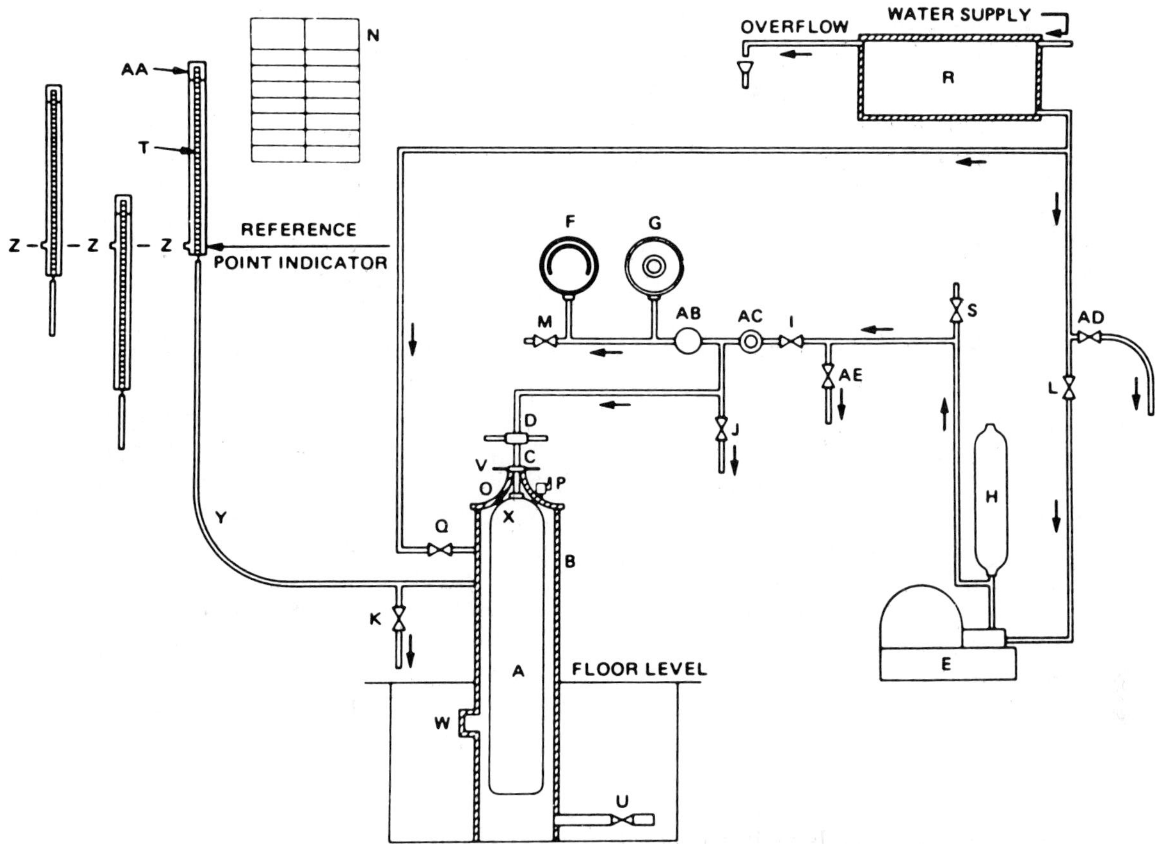

Figure 2-24. Hydrostatic testing apparatus for a medical gas cylinder. A, Cylinder; B, water jacket; C, cylinder connection; D, detachable pressure connection; E, hydraulic pressure source; F, pressure indicating gauge; H, pressure recording gauge; H, pressure surge chamber (optional); I,J,K,L,Q, valves; M, valve (for master gauge in-line testing); N, test data sheet O, water jacket cover; P, pet cock; R, water reservoir (optional); S, safety relief device; T, burrette (reading in cubic centimeters); U, clean-out valve (optional); V, wing nut; W, safety port or other suitable means of relief or containment. (From Klein PE. Health Care Facilities Handbook. 4th Ed. National Fire Protection Association. Quincy, MA 1993)

pressure in the large cylinder can cause rapid recompression of gas in the small cylinder with resultant high temperatures. Temperatures can rise high enough to ignite combustible materials and oxidize metal. Overfilling may also occur, causing cylinder and/or regulator damage. Other risks include contamination of gases and inadvertent mixing (eg, filling an oxygen cylinder with air could have disastrous consequences).

Determining Duration of Cylinder Gas Flow

Determining the volume of gas remaining in a cylinder and the duration of use left at a given flow are important skills of the respiratory care practitioner.

Calculating remaining cylinder volume can be accomplished by measuring pressure and weight of the cylinder (Fig. 2-25). A gas stored partially in liquid form can have cylinder volume measured best by weight. Nonliquefied gases show a reduction in pressure commensurate with the change in volume.

Conversion Factors

In emergencies and during transport it is important to know how long a cylinder will last at a given flow. This is accomplished by determining the volume in the cylinder, as reflected by pressure and a conversion factor. The conversion factor refers to the conversion of cubic feet into liters: 1 cu ft of gas = 28.3 L. The conversion factor for each size cylinder is different but can be calculated using the formula in Equation Box 2-2. Cylinder sizes and conversion factors are listed in Table 2-8. Once the conversion factor is known, duration of flow can be determined from cylinder pressure (psig) and gas flow (L/min), as shown in Equation Box 2-3.

Hazards

By far the most common hazards associated with cylinders are the result of human error. The majority of these events are related to mislabeling and inappropriate use.

Numerous cases have been reported in which cylinders were connected to the wrong yokes.[73–82] The Pin Index Safety System should prevent this problem, but poor manufacturing and customer alteration contribute to this continuing problem. Additionally, pins can be bent, broken, or removed and index holes can become worn and enlarge. In the latter case, a yoke for oxygen (pins 2 and 5) can be forced onto a cylinder of nitrous oxide (pins 3 and 5). The result would be disastrous.

Delivery of the improper gas has also been reported owing to incorrect labeling,[83,84] incorrect coloring,[85] incorrect filling,[86–89] and improperly installed valves.[90–92]

Equation Box 2-2: Gas Cylinder Conversion Factors

$$\text{Conversion factor} = \frac{\text{Cubic feet of gas full cylinder} \cdot 28.\,3\ \text{L/ft}^3}{\text{Full cylinder pressure (psig)}}$$

For an E cylinder the conversion factor would be calculated based on a full-cylinder volume of 22 cubic feet and a full-cylinder pressure of 2200 psig.

$$\text{E cylinder conversion factor} = \frac{22\ \text{cu ft} \cdot 28.3\ \text{L/cu ft}}{2200\ \text{psig}}$$

$$= 0.28\ \text{L/psig}$$

Conversion factors for other cylinder sizes can be calculated in the same manner.

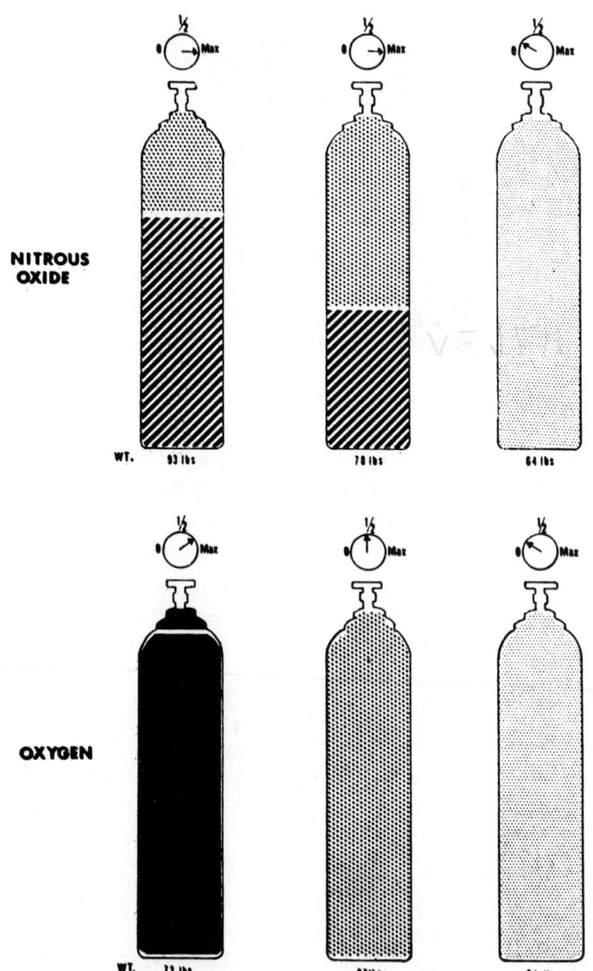

Figure 2-25. The relationship between cylinder weight, pressure, and contents. A gas stored partially in liquid (nitrous oxide) form will show a constant pressure (if temperature is constant) until all the liquid has evaporated. At this point, cylinder volume will be directly related to pressure. A nonliquefied gas (oxygen) will show a steady decline in pressure as the cylinder is evacuated. Each cylinder, however, will show a steady decline in weight as gas is discharged. (From Dorsch JA, Dorsch SE. Understanding Anesthesia Equipment. Baltimore: Williams & Wilkins, 1991)

Blogg and Colvin[93] reported a group of apparently empty cylinders in which blocked cylinder valves prevented access to cylinder contents. Other authors have reported damage to a cylinder valve when the yoke-retaining screw was screwed into the safety relief device.[94,95] If the retaining screw is placed into the safety release valve instead of the conical depression, the cylinder's contents will be released into the room. Cylinder contamination with oil and water has been reported.[96–99] Contamination with oil is particularly hazardous and has been associated with fires.[100] Other contaminants may be introduced during cylinder filling. Medical-grade oxygen must be 99% pure according to USP standards. The remaining 1% (10,000 ppm), must contain not more than 300 ppm of carbon dioxide, 10 ppm of carbon monoxide, and 5 ppm of nitrogen. No other standards exist for the remaining 9,685 ppm.[101] This leaves room for significant impurities to be present in an oxygen cylinder. In general, gas from a cylinder should not have any odor and should not result in discoloration of equipment. Clutton-Brock[102] has reported accidental poisoning in two patients due to contamination of nitrous oxide cylinders with higher oxides of nitrogen.

Improper handling and storage of high-pressure gas cylinders can result in rapid escape of gas, turning the cylinder into a dangerous projectile. If a cylinder

TABLE 2-8. Conversion Factors of Gas Cylinders

Size	Conversion Factor
D	0.16
E	0.28
G	2.41
H	3.14

Equation Box 2-3: Duration of Flow for Oxygen Cylinders

$$\text{Time remaining (min)} = \frac{\text{Cylinder Pressure (psig)} \cdot \text{conversion factor}}{\text{Flow (L/min)}}$$

For example, a full E cylinder of oxygen (2200 psig) used to transport a patient receiving 3 L/min will last:

$$\frac{2200 \text{ psig} \cdot 0.28 \text{ L/psig}}{3 \text{ L/min}} = 205 \text{ minutes}$$

$$= 3 \text{ hours, } 25 \text{ minutes}$$

without its protective cap (Fig. 2-26) is dropped, the valve may break off, rocketing the cylinder in the opposite direction of gas flow. Finch[103] reported a case of a cylinder valve being ejected from a cylinder when the packing nut was accidentally loosened instead of the valve stem.

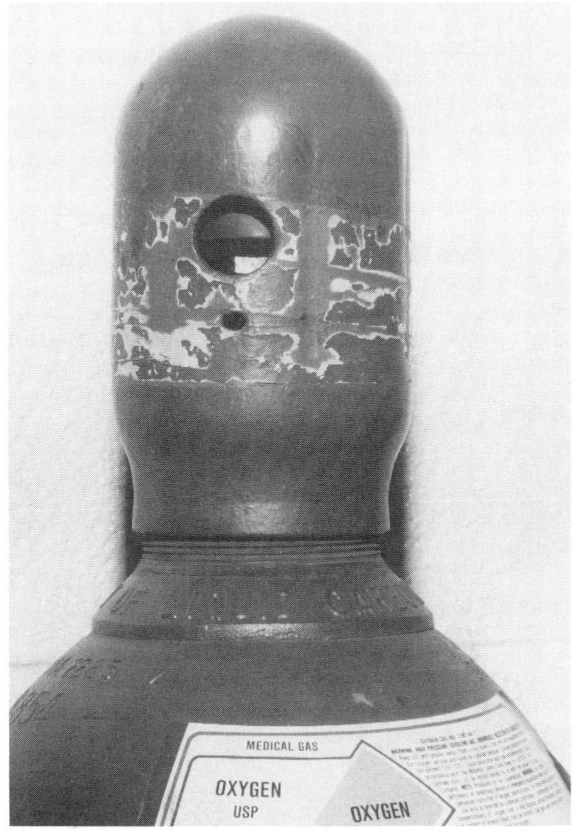

Figure 2-26. H-cylinder with protective cap in place.

Liquid Oxygen Containers

Liquid oxygen containers are smaller versions of bulk systems that are used in home oxygen therapy and during patient transport. Liquid oxygen containers may be advantageous to compressed gas cylinders in certain situations. Liquid systems are more compact, require fewer refills, and operate at lower pressures.

Description

Home liquid systems typically consist of a larger stationary or reservoir unit and a smaller portable or receiving unit (Fig. 2-27). The reservoir system is similar to the hospital bulk system, having pressure relief valves, a vaporizing coil, and a "thermos bottle" construction to maintain the required low temperature (Fig. 2-28). Most liquid systems operate around 20 psig.

The stationary unit can be used to directly deliver oxygen to the patient or to fill the portable unit. During normal operation the flow control valve is open to deliver gas to the patient. This creates a pressure gradient between the gas-filled upper section of the container (often called the head pressure) and atmospheric pressure. Gas flows through the economizer valve through warming coils and out the flow control valve to the patient. The warming coils help increase gas temperature before reaching the patient. As gas flow continues, the head pressure declines steadily. When the head pressure falls below 0.5 psig, the economizer valve closes and liquid oxygen is drawn up the liquid withdrawal tube through the vaporizing and warming coils where it becomes a gas. The economizer valves allow a constant flow of oxygen to the patient.

When the reservoir is not in use, ambient temperature will increase evaporation of liquid until the head pressure causes the primary relief valve to open (about 2 psig above operating pressure). If the primary relief fails, the secondary relief valve will vent gas to atmosphere at 10 psig above operating pressure. This safety process will cause a liquid system to empty regardless of whether it is used or not.

The portable unit is also a Dewar container and weighs 5 to 15 pounds (Fig. 2-29). The portable unit is filled from the stationary unit and carried or carted by the patient or caregiver during use. Like the stationary unit, the portable unit has a primary and secondary relief valve and a fill tube. Gas travels from the pressure head through the warming coils to the flow control valve.

Safety

The DOT, CGA, and NFPA have regulations governing liquid oxygen use similar to those for cylinders and hospital systems. These are summarized below.

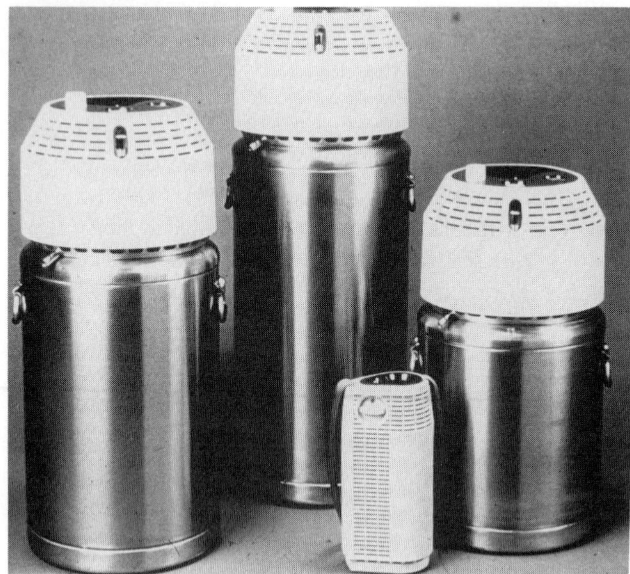

Figure 2-27. Three typical liquid stationary units and a portable unit.

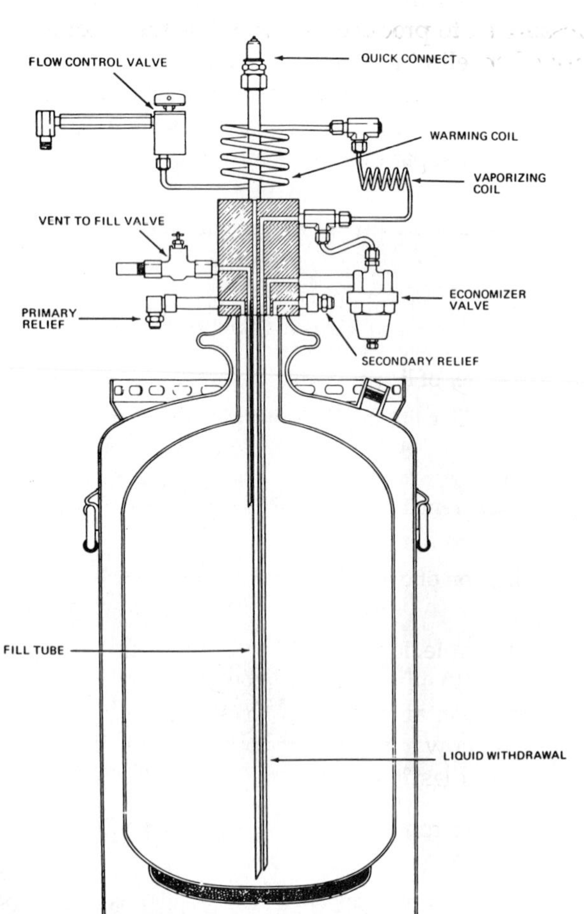

Figure 2-28. A stationary liquid oxygen container. (Courtesy of Puritan-Bennett Corp, Kansas City, MO)

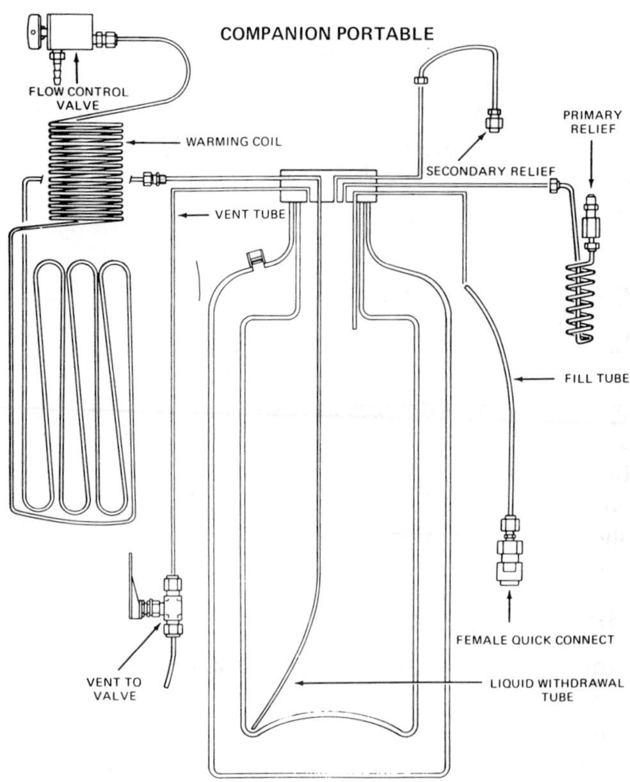

Figure 2-29. A portable liquid oxygen container (Courtesy of Puritan-Bennett Corp, Kansas City, MO)

Storage

- Stationary and portable units should be kept in the open in a cool, dry, well-ventilated area. Containers should not be stored in a closet.
- Stationary and portable units should not be stored near a heat source (eg, space heater, radiator).
- Stationary units should be stored in an upright position.

Safe Use

- Contact between liquid oxygen and skin should be avoided. Severe burns may result.
- If spilled, liquid oxygen should be allowed enough time to evaporate.
- No organic or combustible materials (oil-based lubricants) should come in contact with the containers or their outlets.
- Moisture should be removed to prevent freezing of valves and couplings.
- Containers should be handled carefully to avoid physical damage.
- Markings and labels on containers must be legible and unaltered.
- Under no circumstances should the pressure relief valves be adjusted or tampered with.

Transfilling

Transfilling a liquid oxygen container should take place in a well-ventilated area using equipment that complies with CGA requirements. Equipment should use the appropriate CGA or manufacturer specific connections. The transfilling system should contain its own pressure relief valve.

Calculating Duration of Flow

Like cylinders containing some liquid, the only way to determine duration of flow from a liquid container is by weight. Most devices have a system to monitor liquid level, but this is not useful for determining duration. Some systems have integral scales to facilitate weighing. Calculating duration of flow is done as shown in Equation Box 2-4.

Hazards

Liquid oxygen systems are a fire hazard if equipment is contaminated with oil, grease, or combustible material. Vaporization of spilled liquid oxygen can result in an oxygen-enriched atmosphere and increase the likelihood of fire.

Improperly maintained or malfunctioning pressure relief valves may lead to over-pressure accidents. Condensation from vaporization can freeze, disabling valves and couplings.

Burns from spilled liquid oxygen have been reported.[104] Care should be exercised during transfilling to prevent contact with skin.

Massey and co-workers[105] have reported inaccurate flow delivery by liquid systems used in the home. Practitioners should verify that systems provide the prescribed flow.

Portable Air Compressors

Portable air compressors are small versions of the large systems typically used in hospital supply systems. These systems compress room air using a piston, piston and diaphragm, or rotary motor. Compressors are used in the home to power nebulizers and to provide an air source for ventilators. Piston and diaphragm compressors usually provide low pressures and moderate flow rates and are suitable for home nebulizer therapy. Piston and rotary compressors are required to produce the pressures (45–55 psig) and flow rates (60–80 L/min) to power a ventilator. Compression of ambient air can produce significant amounts of condensation. A system to dry the air or collect condensate should be used to prevent delivery of air high in water content to ventilators. Water vapor can cause damage to blenders, solenoids, and other electric and mechanical components.

Oxygen Concentrators

Oxygen concentrators are electronic devices that use specialized filters to eliminate other gases from room air and "concentrate" the oxygen for delivery to the patients. Oxygen concentrators either operate using a molecular sieve or a permeable plastic membrane.

Molecular Sieve Concentrator

These are the most popular devices and their principle of operation is similar. Specific devices may use more or fewer sieve beds and deliver a different percentage. Concentrators draw ambient air through a filtering system using an air compressor (see Fig. 2-29). Gas travels through a heat exchanger to dissipate heat created during compression to a solenoid valve. Gas is then directed to the two molecular sieve beds where oxygen is concentrated. This type of concentrator is known as a pressure swing cycle concentrator because the solenoid valve allows one of the sieve beds to be pressurized to produce oxygen while the other is pressurized to eliminate nitrogen and other trace gases. Each sieve bed contains a granular zeolite crystal. Zeolite contains an array of small particles (about 5 Å in diameter) that separate gases according to their size and

Equation Box 2-4: Duration of Flow for Liquid Oxygen

One liter of liquid oxygen weighs 2. 5 lb (1. 1 kg)

One liter of liquid oxygen produces 860 L of gaseous oxygen

$$\text{Gas remaining} = \frac{\text{liquid weight (lb)} \times 860}{2.5\ \text{lb/L}}$$

$$\text{Duration of contents (min)} = \frac{\text{Gas remaining (L)}}{\text{Flow L/min}}$$

For example, if a patient fills a portable container with 4 lb of liquid oxygen from the stationary container and requires a flow of 4 L/min, how long will the oxygen in the portable container last?

$$\text{Gas remaining} = \frac{4\ \text{lb} \times 860}{2.5\ \text{lb/L}} = 1376\ \text{L}$$

$$\text{Duration of contents} = \frac{1376\ \text{L}}{4\ \text{L/min}} = 344\ \text{minutes}$$

$$= 5\ \text{hours, } 44\ \text{minutes}$$

polarity. Zeolite in a concentrator traps nitrogen, water, carbon dioxide, carbon monoxide, and hydrocarbons while allowing oxygen to pass through. Pressuring the sieve beds helps increase the amount of gas absorbed.

Air is first pressurized in one sieve bed to increase nitrogen absorption. As oxygen passes through, a portion is stored in the product tank. The remaining oxygen is diverted to the second sieve bed to eliminate nitrogen absorbed from the previous cycle. When the first sieve bed becomes saturated with nitrogen, it is exhausted to the room, decreasing the pressure. This reduces nitrogen content and prepares the bed for another cycle. Simultaneously, oxygen from the opposite sieve bed flows to the first sieve bed (due to the pressure difference), which helps remove nitrogen. This process is cycled every 10 to 30 seconds, and oxygen is produced for delivery to the patient as well as regeneration of the sieve beds.

Oxygen in the product tank is maintained at less than 10 psig and is delivered to the patient after traveling through a bacteria filter and flowmeter. Oxygen delivery percentage is inversely proportional to flow. At low flow rates, less than 2 L/min, an oxygen concentration of 95% to 97% is produced. At flow rates of 3 to 5 L/min, concentration falls to 86% to 93%, depending on the manufacturer.

Oxygen Enricher

The oxygen enricher uses a 1-μm thick plastic membrane that separates gases according to their diffusion rates (Fig. 2-30). Oxygen and water vapor diffuse more quickly, allowing delivery of a gas containing 40% oxygen. A vacuum pump draws room air through the membrane and delivers the oxygen-enriched gas to a condensing coil where excess water vapor is removed. Gas is then delivered to the patient through a flowmeter. Interestingly, the gas is also delivered at three times ambient humidity. To deliver equivalent oxygen compared with a concentrator, the manufacturer recommends a flow three times greater. If a patient was receiving oxygen at 2 L/min from a cylinder or concentrator, the oxygen enricher would be set to deliver 6 L/min. (Fig. 2-31).

Regulatory Agencies

A number of agencies regulate medical gases, gas distribution systems, and gas containers. These agencies, as well as agencies that have no regulatory authority but make recommendations, are shown below.

- Department of Transportation (DOT): provides regulatory control over handling and shipping of compressed gas cylinders.
- Department of Health and Human Services (DHHS) Food and Drug Administration (FDA): regulates devices for medical use and purity of medical gases.
- Occupation Safety and Health Administration (OSHA): regulates occupational safety related to medical gases.
- Compressed Gas Association (CGA): makes recommendations and specifications for manufacture and safety systems for medical gases and gas distribution systems.
- National Fire Protection Agency (NFPA): makes recommendations for safety concerning storage and distribution of medical gases.
- International Standards Organization (ISO): recommends standards of manufacturing and safety systems.
- American National Standards Institute (ANSI): coordinates standards for health devices.
- Canadian Standards Association (CSA): independent Canadian organization that recommends standards for the safety, quality, and performance of respiratory care equipment.

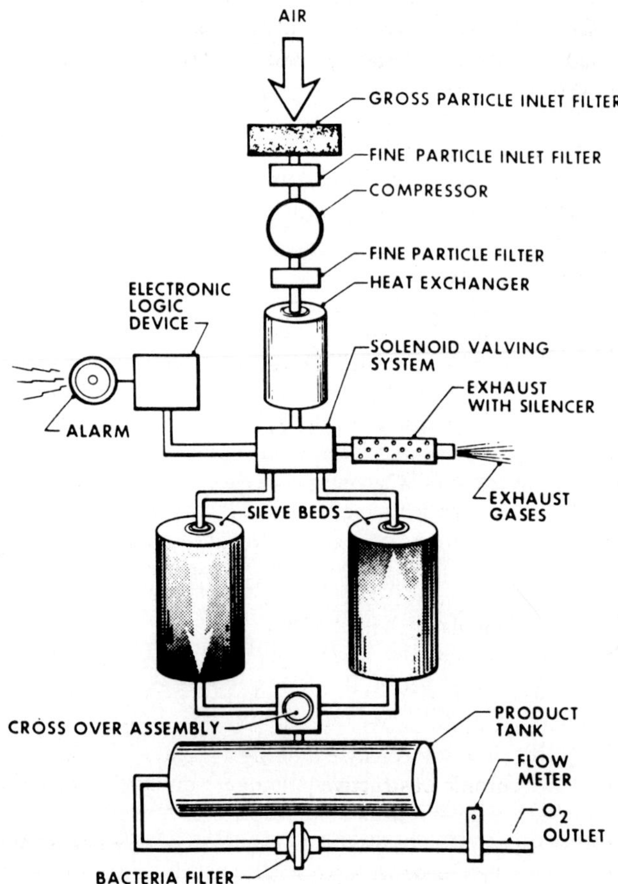

Figure 2-30. Molecular sieve oxygen concentrator. (From Lucas J, Golish J, Sleeper G, O'Rayne J. Home Respiratory Care. Norwalk, CT: Appleton & Lange, 1987)

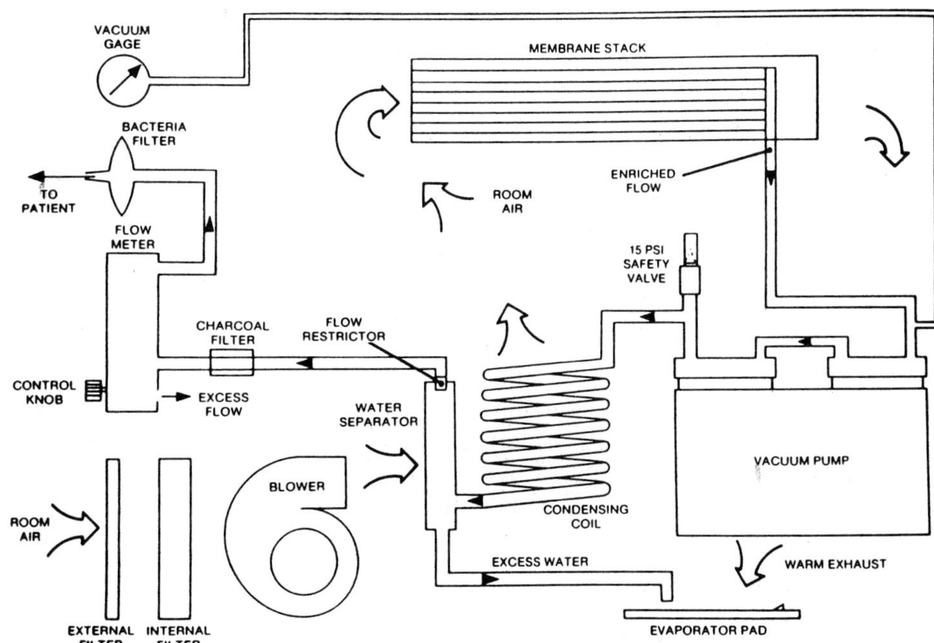

Figure 2-31. Oxygen enrichment device. (Courtesy of The Oxygen Enrichment Co, Schenectady, NY)

AARC Clinical Practice Guideline

Oxygen Therapy in the Home or Extended Care Facility: Indications, Contraindications, Hazards and Complications

Oxygen therapy is the administration of oxygen at concentration greater than that in ambient air with the intent of treating or preventing the symptoms and manifestations of hypoxia.

- Indications:
  - Documented hypoxemia: In adults, children and infants older than 28 days: $Pa_{O_2} \leq 55$ mm Hg or $Sa_{O_2} \leq 88\%$ in subjects breathing room air, or Pa_{O_2} of 56–59 mm Hg or $Sa_{O_2}/Sp_{O_2} \leq 89\%$ in association with specific clinical conditions (cor pulmonale, congestive heart failure, or erythrocythemia with hematocrit > 56%).
  - Some patients may not qualify for oxygen therapy at rest but will qualify for oxygen therapy during ambulation, sleep, or exercise. Oxygen therapy is indicated during these specific activities when Sa_{O_2} is demonstrated to fall to ≤ 88%.
- Contraindications: No absolute contraindications to oxygen therapy exist when indications are present.
- Precautions and/or Possible Complications:
  - In spontaneously breathing hypoxemic patients with chronic obstructive pulmonary disease, oxygen therapy may lead to an increase in Pa_{CO_2}
  - Undesirable results or events may result from noncompliance with physician's orders or inadequate instruction in home oxygen therapy.
  - Complications may result from use of nasal cannulae or transtracheal catheters.
  - Fire hazard is increased in the presence of increased oxygen concentrations.
  - Bacterial contamination is associated with certain nebulizers and humidification systems.
  - Possible physical hazards can be posed by unsecured cylinders, ungrounded equipment, or mishandling of liquid oxygen. Power and equipment failure can lead to inadequate oxygen supply.

(Adapted from AARC Clinical Practice Guideline, published in August, 1992, issue of Respiratory Care; see original publication for complete text)

AARC Clinical Practice Guideline

Oxygen Therapy in the Acute Care Hospital: Indications, Contraindications, Hazards and Complications

Oxygen therapy is the administration of oxygen at concentrations greater than that in ambient air with the intent of treating or preventing the symptoms and manifestations of hypoxia.

- Indications:
  - documented hypoxemia; in adults, children, and infants older than 28 days, arterial oxygen tension <60 mm Hg or arterial oxygen saturation <90% in subjects breathing room air or with Pa_{O_2} and/or Sa_{O_2} below the desirable range for specific clinician situation; in neonates, Pa_{O_2} 50 mm Hg or Sa_{O_2} <88% or capillary oxygen tension <40 mm Hg.
  - an acute care situation is which hypoxemia is suspected—substantiation of hypoxemia is required

within an appropriate period of time following initiation of therapy
   - severe trauma
   - acute myocardial infarction
   - short term therapy (eg, post anesthesia recovery)
- Contraindications: no specific contraindications to oxygen therapy exist when indications are judged to be present.
- Precautions and/or Possible Complications:
   - with $PaO_2 \geq 60$ mm Hg, ventilatory depression may occur in spontaneously breathing patients with elevated $PaCO_2$
   - with $FIO_2 \geq 0.5$, absorption atelectasis, oxygen toxicity, and/or depression of ciliary and/or leukocytic function may occur
   - in premature infants, $PaO_2 > 80$ mm Hg should be avoided because of the possibility of retinopathy of prematurity; increased PaO_2 can contribute to closure or constriction of the ductus arteriosus (a possible concern in infants with ductus-dependent heart lesions)
   - supplemental oxygen should be administered with caution to patients suffering from paraquat poisoning and to patients receiving bleomycin
   - during laser bronchoscopy, minimal levels of supplemental oxygen should be used to avoid intratracheal ignition
   - fire hazard is increased in the presence of increased oxygen concentrations
   - bacterial contamination associated with certain nebulizer and humidification systems is a possible hazard

(Adapted from AARC Clinical Practice Guideline, published in December, 1991, issue of Respiratory Care; see original publication for complete text)

References

1. Klein BR. Health Care Facilities Handbook, 3rd ed. Quincy, MA: National Fire Protection Association, 1990.
2. Compressed Gas Association. Handbook of Compressed Gases, 2nd ed. New York: CGA, 1990.
3. Canadian Standards Association. Nonflammable Medical Gas Piping Systems (CSA Z305.1-M1984). Toronto: CSA, 1984.
4. International Organization for Standardization. Terminal Units for Use in Medical Pipeline Systems (ISO 9170:1990[E]). Geneva: ISO, 1990.
5. International Organization for Standardization. Oxygen Concentrators for Medical Use—Safety Requirements (ISO 8359: 1988[E]). Geneva: ISO, 1988.
6. Feeley TW, Hedley-Whyte J. Bulk oxygen and nitrous oxide delivery systems: Design and dangers. Anesthesiology 1976;44: 301–305.
7. Canadian Standards Association. Qualification Requirements for Agencies Testing Nonflammable Medical Gas Piping Systems (CSA Z305.4-1077). Toronto: CSA, 1977.
8. Bancroft ML, du Moulin GC, Hedley-Whyte J. Hazards of hospital bulk oxygen delivery systems. Anesthesiology 1980;52: 504–510.
9. Modification of medical gas systems. Health Devices 1980;9: 181–185.
10. Wright CJ, Bostock F. Pipeline hazards—a simple solution. Anaesthesia 1978;33:759.
11. Johnson DL, Central oxygen supply versus mother nature. Respir Care 1975;20:1043–1044.
12. Chi OZ. Another example of hypoxic gas mixture delivery. Anesthesiology 1985;62:543–544.
13. Russell EJ. Oxygen supply at risk. Anaesth Intensive Care 1985;13:216–217.
14. Mystery of turned-off hospital oxygen supply solved by Denver police. Biomed Safe Stand 1987;17:18–19.
15. MacWhirter GI. An anesthetic pipe line hazard. Anaesthesia 1978;33:639.
16. Gibson OB. Another hazardous pipeline isolator valve. Anaesthesia 1979;34:213.
17. Black AE. Extraordinary oxygen pipeline failure. Anaesthesia 1990;45:599.
18. Francis RN. Failure of nitrous oxide supply to theatre pipeline system. Anaesthesia 1990;45:880–882.
19. Carley RH, Haughton IT, Park GR. A near disaster from piped gases. Anaesthesia 1984;39:891–893.
20. Feeley TW, McClelland KJ, Malhotra IV. The hazards of bulk oxygen delivery systems. Lancet 1975;1:1416–1418.
21. Janis KM. Sudden failure of ceiling oxygen connector. Can Anaesth Soc J 1978;25:155.
22. Krenis LJ, Berkowitz DA. Errors in installation of a new gas delivery system found after certification. Anesthesiology 1985;62:677–678.
23. Craig DB, Culligan J. Sudden interruption of gas flow through a Schrader oxygen coupler unit. Can Anaesth Soc J 1980;27: 175–155.
24. Chung DC, Hunter DJ, Pavan FJ. The quick-mount pipeline connector: Failure of a "fail-safe" device. Can Anaesth Soc J 1986;33:666–668.
25. Mather SJ. Put not your trust in: A case of pipeline failure during routine anaesthesia. Anaesth Points West 1969:2:21–22.
26. Puritan-Bennett quick connect valves for medical gases: Canadian medical devices alert warns of possible cracks. Biomed Safe Stand 1984;14:52–53.
27. Morrison AB. Puritan-Bennett Quick Connect Valves for Medical Gases: Medical Devices Alert. Ottawa: Health and Welfare Canada, April 9, 1984.
28. Anderson B, Chamley D. Wall outlet oxygen failure. Anaesth Intes Care 1987;15:468–469.
29. Arrowsmith LWM. Medical gas pipelines. Eng Med 1979;8: 247–249.
30. Anderson WR, Brock-Utne JG. Oxygen pipeline supply failure: A coping strategy. J Clin Monit 1991;7:39–41.
31. Sprague DH, Archer GW. Intraoperative hypoxia from an erroneously filled liquid oxygen reservoir. Anesthesiology 1975;42: 360–362.
32. Paul DL, Pipeline failure. Anaesthesia 1989;44:523.
33. Holland R. Foreign correspondence: ``Wrong gas'' disaster in Hong Kong. APSK Newslett 1989;4:26.
34. Smith FP. Multiple deaths from argon contamination of hospital oxygen supply. J FSCA 1987;32:1098–1102.
35. O_2-N_2O mix-up leads to probe into deaths of two patients. Biomed Safe Stand 1981;11:123–124.
36. Eichhorn JH, Bancroft ML, Laasberg L, et al. Contamination of medical gas and water pipelines in a new hospital building. Anesthesiology 1977;46:286–289.
37. Tingay MG, Ilsley AH, Willis RJ, et al. Gas identity hazards and major contamination of the medical gas system of a new hospital. Anaesth Intensive Care 1978;6:202–209.
38. Interchanged oxygen and nitrous oxide lines caused death, suit charges. Biomed Safe Stand 1980;10:28–29.
39. Undetected crossed air—oxygen lines may have contributed to deaths of 7. Biomed Safe Stand 1982;12:41.
40. Cross-connected anesthesia supply lines allegedly result in two deaths: Negligence suits filed. Biomed Safe Stand 1984;14:15–16.
41. Medical gas/vacuum systems. Technol Anesth 1987;7:1–2.
42. Emmanuel ER, Teh JL. Dental anaesthetic emergency caused by medical gas pipeline installation error. Aust Dent J 1983;28: 79–81.
43. LeBourdais E. Nine deaths linked to cross-contamination: Sudbury General inquest makes hospital history. Dimens Health Serv 1974;51:10–12.
44. Sato T. Fatal pipeline accidents spur Japanese standards. APSK Newslett 1991;6:14.

45. Dinnick OP. Medical gases-piping problems. Eng Med 1979;8: 243–247.
46. Installation of oxygen system probed in nitrous oxide death suit. Biomed Safe Stand 1980;10:41–42.
47. Fittings, quick-connect. Technol Anesth 1982;3:4.
48. Crossed N_2O and O_2 lines blamed for outpatient surgery death. Biomed Safe Stand 1992;22:13.
49. Crossed connections in medical gas systems. Technol Anesth 1984;5:3.
50. Fittings/adapters, pneumatic, quick connect. Technol Anesth 1990;11:11.
51. Klein SL, Lilburn K. An unusual case of hypercarbia during general anesthesia. Anesthesiology 1980;53:248–250.
52. Lane GA. Medical gas outlets: A hazard from interchangeable "quick connect"couplers. Anesthesiology 1980;52:86–87.
53. Misconnection of O_2 line to CO_2 outlet claimed in death. Biomed Safe Stand 1991;21:92–93.
54. Ziecheck HD. Faulty ventilator check valves cause pipeline gas contamination. Respir Care 1981;26:1009–1010.
55. Bageant RA, Hoyt JW, Epstein RM. Error in a pipeline gas concentration: An unanticipated consequence of a defective check valve. Anesthesiology 1981;54:166–169.
56. Jenner W, Geroge BF. Oxygen–air shunt syndrome strikes again. Respir Care 1982;27:604.
57. Karmann U, Roth F. Prevention of accidents associated with air–oxygen mixers. Anaesthesia 1982;37:680–682. 58.
58. Thorp JM, Railton R. Hyposia due to air in the oxygen pipeline. Anaesthesia 1982;37:683–687.
57. Bourns Bear 1 ventilator. Health Devices 1983;12:167–168.
60. Bedsole SC, Kempf J. More faulty Bear check valves. Respir Care 1984;29:1159.
61. Shaw A, Richardson W, Railton R. Malfunction of air-mixing valves. Anaesthesia 1985;40:711.
62. Shaw R, Beach W, Metzler M. Medical air contamination with oxygen associated with the Bear 1 and 2 ventilators. Crit Care Med 1988;16:362.
63. Weightman WM, Fenton-May V, Saunders R, et al. Functionally crossed pipelines: An intermittent condition caused by a faulty ventilator. Anaesthesia 1992;47:500–502.
64. Bushman JA, Clark PA. Oil mist hazard and piped air supplies. Br Med J 1967;3:588–590.
65. Gilmour IJ, McComb C, Palanium RJ. Contamination of a hospital oxygen supply. Anesth Analg 1990;71:302–304.
66. Lackore LK, Perkins HM. Accidental narcosis: Contamination of compressed air system. JAMA 1970;211:1846–1847.
67. RB. Contaminated "medical" air. Respir Care 1972;17:125.
68. Conely JIM, Railton R, MacKenzie AI. Ventilator problems caused by humidity in the air supplied from simple compressors. Br J Anaesth 1981;53:549—550.
69. McAdams SA, Barnes W. Air compressor failure complicating mechanical ventilation. Respir Care 1983;28:1601.
70. Bjerring P, Oberg B. Bacterial contamination of compressed air for medical use. Anaesthesia 1986;41:148-150.
71. Warren RE, Newsom SWB, Matthews JA, et al. Medical grade compressed air. Lancet 1986;1:1438.
72. Bjerring P, Oberg B. Possible role of vacuum systems and compressed air generators in cross-infection in the ICU. Br J Anaesth 1987;59:648–650.
73. Patient dies after oxygen tank is replaced with carbon dioxide: Investigation clears hospital. Biomed Safe Stand 1983;13:5–6.
74. Misconnection of oxygen regulator to nitrogen cylinder could cause death. Biomed Safe Stand 1988;18:90–91.
75. Nonstandard user modification of gas cylinder pin indexing. Technol Anesth 1989;10:2.
76. Medical gas cylinders. Technol Anesth 1991;12:12.
77. Goebel WM. Failure of nitrous oxide and oxygen pin-indexing. Anesth Prog 1980;27:188–191.
78. Hogg CE. Pin-indexing failures. Anesthesiology 1973;38:85–87.
79. MacMillan RR, Marshall MA. Failure of the pin index system on a Cape Waine Ventilator. Anaesthesia 1981;36:334–335.
80. Mead P. Hazard with cylinder yoke. Anaesth Intensive Care 1981;9:79–80.
81. Orr IA, Hamilton L. Entonox hazard. Anaesthesia 1985;40:496.
82. Upton LG, Robert EC Jr. Hazard in administering nitrous oxide analgesia: Report of a case. J Am Dent Assoc 1977; 94: 696–697.
83. Boon PE. C-size cylinders. Anaesth Intensive Care 1990;18: 586–587.
84. Sawhney KK, Yoon YK. Erroneous labeling of a nitrous oxide cylinder. Anesthesiology 1983;59:260.
85. Feeley TW, Bancroft ML, Brooks RA, et al. Potential hazards of compressed gas cylinders: A review. Anesthesiology 1978; 48:72–74.
86. Medical gas cylinders. Technol Anesth 1986;7:8.
87. Nitrous oxide cylinders found to contain carbon dioxide. Biomed Safe Stand 1990;20:84.
88. Menon MRB, Lett Z. Incorrectly filled cylinders. Anaesthesia 1991;46:155–156.
89. Jawan B, Lee JH. Cardiac arrest caused by an incorrectly filled oxygen cylinder: A case report. Br J Anaesth 1990;64:749–751.
90. Jayasuriya JP. Another example of Murphy's law: Mix up of pin index valves. Anaesthesia 1986;41:1164.
91. Steward DJ, Sloan IA. Additional pin-indexing failures. Anesthesiology 1973;39:355.
92. Russell WJ. Industrial gas hazard. Anaesth Intensive Care 1985;13:106.
93. Blogg CE, Colvin MP. Apparently empty oxygen cylinders. Br J Anaesth 1977;49:87.
94. Fox JWC, Fox EJ. An unusual occurrence with a cyclopropane cylinder. Anesth Analg 1968;47:624–626.
95. Milliken RA. Correspondence. Anesth Analg 1971;50:775.
96. Herlihy WJ. Report: Contamination of medical oxygen. Anaesth Intens Care 1973;1:240–241.
97. Rendell-Baker L. Purity of oxygen. USP. Anesth Analg 1980;59:314–315.
98. Coveler LA, Lester RC. Contaminated oxygen cylinder. Anesth Analg 1989;69:674–676.
99. Oxygen cylinders recalled because of oil contamination. Biomed Safe Stand 1991;21:20.
100. Ito Y, Horikowa H, Ichiyanagi K. Fires and explosions with compressed gases: Report of an accident. Br J Anaesth 1965;37: 140–141.
101. Bassell GM, Rose DM, Bruce DL. Purity of USP medical oxygen. Anesth Analg 1979;58:441–442.
102. Clutton-Brock J. Two cases of poisoning by contamination of nitrous oxide with higher oxides of nitrogen during anesthesia. Br J Anaesth 1967;39:388–392.
103. Finch JS. A report on a possible hazard of gas cylinder tanks. Anesthesiology 1970;33:467.
104. Valves may open and release liquid oxygen. Biomed Safe Stand 1990;20:20–21.
105. Massey LW, Hussey JD, Albert RK. Inaccurate oxygen delivery in some portable liquid oxygen devices. Am Rev Respir Dis 1988;137:204–205.

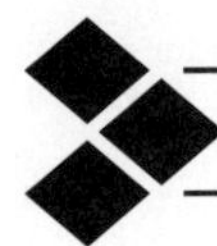
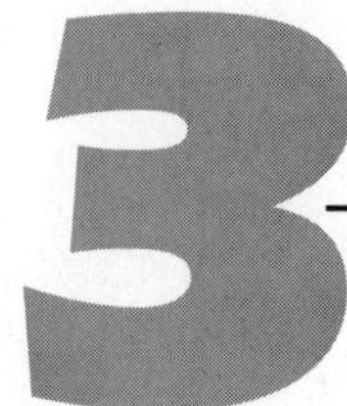

Gas Delivery Systems: Regulators, Flowmeters, and Therapy Devices

Richard D. Branson

OBJECTIVES

1. Describe the function of regulators.
2. Describe the operation and use of flowmeters.
3. Differentiate between pressure-compensated and non–pressure-compensated flowmeters.
4. Describe the types of flow-regulating devices.
5. Explain the difference between variable-performance oxygen therapy devices and fixed-performance oxygen therapy devices.
6. Describe the placement, problems, and performance of variable-performance and fixed-performance oxygen therapy devices.
7. Describe the methods of blending air and oxygen.
8. Describe the operation and use of air–oxygen blenders.

KEY TERMS

Bourdon flowmeter
Bourdon gauge
combustible
compressor
flowmeter
flow restrictor
French scale
NFPA
oxygen concentrator (enricher)
oxygen delivery system:
fixed-performance oxygen delivery system
variable-performance oxygen delivery system
oxygen proportioner
proportioning valve
Thorpe tube

Introduction

Medical gases delivered to the bedside by means of cylinders or piping systems must be regulated and controlled before delivery to the patient. Devices for regulating pressure, controlling flow, and administering gases are common tools of the respiratory care practitioner. A detailed knowledge of the operation and trouble shooting of these devices is paramount for safe and effective application.

In this chapter the focus is on the devices used in regulation and control of medical gases and on the equipment used to deliver medical gases to the patient.

Regulators

Regulators, or pressure-reducing valves, are devices that reduce pressure by using opposing forces (gas pressure and spring tension) separated by a flexible diaphragm. Regulators are used extensively in gas distribution systems and mechanical ventilators to maintain a constant gas pressure traveling to precision flow valves. Regulators are also commonly used to reduce gas pressure from cylinders (2200 psig) to a lower, working pressure of 50 psig. Since cylinders have declining pressure during use (as gas is withdrawn), regulators are required to maintain a constant gas pressure output.

Regulators are divided into direct-acting and indirect-acting devices. Frequently, regulators are also divided into single-stage, dual-stage and multistage devices. The principle of operation for dual-stage and multistage regulators is the same as for a single-stage regulator. As the names imply, a dual-stage regulator is simply two single-stage regulators in series, while a multistage regulator is three or more single-stage regulators in series. Multistage regulators allow greater accuracy in maintaining pressure.

A direct-acting, single-stage regulator is shown in Figure 3-1 in both the closed and open positions. Gas at high pressure enters the high-pressure chamber at the bottom left. In the closed position, the diaphragm is in a neutral (horizontal) position and the poppet or valve thrust pin closes the communication between the high-pressure (bottom) and low-pressure (top) chambers. In this position the spring tension in the high-pressure chamber is greater than the main spring tension in the low-pressure chamber. As the adjusting screw is tightened, the diaphragm is displaced downward, pushing the valve thrust pin away from the communication between the chambers. Gas then flows around the thrust pin and into the low-pressure chamber. The gas pressure then opposes the pressure exerted by the adjusting screw. Gas from the low-pressure chamber can flow through the outlet to a flow-controlling device. Gas continues to flow until the gas supply is exhausted or gas flow is turned off downstream of the regulator. When gas is turned off downstream, pressure against the diaphragm will increase and along with pressure from the sealing spring will push the valve thrust pin into a closed position. While gas is flowing, the gas pressure and spring tension are in equilibrium but the pressures are not equal. Spring tension remains greater than gas supply pressure. If supply pressure falls, spring tension displaces the diaphragm farther, increasing gas flow into the low-pressure chamber and maintaining a constant outlet pressure. A pressure relief valve is required for each stage of a regulator. Figure 3-1 shows a spring-disk pressure relief valve as an integral part of the regulator. Pressure relief valves are typically set at a pressure 50% greater than working pressure and prevent damage to equipment placed downstream. If pressure exceeds the threshold value, the disk is lifted from its seat and excess gas is vented to atmosphere. If gas pressure returns to normal, the disk reseats and the

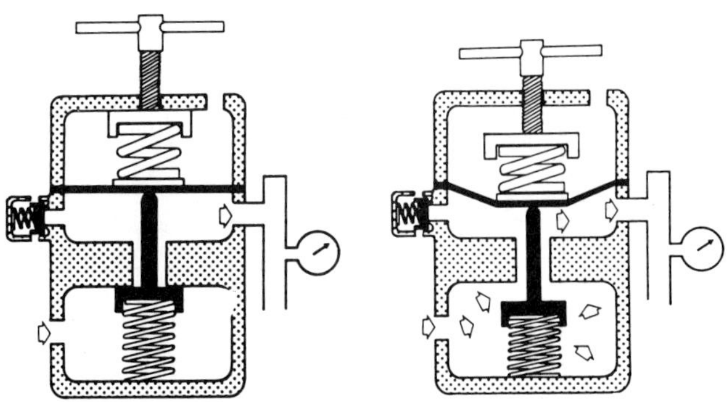

Figure 3-1. A direct-acting regulator or pressure-reducing valve in the closed (left) and open (right) positions.

regulator continues to operate. Overpressure typically results from water or other contaminants introduced from the gas supply.

Figure 3-2 is an indirect-acting regulator shown in the closed and open positions. Like the direct-acting valve, in the closed position the diaphragm is in a neutral position and the sealing spring tension keeps the valve thrust pin closed. When the adjusting screw is tightened, the main spring tension overcomes the sealing spring tension, forcing the valve thrust pin downward. Gas flows around the thrust pin and into the low-pressure chamber where it opposes mainspring tension under the diaphragm. When downstream flow is turned off, gas pressure forces the diaphragm upward, closing the valve thrust pin. Like the direct-acting device, the indirect-acting regulator maintains a fairly constant outlet pressure by balancing spring tension and gas pressure.

The devices shown in Figure 3-1 and 3-2 are adjustable regulators. All adjustable regulators are equipped with a pressure gauge to indicate the set pressure. Nonadjustable regulators are used in some ventilators and do not require a pressure gauge.

A typical pressure-reducing valve for an H-cylinder is shown in Figure 3-3. The regulator is connected to the cylinder by an American Standard connection. A gauge is mounted above, and the pressure relief valve protrudes from below. The gas outlet is to the left. This type of regulator is adjustable by removing the nut on the front of the assembly and turning the adjusting screw with an Allen wrench. Adjustment of a regulator should only be attempted by a qualified individual.

Pressure gauges for regulators are typically Bourdon gauges. Figure 3-4 depicts a Bourdon gauge with the gas flow turned off (top) and with increasing pressure (bottom). Gas from the regulator travels into a coiled metal tube. As gas pressure increases, the coiled tube attempts to straighten. A series of gears are attached to the end of the coiled tube, and an indicator needle is attached to the final gear. As the tube

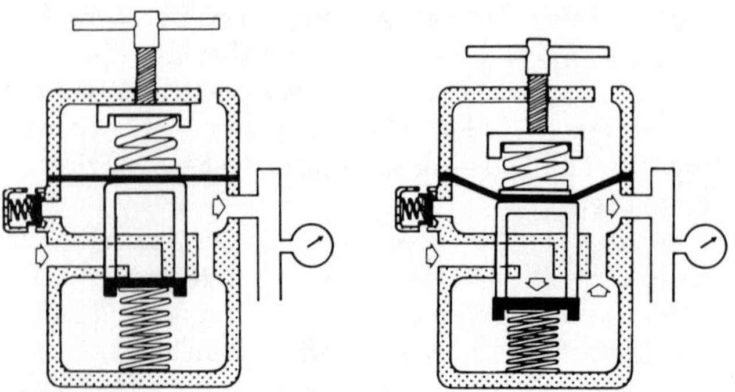

Figure 3-2. An indirect-acting regulator or pressure-reducing valve in the closed (left) and open (right) positions.

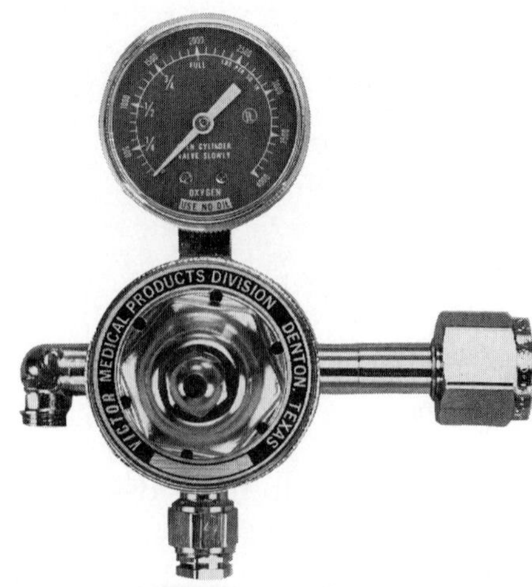

Figure 3-3. A pressure-reducing valve for an H-cylinder, with a gauge (top), American Standard connection (right), and pressure relief valve (bottom).

straightens, the gears move, causing the indicator needle to display the pressure. As gas pressure falls, the tube moves back toward its coiled shape and the gears move the needle in a counterclockwise position. Figure 3-5 shows two Bourdon gauges with the coiled tubes, gears, and needle indicators exposed. The gauge on the right has a stainless steel coiled tube and measures pressure in a cylinder. The gauge on the left has a softer copper coil and is used to indicate flow (discussed later in this chapter).

Regulators require routine maintenance to ensure proper function. Movement of springs and diaphragms causes wear, and these parts require replacement over time. Contaminated gas can introduce debris into the regulator and cause corrosion, preventing normal regulator function. Foreign objects introduced into the regulator can prevent proper seating of the valve. Cracking cylinder valves to eliminate dust before attaching the regulator helps prevent regulator contamination. Petroleum-based lubricants should never be used on regulators because of the fire hazard associated with oxygen delivery.[1] Box 3-1 is a summary of regulations regarding regulators.

Flowmeters

Flowmeters are devices used to control and indicate gas flow, typically in liters per minute (volume per unit time). Flowmeters are simple devices but serve the same function for medical gases that intravenous infusion pumps do for parenteral medications. Gas supply to flowmeters usually originates from a regulator attached to a cylinder or from a station outlet at the end of the medical gas distribution system. Inlet pressure to a flowmeter is relatively constant at 50 psig.

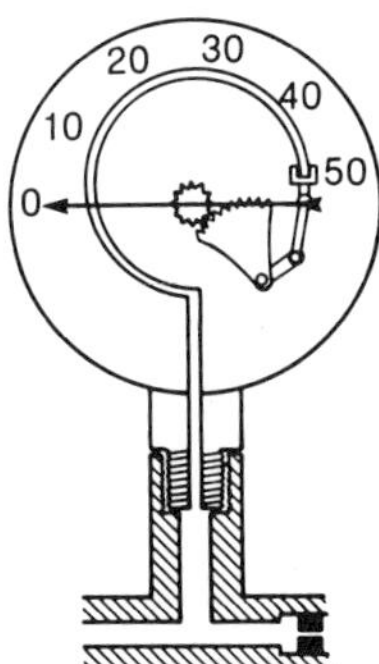

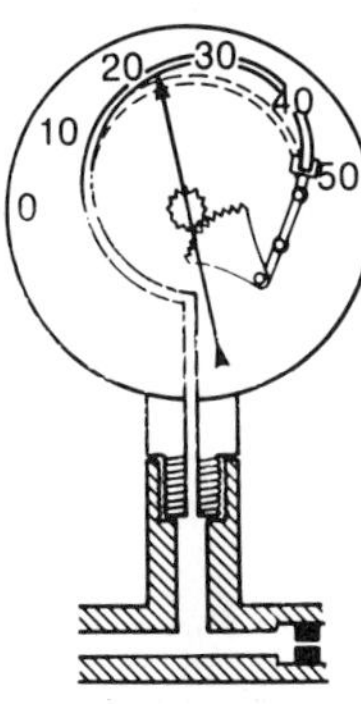

Figure 3-4. A Bourdon gauge used to measure pressure in a regulator. As pressure increases (bottom) the coiled tube straightens. This upward movement of the coil causes the gear mechanism to move. As the gears turn, the needle rises to indicate the resulting pressure.

Box 3-1
Summary of NFPA Regulations Regarding Regulators (Pressure-Reducing Valves)

- A regulator must be used on a high-pressure cylinder.
- It is hazardous to connect a flow-controlling device to a cylinder without a regulator.
- Regulator connections should comply with the Index Safety System, American Standard, or Diameter Index Safety System of noninterchangeability.
- Regulators used for oxygen should be labeled "Oxygen—Use No Oil."
- Regulators should be permanently labeled with the name of the gas it is intended for.
- Regulators must be on a preventative maintenance program.
- Regulators should be cleaned with a cloth and mild soap or disinfectant.

All flowmeters operate by restricting flow with a fixed or variable orifice. Flow through an orifice is governed by the principles described below.

Flow through an orifice is directly proportional to the square root of the pressure difference across the orifice.[2]

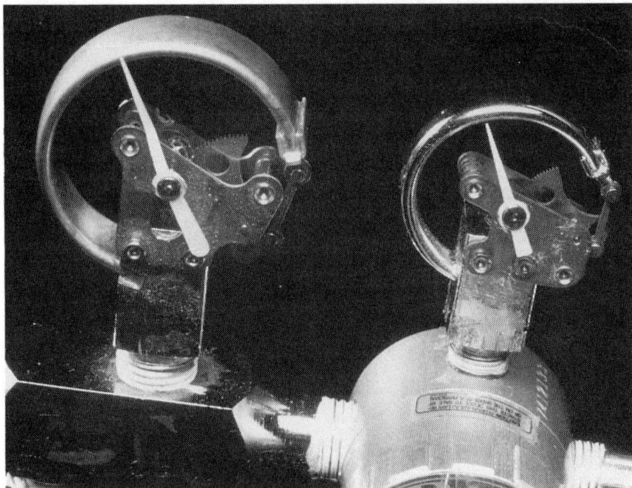

Figure 3-5. Bourdon gauges used to monitor pressure and flow.

$$\text{Flow} \propto \sqrt{P_1 - P_2}$$

where P_1 is the source pressure driving gas through the orifice and P_2 is the downstream pressure, usually equivalent to atmospheric pressure. Altering P_2 by attaching any device with a smaller orifice than the outlet will cause the P_1-P_2 difference and flow to diminish. Clinically, this can happen when tubing from a flowmeter is kinked or an air-entrainment mask is used. Bourdon gauge and non–pressure-compensated Thorpe tube flowmeters are examples of devices that control gas flow based on a fixed orifice and variable pressure.

At a constant pressure (P_1-P_2), flow through an orifice is directly proportional to the square of the diameter opening.

$$\text{Flow} \propto \text{diameter}^2$$

In this instance, flow increases or decreases exponentially as the diameter of the orifice is increased or decreased. This is typically accomplished by opening or closing a needle valve. Flowmeters that use a constant pressure and variable orifice are known as pressure-compensated Thorpe tube flowmeters. Thorpe tube flowmeters are the most commonly used devices to regulate gas flow.

Devices that use a constant pressure and fixed orifice to control flow are known as flow restrictors. Flow restrictors are governed by the principle of proportionality between flow and orifice diameter.

The last principle associated with flowmeters is related to density of the gas. Flow through an orifice is inversely proportional to the square root of gas density.

$$\text{Flow} \propto \frac{1}{\sqrt{\text{density}}}$$

Simply stated, at a constant pressure and constant orifice diameter, gas flow increases as gas density decreases and gas flow decreases as density increases.

This principle explains why flowmeters must be labeled for the gas intended to be controlled. The difference in gas density between air and oxygen is small enough that flow readings are not significantly different. However, use of an oxygen flowmeter to deliver heliox (helium 80%, oxygen 20%) results in clinically important inaccuracies.

The density of oxygen is 1.43 g/L, and the density of an 80%/20% heliox mixture is 0.43 g/L. If an oxygen flowmeter is used to deliver the heliox mixture, then the actual flow can be determined from the indicated flow and the square root of the gas density. For example, at an indicated flow on an oxygen flowmeter of 1 L/min from a cylinder of 80%/20% heliox, the actual flow is 1.8 L/min. This is illustrated in Equation Box 3-1.

This relationship of oxygen to heliox (1 L/min of indicated oxygen flow equals 1.8 L/min actual heliox flow) allows the flow to be easily calculated. Purchase of flowmeters calibrated for different heliox mixtures would be cost prohibitive.

Density of a gas can also be effected by temperature and barometric pressure. A flowmeter calibrated at sea level will demonstrate a 1% error in indicated flow for every 1000 ft in altitude. This difference can be important during air transport and in cities at high altitudes. The differences can be calculated using the formula in Equation Box 3-2. For the most part, changes in density due to decreased barometric pressure are clinically unimportant.

Flow Restrictors

The simplest flowmeters are known as flow restrictors. Flow restrictors rely on a constant pressure and fixed orifice diameter to precisely meter flow from a 50-psig pressure source. Flow restrictors do not have a gauge to indicate flow. Most flow restrictors provide a single flow (Fig. 3-6), and if a change in flow is necessary, another restrictor is used. An adjustable restrictor (Fig. 3-7) allows the operator to select several flow rates by rotating a knob that changes the size of the orifice outlet. Figure 3-8 shows an adjustable flow restrictor connected to a regulator and small cylinder yoke.

Flow restrictors are most often used in home care with oxygen concentrators and portable systems. Other uses include emergency care to provide a constant flow to resuscitation equipment. Advantages of flow restrictors include non–gravity-dependent operation and prevention of inadvertent changes in prescribed flow.

Flow restrictors are reliable and require no maintenance because there are no moving parts. Since no gauge is provided, the actual flow from flow restrictors should be checked periodically. The most common cause of inaccurate flow is alteration of the $P_1 - P_2$ relationship. This can result from an inlet pressure less than or greater than 50 psig, connection of a device with a narrower orifice downstream of the flow restrictor, or any situation causing downstream backpressure. Debris or moisture from contaminated gas supplies may alter the diameter of the flow restrictor, causing inaccurate flow rates.

Bourdon Gauge Flowmeters

The Bourdon gauge has been previously described and is shown in Figure 3-4. Bourdon gauges use a

Equation Box 3-1: Effect of Gas Density on Accuracy of Oxygen Flowmeter When Using Heliox

$$\text{Actual flow} = \text{Indicated flow} \times \frac{\sqrt{\text{density of oxygen}}}{\sqrt{\text{density of heliox}}}$$

$$\text{Actual flow} = 1 \times \frac{\sqrt{1.43}}{\sqrt{0.43}}$$

$$\text{Actual flow} = 1 \times \frac{1.20}{0.66}$$

$$\text{Actual flow} = 1.8\ \text{L/min}$$

Equation Box 3-2: Effect of Barometric Pressure on Accuracy of Oxygen Flowmeter

$$\text{Actual flow (L/min)} = \text{Indicated flow (L/min)} \times \frac{P_B\ \text{sea level}}{P_B\ \text{local}}$$

In the case of a patient traveling with oxygen at 2 L/min on an aircraft that maintains cabin pressure equivalent to 7500 ft ($P_B = 573$), then

$$\text{Actual flow (L/min)} = 2\ \text{L/min} \times \frac{760\ \text{mm Hg}}{573\ \text{mm Hg}}$$

$$\text{Actual flow (L/min)} = 2\ \text{L/min} \times 1.326$$

$$\text{Actual flow (L/min)} = 2.65\ \text{L/min}$$

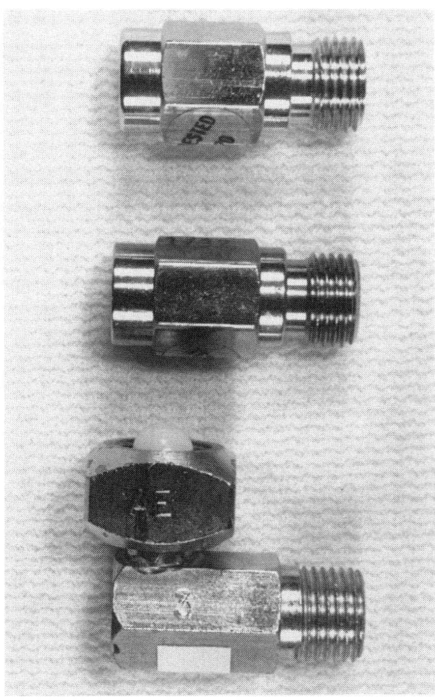

Figure 3-6. Different sizes of single-flow flow restrictors.

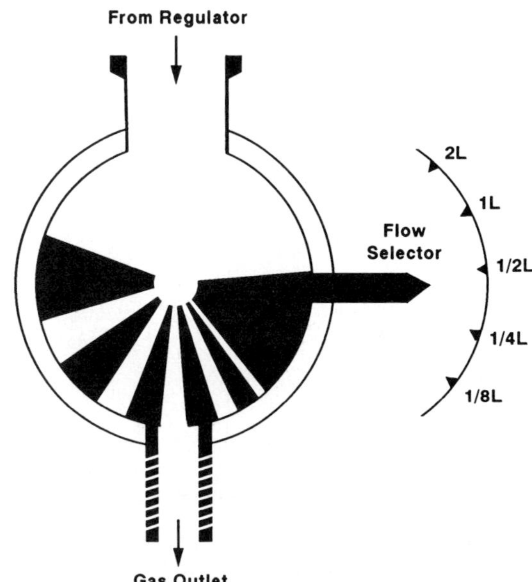

Figure 3-7. Adjustable flow restrictor. Changing the orifice size for gas flow regulates flow rate.

fixed orifice and variable pressure to control flow. When a Bourdon gauge is used to control flow, a fixed orifice is placed downstream of the gauge. The gauge then measures back-pressure (P_1) and indicates flow based on the known diameter of the forward orifice. Bourdon gauges are always used in conjunction with an adjustable pressure regulator.

Bourdon gauge flowmeters are useful during transport because flow can be accurately displayed regardless of cylinder position. These flowmeters are improvements over flow restrictors because there is an indication of flow and flow is selectable over a continuous range. This type of flowmeter is frequently used to control flow to oxygen delivery devices from a cylinder.

Because the Bourdon gauge measures pressure to indicate flow, a change in downstream pressure (P_2) will result in inaccurate flow readings. If a kink occurs in the oxygen tubing connected to the flowmeter, back-pressure P_2 will increase. As back-pressure increases, the hollow, metallic tube in the Bourdon gauge will attempt to straighten, indicating an increase in flow. The actual flow will decrease as the P_1-P_2 difference falls. A Bourdon gauge will indicate a flow higher than actually delivered whenever significant resistance is present downstream of the outlet. In fact, the Bourdon gauge will continue to indicate flow even when the outlet is completely obstructed!

Bourdon gauges should not be used with nebulizers or other devices that increase downstream pressure. A Bourdon gauge flowmeter attached to a regulator for an H-cylinder is shown in Figure 3-9.

Thorpe Tube Flowmeters

Thorpe tube flowmeters are the most frequently used devices to control flow. These flowmeters operate using a variable orifice and constant pressure. Thorpe tube flowmeters are connected to a pre-set pressure-reducing valve or station outlet providing 50 psig.

A Thorpe tube flowmeter consists of a needle valve, a tapered transparent tube with a calibrated scale, and a float. The needle valve is responsible for controlling flow, while the tube and float serve to measure the flow provided. Figure 3-10 shows a schematic of a Thorpe tube flowmeter.

Gas from a 50-psig source enters the Thorpe tube from a regulator or station outlet. If the needle valve is

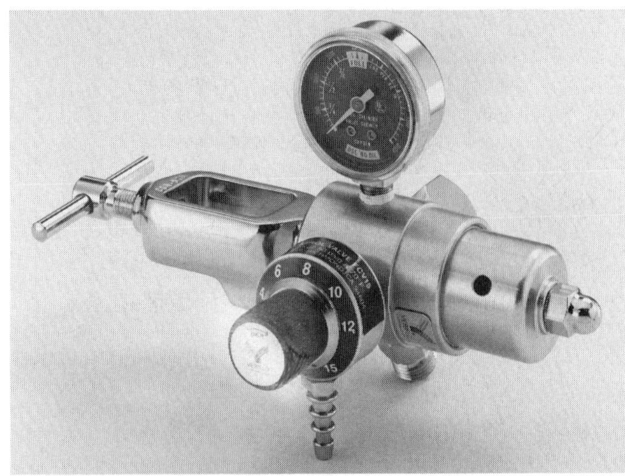

Figure 3-8. Adjustable flow restrictor for metering gas flow from an E-cylinder. (Courtesy of Veriflow Corporation)

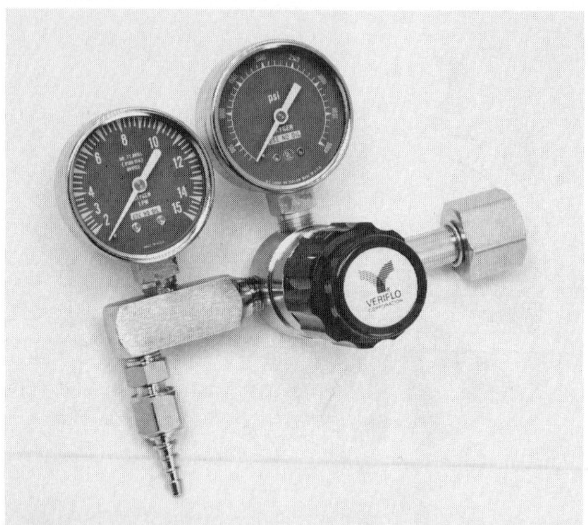

Figure 3-9. Bourdon gauge flowmeter and Bourdon gauge regulator (pressure-reducing valve) used to indicate cylinder pressure and flow from an H-cylinder. (Courtesy of Veriflo Corporation)

closed, flow is prevented. As the needle valve is opened, gas travels through the tube, lifting the float and exiting past the needle valve. The position of the float is related to its weight, gravity, width of the tube, and gas flow. When the needle valve is opened, the pressure difference (P_1-P_2) causes the float to rise. As the float rises up the widening tube, the space available for gas flow (orifice size) past the float increases. As flow is increased, the float rises and orifice size increases, while as flow is decreased the float falls and orifice size diminishes.

Thorpe tube flowmeters are separated into pressure-compensated and non–pressure-compensated devices. Pressure-compensated devices are used in respiratory care and are distinguished by placement of the needle valve downstream of the Thorpe tube. This maintains pressure in the Thorpe tube down to the needle valve at 50 psig.

Pressure-compensated flowmeters allow accurate flow readings regardless of downstream pressure. If a device with a high resistance is connected to a pressure-compensated flowmeter and the P_1-P_2 difference is altered, the float indicates the true flow. The downstream resistance only increases pressure distal to the needle valve. If back-pressure were to exceed 50 psig, flow would cease. Compensated flowmeters will provide accurate readings if (1) the inlet pressure is constant at 50 psig, (2) the Thorpe tube remains in an upright position, and (3) the flow setting is less than flow from the gas source. A pressure compensated flowmeter is shown in Figure 3-11.

Uncompensated Thorpe tube flowmeters have a needle valve between the gas source and the Thorpe tube. Gas flow through the Thorpe tube is controlled by the needle valve, and tube pressure is near atmospheric pressure.

If a restriction is placed downstream of an uncompensated flowmeter, pressure in the Thorpe tube increases back to the needle valve. As P_2 rises, the float assumes a position in the Thorpe tube, lower than the actual flow. Uncompensated flowmeters are used in some anesthesia machines and in laboratory instruments.

A simple test identifies pressure-compensated flowmeters from non–pressure-compensated devices. Turn the needle valve off and connect the flowmeter to a 50 psig gas source. If the float "jumps," the flowmeter is compensated. Because the needle valve is downstream of the float, the tube will be pressurized to 50 psig down to the needle valve. This requires that gas travel around the float. When pressure reaches an

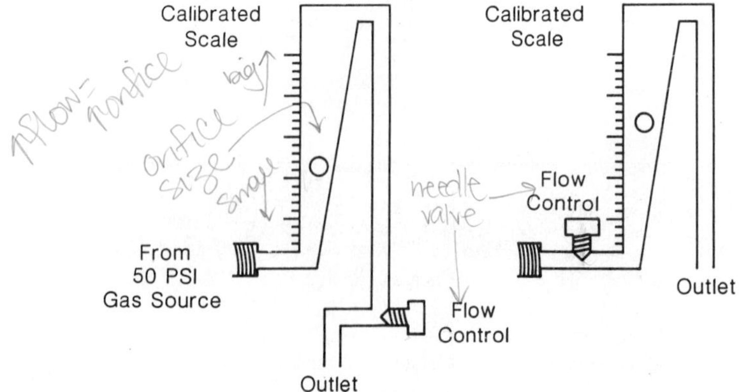

Figure 3-10. Pressure-compensated Thorpe tube flowmeter (left) and a non–pressure-compensated Thorpe tube flowmeter (right).

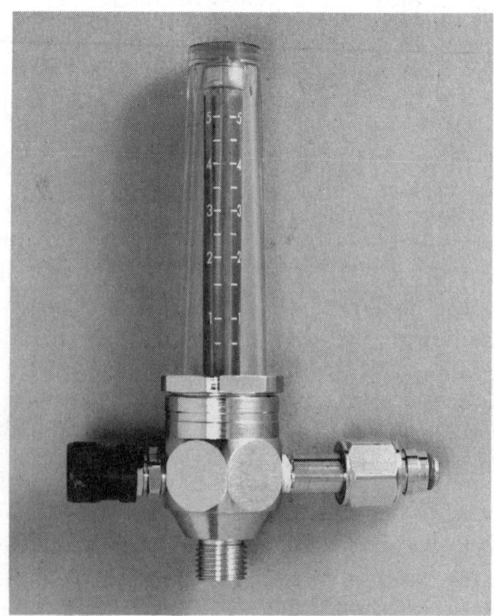

Figure 3-11. Pressure-compensated Thorpe tube flowmeter.

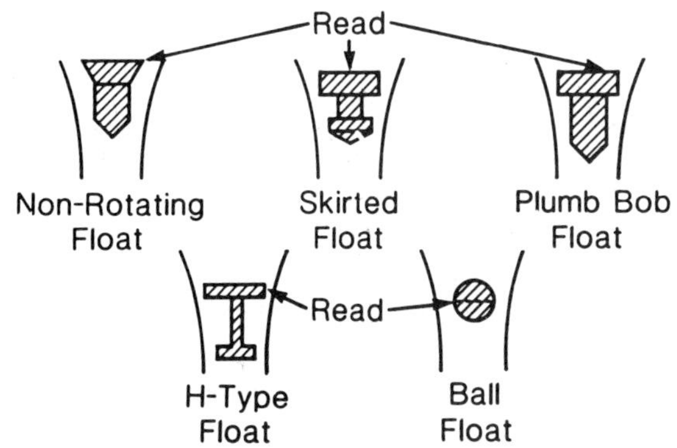

Figure 3-12. Types of floats used in flowmeters. All floats except the ball float should be read at the top of the float. The ball float should be read at its center.

equilibrium, because the needle valve is closed, the float returns to its resting position.

The float in a flowmeter is usually a ball, although many other types are used in anesthesia and in older devices. Accurate reading requires sighting the center of the ball at eye level. Figure 3-12 depicts several types of floats and the appropriate site for reading flow.

Inaccurate flow readings may be the result of contamination with water or debris, cracked tubes, faulty O-rings, and worn needle valves and seats. Periodic testing of indicated flow against a rotameter should be accomplished regularly and whenever a device appears damaged.

Characteristics of flowmeters are compared in Table 3-1.

Cylinder Regulators

Besides regulators that regulate pressure, a regulator is often described as the combination of a pressure-reducing valve and a flow-controlling device. These devices operate using the same principles previously described. In clinical practice, the term *regulator* usually means a pressure-reducing valve and flowmeter used to measure cylinder pressure and control gas flow. A regulator for an H-cylinder with a Bourdon flowmeter is shown in Figure 3-13, and a regulator for an E-cylinder with a Thorpe tube flowmeter is shown in Figure 3-14.

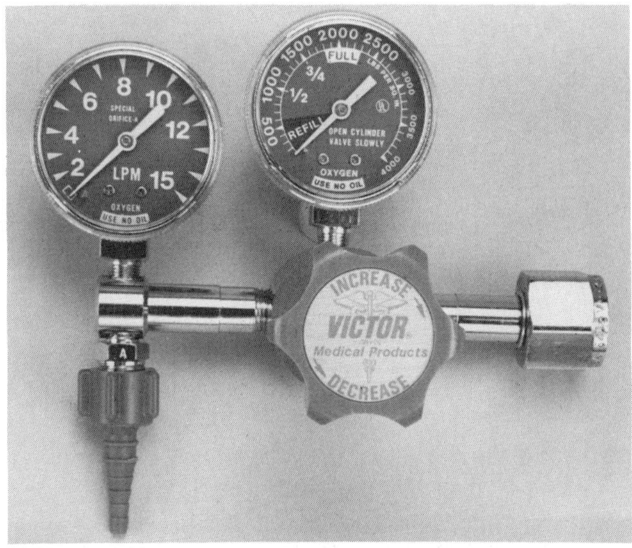

Figure 3-13. A regulator for use with an H-cylinder. The first Bourdon gauge measures cylinder pressure, the second indicates flow. (Courtesy of Victor Medical Products)

Oxygen Therapy Devices

Oxygen therapy is one of the cornerstones of respiratory care. Yet despite the fact that oxygen has been delivered to patients with lung disease for almost a century, it is commonly delivered in imprecise concentrations. Because oxygen is "unseen" it has often been relegated to a status considerably less than the potent drug that it is. Severinghaus and Astrup[3] have eloquently described the current status of oxygen:

> Oxygen is addicting; in its grip are all the mitochondria-rich eukaryotes who learned to depend on it

TABLE 3-1. Characteristics of Flowmeters

Flowmeter	Principle	Gauge	Measurement	Effects of Increasing Downstream Pressure
Flow restrictor	Fixed orifice Constant pressure	No	None	Decrease flow
Bourdon gauge	Fixed orifice Variable pressure	Yes	Pressure, indicates flow	Decrease flow Gauge overestimates flow
Pressure-compensated Thorpe tube	Variable orifice Constant pressure	Yes	Flow	Decrease flow Gauge accurately measures flow
Non–pressure-compensated Thorpe tube	Variable orifice Constant pressure	Yes	Flow	Decrease flow Underestimates actual flow

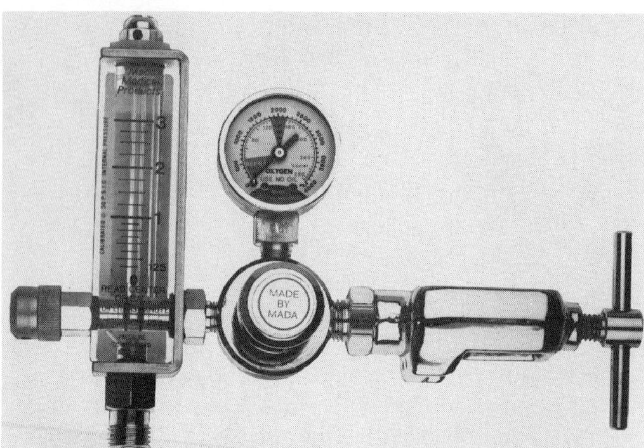

Figure 3-14. A regulator for use with an E-cylinder using a Thorpe tube flowmeter. (Courtesy of MADA)

> during the past 1.4 billion years. This, the first atmospheric pollutant, is the waste product of stromatolites (formation of algal plankton), which excreted it at least 2.3 billion years ago. Since then all sediments have been rusted or oxidized. Oxygen is toxic. It rusts a person in a century or less. With oxygen came the danger and blessing of fire. If introduced today, this gas might have difficulty getting approved by the Food and Drug Administration.

Oxygen therapy devices are typically classified into two groups, low-flow, or variable-performance, equipment and high-flow, or fixed-performance, equipment. The status of oxygen therapy in the hospital has been well established for many years, and few changes have occurred in the past decade.

Low-flow, or variable-performance, equipment delivers oxygen at a fixed flow that only represents a portion of the patient's inspired gas. The term *variable performance* relates to the fact that as the patient's ventilatory pattern changes, delivered oxygen is diluted with room air. This results in a widely variable and fluctuating fraction of inspired oxygen concentration (F_{IO_2}). In fact, despite some commonly published figures for delivered F_{IO_2} at given flow rates, the actual F_{IO_2} delivered to the patient is neither precise or predictable.

High-flow, or fixed-performance, equipment provides all the patient's inspired gas with a precisely controlled F_{IO_2}. When applied appropriately, the F_{IO_2} delivered to the patient is therefore constant, regardless of ventilatory pattern. Fixed performance devices include air-entrainment masks, large-volume aerosol systems, and large-volume humidifier systems.

The following describes the various oxygen delivery devices, their placement, problems, and performance. A review of the pertinent literature for each is also provided. Historical notes are left out in the interest of brevity. Interested readers are referred to the article by Leigh.[4]

Variable Performance Equipment

Nasal Catheter

DESCRIPTION. The nasal catheter is the simplest of oxygen delivery devices. It is a soft, plastic, blind-end tube with numerous side holes at the distal tip (Fig. 3-15). Nasal catheters typically come in French sizes, which is an odd reference to the outside diameter (OD) of the device. A French (F) size is three times the OD, with typical adult sizes being 12F to 14F. Oxygen is delivered to the nasal catheter from a bubble humidifier through oxygen tubing.

PLACEMENT. Before use, the patency of the catheter should be confirmed and the catheter liberally lubricated with a water-soluble lubricant. The catheter is placed in the external naris and advanced along the floor of the nasal cavity into the oropharynx, stopping just behind the uvula. Appropriate size should be determined to prevent unnecessary trauma during insertion. Size can be determined by inspection of the external naris and by measurement of the distance between the tip of the nose and the external ear.

Appropriate placement is best confirmed by visual inspection of the catheter tip in the oropharynx. This is accomplished using a tongue blade and flashlight. During insertion, advance the catheter into the oropharynx until it appears below the uvula. After identifying the catheter tip, withdraw the catheter until the tip of the catheter is no longer seen. If placement is difficult, the opposite naris should be used. Once proper placement is achieved, the catheter should be secured to the nose with tape.

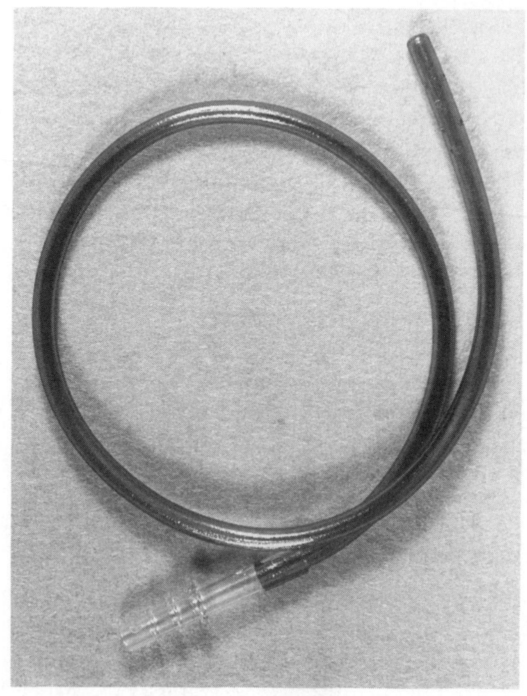

Figure 3-15. An adult nasal catheter.

PROBLEMS. Pain and discomfort during insertion are common problems. In the presence of nasal pathology, including nasal polyps, deviated septum, and nasal congestion, placement may be particularly traumatic or impossible. Bleeding is a common complication resulting from mucosal irritation. Patients with coagulation disorders should not have a nasal catheter placed.

Migration of the catheter into the esophagus with subsequent gastric insufflation represents another potential complication. A stomach full of oxygen is uncomfortable for the patient and impedes ventilation. Routine changing of the catheter is required to prevent blockage of the side holes with secretions and subsequent cessation of oxygen flow. A buildup of secretions around the catheter can also prove problematic during removal.

PERFORMANCE. Nasal catheters have been used for adults as well as infants.[5] In adults, nasal catheters provide a relatively low FIO_2.[6] Gibson and associates[6] found that at 3 L/min the nasal catheter provided an FIO_2 of 0.23. At a flow of 15 L/min, an FIO_2 of 0.44 was found. Kory and co-workers[7] measured an FIO_2 of 0.69 to 0.82 using flow rates from 6 to 10 L/min.

The increase in FIO_2 associated with a nasal catheter is directly related to gas flow and is enhanced at low flow rates by using the nasopharynx and oropharynx as a reservoir for oxygen. Like all variable performance equipment, delivered FIO_2 will vary with a change in respiratory rate or tidal volume.

Nasal catheters are infrequently used today. Because placement is intranasal, complications and discomfort are much greater than for a nasal cannula. The major advantage of the nasal catheter is that it can be securely placed in obtunded patients. The long list of disadvantages, including discomfort, difficulty in insertion, and bleeding, cause the nasal catheter to be a last choice device.

Nasal Cannula

DESCRIPTION. The nasal cannula is the most commonly used oxygen therapy delivery device. It consists of a blind-end tube with two protruding "nasal prongs" that rest in the external naris. Cannulae come in a variety of designs for more comfortable or inconspicuous application. These include devices with elastic bands encircling the head, a lariat style that attaches above the ears and under the chin, and tubing incorporated into eyeglasses. Regardless of the design, the principle of oxygen delivery is the same.

Cannulae are connected to an oxygen flowmeter through oxygen tubing without a humidification device when flow is less than 4 L/min. At higher flow rates, a bubble humidifier may be used to prevent nasal drying.[8–10]

PLACEMENT. Nasal cannulae are easily placed regardless of the style (Fig. 3-16). Attention should be paid to patient comfort by eliminating twisting and kinking in the tubing and ensuring the adjustable portion is not too tight. Long-term use can cause pressure sores above the ears, under the chin, and above the upper lip.

PROBLEMS. The nasal cannula is relatively problem free. Twisted or kinked tubing and tubing disconnected from the oxygen source are the most common problems. Pressure sores can develop at areas of prolonged contact between the cannula and the patient's skin. Gauze or foam padding can be placed between the cannula and irritation sites.

PERFORMANCE. A nasal cannula is used with oxygen flow rates of 1 to 6 L/min in adults and as low as 1/16 L/min in infants. The exact FIO_2 delivered with a nasal cannula has been measured and predicted using a variety of methods and a wider variety of results.

Shapiro and associates have devised a method to predict FIO_2 provided by variable performance equipment using a host of assumptions and a simplified equation.[11] This equation assumes that (1) the anatomic reservoir is 50 mL; (2) the anatomic reservoir is filled with 100% oxygen before inspiration; and (3) ventilatory pattern (tidal volume, frequency, and inspiratory–expiratory ratio) is constant.[11] Equation Box 3-3 demonstrates the use of this equation assuming a tidal volume of 500 mL, inspiration–expiration ratio of 1:2, frequency of 20 breaths per minute, and inspiratory time of 1.0 second. Perhaps the most important lesson learned from this equation is the wide range of FIO_2 values delivered at any given constant flow of oxygen.

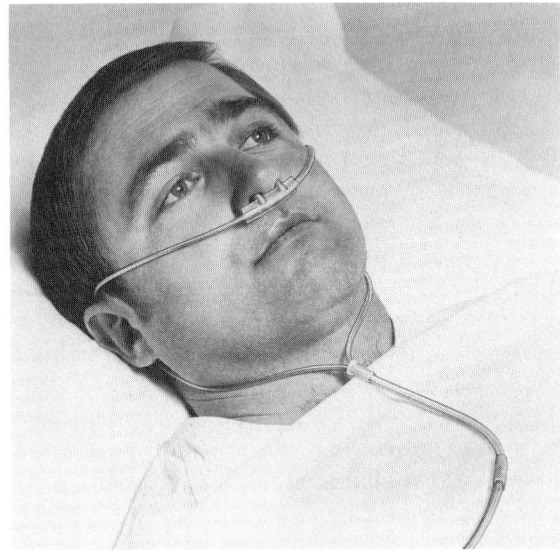

Figure 3-16. A lariat-style nasal cannula on a patient. (Courtesy of Hudson-RCI, Temecula, CA)

Equation Box 3-3: Estimation of F_{IO_2} from Low-Flow Systems

Cannula—6 L/min	V_T—500 mL
Mechanical reservoir—none	I:E—1:2
Anatomic reservoir—50 mL	f—20/min
100% O_2 provided/s— 100 mL	Inspiratory time— 1 s

Volume of O_2 inspired
50 mL anatomic reservoir
100 mL flow/s
70 mL from room air
220 mL O_2 inspired

Because 150 mL of 100% O_2 is inspired, the remainder of V_T is room air (350 mL), 20% of 350 mL = 70 mL, amount of O_2 in in room air inspired.

$$F_{IO_2} = \frac{220\ mL(O_2)}{500\ mL(V_T)} = 0.44$$

If V_T is decreased to 250 mL, volume O_2 inspired is

50 mL anatomic reservoir
100 mL flow/s
20 mL from room air (20% of 250 − 150)
170 mL O_2 inspired

$$F_{IO_2} = \frac{170\ mL\ (O_2)}{250\ mL(V_T)} = 0.64$$

If V_T increased to 1000 mL, volume O_2 inspired is

50 mL anatomic reservoir
100 mL flow/s
170 mL room air (20% of 1000 − 150)
320 mL O_2 inspired

$$F_{IO_2} = \frac{320\ mL\ (O_2)}{1000\ mL\ (V_T)} = 0.32$$

Several authors have attempted to quantify the F_{IO_2} delivered with the nasal cannula. Gibson and others measured tracheal oxygen concentrations by means of a transtracheal catheter in two subjects.[6] Both subjects had tracheal F_{IO_2} measured with a mass spectrometer during "quiet" (f = 16 breaths per minute, tidal volume = 400 mL, minute ventilation = 6.42 L/min), "normal" (f = 17 breaths per minute, tidal volume = 690 mL, minute ventilation = 11 L/min), and "hyperventilation" (f = 14 breaths per minute, tidal volume = 1400 mL, minute ventilation = 19.5 L/min). Using a nasal cannula at 1, 2, 3, 5, 10 and 15 L/min, they reported little variation in F_{IO_2} at low flow rates, yet wide variations at high flow rates (Table 3-2).

Schacter and associates studied delivered F_{IO_2} during oxygen delivery in patients in intensive care unit settings.[12] They found similar concentrations to the study of Gibson and colleagues[6] (see Table 3-2). More recently, Ooi and associates[13] studied F_{IO_2} delivered through the nasal cannula using a model of the respiratory system. Their model consisted of a face shield from a resuscitation mannequin attached to a rubber test lung through tubing that approximated tracheal volume. The test lung was placed inside a rigid container, creating a bag-in-the-box system. A ventilator producing a sine wave was connected to the container, and inspiratory flow was varied from 12 to 40 L/min at a constant rate and volume. Ooi and associates[13] found that delivered F_{IO_2} varied 13% to 40% at a given oxygen flow when inspiratory flow varied from 12 to 40 L/min (see Table 3-2).

The nasal cannula is typically used to deliver oxygen to stable patients postoperatively and to patients requiring long-term therapy. Its use to combat hypoxemia in critically ill patients is unwarranted owing to the uncontrollable and widely variable F_{IO_2}. Theoretically, the nasal cannula increases F_{IO_2} by 0.04 for every liter of oxygen flow. Flow is typically set between 1 and 6 L/min. Flow above 6 L/min adds little to increased F_{IO_2} and may produce patient discomfort, including nasal dryness and bleeding. The cannula is generally considered comfortable and well tolerated by the patient.

Cannulae have been successfully used for infants by Vain and co-workers.[14] These investigators found that hypopharyngeal F_{IO_2} values while infants were breathing 0.25, 0.5, 0.75, and 1 L/min were 0.35, 0.45, 0.60, and 0.68, respectively. Oxygen delivered to a nasal cannula for an infant should be controlled by a pressure-compensated, Thorpe tube flowmeter calibrated from 1 to 3 L/min in 0.25-L increments. The maximum flow to a nasal cannula used with an infant should be 2 L/min.

Cannula Modifications

The popularity of nasal cannulae for long-term oxygen therapy has led to discovery of certain device limitations. First among these is the fact that patient ventilation is rhythmic while cannula flow is constant. This means that during expiration, which is commonly three to five times longer than inspiration, oxygen flow is "wasted" to the room. In an attempt to eliminate this "waste" and reduce the cost of oxygen delivery, several devices have been developed. These devices are often called oxygen-conserving devices.

Reservoir Cannula

DESCRIPTION. Two types of reservoir cannulae are available. The first is the moustache-style cannula (Fig. 3-17). The reservoir cannula contains a soft, inflatable reservoir with a volume of approximately 20 mL (Fig. 3-18). During patient exhalation, oxygen flow fills the expandable reservoir. During early inspiration, the patient inspires from the reservoir (causing

TABLE 3-2. Oxygen Concentrations Delivered by the Nasal Cannula

		F_{IO_2}		
Flow (L/min)	**Theoretical**	Gibson et al.[6]	Schacter et al.[12]	Ooi et al.[13]
1	0.24	0.22	0.23	0.25–0.38
2	0.28	0.21–0.22	0.24	0.29–0.52
3	0.32	0.224–0.236	0.25	0.33–0.61
4	0.36	—	0.26	0.38–0.70
5	0.40	0.238–0.254	—	—
6	0.44	—	—	0.44–0.83
8	—	—	—	0.50–0.90
10	—	0.301–0.462	—	—
15	—	0.362–0.609	—	—

the reservoir to begin to empty) and from the continuous flow. The addition of this small volume of oxygen increases the delivered F_{IO_2} by delivering a bolus of oxygen during early inspiration when patient demand is greatest. Once the reservoir is depleted, the continuous flow operates like a conventional nasal cannula.

PLACEMENT. The reservoir cannula rests directly beneath the nose and is secured by adjusting the lariat-style tubing below the chin.

PROBLEMS. Reservoir cannulae suffer all of the drawbacks seen with conventional cannulae. The major difference between the devices are patient comfort and patient acceptance of appearance. The moustache-style cannula is larger, heavier, and more obvious than the traditional cannula. Patients may decline to use the device because of its obtrusive appearance.

PERFORMANCE. Because the reservoir cannula provides more oxygen during the beginning of inspiration, it can achieve oxygenation equivalent to a conventional nasal cannula, but at a lower flow.[15–20] Several investigations have demonstrated that, compared with a conventional cannula, the reservoir cannula produces equivalent oxygen saturation at the continuous flow setting. In general, the lower the required continuous flow, the greater the savings.

Pendant Reservoir Cannula

DESCRIPTION. The pendant reservoir cannula (Fig. 3-19) uses a reservoir that is worn on the chest like a pendant. The portion of the cannula attached beneath the patient's nose appears identical to the conventional nasal cannula except that the cannula and connecting tubing are larger in diameter. During expiration, some of the patient's expired gas enters the cannula tubing (Fig. 3-20*A*). The pendant contains an

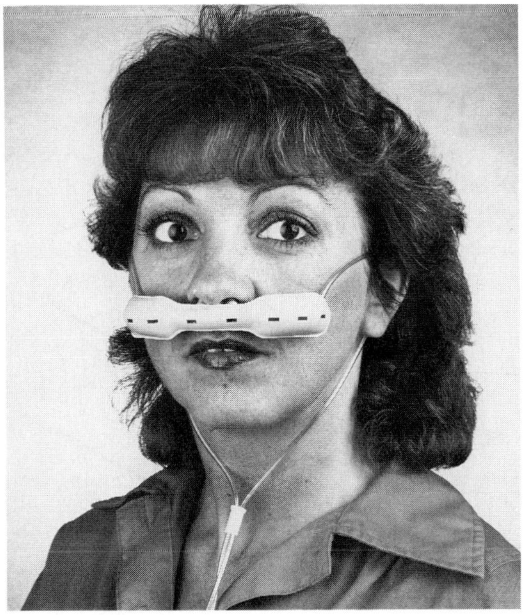

Figure 3-17. Moustache-style reservoir cannula. (Courtesy of Chad Therapeutics, Chatsworth, CA)

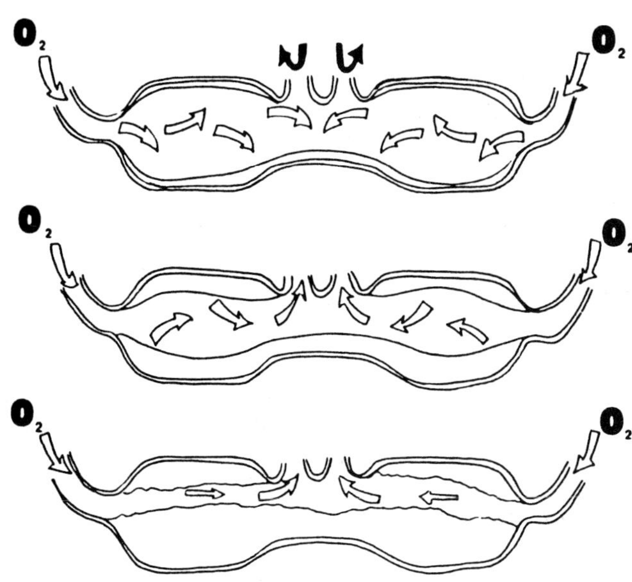

Figure 3-18. Function of the reservoir cannula.

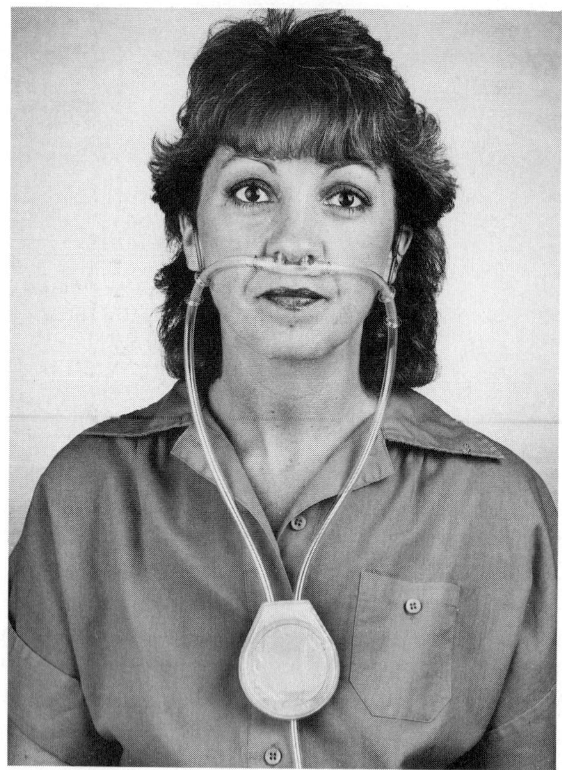

Figure 3-19. Pendant reservoir cannula. (Courtesy of Chad Therapeutics, Chatsworth, CA)

inflatable reservoir with a volume of approximately 40 mL. As oxygen flow opposes patient expiration, the reservoir expands and forces gas up the cannula tubing. This tubing contains a volume of oxygen nearly equivalent to that of the reservoir cannula (20 mL). During early inspiration (see Fig. 3-20*B*) the gas stored in the tubing acts as a reservoir of oxygen. As inspiration continues, the pendant reservoir is depleted (see Fig. 3-20*B*) and the cannula begins to function like a conventional cannula. The volume of gas in the reservoir is depleted relatively late in the inspiratory phase and does not appear to contribute significantly to improved oxygenation. The majority of the benefit appears to come from the oversized tubing between the patient and the pendant.[21–23]

Like the reservoir cannula, the reservoir pendant allows for equivalent oxygen saturation at lower oxygen flow rates. This decreases the cost of oxygen therapy and increases the duration of portable supplies.

PLACEMENT. The pendant reservoir attaches to the patient in a manner similar to the conventional cannula. Supporting the pendant or hiding it behind a scarf may aid in patient acceptance.

PROBLEMS. The pendant reservoir cannula is associated with the same problems seen with a traditional cannula. Tubing size makes the pendant cannula more obtrusive, but less so than the moustache-style cannula. Patients may still find the appearance of the pendant unattractive. The extra size and weight of the entire pendant device may increase the risk of pressure sores and skin irritation.

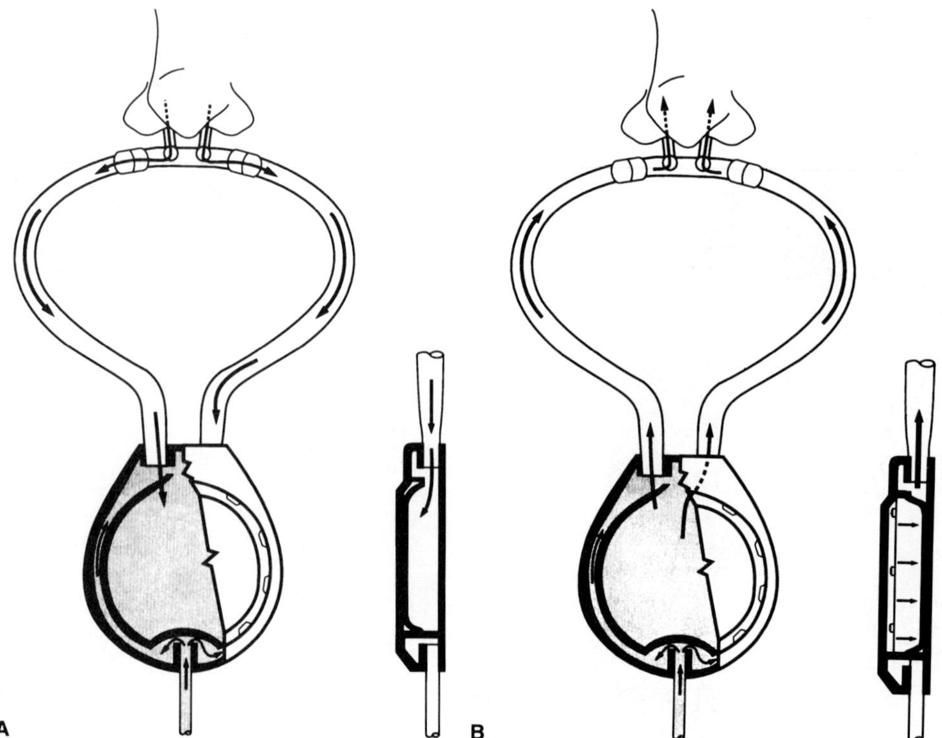

Figure 3-20. Function of the pendant reservoir cannula during expiration (A) and inspiration (B) in front and side views.

PERFORMANCE. Like the moustache-style cannula, the pendant reservoir cannula is capable of providing similar oxygenation at the flow used with a conventional cannula.[21–24] The reasons for improved oxygenation are equivalent to those of the moustache-style cannula.

Electronic Demand Pulsed-Dose Oxygen Delivery

DESCRIPTION. Electronic demand pulsed-dose oxygen therapy can be used in conjunction with a cannula, reservoir cannula, or transtracheal catheter. Pulsed-dose oxygen systems work by detecting patient effort and only providing gas during inspiration.[24–28]

Pulsed-dose oxygen devices take the place of a flowmeter during oxygen therapy (Fig. 3-21). This device allows the operator to select the gas flow and the mode of operation (most devices can provide continuous flow if desired). During expiration, the demand device is referenced to atmospheric pressure (Fig. 3-22A). When the patient initiates an inspiration, flow is drawn through the flow sensor. Once the flow sensor detects patient effort, the solenoid valve opens and provides a "pulsed dose" of oxygen at the selected flow setting (see Fig. 3-22B). Operation is typically controlled by a battery-operated fluidic valve.[24]

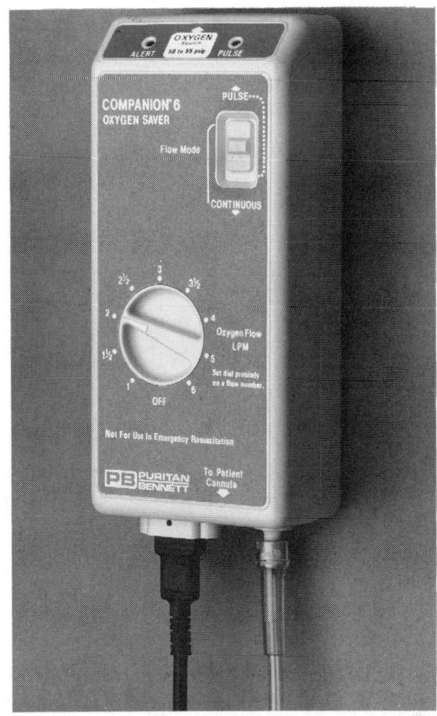

Figure 3-21. An electronic pulsed-demand oxygen delivery system. (Courtesy of Puritan-Bennett Corp, Kansas City, MO)

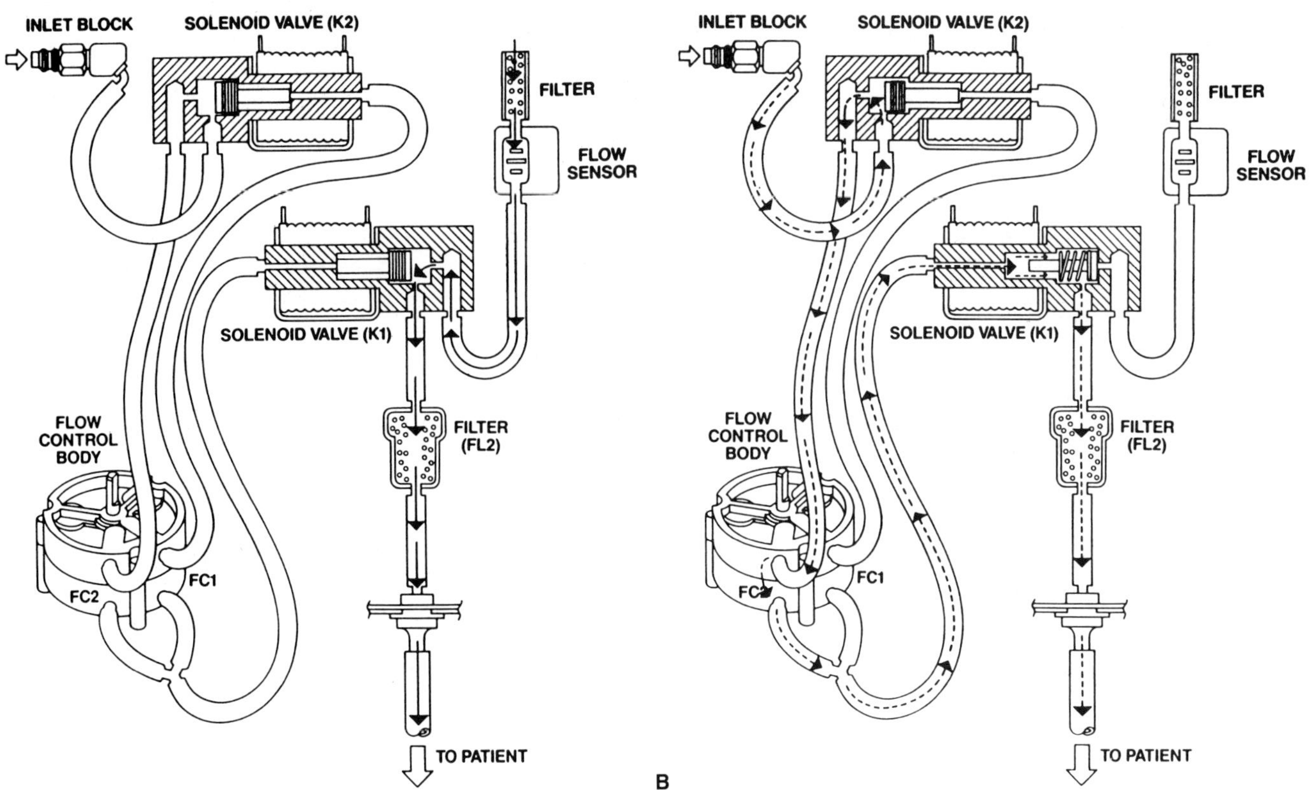

Figure 3-22. Electronic pulsed-demand oxygen system during expiration (A) and inspiration (B). (Courtesy of Puritan-Bennett Corp, Kansas City, MO)

PLACEMENT. Pulsed-dose devices are connected to 50-psig gas sources, including station outlets, cylinders, and liquid systems. The device takes the place of a standard flowmeter.

PROBLEMS. Technical problems with pulsed-dose oxygen therapy devices include disconnection, improper placement preventing sensing of patient effort, and device failure. Cost for the device is also a concern and must be balanced against the savings in oxygen. Many systems have alarms to alert the operator that sensing has not occurred over a pre-set time limit.

PERFORMANCE. Advantages of pulsed-dose oxygen systems include reduced oxygen use with subsequent decreased oxygen costs and longer life of portable sources. Equivalent oxygenation can also be accomplished at lower flow rates.[24–30]

Transtracheal Oxygen Catheters

DESCRIPTION. Transtracheal oxygen catheters deliver oxygen directly into the trachea through small-bore catheters (Fig. 3-23). Direct delivery into the trachea prevents dilution of oxygen with room air as seen with other appliances and fills the upper respiratory tract with oxygen.

PLACEMENT. The SCOOP catheter is the most popular transtracheal oxygen system and is used here for description of catheter placement. After preparing the patient, a small incision is made in the skin under sterile technique. This procedure is done in the hospital with the use of local anesthesia. A tracheal stent is advanced through the incision into the trachea. This stent remains in place for 1 week to facilitate tract formation. The inner lumen of the passageway begins to form a permanent communication between the trachea and the outer skin. This is known as the "tract." After the first week the stent is removed over a guide wire and a 9F (3.0 mm OD) catheter is inserted over the wire into the tract. The catheter is held in place with a neck chain attached to an external flange.

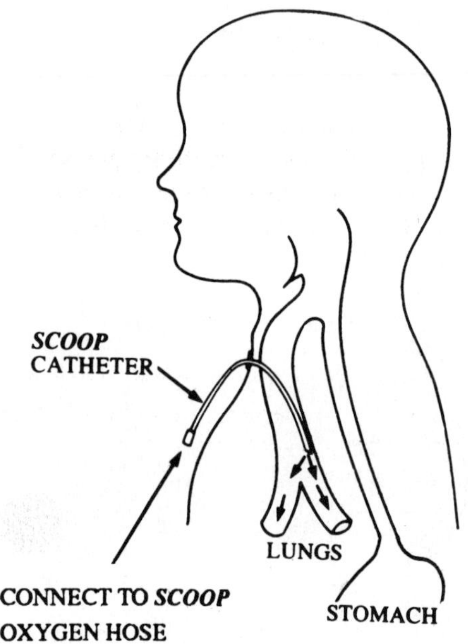

Figure 3-23. SCOOP catheter for transtracheal oxygen therapy. (Courtesy of Transtracheal Systems, Greenwood Village, CO)

PROBLEMS. Reports of subcutaneous emphysema, infection, hemoptysis, malposition, mucous obstruction, and shearing of the catheter have all appeared as complications of transtracheal oxygen therapy. The most common problem is mucous obstruction and creation of a "mucus ball" at the tip of the catheter. Care of the catheter, including instillation of saline and use of a cleaning rod to clear the catheter lumen, appears to prevent these problems.

PERFORMANCE. Transtracheal systems have been shown to increase oxygenation compared with conventional oxygen therapy with a nasal cannula at equivalent flow rates or provide equivalent oxygenation at lower flow rates.[31–36] Patient acceptance is also reported to be improved because of the relatively hidden appearance of the equipment. Reduced oxygen usage, reduced costs, and increased life of portable gas sources have all been reported with transtracheal oxygen therapy.[31–36] It has been estimated that a reduction in oxygen flow of 50% can be obtained with use of transtracheal oxygen therapy. Combining transtracheal delivery with demand pulsed-dose oxygen can further increase savings.

Masks

Simple Mask

DESCRIPTION. The simple mask is a disposable lightweight plastic that increases F_{IO_2} by increasing the available reservoir. With a cannula, the oxygen reservoir consists of the anatomic deadspace. The simple mask increases the size of the reservoir by adding the volume of the mask, covering the nose and mouth (Fig. 3-24). Oxygen is delivered to the simple mask through standard oxygen tubing at a flow rate of 5 to 12 L/min. The size of the mask varies among manufacturers. Because the flow generated will not meet patient demands, the mask allows room air to be drawn in around the mask edges and through side ports. A bubble humidifier is typically used with a simple mask.

PLACEMENT. Simple masks are held in place over the patient's nose and mouth with an adjustable elastic strap. The elastic band should be tightened so the mask stays in place despite patient movement. A tight seal is unnecessary. A thin, malleable metal strip is

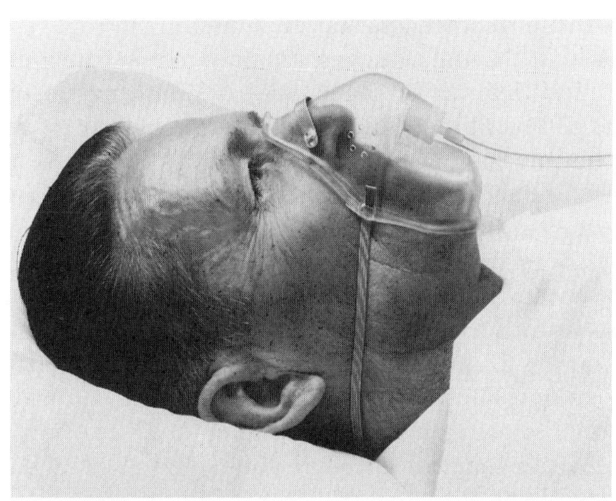

Figure 3-24. Simple mask applied to a patient. (Courtesy of Hudson-RCI, Temecula, CA)

often placed on the mask at the bridge of the nose to aid in securing the mask.

PROBLEMS. Patients wearing a mask may complain of claustrophobia, being hot, or pain at the site of mask application. Long-term use can result in development of skin irritation and pressure sores.

The mask muffles speech, which can be a problem for patients as well as caregivers. Eating and drinking are also difficult. Vomiting into the mask and aspiration is a potential problem.

PERFORMANCE. Simple masks are variable performance devices. The actual FIO_2 will vary with mask fit, flow, and patient respiratory pattern. The available FIO_2 is generally thought of as 0.30 to 0.60.[37] Like the nasal cannula, investigations into the operation of the simple mask have yielded a wide variety of results.

Gibson and colleagues[6] found that FIO_2 values of 0.82 to 0.88 were delivered at a flow of 15 L/min. Redding and associates[38] studied normal volunteers using a variety of oxygen delivery devices. This study deserves particular attention, if for no other reason, the method used to determine FIO_2. These researchers solicited five normal volunteers from their respiratory therapy department to participate in a study. Each had a radial arterial line placed to monitor PaO_2. Volunteers were then delivered oxygen at precise oxygen concentrations from a high-flow blender and tight-fitting mask. Arterial blood was drawn and PaO_2 was plotted against FIO_2 for each volunteer. Using regression analysis by the method of least squares, a fitted line was plotted. Samples for blood gas analysis were then drawn while volunteers breathed from five types of oxygen masks. These values were then used to determine FIO_2 by placement of data points on the fitted lines. Using this unique approach, Redding and associates[38] found that at a flow of 6 L/min, FIO_2 ranged from 0.38 to 0.46. No control or measurements of breathing depth or frequency were made. Bethune and Collis[39] studied the FIO_2 delivered by simple masks and were among the first to suggest that a minimum flow was necessary to prevent rebreathing of carbon dioxide (CO_2). They found that at flow rates of 1 to 8 L/min an FIO_2 of 0.21 to 0.60 was delivered at a tidal volume of 500 mL and an FIO_2 of 0.21 to 0.43 was delivered at a tidal volume of 1000 mL.[40]

Milross and associates[41] studied the Hudson Oxy-one face mask under laboratory conditions. They had a single, trained volunteer, placed in a body plethysmograph, breathe at tidal volumes of 0.3, 0.6, and 1.2 L. The volunteer breathed through the plethysmographic mouthpiece. On the opposite side of the mouthpiece, the face mask was fitted to a plaster of paris model of the volunteer's face. Oxygen concentration was measured between the mask and the volunteer. At a constant frequency of 15 breaths per minute, tidal volume was varied as described and the mask was placed "tightly" or "loosely" on the face. Table 3-3 depicts the study's results. Milross and associates[41] concluded that delivered FIO_2 with a simple mask is reliable and predictable as long as the mask is fitted properly to the face. However, they point out that position of the mask is difficult to control and changes in the inspiratory to expiratory ratio may alter their results.

It is generally stated that a minimum flow of 5 L/min is necessary to prevent rebreathing of CO_2. This has been confirmed by Jensen and co-workers.[42] By studying normal volunteers, they found that at flow rates of less than 5 L/min, minute ventilation increased to maintain a constant $PaCO_2$. Simple masks are typically used for short periods of time in the recovery room or the emergency department when a nasal cannula is insufficient.

Partial Rebreathing Reservoir Mask

DESCRIPTION. Partial rebreathing reservoir masks are simple masks with the addition of a 600- to 800-mL reservoir below the patient's chin (Fig. 3-25). The

TABLE 3-3. FIO_2 Delivered at Flows of 2 to 8 L/min

	Minute Ventilation (L/min)					
	Loose Fitting			Tight Fitting		
Flow (L/min)	5	12	20	5	12	20
2	0.36	0.31	0.28	0.47	0.31	0.27
4	0.46	0.37	0.33	0.60	0.41	0.33
6	0.47	0.40	0.35	0.72	0.50	0.40
8	0.46	0.42	0.38	0.77	0.59	0.46

From Milross J, Young IH, Donnelly P. The oxygen delivery characteristics of the Hudson Oxy-one face mask. Anaesth Intens Care 1989;17:180–184.

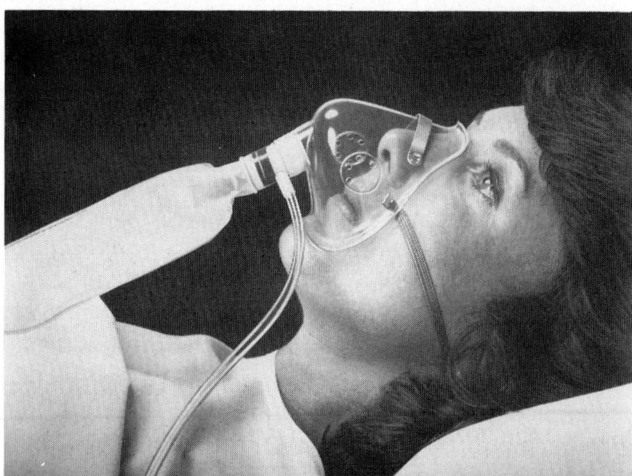

Figure 3-25. Partial rebreathing reservoir mask applied to a patient. (Courtesy of Hudson-RCI, Temecula, CA)

reservoir further extends that provided by the anatomic space and mask volume. Oxygen flow is provided from a bubble humidifier at a flow that keeps the reservoir bag at least half full during inspiration (usually 8 to 15 L/min). The oxygen is attached between the mask and the reservoir. The term partial rebreathing refers to the fact that the first one third of expired gas enters the reservoir bag. This is gas from the anatomic reservoir so it is high in oxygen and contains little CO_2. As the bag fills from the oxygen flow and first third of expiration, the remaining expired gas exits the exhalation ports of the mask.

PLACEMENT. The partial rebreathing mask is fitted in the same fashion as a simple mask. Care should be taken to not restrict filling and emptying of the reservoir.

PROBLEMS. The only new problem presented by the partial rebreathing mask is the need to adjust flow as patient demand changes. A quietly breathing patient receiving 10 L/min may deflate the reservoir during a period of anxiety. In these instances, flow must be adjusted accordingly.

PERFORMANCE. Although some authors might consider the partial rebreathing mask a fixed performance device, the ability to entrain room air around mask edges and through side ports clearly makes it a variable performance piece of equipment. At flow rates of 6 to 10 L/min the partial rebreathing mask is generally thought to deliver an F_{IO_2} from 0.40 to 0.70.[37]

Few studies have measured F_{IO_2} delivered with the partial rebreathing mask. Kory and colleagues[7] found that at flow rates of 6 to 10 L/min the partial rebreathing mask delivered F_{IO_2} values from 0.35 to 0.60. As with any low-flow system, delivered F_{IO_2} can be expected to change as ventilatory pattern and oxygen flow are altered.

Non-Rebreathing Reservoir Mask

DESCRIPTION. The non-rebreathing reservoir mask is a modification of the partial rebreathing design (Fig. 3-26). At first glance, the differences may be imperceptible. The non-rebreathing mask incorporates one-way valves over one of the mask side ports and above the reservoir bag (Fig. 3-27). The one-way valve over the reservoir bag prevents expired gas from entering. The one-way valve over the side port limits entrainment of room air. In the past, as shown in Figure 3-27, both sideports were covered with one-way valves. Recently manufactured devices typically use only one, to allow room air to enter more easily if gas flow is inadvertently disconnected. Masks that use two one-way valves have a safety valve to allow ambient air to enter the mask in the event gas flow is interrupted.

PLACEMENT AND PROBLEMS. Placement is the same for the non-rebreathing mask as it is for the partial rebreathing mask. Additional problems are associated with the one-way valves. The combined effects of time and moisture can cause one-way valves to stick in an open or closed position.

PERFORMANCE. Oxygen flow should be set such that the reservoir bag does not collapse during inspiration. This typically requires a minimum flow of 10 L/min and often flow rates of more than 15 L/min are necessary. It is generally accepted that F_{IO_2} delivered with a non-rebreathing mask is 0.60 to 0.80.[37]

Redding and co-workers[38] found an F_{IO_2} of 0.57 to 0.70 was delivered when oxygen flow was set greater than patient minute ventilation. Previous reports describing F_{IO_2} values near 1.0 using a non-rebreathing mask should be viewed with caution.[43] They frequently refer to the Boothby-Lovelace-Bulbulian (BLB) masks, which were tight-fitting, nondisposable masks with spring-loaded expiratory valves that completely prevented entrainment of room air. Today's disposable devices cannot achieve similar results. Non-

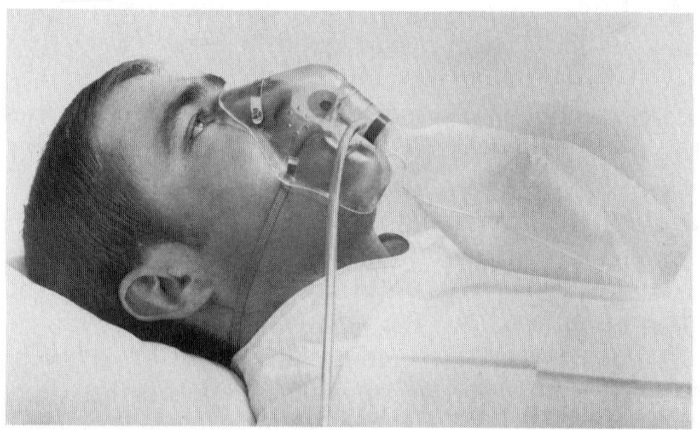

Figure 3-26. Non-rebreathing reservoir mask applied to a patient. (Courtesy of Hudson-RCI, Temecula, CA)

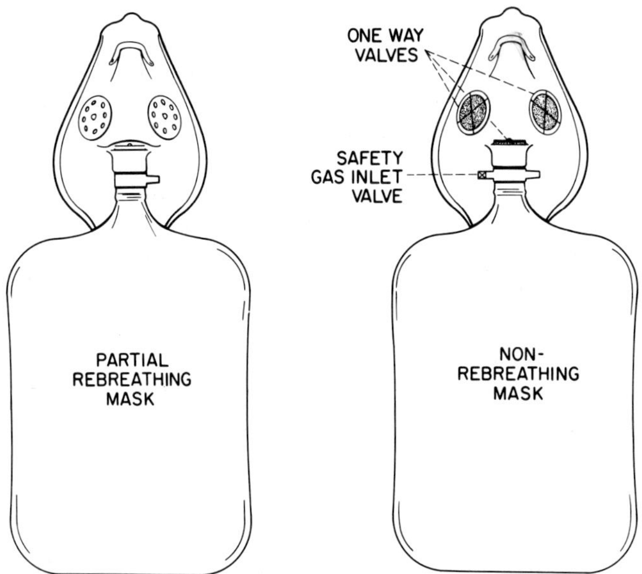

Figure 3-27. Partial rebreathing and non-rebreathing mask showing placement of one-way valves. (From Kacmarek RM. Methods of oxygen delivery in the hospital. Probl Respir Care 1990;3:563–574)

rebreathing masks should be reserved for short-term use when the highest possible FIO_2 is desired.

Fixed Performance Devices

Air-Entrainment Masks

DESCRIPTION. Frequently mislabeled as "Venturi masks" owing to mistaken operating principles, air-entrainment masks are the most frequently studied oxygen therapy devices.[44–58] Campbell[50] developed the original air-entrainment mask in 1960. His system was large and bulky and included a series of small exhaust holes in the mask. Commercially available designs are based on Campbell's original description.

An air-entrainment mask consists of the mask, a jet nozzle, and entrainment ports (Fig. 3-28). Oxygen under pressure is delivered through the jet nozzle just below the mask. As gas travels through the jet nozzle, its velocity increases dramatically. On exiting the nozzle, the gas at high velocity entrains or drags ambient air into the mask. This is not due to the Bernoulli or Venturi principle but to viscous shearing forces between the gas traveling through the nozzle and the stagnant ambient air.[45] The delivered FIO_2 is dependent on the size of the nozzle, size of the entrainment ports, and oxygen flow. Commercially available systems use either interchangeable jet sizes, adjustable entrainment ports, or a combination of the two (Fig. 3-29). Typically, an air-entrainment mask has six to eight FIO_2 settings as well as minimum suggested oxygen flow rates for each setting (Table 3-4).

Bubble humidifiers provide very little additional humidification when used with air-entrainment masks and often result in the pressure release valve being activated. This is due to the comparatively small oxygen flow versus entrained flow. Alternatively, humidity can be increased by using aerosol collars that surround the entrainment ports. The dry oxygen then entrains air from an aerosol system, increasing humidity delivered to the patient. Because the addition of aerosol particles to room air increases gas density, entrained volume falls, and delivered FIO_2 increases slightly.

PLACEMENT. The air-entrainment mask is secured to the patient using an adjustable, elastic band.

PROBLEMS. The only additional problem associated with the air-entrainment mask is obstruction of the en-

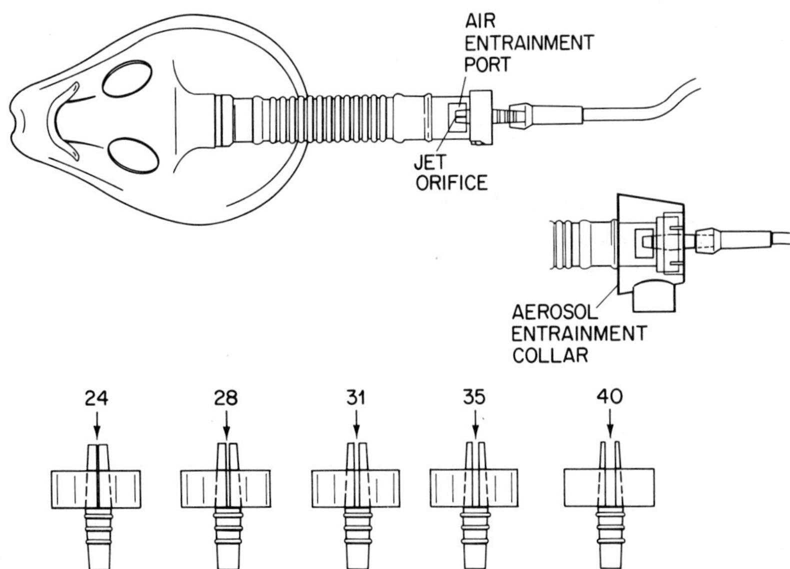

Figure 3-28. An air-entrainment mask that uses interchangeable jet orifices to change FIO_2. (From Kacmarek RM. Methods of oxygen delivery in the hospital. Probl Respir Care 1990;3:563–574)

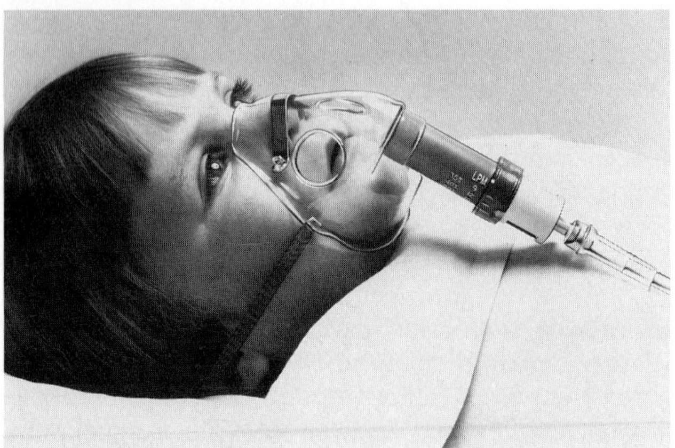

Figure 3-29. Air-entrainment mask with an adjustable entrainment orifice and fixed jet orifice. (Courtesy of Hudson-RCI, Temecula, CA)

TABLE 3-4. Set F_{IO_2}, Minimum Flow Requirements, Outputs, and Entrainment Ratios for an Air-Entrainment Mask

F_{IO_2} Setting	Minimum Oxygen Flow (L/min)	Entrainment Ratio O_2:Air	Total Flow (L/min)
0.24	4	1:25	104
0.28	4	1:10	44
0.31	6	1:7	48
0.35	8	1:5	48
0.40	8	1:3	32
0.50	12	1:1.7	32
0.60	12	1:1	24
0.70	12	1:0.6	19

trainment port by sheets, gowns, and other materials. Obstruction of this port decreases total flow dramatically and increases F_{IO_2}.

PERFORMANCE. At F_{IO_2} values less than 0.35 the air-entrainment mask can function as a fixed performance system because total flow is sufficient. However, at F_{IO_2} greater than 0.35 the total flow falls below 40 L/min, causing the air-entrainment mask to be considered a variable performance device.

The accuracy of air-entrainment masks has been studied by numerous investigators. Campbell and Minty[49] have criticized commercially available air-entrainment masks because the mask volume is insufficient. They point out that as patient demand for flow increases, room air may be drawn in around the mask. In this instance, masks with larger volumes act as reservoirs for blended gas, keeping F_{IO_2} constant. Cohen and associates[48] monitored F_{IO_2} inside the mask of four air-entrainment masks in a laboratory study. They found a small but measurable difference between set and delivered F_{IO_2}. These differences were exaggerated by rainout from an aerosol entrainment system.

Woolner and Larkin[56] studied the Hudson Multivent mask in the laboratory to determine its ability to deliver a precise F_{IO_2}. Using a model face connected to a pneumotachograph and mouthpiece they measured F_{IO_2} during quiet breathing and with varying peak inspiratory flow. They found that a group of five masks delivered accurate F_{IO_2} values at the 0.24, 0.26, and 0.28 settings. At the 0.30 setting and above, F_{IO_2} accuracy diminished. As oxygen flow was increased, the F_{IO_2} accuracy at the 0.30 and 0.35 setting improved, but at the 0.50 setting delivered F_{IO_2} only averaged 0.39. Woolner and Larkin also demonstrated that as peak inspiratory flow increased to 200 L/min, F_{IO_2} fell dramatically. They concluded that for accurate F_{IO_2} delivery, total gas flow must be 30% greater than peak inspiratory flow at settings less than 0.30. Above the 0.30 setting, Woolner and Larkin concluded the air-entrainment mask is a variable performance device.

Fracchia and Torda[57] studied five different air-entrainment masks and found that those with larger volume masks and extension tubes between the jet and mask provided more reliable and consistent F_{IO_2} values. Cox and Gillbe[55] investigated the ability of five air-entrainment masks to provide reliable F_{IO_2} values under laboratory conditions. They calculated the mean difference in delivered F_{IO_2} from set F_{IO_2} at tidal volumes of 0.25 L, 0.5 L, and 0.75 L. In agreement with other investigators, they found large-volume masks provided more precise F_{IO_2} delivery. They also suggested the aviation-style masks typically used are disadvantageous owing to the delivery of gas at a right angle to the face. The original design by Campbell delivered gas directly at the face. Cox and Gillbe concluded that for air-entrainment masks to deliver precise F_{IO_2} values, mask volume must be a minimum of 300 mL.

Hill and associates[54] found mask volume was only important if patient demand exceeded total flow. They suggested low-volume masks with high flow rates were preferable to high-volume masks with lower flow rates. Lyew and colleagues[47] have modified air-entrainment masks to entrain additional oxygen so that any number of F_{IO_2} values may be obtained. The clinical usefulness of this concept has not yet been tested.

Air-entrainment masks are ideally suited for providing precise F_{IO_2} delivery to patients requiring less than 0.35 oxygen. Patients with chronic lung disease who may hypoventilate when exposed to high F_{IO_2} values are also candidates for air-entrainment mask use. The air-entrainment mask is intended for patients with high or changing ventilatory demands. Its use

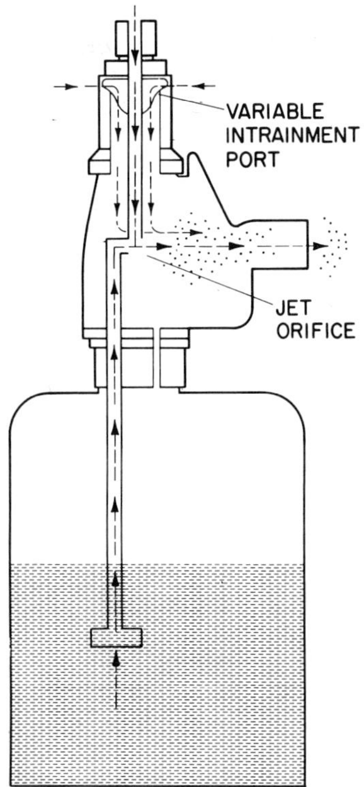

Figure 3-30. Large volume aerosol system with variable entrainment port to adjust F_{IO_2}. (From Kacmarek RM. Methods of oxygen delivery in the hospital. Probl Respir Care 1990;3:563–574)

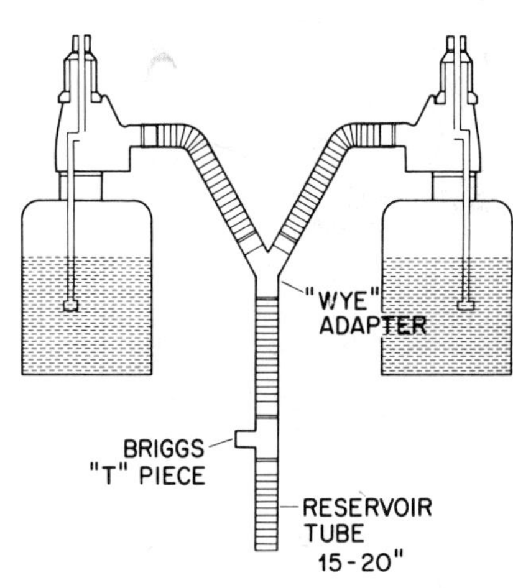

should be limited to these instances due to its high cost compared with variable performance equipment.

Large-Volume Aerosol and Humidifier Systems

DESCRIPTION. Large-volume aerosol systems use air-entrainment nebulizers alone or in tandem (Fig. 3-30) to provide gas to face masks, face tents, T-pieces, tracheostomy collars, and head hoods (Fig. 3-31). Nondisposable aerosol systems usually offer F_{IO_2} values of 0.40, 0.60, and 1.0, while disposable systems offer a continuous adjustment with six to eight settings calibrated from 0.28 to 1.0. These systems use a constant jet nozzle size with a variable size entrainment port to change F_{IO_2}.

PLACEMENT. Placement varies with the device used. Most systems use an elastic band (Figs. 3-32 and 3-33). The T-piece connects directly to the artificial airway.

PROBLEMS. The most common problem with the system is inadequate flow. The respiratory care practitioner should observe the patient to ascertain that flow is sufficient. If mist from the aerosol escapes the oxygen delivery device during inspiration, flow is generally considered sufficient.

Water collecting in the delivery tubing can increase back-pressure and prevent air entrainment. Condensation in the tubing increases delivered F_{IO_2} and should be removed as needed.

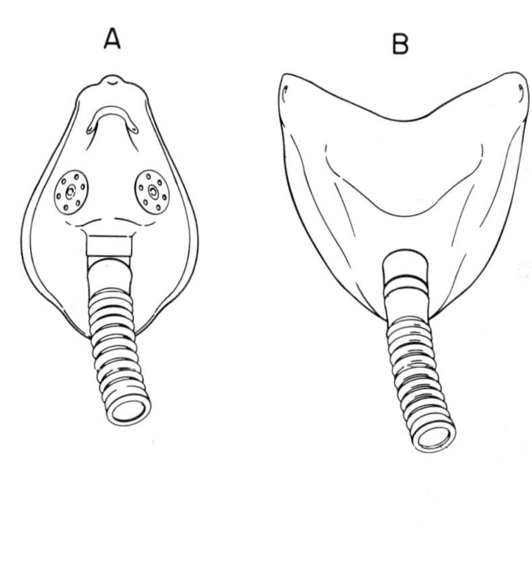

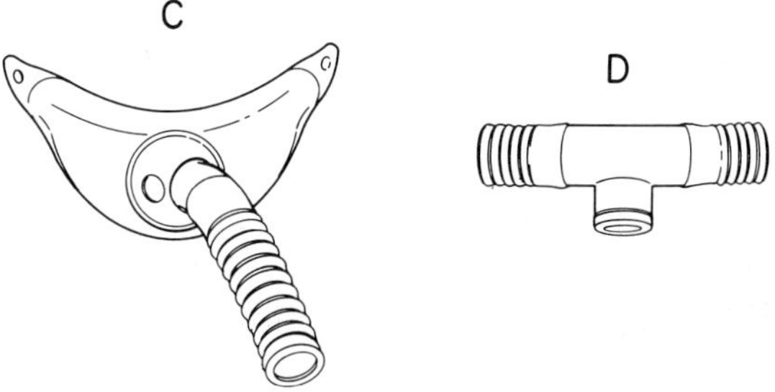

Figure 3-31. (A.) Aerosol mask. (B.) Face tent. (C.) Tracheostomy collar. (D.) T-piece. All are used to deliver oxygen from a large-volume aerosol system. (From Kacmarek RM. Methods of oxygen delivery in the hospital. Probl Respir Care 1990;3:563–574)

PERFORMANCE. Foust and co-workers[59] studied jet nebulizers in tandem with an aerosol face mask under laboratory conditions. Using tidal volumes from 0.2 to 0.9 L and frequencies from 20 to 40 breaths per minute, they measured FIO_2 delivered to a lung model from tandem aerosols set at FIO_2 values of 0.60, 0.80, and 1.0. Essentially their results demonstrated that under conditions of high ventilatory demand, these systems become variable performance devices. This is particularly evident when data from the 0.80 and 1.0 setting are compared. Despite the increase in set FIO_2 values, delivered FIO_2 falls. This is due to the overall decrease in delivered flow resulting in entrainment of room air around the mask. These investigators recommended that when precise FIO_2 values are necessary, a high-flow humidifier system is preferred.

Kuo and colleagues[60] compared large-volume aerosol systems to humidifier systems in 30 patients receiving oxygen therapy. They found that at similar FIO_2 values, PaO_2 fell when patients were on aerosol therapy. This was attributed to the adverse effects of aerosol therapy on lung function. However, these researchers did not measure delivered FIO_2 and therefore may have overlooked the findings of Foust and co-workers.[59] It is doubtful the changes in PaO_2 in this study were due to aerosol deposition. Rather, it is likely that delivered FIO_2 was less with the air-entrainment nebulizer than the large-volume humidification system.

Large-volume humidifier systems are the preferred method of delivering precise FIO_2 values at high flow rates. Figure 3-34 depicts the system described by Foust and co-workers.[59] Gas can originate from a blender, air–oxygen flowmeter, or a venturi system, such as the Downs flow generator. All these devices are capable of delivering gas in excess of 100 L/min. Gas is then directed through a heated humidifier, such as those used for mechanical ventilation. Standard 22 mm ID tubing connects the humidifier to the aerosol mask. A reservoir is often placed in line. The system depicted in Figure 3-34 was capable of delivering an FIO_2 of 100% under all laboratory conditions studied by Foust and co-workers.[59]

Oxygen Hoods and Tents

Oxygen hoods are used to deliver oxygen to infants who are too small to use a mask. Hoods allow care to be delivered without removing the infant from oxygen and allow the infant greater comfort. Hoods typically receive oxygen from a blender or high-flow humidification system. Flow is set at 10 to 15 L/min to provide a constant flow through the hood, maintain a constant FIO_2, and wash out CO_2.

Tents use a frame and large, soft plastic material to enclose the patient. Tents receive oxygen from a high-flow aerosol system and are almost exclusively used in pediatrics. Control of FIO_2 in a tent is difficult owing to the large volume and frequent opening of the enclosure.

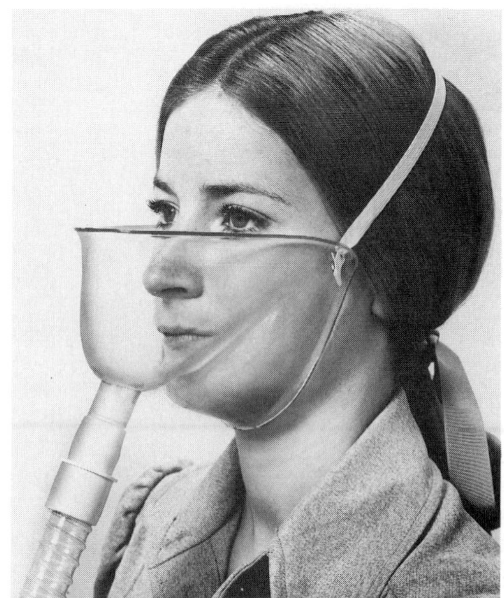

Figure 3-32. Oxygen delivered by face tent. (Courtesy of Hudson-RCI, Temecula, CA)

Mixing Air and Oxygen

Air and Oxygen Flowmeters

Two flowmeters, one air and one oxygen, can be used to deliver precise oxygen concentrations. Gas should be humidified before being delivered to the patient but can be delivered through any of the masks previously described or a head hood. Calculating FIO_2 from known flow rates of air and oxygen is fairly easy, remembering that air is 0.21 oxygen. See Equation Box 3-4.

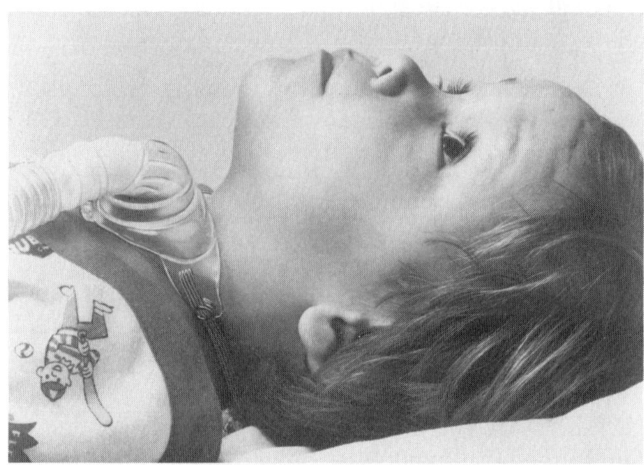

Figure 3-33. Oxygen delivered by tracheostomy collar. (Courtesy of Hudson-RCI, Temecula, CA)

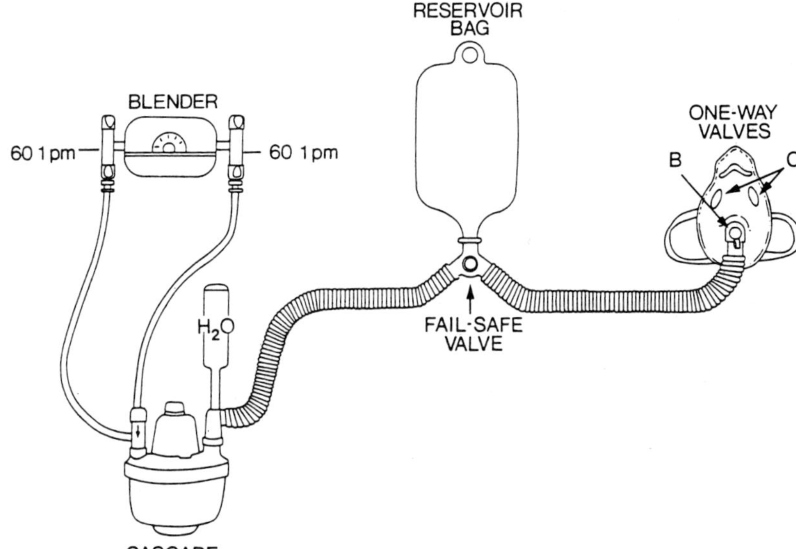

Figure 3-34. High-flow humidification system for delivering precise FIO_2 values. (From Foust GN, Potter WH, Wilson MD, Golden EB. Shortcomings of using two jet nebulizers in tandem with an aerosol face mask for optimal oxygen therapy. Chest 1991;99:1346–1351)

Air–Oxygen Blenders

Air–oxygen blenders (Fig. 3-35) use 50-psig sources of air and oxygen to deliver precise FIO_2 values. Blenders are compact and convenient but expensive compared with using two flowmeters.

Blenders have three sections where distinct functions are performed. These are the alarm module, pressure-balancing module, and proportioning module.

Air and oxygen enter the alarm module (Fig. 3-36) at 50-psig from cylinders or station outlets. Because a blender operates pneumatically, the two inlet pressures must be within 10 psig of each other. If the pressure difference is greater than 10 psig, accuracy of FIO_2 will be compromised.

Gas passes into the alarm module where the gas pressures are set in opposition. If one pressure is 10 psig greater than the other, gas escapes through the central channel and travels through the alarm reed. Gas escaping the small hole covered with the reed creates a high-pitched alarm, warning the operator. The alarm module also contains check valves to prevent cross-contamination of gases. Instances have been reported in which a blending system not in use was connected to a gas piping system and air flowed into the oxygen line through a faulty check valve.[61,62]

From the alarm module, gas travels to the pressure-balancing module (Fig. 3-37). The pressure-balancing module uses one or two diaphragms on a spool to balance the air and oxygen pressures. If air pressure is greater than oxygen pressure, the diaphragm moves toward the lower oxygen pressure.

Equation Box 3-4: Technique for Mixing Air and Oxygen

$$FIO_2\text{ (total flow)} = O_2\text{ flow} + \text{air flow } (0.21)$$

Example: At an oxygen flow of 20 L/min and an air flow of 40 L/min, what is the total flow and FIO_2?

$$FIO_2\text{(total flow)} = 20\text{ L/min} + 40\text{ L/min } (0.21)$$

$$FIO_2(20\text{ L/min} + 40\text{ L/min}) = 20\text{ L/min} + 8.4\text{ L/min}$$

$$FIO_2(60\text{ L/min}) = 26.4\text{ L/min}$$

$$FIO_2 = \frac{26.4\text{ L/min}}{60\text{ L/min}}$$

$$FIO_2 = 0.47$$

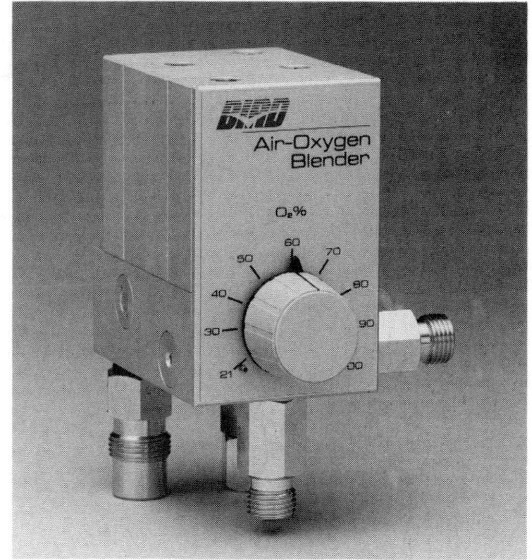

Figure 3-35. Bird air–oxygen blender. (Courtesy of Bird Products Corp, Palm Springs, CA)

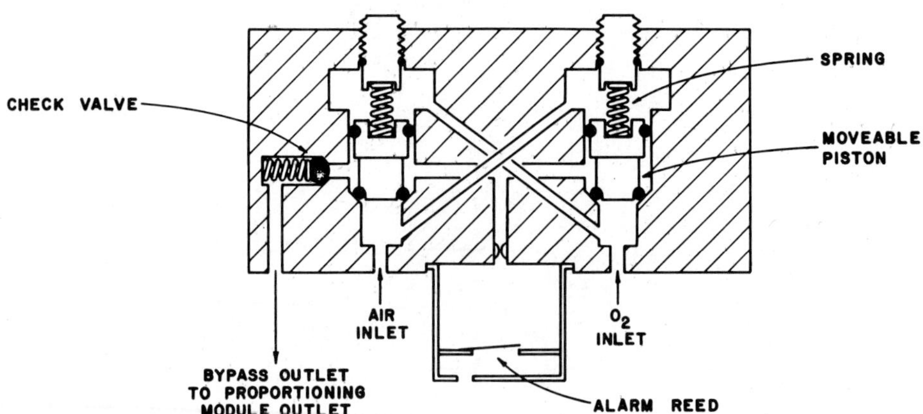

Figure 3-36. Alarm module from a Sechrist blender. (Courtesy of Sechrist Industries, Anaheim, CA)

This module allows pressures to be reduced and closely matched.

Gas then travels to the proportioning module (Fig. 3-38), where air and oxygen at equivalent pressures are metered in proportion to the desired F_{IO_2}. Clockwise movement of the control knob decreases F_{IO_2} by increasing the area for gas from the air source to flow to the outlet. Counterclockwise movement increases F_{IO_2} by allowing greater oxygen flow and less air flow. All these components working in unison are shown in Figure 3-39.

Evaluations of blenders demonstrate that accuracy is improved when inlet pressures are matched.[63,64] Problems with blenders are usually caused by contamination from gas sources. Particulate matter, water, and subsequent corrosion can prevent check valves from seating and diaphragms from moving properly. Filters at gas inlets can help alleviate these problems.

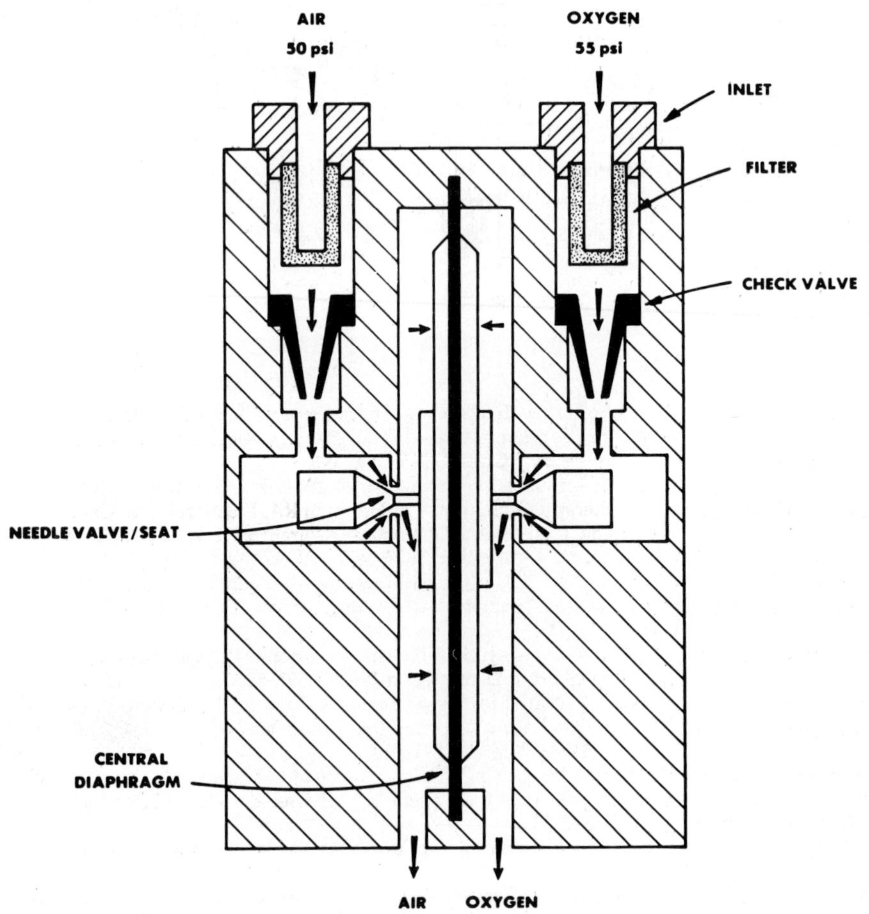

Figure 3-37. Pressure-balancing module from a Sechrist blender. (Courtesy of Sechrist Industries, Anaheim, CA)

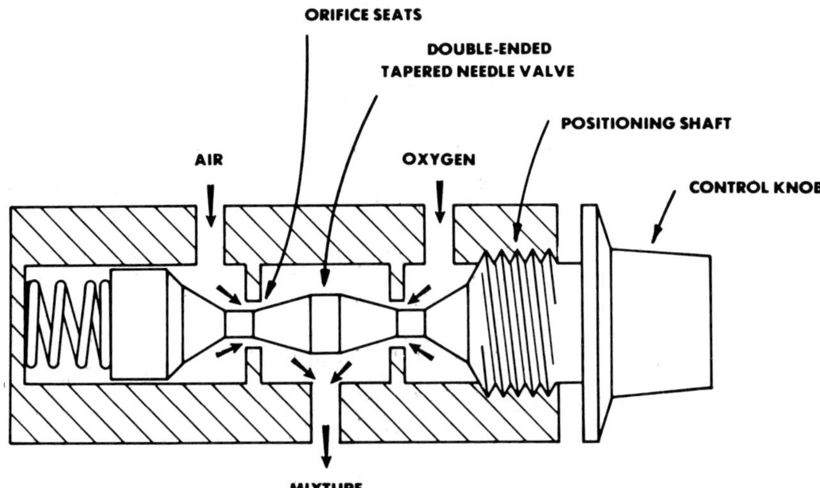

Figure 3-38. Proportional module from a Sechrist blender. (Courtesy of Sechrist Industries, Anaheim, CA)

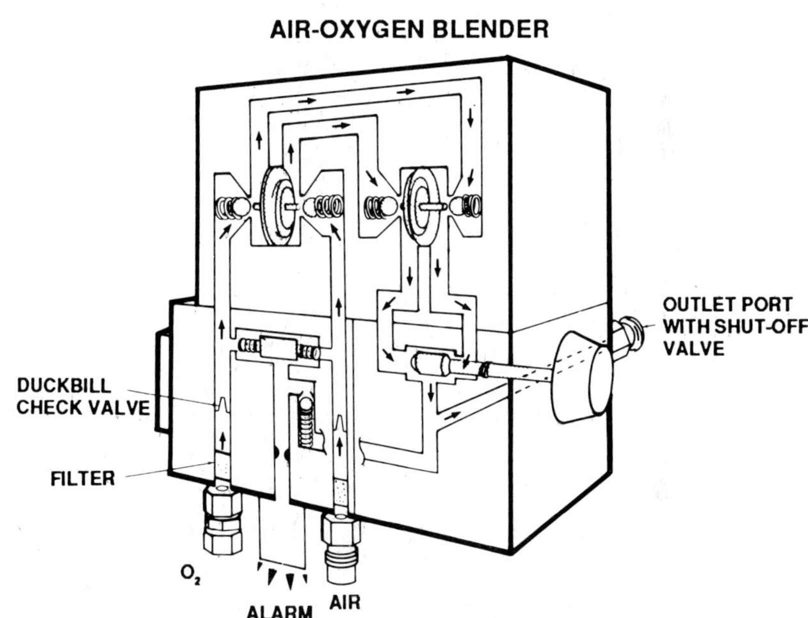

Figure 3-39. A Bird blender showing all modules working in unison. (Courtesy of Bird Products Corp, Palm Springs, CA)

References

1. Klein BR. Health Care Facilities Handbook, 4th ed. Quincy, MA: National Fire Protection Agency, 1993.
2. Duffin J. Physics for anaesthetists. Springfield, IL: Charles C Thomas, 1976.
3. Severinghaus JW, Astrup PB. History of blood gas analysis: IV. Leland Clark's oxygen electrode. J Clin Monit 1986;2:125–139.
4. Leigh JM. The evaluation of oxygen therapy apparatus. Anaesthesia 1974;29:462–485.
5. Guilfoile T, Dabe K. Nasal catheter oxygen therapy for infants. Respir Care 1981;26:35–39.
6. Gibson RL, Comer PB, Beckham RW, McGraw CP. Actual tracheal oxygen concentrations with commonly used oxygen equipment. Anesthesiology 1976;44:71–73.
7. Kory RC, Bergman JC, Sweet RD, Smith JR. Comparative evaluation of oxygen therapy techniques. JAMA 1962;179:123–128.
8. American Association for Respiratory Care. Clinical Practice Guideline: Oxygen therapy in the acute care hospital. Respir Care 1991;36:1410–1411.
9. Estey W. Subjective effects of dry versus humidified low flow oxygen. Respir Care 1980;25:1143–1144.
10. Campbell EJ, Baker D, Crites-Silver P. Subjective effects of humidification of oxygen for delivery by nasal cannula: A prospective study. Chest 1988;93:289–293.
11. Shapiro BA, Harrison RA, Kacmarek RM, Cane RD. Oxygen therapy. In: Shapiro BA, Harrison RA, Kacmarek RM, Cane RD, eds. Clinical Application of Respiratory Care, 3rd ed. Chicago: Year Book Medical Publishers, 1985;176–191.
12. Schacter EN, Littner MR, Luddy P, et al. Monitoring of oxygen delivery systems in clinical practice. Crit Care Med 1980;8:405–409.
13. Ooi R, Joshi P, Soni N. An evaluation of oxygen delivery using nasal prongs. Anesthesia 1992;47:591–593.
14. Vain NE, Prudent LM, Stevens DP, et al. Regulation of oxygen concentration delivered to infants by nasal cannulas. Am J Dis Child 1989;143:1458–1465.
15. Tiep BL, Lewis ML. Oxygen conservation and oxygen-conserving devices in chronic lung disease: A review. Chest 1987;92:-263–273.
16. Tiep BL. New portable oxygen devices. Respir Care 1987;32:106–112.
17. Tiep BL, Nicotra B, Carter T, et al. Evaluation of a low flow oxygen conserving cannula. Am Rev Respir Dis 1984;130:500–502.

18. Moore-Gillon JC, Geddes DM. An oxygen conserving nasal cannula. Thorax 1985;40:817–819.
19. Hussey JD, Massey LA, Lakshminarayan S. Evaluation of the effect of a reservoir cannula on oxygen saturation during rest and exercise in patients with COPD. Respir Care 1985;30:885.
20. Soffer M, Tashkin DP, Shapiro BJ, et al. Conservation of oxygen supply using a reservoir nasal cannula in hypoxemic patients at rest and during exercise. Chest 1985;88:663–668.
21. Evans TW, Waterhouse JC, Suggett AJ, et al. A conservation device for oxygen therapy in COPD. Eur J Respir Dis 1988;1:959–960.
22. Collard P, Wautalet F, Delwiche JP. Improvement of oxygen delivery in severe hypoxaemia by a reservoir cannula. Eur J Respir Dis 1989;2:778–781.
23. Tiep BL, Burns M, Herrera J. A new pendent oxygen-conserving cannula which allows pursed lips breathing. Chest 1989;95: 857–860.
24. Shiyeoka JW. Bonekat WH. The current status of oxygen conserving devices. Respir Care 1985;30:833-836.
25. Franco MA, Conner SA, Gougenheim C. Pulse dose oxygen delivery system. Respir Care 1985;30:888–889.
26. McDonnell TJ, Wanger JS, Senn S, et al. Efficacy of pulsed oxygen delivery during exercise. Respir Care 1986;31:883–888.
27. Bower JS, Brook CJ, Zimmer K, et al. Performance of a demand oxygen saver system during rest, exercise, and sleep in hypoxemic patients. Chest 1988;94:77–80.
28. Kerby GR, O'Donahue WJ, Romberger DJ, et al. Clinical efficacy and cost benefit of pulse flow oxygen in hospitalized patients. Chest 1990;97:369–372.
29. Tiep BL, Christopher KL, Spofford BT, et al. Pulsed nasal and transtracheal oxygen. Chest 1990;97:364–368.
30. Carter R, Tashkin D, Diahed B, et al. Demand oxygen delivery for patients with restrictive lung disease. Chest 1989;96: 1307–1311.
31. Heimlich HJ. Respiratory rehabilitation with transtracheal oxygen system. Ann Otol Rhinol Laryngol 1982;91:643–647.
32. Banner NR, Govan JR. Long term transtracheal oxygen delivery through microcatheter in patients with hypoxaemia due to chronic obstructive airways disease. Br Med J 1986; 293:111–114.
33. Hoffman LA, Johnson JT. Wesmiller SW, et al. Transtracheal delivery of oxygen: Efficacy and safety for long-term continuous therapy. Ann Otol Rhinol Laryngol 1991;100:108–115.
34. Christopher KL, Spofford BT, Brannin PK, et al. Transtracheal oxygen therapy for refractory hypoxemia. JAMA 1986;256:- 494–497.
35. Heimlich HJ, Carr GC. The Micro-Trach: A seven-year experience with transtracheal oxygen therapy. Chest 1989;95: 1008–1012.
36. Walsh DA, Gouan JR. Long-term continuous domiciliary oxygen therapy by transtracheal catheter. Thorax 1990;45:478–781.
37. Kacmarek RM. Methods of oxygen delivery in the hospital. Probl Respir Care 1990;3:563–574.
38. Redding JG, McAfee PD, Parham AM. Oxygen concentrations received from commonly used delivery systems. South Med J 1978;71:169–172.
39. Bethune DW, Collis JM. The evaluation of oxygen masks. Anaesthesia 1967;22:43–54.
40. Bethune DW, Collis JM. Evaluation of oxygen therapy equipment. Thorax 1967;22:221–225.
41. Milross J, Young IH, Donnelly P. The oxygen delivery characteristics of the Hudson Oxy-one face mask. Anaesth Intens Care 1989;17:180–184.
42. Jensen AG, Johnson A, Sandstedt S. Rebreathing during oxygen treatment with face mask. Acta Anaesth Scand 1991; 35:289–292.
43. Boothby WM, Lovelace WR, Bulbulian A. The BLB oxygen inhalation apparatus: Improvements in design and efficiency by studies on oxygen percentages in alveolar air. Proc Mayo Clin 1940;15:194–206.
44. Hudes ET, Marans HJ, Hirano GM, et al. Recovery room oxygenation: A comparison of nasal catheters and 40 percent oxygen masks. Can J Anaesth 1989;36:20–24.
45. Scacci R. Air-entrainment masks: Jet mixing is how they work; The Bernoulli and Venturi principles are how they don't. Respir Care 1979;24:928–931.
46. Friedman SA, Weber B, Briscoe WA, et al. Oxygen therapy: Evaluation of various air-entraining masks. JAMA 1974;228:474–478.
47. Lyew MA, Holland AJ, Metcalf IR. Combined air and oxygen entrainment. Anaesthesia 1990;45:732–735.
48. Cohen JL, Demers RR, Sakland M. Air-entrainment oxygen masks: A performance evaluation. Respir Care 1977;22:277–282.
49. Campbell EJM, Minty KB. Controlled oxygen therapy at 60% concentration. Lancet 1976;2:1199–1203.
50. Campbell EJM. A method of controlled oxygen administration which reduces the risk of carbon dioxide retention. Lancet 1960;2:12–14.
51. Campbell EJM. Apparatus for oxygen administration. Br Med J 1963;2:1269–1270.
52. Campbell EJM, Gebbie J. Masks and tents for providing controlled oxygen concentrations. Lancet 1966;1:468–469.
53. Speir WA, Kaplan H, Weir M, Ellison L. Oxygen concentration delivered with in-line humidification. JAMA 1971;216:879–880.
54. Hill SL, Barnes PK, Hollway T, Tennant R. Fixed performance oxygen masks: An evaluation. Br Med J 1984;288:1261–1263.
55. Cox D, Gillbe C. Fixed performance oxygen masks. Anaesthesia 1981;36:958–964.
56. Woolner DF, Larkin J. An analysis of the performance of a variable Venturi-type oxygen mask. Anaesth Intens Care 1980; 8:44–51.
57. Fracchia G, Torda TA. Performance of Venturi oxygen delivery devices. Anaesth Intens Care 1980;8:426–430.
58. Canet J, Sanchis J. Performance of a low flow O_2 Venturi mask: Diluting effects of breathing pattern. Eur J Respir Dis 1984;65: 68–73.
59. Foust GN, Potter WH, Wilson MD, Golden EB. Shortcomings of using two jet nebulizers in tandem with an aerosol face mask for optimal oxygen therapy. Chest 1991;99:1346–1351.
60. Kuo CD, Lin SE, Wang JH. Aerosol, humidity and oxygenation. Chest 1991;99:1325–1356.
61. Ziecheck HD. Faulty ventilator check valves cause pipeline gas contamination. Respir Care 1981;26:1009–1010.
62. Jenner W, George BG. Oxygen-air shunt syndrome strikes again. Respir Care 1982;27:604.
63. Emergency Care Research Institute: Oxygen-air proportioners. Health Devices 1985;14:263–284.
64. Scott LR, Benson MS, Pierson DJ. Performance of five air–oxygen blenders under simulated clinical conditions. Respir Care 1986;31:31–36.

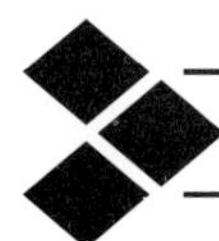
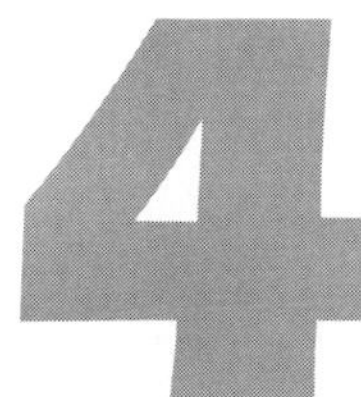

Clinical Hyperbaric Oxygen Chambers and Related Respiratory Care Equipment

David A. Desautels
John M. Graybeal

OBJECTIVES

1. Explain the effects of supra-atmospheric pressure on gas volume, density, and solubility.
2. Explain the effects of hyperbaric oxygen on oxygen delivery.
3. Compare monoplace and multiplace chambers.
4. Describe systems to deliver gases to the patient in a hyperbaric chamber.
5. Describe the problems associated with mechanical ventilation in a hyperbaric chamber.
6. Describe methods for monitoring patient oxygenation and ventilation during hyperbaric oxygen (HBO) treatment.
7. Explain fire and safety hazards associated with HBO and methods of prevention.
8. Describe the patient's experience of undergoing compression.
9. List the diseases that may respond to HBO treatment.

Richard D. Branson: RESPIRATORY CARE EQUIPMENT,

KEY TERMS

atmosphere's absolute (ATA)	hyperbaric	hypobarism
decompression illness	hyperbaric chamber	monoplace chamber
feet of sea water (FSW)	hyperbaric oxygenation	multiplace chamber
Henry's law		

Introduction

Hyperbaric medicine is a rapidly growing field especially suited for the respiratory care practitioner. With a special familiarity of the gas laws and a specific working knowledge of gas delivery systems, it is natural that the respiratory care practitioner contributes in a significant way to the field of hyperbaric medicine.

In this chapter we discuss hyperbaric oxygen (HBO) and the equipment used to administer this unique form of therapy. HBO consists of both the elevated environmental pressure and the administration of oxygen during this increased pressure. The basic function of the increased environmental pressure on both physical and physiologic principles warrants special consideration and therefore is discussed first. A discussion of the equipment commonly used in HBO, both for compression and oxygen delivery, follows. Monitoring, of both oxygenation and ventilation, is discussed at the end of the chapter.

History of Hyperbaric Medicine

The history of hyperbaric medicine is long and tenuous. Beginning as early as 1662, a British physician named Henshaw made a "domicilium," which he used to treat large categories of diseases. He used high-pressure (compressed) gas in the "domicilium" for acute disease and low-pressure (rarefied) gas in the "domicilium" for chronic disease. This domicilium was used to aid digestion, promote insensible respiration, help breathing and expectoration, and in general help most lung diseases. Little was done to follow this up until the late 19th century when chambers became "faddish," attracting persons from all over Europe to centers such as Bertin's in 1855. Even mobile chambers with operating rooms were used with some success to reduce cyanosis, vomiting, and postanesthetic problems by Fontaine in 1879. The greatest boost for hyperbaric therapy came with Paul Bert, the father of pressure physiology. Bert did most of his experiments on himself in a chamber he could operate from the inside. His classic publication "La Pression Barométrique" chronicles his work on oxygen/nitrous oxide anesthesia under pressure, oxygen toxicity under pressure, and plant growth under pressure.[1]

The first chamber in the United States was in Rochester, New York. It was quickly followed by a chamber in New York City built by J. L. Corning in 1891. Corning was also the first person to do spinal anesthesia at atmospheric pressure and the first to experiment on the spinal cord under pressure. Hyperbaric medicine peaked just after the turn of the century with O. L. Cunningham's "hyperbaric hotel." Measuring five stories high and 64 feet in diameter, this facility was built by Cunningham in Kansas City in 1928. After this extraordinary use, hyperbaric medicine died out until the early 1960s when Boerema described how HBO could be used to support life without hemoglobin and stop the spread of gas gangrene. This resurgence was short lived, however, because of spurious work on senility and impotence in the mid-1960s. Seeing a need for control, a group of interested physicians banded together in 1967 to form the Undersea Medical Society (UMS). These physicians were largely military physicians interested in the field of diving medicine, and it took some time before the committee on Hyperbaric Oxygenation from the UMS adopted a comprehensive list of diseases divided into categories considered experimental and accepted for treatment in 1970. In 1987, the name of the UMS was changed to the Undersea and Hyperbaric Medical Society to reflect the range of clinician involvement. This organization has restored credibility to the field of hyperbaric medicine. Now Medicare and Medicaid as well as most third-party payers follow guidelines set down by this organization.

Basic Physical and Physiologic Principles

Pressure is the force per unit area and can be measured in units of pounds per square inch (psi), millimeters of mercury (mm Hg or torr), centimeters of water (cm H_2O), feet of sea water (FSW), atmospheres absolute (ATA), as well as many others. By tradition, from the diving literature, pressure is usually expressed in FSW and psi, although the use of ATA is becoming more popular (Table 4-1). Throughout this chapter ATA units are used.

The increased environmental pressure exerted during HBO will have effects on several physical princi-

TABLE 4-1. Pressure Conversion Units

FSW	psig	psia	ATA	mm Hg	cm H_2O
0	0	14.7	1	760	1033
33	14.7	29.4	2	1520	2066
66	29.4	44.1	3	2280	3099
99	44.1	58.8	4	3040	4132
132	58.8	73.5	5	3800	5165
165	73.5	88.2	6	4560	6198

ples. The amount of pressure applied will effect the volume (Boyle's law) of substances in the chamber, most notably gases. Liquids are much less compressible and therefore are not affected to the same extent as gases. Boyle's law states that when temperature remains constant the volume occupied by a given molecular quantity of a gas is inversely proportional to the pressure exerted on the gas. When applied to the hyperbaric environment this law has important implications. If a sealed 1-L bag of air is placed into a hyperbaric chamber and compressed to 2 ATA it will now occupy only 0.5 L (Fig. 4-1), although the number of moles (the molecular quantity) of air within the bag will remain the same. In the same way, a "bubble" of gas within the blood would occupy a proportionately smaller volume when exposed to a hyperbaric environment. If the molecular quantity of gas remains unchanged and the volume that the gas occupies becomes smaller, than the relative density of the gas must increase. This becomes important in the function of gas delivery systems (especially mechanical ventilators) in the hyperbaric chamber and is discussed in more detail later.

Another important consequence of the increased pressure during HBO is explained by Gay-Lussac's law. Assuming the volume of the hyperbaric chamber remains constant, the temperature within the chamber will vary directly with pressure within the chamber. During compression, heat is generated. The opposite occurs during decompression. Dalton's law of partial pressures is also important during the elevated pressure of HBO. The fractional concentrations of a given gas mixture will remain the same, but the partial pressure exerted by a specific gas (within the mixture) will be increased by the same factor as the total pres-

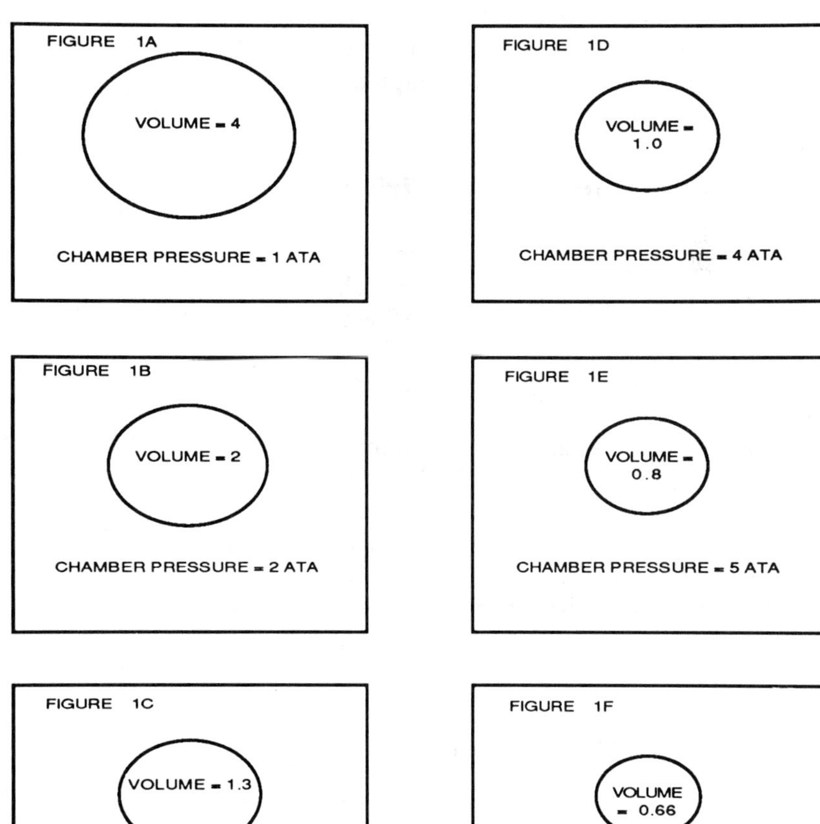

Figure 4-1. The effect of increasing chamber pressure on a "bubble." The six panels show the relative change in volume of a bubble as it is exposed to compression to 6 ATA.

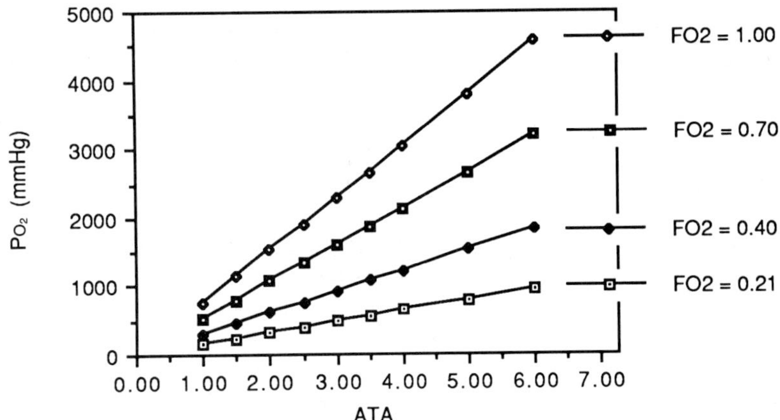

Figure 4-2. Increasing partial pressures exerted by oxygen in four different gas mixtures at increasing chamber pressures (1–6 ATA).

sure exerted within the chamber. This explains how it is possible to deliver 1 ATA (760 mm Hg) of oxygen, the equivalent of pure oxygen at sea level, using a gas mixture containing only 20% oxygen at a chamber pressure of 5 ATA. Although the fractional concentration of oxygen in compressed air remains the same, as chamber pressure increases the partial pressure of oxygen (or any gas) will increase. This allows the generation of a much higher oxygen tension in the alveolus and in the arterial blood. Figure 4-2 shows the increasing partial pressure of oxygen as chamber pressures are increased during HBO therapy. This high partial pressure of oxygen in the breathing mixture causes a large gradient to develop, which allows a more rapid clearance of nitrogen and other inert gases from the body through the lungs (sometimes referred to as the off-gassing principle). This elevation of the partial pressure of oxygen is thought to be responsible for the other physiologic beneficial effects of HBO. Because of this increased partial pressure of oxygen, there is a greatly increased risk of combustion within the chamber. Oxygen, although not directly flammable, is necessary to support combustion. The more oxygen present (partial pressure), the faster the rate of combustion. The hazard of combustion and the safety requirements necessary in a chamber are discussed later.

The pressure exerted on a gas also effects its solubility. The absolute quantity of a gas dissolved in a liquid is a function of the solubility coefficient for the specific gas and diluent in question (Table 4-2). The relative amount of a gas dissolved in a liquid however, varies directly with the pressure exerted by the gas over the liquid. An example of this principle relevant to HBO involves the oxygen-carrying capacity of blood. During normobaric conditions the greatest portion of oxygen carried within the blood is bound to the hemoglobin molecules. A healthy adult breathing room air, at sea level would have approximately 20.4 mL/dL of oxygen bound to hemoglobin (assuming hemoglobin = 15 g/dL) while only 0.315 mL/dL is carried in the dissolved form (assuming PaO_2 = 105 mm Hg) in the plasma. For every 333 mm Hg of pressure exerted by dissolved oxygen in the plasma, there is an additional 1 mL/dL of oxygen carried. Figure 4-3 shows the relationship between increased pressure and the amount of dissolved oxygen (in proportion to that carried on hemoglobin) carried in the blood. When the partial pressure of oxygen reaches 4 ATA, approximately one-third of the total quantity of oxygen carried by the blood is in the dissolved form.

TABLE 4-2. Solubility Coefficients of Three Common Gases at 37°C

Gas	Solubility (mL/mL plasma/atm)
Oxygen	0.0214
Nitrogen	0.067
Carbon dioxide	0.53

Types of Hyperbaric Chambers

There are two general types, or classifications, of high-pressure (hyperbaric) chambers. The division is based solely on the number of occupants, both patients and attendants, that the chamber is capable of supporting. A hyperbaric chamber is either a monoplace or a multiplace style. Treatment protocols vary somewhat depending on the type of chamber available at a particular institution.

Multiplace Chambers

A multiplace chamber is any chamber that has positions and gas delivery systems (which provide a source of gas for respiration separate from that used to compress the chamber) for more than one patient.

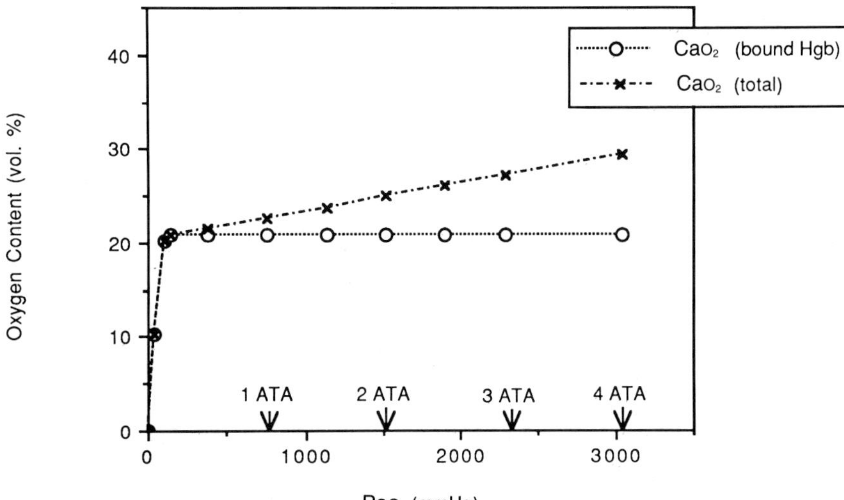

Figure 4-3. Relationship between increased pressure and the amount of dissolved oxygen (in proportion to that carried on the hemoglobin) carried in the blood.

Most multiplace chambers are custom designed for each individual facility, allowing for a wide range of multiplace chamber styles and sizes. One of the largest of these in the United States actually combines several interconnected multiplace chambers and is located at Duke University (Fig. 4-4). In addition to the wide range of styles and sizes available, the range of uses varies and includes clinical therapy, industrial (offshore diving) uses, and research protocols. Figure 4-5 shows a commercially available multiplace chamber.

Although the overall size may vary, the design concept is one of a large cylinder divided into at least two sections. One of these sections is considerably smaller than the other (called the entry compartment); its primary function is to allow passage of attendants, other health care providers, and needed supplies in and out of the high-pressure environment without loss of pressure within the main compartment. The large amount of available room within the multiplace chamber allows for a great deal of flexibility. Treatment schedules can be arranged that allow either multiple patients and a few attendants or one (more acutely ill) patient and a larger number of attendants. Equipment for

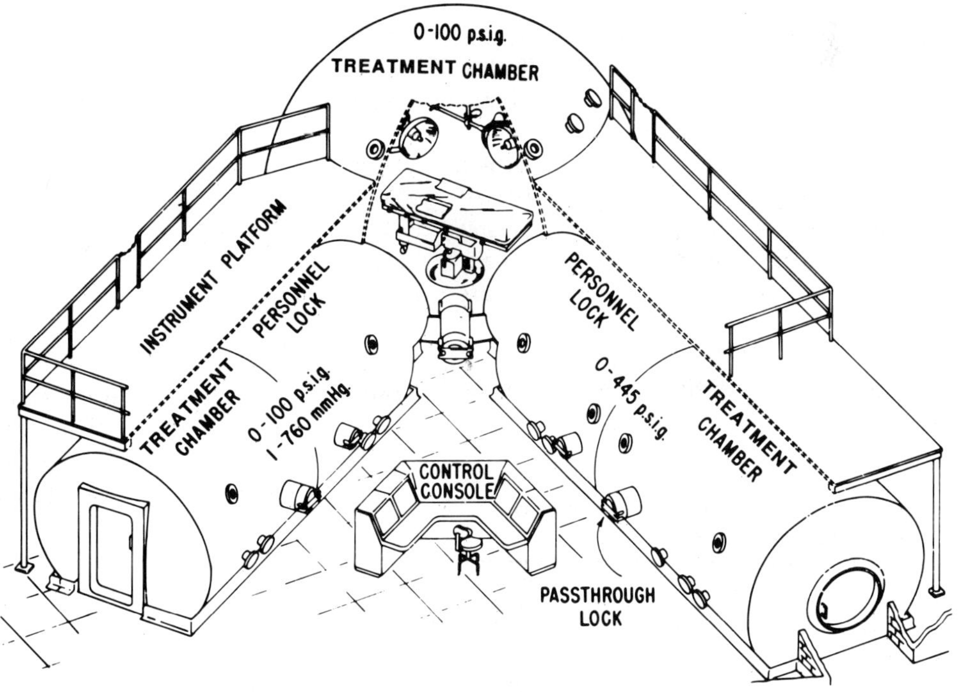

Figure 4-4. Multiplace hyperbaric oxygen facilities at Duke University. (Courtesy of Duke University)

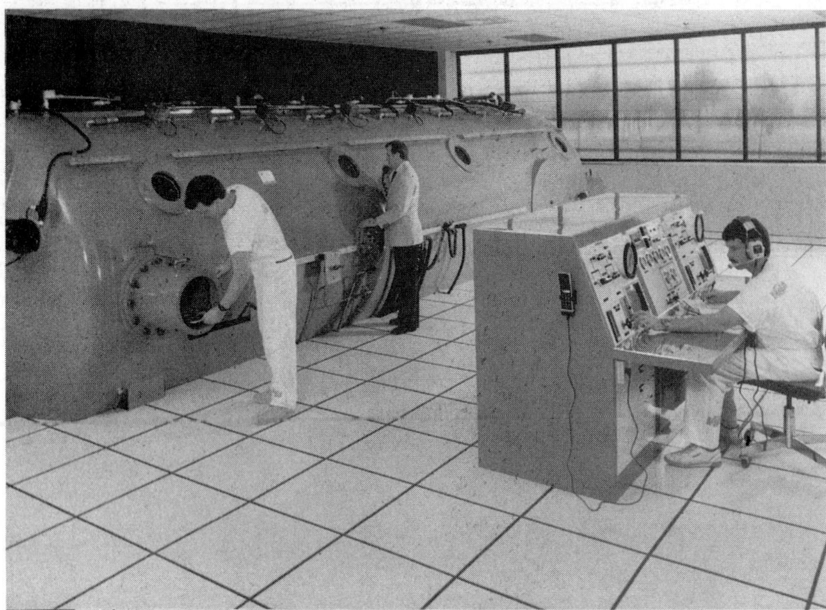

Figure 4-5. Multiplace hyperbaric chamber. (Courtesy of Perry Baromedical Services, Riviera Beach, FL)

patient care can be placed inside the chamber, after having been tested for air space compression (the presence of air spaces within the device that could cause it to implode during compression) and electrical and fire safety.

Monoplace Chambers

A monoplace chamber is designed for a single occupant. There are several companies manufacturing this style of chamber. The outward appearance of these chambers can be vastly different, but the general operating principles are similar (Fig. 4-6). Table 4-3 details the specifications of currently available monoplace hyperbaric chambers. Frequently, the only gas available for patient respiration is the atmospheric gas used to compress the chamber. In some of the newer designs there is a provision for a respiration gas source separate from the compression gas source. Connection must be made to the outside so that patients may be monitored and provided with intravenous administration and ventilation. All devices operated from the outside must have the ability to increase their working pressure above that of the chamber. The increased acuity of patients being treated with HBO has shown the importance of an inside at-

(text continues on page 81)

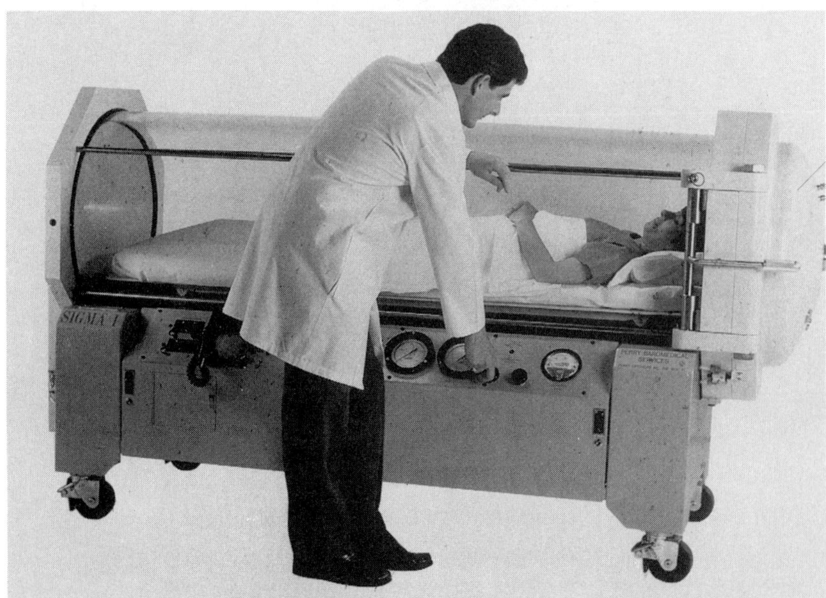

Figure 4-6. Monoplace hyperbaric chamber. (Courtesy of Perry Baromedical Services, Riviera Beach, FL)

TABLE 4-3. Specifications of Monoplace Chambers

Chamber	Maximum Pressure (ATA)	Maximum Compression Rate (psi/min)	Emergency Decompression Rate (psi/min)	Gas Supply Pressure (psi)/ Peak Flow (L/m)	Power Supply (VAC)	Materials of Construction	Weight (kg)	Dimensions (meters) Height	Length Open	Length Closed	Width	Internal Diameter	Address
Drager HTK 1200	3.0	7.4	59	O_2: 74–150/50–900 Air: 74–150/80	220/110	Steel	1120	1.36	5.25	3.03	1.88	0.9	Dragerwerk AG Lubeck, Werk Druckkammertechnik Auf Dem Braggersand 17, Postfach 150 149, D-2400 Lubeck-Travemunde, Federal Republic of Germany
Environmental Tectonics Corporation Bara-Med Amp-100	3.0	5	30	50–70/60–400	120	Single acrylic	544	1.40	5.33	2.59	1.016	0.76	Environmental Tectonics Corporation, County Line Industrial Park, Southampton, PA 18966
HYOX													HYOX Systems Limited, Pressure Products House, Westhill Industrial Estate, Westhill, Aberdeen A83 6TQ
CHU3/OC	3.0	3.0	60	60/300	220/120	Double acrylic	405	1.17	4.27	2.13	0.99	0.59	
CHU4/OC	4.0	3.0	60	60/300	220/120	Double acrylic	405	1.17	4.27	2.13	0.99	0.59	
HTU	2.0	3.0	60	O2:300 Inboard air compressor	220/110	Steel	800	1.36	3.53	2.28	0.82	NA	
Perry Sigma 1	3.04	5	60	50–70/120–300	115	Double acrylic	454	1.35	4.35	2.44	0.89	0.64	Perry Baromedical Service, 275 West 10th Street, Riviera Beach, FL 33404
Reneau	6.0	14.7	14.7	O_2: 50/60 Air: 50–150/283 N_2: 50–150/283	120	Steel	2359	1.55	5.16	3.33	1.07	0.90	Reneau, Inc., 12701 Executive Drive, Suite 608, Stafford, TX 77477
Sechrist 25008	3.0	5	60	50–70/249–380	120	Double acrylic	438	1.27	4.60	2.41	0.9	0.64	Sechrist Industries, Inc., Medical Products, 2820 Gretta Lane, Anaheim, CA 92806

From Moon RE, Camporesi EM. Clinical Applications of Hyperbaric Oxygen. Problems in Respiratory Care 1991; 4:176.

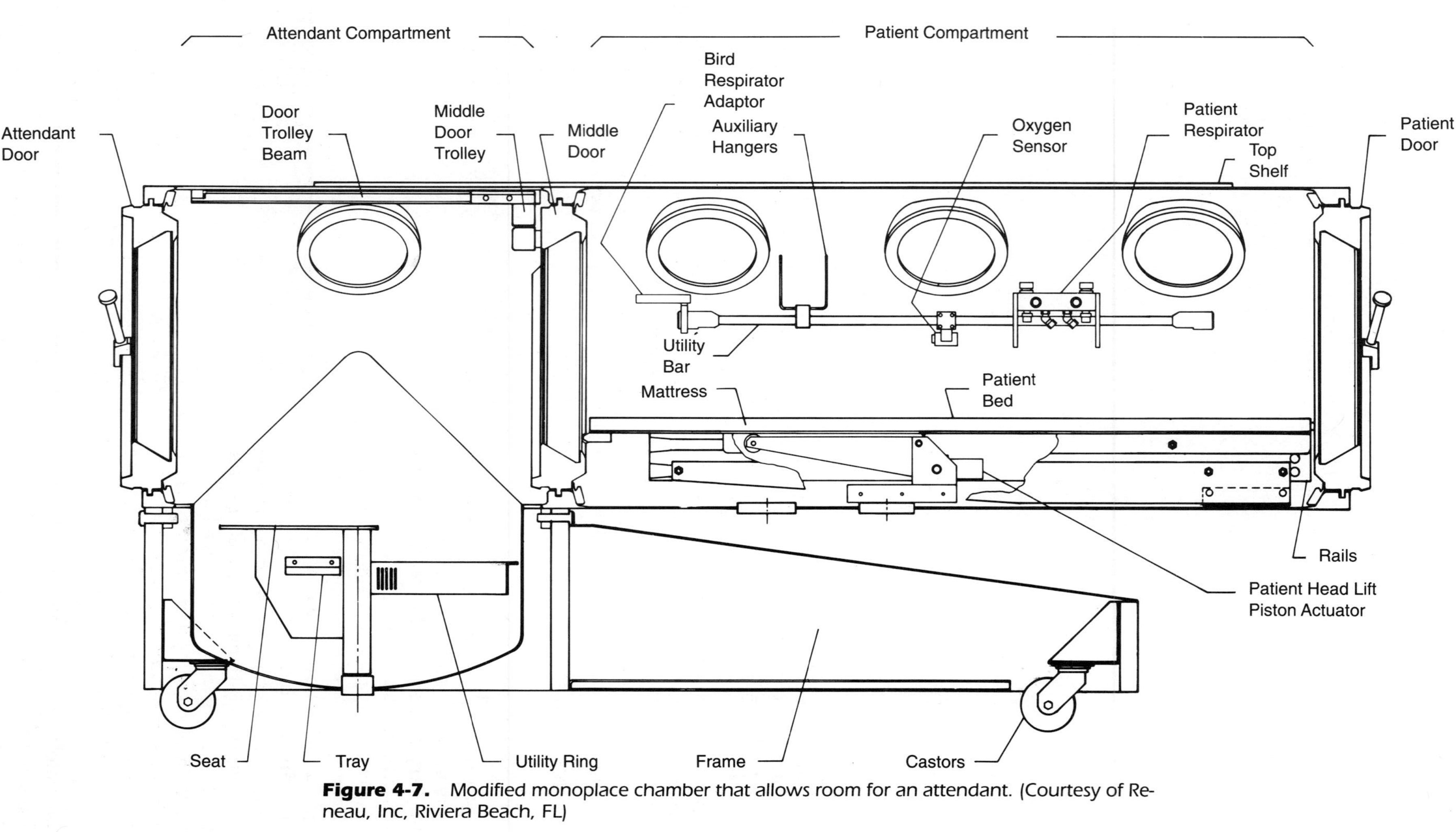

Figure 4-7. Modified monoplace chamber that allows room for an attendant. (Courtesy of Reneau, Inc, Riviera Beach, FL)

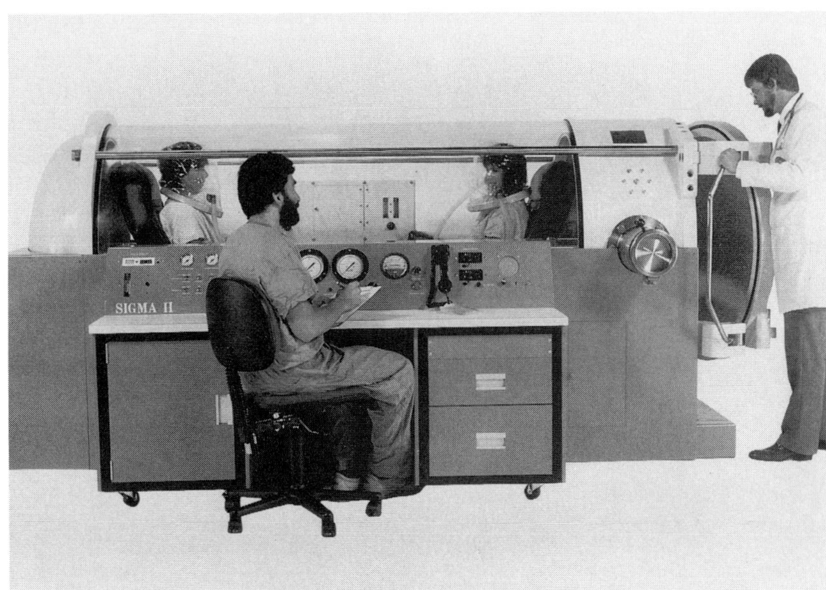

Figure 4-8. Modified monoplace chamber that allows treatment of two patients. (Courtesy of Perry Baromedical Services, Riviera Beach, FL)

tendant. To address this need, some companies have designed a modified monoplace chamber, having room for an attendant (usually through a separate entrance) in addition to the patient receiving treatment. Figures 4-7 and 4-8 show a typical example of this modified monoplace design. An additional feature of this design is the inclusion of a separate source of respiration gas.

Gas Delivery Systems

Respiration Gas Supply

When a multiplace chamber is used, during chamber pressurization the patient would be asked to breathe pure oxygen for varying periods of time, depending on which treatment schedule is being used (a treatment schedule commonly used to treat simple decompression sickness is included in Table 4-4). Oxygen is supplied for this purpose from a separate gas source with individual breathing devices located within the chamber. Breathing gas mixtures can be delivered with either a tight-fitting face mask or a soft shell oxygen tent, similar to an oxyhood used for infants (Fig. 4-9). Both of these systems require close control of both inspiratory and expiratory gas flows. The inspiratory flow requires a driving pressure greater than the internal pressure of the chamber. Generally, the source of oxygen is maintained at a pressure approximately 50 psig greater than the maximum internal pressure of the chamber. A tight-sealing system is necessary to limit the amount of oxygen that exists in the system, thereby contaminating the chamber environment. A shutoff valve is also required to prevent unnecessary oxygen leakage into the chamber while the system is not in use. Many multiplace chambers use a tight-fitting aviator's mask, which incorporates a demand valve system, for this purpose. Exhaled gas is then directed through the chamber hull to the external environment. This is done for two reasons, to help control the leakage of oxygen into the chamber and to control the internal carbon dioxide concentration.

There are a wide variety of treatment tables in clinical use. It is important that all caregivers involved with a specific patient be aware of the treatment table being used and all modifications that are being employed.

TABLE 4-4. Sample Treatment Table

Depth (feet)	Time (minutes)*	Breathing Media	Elapsed Time (hr:min)
60	20	Oxygen	0:20
60	5	Air	0:25
60	20	Oxygen	0:45
Traveling	30	Oxygen	1:15
30	5	Air	1:20
30	20	Oxygen	1:40
30	5	Air	1:45
Surfacing	30	Oxygen	2:15

*Does not include descent time. Adapted from Navy Decompression Table 5. In: U.S. Navy Diver's Handbook. U.S. Government Printing Office. Washington, D.C., 1985.

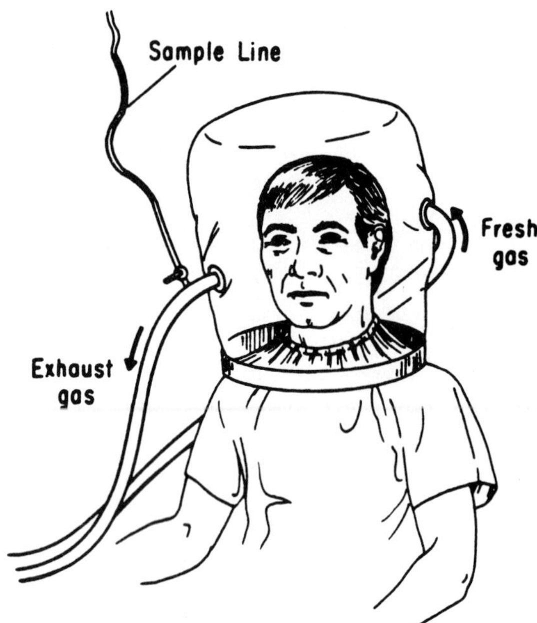

Figure 4-9. Head tent used to deliver oxygen to awake patients in multiplace chambers. Oxygen flow at a rate of 30 to 60 L/min delivered at pressure will usually maintain head tent oxygen concentrations greater than 98% and carbon dioxide concentrations less than 0.1%. Patient treatment gas may be monitored with a sample line, preferably connected to the expired limb of the circuit. This will also facilitate the detection of leaks. (From Moon RE, Camporesi EM. Operational use and patient monitoring in a multiplace hyperbaric chamber. In: (Problems in Respiratory Care), Philadelphia, PA: J. B. Lippincott; 1991; 4(2).

Chamber Compression Gas Supply

Large volumes of gas are required to compress a chamber. For each ATA increase in pressure, 1 complete volume (internal volume of chamber) needs to be added to the chamber. The storage pressure of this gas will then determine the maximum rate of compression that the chamber can achieve. Frequently, large volume air compressors are used for this purpose, with an attached gas reservoir. Safety dictates that an additional backup reservoir of gas, often in the form of a "bank" of gas cylinders, is maintained in case of electrical or mechanical failure of the compressor. The reservoir should be large enough to maintain chamber pressure during all necessary decompression stops during a decompression schedule, safely allowing all interior subjects to exit.

In addition to maintaining chamber pressure, compressed gas is consumed during ventilation of the chamber interior. Ventilation of the chamber is required to maintain a low oxygen concentration (as close to 21% as possible), a low carbon dioxide concentration, and a comfortable temperature within. Elevated carbon dioxide concentrations have important physiologic consequences during hyperbaric exposure just as during normobaric conditions. In addition to the expected side effects of increased inhaled carbon dioxide concentrations, central nervous system (CNS) oxygen toxicity triggering may be increased.

Box 4-1 lists several constants that are useful when calculating the volume of gas required for chamber ventilation. Box 4-2 demonstrates the proper method for calculating chamber ventilation rates. The importance of adequate chamber ventilation is increased as the internal volume of the chamber decreases.

Mechanical Ventilation Systems

Although most patients receiving multiple HBO treatments are breathing spontaneously, there are many acute patients (those with carbon monoxide poisoning

Box 4-1
Constants for Chamber Ventilation Rate

Breathing air or an air–helium mixture:
- 2 acfm per subject at rest
- 4 acfm per subject at work

Breathing oxygen by mask or ventilator:
- 12.5 acfm per subject at rest
- 25 acfm per subject at work

Interrupted ventilation:
- Twice the calculated acfm for twice the interrupted period. Resume normal rate after that time.

acfm, actual cubic feet per minute; scfm, surface cubic feet per minute.

Box 4-2
Sample Calculation for Chamber Ventilation Requirements

Three subjects in a chamber pressurized to 6 ATA, two at work breathing air, and one at rest breathing oxygen with overboard dump system.

4 acfm = air breathing, at work per subject
12.5 acfm = oxygen breathing, at rest per subject
[(4 acfm · 2) + (12.5 acfm · 1)] = 6 ATA = scfm
= 123 scfm of ventilation gas

acfm, actual cubic feet per minute; scfm, surface cubic feet per minute.

and unconscious patients with gas embolism) who require assisted ventilation during the HBO treatment. At present there are few, if any, mechanical ventilators that have been shown to function properly under high-pressure conditions.[2–8]

There are two major problems associated with use of mechanical ventilators in a hyperbaric environment. The first is the increased environmental pressure at which they must operate. The maximum peak airway pressure of most mechanical ventilators in clinical use is within the 120 cm H_2O range or 88.3 mm Hg (at normal atmospheric pressure). Although the pressure gradient for ventilation remains the same, at increased environmental pressure the absolute pressure within the ventilation system is greatly increased. The ventilator requires a higher operating pressure, but peak inspiratory pressure remains the same.

The second (and more serious) problem is the increased density of the ventilating gases during high pressure exposure. Recall that as pressure increases the volume of a given quantity of gas decreases, thereby increasing its density. When the density of a ventilating gas increases, the resistance to flow of that gas through a tube also increases. Depending on the cycling mechanism of the ventilator in question, this will cause significant alterations in the tidal volume, inspiratory time, inspiratory flow rate, or the minute volume delivered. Several mechanical ventilators have been evaluated in the high-pressure environment. Table 4-5 summarizes the results of these tests. Although the response range is wide, there is a general pattern of decreasing tidal volume and gas flow rate. Several other ventilators have been anecdotally reported with variable results. Data are lacking with these reports. Caution must, therefore, be exercised whenever a patient is mechanically ventilated in the high-pressure environment. A therapist, knowledgeable in both mechanical ventilation and high-pressure physics, should be present whenever a patient requiring mechanical ventilation is in the HBO chamber.

Careful monitoring of the mechanical ventilation system (including the patient) is important. Endotracheal tube cuffs will be affected according to Boyle's law. The respiratory care practitioner must inflate and deflate the cuff as pressure is increased and decreased. Continuous monitoring of the respiratory rate and tidal volume must be accomplished. Respiratory rate can easily be counted and should be maintained constant. Changes in gas flow rates can cause inspiratory-expiratory ratios to vary during compression and should therefore be carefully monitored. Monitoring of tidal volume and minute ventilation is more difficult. Both the Wright respirometer and the Boehringer spirometer have been used in the hyperbaric chamber. The accuracy of both has been shown to be affected by the increased pressure within the chamber. This is most likely due to the increased gas density. Calibration values have been published but are widely variable between individual devices of the same brand. Each individual device should be calibrated in the hyperbaric environment with a known quantity of gas before its use is accepted in the clinical setting.

Monitoring of Oxygenation and Ventilation

The use of the transcutaneous oxygen monitor is widely accepted in the HBO chamber. Information can be gained about overall patient oxygenation and also specifically about oxygenation at the probe location. This is useful in monitoring of ischemic tissue and its response to HBO. Both the level and the duration of elevation of the tissue oxygen can be monitored with these devices. The response of a problem wound to the increased oxygen available during HBO can easily be evaluated with these devices. Care must be taken not to burn the patient with prolonged application of the electrode at one site. Most moni-

TABLE 4-5. Mechanical Ventilator Responses in High-Pressure Environments

Ventilator*	Tidal Volume	Minute Ventilation	Respiratory Rate	Inspiratory Time	Reference
Monaghan 225	d	d	d	—	3
Emerson pneumatic	o	o	o	—	4
IMV bird	d	d	d	—	4,5
Mark 2 bird (modified)	d	d	o	—	4,5
Urgency bird	d	d	d	—	4
Oxford-Penlon	o	o	o	o	6,8
Sechrist 500A	d	d	d	i	7

d, decreased; o, unchanged; i, increased; —, not reported.

*Several other ventilators have been anecdotally reported with variable results (favorable or unfavorable). Data are not included with these reports. For these reasons caution must be exercised whenever a patient is mechanically ventilated in the high-pressure environment.

tors need to be modified by the manufacturer to incorporate the higher levels of oxygenation seen during HBO therapy .

Arterial blood gas analysis, providing useful information concerning both oxygenation and ventilation, must be handled with great care. Some centers have adapted their analyzer to the high-pressure environment. Although this may be handy in critical situations, it is not necessary. The blood sample can be removed from the chamber and directly analyzed. Care must be exercised to accomplish this before the gases, dissolved in solution, come out of solution. The electronic output of most analyzers requires modification to compensate for the increased levels of oxygen dissolved in the blood.

Monitoring of the adequacy of ventilation is somewhat more difficult. Gas withdrawal systems (for $PetCO_2$), such as a mass spectrometer, are designed to function at normal ambient pressure. When monitoring is performed through the chamber hull, a pressure reduction system is required. This can be accomplished with a regulated "Y" valve placed just before the measuring device, allowing excess gas to dump to the atmosphere.

Fire and Safety Issues

Although the requirements for chamber safety vary somewhat, depending on the type of chamber in question, the general principles remain the same. The American Society of Mechanical Engineers (ASME) has set forth standards describing the materials, the design and fabrication process, and the inspection and testing necessary for certification as a pressure vessel for human occupancy.[9] All clinical chambers must be so certified. Chapter 19 of the National Fire Protection Agency's NFPA 99 fire safety code describes the requirements for safe installation and operation of a HBO facility. Both of these documents should be reviewed carefully by anyone involved in the operation of a hyperbaric facility.

Chamber fires are a reality. Recall that oxygen supports combustion. The higher the fractional concentration of oxygen present, the faster the combustion rate for a given material. Chamber fires occurring in monoplace chambers, which almost always use oxygen as the compression gas, are tragic. Absolutely all sources of ignition must be removed. Special attention must be given to children's sparking toys. The simplest electric source can spark and the resultant fire can quite rapidly consume every flammable object in the chamber, including the patient. A chamber fire in a multiplace chamber has been reported by Youn and co-workers.[10] Cotton blankets, warmed in a microwave, were passed through the medication lock for patient use. After compression in the medication lock and exposure to the chamber environment (maintained with compressed air) the blanket began to burn with open flame. Fortunately no patients or attendants were injured. This underscores the need for frequent review of fire codes and safety procedures. Some simple rules to follow for safe chamber operation are listed below:

- If possible, maintain the fractional concentration of oxygen less than 23.5%. Most monoplace chambers are compressed with 100% oxygen.
- Keep all combustible substances out of the chamber, including newspapers (these are particularly flammable) and other reading materials.
- Remove all ignition sources possible. Whenever possible, use pneumatically driven equipment and have all equipment checked for electrical safety.
- Never use oil on any oxygen fitting or any piece of chamber equipment.
- When in doubt, keep it out!

The possibility of spontaneous ignition increases as chamber pressure increases. Even some hydrocarbons are capable of spontaneous ignition at pressure.

Patient Experience During Compression

Patients experience a hot, noisy environment during compression. Heat is generated from the increasing pressure (Gay-Lussac's law). Noise results from the air passing through the pipes en route to the chamber. Pressure on the ears is from the effect of Boyle's law. The volume of air in the middle ear, which is a closed space, is at atmospheric pressure. As chamber pressure is increased, the tympanic membrane is pushed inward, attempting to fill the middle ear space. Once air at chamber pressure is passed through the eustachian tube to the middle ear, during a Valsalva maneuver, the tympanic membrane is returned to normal and the discomfort is relieved. This compression phenomenon effects all air spaces in the patient (middle ear, sinuses, lung, and gut) as well as devices attached to the patient (eg, intravenous lines, endotracheal tube cuffs, blood pressure cuffs, ventilator systems, vials, and bottles).

Conversely, Boyle's law also affects all spaces during decompression. Air compressed at pressure inside air spaces must expand or vent to the environment as chamber pressure is reduced. As an example, if a patient is compressed to 3 ATA, breathing sponta-

Box 4-3
Indications for Hyperbaric Oxygen Therapy

1. Air or gas embolism
2. Carbon monoxide poisoning and smoke inhalation, carbon monoxide complicated by cyanide poisoning
3. Clostridial myonecrosis (gas gangrene)
4. Crush injury, compartment syndrome, and other acute traumatic ischemias
5. Decompression sickness
6. Enhancement of healing in selected problem wounds
7. Exceptional blood loss (anemia)
8. Necrotizing soft tissue infections (subcutaneous tissue, muscle, fascia)
9. Osteomyelitis (refractory)
10. Radiation tissue damage (osteoradionecrosis)
11. Skin grafts and flaps (compromised)
12. Thermal burns

From Hyperbaric Oxygen Therapy: A Committee Report. Bethesda, MD: Undersea and Hyperbaric Medical Society, revised 1992.

neously, then brought directly to the surface without exhaling, the patient's lungs would now have the equivalent of three lungs full of air at the surface. This overexpansion would stretch and tear the lung, expelling air into the bloodstream and resulting in a gas embolism, which is often fatal.

Other problems the patient and attendants may be exposed to include decompression illness and CNS oxygen toxicity. Strict adherence to the proper treatment schedules will minimize the occurrence of CNS oxygen toxicity. If it should occur, the oxygen supply can simply be removed from the patient. This should relieve the symptoms (muscle twitching and convulsions). Decompression illness is a problem of prolonged, repeated exposures to pressure followed by an inadequate degassing time. Increased partial pressures of nitrogen saturate the tissue during compression. Returning to the surface without allowing that tissue to desaturate will result in nitrogen coming out of physical solution and forming bubbles, much like soft drinks do when they are opened and carbon dioxide bubbles out of solution. These bubbles can cause many different symptoms, depending on the tissue involved. Symptoms, related to ischemia of the involved area are most commonly pain (type I) or neurologic symptoms (type II). Treatment involves recompression until symptoms are relieved, followed by slow decompression on the appropriate schedule.

Box 4-4
Relative Contraindications of Hyberbaric Oxygen Therapy

Concurrent viral infection
Congenital spherocytosis
Sinusitis
Obstructive bronchial disease
Confinement anxiety
P_{CO_2} greater than 60 mm Hg
Epilepsy
Pneumothorax*

*This is the only absolute contraindication.

Diseases Treated by Hyperbaric Therapy

HBO therapy has been used to treat a wide variety of diseases and maladies. And although the importance of HBO treatment in cases of diving accidents is well known, its other medical uses have been questioned. Box 4-3 is a list of disorders and diseases that are considered treatable by the use of HBO. The contraindications to HBO are given in Box 4-4.

References

1. Jacobson JH, Morsch JHC, Rendell-Baker L. The historical perspective of hyperbaric therapy. Ann NY Acad Sci 1965;117: 651–670.
2. Moon RE, Camporesi EM. Clinical Applications of Hyperbaric Oxygen. Problems in Respiratory Care 1991; 4:176.
3. Moon RE, Bergquist LV, Conklin B, Miller JN. Monaghan 225 ventilator use under hyperbaric conditions. Chest 1986;89: 846–851.
4. Gallagher TJ, Smith RA, Bell GC. Evaluation of mechanical ventilators in a hyperbaric environment. Aviat Space Environ Med 1978;49:375–376.
5. Gallagher TJ, Smith RA, Bell GC. Evaluation of the IMV Bird and the modified Mark 2 Bird in a hyperbaric environment. Respir Care 1977;22:501–504.
6. Blanch PB, Desautels DA, Gallagher TJ. Mechanical ventilator function under hyperbaric conditions. Undersea Biomed Res 1989;16(s):17.
7. Weaver LK, Greenway L, Elliott CG. Performance of the Sechrist 500A hyperbaric ventilator in a monoplace hyperbaric chamber. J Hyperbaric Med 1988;3:215–225.
8. Saywood AM, Howard R, Goad RF, Scott C. Function of the Oxford ventilator at high pressure. Anaesthesia 1982;37:740–744.
9. American Society of Mechanical Engineers. ANSI/ASME safety standard for pressure vessels for human occupancy. New York: American Society of Mechanical Engineers, PHVO-I, 1974.

10. Youn BA, Gordon D, Moran C. Fire in the multiplace hyperbaric chamber. J Hyperbaric Med 1989:4;63–67.

Additional Reading

Bardin H, Lambertsen CJ. A Quantitative Method for Calculating Pulmonary Toxicity: Use of the "Pulmonary Toxicity Dose" (UPTD). Institute for Environmental Medicine Report, 1970.

Camporesi EM, Moon RE. Management of critically ill patients in the hyperbaric environment. J Hyperbaric Med 1987;2:195–198.

Clark JM, Lambertsen CJ. Rate of development of pulmonary oxygen toxicity in men during oxygen breathing at 2.0 ATA. J Appl Physiol 1971:30;739–753.

Hart GB, Lee WS, et al. Complications of repetitive hyperbaric therapy. Presented before the 5th International Congress. 1974;2: 867–873.

Kindwall EP, Goldman RW. Hyperbaric Medicine Procedures: St. Lukes Hospital, Milwaukee, Wisconsin.

Kindwall EP, Goldman EW, Thombs PA. Monoplace vs multiplace chamber in the treatment of diving diseases. J Hyperbaric Med 1988:3;5–10.

Meyer GW, Hart GB, Strauss MB. Noninvasive blood pressure monitoring in the hyperbaric chamber: A new technique. J Hyperbaric Med 1989:4;211–216.

Myers RAM, ed. Hyperbaric Oxygen Therapy: A Committee Report. Bethesda, MD, Undersea and Hyperbaric Medical Society, 1986.

Rockswold GL, Ford E, Anderson JR, et al. Patient monitoring in the monoplace hyperbaric chamber. Hyperbaric Oxygen Rev 1985:6;161–168.

Sheffield PJ, Stork RL, Morgan TR. Efficient oxygen mask for patients undergoing hyperbaric oxygen therapy. Aviat Space Environ Med 1977:48;132–137.

Yarborough OD, Behnke AR. The treatment of compressed air illness utilizing oxygen. J Indust Hyg Toxicol 1039:21;213–218.

Wolf HK, Moon RE, Mitchell PR, et al. Barotrauma and air embolism in hyperbaric oxygen therapy. Am J Forensic Med Pathol 1990:11;149–153.

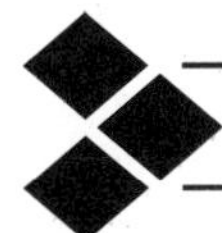
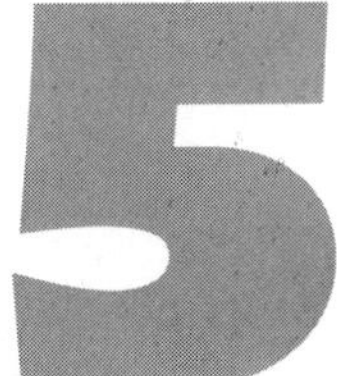

Humidification: Humidifiers and Nebulizers

Dean R. Hess
Richard D. Branson

OBJECTIVES

1. Explain the efficiency of the upper airway in heating and humidifying inspired gases.
2. Compare water vapor pressure, absolute humidity, and relative humidity.
3. Describe the principle of operation of a psychrometer.
4. Define humidity deficit and dew point.
5. Describe factors that influence penetration and deposition of aerosols in the respiratory tract.
6. Compare the principle of operation of passover humidifiers, bubble humidifiers, bubble diffuser humidifiers, jet diffuser humidifiers, and jet humidifiers.
7. Describe the factors that affect the performance of low-flow humidifiers.
8. Describe the principle of operation of servo-controlled and heated wire humidifiers.
9. Compare the principle of operation of the following types of high-flow humidifiers: heated passover, bubble, cascade, wick, vapor phase.
10. Compare the following types of artificial noses: heat and moisture exchangers, heat and moisture exchanging filters, hygroscopic condenser humidifiers, hygroscopic condenser humidifier filters.
11. List instances in which artificial noses should not be used.
12. Compare atomizers and nebulizers.
13. Describe factors that affect performance of small-volume medication nebulizers.
14. Describe the correct use of metered-dose inhalers.
15. Describe the dry powder inhaler.
16. Describe the principle of operation of spinning disk nebulizers, pneumatic jet nebulizers, Babington nebulizers, ultrasonic nebulizers, and small-particle aerosol generators.
17. Discuss issues related to caregiver protection when using ribavirin.
18. List factors that affect aerosol bronchodilator administration during mechanical ventilation.

KEY TERMS

absolute humidity
aerosol
artificial nose
atomizer
Babington nebulizer
bland aerosol therapy
bubble diffuser humidifier
bubble humidifier
cascade humidifier
dew point
dry powder inhaler
heat and moisture exchanger
heat and moisture exchanging filter
heated passover humidifier
heated wire
high-flow humidifier
humidity
humidity deficit
hygrometer
hygroscopic
hygroscopic condenser humidifier
hygroscopic condenser humidifier filter
inertial impaction
isothermic saturation boundary
jet diffuser humidifier
jet humidifier
low-flow humidifier
mass median aerodynamic diameter
metered-dose inhaler
passover humidifier
pneumatic jet nebulizer
psychrometer
relative humidity
sedimentation
servo-controlled
small-particle aerosol generator
small-volume medication nebulizer
spinning disk nebulizer
ultrasonic nebulizer
vapor phase humidifier
water vapor
water vapor pressure
wick humidifier

Introduction

Administration of humidity and aerosols is a common task of the respiratory care practitioner. Humidification of inspired gases is necessary when artificial airways are used. Aerosols are used to humidify the inspired gases, to deliver medications into the respiratory tract, and to deliver bland aerosols. The following discussion is on the types of equipment used for humidity and aerosol therapy.

Physical Properties

Humidity is water that is present in a gas mixture as a vapor. Water vapor is sometimes called molecular water. Evaporation of water from liquid phase to gaseous phase requires energy, and for this reason an unheated humidifier will be cooler than the ambient temperature. The maximal amount of water vapor that can be present in a gas mixture is determined by the temperature of the gas. Increasing the temperature increases the ability of the gas to hold water vapor, and vice versa. A gas mixture that is holding all of the water vapor that it is capable of holding is said to be saturated. If the temperature of a gas mixture that is saturated with water vapor is decreased, the excess water will condense. This commonly occurs when a gas cools as it is delivered from a heated humidifier though tubing to the patient. Water condenses inside the tubing, which is referred to as "rain-out." The temperature at which a gas mixture becomes saturated with water vapor is called the dew point. The amount of water vapor in a gas mixture is measured as water vapor pressure, absolute humidity, or relative humidity.

Water vapor molecules, like all gas molecules, exert a partial pressure. The partial pressure of water vapor is called water vapor pressure (PH_2O), which is temperature dependent (Table 5-1). Absolute humidity is the actual mass of water present in a given volume of gas and is measured in grams per cubic meter

TABLE 5-1. Absolute Humidity and Water Vapor Pressure at Various Temperatures if the Gas is Completely Saturated with Water

Temperature (°C)	Absolute Humidity (mg/L)	Water Vapor Pressure (PH_2O)
0	4.85	4.6
5	6.8	6.5
10	9.4	9.2
15	12.8	12.8
16	13.6	13.6
17	14.5	14.5
18	15.4	15.5
19	16.3	16.5
20	17.3	17.5
21	18.4	18.6
22	19.4	19.8
23	20.6	21.0
24	21.8	22.3
25	23.0	23.7
26	24.4	25.1
27	25.8	26.7
28	27.2	28.3
29	28.8	29.9
30	30.4	31.7
31	32.0	33.6
32	33.8	35.5
33	35.6	37.6
34	37.6	39.8
35	39.6	42.0
36	41.7	44.4
37	43.9	46.9
38	46.2	49.5
39	48.6	52.3
40	51.1	55.1
41	53.7	58.1
42	56.5	61.3
43	59.5	64.6
44	62.5	68.1
100	598.0	760.0

Equation Box 5-1: Relative Humidity

$$\%\text{ relative humidity} = \frac{\text{content}}{\text{capacity}} \cdot 100\%$$

From Table 5–1, it can be seen that the capacity at 22°C is 19.4 mg/L. If the actual humidity content is 10 mg/L, then the % relative humidity is

$$\%\text{ relative humidity} = \frac{10}{19.4} \cdot 100 = 51.5\%$$

As another example, if the % relative humidity is 80% at 32°C, then the water content is

$$\text{content} = \frac{\%\text{ relative humidity} \cdot \text{capacity}}{100}$$

$$= \frac{(80 \cdot 33.8)}{100} = 27\text{ mg}$$

If the relative humidity and temperature are known, the absolute humidity and water vapor pressure can be calculated. For example, at a relative humidity of 40% and a temperature of 24°C, absolute humidity will be 8.7 mg/L and P_{H_2O} will be 8.9 mm Hg.

(g/m^3) or milligrams per liter (mg/L) (see Table 5-1). Relative humidity is the actual amount of water present in a gas divided by the capacity of the gas to hold water at a given temperature. See Equation Box 5-1. At normal body temperature (37°C) and 100% relative humidity, absolute humidity is 43.9 mg/L, and P_{H_2O} is 47 mm Hg.

Relative humidity is measured by a hygrometer (Fig. 5-1) or psychrometer. A psychrometer uses two thermometers to measure relative humidity. One of the thermometers is dry, and the other is saturated with water. The difference between the temperatures of the two thermometers is used to calculate relative humidity. A sling psychrometer (Fig. 5-2) allows the thermometers to be whirled by hand to provide the necessary ventilation of the dry bulb and wet bulb. Hygroscopic hygrometers use a hygroscopic chemical to absorb water vapor, and the relative humidity is determined gravimetrically (by weighing). An electric hygrometer uses a transducing element whose electrical properties are determined by water vapor content. A diffusion hygrometer measures the diffusion of water vapor through a porous membrane. A spectral hygrometer measures the absorption spectra of water.

Some electric hygrometers have a sensor that is small enough to be placed into a respiratory breathing circuit. An example is the Thunder Scientific BR-101B-SS (Fig. 5-3). This sensor is constructed of a semiconducting molecular diffusion barrier. When water vapor diffuses into the sensor, the conductivity of the device changes, which is translated into a display of relative humidity.

Particulate water suspended in a gas is called an aerosol. An aerosol is characterized by the size of its particles, which are usually referred to in units of mass median aerodynamic diameter (MMAD). MMAD is the particle size that evenly separates the mass of the particles. In other words, MMAD is the particle size above which 50% of the mass of the particles is found (and also below which 50% of the particles are found). To appreciate this idea, one must understand the relationship between the size of a particle and its mass, which is given by the geometric equation for the volume of a sphere. See Equation Box 5-2. The variability of particle size within an aerosol is stated as its geometric standard deviation (GSD).

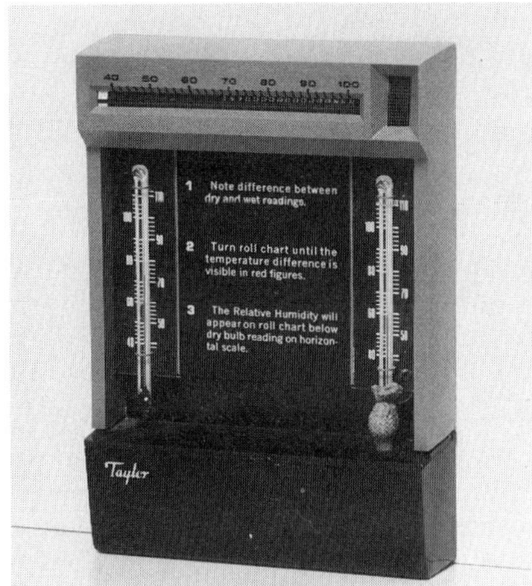

Figure 5-1. Dry bulb–wet bulb hygrometer used to measure ambient humidity.

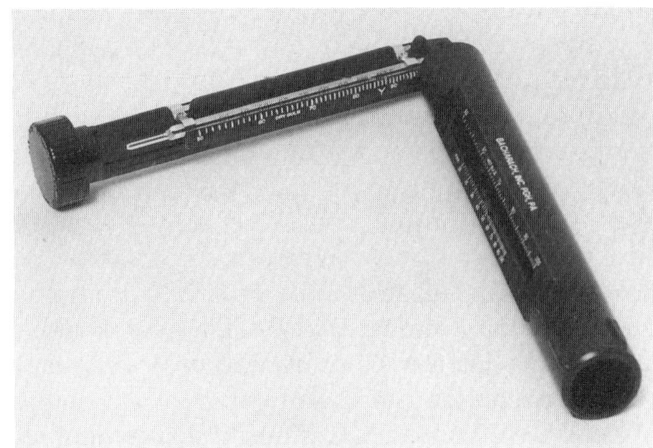

Figure 5-2. Sling psychrometer.

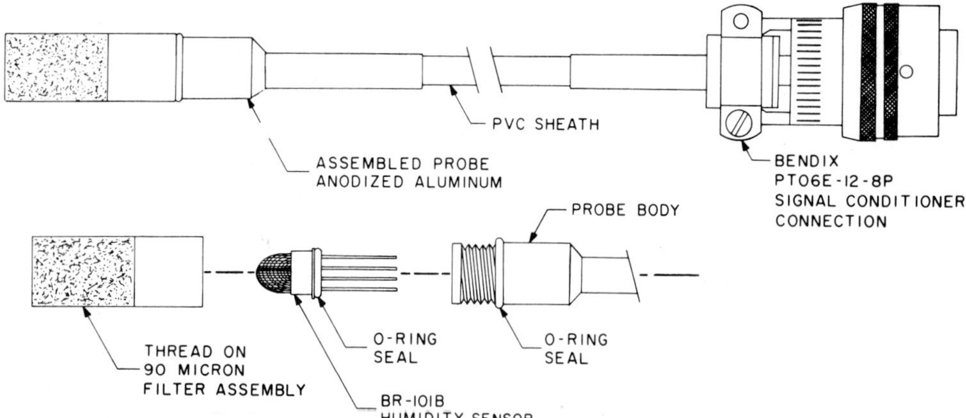

Figure 5-3. Thunder Scientific BR-101B-SS relative humidity sensor. (Courtesy of Thunder Scientific, Albuquerque, NM)

Physiologic Principles

Humidity therapy is commonly used to prevent the humidity deficit that can result from breathing a dry gas. A humidity deficit is the amount of humidity that is not present in the inspired gases and thus needs to be supplied by the body (primarily the upper airway). The output of any therapeutic gas delivery system should match the inspiratory conditions occurring at its point of entry into the respiratory system (Fig. 5-4).[1,2] If the level of heat and humidity is less than this, a humidity deficit may be produced. If the level of heat and humidity is greater than this, fluid overload and patient discomfort may be produced. Ideally, gases delivered to the nose and mouth (eg, cannula, mask) should be heated and humidified to room conditions. Gas delivered to the oropharynx should range from 29°C to 32°C at about 95% relative humidity. Gas bypassing the upper respiratory tract (through endotracheal tubes and tracheostomy tubes) should be heated to 32°C to 34°C at about 100% relative humidity.

Aerosols are used to overcome a humidity deficit, for the delivery of medications into the respiratory tract, and for bland aerosol therapy.[3] Bland aerosol therapy refers to the delivery of large volumes of saline or water into the respiratory tract to decrease inflammation of the upper airway (eg, croup, postextubation laryngeal edema), to liquefy lower respiratory tract secretions and thus aid in bronchial hygiene, and for sputum induction.

Equation Box 5-2: Relationship Between Volume and Radius for an Aerosol Particle

The volume of a sphere is determined as

$$V = \frac{4}{3} \pi r^3$$

where V is the volume of the sphere (the aerosol particle) and r is the radius of the sphere (aerosol particle). As indicated by this relationship, there will be very few particles with a diameter greater than the mass median aerodynamic diameter (MMAD). In other words, most of the particles will have a diameter less than the MMAD.

If an aerosol particle has a diameter of 4 μm (radius, 2 μm), its volume is 25.12 cubic μm. If the particle size decreases to 2 μm (radius, 1 μm), its volume decreases to 4.19 μm^3. Thus, a decrease in radius to 50% results in a decrease in volume to 17%.

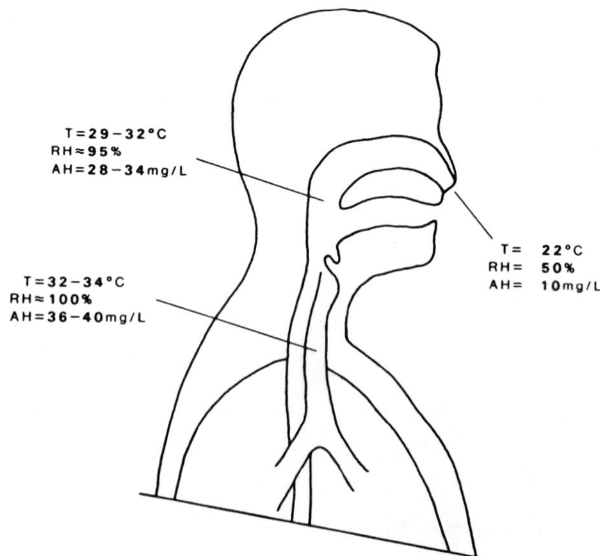

Figure 5-4. The temperature and relative humidity of air entering the respiratory tract at nose, oropharynx, and trachea, assuming a room temperature of 22°C and a relative humidity of 50%. (From Chatburn RL, Primiano FP. A rational basis for humidity therapy [editorial]. Respir Care 1987;32:249–254)

Several factors influence the penetration and deposition of aerosols in the respiratory tract, as described below.[4,5]

- *Sedimentation* is the deposition of aerosol in the lungs because of the effect of gravity. Stokes' law states that the rate of sedimentation is determined by the density and the diameter of the aerosol particle. See Equation Box 5-3. The larger the particle, the greater is the effect of gravity.
- *Inertial impaction* refers to the tendency of aerosol particles to be deposited when the gas stream changes directions. Thus, aerosol particles tend to be deposited at the bifurcations of airways.
- *Diffusion* is the deposition of very small particles because of the brownian movement surrounding gas molecules.
- The *physical nature of aerosol particles* affects their tendency to become larger or smaller as they penetrate the respiratory tract. Hygroscopic particles tend to take on water and thus become larger. Hypotonic particles tend to lose water and become smaller, whereas hypertonic particles tend to grow as they penetrate the respiratory tract. If an aerosol particle passes into a warm humid gas stream, it will tend to take on water and become larger.
- *Ventilatory pattern* affects aerosol penetration and deposition. Aerosol penetration and deposition improves significantly if a slow, rather than a fast, inspiratory flow rate is used. The volume of aerosol deposited in the lung can be improved by an increase in volume of inhalation, and an inspiratory breath hold will improve aerosol deposition in the lung. The optimal inspiratory pattern during therapeutic aerosol administration is a maximal slow inspiration of 5 to 6 seconds followed by an inspiratory hold of 10 seconds.
- *Pathologic obstruction* of airways decreases the penetration of aerosol into the lungs.
- An important determinant of aerosol penetration in the lungs is the *size of the particles*. Particles greater than 5 μm in diameter do not penetrate the nose. Particles in the 5- to 10-μm range can enter the lower respiratory tract with mouth breathing. Particles of 1- to 5-μm deposit in the lung periphery, with maximal deposition of particles in the 2- to 4-μm range. Particles smaller than 1 μm are very stable and may be exhaled rather than deposited in the lung. Most of the aerosol delivered from a therapeutic aerosol generator is not deposited in the lung. The majority (about 80%) is deposited in the upper respiratory tract. Only about 10% is deposited in the lung, and the remaining 10% is exhaled.

Equation Box 5-3: Stokes' Law

According to Stokes' law

$$\text{sedimentation} \propto D \cdot d^2$$

where D is the density of the particle and d is the diameter of the particle. If density doubles, sedimentation will also double. If the diameter of the particle doubles, sedimentation will quadruple.

Humidity and aerosol therapy is associated with several complications.[3,6] These include contamination of the lower respiratory tract, fluid overload, and increased volume of respiratory secretions. Cool aerosols can irritate the airways, resulting in an increase in airways resistance. For this reason, molecular high humidity rather than aerosol therapy should be used for humidification in patients with reactive airways.[7]

Low-Flow Humidifiers

Several types of humidifiers are used primarily for low-flow (≤ 10 L/min) applications. These include unheated passover humidifiers, bubble humidifiers, bubble diffuser humidifiers, jet diffuser (underwater jet) humidifiers, and jet humidifiers. These humidifiers are very inefficient, and their efficiency is roughly in the order listed in the previous sentence.

The bubble humidifier (Fig. 5-5) directs the flow of gas through a stem beneath the surface of the water reservoir to produce gas bubbles that rise to the water's surface. While the gas is in contact with the water, evaporation occurs to increase the relative humidity of the gas. When the bubbles reach the surface of the reservoir, the gas flows into the gas delivery system to the patient.

A diffuser can be added to the bottom of the stem of a bubble humidifier to produce a bubble diffuser humidifier (Fig. 5-6). The diffuser is a microgrid and is often constructed of a porous metal or plastic material. The purpose of the diffuser is to produce smaller bubbles and thus increase the total gas–water interface to increase the relative humidity.

A jet diffuser (Fig. 5-7) adds a jet to the stem immediately proximal to the diffuser. An opening lateral to the jet allows water to be entrained as the high-velocity, low-pressure gas exits the jet. In this device, water is drawn into the gas stream, which partially humidifies the gas before it passes through the diffuser and bubbles up the water reservoir.

A jet humidifier (Fig. 5-8) uses Bernoulli's principle. The gas exits the jet at a high velocity and low lateral pressure. This draws water up a capillary tube. As the water leaves the capillary tube, it is broken into an aerosol, which then evaporates to humidify the gas.

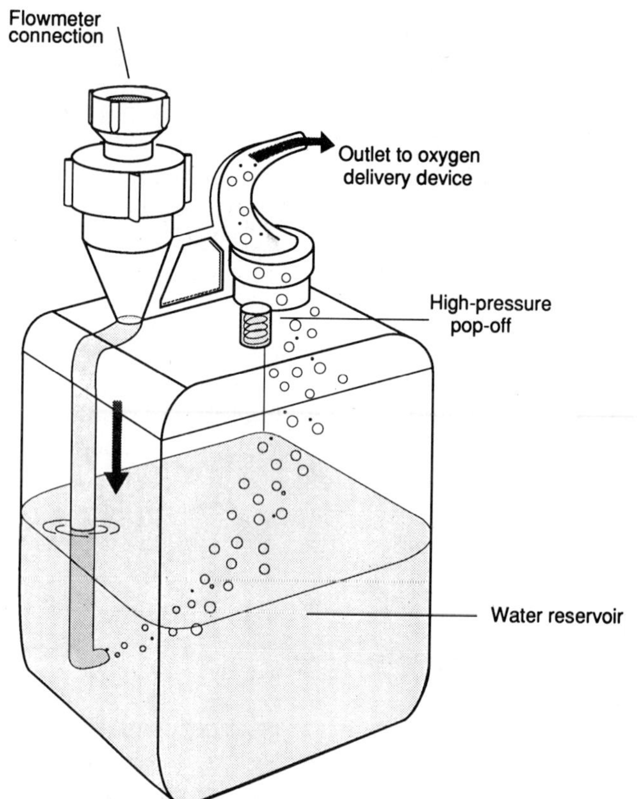

Figure 5-5. Bubble humidifier.

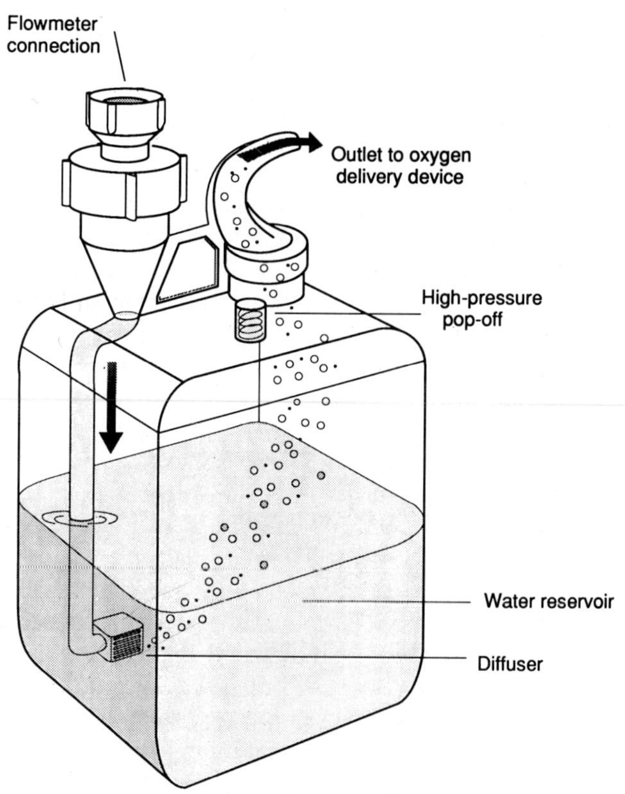

Figure 5-6. Bubble diffuser humidifier.

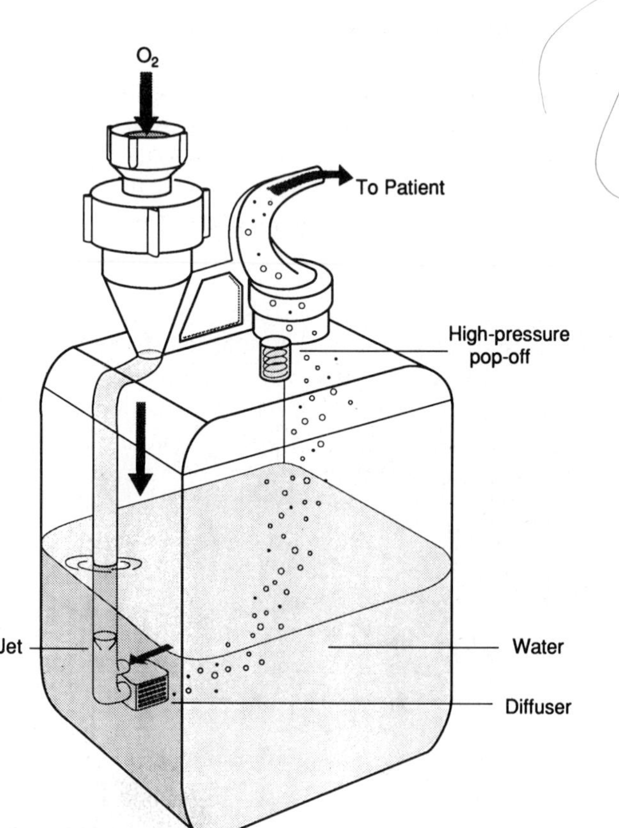

Figure 5-7. Jet diffuser.

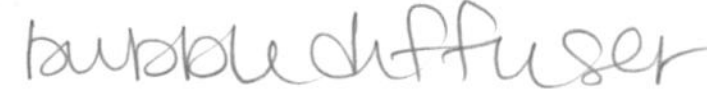

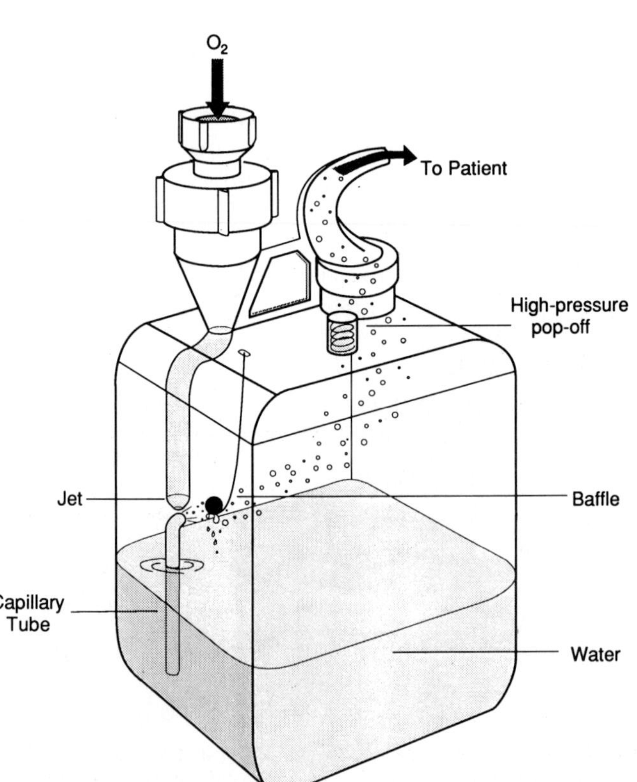

Figure 5-8. Jet humidifier.

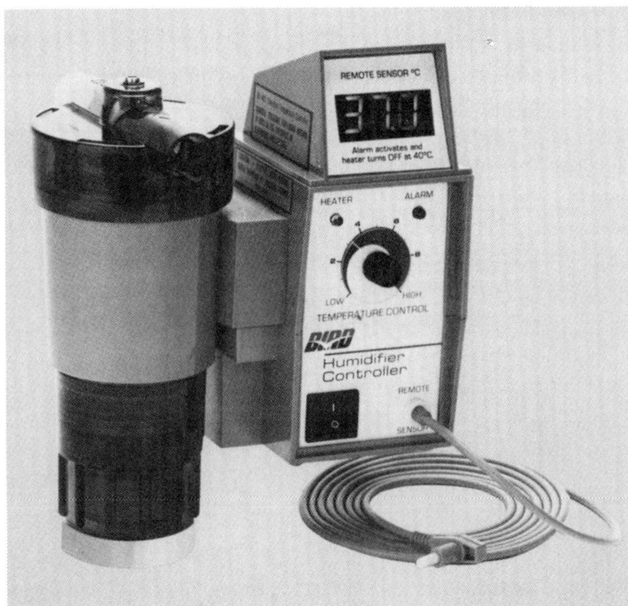

Figure 5-20. Bird wick humidifier. (Courtesy of Bird Products Corp, Palm Springs, CA)

midifiers are servo-controlled and include alarms. The Fisher and Paykel humidifier also uses a heated wire in the tubing leading to the patient.

The Marquest SCT 2000 heated humidifier has a separate heater/control unit and humidifying chamber (Fig. 5-23). The system can use either a simple heated passover humidification chamber or a heated wick humidifier chamber. The humidification chamber is disposable and is available in adult, pediatric, and neonatal sizes. The humidifier temperature is servo-controlled to the desired temperature at the patient's airway and allows the user to select both temperature and relative humidity settings. The system uses a heated wire circuit to minimize condensation.

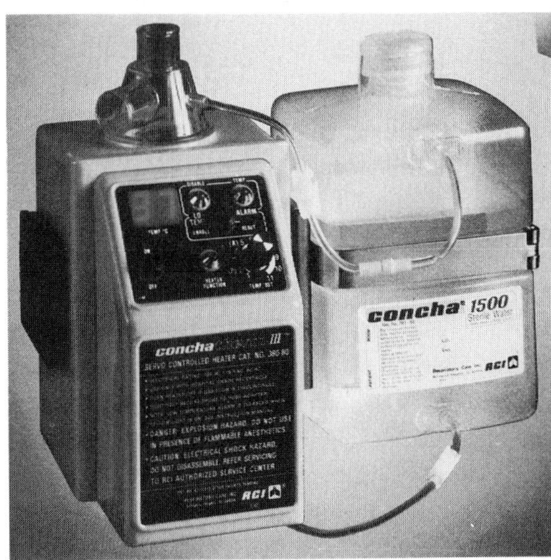

Figure 5-21. Hudson-RCI Conchatherm. (Courtesy of Hudson-RCI, Temecula, CA)

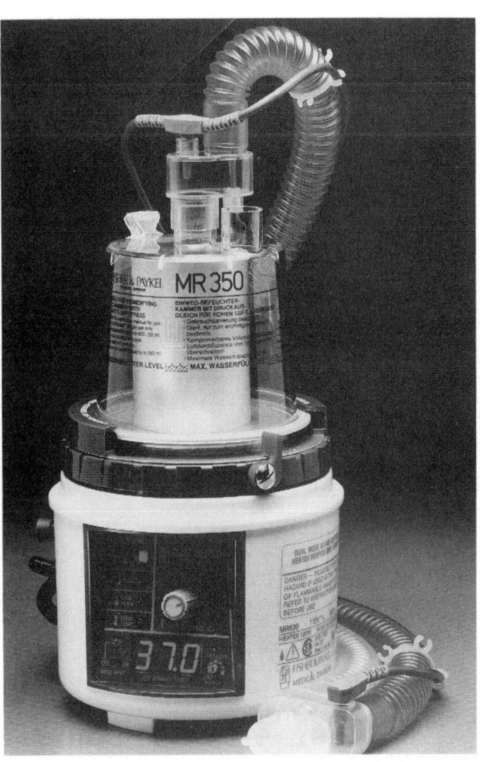

Figure 5-22. Fisher and Paykel MR600. (Courtesy of Baxter Medical, Valencia, CA)

The system also features a number of alarms, including high and low temperature protection.

The BEAR VH820 is an efficient heated passover humidifier. It has separate humidifier and control modules (Fig. 5-24). The humidifier module has a large spiral surface area (Figure 5-25). A small amount of water is heated, and the water vapor that coats the interior of the module is carried to the patient by the gas flow. The temperature at the patient's airway is servo-controlled. Heat loss and condensation are minimized by use of a heated wire circuit. An automatic water filling system keeps the internal compliance

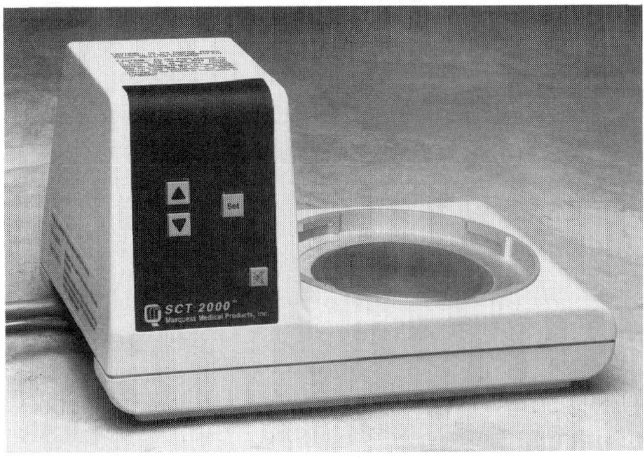

Figure 5-23. Marquest SCT 2000 heated humidifier. (Courtesy of Marquest Medical, Valencia, CA)

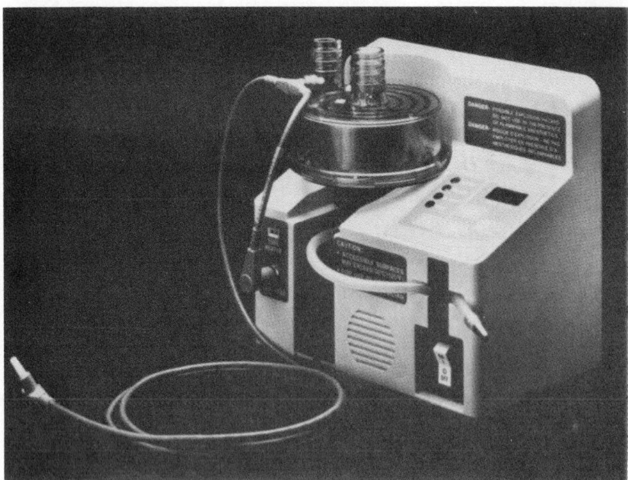

Figure 5-24. Bear VH820 humidifier. (Courtesy of Bear Medical Corp, Riverside, CA)

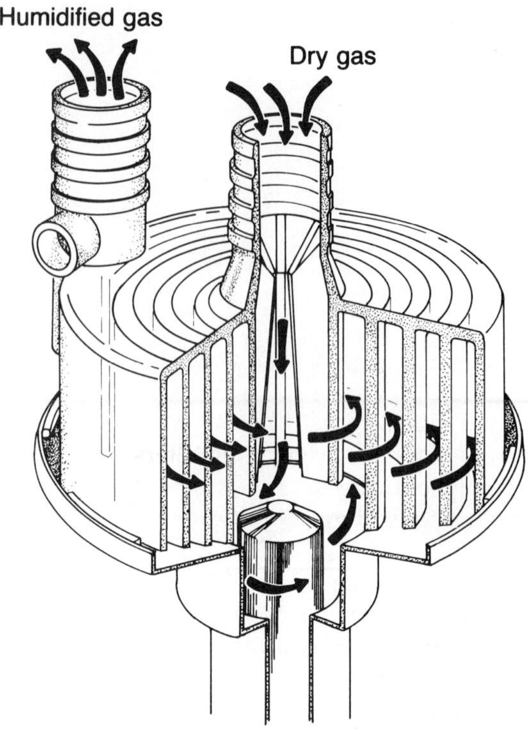

Figure 5-25. Flow-through spiral surface of Bear VH820. (Courtesy of Bear Medical Corp, Riverside, CA)

constant. This humidifier also has a comprehensive alarm system.

The Inspiron Vapor Phase humidifier is a servo-controlled unit that uses a hydrophobic filter (Fig. 5-26). Water is heated under the filter, and the water vapor passes through the hydrophobic filter to humidify the gas (Fig. 5-27). The hydrophobic filter in this humidifier allows no microbial penetration. Only pure water vapor is permitted to pass through the filter.

Another membrane humidification device is the Oxygen Enrichment Company OE PLUS. The OE PLUS is designed primarily for home oxygen use and produces 6 L/min of 30% to 40% oxygen with 30 to 38 mg/L of water vapor. This system draws room air through a selectively permeable membrane, which enriches the oxygen and water vapor. A heated delivery tube is used to keep the humidified flow to the patient in the vapor phase.

Artificial Noses

Artificial nose is the generic term used to describe several similar humidification devices. By definition, an artificial nose is a passively acting humidifier that collects the patient's expired heat and moisture and returns it during the following inspiration (Fig. 5-28). The material in which the heat and moisture is stored distinguishes the four types of artificial noses:

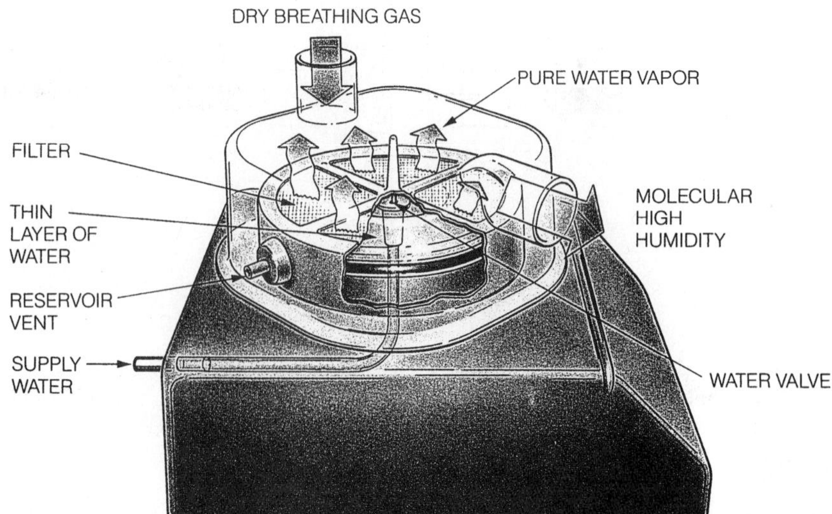

Figure 5-26. Functional diagram of the Inspiron Vapor Phase humidifier. (Courtesy of Inspiron)

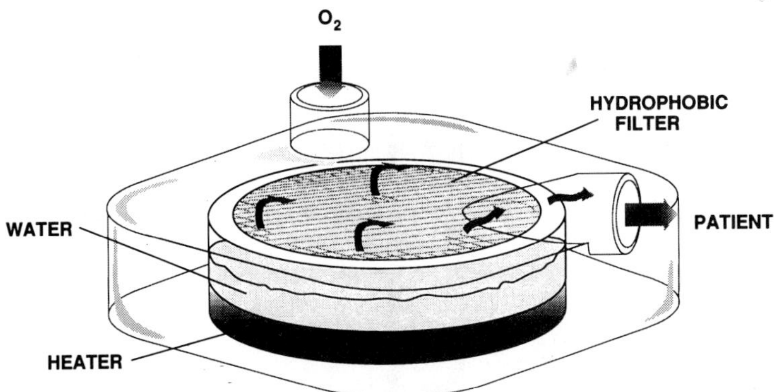

Figure 5-27. Vapor phase humidifier.

- heat and moisture exchangers (HME)
- heat and moisture exchanging filters (HMEF)
- hygroscopic condenser humidifiers (HCH)
- hygroscopic condenser humidifier filters (HCHF)

The HME is the simplest of these devices and was the first used.[19,20] It generally uses a layered aluminum insert with or without an additional fibrous element. Aluminum exchanges temperature quickly, and during expiration condensation forms between the aluminum layers. The retained heat and moisture are returned during inspiration. The HME is the least efficient of artificial noses. Figure 5-29 shows two commercially available HMEs.

The only HMEF is the Pall Conserve (Fig. 5-30). Originally marketed as a bacterial filter, it also functions as an HMEF.[21] Several studies have shown that the Conserve is capable of delivering 18 to 28 mg H_2O/L to the airway.[22–25] It is also an effective bacterial filter. It contains a fibrous insert that is hydrophobic and thus repels water and traps heat and moisture on the patient side of the insert. After prolonged use, condensation can be seen to form inside the housing of the Conserve. The manufacturer recommends that the Conserve be kept perpendicular to the patient such that any of this condensation will be returned to the airway.

The HCH is the most popular type of artificial nose (Fig. 5-31). These devices are all very similar. All use a hygroscopically treated insert that allows efficient exchange of moisture. They differ only in size, shape, and type of insert. Inserts generally consist of polypropylene or paper and are treated with lithium chloride or calcium chloride. Comparative studies have shown that most HCHs are capable of delivering 22 to 30 mg H_2O/L, with the larger devices being the most efficient.[22–25]

Presently, the only HCHF is the Humid-Vent Filter from Gibeck-Dryden (Fig. 5-32). This device uses the hygroscopically treated paper roll with the addition of a thin bacterial filter between the insert and the source of inspired gas.

Table 5-2 compares commercially available artificial noses. These devices are attractive alternatives to heated humidification because of their low cost, passive operation, and ease of use. Additionally, there is some evidence to suggest that use of an artificial nose can reduce the incidence of nosocomial infection and extend the time between ventilator circuit changes.[26,27] Long-term use of artificial noses during mechanical

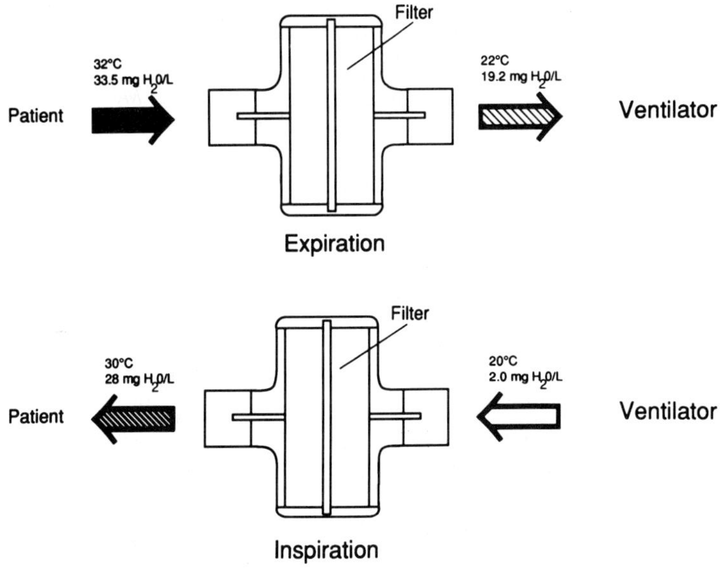

Figure 5-28. Operation of a typical artificial nose. (Top.) Warm, humid gas from the patient passes through the insert where a portion of the heat and moisture are trapped. (Bottom.) During the next inspiration, cool, dry gas enters the insert where the heat and moisture is picked up and returned to the patient.

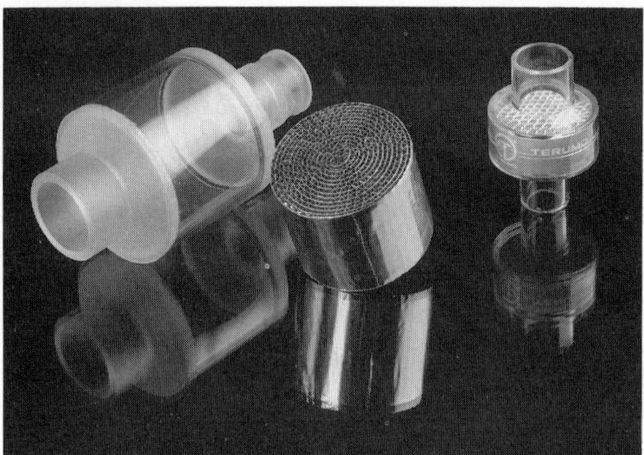

Figure 5-29. The Teurmo Breath-Aid and Dameca HME.

ventilation is controversial. Although the most efficient devices can provide 26 to 28 mg H_2O/L, most authors recommend that patients be evaluated every 24 hours for evidence of inadequate humidification (eg, thick secretions, bronchial casts). If signs of inadequate humidification become evident, heated humidification should be initiated (Fig. 5-33).[28]

Situations in which artificial noses are ideally suited include patient transport (where heated humidification is impractical) and during anesthesia. Spontaneously breathing patients with an artificial airway may also benefit from an artificial nose. Several devices are modified for this purpose (Fig. 5-34). These devices serve a dual purpose in this application. They provide humidity to prevent incrustation of secretions, and they filter the inspired gas of dust and other small particles. There are several instances when artificial noses are contraindicated:

- Patients who produce copious amounts of sputum and require therapeutic humidity. The lack of therapeutic humidity will result in thickening of secretions. Occasionally, the patient will cough secretions into the artificial nose. The presence of secretions in the insert of the artificial nose will significantly increase resistance. If contamination of the artificial nose with secretions occurs, it should be replaced.
- Patients receiving very small or very large tidal volumes. With small tidal volumes, the deadspace of the artificial nose may compromise ventilation and lead to CO_2 retention. With excessively high volumes (>1 L) the ability to humidify gases will be reduced. Most manufacturers provide a range of tidal volumes within which the device should be used.
- Patients with high (>10 L/min) levels of spontaneous minute ventilation. The inserts inside artificial noses will produce a measurable increase in airway resistance. During use, this resistance tends

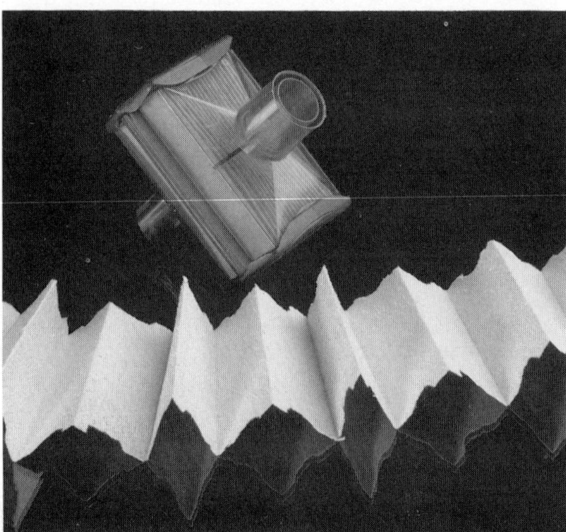

Figure 5-30. The Pall Conserve heat and moisture exchanging filter.

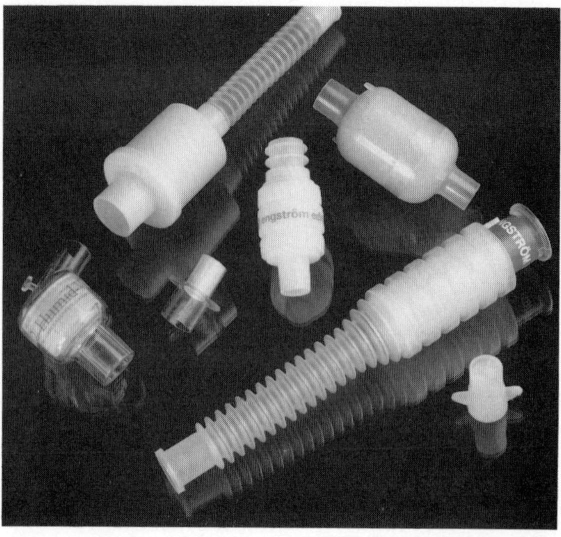

Figure 5-31. Examples of hygroscopic condenser humidifiers.

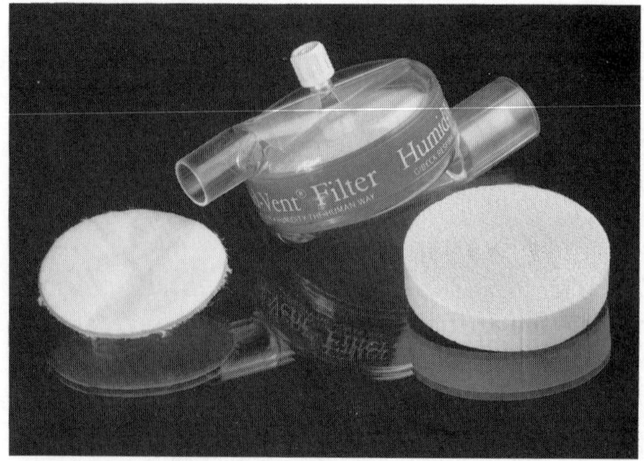

Figure 5-32. The Gibeck-Dryden hygroscopic condenser humidifying filter. (Courtesy of Gibeck-Dryden, Indianapolis, IN)

TABLE 5-2. Comparison of Commercially Available Artificial Noses

Device	Weight (g)	Deadspace (mL)	Type of Insert	Maximum Output (mg H_2O/L)	Tidal Volume Range (mL)
Heat and Moisture Exchangers					
Dameca HME	44	62	Corrugated aluminum roll	16	NS
Vitalograph Vapour Condenser	30		Stainless steel screens	16	NS
Teurmo Breath Aid	14	10	Alternated aluminum and cellulose disks	14	NS
Heat and Moisture Exchanging Filter					
Pall Conserve	47	98	Pleated, multilayered ceramic filter	25	150–1200
Hygroscopic Condenser Humidifiers					
Engstrom Edith	18	89	Polypropylene fiber coated with lithium chloride	27	250–1300
Engstrom Edith 1,000	9	28	Polypropylene fiber coated with lithium chloride	27	250–1000
Gibeck Humid-Vent-1	11	10	Corrugated paper roll coated with calcium chloride	25	50–600
Gibeck Humid-Vent-2	18	25	Corrugated paper roll coated with calcium chloride	26	200–1200
Gibeck Humid-Vent Mini	4	2.4	Corrugated paper roll coated with calcium chloride	30	5–50
Mallinkrodt In-Line Foam Nose	16	60	Polyurethane foam treated lithium chloride	24	NS
Siemens Elema 153	25	70	Hygroscopically treated cellulose sponge and synthetic felt	28	400–1200
Vital Signs HCH	10	42	Spun polypropylene treated with lithium chloride	28	400–1500
Vital Signs Neonatal HCH	4	2	Spun polypropylene treated with lithium chloride	33	5–50
Hygroscopic Condenser Humidifier Filter					
Gibeck-Dryden Humid-Vent Filter	44	63	Corrugated paper roll coated with calcium chloride with bacterial filter	31	300–1500

NS, not specified.

Data from references 20–25.

to increase; and in patients with high minute volumes, this may result in an increased work of breathing.[29,30] These patients should be monitored for signs of respiratory distress.

- Cases in which the expired tidal volume does not traverse the artificial nose (bronchopleural fistula, incompetent intratracheal tube cuffs). For proper function, both cool, dry, inspired gases and warm, moist expiratory gases must travel through the insert. This cycle is necessary for the efficient exchange of heat and water vapor. Patients with bronchopleural fistula and incompetent intratracheal tube cuffs will not have adequate expired volumes through the device, causing this cycle to break down.

Artificial noses should never be used in conjunction with heated humidifiers or nebulizers. This would result in excessive airway resistance and inefficient humidification. At present, use of an artificial nose during mechanical ventilation for less than 72 hours seems prudent, providing the aforementioned problems are considered. Use during transport and anesthesia should be considered routine. Further study is required to determine the use of artificial noses in long-term ventilatory support.

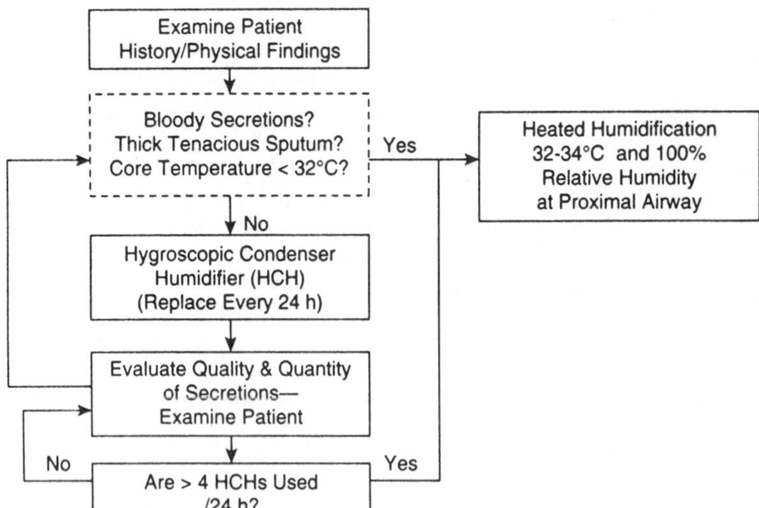

Figure 5-33. University of Cincinnati algorithm for application of an artificial nose.

Atomizers Versus Nebulizers

An atomizer has three primary components (Fig. 5-35): a reservoir containing the liquid to be aerosolized, a capillary tube, and a jet. The capillary tube is adjacent to the jet. As gas passes through the jet orifice, the low lateral pressure draws solution up the capillary tube and the gas stream emerging from the jet breaks the liquid into particles. Atomizers are used most commonly to deliver anesthetic medications to the upper airway during laryngoscopy and bronchoscopy (Fig. 5-36).

The addition of a baffle ball converts an atomizer to a nebulizer (see Fig. 5-36). The baffle ball decreases the size of the particles and produces particles of a more uniform size. Although a baffle can be any structure that acts to screen larger particles by impaction, the nebulizer specifically has a baffle ball. Nebulizers are often classified as either mainstream or sidestream. In the mainstream nebulizer, the main flow of gas passes through the nebulizer. In the sidestream nebulizer, the aerosol is passed from the nebulizer into the main gas flow. A nebulizer also can be classified as slipstream, which is a combination of mainstream and sidestream.

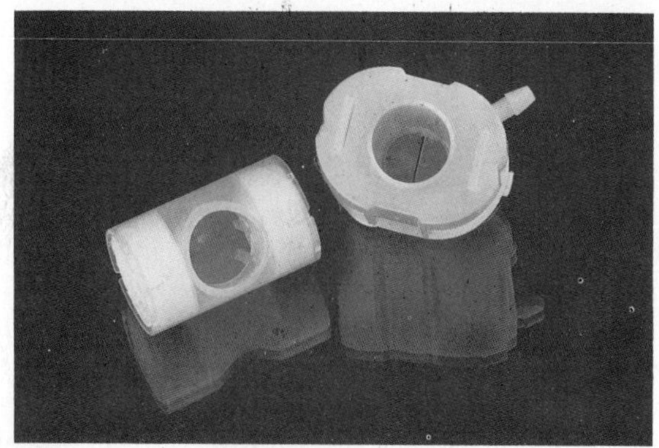

Figure 5-34. Artificial noses used for spontaneously breathing patients with a tracheostomy.

Small-Volume Medication Nebulizers

Small-volume medication nebulizers, or gas-powered hand-held nebulizers, are used for therapeutic aerosol administration (Fig. 5-37). A small volume of active drug and a larger volume of diluent (usually saline or water) is put in the nebulizer, and this solution is then nebulized by a flow of compressed gas (air or oxygen). Some of the solution placed into the nebulizer is trapped in the nebulizer. This trapped solution, sometimes called dead volume, is not available to the patient and is thus wasted.[31–33] To minimize the amount of solution trapped in the nebulizer, a flow of 8 L/min and a diluent volume of 4 mL should be used. A flow of 8 L/min also produces a more therapeutic particle size than that produced at lower flows.

Small-volume medication nebulizers usually operate at a continuous gas flow. This results in wasting of medication during the expiratory phase of the patient. To reduce this wastage of medication, a patient-controlled T-piece can be put in the circuit between the gas delivery tubing and the nebulizer. In this configuration, the solution will be nebulized only during inspiration. However, this may be difficult for some patients to coordinate. A short tube reservoir can be attached to the nebulizer, which may increase the amount of medication delivered to the respiratory tract.[34]

Specially constructed small-volume nebulizers should be used when contamination of the ambient

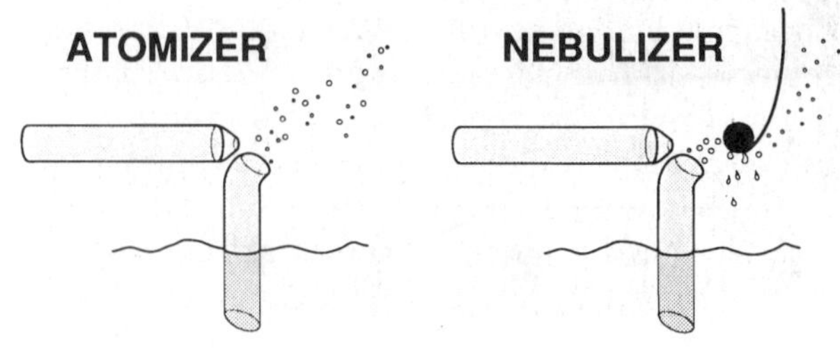

Figure 5-35. Atomizer and nebulizer.

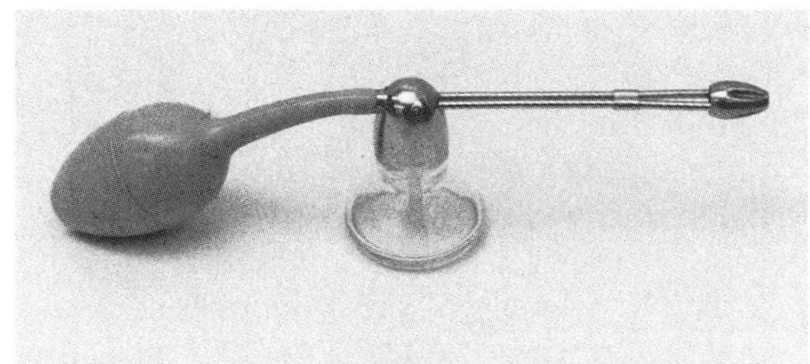

Figure 5-36. Squeeze bulb atomizer.

environment with the aerosolized drug needs to be avoided. The most common example of this is the use of aerosolized pentamidine (Pentam). In these cases, the nebulizer is fitted with one-way valves and filters to prevent gross contamination of the environment. Examples of these devices include the Cadema Aero-Tech II and the Respirgard II (Fig. 5-38). These devices also produce a very small particle size (MMAD, 1–2 μm), which is necessary to improve alveolar deposition of the drug.[35]

Metered-Dose Inhalers

A metered-dose inhaler (MDI) is a convenient means of therapeutic aerosol administration.[36,37] The MDI is commonly used by stable outpatients and is less commonly used for hospitalized patients. The MDI consists of a drug-filled canister that is fitted to a mouthpiece actuator (Figs. 5-39 and 5-40). Activation by compression of the canister into the mouthpiece results in release of a unit dose of medication. The amount of drug remaining in an MDI can be estimated by weighing or by placing it into a pan of water (Fig. 5–41).

Correct use of an MDI requires patient coordination and practice. It is usually necessary for the respiratory care practitioner to teach the patient the correct method of use of an MDI, because most patients have difficulty learning to use an MDI correctly by reading the package insert. Before activation, the cap is removed from the mouthpiece and the MDI is shaken. The canister must be held upright for activation. The MDI is activated near the beginning of a slow (ideally, 5 to 6 seconds), deep inspiration through the mouth. The patient should be encouraged not to forcibly exhale before beginning the deep breath during which the MDI is activated. At the end of the deep inspiration, the patient should be encouraged to hold his or her breath for as long as 10 seconds and then exhale slowly. The MDI is activated only once for each deep breath. If more than one puff is prescribed, the patient should wait several minutes before administering the next puff. The tongue should be positioned so that it does not obstruct the flow of aerosol through the mouth. To avoid complications due to pharyngeal deposition of the steroids discharged from the MDI, the patient should be encouraged to rinse the mouth and pharynx if these drugs are used.

For patients with arthritic hands, a VentEase device is available that aids in activation of the MDI (Fig. 5-42). A variety of MDI auxiliary devices are also available to overcome problems due to patient coordination and pharyngeal deposition.[38–41] The most commonly used of these are shown in Figure 5-43. Some of these devices provide auditory feedback to achieve a

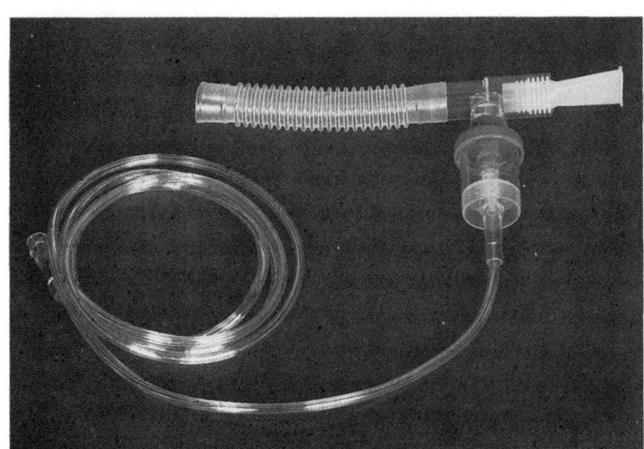

Figure 5-37. Small-volume medication nebulizer.

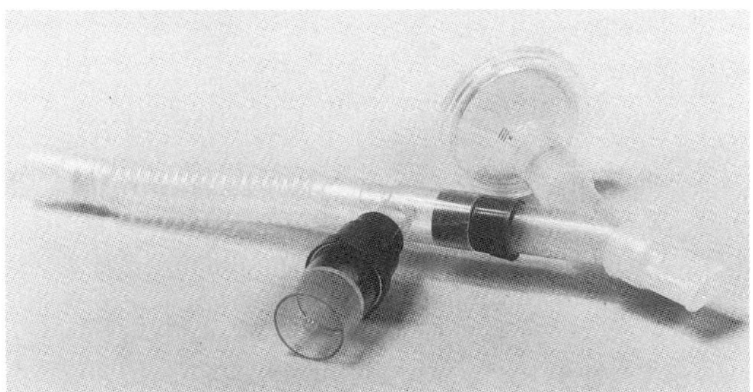

Figure 5-38. Respirgard II nebulizer system.

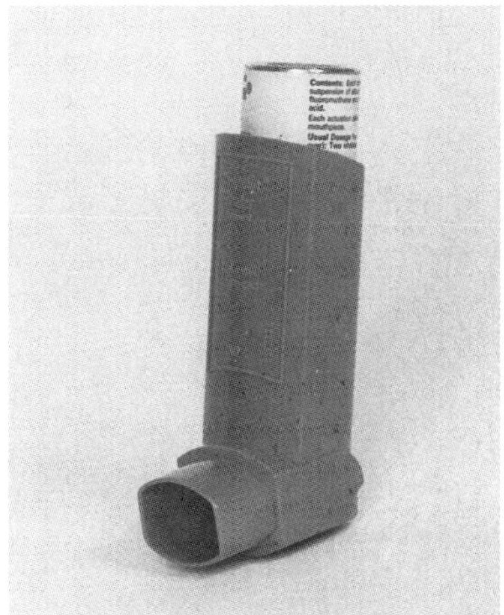

Figure 5-39. Metered-dose inhaler.

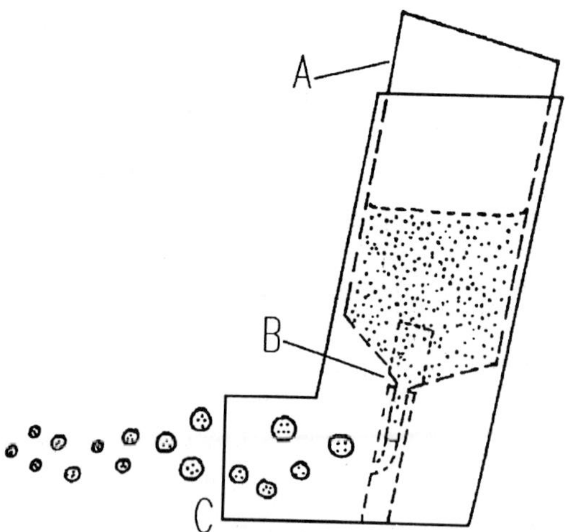

Figure 5-40. Metered-dose inhaler. (A.) Canister. (B.) Metering chamber. (C.) Mouthpiece.

slow inspiratory flow rate, and the InspirEase also provides visual and tactile feedback to help the patient in achieving a targeted volume. Breath-actuated MDIs are available and may be useful for some patients with poor hand–breath coordination.

Dry Powder Inhalers

Spinhalers and rotahalers (Figs. 5-44 and 5-45) are used to dispense a dry powdered drug into the airway.[41] The Spinhaler is used for the administration of cromolyn sodium (Intal), and the Rotahaler is used for administration of albuterol (Ventolin). In both cases, a capsule of powdered drug is placed into the device.

The Spinhaler punctures holes in the capsule with a pair of needles. The Spinhaler is breath activated, and inhaling through the device causes a rotor to rotate rapidly, which disperses the powdered drug into the air stream. The Rotahaler separates the capsule by a twisting motion. When the patient inhales through the device, the powder is dispersed into the gas stream and delivered into the respiratory tract.

An advantage of a dry powder inhaler over the MDI is that the device is breath actuated. A major disadvantage of these devices is that the capsule must be added to the device before it is used. Use of the dry powder inhaler also differs from the MDI in that the patient should be instructed to use a fast inhalation, rather than a slow inhalation as is desirable for the MDI.

Spinning Disk Nebulizers

The spinning disk nebulizer, or centrifugal force nebulizer, is used as a room humidifier to increase the ambient relative humidity (Fig. 5-46). This device is electrically powered and uses the principle of the Archimedean screw. A disk rotates around a hollow shaft that is immersed into a water reservoir. As the disk spins, water is drawn through the hollow shaft and out an opening onto the disk. The water is hurled against a series of baffles, which break it into smaller particles. Blades on the disk create an air current, which carries the smaller particles into the room. These room nebulizers are not commonly recommended because they can be a source of bacterial contamination of the environment.

Pneumatic Jet Nebulizers

A commonly used large-volume nebulizer is the jet (or mechanical) nebulizer (Fig. 5-47). This type of nebulizer is used for bland aerosol therapy and to increase

(text continues on page 107)

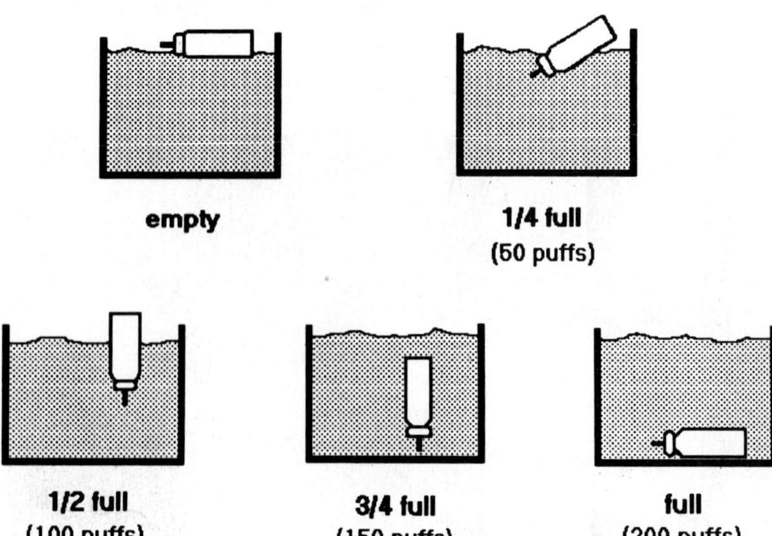

Figure 5-41. Placing the metered-dose inhaler into a pan of water can be used to estimate the amount of drug remaining. If the canister is full, it will sink to the bottom. If it is empty, it will float.

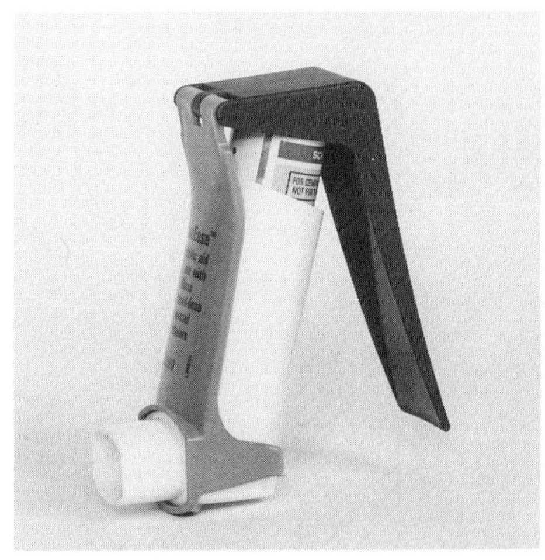

Figure 5-42. Metered-dose inhaler with VentEase.

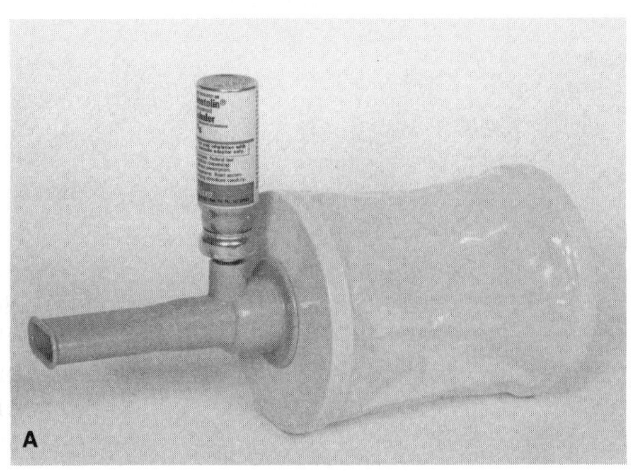

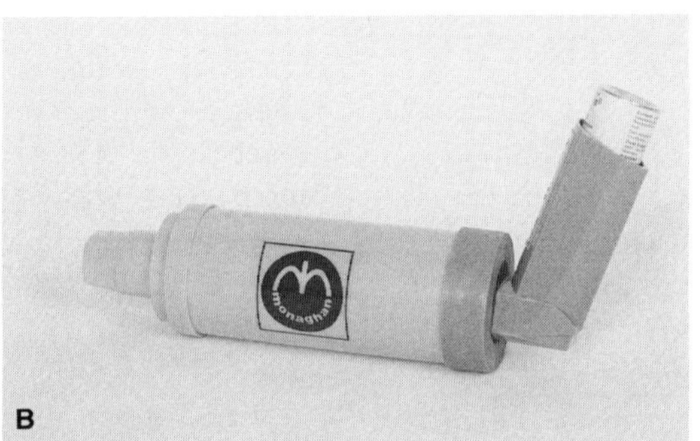

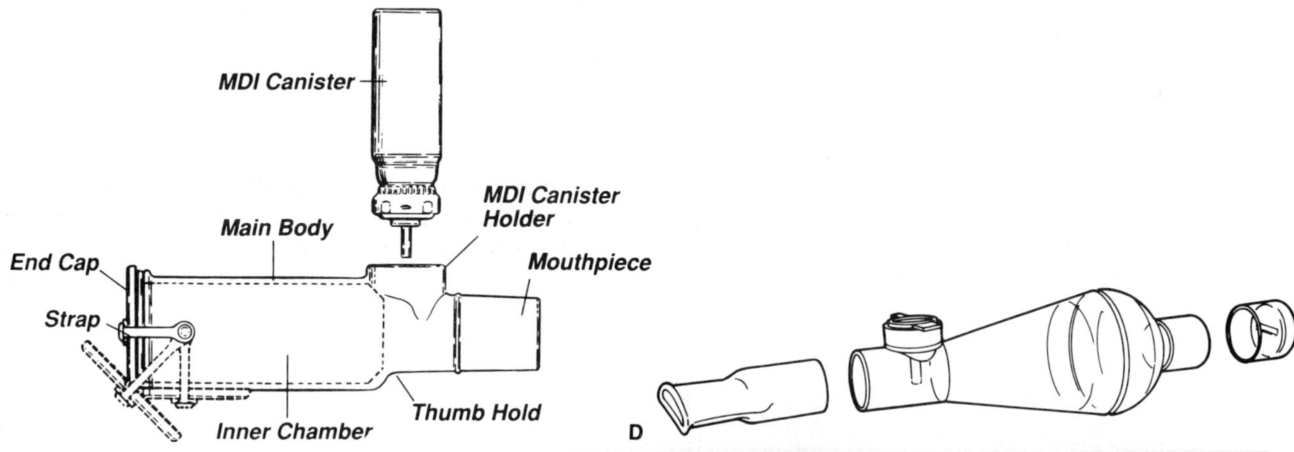

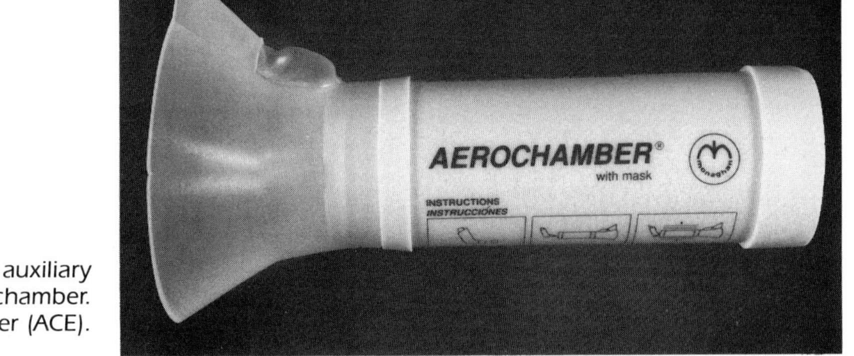

Figure 5-43. Metered-dose inhaler auxiliary spacer devices. (A.) InspirEase. (B.) Aerochamber. (C.) OptiHaler. (D.) Aerosol Cloud Enhancer (ACE). (E.) Aerochamber with mask.

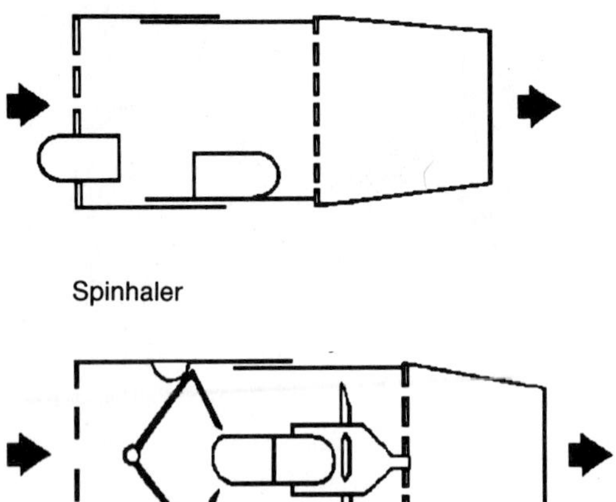

Figure 5-44. Rotahaler and spinhaler.

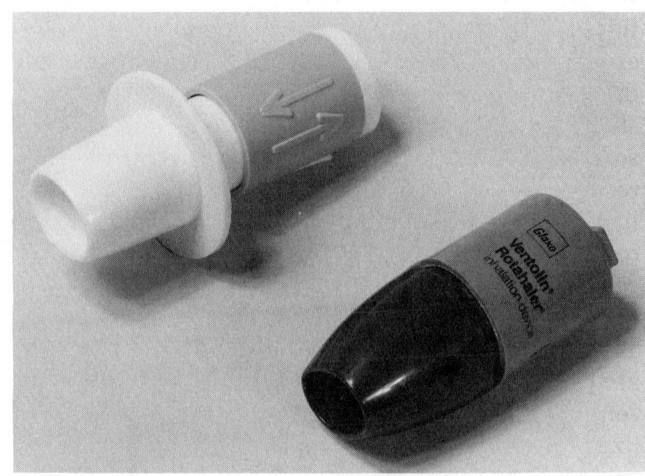

Figure 5-45. Spinhaler (left) and rotahaler (right).

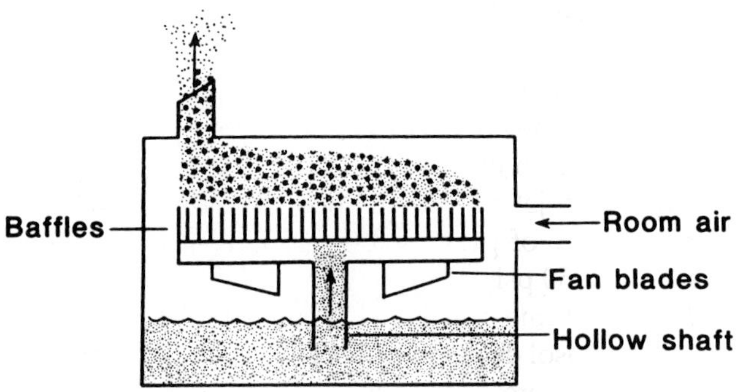

Figure 5-46. Spinning disk nebulizer.

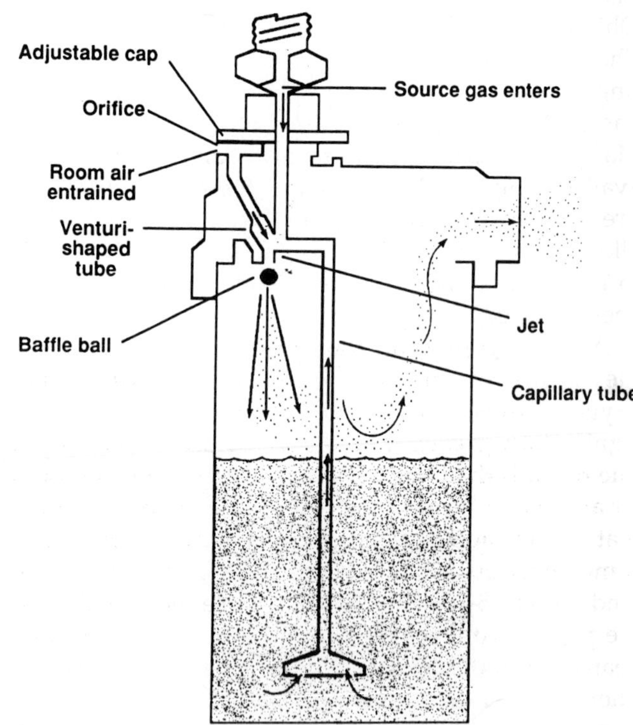

Figure 5-47. Pneumatic jet nebulizer.

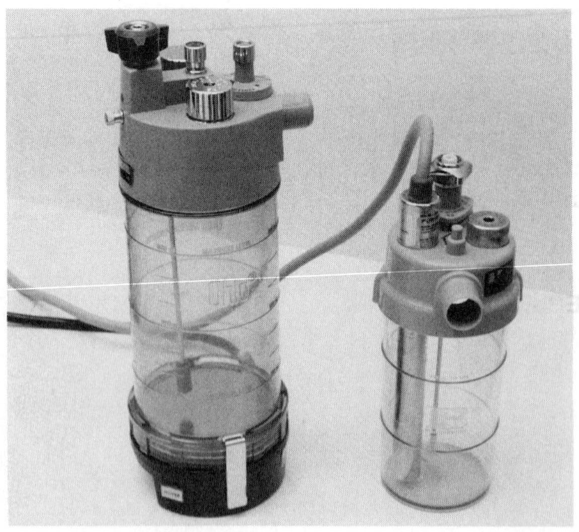

Figure 5-48. Ohio Deluxe (left) and Puritan All-Purpose (right) nebulizers.

the inspired humidity of patients with artificial airways. In this device, a high-pressure gas is directed through a jet orifice, resulting in creation of a low lateral pressure (Bernoulli's principle). This low pressure draws water up a capillary tube, where the gas stream shatters it and breaks it into small particles. The aerosol is then thrown against a baffle ball, which further reduces the size of the particles. The jet of this nebulizer is also used to entrain room air. This mixing of room air with source oxygen is used to adjust the concentration of oxygen to the patient and the total flow of gas to the patient. For example, a nebulizer set at 40% will increase the total flow fourfold and the aerosol output by 50% (as compared with the 100% setting). However, as the oxygen setting on the nebulizer decreases, the density of the aerosol also decreases because the increase in flow is greater than the corresponding increase in aerosol production.

Jet nebulizers are available as disposable and nondisposable models. Two nondisposable nebulizers that have been commonly used in the past are the Ohio Deluxe and the Puritan All-Purpose (Fig. 5-48). The Ohio Deluxe nebulizer has oxygen dilution settings of 40%, 60%, and 100%. The Puritan All-Purpose has oxygen dilution settings of 40%, 70%, and 100%. Many disposable jet nebulizers are also commercially available (Fig. 5-49), and some of these are available as prefilled units. Many of the disposable nebulizers allow the oxygen concentration to be varied from 30% to 100%. Evaluations of pneumatic jet nebulizers have been reported.[42,43]

As the oxygen setting on a jet nebulizer is increased, the total flow to the patient is decreased. With higher oxygen settings, the patient's inspiratory flow may be significantly greater than the flow from the nebulizer. The result is that the patient breathes in ambient room air and may have an actual FIO_2 considerably less than that set on the nebulizer. To overcome this problem, some practitioners hook two nebulizers together in tandem (Fig. 5-50).[44,45] This will double the total flow to the patient. Another alternative is to use a high-flow heated humidifier rather than a nebulizer system. There are also high-flow jet nebulizers that are commercially available. If water accumulates in the tubing leading from a nebulizer system, the resistance to flow will increase. This will have two undesirable effects. First, it will decrease the flow of gas to the patient. Second, it will place back-pressure on the nebulizer, which will decrease the amount of room air entrained and thus increase the delivered oxygen concentration.

Many commercially available jet nebulizers can be heated to increase their humidity output. This can be accomplished in several ways. The water in the reservoir can be heated with an immersion heater, by wrapping a heater around the reservoir, or by placing a heater under the base of the reservoir. Alternatively, the aerosol can be heated as it leaves the nebulizer.

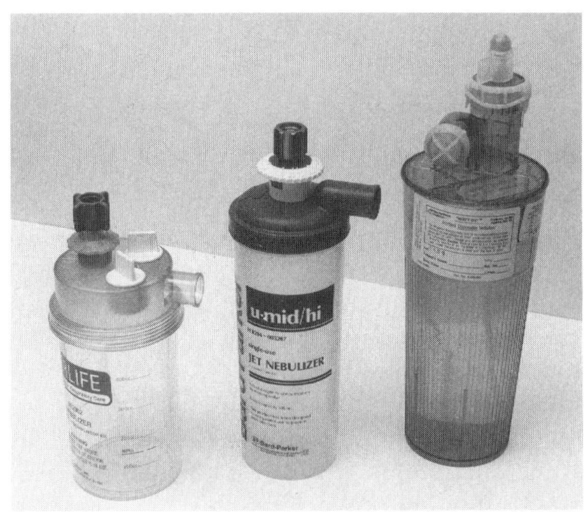

Figure 5-49. Disposable pneumatic jet nebulizers.

Particles produced by a jet nebulizer range from 2 to 20 μm, with 40% to 50% of the particles in the 2- to 4-μm range. The total output of a jet nebulizer is 30 to 50 mg/L, depending on gas flow, air entrainment, and whether the nebulizer is heated. Most jet nebulizers are designed to operate at an oxygen flow of 8 to 15 L/min. The jet orifice of most nebulizers will not allow a flow of greater than 15 L/min at a driving pressure of 50 psig.

Large-volume nebulizers are also available for therapeutic aerosol delivery. These are used for continuous beta-agonist aerosol therapy and offer the convenience of not needing to frequently refill the nebulizer cup during this therapy.

Babington Nebulizers

The Babington (or hydrodynamic) nebulizer produces a dense aerosol with an MMAD of 3 to 5 μm and output of 60 to 70 mg/L.[3] A high-pressure gas source enters the nebulizer and is split into two directions (Fig.

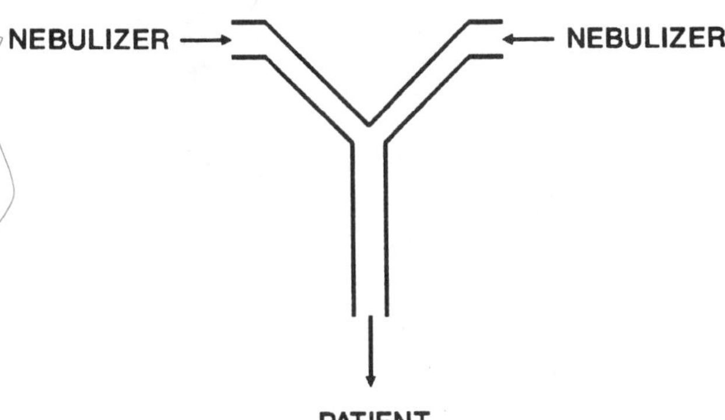

Figure 5-50. Jet nebulizers can be used in tandem to increase total flow to the patient.

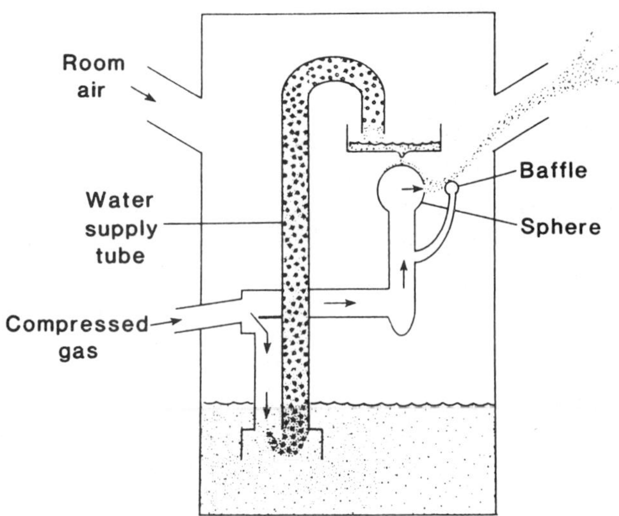

Figure 5-51. Babington nebulizer.

5-51). Part of the gas travels into the water reservoir and forces water up a capillary tube, where it flows into a container and drips over a hollow glass sphere. The remaining flow is forced through a small opening in the glass sphere, where it strikes the water and produces an aerosol. The aerosol is then thrown against a baffle, which further reduces the size of the particles. Similar to the jet nebulizer, the oxygen concentration can be varied from about 30% to 100%. Examples of the Babington nebulizer are the Hydro-Sphere and Solosphere (Fig. 5-52).

Ultrasonic Nebulizers

The ultrasonic nebulizer (Fig. 5-53) uses a piezoelectric transducer to produce ultrasonic waves that pass through the solution to be aerosolized.[3] At the surface

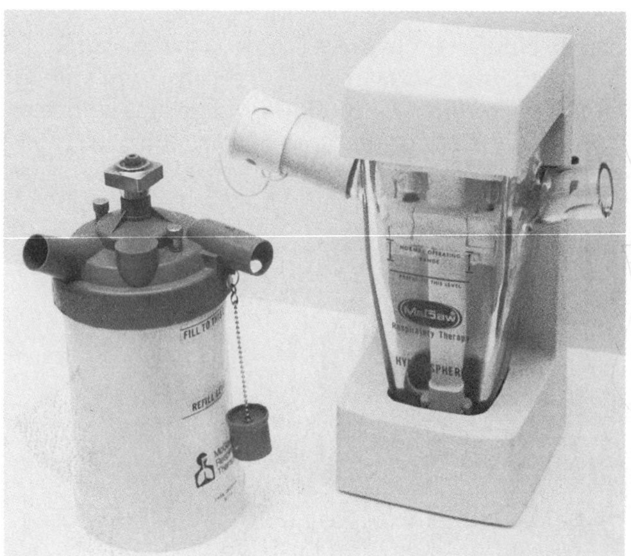

Figure 5-52. Hydrosphere (right) and Solosphere (left) nebulizers.

of the solution, these ultrasonic waves create an aerosol. The ultrasonic nebulizer creates particle sizes of 1 to 10 μm, with an MMAD of 3 μm. The output of the ultrasonic nebulizer is 60 to 100 mg/L.

There are three parts of the ultrasonic nebulizer: the power unit, the transducer, and a fan. The power unit converts electrical energy to high-frequency ultrasonic waves at a frequency of 1.3 to 1.4 MHz. The frequency of the ultrasonic waves determines the size of the particles, with an inverse relationship between frequency and particle size. The frequency is not user adjustable and is controlled by the Federal Communications Commission (FCC) because this frequency is in the range of radio waves. The power unit also controls the amplitude of the ultrasonic waves. This is user adjustable, with an increase in amplitude resulting in an increase in output from the ultrasonic nebulizer. The ultrasonic waves are carried from the power unit to the transducer by a radiofrequency cable.

The transducer in the ultrasonic nebulizer is usually ceramic and is piezoelectric. This means that it changes shape when high-frequency radio waves are applied to it. Specifically, the transducer vibrates at the frequency of the ultrasonic waves applied to it. The transducer is found in two shapes (Fig. 5-54). The concave transducer focuses the ultrasonic waves to point just above the solution level. Ultrasonic nebulizers that use a concave transducer have a higher output but require a constant level of solution for proper operation. If a flat transducer is used, it can be covered with stainless steel, which increases the output of the ultrasonic nebulizer. The conversion of ultrasonic energy to mechanical energy by the transducer results in heat production. This heat is absorbed by the solution over the transducer.

In some models of ultrasonic nebulizers, the solution to be nebulized is placed directly over the transducer. In others, the solution to be nebulized is placed into a nebulization chamber and a water couplant chamber is placed between the transducer and the medication chamber. Ultrasonic waves are transmitted to the nebulization chamber. A fan is used to deliver the aerosol produced by the ultrasonic nebulizer to the patient. This fan usually produces a flow of about 30 L/min. Commercially available ultrasonic nebulizers include the Devilbiss, Mist-O_2-Gen, and Puritan-Bennett (Figs. 5-55 and 5-56). Hand-held ultrasonic nebulizers are also commercially available for aerosol medication delivery, but these are not commonly used.

Small-Particle Aerosol Generator

The Small-Particle Aerosol Generator (SPAG) is used specifically to aerosolize ribavirin (Virazole). The device consists of a nebulizer and a drying chamber

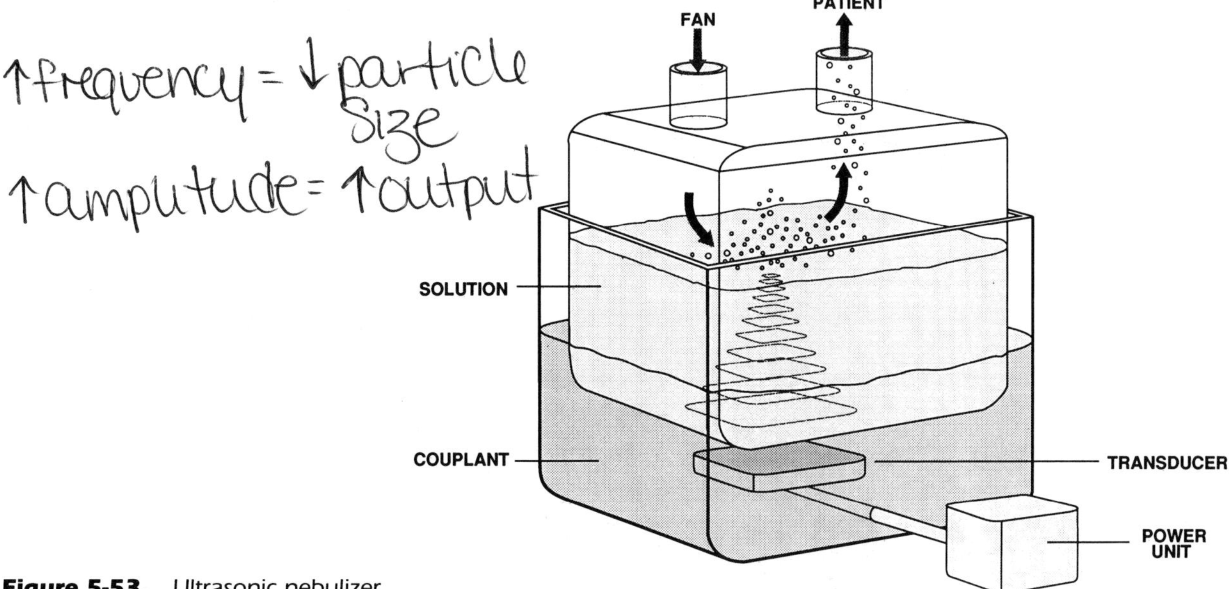

Figure 5-53. Ultrasonic nebulizer.

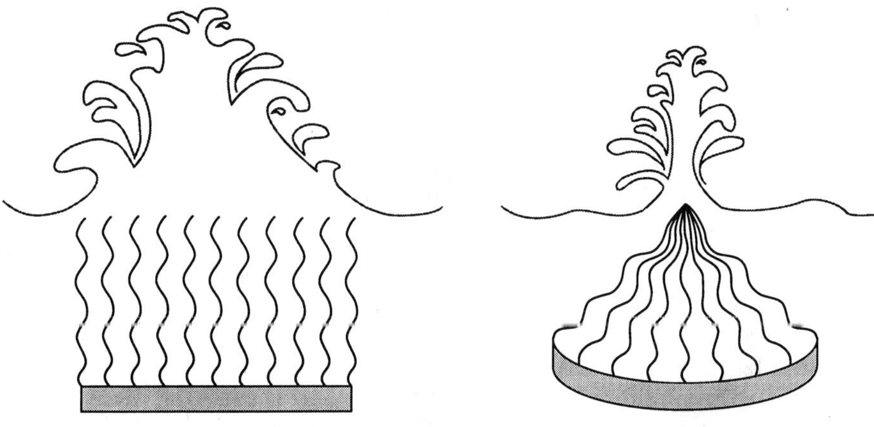

Figure 5-54. Concave (left) and flat (right) transducers.

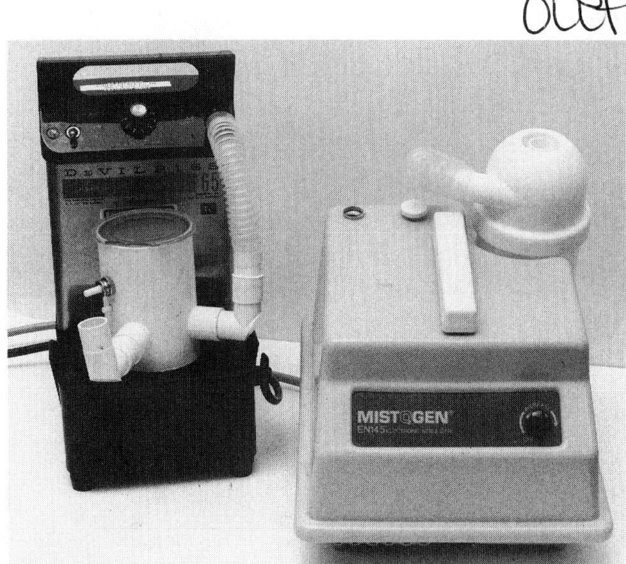

Figure 5-55. Devilbiss (left) and Mist-O_2-Gen (right) ultrasonic nebulizers.

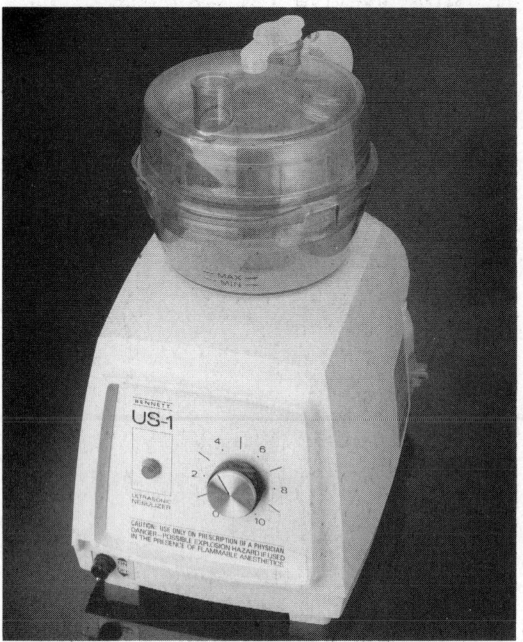

Figure 5-56. Puritan-Bennett ultrasonic nebulizer. (Courtesy of Puritan-Bennett Corp, Kansas City, MO)

(Fig. 5-57). The MMAD of particles produced is about 1.3 μm. A pressure of 25 psig is set on the regulator at the front of the device, the nebulizer flow is set at 6 to 10 L/min, and the drying chamber flow is set at 3 to 8 L/min. The ribavirin aerosol is delivered to a mask, oxyhood, tent, or ventilator.[46] Because of the potentially deleterious effects of this drug to the health of normal persons, care should be taken to avoid gross ambient environmental contamination with the aerosol.

Because ribavirin is teratogenic in small mammals, there are concerns about the potential adverse effects of this drug on health care workers.[47] For this reason, a vacuum scavenging system should be used when ribavirin is administered.[48,49] Such a system is shown in Figure 5-58. This is a double-enclosure system, with a ribavirin administration oxygen hood inside an oxygen tent. Two high-flow vacuum scavenging systems aspirate ribavirin from the system through high-efficiency particulate air filters at a total flow greater than 350 L/min. When the system is entered to care for the child, the following steps are followed: (1) turn on secondary oxygen

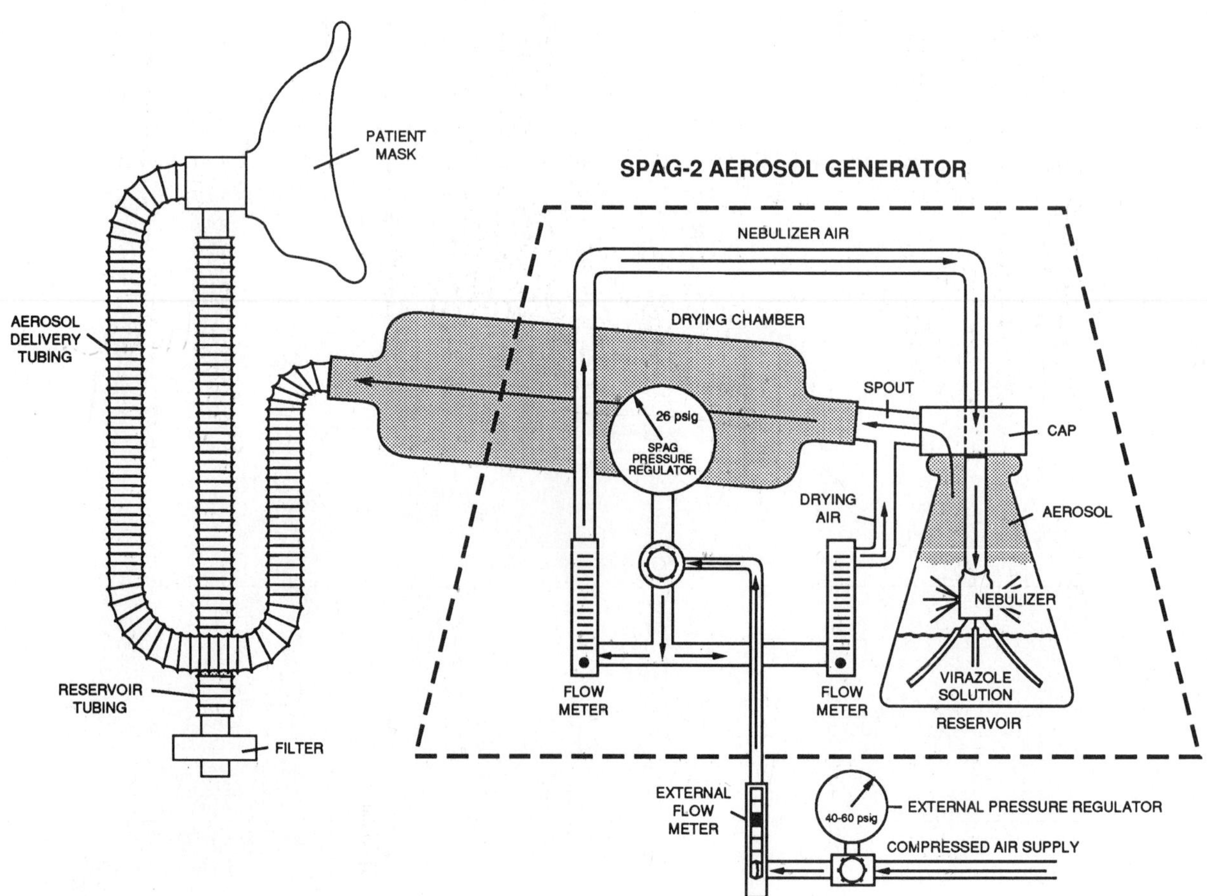

Figure 5-57. Small-particle aerosol generator (SPAG). (Courtesy of ICN Pharmaceuticals)

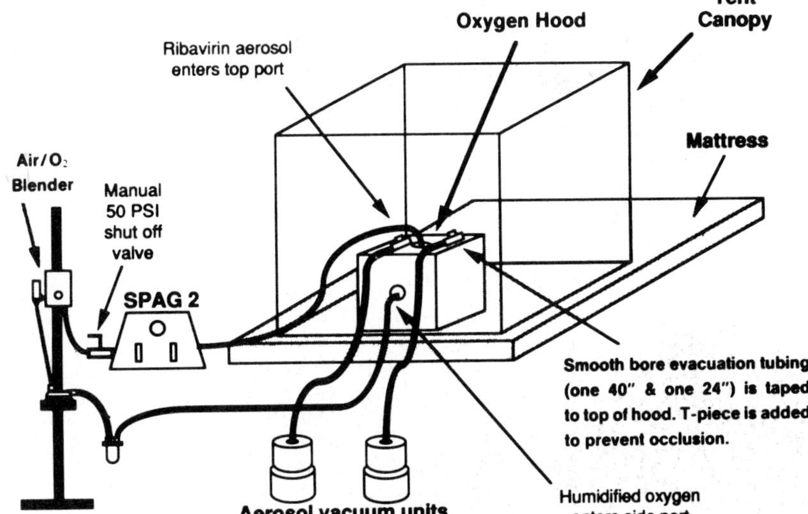

Figure 5-58. Double-tent, double-vacuum scavenging system used for the administration of ribavirin to spontaneously breathing infants. (From Charney W, Corkery KJ, Kraemer R. Engineering and administrative controls to contain aerosolized ribavirin: Results of simulation and application to one patient. Respir Care 1990;35:1042–1048)

source, (2) turn off SPAG unit, (3) wait 5 minutes, and (4) enter tent. When the child is placed into the tent, the following steps are followed: (1) place child into ribavirin hood, (2) seal tent with blanket, (3) turn on SPAG unit, and (4) turn off secondary oxygen source.

Aerosol Bronchodilator Administration During Mechanical Ventilation

Aerosol bronchodilators are commonly administered to mechanically ventilated patients. Pulmonary deposition of aerosols during mechanical ventilation is typically less than 5%, as compared with approximately 10% in ambulatory patients. Although pulmonary deposition is lower in mechanically ventilated patients, a physiologic response to inhaled bronchodilators can be demonstrated in these patients. In mechanically ventilated patients, inhaled bronchodilators can be administered by nebulizer or MDI.[50]

Many factors are known to affect pulmonary deposition when nebulizers are used during mechanical ventilation.[51–56]

- *Endotracheal tube size:* Aerosol deposition is decreased with smaller endotracheal tubes. This particularly becomes an issue with infants and children.
- *Nebulizer placement:* When a nebulizer is used in a ventilator circuit, it can be placed at the ventilator Y-piece (Fig. 5-59) or at some point in the circuit between the ventilator and the Y-piece (Fig. 5-60). More medication is delivered to the patient if the nebulizer is placed between the ventilator and the patient (approximately 18 inches from the Y-piece).[51]
- *Type of nebulizer and fill volume:* As with sponta-

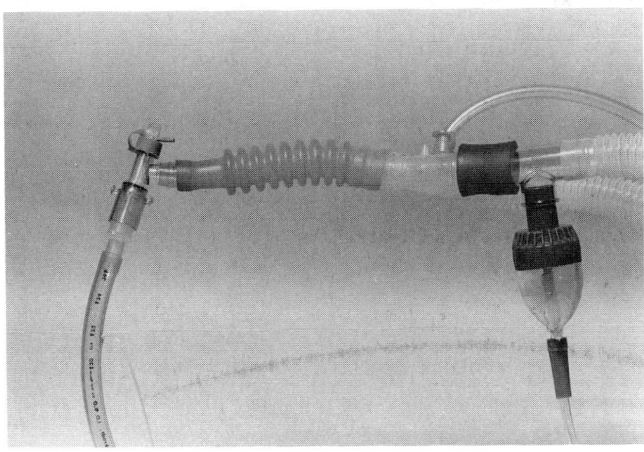

Figure 5-59. Placement of nebulizer at the ventilator Y-piece during mechanical ventilation.

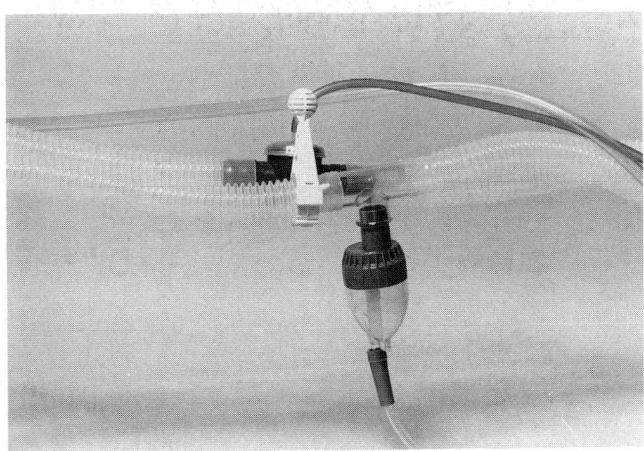

Figure 5-60. Placement of nebulizer between the ventilator and the Y-piece during mechanical ventilation.

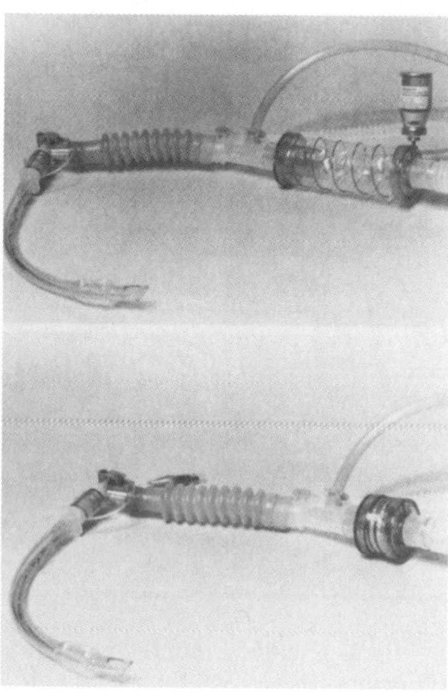

Figure 5-61. Chamber-style metered-dose inhaler adapter in ventilator circuit.

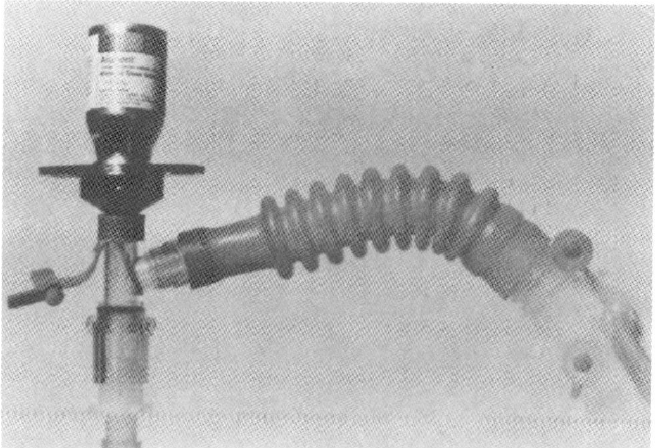

Figure 5-63. Elbow-style metered-dose inhaler adapter in ventilator circuit.

neously breathing patients, the choice of nebulizer brand and fill volume affects the amount of medication delivered to the patient.

- *Presence of a humidification device:* Because a humidifier in the ventilator circuit decreases aerosol delivery by about 50%, it is desirable to bypass the humidifier during therapeutic aerosol administration. If an artificial nose is used, it should be removed during aerosol therapy.[55]
- *Treatment time:* It is reasonable to expect greater pulmonary deposition with longer treatment times.
- *Duty cycle:* Increasing the duty cycle (ie, the inspiratory time and decreasing the respiratory rate) increases aerosol delivery into the lungs.
- *Choice of ventilator:* With some ventilators, the nebulizer can be powered by a nebulizer control on the ventilator. It has been shown that this control works better on some ventilators than others.[56]

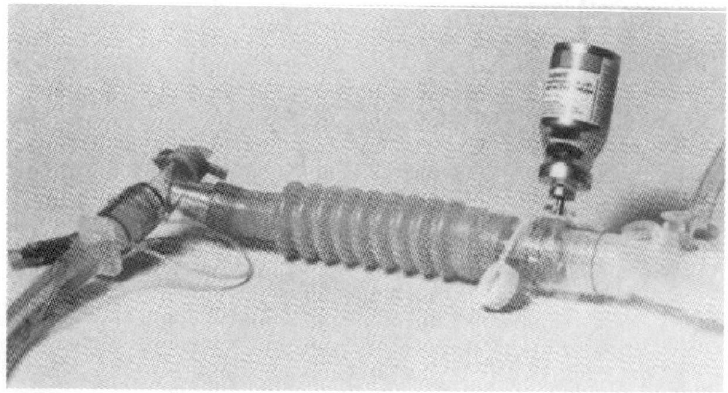

Figure 5-62. In-line style metered-dose inhaler adapter in ventilator circuit.

There are several commercially available adapters that allow an MDI to be placed into a ventilator circuit.[50,57-59] These include chamber (reservoir, spacer) devices, in-line devices, and elbow devices. The chamber/spacer devices fit into the inspiratory limb of the circuit (Fig. 5-61) and act as an aerosol reservoir. The in-line devices can be attached at any point along the inspiratory limb of the circuit (Fig. 5-62), and the elbow devices attach directly to the endotracheal tube (Fig. 5-63). Although the chamber devices may deliver a higher dose per puff than the other styles,[57-60] any of these devices may be effective if the number of puffs is titrated to the desired physiologic effect.[61]

AARC Clinical Practice Guideline

Bland Aerosol Administration: Indications, Contraindications, Hazards, and Complications

Bland aerosol is the delivery of sterile water or hypotonic, isotonic, or hypertonic saline in aerosol form. Bland aerosol administration may be accompanied by oxygen administration.

- Indications:
  - the presence of upper airway edema (laryngotracheobronchitis, subglottic edema, postextubation edema, postoperative management of upper airway)
  - the presence of a bypassed upper airway
  - the need for sputum specimens
- Contraindications:
  - bronchospasm
  - history of airway hyperresponsiveness

- Hazards/Complications:
  - wheezing or bronchospasm
  - bronchoconstriction when an artificial airway is employed
  - infection
  - overhydration
  - patient discomfort
  - caregiver exposure to droplet nuclei of *Mycobacterium tuberculosis* or other airborne contagion produced as a consequence of coughing, particularly during sputum induction

(Adapted from AARC Clinical Practice Guideline, published in December, 1993, issue of Respiratory Care; see original publication for complete text)

AARC Clinical Practice Guideline

Selection of Aerosol Delivery Device: Indications, Contraindications, Hazards and Complications

An aerosol delivery device is used to administer pharmacologically active aerosol to the lower respiratory tract. The device selected should produce particles with a mass median aerodynamic diameter of 2–5 microns.

- Indications: An aerosol delivery device is used to deliver an aerosol to the lower airways, including beta adrenergic agents, anticholinergic agents, anti-inflammatory agents, mediator-modifying agents, and mucokinetics.
- Contraindications:
  - No contraindications exist to the administration of aerosols by inhalation
  - Contraindications related to the substances being delivered may exist. Consult the package insert for product-specific contraindications.
- Hazards/Complications:
  - Malfunction of the device and/or improper technique may result in underdosing
  - The potential exists for malfunction of device and/or improper technique to result in overdosing
  - Complications of specific pharmacologic agents may occur
  - Cardiotoxic effects of Freon have been reported as an idiosyncratic response that may be a problem with excessive use of metered-dose inhaler
  - Freon may effect the environment by its effect on the ozone layer
  - Repeated exposure to aerosols has been reported to produce asthmatic symptoms in some caregivers

(Adapted from AARC Clinical Practice Guideline, published in August, 1992, issue of Respiratory Care; see original publication for complete text)

AARC Clinical Practice Guideline

Humidification During Mechanical Ventilation: Indications, Contraindications, Hazards and Complications

Humidification during mechanical ventilation can be accomplished using either a heated humidifier or heat and moisture exchanger. The device should provide a minimum of 30 mg/L of delivered gas at 30°C.

- Indications: Humidification of inspired gas during mechanical ventilation is mandatory when an endotracheal tube is present.
- Contraindications: There are no contraindications to providing physiologic conditioning of inspired gas during mechanical ventilation. A heat and moisture exchanger is contraindicated under some circumstances:
  - patients with thick, copious, or bloody secretions
  - patients with an expired tidal volume less than 70% of the delivered tidal volume
  - patients with a body temperature less than 32°C
  - patients with high spontaneous minute ventilation (>10 L/min)
  - a heat and moisture exchanger must be removed from the patient circuit during aerosol treatments when a nebulizer or inhaler is placed in the patient circuit
- Hazards/Complications:
  - potential for electrical shocks (heated humidifiers)
  - hyperthermia with heated humidifiers and hypothermia with heat and moisture exchangers or heated humidifiers
  - thermal injury to the airway from heated humidifiers; burns to the patient and tubing meltdown if heated wire circuits are covered or circuits and humidifiers are incompatible
  - underhydration and impaction of secretions
  - hypoventilation and/or alveolar gas trapping due to mucus plugging of airways
  - increased work of breathing due to mucus plugging of airways
  - increased resistive work of breathing through the humidifier
  - hypoventilation due to increased dead space of heat and moisture exchanger
  - inadvertent overfilling resulting in unintentional tracheal lavage
  - aerosolization of contaminated condensate into the environment
  - potential for burns to caregivers
  - inadvertent tracheal lavage from pooled condensate in the patient circuit
  - elevated airway pressures due to pooled condensate
  - patient-ventilator dysynchrony and improper ventilator performance due to pooled condensate in the circuit
  - ineffective low-pressure alarm during disconnection due to resistance through heat and moisture exchanger

(Adapted from AARC Clinical Practice Guideline, published in August, 1992 issue of Respiratory Care; see original publication for complete text)

References

1. Chatburn RL, Primiano FP. A rational basis for humidity therapy (editorial). Respir Care 1987;32:249–254.
2. Branson RD. Humidification: A dry subject but . . . (editorial). Respir Care 1987;32:731–732.
3. Branson RD, Seger SM. Bland aerosol therapy. In: Kacmarek RM, Stoller JK, eds. Current Respiratory Care. Toronto: BC Decker, 1988:24–28.
4. Stuart BO. Deposition of inhaled aerosols. Arch Intern Med 1973;131:60–73.
5. Morrow PE. Aerosol characterization and deposition. Am Rev Respir Dis 1974;110:88–99.
6. Graff TD. Humidification: Indications and hazards in respiratory therapy. Anesth Analg 1975;54:444–448.
7. Bakow ED, Vincent JE, Evans RN, Galgon JP, Smith RW. Molecular high humidity in the weaning of patients from mechanical ventilation: A case report. Respir Care 1978;23:281–285.
8. Dolan GK, Zawadzki JJ. Performance characteristics of low-flow humidifiers. Respir Care 1976;21:393–403.
9. Darin J, Broadwell J, MacDonell R. An evaluation of water-vapor output from four brands of unheated, prefilled bubble humidifiers. Respir Care 1982;27:41–50.
10. Darin J. The need for rational criteria for the use of unheated bubble humidifiers (editorial). Respir Care 1982;27:945–947.
11. Estey W. Subjective effects of dry versus humidified low flow oxygen. Respir Care 1980;25:1143–1144.
12. Hess D, Figaszweski E, Henry D, et al. Subjective effects of dry versus humidified low-flow oxygen on the upper respiratory tract. Respir Ther 1982(Nov/Dec):71–75.
13. Campbell EJ, Baker D, Crites-Silver P. Subjective effects of humidification of oxygen for delivery by nasal cannula. Chest 1988;93:289–293.
14. Golar SD, Sutherland LLA, Ford GT. Multipatient use of prefilled disposable oxygen humidifiers for up to 30 days: Patient safety and cost analysis. Respir Care 1993;38:343–347.
15. Miyao H, Hirokawa T, Miyasaka K, Kawazoe T. Relative humidity, not absolute humidity, is of great importance when using a humidifier with a heating wire. Crit Care Med 1992; 20:674–679.
16. Chatburn R. Physiologic and methodologic issues regarding humidity therapy (editorial). J Pediatr 1989;114:416–420.
17. Rhame FS, Streifel A, McComb C, Boyle M. Bubbling humidifiers produce microaerosols which can carry bacteria. Infect Control 1986;7:403–407.
18. Goularte TA, Manning MT, Craven DE. Bacterial colonization in humidifying cascade reservoirs after 24 and 48 hours of continuous mechanical ventilation. Infect Control 1987;8:200–203.
19. Shanks CA. Clinical anesthesia and the multiple gauze condenser humidifier. Br J Anaesth 1974;46:773–777.
20. Mapelson WW, Morgan JG, Hillard ER. Assessment of condenser humidifiers with special reference to the multiple gauze model. Br Med J 1963;1:300–305.
21. Chalon J, Markham JP, Ali MM, Ramanthan S, Turndorf H. The Pall Ultipor breathing circuit filter: An efficient heat and moisture exchanger. Anesth Analg 1984;63:366–370.
22. Weeks DB, Ramsey FM. Laboratory investigation of six artificial noses during endotracheal anesthesia. Anesth Analg 1983;62: 753–758.
23. Branson, RD, Hurst JM. Laboratory evaluation of moisture output of seven airway heat and moisture exchangers. Respir Care 1987;32:741–747.
24. Shelly M, Bethune DW, Latmer Rd. A comparison of five heat and moisture exchangers. Anaesthesia 1986;11:527–532.
25. Walker AKY, Bethune DW. A comparative study of condenser humidifiers. Anaesthesia 1976;31:1086–1093.
26. Gallagher J, Strangeways JEM, Allt-Graham J. Contamination control in long-term ventilation. Anaesthesia 1987;42:476–481.
27. Stange K, Bydgeman S. Do moisture exchangers prevent patient contamination of ventilators? Acta Anaesth Scand 1980;24: 487–490.
28. Branson RD, Davis K, Campbell RS, Porembka DT. Humidification in the intensive care unit: Prospective study of a new protocol utilizing heated humidification and a hygroscopic condenser humidifier. Chest 1993;104:1800–1805.
29. Ploysongsang Y, Branson RD, Rashkin MC, Hurst JM. Pressure flow characteristics of commonly used heat-moisture exchangers. Am Rev Respir Dis 1988;138:675–678.
30. Ploysongsang Y, Branson RD, Rashkin MC, Hurst JM. Effect of flow rate and duration of use on the pressure drop across six artificial noses. Respir Care 1989;34:902–907.
31. Hess D, Horney D, Snyder T. Medication-delivery performance of eight small-volume, hand-held nebulizers: Effects of diluent volume, gas flow rate, and nebulizer brand. Respir Care 1989;34: 717–723.
32. Kradjan WA, Lakshminarayan S. Efficiency of air compressor-driven nebulizers. Chest 1985;87:512–516.
33. Clay MM, Pavia D, Newman SP, Lennard-Jones T, Clarke SW. Assessment of jet nebulizers for lung aerosol therapy. Lancet 1983;2:592–594.
34. Pisut FM. Comparison of medication delivery by T-nebulizer with inspiratory and expiratory reservoirs. Respir Care 1989;34: 985–988.
35. Corkery KJ, Luce JM, Montgomery AB. Aerosolized pentamidine for treatment and prophylaxis of *Pneumocystis carinii* pneumonia: An update. Respir Care 1988;33:676–685.
36. Hess D. Aerosolized drug delivery: Technical aspects. In: Kacmarek RM, Stoller JK, eds. Current Respiratory Care. Toronto: BC Decker, 1988:56–61.
37. Kacmarek RM, Hess D. The interface between patient and aerosol generator. Respir Care 1991;36:952–976.
38. Konig P. Spacer devices used with metered-dose inhalers. Breakthrough or gimmick? Chest 1985;88:276–284.
39. Newman SP. Aerosol deposition considerations in inhalation therapy. Chest 1985;88:152S–160S.
40. Sackner MA, Kim CS. Auxiliary MDI aerosol delivery systems. Chest 1985;88:161S–170S.
41. Newman SP. Delivery of therapeutic aerosols. In: Witek TJ, Schacter N, eds. Advances in Respiratory Care Pharmacology. Philadelphia: PA; J.B. Lippincott Co.; 1988.
42. Klein EF, Dinesh DA, Shah NJ, Modell JH, Desautels D. Performance characteristics of conventional and prototype humidifiers and nebulizers. Chest 1973;64:690–696.
43. Hill TV, Sorbello JG. Humidity outputs of large-reservoir nebulizers. Respir Care 1987;32:255–260.
44. Kaye W, Summers JT, Monast R, McEnany MT. Nasal oxygen sampler. Heart Lung 1981;10:679–685.
45. Monast RL, Kaye W. Problems in delivering desired oxygen concentrations from jet nebulizers to patients via face tents. Respir Care 1984;29:994–1000.
46. Demers RR, Parker J, Frankel LR, Smith DW. Administration of ribavirin to neonatal and pediatric patients during mechanical ventilation. Respir Care 1986;31:1188–1195.
47. Kacmarek RM. Ribavirin and pentamadine aerosols: Caregiver beware! (editorial). Respir Care 1990;35:1034–1036.
48. Charney KJ, Corkery KJ, Kraemer R. Engineering and administrative controls to contain the delivery of aerosolized ribavirin: Results of simulation and application to one patient. Respir Care 1990;35:1042–1048.
49. Kacmarek RM, Kratohvil J. Evaluation of a double-enclosure double-vacuum unit scavenging system for ribavirin administration. Respir Care 1992;37:37–45.
50. Hess D. How should bronchodilators be administered to patients on ventilators? Respir Care 1991;36:377–394.
51 Hughes JM, Saez J. Effects of nebulizer mode and position in a mechanical ventilator circuit on dose delivery. Respir Care 1987;32:1131–1135.
52. Ahrens RC, Ries RA, Popendorf W, Wiese J. The delivery of therapeutic aerosols through endotracheal tubes. Pediatr Pulmonol 1986;2:19–26.
53. O'Riordan TG, Greco MJ, Perry RJ, Smaldone GC. Nebulizer function during mechanical ventilation. Am Rev Respir Dis 1992;145:1117–1122.
54. Quinn WW. Effect of a new nebulizer position on aerosol delivery during mechanical ventilation: A bench study. Respir Care 1992;37:423–431.
55. O'Doherty MJ, Thomas SHL, Page CJ, Treacher DF, Nunan TO. Delivery of nebulized aerosol to a lung model during mechanical ventilation: Effect of ventilator settings and nebulizer type,

eters. Silicone is expensive but can be autoclaved; tissue will not adhere to it, and it will not react with body tissues. The material used to manufacture endotracheal tubes is implant tested, meaning that it is nonreactive to tissue. The construction of an endotracheal tube is standard (Fig. 6-13). The distal end is beveled and rounded to minimize trauma on insertion. Many endotracheal tubes also have a Murphy eye that allows passage of gas through it if the end becomes occluded by secretions or the wall of the patient's airway. Some endotracheal tubes do not have the Murphy eye, and these are called McGill tubes. A cuff is present near the distal end of the tube that can be inflated by a pilot tube that extends past the proximal end of the tube and terminates with a pilot balloon and spring-loaded valve. Molded into the tube is a radiopaque line that allows for ready visualization of the tube on radiography. The tube contains markings for inside diameter (ID) and outside diameter (OD) in millimeters, distance from the distal tip in centimeters, manufacturer's name or mark, whether the tube is for oral or nasal use (an oral tube has a 45-degree angle at the tip, a nasal or oral-nasal tube has a 60-degree angle), an indication that the tube conforms to the standards of the American National Standards Institute (ANSI) Z79 committee, and an indication that the tube material has been implant tested (IT). The proximal end of the tube is fitted with a standard 15-mm OD connection for respiratory and anesthesia equipment.

There are many variations in the design of the endotracheal tube. The "anode tube" contains a steel reinforcing wire that is wound spirally within the wall of the tube. This allows the tube to be made of a softer material yet prevents kinking when the tube must be bent at an angle to clear the surgical field. Since the wire makes the tube visible on radiography, these tubes do not have a radiopaque line. Instead, there are two rectangular marks located 1 and 2 cm above the cuff on smaller tubes (less than 6.5 mm ID) and 2 and 4 cm above the cuff on larger tubes (greater than 6.0 mm ID). These marks allow the clinician to reference the location of the endotracheal tube tip.

Another type of endotracheal tube is the Rae tube, which is available in oral and nasal types, with or without a cuff. These tubes feature a preformed curve that directs the airway connection away from the surgical field (Fig. 6-14). The curve on the Rae tube allows the airway and anesthesia equipment to be positioned away from the operative field for some surgical procedures. However, use of the Rae tube makes it difficult to suction the airway. Mallinckrodt Critical Care manufactures a tube called the Endotrol that enables the user to control the direction of the distal endotracheal tube tip during intubation by pulling a loop that is found near the proximal end of the tube (Fig. 6-15). Mallinckrodt Critical Care also manufactures the Hi-Lo Jet tube for high-frequency jet ventilation. Besides the pilot tube for the cuff, this tube has a monitoring/irrigation lumen that enters the tube at the tip and an insufflation lumen that enters approximately 2.5 cm before the tip (Fig. 6-16). Recognizing the increased use of laser surgery, Mallinckrodt Critical Care also manufactures a flexi-

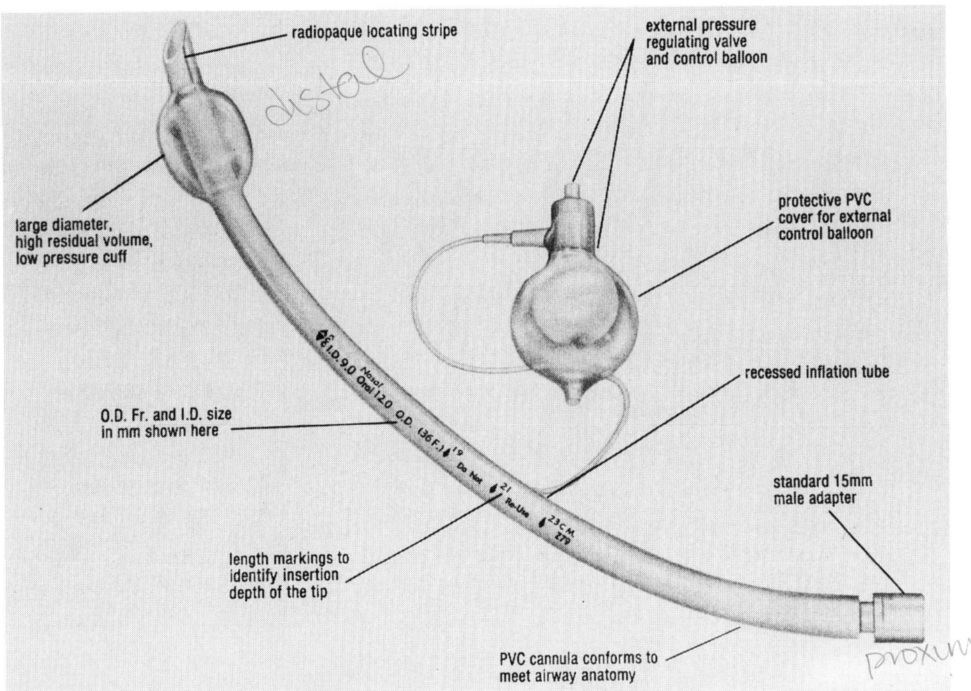

Figure 6-13. Lanz endotracheal tube. (Courtesy of Mallinckrodt Critical Care, Glen Falls, NY)

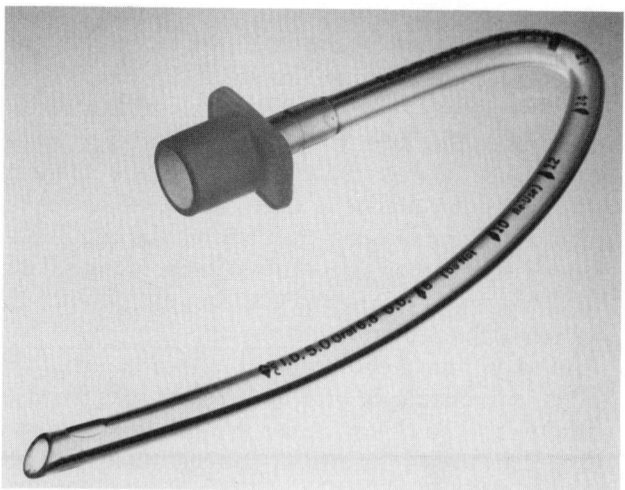

Figure 6-14. Rae tube.

ble, spiral stainless steel tube called the Laser-Flex. If the laser beam accidentally comes into contact with the tube, the result is simply a reflection of a diffused beam (Fig. 6-17).

The Cole tube has a distal tapered end (Fig. 6-18). It is available only in neonatal and pediatric sizes and was designed to avoid endobronchial intubation. However, Cole tubes are no longer commonly used because they fail to prevent endobronchial intubation and may be damaging to the vocal cords. Straight (untapered) cuffless endotracheal tubes are most commonly used with the neonate, and some of these have a line indicating the approximate level of the vocal cords. The Bard TRACHMATE neonatal/pediatric endotracheal tube contains an encapsulated magnetic metal marker, and a battery-operated sensing instrument is used that produces an audiovisual

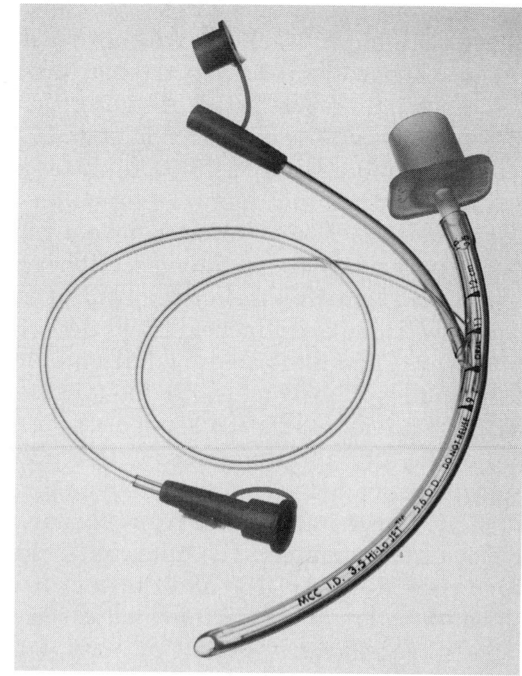

Figure 6-16. Hi-Lo Jet tube. (Courtesy of Mallinckrodt Critical Care, Glen Falls, NY)

signal that correlates with the proximity of the tube marker to the instrument.

Several tubes are available for selective endobronchial intubation. Sheridan makes one for cannulating the left mainstem bronchus. Mallinckrodt Critical Care makes separate tubes for selective intubation of each mainstem bronchus (Fig. 6-19). Rusch manufactures a Carlens tube, designed to enter the left mainstem bronchus (Fig. 6-20), and the White tube designed to enter the right mainstem bronchus (Fig. 6-21). The Carlens and White tubes have a tracheal hook. A similar tube, the Robertshaw, is designed to enter a mainstem bronchus but does not

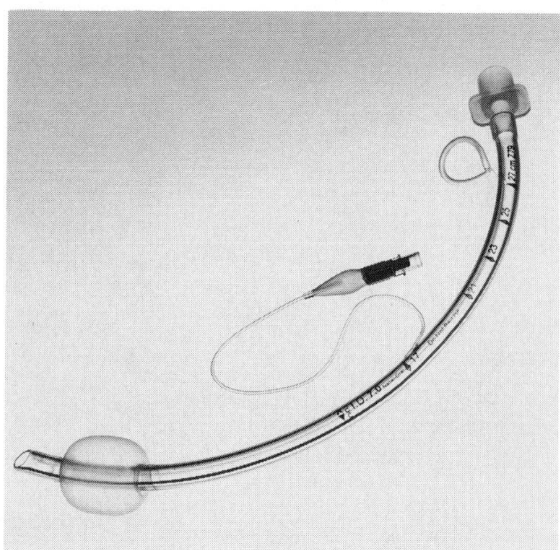

Figure 6-15. Endotrol tube. (Courtesy of Mallinckrodt Critical Care, Glen Falls, NY)

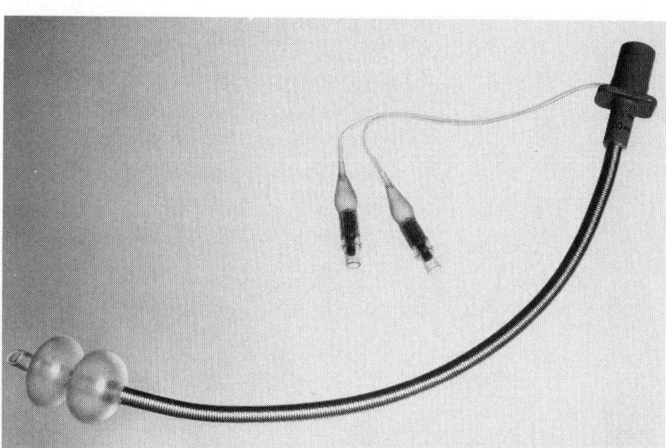

Figure 6-17. Laser-Flex tube. (Courtesy of Mallinckrodt Critical Care, Glen Falls, NY)

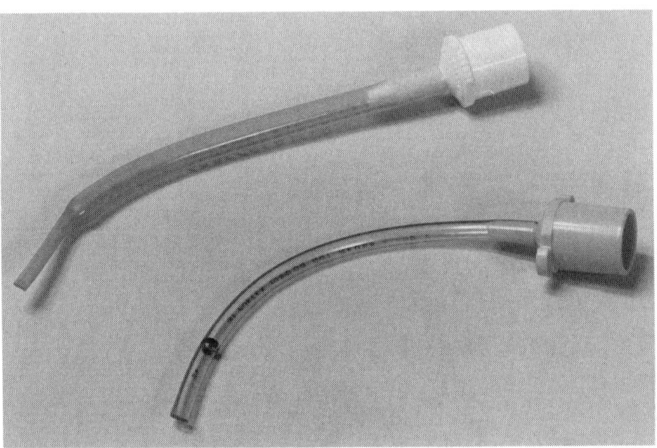

Figure 6-18. Cole tube (left) and infant cuffless straight tube (right).

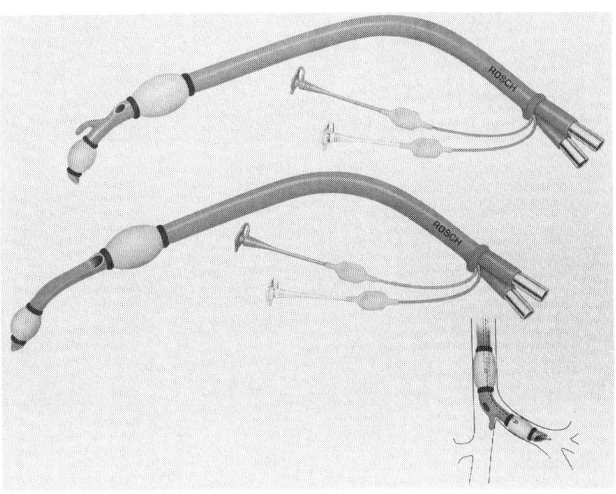

Figure 6-20. Carlens tube (top) and Robertshaw tube (bottom). (Courtesy of Rusch, New York, NY)

have the carinal hook. Because of their large size, endobronchial tubes are difficult to insert. These tubes are used during thoracic surgery (such as pneumonectomy), independent lung ventilation, or bronchospirometry.

Equipment for Insertion of Endotracheal Tubes

Equipment used to perform orotracheal and nasotracheal intubation is listed in Box 6-2.

Laryngoscope

The primary piece of equipment used to insert an endotracheal tube is the laryngoscope. It has two principal parts: the handle and the blade. There are also single-piece disposable laryngoscopes. The handles, regardless of manufacturer, are similar. They are powered by two batteries (D, C, or AA).

Laryngoscope blades are of two types: straight and curved. The straight blade is designed to directly lift the epiglottis to allow visualization of the vocal cords. Two types of straight blades are the Wisconsin and Miller (Fig. 6-22). The Wisconsin blade has a curve of slightly larger radius along the longitudinal axis and is straight for its entire length. The Miller blade has a slight curve at the tip and a slight ridge at the tip. The curved or Macintosh blade (Fig. 6-23) is inserted into the vallecula to lift the epiglottis indirectly. The blade used depends on personal preference.

Infants are usually intubated more easily with a straight blade. The straight blade, by lifting the epiglottis directly, does not disturb the larynx, whereas the curved blade will sometimes move the larynx with the

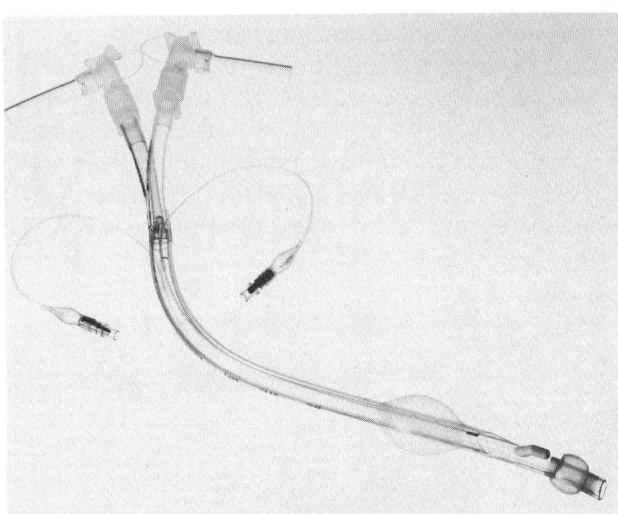

Figure 6-19. Mallinckrodt endobronchial tube. (Courtesy of Mallinckrodt Critical Care, Glen Falls, NY)

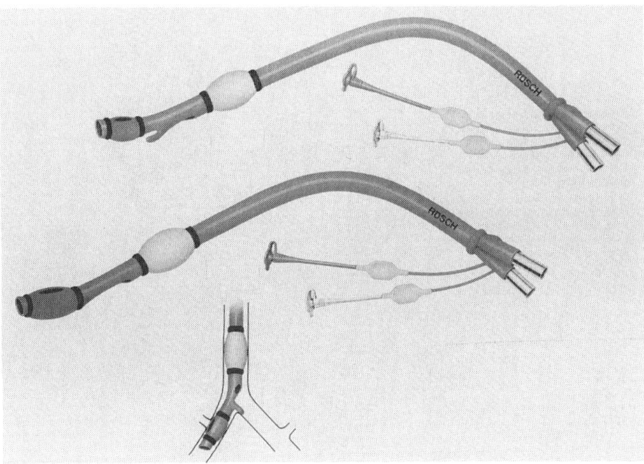

Figure 6-21. White tube (top) and Robertshaw tube (bottom). (Courtesy of Rusch, New York, NY)

Box 6-2
Equipment for Oral and Nasal Intubation

Laryngoscope handles and blades
Endotracheal tubes, assorted sizes
Tape or commerical tube fixation device
Magill forceps
Syringe
Stylet
Suction
Manual resuscitator/oxygen
Water-soluble lubricant
Stethoscope
Benzoin tincture
Sedatives and/or paralyzing agents

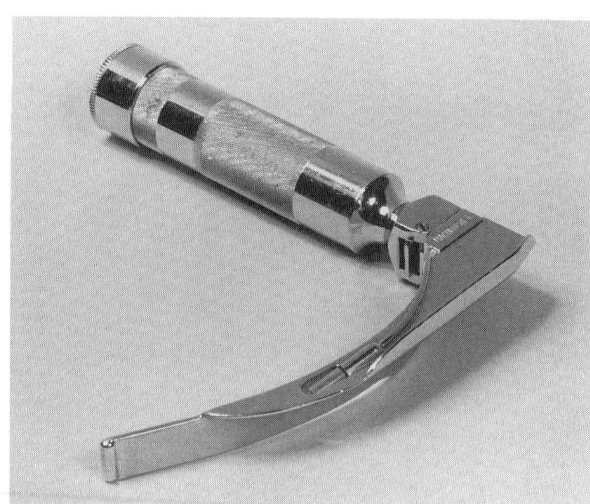

Figure 6-23. Laryngoscope with Macintosh blade.

epiglottis. Also, the epiglottis of the infant is large and floppy and may require the direct lifting of the straight blade.

Proper Size Tube

The tube size for a neonate is 2.5 to 3.0 mm. This increases to 3.5 mm at 6 months, 4.5 mm at 1 year, and 5.0 mm at 2 years. After that age, the size increases by 0.5 mm for every 2 years up to age 14.[26] In general, a tube with an internal diameter of 7.0 to 8.5 mm is used with adult females (14 years of age and older), and a tube of 8.0 to 9.5 mm is used with adult males. As a rule, the largest diameter tube possible should be inserted. According to Poiseuille's law (see Chapter 1), resistance varies inversely with the fourth power of the radius of the tube. If radius decreases by 16% (roughly equivalent to going from a 6.0-mm ID tube to a 5.0-mm ID tube), the resistance *doubles*.

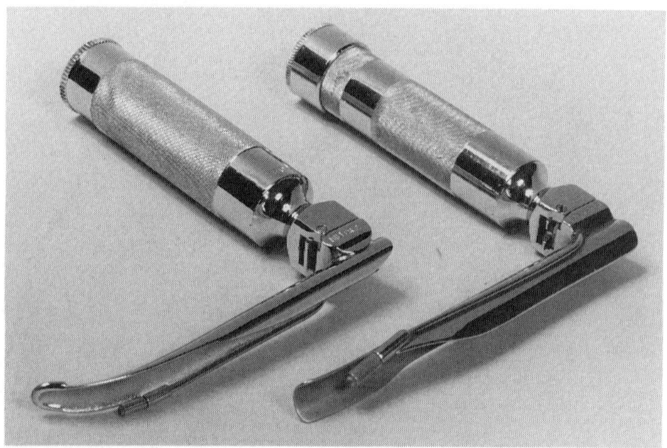

Figure 6-22. Laryngoscopes with straight blades: Wisconsin (left) and Miller (right).

Magill Forceps

Magill forceps (Fig. 6-24) enable one to manipulate the endotracheal tube tip without blocking one's view. They are useful for removal of a foreign object and for nasal intubation. Although nasal intubation is usually performed blindly, it can be accomplished with direct visualization of the cords and advancement of the tube with Magill forceps (Fig. 6-25).

Other Equipment

Sterile water-soluble lubricant should be used on the tip of the endotracheal tube to facilitate its passage through the upper airway. For a nasal intubation, the use of 2% lidocaine jelly makes the insertion more comfortable. A lubricant with a petroleum or other chemical base (such as Vaseline) should be avoided because it may cause a chemical pneumonitis.

A syringe should be readily available during intubation so that the cuff can be inflated and the patient ventilated once the tube is inserted. A stylet (Fig. 6-26) is useful when the curvature of the tube does not match that of the patient's upper airway. A stylet should not be used for nasal intubation and should be lubricated to facilitate removal after intubation. Suction should be immediately available to clear the airway of secretions

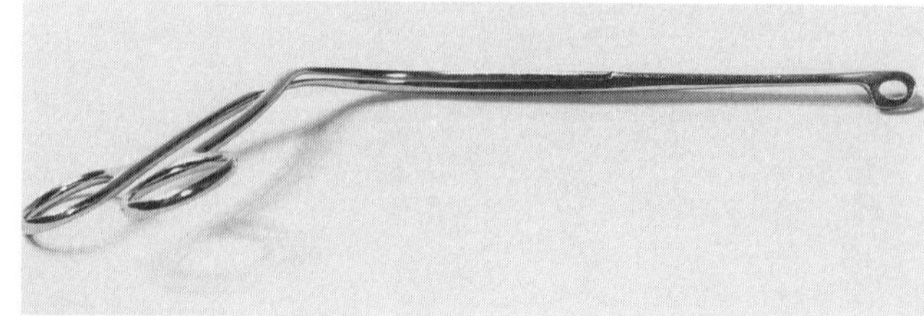

Figure 6-24. Magill forceps.

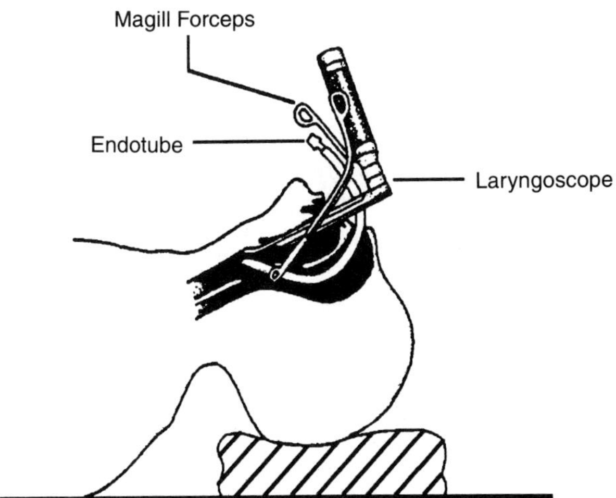

Figure 6-25. Use of Magill forceps during nasal intubation.

during intubation, and suctioning of the trachea also may be necessary after the tube is inserted. A self-inflating manual resuscitator also should be available to manually ventilate through a mask while the intubation equipment is being prepared and to manually ventilate after intubation. An important piece of equipment for endotracheal intubation is the stethoscope, which is used to confirm proper position of the tube. A CO_2 detector is also useful to confirm endotracheal (rather than esophageal) intubation (see Chapter 9).

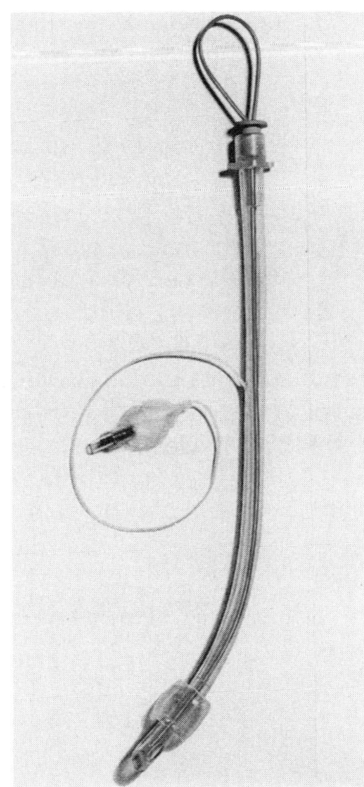

Figure 6-26. Stylet for intubation.

Technique of Endotracheal Intubation

Placement of an endotracheal tube should only be attempted by a trained practitioner. Before intubation, adequate ventilation and oxygenation should be ensured. The necessary equipment should be assembled and tested. Once all is ready, the head should be placed in the "sniffing" position and the mouth opened using the crossed-finger technique. The laryngoscope blade is then inserted on the right side of the mouth, advanced the proper depth, and moved into the midline. The laryngoscope is then *lifted* and positioned to visualize the vocal cords. With the curved blade, the laryngoscope should be placed into the vallecula (Fig. 6-27). The straight blade is used to lift the epiglottis directly (Fig. 6-28). An assistant can pull gently at the right corner of the mouth to increase the field of vision and also place gentle pressure on the larynx. Cricoid pressure is also useful to move an anterior larynx into better position for visualization and to close the esophagus to prevent regurgitation. Once the larynx is visualized, the tube is inserted until the practitioner sees the cuff pass through the vocal cords.

For nasal intubation, the endotube should be well lubricated before insertion. Nasal intubation can be performed blindly or by direct visualization using a Magill forceps (see Fig. 6-25). A stylet should not be used, and a smaller tube may be necessary with nasal intubation.

After inflating the cuff, a manual resuscitator is connected and ventilation is provided. Auscultation and exhaled carbon dioxide monitoring are used to confirm proper placement of the tube. The best place to auscultate is over the bases, because right mainstem intubation may obstruct the right upper lobe as well as the entire left lung. If the breath sounds are not equal, the cuff should be deflated, the tube withdrawn 1 to 2

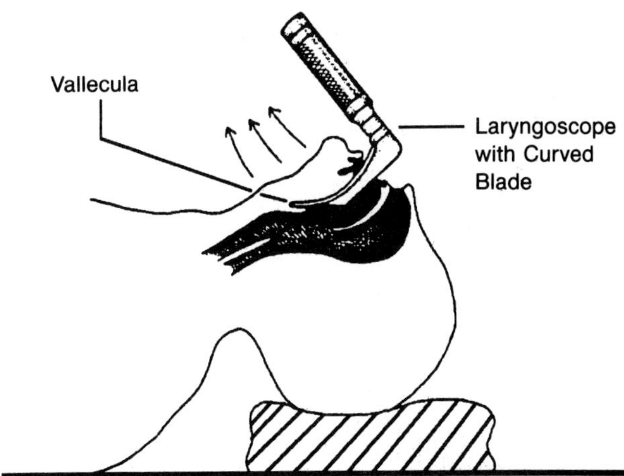

Figure 6-27. Curved laryngoscope blade in vallecula.

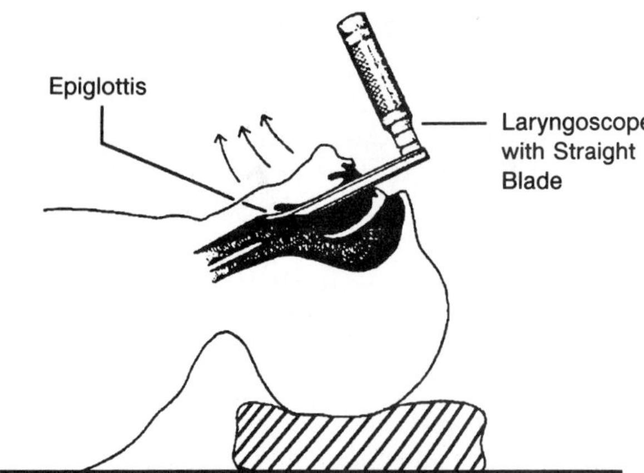

Figure 6-28. Straight laryngoscope blade under epiglottis

cm, the cuff reinflated, and breath sounds reevaluated. When proper placement of the tube has been confirmed, it should be secured in place.

Maintenance of Endotracheal Tubes

The tube should be retaped if the tape is excessively soiled (for aesthetic reasons) or if the tape is no longer holding the tube in place. Adequate humidification and heating of the inspired gases should be provided (see Chapter 5). The cuff should be maintained at the proper state of inflation, using either minimal leak technique or minimal occlusion pressure technique. With the minimal leak technique, a volume of air is added to the cuff so that a small leak occurs near the end of a positive pressure breath. With the minimal occlusion pressure technique, a volume of air is added to the cuff so that the leak barely disappears at end-inhalation during a positive-pressure breath. It is common practice in many hospitals to routinely measure the pressure in the cuff required for minimal leak or minimal occlusion. With the Kamen-Wilkinson tube, it is not possible to measure cuff pressure.

Flexible Fiberoptic Laryngoscopes and Lighted Stylets

A fiberoptic laryngoscope is used for patients who are difficult to intubate (Fig. 6-29). It can also be used for assessing endotracheal tube position, changing endotracheal tubes, removing secretions, and assessing laryngeal and tracheal damage.[27,28] The fiberoptic laryngoscope is composed of the following parts:

- light source, usually contained in the handle
- body, containing the eye piece and tip control knob
- flexible insertion portion, containing the fiberoptic bundles
- working channel (not present in all units), used to remove secretions
- the tip cable, which allows movement of the tip

Also available is the stylet fiberoptic laryngoscope, composed of a handle, body, and stylet. The distal portion of the stylet is malleable. To intubate with the flexible laryngoscope, the tube is first threaded over the laryngoscope. The scope is then passed into the trachea, and the tube is passed over the scope into place.

Battery-powered lighted stylets are available in both rigid and flexible styles.[29-31] The rigid style is used for blind oral intubation, and the flexible style is used for blind nasal intubation (Fig. 6-30). Placement of the tube in the trachea results in a bright glow in the anterior neck at the midline (Fig. 6-31). The flexible lighted stylet also can be used to confirm correct placement of the endotracheal tube.

Tracheal Tube Changers

It is sometimes necessary to change an endotracheal tube. Such situations include damage to the cuff or pilot tube, and the necessity of placing a larger tube (fiberoptic bronchoscopy). There are two products that minimize the risk of this procedure, the T.T.X. Tracheal Tube Exchanger and the JEM 400 Endotracheal Tube Changer (Fig. 6-32). The T.T.X. comes in three sizes to

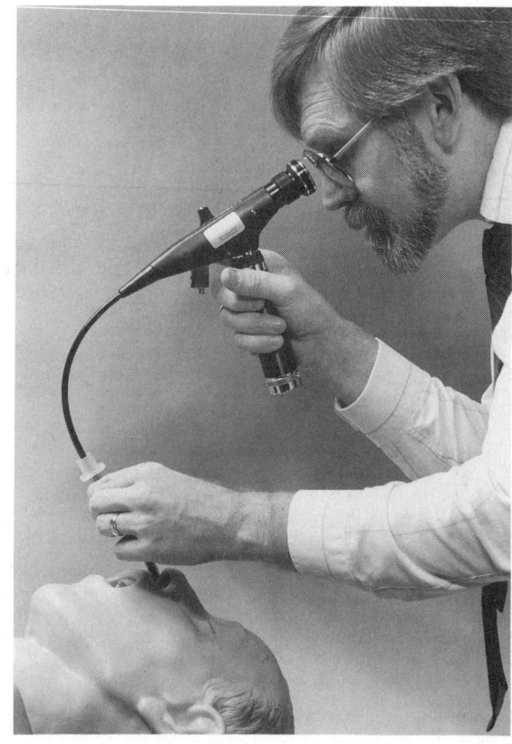

Figure 6-29. Fiberoptic laryngoscope used to intubate.

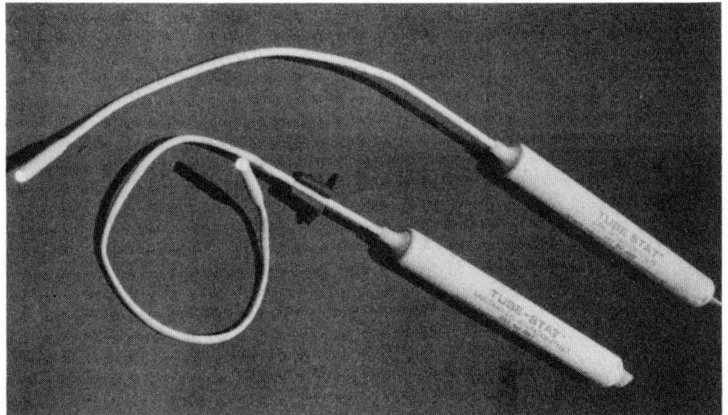

Figure 6-30. Rigid and flexible light stylets for intubation.

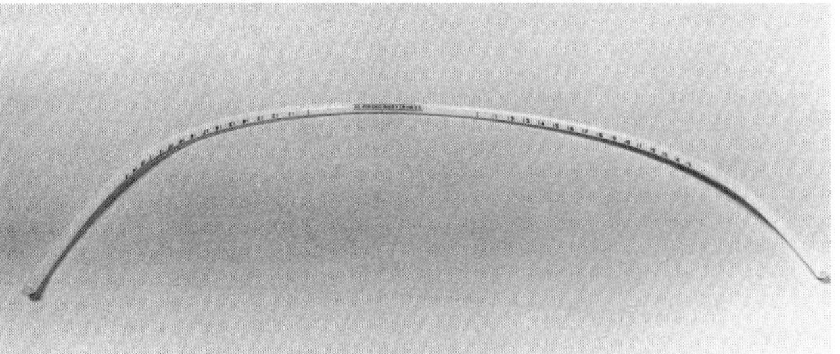

Figure 6-32. JEM 400 Endotracheal Tube Changer.

cover tubes from 4.0 to 10.0 mm ID. The JEM 400 can be used only on tubes larger than 7.5 mm ID. These function in a manner analogous to a guidewire used to change an intravascular catheter. The tube changer is inserted into the tube that is already in the patient. Guide marks on the tube changer allow the practitioner to judge how far it should be inserted. The cuff on the tube is deflated, the tube is withdrawn, and the new tube is advanced over the changer until the proper guide mark is visible. Both manufacturers state that these changes can be effected under usual circumstances in 30 to 120 seconds.

Tracheostomy Tubes

A tracheostomy tube has several advantages over oral or nasal endotracheal tubes. Suctioning is facilitated, it is better tolerated by the conscious patient, fixation of the tube is easier, eating and even speaking (with the proper tube) are possible, and changing the tube is easier.

While the tracheostomy tube has many advantages over other airway devices, the fact that a surgical procedure is required to insert it leads to many potential complications (Box 6-3).[26] A tracheostomy is used when endotracheal intubation is impossible (complete upper airway obstruction) or undesirable (acute epiglottitis). A tracheostomy is also used when a long-term airway is needed, and it is usually considered after 10 to 14 days of intubation.

The tracheostomy tube is designed to pass through a surgically placed tracheal stoma and has four parts: the inner cannula, the outer cannula, the obturator, and the cuff (if one is used). The inner cannula can be removed to clean secretions and blood from the interior surface without removing the entire tube. With some tubes (eg, Shiley), a disposable inner cannula can be used. Some practitioners believe that an inner cannula that is frequently replaced may decrease the risk of nosocomial infection associated with tracheostomy. However, many hospitals do not use tracheostomy tubes with an inner cannula. The obturator prevents blood or mucus from entering the tube as it is being inserted and provides a smoothly tapered surface to facilitate introduction of the tube into the airway. It is removed when the tube is in the proper position.

Tracheostomy tubes were originally metal and were made of sterling silver or stainless steel (Fig. 6-33). The cuff on metal tubes is a separate item and as such has the potential to slip over the end of the tube, thus oc-

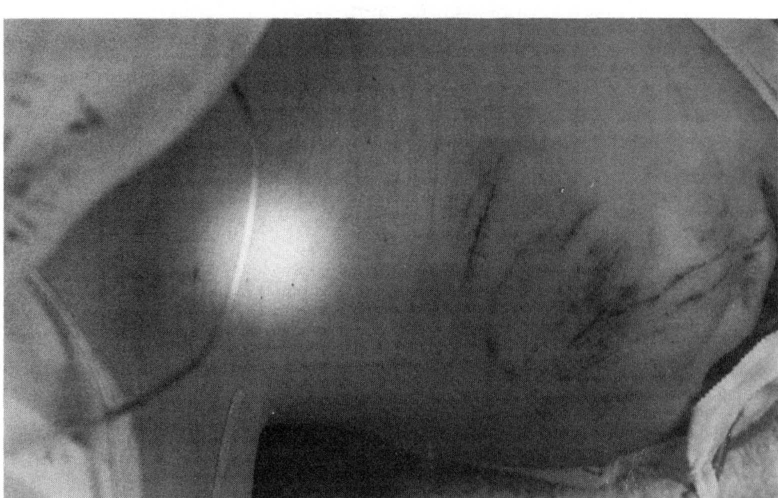

Figure 6-31. Light produced from light stylet with endotube in trachea.

Box 6-3
Complications of Tracheostomy

Early
Hemorrhage
Apnea, cardiac arrest
Hypotension
Obstruction, displaced tube
Subcutaneous emphysema
Pneumothorax, pneumomediastinum
Aspiration and atelectasis
Recurrent laryngeal nerve damage
Tracheoesophageal fistula
Aerophagia

Late
Hemorrhage
Obstruction
Tracheitis
Pneumonia
Wound infection
Subglottic edema
Tracheal stenosis
Dysphagia
Tracheoesophageal fistula
Persistent tracheocutaneous fistula
Difficult decannulation
Unsightly scar

cluding the airway. For this reason and others, such as lack of ability to conform to the airway anatomy, metal tubes are seldom used.

Tracheostomy tubes made from a plastic, such as PVC or silicone, are more satisfactory. Several manufacturers manufacture tracheostomy tubes. These tubes have a standard 15-mm connector, a neck plate for securing the tube to the patient, and a cuff (Fig. 6-34).

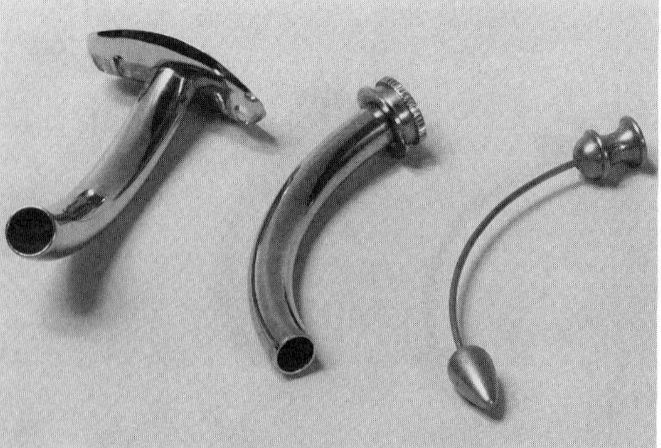

Figure 6-33. Metal tracheostomy tube with inner cannula and obturator.

Several manufacturers also produce a fenestrated tube (Figs. 6-35 and 6-36).[32] Fenestrated tubes may have a single fenestration or several fenestrations. The fenestration (or window) is cut on the cephalad side of the tube. With the inner cannula removed, the patient can breathe through the upper airway. During suctioning, the inner cannula should be replaced to ensure proper direction of the suction catheter. To ensure that the patient breathes only through his or her upper airway, a decannulation plug is used to occlude the external opening of the tube.

Cuffless tracheostomy tubes are also available in both fenestrated and nonfenestrated models. The nonfenestrated tube has three different inner cannulas: one with a 15-mm connector for humidification or ventilation (although not very satisfactory ventilation); one with a low-profile connection that is open; and one with a low-profile connection that is closed. The fenestrated tube has inserts similar to its cuffed sibling: an inner cannula with a 15-mm connector and a red decannulation plug; it also comes with the open connector with a low profile. There are also neonatal and pediatric tracheostomy tubes and laryngectomy tubes.

In the past, Mallinckrodt manufactured a tracheostomy tube called the Pitt Speaking Tube. This had an opening, located above the cuff, that was supplied with a flow of air or oxygen through the patient's vocal cords to allow speech (Fig. 6-37). The COMMUNItrach 1 (Fig. 6-38) has several ports above the cuff from which gas flows into the upper airway. The manufacturer recommends a gas flow of 6 to 8 L/min. It is available in sizes 7 and 9 mm.

Sometimes it is difficult to remove respiratory equipment from the tracheostomy tube. Several manufacturers supply a tracheal tube wedge (Fig. 6-39), which can be placed between the equipment and the tube to dislodge the respiratory equipment.

Cuffs

Most manufacturers use a cuff that is inflated using a syringe. A spring-loaded valve on the pilot balloon maintains cuff inflation when the syringe has been removed. The pilot balloon functions to show an "inflated" or "not inflated" condition of the cuff. It is impossible to judge the pressure within the cuff by squeezing the pilot balloon. The desired characteristics of the cuff are high residual volume and low pressure (called a high-volume/low-pressure cuff). The cuff is wrinkled when deflated. The cuff is nearly cylindrical in shape when inflated, which provides a large surface area for contact with the trachea. With this cuff, a seal can be produced with minimal pressure on the tracheal mucosa, and thus minimal ischemic injury to the tracheal wall. Older, high-

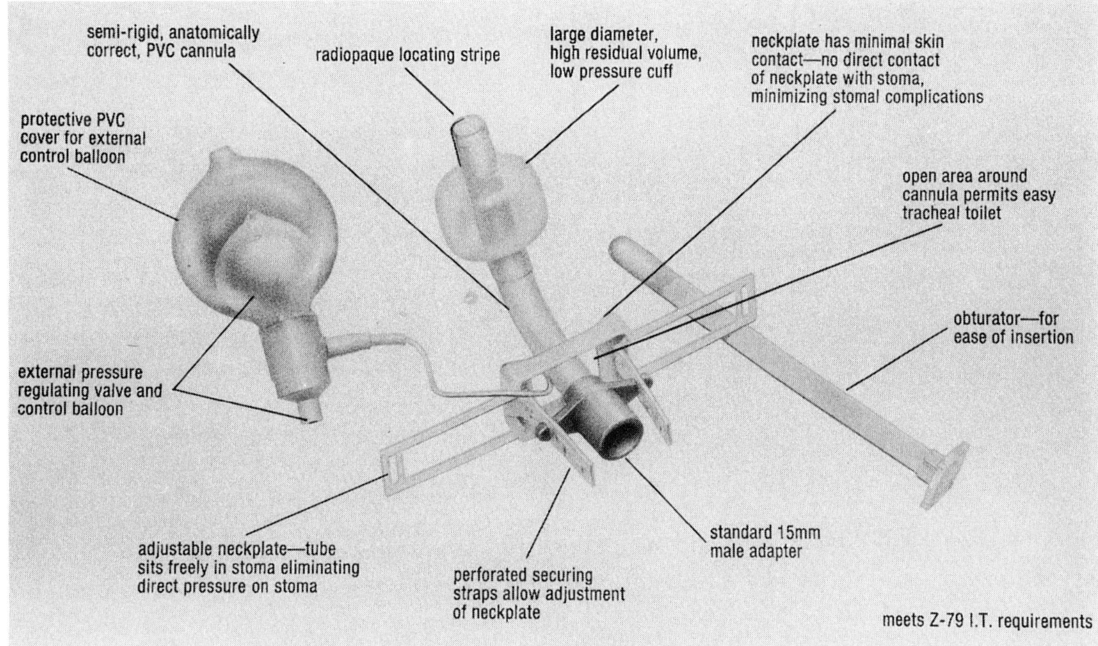

Figure 6-34. Lanz tracheostomy tube. (Courtesy of Mallinckrodt Critical Care, Glen Falls, NY)

pressure/low-volume cuffs (Fig. 6-40) lie against the tube when deflated and assume a donut shape when inflated. They require a higher pressure on the tracheal wall to obtain a seal than the low-pressure cuffs. High-volume/low-pressure cuffs are preferred because they produce less tracheal wall damage, but they are associated with a greater risk of aspiration.[33–36] Although a cuffed airway usually prevents massive aspiration, it should be appreciated that aspiration of pharyngeal secretions commonly occurs in intubated patients.

Lanz features a pressure-controlling pilot balloon. It is easily recognized by the presence of the large, floppy PVC cover over the pilot balloon (see Figs. 6-13 and 6-34). The compliance of the pilot balloon limits the pressure in the cuff to 20 to 25 mm Hg. Shiley uses a pop-off valve that limits cuff pressure to 25 mm Hg (Fig. 6-41).

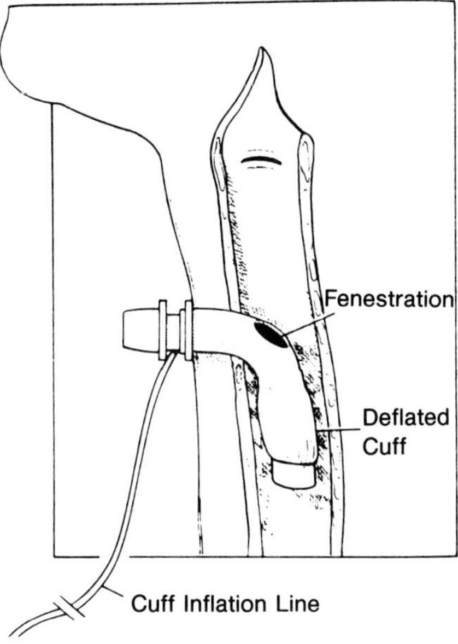

Figure 6-35. Fenestrated tracheostomy tube. (From Wilson DJ. Airway management of the ventilator-assisted individual. In: Gilmartin ME, Make BJ, eds. Mechanical ventilation in the home. Probl Respir Care 1988;1:192–203)

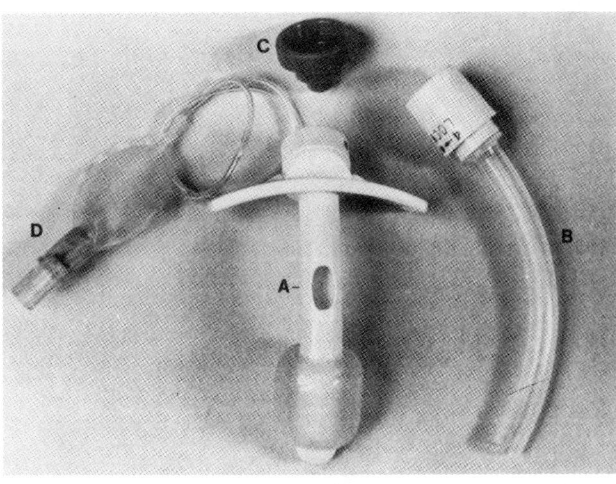

Figure 6-36. Shiley fenestrated tracheostomy tube. (A.) Fenestration. (B.) Inner cannula. (C.) Decannulation plug. (D.) Cuff inflation line. (From Wilson DJ. Airway management of the ventilator-assisted individual. In: Gilmartin ME, Make BJ, eds. Mechanical ventilation in the home. Probl Respir Care 1988;1:192–203)

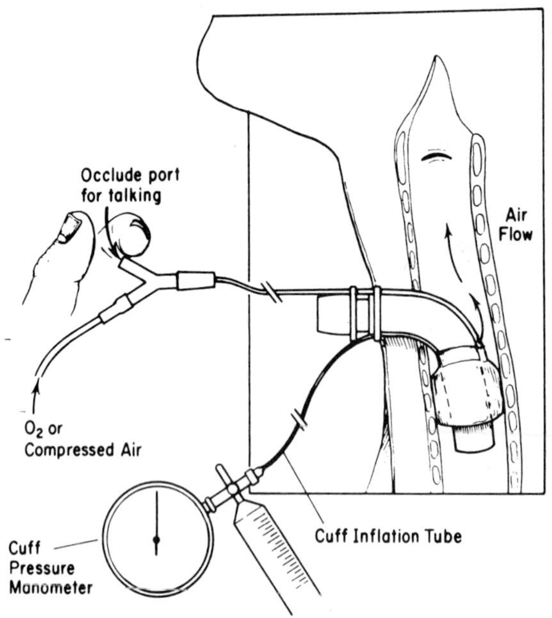

Figure 6-37. Schematic of speaking trach tube. (From Wilson DJ. Airway management of the ventilator-assisted individual. In: Gilmartin ME, Make BJ, eds. Mechanical ventilation in the home. Probl Respir Care 1988;1:192–203)

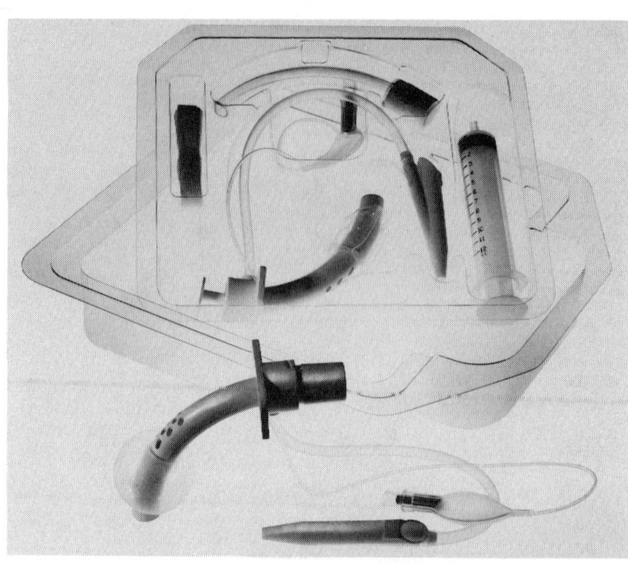

Figure 6-38. COMMUNItrach tube. (Courtesy of Implant Technologies)

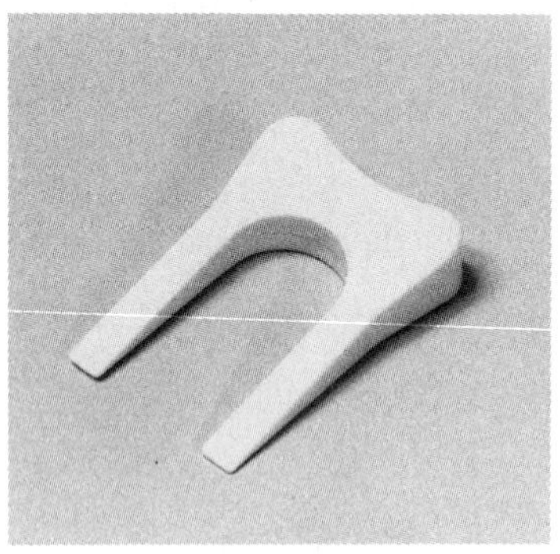

Figure 6-39. Tracheal wedge.

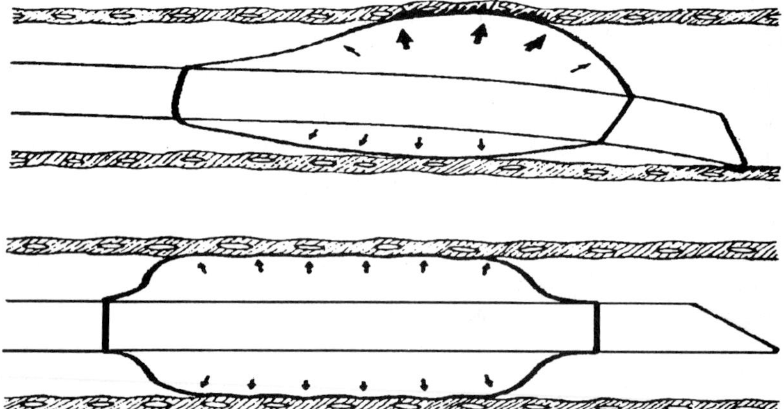

Figure 6-40. High-volume low-pressure cuff (bottom) and high-pressure low-volume cuff (top).

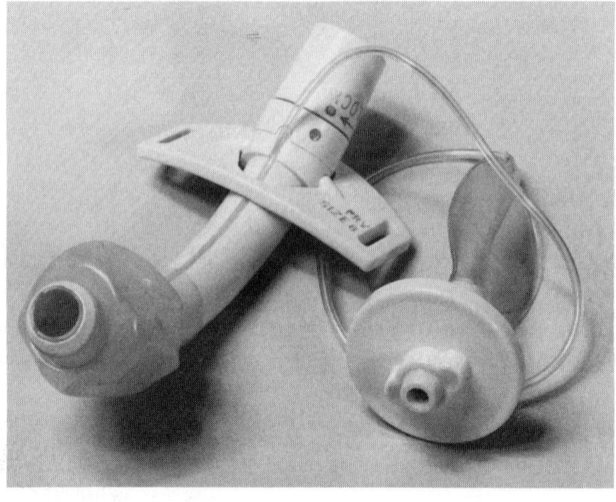

Figure 6-41. Shiley tracheostomy tube with pressure pop-off.

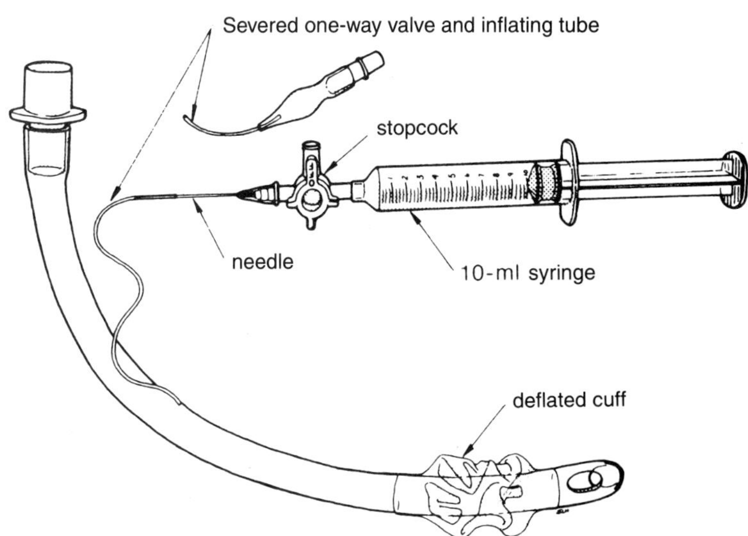

Figure 6-42. Use of a blunt needle to repair a severed pilot tube. (From Sills J. An emergency cuff inflation technique. Respir Care 1986;31: 199–201)

Occasionally, the pilot tube may be severed, removing the spring-loaded valve and pilot balloon. When this happens, a short blunt needle can be passed into the pilot tube, and a stopcock can then be attached to the needle hub to add and maintain air in the cuff until the tube is replaced (Fig. 6-42).[37]

Distinct from the other two types of tracheal tube cuffs is the Kamen-Wilkinson Fome-Cuff, often called the foam cuff (Fig. 6-43).[38] This cuff contains polyurethane foam that expands when the pilot tube is open to the atmosphere. It operates in a fashion opposite to that of the other cuffs. For insertion, the cuff is actively deflated by use of a syringe to remove the air. After insertion, the pilot tube is opened and the cuff expands until it contacts the tracheal wall. One feature that differentiates this cuff from the others is that as the cuff expands, the pressure it exerts on the trachea *decreases*. This means that the smaller the tube with respect to the airway, the less pressure is exerted on the airway wall. The pressure cannot be measured directly but is determined by evacuating the residual air from the cuff once it is in place and referring to a chart that is supplied by the manufacturer.

The pilot tube of a Kamen-Wilkinson tube is distinct from all other tubes because it lacks a pilot balloon.

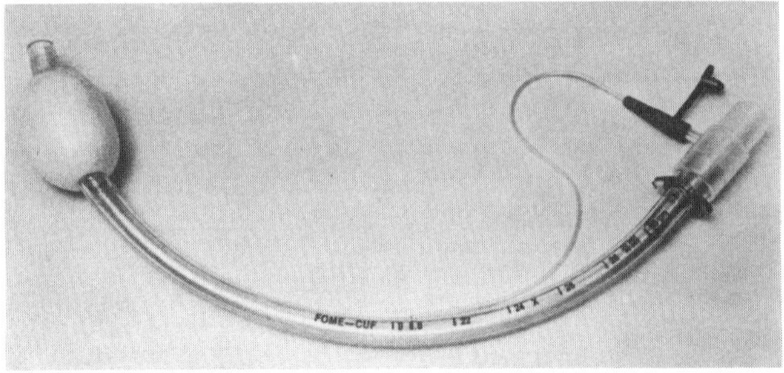

Figure 6-43. Kamen-Wilkinson Fome-Cuff. (Courtesy of Bivona, Gary, IN)

Also, the pilot tube for this airway should *never* be plugged. If air is added and the tube left plugged, it is converted to a "high pressure" cuff, with possible damage to the trachea. Kamen-Wilkinson tubes tend to leak if peak ventilatory pressure exceeds roughly 40 cm H_2O. To eliminate this problem, the manufacturer supplies a T-connector that allows pressurization of the cuff during the delivery of a positive-pressure breath. A concern regarding the Kamen-Wilkinson tube is its removal, especially in the situation in which the pilot tube has been damaged or cut. In this case, the tip of an 18- or 20-gauge needle is inserted into the remaining pilot tube so that the cuff can be deflated. However, it may not be necessary to deflate the cuff before removing the tube. Kamen, the developer of the tube, suggests that the cuff will deflate if the tube is removed slowly. It may be preferable to remove it without deflating the cuff, since this will prevent secretions that have pooled above the cuff from being aspirated into the trachea.[39]

Cuff Pressure Measurement

Cuff pressure can be measured using a manometer, stopcock, and 10-mL syringe (Fig. 6-44). Air is added or taken out of the cuff until a minimal leak or minimal occlusion is obtained. Minimal leak or minimal occlusion can be determined by auscultation over the trachea. The cuff pressure is then measured at end-exhalation. Care must be taken to avoid deflation of the cuff and aspiration of secretions above the cuff during this measurement. After the cuff pressure is measured, the stopcock is removed from the spring loaded valve to seal the air in the cuff. If the spring loaded valve is faulty, the stopcock can remain in place and be turned to seal air in the cuff. Ideally, the cuff pressure should not exceed 20 mm Hg (25 cm H_2O). Reasons for a high cuff pressure include use of a

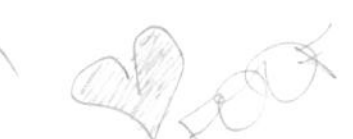

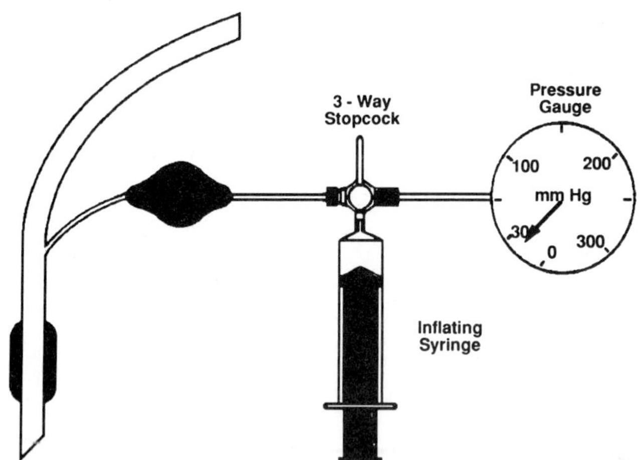

Figure 6-44. Cuff pressure measurement.

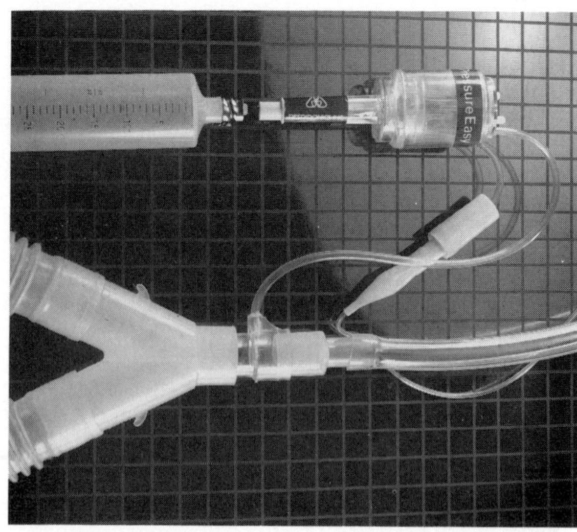

Figure 6-46. Respironics PressureEasy system. (Courtesy of Respironics, Murrysville, PA)

high-pressure cuff, use of a tube that is too small, dilation of the tracheal wall, and inflation of the cuff in the larynx or pharynx (in the case of an endotube).

Several devices are manufactured to measure or control cuff pressure. For measuring the pressure, Posey makes the Tracheal Cuff Inflation & Monitor (Fig. 6-45). It contains a manometer that is calibrated in centimeters of water, a bulb to inflate the cuff, and a valve to bleed air from the cuff. It is small and convenient, with a hook that enables it to be hung on a pocket. It also contains minimal deadspace so that the cuff does not deflate when the monitor is attached.

Respironics manufactures the PressureEasy (Fig. 6-46), which maintains a low pressure in the cuff while ensuring a seal during a positive-pressure breath. There is a diaphragm and spring that maintains the cuff at a pressure less than 27 cm H_2O. There is also a line that connects to the endotracheal tube or tracheostomy tube through a T-connector. This increases the pressure inside the cuff by an amount equal to the airway pressure, thus preventing the loss of tidal volume.

The Cuff-Mate is available from DHD Medical Products. The Cuff-Mate (Fig. 6-47) is a pocket-sized device that allows the user to inflate and deflate the cuff and to measure the volume added to the cuff. It also features an indicator light that alerts the user to cuff pressures above recommended safety limits. The Cuff-Mate 2 is also now available. It does all that the Cuff-Mate does, plus it has a digital display of cuff pressure in centimeters of water. The Cuff-Gauge is available from InterMed (Fig. 6-48). The Cuff-Gauge is a pocket-sized, battery-operated cuff inflator, deflator, and manometer. It provides a digital display of cuff pressure and measures inflation volume.

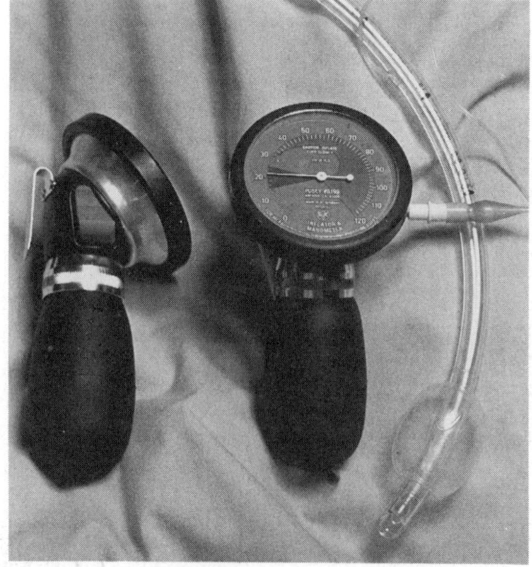

Figure 6-45. Posey cuff pressure measurement system.

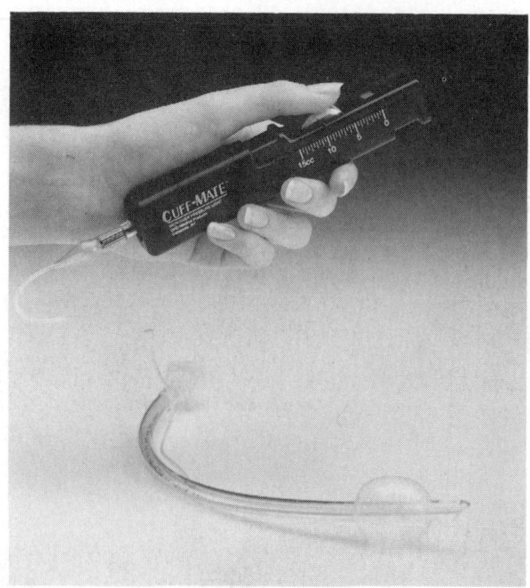

Figure 6-47. DHD Cuff-Mate. (Courtesy of DHD Medical Products, Canastota, NY)

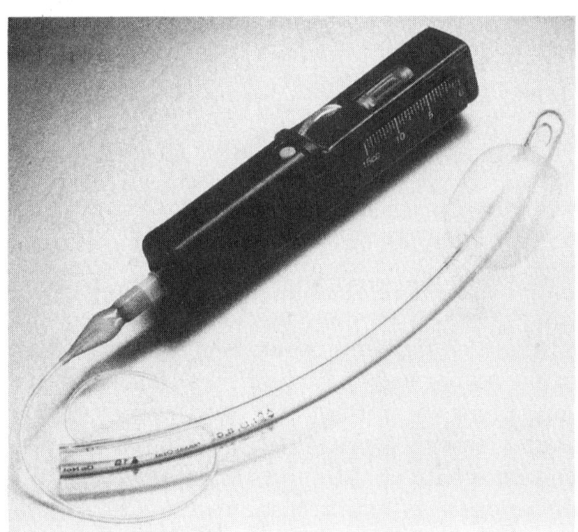

Figure 6-48. InterMed Digital Cuff-Gauge. (Courtesy of InterMed, Mentor, OH)

Stomal Maintenance Devices

There are two similar devices that are used to maintain the patency of the tracheal stoma without impinging on the lumen of the airway. They are used in cases when it is thought that periodic suctioning will be needed, during the process of weaning from a tracheostomy when it is believed the patient may not be able to tolerate decannulation, and in patients who may require repeated tracheostomy (eg, those with myasthenia gravis or chronic obstructive pulmonary disease).

One of these devices is the Olympic Trach-Button. It has a cannula with spacers and a closure plug (Fig. 6-49). The cannula is available in lengths from 9 to 14 mm in 1-mm steps. Each diameter is available in two lengths: 27 and 40 mm. The five spacers provided are of 1-, 2-, 4-, 7-, and 10-mm thickness. By using any two of these spacers with the proper length cannula, stomas from 15 to 40 mm in length can be fitted.

The other airway access device is the Kistner tube. This has a cannula with a flange on the end, a series of ridges, a movable flange, and a cap with a one-way valve inside. For insertion, a curved clamp is used to pinch the flange from the inside of the cannula. Once the cannula is inserted, the clamp is removed and the flange expands to anchor the cannula. The movable flange can then be moved to a different ridge as appropriate to stabilize the tube. Once the tube has been inserted, the cap is placed on the end. This cap has a one-way valve that allows inspiration through the valve but permits exhalation only through the patient's upper airway. Consequently, the patient will be able to talk and cough and expectorate secretions.

The one-way valve on the Kistner tube will not fit a standard 15-mm connector on a tracheostomy tube. Until early in 1986, a patient with a tracheostomy had to place a finger over the opening of the tracheostomy tube to talk. Then Muir invented the Passy-Muir Tracheostomy Speaking Valve. This device fits to the 15-mm connector of the tracheostomy tube and allows the patient to talk without significant exertion or having to cover the opening with a finger each time he or she speaks. The Passy-Muir Tracheostomy Speaking Valve is a one-way valve. It attaches to a tracheostomy tube, opens on inspiration to allow air to pass into the

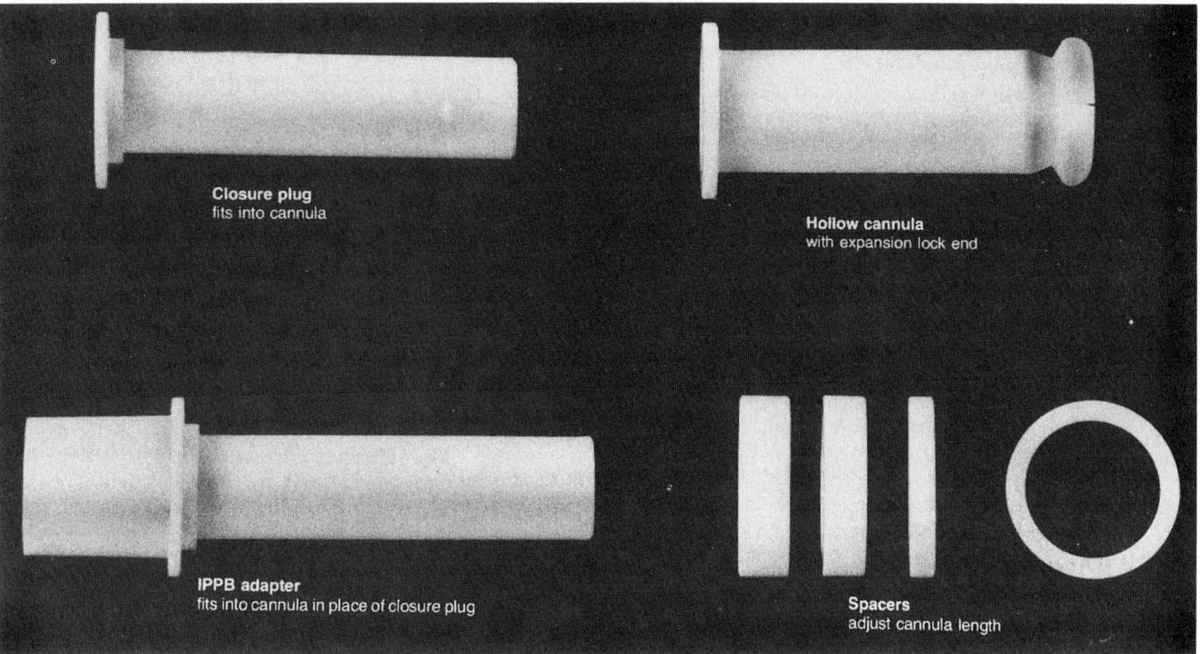

Figure 6-49. Olympic Trach-Button. (Courtesy of Olympic Medical, Seattle, WA)

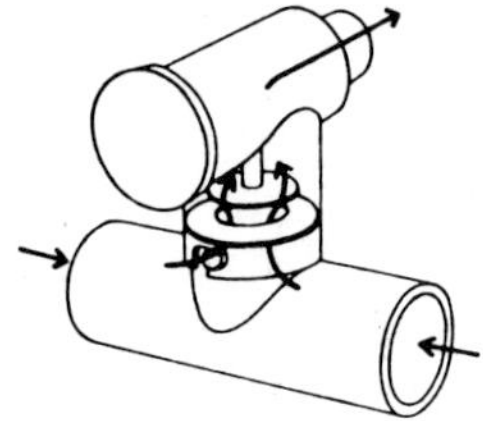

Inhalation
Spring-loaded, one-way valve remains open during inhalation.

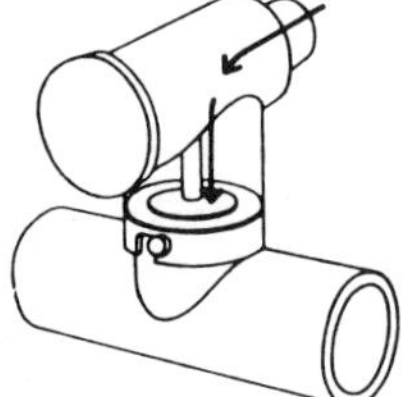

Exhalation
One-way valve closes, forcing air and mucus up trachea and past vocal cords.

Figure 6-50. Olympic Trach-Talk. (Courtesy of Olympic Medical, Seattle, WA)

lungs, and closes on expiration to direct air past the vocal cords and allow speech. The Passy-Muir valve must always be used with the cuff on the tracheostomy tube deflated.

The Olympic (Seattle, WA) Trach-Talk is a T-tube with a one-way valve that attaches to any tracheostomy tube to allow the patient to speak (Fig. 6-50). The Trach-Talk has both a 9-mm and a 15-mm connection that will enable it to fit any tracheostomy tube connector (the adaptor can be reversed and the suctioning cap placed on the other end). If the patient needs to be suctioned while the Trach-Talk is attached, this can be accomplished by removing the suctioning cap.

Before the Passy-Muir valve or Trach-Talk is applied, the patient should be suctioned while the cuff is deflated on the tracheostomy tube, since there may be secretions pooled above the cuff that may be aspirated into the airway. A sign should be posted above the patient's bed advising that the cuff should *not* be inflated when these devices are in use. Additionally, a patient with a Kamen-Wilkinson cuff should *never* have these devices applied.

Tube Fixation Devices

Several manufacturers make devices to secure an endotracheal tube in place. Olympic makes the Endolok (Fig. 6-51), Mallinckrodt makes the Tracheal Tube Restraint, Dale makes the Endotracheal Tube Holder, Posey makes the Endo-Fix, and Respironics makes the SecureEasy (Fig. 6-52). Each of these fastens the tube to the patient without the use of adhesive. These devices have several advantages over tape. They are easier to remove for mouth and skin care, they are less likely to cause allergic reactions, and they may be faster to apply. Balanced against these advantages is the disadvantage of cost. The decision to use these devices rather than adhesive tape to secure an endotracheal tube is a matter of institutional bias.

For tracheostomy tubes, Exidyne makes the Martin Trach-Secure. This consists of a padded tape that has Velcro at its ends. The tape is passed behind the patient's head, through the slits in the neck plate of the tube, and folded back on itself to secure the tracheostomy tube. Advantages of this over conventional cloth tape are that there is no need to use scissors, it is rapid to apply, it can be applied by one person, it is readily adjustable, and the elastic properties of the foam permit stretching to accommodate swelling of the neck or movement of the patient.

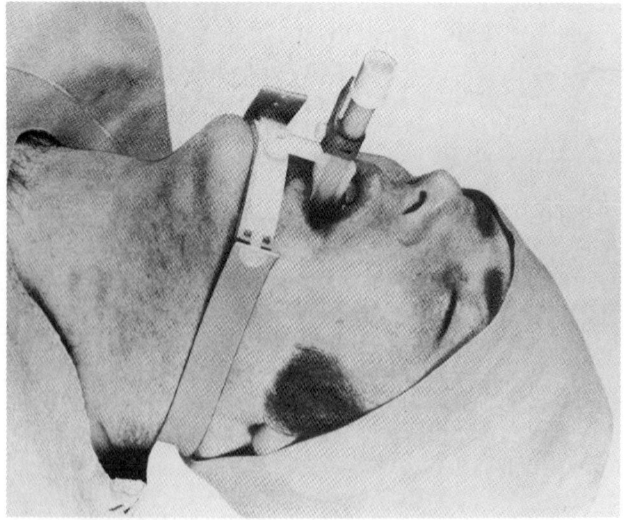

Figure 6-51. Olympic Endolok. (Courtesy of Olympic Medical, Seattle, WA)

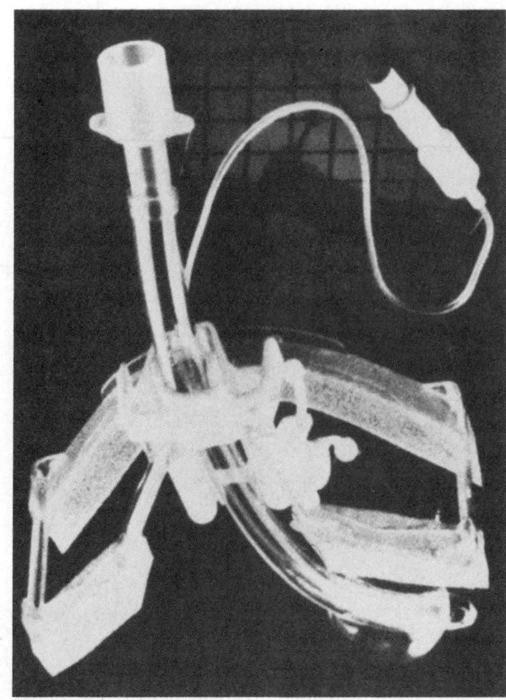

Figure 6-52. Respironics SecureEasy. (Courtesy of Respironics, Murrysville, PA)

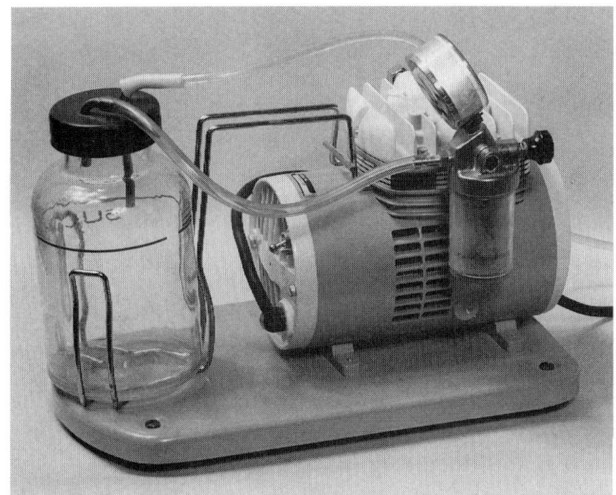

Figure 6-53. Portable suction machine.

Suction Equipment

Suction is used to aspirate secretions from the airway of the patient. A suction system has a vacuum source, a vacuum regulator, a trap bottle, a connecting tubing, and a suction catheter. The vacuum source may be either a hospital piped vacuum system or a portable vacuum pump. The portable vacuum pump (Fig. 6-53) is a diaphragm pump that works in the reverse of a diaphragm air compressor. For field and transport use, battery-operated suction devices are available (Impact Medical, West Caldwell, NJ) (Fig. 6-54). The vacuum source also may be a Venturi suction device (Fig. 6-55), which attaches to a 50-psig gas source and produces suction by control of gas flow through a jet.

A regulator is used to control the amount of pressure applied to the airway. A regulator that attaches to wall vacuum (Fig. 6-56) may control suction by partially obstructing the flow through it (Fig. 6-57) or by using a spring-loaded valve that limits the suction pressure. A portable suction machine uses a bleed-in valve to control suction. The greater the amount of flow drawn in through a needle valve from the room, the less suction is applied to the patient's airway (Fig. 6-58).

A trap bottle is used to collect the secretions removed from the airway so that they do not contaminate the vacuum regulator or suction machine. The trap bottle is usually equipped with a system to interrupt suction when it is full.

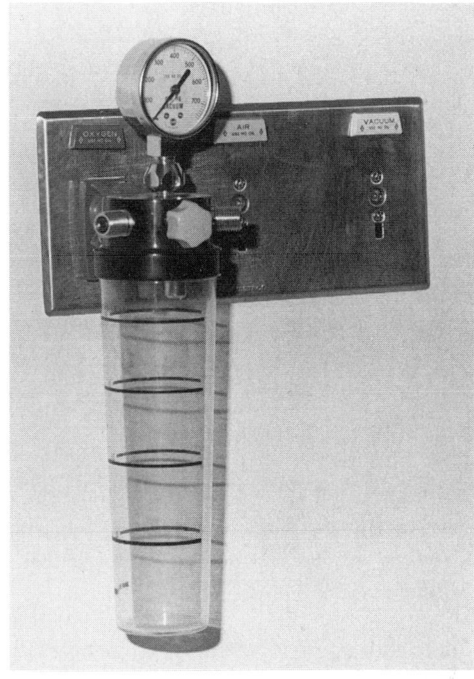

Figure 6-55. Venturi suction device.

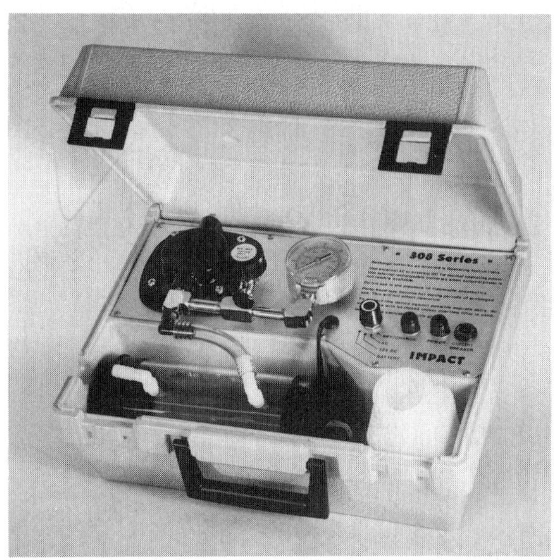

Figure 6-54. Impact battery-operated suction machine. (Courtesy of Impact Medical, West Caldwell, NJ)

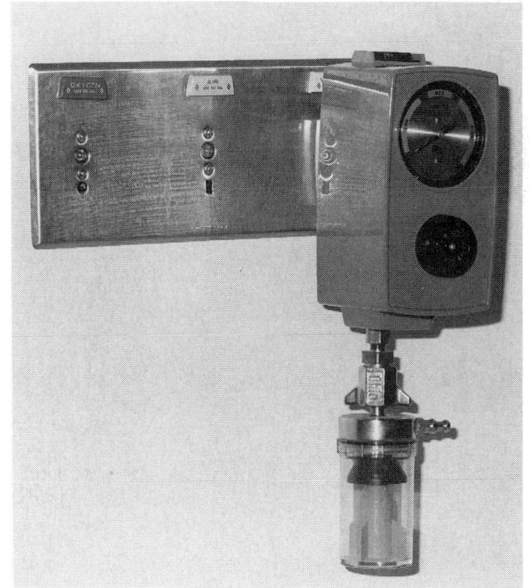

Figure 6-56. Vacuum regulator.

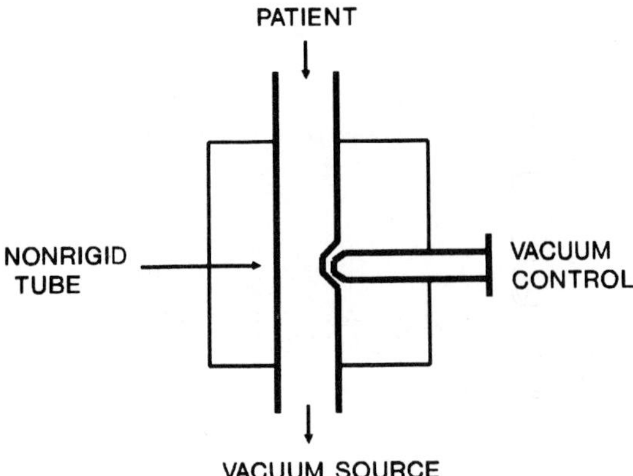

Figure 6-57. Operation of vacuum regulator.

The suction catheter is the part of the system that enters the airway of the patient. Several general features apply to all suction catheters.

- The catheter should be long enough to enter the mainstem bronchi. It is usually 22 inches long.
- The suction catheter should have some means to interrupt vacuum. Most have a thumb port at their proximal end, the internal diameter of which should be larger than the internal diameter of the catheter to prevent any residual vacuum when the thumb port is open.
- The catheter should be flexible enough to prevent damage to the airway mucosa but rigid enough to allow passage through an artificial airway.
- The catheter should effectively remove mucus with a pressure that does not damage the tracheal mucosa.
- The catheter should have smooth, molded ends to prevent airway mucosal damage.

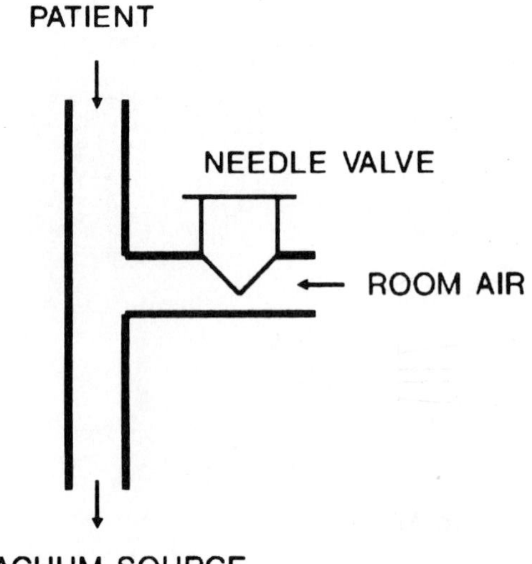

Figure 6-58. Bleed-in valve used on portable suction device.

- The catheter should have minimal frictional resistance when passed through an artificial airway.

Many catheter tips are commercially available. Although each manufacturer suggests that its catheter tip is safer than the others, correct technique is more important than catheter design in affecting complications due to suctioning.[40,41]

Suction catheter tips can be either straight or curved (Fig. 6-59). The curved-tip catheter is available in two designs, the Coude and the Bronchitrac. These catheters are designed to increase the possibility of the catheter entering the left bronchus. Curved-tip catheters are more effective in entering the left bronchus in tracheostomy patients than intubated patients.[42] The use of a curved-tip catheter will not result in 100% entry of the catheter into the left bronchus, although it does increase the possibility of left bronchial entry.

Suction catheters are available in a variety of sizes. Suction catheter size is determined by outside diameter in French size. French size refers to the external circumference of the tube. Because circumference equals 3.14 (π) times diameter, the outside diameter of the catheter can be estimated by dividing the French size by 3. As a rule, the outside diameter of a suction catheter should not exceed one-half to two-thirds of the inside diameter of the artificial airway. In adult patients, French size 14 is usually suitable.

Commercially available suction kits (Fig. 6-60) are available from many manufacturers. These kits include gloves, a sterile cup to rinse the catheter, and a sterile field. Other equipment needed to suction a patient's airway include a mask and goggles or face shield.

The Yankauer tip, or tonsil suction, is a rigid suction device used to suction the upper airway (Fig. 6-61). It should never be passed into the lower respiratory tract. It is available in transparent and opaque designs, with and without a thumb port.

Closed suction systems (Fig. 6-62) are available from several manufactures. These allow ventilated patients to be suctioned without disconnecting the patient from the ventilator. This may reduce the risk of cross-contamination, desaturation due to ventilation disconnection, or both. However, this has not been scientifically proven.[43,44] These devices can be attached for a period up to 24 hours. They are available in both straight-tip and curved-tip designs. Many swivel adapters for endotracheal tubes also have a port that can be used for suctioning (Fig. 6-63).

A specialized closed suction system is the Jinotti oxygen insufflation catheter. This is a dual-lumen catheter, which can be used to suction secretions and to deliver oxygen between suction procedures (Fig. 6-64).[45]

In infants, pneumothorax has been reported secondary to endotracheal suctioning.[46–49] Because of this, it has been recommended that deep trachea suctioning

(text continues on page 141)

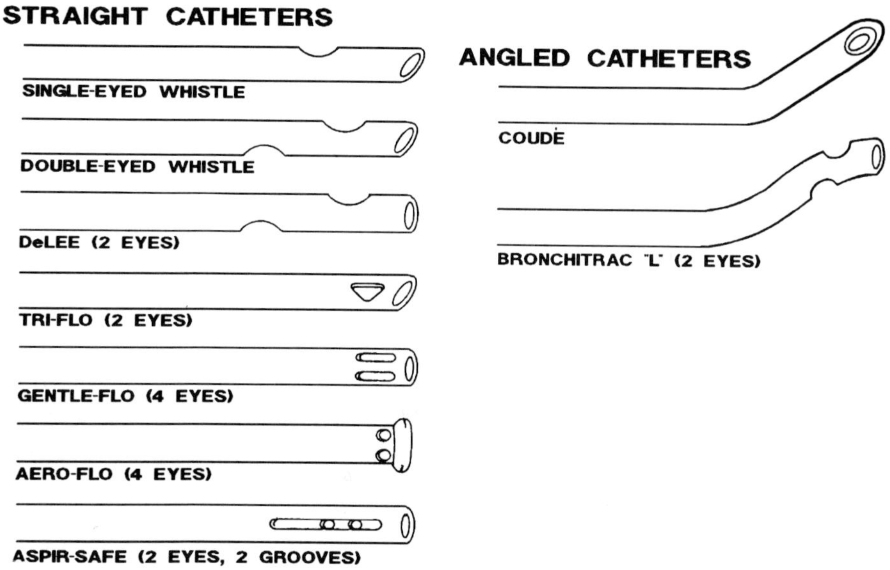

STRAIGHT CATHETERS
SINGLE-EYED WHISTLE
DOUBLE-EYED WHISTLE
DeLEE (2 EYES)
TRI-FLO (2 EYES)
GENTLE-FLO (4 EYES)
AERO-FLO (4 EYES)
ASPIR-SAFE (2 EYES, 2 GROOVES)
ANGLED CATHETERS
COUDE
BRONCHITRAC "L" (2 EYES)

Figure 6-59. Suction catheter tip designs.

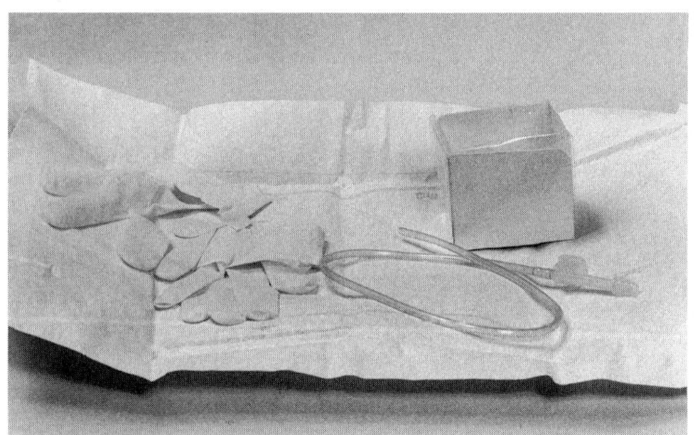

Figure 6-60. Disposable suction catheter kit.

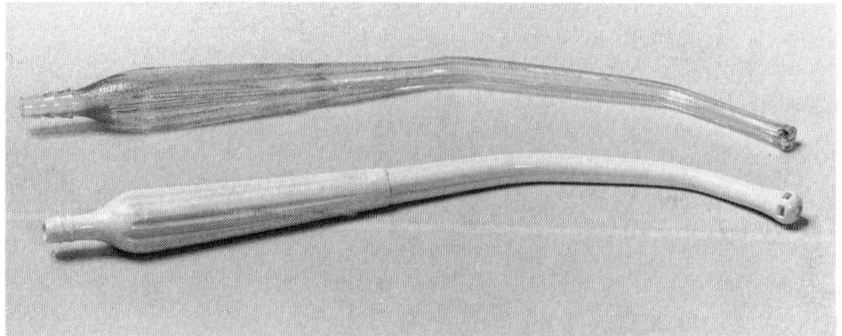

Figure 6-61. Yankauer tip suction devices.

IRRIGATION PORT
LOCK-UNLOCK CONTROL VALVE
LOCK
SUCTION CONNECTION
CATHETER IN SLEEVE
T-PIECE

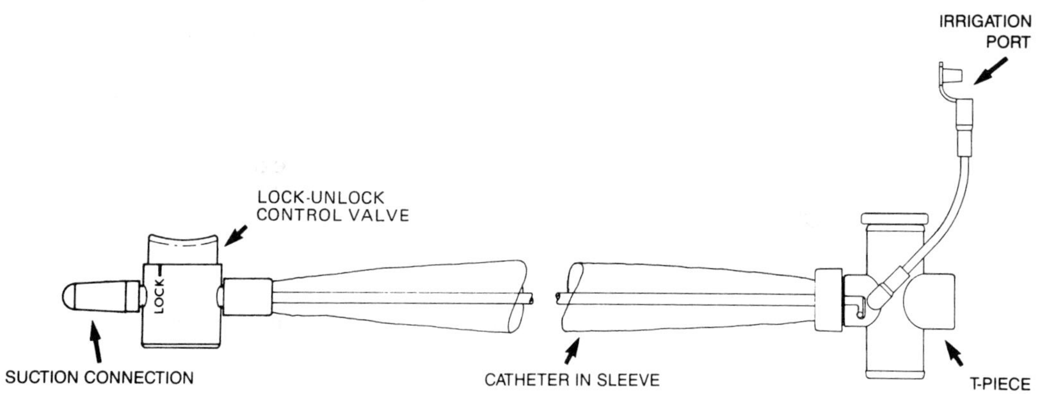

Figure 6-62. Ballard closed suction system. (Courtesy of Ballard, Midvale, UT)

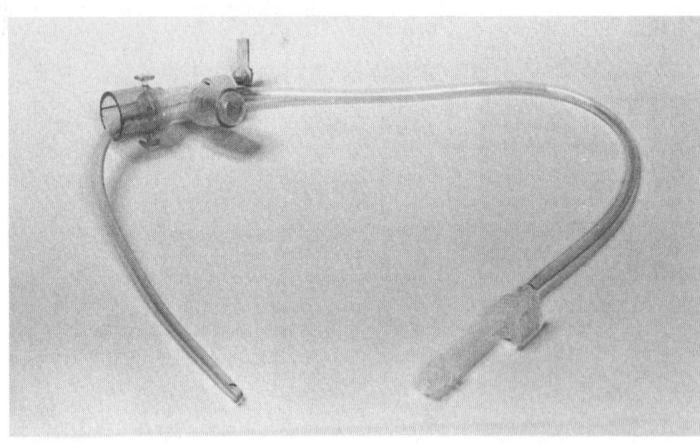

Figure 6-63. Catheter through suction port of swivel adaptor.

To Suction: Valve tabs in closed position

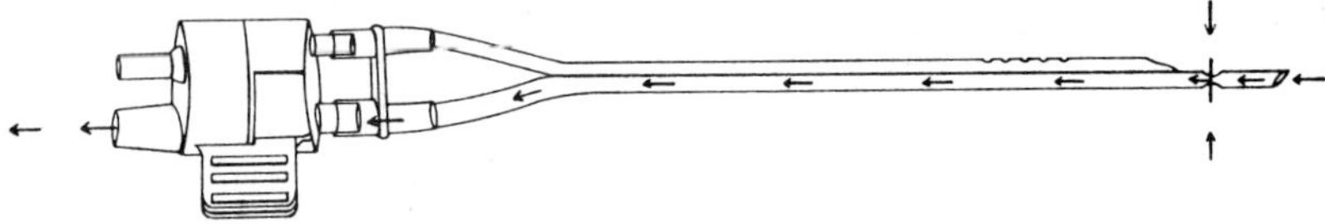

To Supply Oxygen: Valve tabs in open position

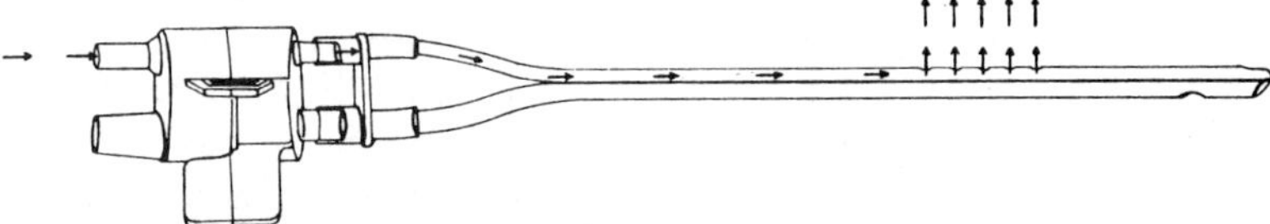

To Instill Tracheal Lavage Fluid: Inject fluid with luer tip syringe through oxygen tubing connection

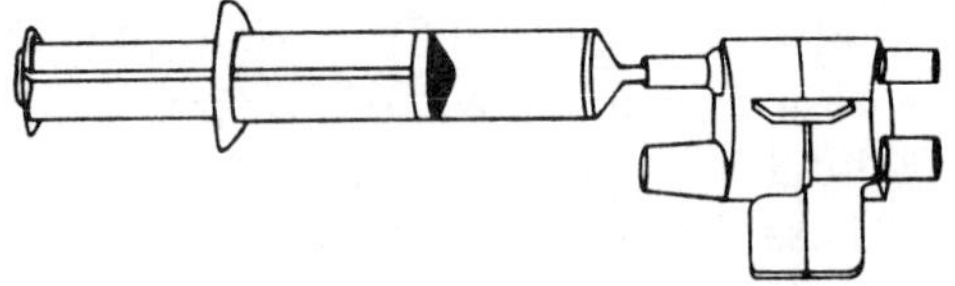

Figure 6-64. Jinotti oxygen insufflation catheter. (Courtesy of American Pharmaseal Co, Valencia, CA)

TABLE 6-1. Maximal Catheter Measurements for Oral Endotracheal Suction of Newborns

Infant Weight (g)	Oral-Carinal Distance (cm)*
500	7
600–1000	8
1100–1500	9
1600–2000	10
2100–2500	11
2600–3000	12
3100–3500	13
3600–4000	14

*To this distance, add the length of endotracheal tube that protrudes from the mouth.

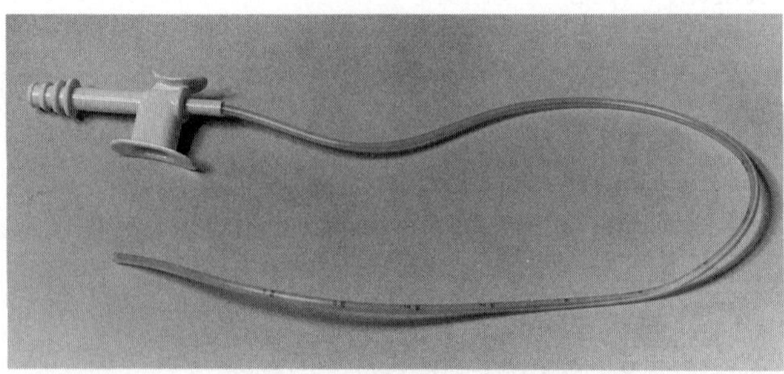

Figure 6-65. Argyle Saf-T-Mark neonatal suction catheter with distance markings. (Courtesy of Sherwood Medical, St. Louis, MO)

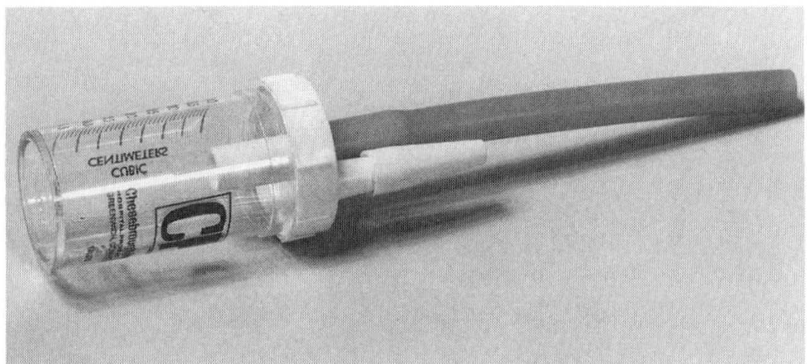

Figure 6-66. Lukens trap.

of the neonate should be avoided. The maximal safe distance to pass a suction catheter through endotracheal tubes has been published for both orocarinal distances and nasocarinal distances. For orotracheal suction, the length of endotracheal tube protruding from the mouth is measured and the length from Table 6-1 is added. The Argyle Saf-T-Mark and some suction catheters from other manufacturers (Fig. 6-65) have distance markings on it as a guide for safe suctioning of the neonate.

A specimen trap can be used to collect sputum during suctioning for laboratory analysis. Commonly used is a Lukens trap (Fig. 6-66), which is placed between the suction catheter and the connecting tubing leading to the trap bottle of the suction system.

Nasal Prongs and Nasal Masks for Positive-Pressure Ventilation

Continuous positive airway pressure (CPAP) is commonly used in the care of neonates with respiratory disease. Although hoods, masks, and endotracheal tubes can be used, neonatal CPAP is often administered by use of nasal prongs. Several types of nasal prongs are available for this use (Fig. 6-67). These include the Argyle, Vesta, Hudson, and Infant Nasal Cannula Assembly (INCA). The Vesta is actually a nasopharyngeal airway for infants. The Argyle and Vesta have a 15-mm adapter to attach respiratory equipment. The Hudson and INCA are supplied with a head strap to allow the system to be secured to the patient (Fig. 6-68). The resistance to breathing through some of these devices is similar to the natural resistance to flow through the nose, but resistance to breathing may increase if small-diameter prongs are used.[50]

In adults, nasal masks are used with nasal CPAP therapy to treat obstructive sleep apnea and with nighttime ventilation to treat chronic respiratory fail-

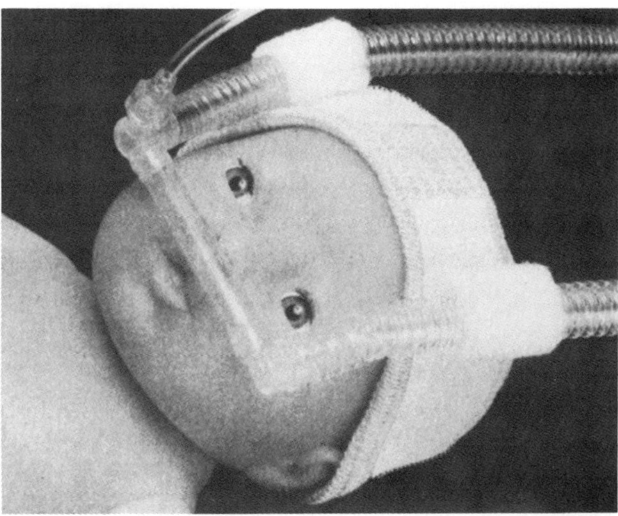

Figure 6-68. Hudson continuous positive airway pressure system secured in place. (Courtesy of Hudson-RCI, Temecula, CA)

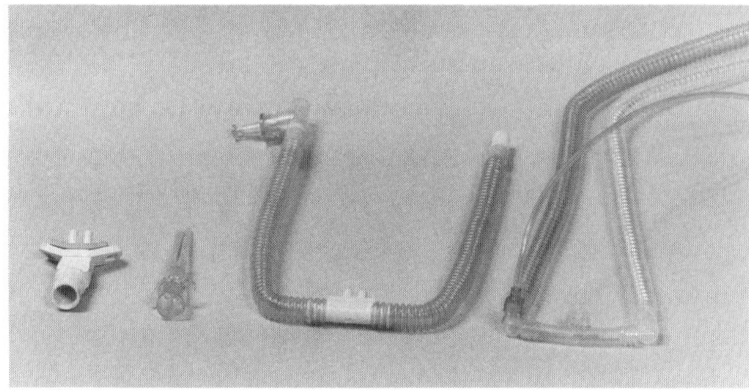

Figure 6-67. Nasal prongs for infant continuous positive airway pressure system (from left): Argyle, Vesta, Hudson, INCA.

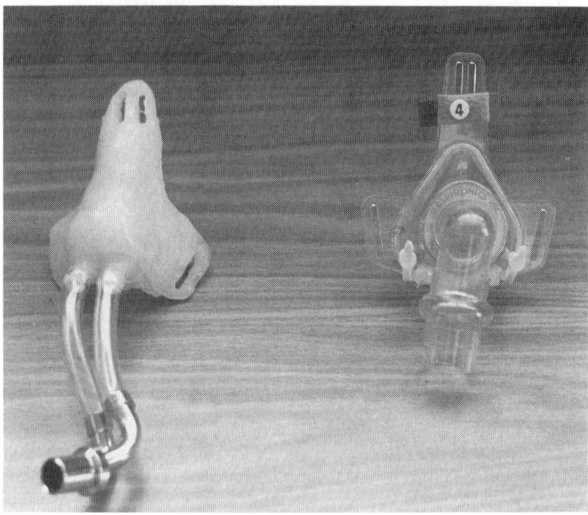

Figure 6-69. Custom-made (left) and commercially available (right, Respironics) nasal masks for positive-pressure breathing.

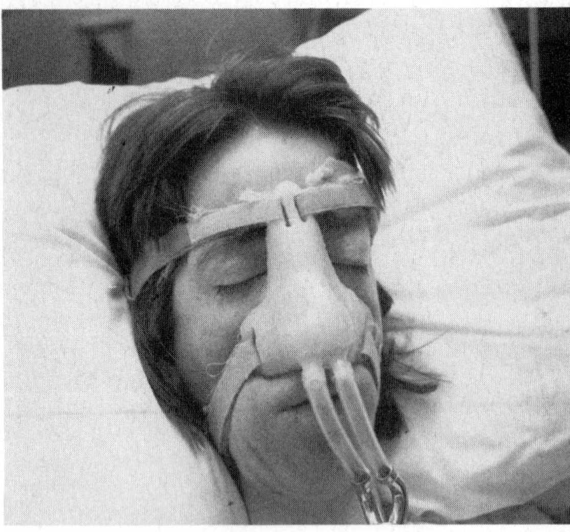

Figure 6-70. Nasal mask in place.

ure. With this therapy, air is prevented from leaking from the mouth because the soft palate and tongue are held together and pushed away from the posterior pharyngeal wall, forming a hermetic seal of the oral cavity. These masks can be either custom made or commercially made (Figs. 6-69 and 6-70).[51]

AARC Clinical Practice Guideline

Nasotracheal Suctioning: Indications, Contraindications, Hazards, and Complications

Nasotracheal suctioning is intended to remove accumulated secretions, blood, vomitus, and other foreign material from the trachea that cannot be removed by the patient's spontaneous cough or other less invasive procedures.

- Indications:
  - inability to clear secretions
  - audible evidence of secretions in the large central airways that persist in spite of the patient's best cough effort
- Contraindications:
  - occluded nasal passages
  - nasal bleeding
  - epiglottitis or croup
  - acute head, facial, or neck injury
  - laryngospasm
  - irritable airway
  - upper respiratory infection
- Hazards and Complications:
  - mechanical trauma
  - hypoxia/hypoxemia
  - cardiac dysrhythmias/arrest
  - bradycardia
  - increase in blood pressure
  - hypotension
  - respiratory arrest
  - uncontrolled coughing
  - gagging/vomiting
  - laryngospasm
  - bronchoconstriction/bronchospasm
  - pain
  - nosocomial infection
  - atelectasis
  - misdirection of catheter
  - increased intracranial pressure

(Adapted from AARC Clinical Practice Guideline, published in August, 1992, issue of Respiratory Care; see original publication for complete text)

AARC Clinical Practice Guideline

Endotracheal Suctioning of Mechanically Ventilated Adults and Children With Artificial Airways: Indications, Contraindications, Hazards, and Complications

Endotracheal suctioning is a component of bronchial hygiene therapy during mechanical ventilation and involves the mechanical aspiration of pulmonary secretions from a patient with an artificial airway in place.

- Indications:
  - the need to remove accumulated pulmonary secretions
  - the need to obtain a sputum specimen to rule out or identify pneumonia or other pulmonary infection or for sputum cytology
  - the need to maintain the patency and integrity of the artificial airway
  - the need to stimulate a patient cough in patients unable to cough effectively secondary to changes in mental status or the influence of medication

- presence of pulmonary atelectasis or consolidation, presumed to be associated with secretion retention

- Contraindications: there are no contraindications to this procedure when it is indicated

- Hazards/Complications:
  - hypoxia/hypoxemia
  - tissue trauma to the trachea or bronchial mucosa
  - cardiac arrest
  - respiratory arrest
  - cardiac dysrhythmias
  - pulmonary atelectasis
  - bronchospasm/bronchoconstriction
  - infection (patient or caregiver)
  - pulmonary hemorrhage/bleeding
  - elevated intracranial pressure
  - interruption of mechanical ventilation
  - hypertension
  - hypotension

(Adapted from AARC Clinical Practice Guideline, published in May, 1993, issue of Respiratory Care; see original publication for complete text)

References

1. Standards and Guidelines for Cardiopulmonary Resuscitation and Emergency Cardiac Care. JAMA 1992;268:2171–2302.
2. Wanner A, Zighelboim A, Sackner MA. Nasopharyngeal airway: A facilitated access to the trachea. Ann Intern Med 1971;75: 593–595.
3. Melker RJ, Gordon AS. The esophageal obturator airway (letter). Chest 1979;76:661–612.
4. McElroy CR. The esophageal obturator airway. J Emerg Nurs 1978;4:358.
5. Don Michael TA. Esophageal obturator airway. Med Instrum 1977;11:331–333.
6. Pilcher DB, DeMeules JE. Esophageal perforation following use of esophageal airway. Chest 1976;69:377–380.
7. Strate RG, Fischer RP. Midesophageal perforations by esophageal obturator airways. J Trauma 1976;16:503–509.
8. Harrison EE, Nord HF, Beeman RW. Esophageal perforation following the use of the esophageal obturator airway. Ann Emerg Med 1980;9:21–25.
9. Johnson KR, Genovesi MG, Lassar KH. Esophageal obturator airway: Use and complication. JACEP 1976;5:36–19.
10. Heide E. Incorrect assembly complicates esophageal obturator airway use (letter). Ann Emerg Med 1980;9:113.
11. McLaughlin AJ Jr, Scott W. Training and evaluation of respiratory therapists in emergency intubation. Respir Care 1981;26: 333–335.
12. Key GK. Use of the esophageal obturator airway. Postgrad Med 1980; 67:189–193.
13. Stewart RD. Iatrogenic intragastric "foreign body" (letter). Chest 1981;80:244.
14. Bartlett RL, Martin SD, Perina D, Raymond JI. The pharyngeotracheal lumen airway: An assessment of airway control in the setting of upper airway hemorrhage. Ann Emerg Med 1987;16: 343–346.
15. Niemann JT, Rosborough JP, Myers R, Scarberry EN. The pharyngeo-tracheal lumen airway: Preliminary investigation of a new adjunct. Ann Emerg Med 1984;13:591–596.
16. Hunt RC, Sheets CA, Shitley TW. Pharyngeal tracheal lumen airway training: Failure to discriminate between esophageal and endotracheal modes and failure to confirm ventilation. Ann Emerg Med 1989;18:947–952.
17. Grigsby JW, Rottman SJ. Prehospital airway management: Esophageal obturator airway or endotracheal intubation? Topics Emerg Med 1981;3:25–29.
18. White RD. Controversies in out-of-hospital emergency airway control: Esophageal obstruction or endotracheal intubation? Ann Emerg Med 1985;13:778.
19. Hammargren Y, Clinton JE, Ruiz E. Standardized comparison of the EOA and endotracheal tube in cardiac arrest. Ann Emerg Med 1984;13:140.
20. Goldenbery IF, Campion BC, Siebold CM, McBride JW. Esophageal gastric tube airway vs. endotracheal tube in prehospital cardiopulmonary arrest. Chest 1986;90:90–96.
21. Shea SR, Mac Donald JR, Gruzinski G. Prehospital endotracheal tube airway or esophageal gastric tube airway: A critical comparison. Ann Emerg Med 1985;14:102–112.
22. Don Michael TA. Comparison of the esophageal obturator airway and endotracheal intubation in prehospital ventilation during CPR. Chest 1985;87:814–819.
23. Pointer JE. Clinical characteristics of paramedics' performance of endotracheal intubation. J Emerg Med 1988;6:505–509.
24. Stewart RD, Peris RM, Winter PM, Pelton GH, Cannon GM. Field endotracheal intubation by paramedical personnel: Success rates and complications. Chest 1984;85:341–345.
25. Pepe PE, Copass MK, Joyce TH. Prehospital endotracheal intubation: Rationale for training emergency medical personnel. Ann Emerg Med 1985;14:1085–1092.
26. Applebaum El, Bruce DL. Tracheal Intubation. Philadelphia: WB Saunders, 1976.
27. Suarez M, Chediak A, Ershowsky P, Krieger B. Evaluation of a flexible catheter in confirming endotracheal tube placement in the intensive care unit. Respir Care 1987;32:81–84.
28. Dietrich KA, Strauss RH, Cabalka AK, Zimmerman JJ, Scanlan KA. Use of flexible fiberoptic endoscopy for determination of endotracheal tube position in the pediatric patient. Crit Care Med 1988;16:884–887.
29. Steward RD, LaRossee A, Stoy WA, Heller MB. Use of a lighted stylet to confirm correct endotracheal tube placement. Chest 1987:92:900–903.
30. Weis FR, Hatton MN. Intubation by use of the light wand: Experience in 253 patients. J Oral Maxillofac Surg 1989;47: 577–580.
31. Yealy DM, Paris PM. Recent advances in airway management. Emerg Med Clin North Am 1989;7:83–89.
32. Wilson DJ. Airway management of the ventilator-assisted individual. In: Gilmartin ME, Make BJ, eds. Mechanical ventilation in the home. Problems in Respiratory Care, vol 1. Philadelphia: JB Lippincott, 1988:192–203.
33. Carroll RG, McGinnis GE, Grenvik A. Performance characteristics of tracheal cuffs. Int Anaesth Clin 1974;12:111–141.
34. Carroll RG. Evaluation of tracheal tube designs. Crit Care Med 1973;1:45–46.
35. Lewis FR, Schlobohm RM, Thomas AN. Prevention of complications from prolonged tracheal intubation. Am J Surg 1978;135: 452–457.
36. Mehta S, Mickiewicz M. Pressure in large volume, low pressure cuffs: Its significance, measurement, and regulation. Intens Care Med 1985;11:267–272.
37. Sills J. An emergency cuff inflation technique. Respir Care 1986;31: 199–201.
38. Kamen JM, Wilkinson CJ. A new low-pressure cuff for endotracheal tubes. Anesthesiology 1971;34:482–485.
39. Kamen JM. More on endotracheal tube cuff deflation (letter). Respir Care 1980;25:16–17.
40. Link WJ, Spaeth EE, Wahle WM, Penny W, Glover JL. The influence of suction catheter tip design on tracheobronchial trauma and fluid aspiration efficiency. Anesth Analg 1976;55: 290–297.
41. Sackner MA, Landa JF, Greeneltch N, Robinson MJ. Pathogenesis and prevention of tracheobronchial damage with suction procedures. Chest 1973;64:284–290.
42. Panacek EA, Albertson TE, Rutherford WF, Fisher CJ, Foulke GE. Selective left endobronchial suctioning in the intubated patient. Chest 1989;95:885–887.
43. Ritz R, Scott LR, Coyle MB, Pierson DJ. Contamination of a multiple-use suction catheter in a closed-circuit system compared to contamination of a disposable, single-use suction catheter. Respir Care 1986;31:1086–1092.

44. Carlon GC, Fox SJ, Ackerman NJ. Evaluation of a closed-tracheal suction system. Crit Care Med 1987;15:522–525.
45. Smith RM, Benson MS, Schoene RB. The efficacy of oxygen insufflation in preventing arterial oxygen desaturation during endotracheal suctioning of mechanically ventilated patients. Respir Care 1987;32:865–869.
46. Bailey C, Kattwinkel J, Teja K, Buckley T. Shallow versus deep endotracheal suctioning in young rabbits: Pathologic effects on the tracheobronchial wall. Pediatrics 1988;82:746–751.
47. Andersib KD, Chandra R. Pneumothorax secondary to perforation of segmental bronchi by suction catheters. J Pediatr Surg 1976;11:687–693.
48. Coldiron JS. Estimation of nasotracheal tube length in neonates. Pediatrics 1968;41:823–828.
49. Grosfield JL, Lemons JL, Ballantine TVN, Schreiner RL. Emergency thoracotomy for acquired bronchopleural fistula in the premature infant with respiratory distress. J Pediatr Surg 1980; 15:416–421.
50. Czervinske M, Durbin CG, Gal TJ. Resistance to gas flow across 14 CPAP devices for newborns. Respir Care 1986;31:18–21.
51. O'Donnell C, Gilmartin ME. Home mechanical ventilators and accessory equipment. In: Gilmartin ME, Make BJ, eds. Mechanical ventilation in the home. Problems in Respiratory Care, vol 1. Philadelphia: JB Lippincott, 1988:217–240.

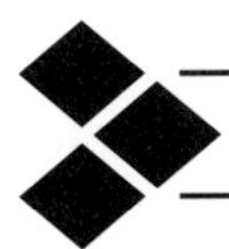

7

Manual and Gas-Powered Resuscitators

Dean R. Hess

OBJECTIVES

1. List the characteristics of an ideal mask for emergency ventilation.
2. Describe the correct use of mouth-to-mask ventilation devices.
3. Distinguish between mouth-to-mask devices and face shield devices.
4. Describe the construction of a bag-valve resuscitator unit.
5. List the characteristics of an ideal bag-valve resuscitator.
6. Compare tube reservoirs, bag reservoirs, and oxygen supply valves for bag-valve resuscitators.
7. Compare spring disk/ball valves, diaphragm/leaf valves, and duck bill valves for bag-valve resuscitators.
8. Describe the construction of a flow-inflating resuscitator.
9. List advantages and disadvantages of oxygen-powered resuscitators.
10. List characteristics of an ideal oxygen-powered resuscitator.

KEY TERMS

bag reservoir
bag-valve resuscitator
face shield device
flow-inflating resuscitator
gastric insufflation
Mapleson circuit
mouth-to-mask devices
mouth-to-mouth technique
non-rebreathing valve
oxygen-powered resuscitator
oxygen reservoir
oxygen supply valve
pressure pop-off
tube reservoir

Richard D. Branson: RESPIRATORY CARE EQUIPMENT,

Emergency Ventilation Devices

Several types of adjuncts are available for emergency ventilation. These include masks, bag-valve resuscitators, flow-inflating resuscitators, oxygen-powered resuscitators, and emergency ventilators. The American Heart Association (AHA), the Emergency Care Research Institute (ECRI), the American Society for Testing and Materials (ASTM), and International Standards Organization (ISO) have published recommendations for the use and evaluation of these devices.[1-9] Because these devices are used with apneic patients, it is imperative that they are used correctly. Misuse of emergency ventilation equipment may have dire consequences for the patient. Thus, respiratory care practitioners must understand how these devices are constructed and how they are used.

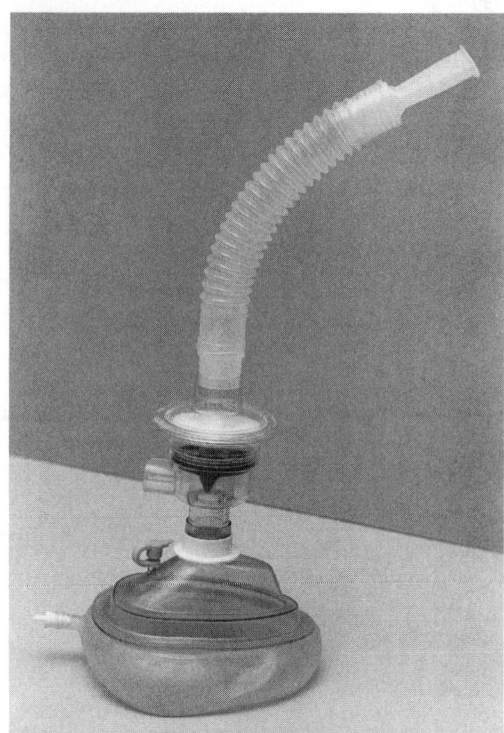

Figure 7-1. Mouth-to-mask ventilation device. Note soft resilient cuff, transparent mask, one-way valve and filter assembly, and oxygen nipple. (Courtesy of Bird/LDS, Carrollton, TX)

Mask Ventilation

A face mask is used for emergency ventilation if an artificial airway is not present. Mask ventilation can be provided using mouth-to-mask technique, bag-valve-mask technique, or an oxygen-powered resuscitator. This section of the chapter focuses on the mouth-to-mask ventilation technique.

Characteristics of an Ideal Mask

ADEQUATE SEAL. The mask should fit tightly against the face to prevent air leaks. This is often accomplished by use of an air-filled resilient cuff. In many cases, the mask is designed using a manufacturer-specific modification of a standard mask design (Fig. 7-1). In other cases, an unusual design has been adopted to facilitate a seal (Fig. 7-2).

OXYGEN INLET. For mouth-to-mask technique, a nipple should be provided to allow administration of supplemental oxygen. The nipple should be fitted with a one-way valve or plug to prevent a gas leak if oxygen is not used.

TRANSPARENCY. The face mask should be constructed of a transparent material. This allows visualization of the nose and mouth and the detection of regurgitation.

STANDARD 15/22 CONNECTOR. The mask should have an adaptor with a 15-mm outside diameter or a 22-mm inside diameter to allow attachment of a one-way valve and filter, resuscitator bag, or oxygen-powered resuscitator.

SIZE. An average size mask should allow it to be used for most adults. Additional sizes should be available for very large or very small adults and for infants and children.

ONE-WAY VALVE OR FILTER. A one-way valve and/or filter should be available to be attached to the mask to protect the rescuer from contamination with the patient's exhaled gas (or vomitus) when mouth-to-mask technique is used. The exhaled gas of the patient should be vented away from the rescuer. The valve (or filter) should not jam in the presence of vomitus or humidity. An extension tube may also be used as an additional barrier between the rescuer and the patient.

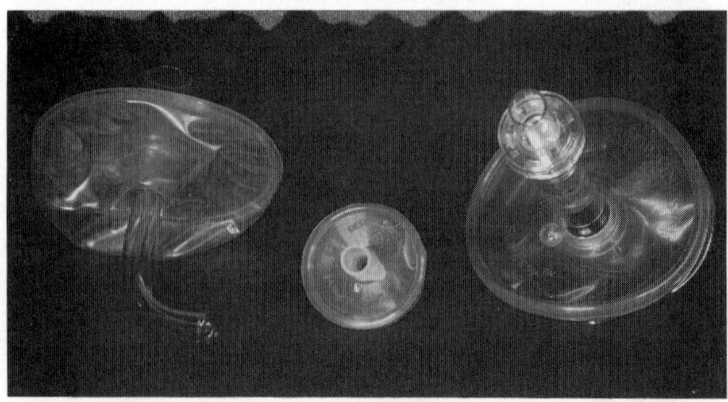

Figure 7-2. SealEasy resuscitation mask. The device on the left is fitted with an oropharyngeal airway, the one in the center is for infant resuscitation, and the one on the right is fitted with a one-way valve. (Courtesy of Respironics, Murrysville, PA)

MINIMAL AIRFLOW RESISTANCE. To prevent rescuer fatigue and improve ventilation of the patient, the valve-filter-extension should have minimal airflow resistance. According to ISO standards,[9] the back pressure produced by the device should be less than 5 cm H_2O at a flow of 50 L/min.

DEADSPACE. The deadspace of the mask should be as small as possible, particularly with infant and pediatric masks.

COST. The mask should be as inexpensive as possible without compromising its quality. In most cases, these are disposable devices intended to be used by a patient and then discarded.

Use of Mouth-to-Mask Devices

Many resuscitation masks are commercially available, and some of these have been objectively evaluated.[7,10–16] Although any tight-fitting resuscitation mask can be used for mouth-to-mask ventilation, several are available primarily for this purpose. Such devices should have a redundant means for protection of the rescuer (eg, one-way valve, filter, and extension tube). Notwithstanding that these devices provide a barrier between the patient and the rescuer, the one-way valves of some do allow back-leak.[17] Although the filter material used in these devices may provide a barrier, it might not be 100% effective in removal of all particles of the size of bacteria and viruses.[18] Mouth-to-mouth technique is not desirable in most circumstances because of the risk of infection to the rescuer by the patient. This has particularly become the case with concerns related to acquired immunodeficiency syndrome and hepatitis B. The Centers for Disease Control and Prevention recommend that a protective barrier always be used between the patient and the rescuer during emergency ventilation procedures.[19] The AHA recommends that mouth-to-mask ventilation be taught to health care providers as part of training in basic cardiac life support,[20] and many hospitals now provide mouth-to-mask ventilation devices at the bedside of all patients.

After respiratory arrest, initial ventilation should begin with mouth-to-mask technique or two-person bag-valve-mask technique (one person holds the mask and opens the airway with two hands, and the second person squeezes the bag with two hands). Mouth-to-mask or two-person bag-valve-mask ventilation should continue until the patient is intubated.

Before intubation, care should also be taken to prevent gastric insufflation. Gastric insufflation is minimized by using slow inspiratory flow rates, which lower pharyngeal pressures[21]; cricoid pressure may be useful.[22,23] Gastric insufflation is also affected by lung compliance and the ventilation device (Fig. 7-3).[24] Gastric insufflation increases with lower lung compliance and is greatest with exhaled gas ventilation (mouth-to-mouth and mouth-to-mask techniques), lower with bag-valve-mask technique, and lowest with mask-and-ventilator methods.

Ventilation volumes using mouth-to-mask technique are superior to the volumes using a bag-valve-mask.[24–32] With mouth-to-mask technique, two hands are used to open the airway and achieve a mask seal. Furthermore, the ventilation volume is limited only by the rescuer's ability to take a deep breath. Even a small person should be able to provide tidal volumes of 800 to 1200 mL using this technique. Because there is usually a large difference between the delivered tidal volume and the rescuer's vital capacity, it is easier to compensate for a mask leak with this technique. In one study, however, it was shown that the volumes delivered using some of these devices are less than the 800 mL recommended by the AHA (Fig. 7-4).[16] In another study, it was shown that the resistance to flow through some of these devices is excessive (Fig. 7-5).[33]

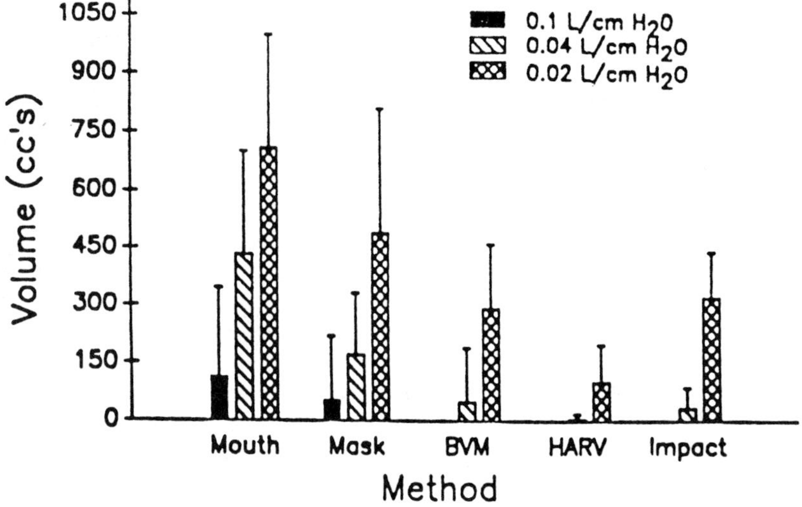

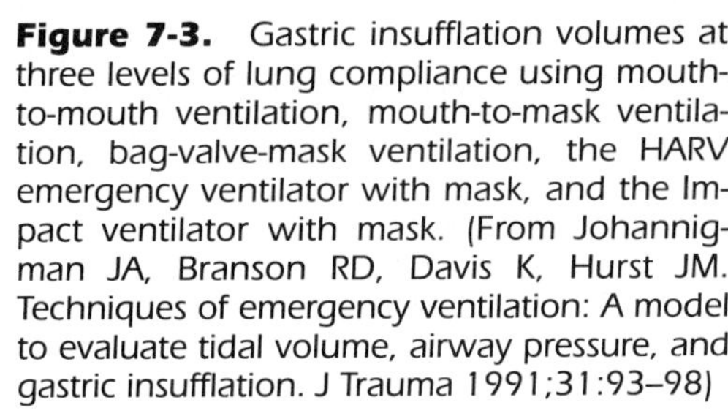
Figure 7-3. Gastric insufflation volumes at three levels of lung compliance using mouth-to-mouth ventilation, mouth-to-mask ventilation, bag-valve-mask ventilation, the HARV emergency ventilator with mask, and the Impact ventilator with mask. (From Johannigman JA, Branson RD, Davis K, Hurst JM. Techniques of emergency ventilation: A model to evaluate tidal volume, airway pressure, and gastric insufflation. J Trauma 1991;31:93–98)

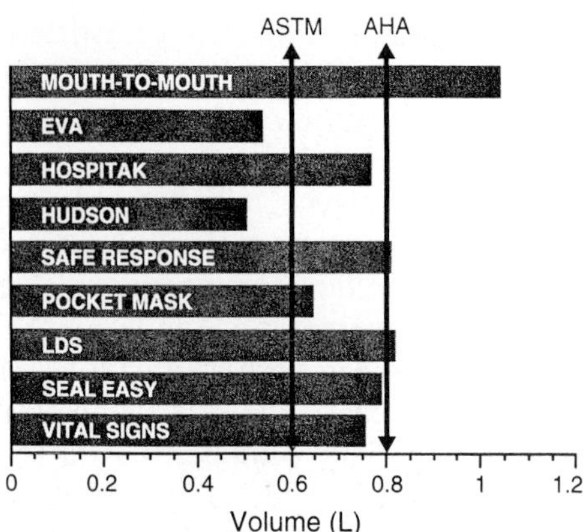

Figure 7-4. Volumes delivered using mouth-to-mouth ventilation and eight mouth-to-mask ventilation devices. (Data from Hess D, Ness C, Oppel, A, Rhoads K. Evaluation of mouth-to-mask devices. Respir Care 1989;34:191–195; redrawn in Barnes TA. Emergency ventilation techniques and related equipment. Respir Care 1992;37:673–694).

It is important that the correct technique for holding the mask is used.[16] The rescuer should be positioned at the head of the patient. The mask is placed over the patient's nose and mouth and held in place with the rescuer's thumbs. The first fingers of each hand are placed under the patient's mandible, and the mandible is lifted as the head is tilted back. The mask is sealed using the rescuer's thumbs (Fig. 7-6). An alternate method is to hold the mask with the thumb and first finger of each hand, and use the other fingers to lift the mandible and hyperextend the head (Fig. 7-7). With either method, both of the rescuer's hands are used to hold the mask and open the patient's airway. In patients with cervical spine injury, the mandible should be lifted without tilting the head. Effective use of these devices requires instruction and supervised practice.[34] Although ventilation volumes with mouth-to-mask technique exceed those of bag-valve-mask technique, it has been suggested that bag-valve-mask technique might be improved with extensive training in this skill.[35,36]

Supplemental oxygen can be administered during exhaled gas ventilation (ie, mouth-to-mouth or mouth-

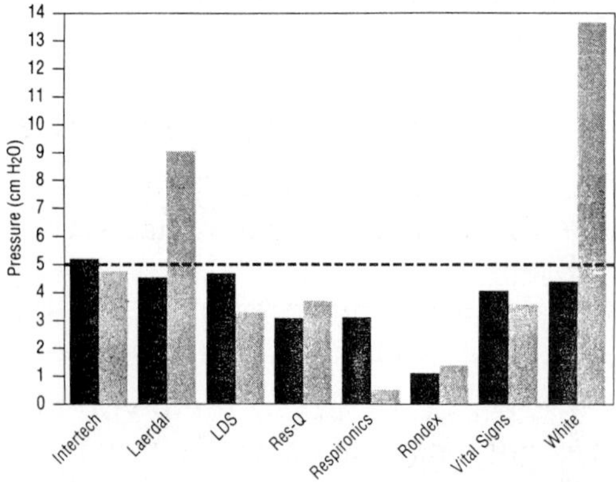

Figure 7-5. Inspiratory (left bar) and expiratory (right bar) back pressures across eight mouth-to-mask ventilation valves at a flow of 50 L/min. The dashed line represents the ISO recommendation of less than 5 cm H_2O at 50 L/min. (Redrawn from Hess D, Simmons M, Slikkers F, Dickerson R. Resistance to flow through the valves of mouth-to-mask ventilation devices. Respir Care 1993;38:183–188)

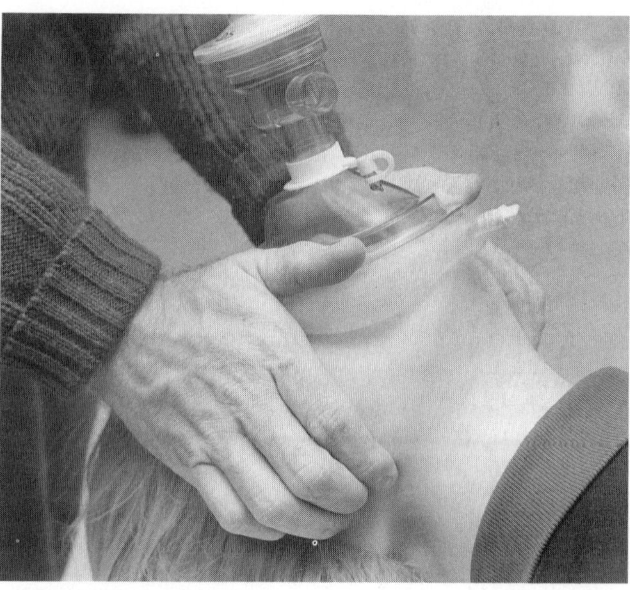

Figure 7-6. Technique used to hold mask during mouth-to-mask technique, with thumbs holding mask in place and airway opened by lifting mandible. (From Hess D, Ness C, Oppel, A, Rhoads K. Evaluation of mouth-to-mask devices. Respir Care 1989;34:191–195)

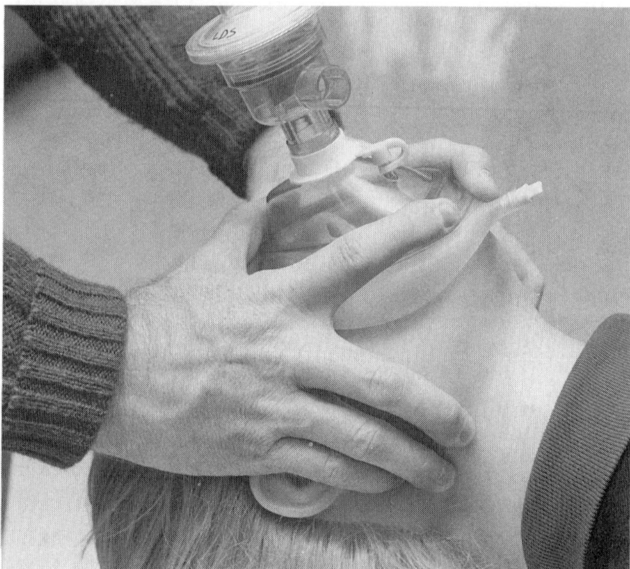

Figure 7-7. An alternate technique for holding mask during mouth-to-mask ventilation, with mask held by thumb and first finger and airway opened by lifting mandible. (From Hess D, Ness C, Oppel, A, Rhoads K. Evaluation of mouth-to-mask devices. Respir Care 1989;34:191–195)

to-mask techniques) by the rescuer breathing oxygen at 8 to 10 L/min by nasal cannula, which delivers about 30% oxygen to the patient (Fig. 7-8).[37] Supplemental oxygen can be added to most commercially available masks for mouth-to-mask technique, which provides a modest increase in F_{IO_2} (Fig. 7-9). If the rescuer inhales oxygen from the oxygen enrichment device of mouth-to-mask ventilation apparatus, relatively high F_{IO_2} values can be delivered (see Fig. 7-9).[38]

Face Shield Devices

Another type of barrier device used for exhaled gas ventilation is the face shield. Face shield devices have a clear plastic sheet and a filter or one-way valve that separates the rescuer from the patient. A seal is made by the rescuer's mouth in a manner similar to that used with mouth-to-mouth technique, and the patient's exhaled gas escapes between the shield and the patient's face. These devices are primarily used by lay persons, and very little has been published regarding their performance. These devices do not have a supplemental oxygen port.

Bag-Valve Resuscitators

The resuscitator bag, attached to either a mask or an endotracheal tube, is commonly used for ventilation during cardiopulmonary resuscitation (CPR). Resuscitator bags are also used for ventilation during transport of the apneic patient and for hyperinflation during endotracheal suctioning.

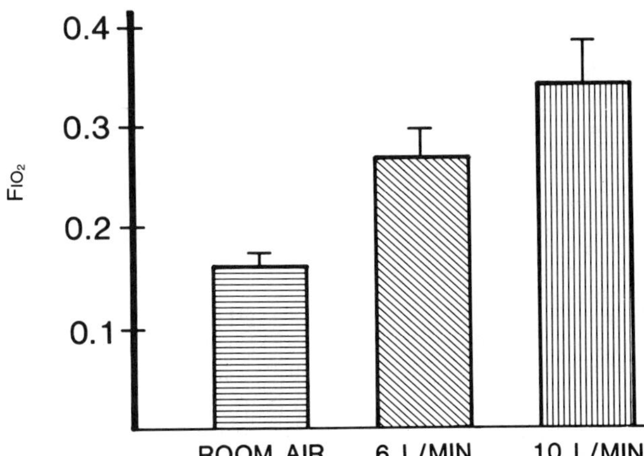

Figure 7-8. Oxygen concentrations delivered during exhaled gas ventilation with the rescuer breathing oxygen at three different flows. (Adapted from Hess D, Kapp A, Kurtek W. The effect on delivered oxygen concentration of the rescuer's breathing supplemental oxygen during exhaled-gas ventilation. Respir Care 1985;30:631–694)

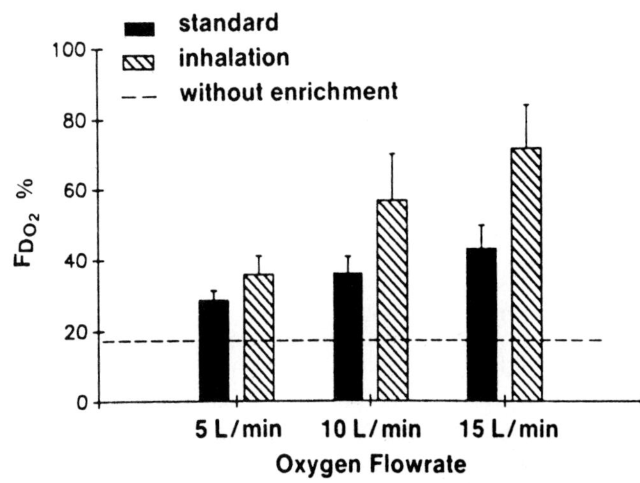

Figure 7-9. Oxygen concentration delivered without supplemental oxygen, using the standard oxygen enrichment device, and with the rescuer inhaling oxygen from the oxygen enrichment device. (From Johannigman JA, Branson RD. Oxygen enrichment of expired gas for mouth-to-mask resuscitation. Respir Care 1991;36:99–103)

Construction of the Bag-Valve Resuscitator Unit

The bag-valve resuscitator consists of a self-inflating bag, an oxygen reservoir, and a non-rebreathing valve (Figs. 7-10 and 7-11). It can be either a reusable device that is sterilized between patients or a disposable single-patient-use device. The bag is squeezed by the operator to ventilate the patient. The volume of this bag varies among manufacturers but ranges from 1.1 to 2.2 L for adults and from 0.2 to 0.9 L for children. One-way valves are used to produce unidirectional flow through the bag, thus drawing gas into the bag (from the atmosphere, oxygen supply, or reservoir) when the bag inflates and directing gas out of the bag to the patient when the bag is compressed.

Characteristics of an Ideal Resuscitator Bag

Criteria for an adequate resuscitator bag are described in general here, and more detailed standards have been published elsewhere.[1,8,9] A number of studies have evaluated the performance of bag-valve resuscitators.[40–60]

DELIVERY OF AN ADEQUATE TIDAL VOLUME. The ASTM recommends a minimum delivered tidal volume of 600 mL for adult resuscitators, 70 to 300 mL for child resuscitators, and 20 to 70 mL for infant resuscitators.[8] However, the AHA recommends that an adult resuscitator be capable of delivering a tidal volume of 800 to 1200 mL.[1] The volume of gas in the bag is not entirely delivered when the bag is compressed. To deliver adequate tidal volumes, the volume of the bag

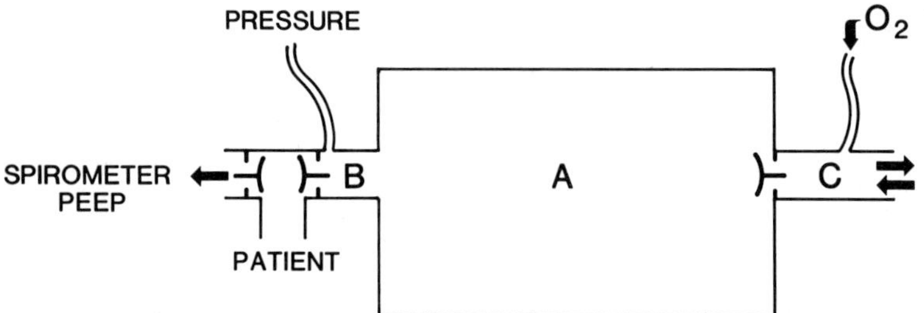

Figure 7-10. Bag-valve resuscitator: A, self-inflating bag; B, non-rebreathing valve; C, oxygen reservoir. See text for details.

should generally be at least twice the desired volume to be delivered (ie, 1600 mL or greater). The construction of the bag should be such that it allows the operator to comfortably squeeze 800 mL or more from the bag with one hand.

The tidal volumes delivered by bag-valve-mask technique are often inadequate (Fig. 7-12).[39] There are four reasons for the low tidal volumes delivered by single-operator bag-valve-mask technique: (1) it is difficult to prevent air leaks around the mask with one hand; (2) it is difficult to maintain an open airway with one hand, even if that hand is large; (3) it is difficult to squeeze an adequate volume (800–1200 mL) out of the bag with one hand, even if that hand is large; and (4) it is difficult to coordinate the delivery of the breath during chest compressions so that gas is delivered into the lungs rather than the stomach.

A number of factors affect the volumes delivered by bag-valve resuscitators (Table 7-1).[50,51,53,54,56–58,61–63] The volume delivery from some commercially available resuscitators has been reported (Table 7-2). As a general rule, two hands should be used to squeeze the resuscitator, and measurement of exhaled tidal volumes may be desirable.[64]

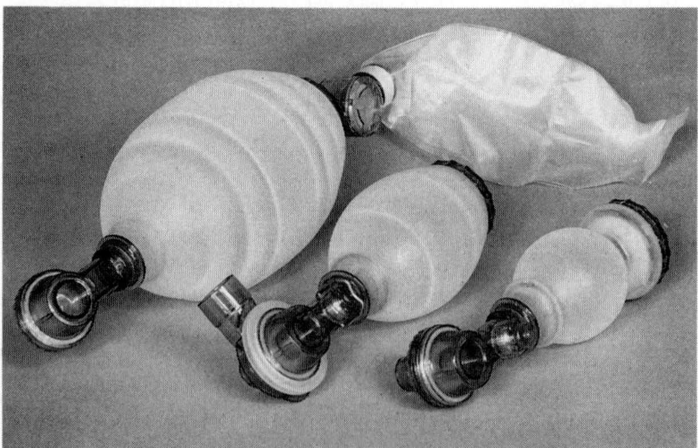

Figure 7-11. Nondisposable adult, pediatric, and infant bag-valve resuscitators. Note the bag oxygen reservoir on the adult resuscitator, the gas collection head (for positive-end expiratory pressure or spirometer) on the pediatric resuscitator, the pop-off on the infant resuscitator, and the lock clip over the pop-off on the pediatric resuscitator.

Little has been published regarding volume delivery when bag-valve-mask devices are used with infants and children. One study found that the volumes delivered during neonatal bag-valve-mask ventilation were inadequate and often less than deadspace volume.[62] However, another study found that infant bag-valve-mask ventilation delivered adequate volumes.[63] During bag-valve ventilation of infants and children, it is important that a bag of adequate volume is used and that the pressure relief valve (if used) does not vent gas to the atmosphere rather than ventilating the patient.

DELIVERY OF AN ADEQUATE FIO_2. The resuscitator should be able to deliver high FIO_2 values, ideally 85% to 100% oxygen during CPR.[1–9] However, when a resuscitator is used for some applications such as transport of an apneic patient, lower FIO_2 values may be desired. Thus, the resuscitator should be able to deliver any desired oxygen concentration from 21% to 100%.

To deliver supplemental oxygen, bag-valve resuscitators are generally designed to accept oxygen flows of 10 to 15 L/min for adults and 5 to 10 L/min for children. It is important that oxygen is not added directly to the resuscitator bag, since this can result in overpressurization of the resuscitator, with possible communication of the pressure to the patient's lungs resulting in barotrauma and hemodynamic compromise.[65,66]

An oxygen reservoir may be used to increase the FIO_2 delivered by the resuscitator bag. This reservoir may be a hollow tube (Fig. 7-13) or an inflatable bag (Fig. 7-14). In some cases, the volume of the tube reservoir is adjustable (poppel tubing). Although the reservoir usually attaches to the rear of the bag, it is attached to the front of the bag in some cases (Figs. 7-15 and 7-16). An inflatable reservoir bag allows the operator to verify that oxygen is flowing to the reservoir.

Modest FIO_2 values are possible without a reservoir, but nearly 100% oxygen can be delivered with a reservoir. To deliver 100% oxygen, the volume of the reservoir should be at least as large as the volume of the resuscitator bag. This can make the resuscitator very clumsy during clinical use, which has encouraged some users to replace the reservoir bag supplied by the manufacturer with a smaller tube reservoir (such as a short length of 22-mm aerosol tubing). These re-

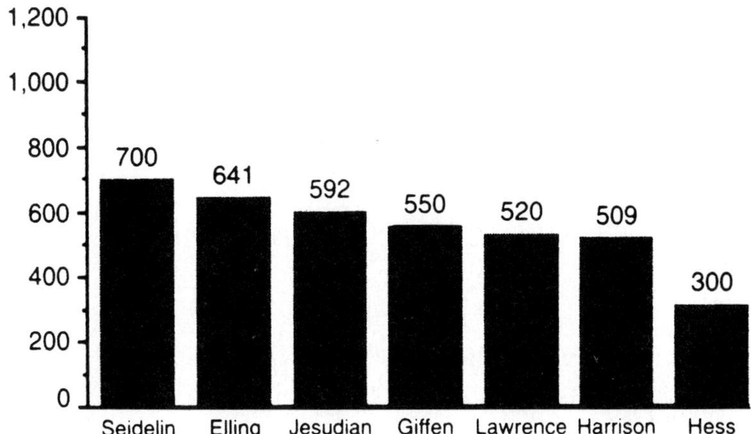

Figure 7-12. Tidal volume by bag-valve-mask from published studies. (From Barnes TA. Emergency ventilation techniques and related equipment. Respir Care 1992;37:673–694)

placement reservoirs may not deliver F_{IO_2} values as high as desired during CPR. If the reservoir is a closed system, one-way valves should be used to vent excess oxygen flow and allow ambient air to enter the reservoir if oxygen flow is insufficient.

If the patient breathes spontaneously, the exhalation valve should close so that the patient breathes oxygen from the bag rather than room air. Most bag-valve resuscitators deliver high F_{IO_2} values at low levels of ventilation. However, the delivered F_{IO_2} tends to drop at higher levels of ventilation. If the reservoir volume is adequate, there is no clinically important difference in delivered F_{IO_2} when tube versus bag reservoirs are used.

With bag-valve devices, the oxygen concentration delivered depends on the construction of the bag, the oxygen flow, the presence of a reservoir or oxygen supply valve, and bag recoil time.[67,68] Bag recoil time should be as long as possible (ie, the rescuer should control bag recoil time so that the bag refills slowly) to minimize the amount to room air drawn into the bag that dilutes the oxygen from the reservoir or oxygen inlet.[67] However, if oxygen flow is great enough (≥15 L/min) and if the volume of the reservoir is great enough (greater than the volume of the bag), bag recoil time becomes less important.

An oxygen supply valve can be used instead of a reservoir (Fig. 7-17), in which case the valve adds 100% oxygen to the bag when it inflates. This valve must be capable of producing high flow rates during

TABLE 7-1. Factors That Affect Tidal Volume During Bag-Valve Ventilation

Factor	Description
Mask versus endotracheal tube	Volumes delivered during bag-valve-mask ventilation are often inadequate
One hand versus two hands	Higher volumes are delivered with two hands rather than one hand squeezing the bag.
Hand size	Higher volumes can be delivered by persons with larger hands.
Lung impedance	Delivered volumes decrease with a decrease in compliance and an increase in resistance.
Resuscitator brand	There are differences for delivered volumes among commercially available resuscitators.
Fatigue	Fatigue does *not* affect delivered volumes, at least for short ventilation periods.
Gloves	Wearing medical gloves does *not* affect delivered tidal volumes.
Operator skill	Rescuer skill and training affect delivered tidal volumes, especially for bag-valve-mask ventilation.

TABLE 7-2. Volumes Delivered by Some Bag-Valve Resuscitators Using a Test Lung with a Compliance of 0.05 L/cm H_2O and a 7-mm Endotracheal Tube

Resuscitator	One Hand Volume* (mean ± SD)	Two Hand Volume* (mean ± SD)
Ambu	0.69 ± 0.09	0.96 ± 0.19
BagEasy	0.76 ± 0.10	1.06 ± 0.22
Hope III	0.81 ± 0.11	0.99 ± 0.20
Hudson	0.72 ± 0.10	0.99 ± 0.15
Laerdal	0.76 ± 0.12	0.96 ± 0.22
PMR	0.69 ± 0.10	0.82 ± 0.15
Pulmanex	0.66 ± 0.10	0.86 ± 0.17
Stat Blue	0.58 ± 0.14	0.71 ± 0.19
1st Response	0.68 ± 0.08	0.90 ± 0.16
Code Blue	0.67 ± 0.10	0.88 ± 0.11
Hospitak	0.48 ± 0.10	0.61 ± 0.07
Mercury	0.65 ± 0.11	0.90 ± 0.16
SPUR	0.67 ± 0.08	0.90 ± 0.16

* Persons squeezing the resuscitators had average-sized hands. Data from Hess D, Goff G, Johnson K. The effect of hand size, resuscitator brand, and use of two hands on volumes delivered during adult bag-valve ventilation. Respir Care 1989;34:805–810; and Hess D, Spahr C. An evaluation of volumes delivered by selected adult disposable resuscitators: The effects of hand size, number of hands used, and use of disposable medical gloves. Respir Care 1990;35:800–805.

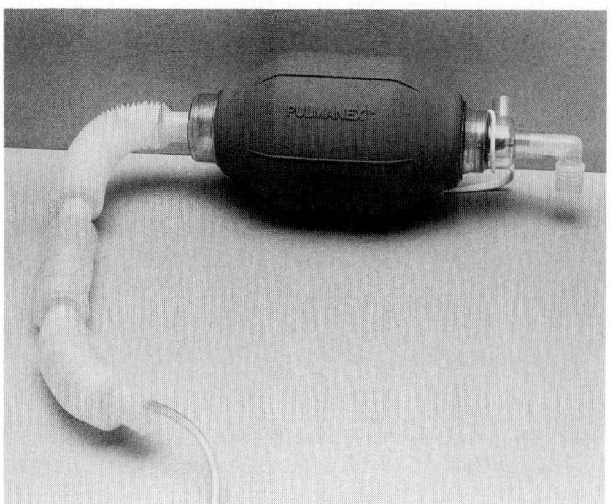

Figure 7-13. Bag-valve resuscitator with hollow tube oxygen reservoir. (Pulmanex resuscitator with poppel tubing; courtesy of Bird/LDS, Carrollton, TX)

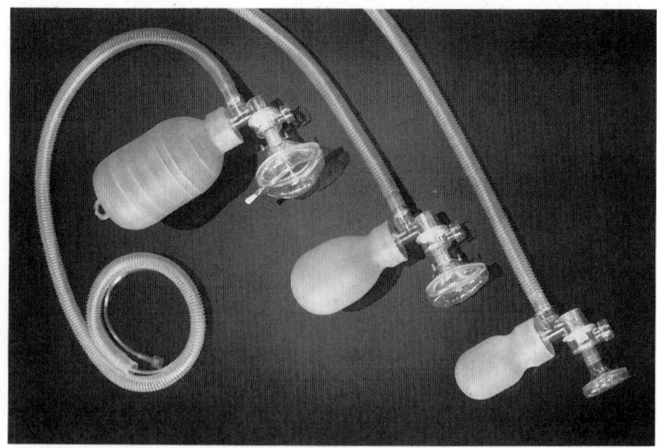

Figure 7-15. Adult, pediatric, and infant resuscitators with tube reservoir at the front of the bag. (Code Blue, Pedi Blue, and Baby Blue; courtesy of Vital Signs, Totowa, NJ)

high-rate ventilation and should allow ambient air to enter the bag if the oxygen supply fails. This device conserves oxygen (ie, only uses oxygen to fill the resuscitator, rather than a continuous flow that wastes oxygen). However, the device adds considerably to the cost of the resuscitator. Advantages of an oxygen supply valve include oxygen conservation, delivery of 100% oxygen (or any desired F_{IO_2} if a blender is used), a less clumsy means of oxygen delivery than a reservoir, and limited atmospheric entrainment during resuscitation in contaminated environments.

VENTILATION AT HIGH RATES. The resuscitator should be capable of ventilation at a rapid frequency, as is sometimes required during resuscitation. This is particularly important for neonatal and pediatric resuscitators. The ability of the resuscitator to deliver high respiratory rates is related to bag recoil time; a faster recoil allows a more rapid respiratory rate. In adults, however, it may be more important to be able to deliver an adequate tidal volume rather than a high respiratory rate.

SELF-INFLATING. The resuscitator should not require gas flow to inflate the bag. Thus, it can be used for ventilation when oxygen is not available or when supplemental oxygen is not desired. The bag should also reinflate rapidly to allow ventilation at high respiratory rates.

FEEL OF RESISTANCE AND COMPLIANCE. The resuscitator bag should allow the operator to feel changes in airway pressure such as might occur with changes in the patient's airway resistance or lung compliance.

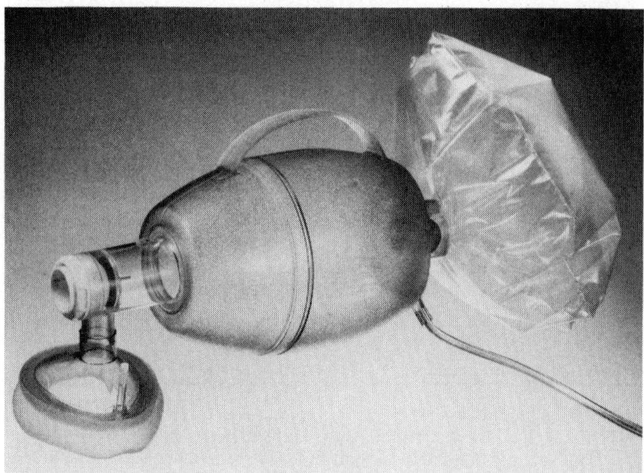

Figure 7-14. Bag-valve resuscitator with inflatable bag reservoir. (Courtesy of Ambu SPUR, Hanover, MD)

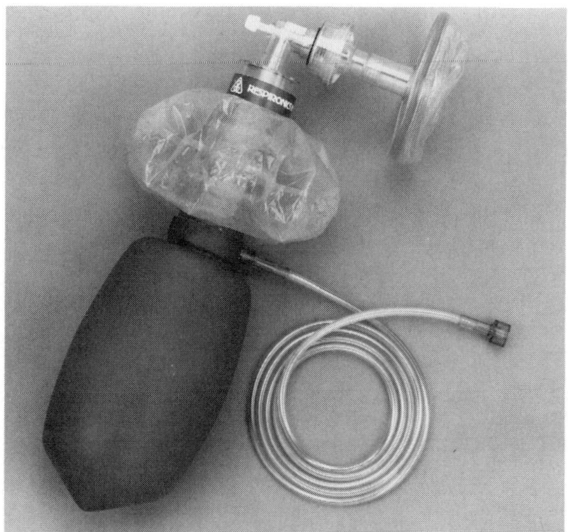

Figure 7-16. BagEasy resuscitator with inflatable bag reservoir at the front of the bag. (Courtesy of Respironics, Murrysville, PA)

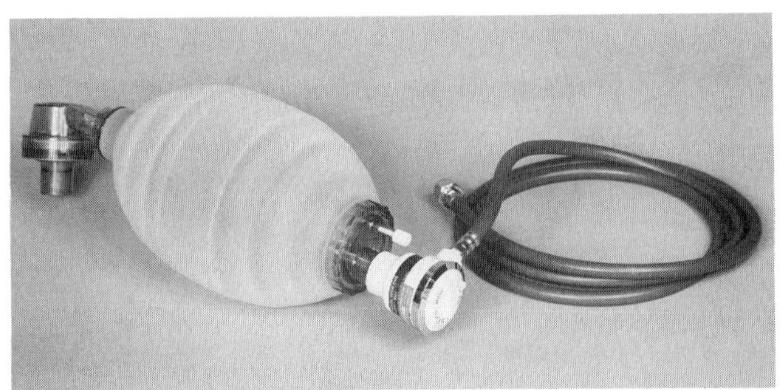

Figure 7-17. Bag refill-valve attached to Laerdal bag. (Courtesy of LSP, Irvine, CA)

The compliance of the bag material is greater for some resuscitators than others, which could make it more difficult to sense changes in patient resistance and compliance. A poorly compliant bag material (ie, stiff) may result in lower delivered tidal volumes and operator fatigue.

NON-REBREATHING VALVE. The non-rebreathing valve is used to direct flow to the patient when the bag is squeezed and to direct flow away from the bag to the atmosphere during exhalation. Numerous valve designs are available to accomplish this; these include spring disk/ball valves, diaphragm/leaf valves, and duck bill valves (Fig. 7-18). The non-rebreathing valve should allow attachment of a spirometer or positive end-expiratory pressure (PEEP) valve, allow for the attachment of a manometer to monitor airway pressure, and include a pop-off in pediatric models.

The resuscitator bag should use a true non-rebreathing valve to prevent exhalation into the bag and subsequent rebreathing of exhaled gas.[69] This valve should have a low resistance so that it does not impede exhalation, and the valve should not jam with high flow rates. According to ISO standards,[9] the back-pressure produced by the device should be less than 5 cm H_2O at a flow rate of 50 L/min. Valve resistance has been evaluated and found to be excessive in some resuscitators (Fig. 7-19).[57] Valve resistance may be particularly problematic during spontaneous breathing through the resuscitator.[54,60] The deadspace of this valve should be as small as possible and should not exceed 30 mL for adults, 15 mL for children, and 7 mL for infants.[8] The non-rebreathing valve should be transparent.

PRESSURE POP-OFF/PRESSURE MONITOR. Adult resuscitator bags should not have a pop-off because high ventilation pressures are often required during CPR.[70] During adult resuscitation, a pop-off will limit the volume delivered to the patient. Because pulmonary barotrauma is recognized as a hazard of emergency ventilation,[65,66,71–73] ventilating pressures during CPR must be adequate but not excessive. For infant and pediatric resuscitator bags, a 40-cm H_2O pop-off should be available, but it should be easy to occlude if higher ventilating pressures are required.[8] Ideally, the pop-off should have minimal flow resistance.

For adult, pediatric, and infant units, it should be possible to attach a pressure manometer to monitor airway pressure. A nipple adaptor can be connected

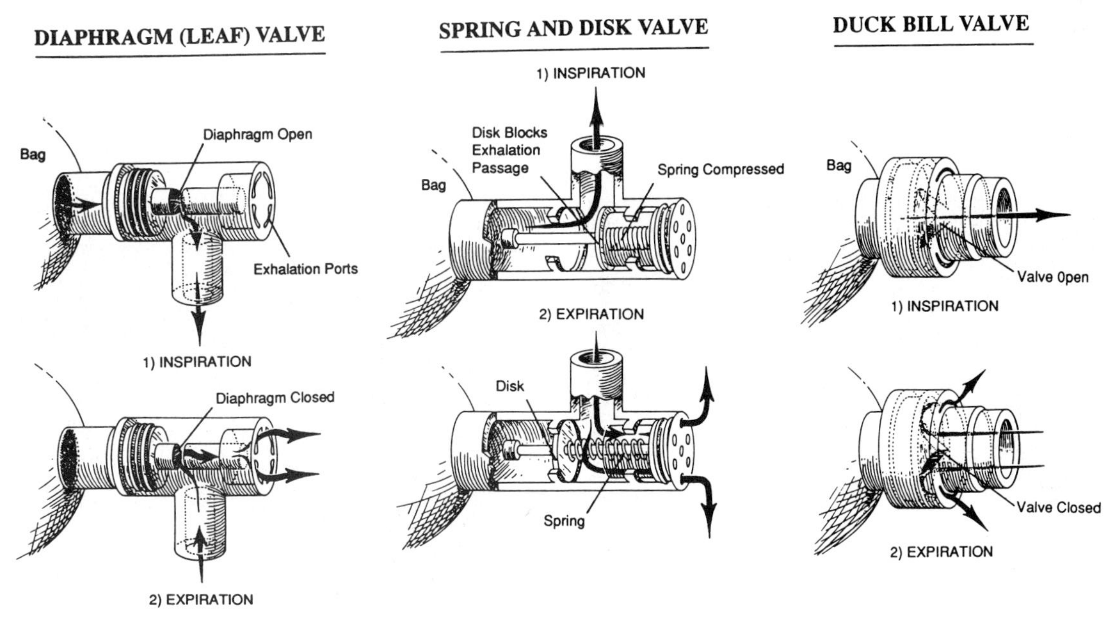

Figure 7-18. Non–rebreathing valves commonly used with bag-valve resuscitators: left, diaphragm or leaf valve; center, spring and disk valve; right, duck bill valve.

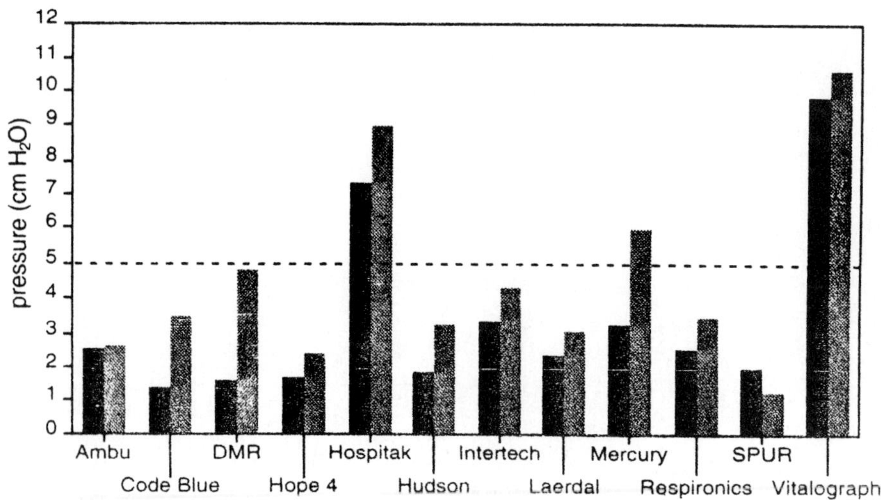

Figure 7-19. Inspiratory (left bar) and expiratory (right bar) back pressures across the valves or 12 bag-valve resuscitators; back pressure should be less than 5 cm H_2O at this flow (dashed line). (Redrawn from Hess D, Simmons M. An evaluation of the resistance to flow through the patient valves of twelve adult manual resuscitators. Respir Care 1992;37:432–438)

between the resuscitator and the patient to attach a manometer (Fig. 7-20).

ATTACHMENT FOR SPIROMETER AND PEEP. The exhalation port should allow a spirometer (Fig. 7-21) or PEEP valve (Fig. 7-22) to be easily attached.[74–79] In some resuscitators, a PEEP valve is manufactured as part of the device. If a PEEP valve is an integral part of the resuscitator, it should be a threshold resistor with low flow resistance.[80,81] A device that produces PEEP by use of expiratory retard is unacceptable. A PEEP device manufactured specifically for resuscitator bags is commercially available (Fig. 7-23).

STANDARD 15/22 ADAPTOR. The patient adaptor should have a standard 15-mm inside diameter and a 22-mm outside diameter to allow it to be connected to either a mask or an artificial airway. The patient adaptor should swivel (ideally 360 degrees) to allow the user to change the angle of operation without excessive torque on the endotracheal tube or mask. A short flex-tube can also be added to the patient adaptor of the resuscitator to decrease traction on the artificial airway.

LIGHTWEIGHT. The resuscitator bag should be light enough so that it can be used with one hand for extended periods of time without fatigue. The size and shape of the resuscitator should allow it to be easily used with one hand.

CLEANING AND STERILIZATION. The resuscitator bag should be easy to disassemble for cleaning, and the number of component parts should be as few as possible. It should not be possible to accidentally interchange parts. Ideally, it should be possible to sterilize the resuscitator using liquid sterilization, ethylene oxide, or steam autoclave. Some units are not intended for sterilization, and are single-patient-use disposable units. Use of disposable units minimizes the risk of misassembly, loss of components, and cross-contamination. Disposable units also decrease costs associated with equipment sterilization and spare parts inventory. If a resuscitator is designed for single-patient-

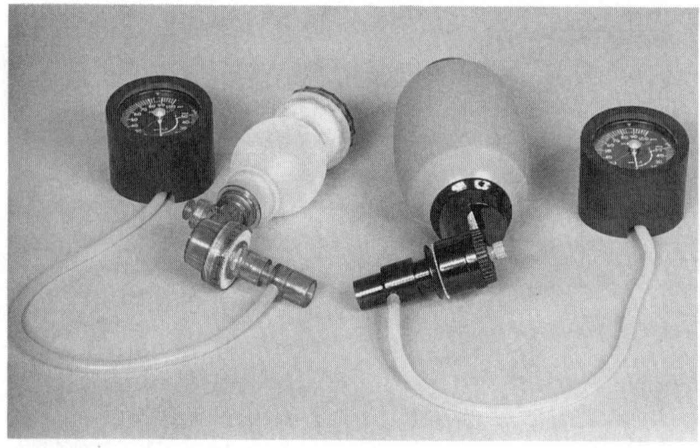

Figure 7-20. Manometer attached to Laerdal and PMR resuscitator bags.

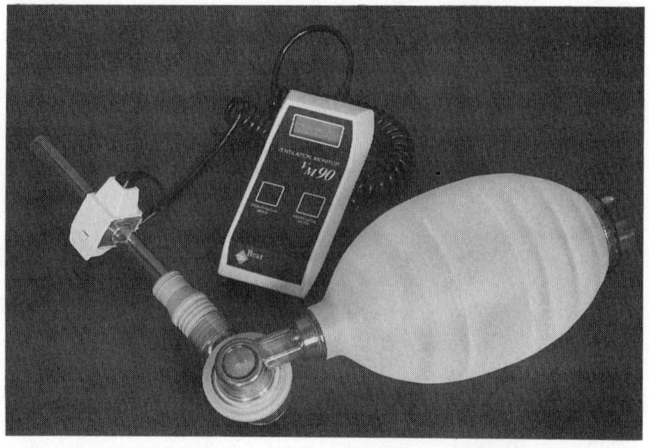

Figure 7-21. Spirometer attached to Laerdal resuscitator.

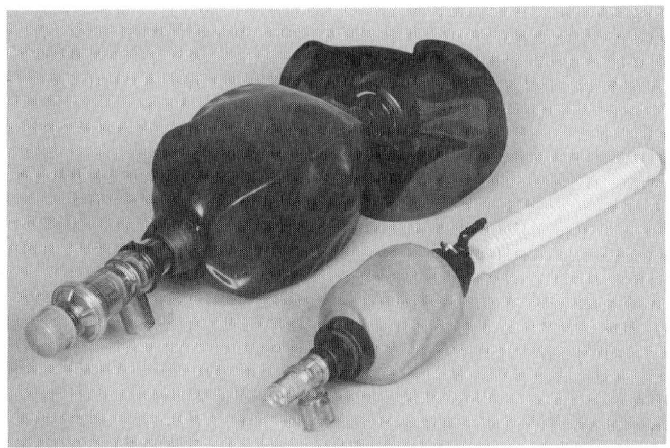

Figure 7-22. Ambu adult and infant resuscitators. Note PEEP valve attached to adult resuscitator.

use, it is not prudent to attempt to sterilize the device for reuse.

PERFORMANCE UNDER ADVERSE CONDITIONS. The unit should be able to withstand adverse conditions such as those that might occur during resuscitation. The valves should not jam in the presence of vomitus, humidity, or low temperatures. The bag material should perform adequately under conditions of low temperature, such as might occur during emergency field resuscitation in mid-winter. The ability of some resuscitators to perform under adverse conditions of temperature and altitude has been reported.[53]

RUGGED. The unit should be able to withstand the rigors of emergency use, such as being dropped from a bed or litter to the floor. The unit should not spontaneously disassemble during routine use.

OPERATOR MANUAL. A detailed operator's manual should be provided by the manufacturer that describes use and operation of the unit, disassembly and reassembly, and sterilization procedures.

COST. Because of concerns regarding health care costs, the resuscitator should be as inexpensive as possible without compromising its quality.

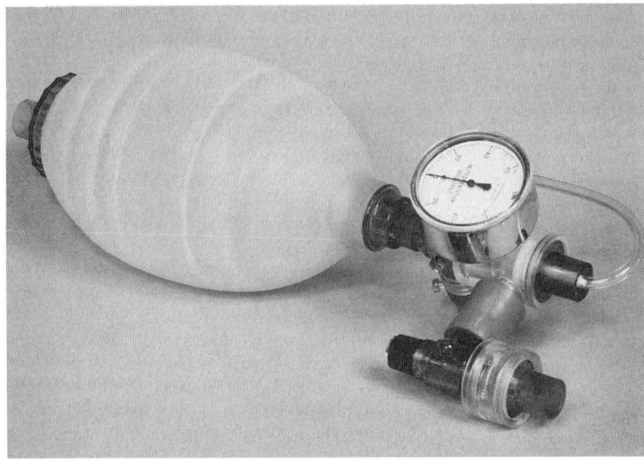

Figure 7-23. PEEP device attached to Laerdal resuscitator. (Courtesy of Instrumentation Industries, Bethel Park, PA)

Nonemergency Use of Bag-Valve Resuscitators

Bag-valve resuscitators are most commonly used to provide ventilation to apneic patients. However, they can also be used for hyperinflation during airway suctioning and during patient transport.

In some hospitals, it is accepted practice to use a resuscitator for hyperinflation during suctioning. If a resuscitator is used for this purpose, it is important that the bag be capable of delivering nearly 100% oxygen, that high tidal volumes can be delivered, and that PEEP can be used (if PEEP is set on the ventilator). If attention is not directed to these factors, the resuscitator may actually hypoventilate and hypo-oxygenate the patient. It is often preferable to hyperinflate and hyperoxygenate the patient using 100% oxygen and sigh volumes with the patient connected to the ventilator.[82–84] Resuscitators may also be used to provide ventilation during transport of apneic patients. In these cases, it is desirable to monitor tidal volumes and airway pressures.

When resuscitators are used with infants, airway pressures should be monitored to lessen the risk of barotrauma. The pressure pop-off provided on resuscitators may not be accurate or reliable.[85,86] It may also be preferable to provide flow to these resuscitators from an air–oxygen blender rather than 100% oxygen, so that any desired F_{IO_2} can be delivered to lessen the risks associated with high F_{IO_2} values in infants. A modification of the Laerdal infant resuscitator to deliver continuous positive airway pressure (CPAP) and PEEP has been described.[87]

Flow-Inflating Bags

Although flow-inflating bags are used in anesthesia and neonatal care, they are not commonly used in adult respiratory care.[88,89] These continuous-flow semiopen breathing systems lack a non-rebreathing valve. An example is the Mapleson circuit, which is designated "A" through "E," depending on the location of the oxygen flow relative to the patient and the exhalation port (Fig. 7-24). A variation of the Mapleson "E" circuit is the Jackson-Rees modification of the Ayre's T-piece, in which a gas reservoir bag with an adjustable bleed-off is added to the expiratory limb (Fig. 7-25). This circuit consists of a thin-walled anesthesia bag, an endotracheal tube or mask connector, a fresh

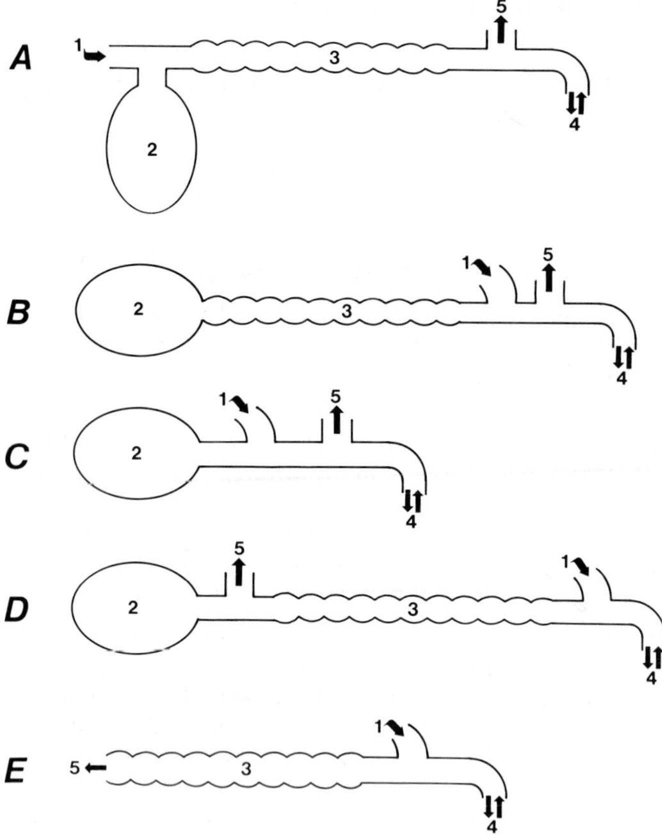

Figure 7-24. (A.) through (E.) Mapleson circuits: 1, oxygen inlet; 2, reservoir bag; 3, flex tube; 4, patient connection; 5, outlet. See text for details.

gas (oxygen) hose, and a bleed-off at the tail of the bag. Inflation of the bag is controlled primarily by oxygen flow and also by the bleed-off. The oxygen flow and the bleed-off control not only bag inflation but also the pressure in the bag; thus the bag can be used to provide CPAP or PEEP as well as ventilation. The bag can be fitted with a manometer and a pressure pop-off. Because the patient exhales into the bag, the oxygen flow must be great enough to prevent accumulation of carbon dioxide. Also, the bleed-off can produce significant resistance to exhalation. A major disadvantage of flow-inflating ventilation circuits is that they can only be used if a source of compressed gas is available. Commercially available flow-inflating systems are also available (Fig. 7-26).

Oxygen-Powered Resuscitators

Oxygen-powered resuscitators (Fig. 7-27) are commonly used by paramedics and the emergency personnel in the field. These devices are powered by a 50-psig oxygen source and cannot be used in the absence of a pressurized gas source. Oxygen-powered resuscitators deliver 100% oxygen when the device is triggered by the operator (resuscitator function) or when triggered by the patient (demand-valve function). They can be used with a face mask or an artificial airway. Unlike mouth-to-mouth, mouth-to-mask, and bag-valve techniques, the oxygen-powered resuscitator does not allow the operator to sense the pressure required to ventilate the patient (ie, changes in resistance and compliance). These devices are frequently associated with gastric insufflation. There has also been a reported case of traumatic pneumocephalus associated with an oxygen-powered resuscitator.[90] These types of resuscitators should be used with caution in pediatric patients and should not be used by untrained individuals. Oxygen-powered resuscitators have been associated with both overventilation[91] and underventilation.[92]

Characteristics of an Ideal Oxygen-Powered Resuscitator

FLOW, PRESSURE, AND OXYGEN CONCENTRATION. Although high flow rates may be necessary with tachypneic spontaneously breathing patients, the flow rate should be limited to 40 L/min when used with a mask to prevent gastric insufflation.[1] The pressure delivered by the oxygen-powered resuscitator should be limited to 60 cm H_2O, and an audible alarm should alert the operator if the pressure limit is reached.[1] The oxygen-powered resuscitator should deliver 100% oxygen.

PERFORMANCE UNDER ADVERSE CONDITIONS. The unit should withstand adverse conditions that might occur during resuscitation such as vomitus, humidity, and low temperature. The unit should be able to withstand the rigors of emergency use.

STANDARD 15/22 ADAPTOR. The patient adaptor should have a standard 15-mm inside diameter and 22-mm outside diameter to allow it to be connected to either a mask or an artificial airway.

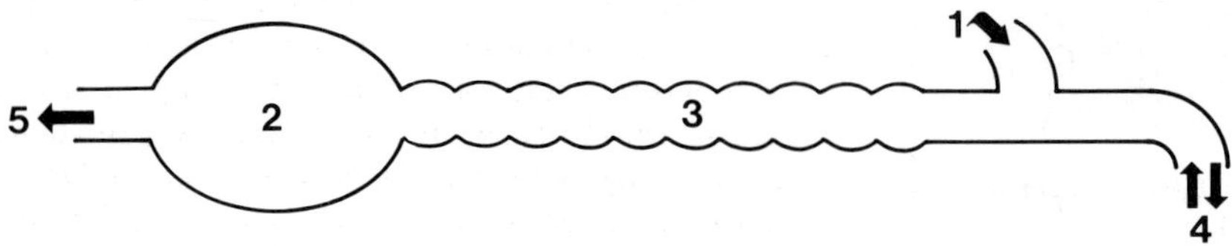

Figure 7-25. Jackson-Rees Modification of the Ayre's T-piece: 1, oxygen inlet; 2, reservoir bag; 3, flex tube; 4, patient connection; 5, outlet. See text for details.

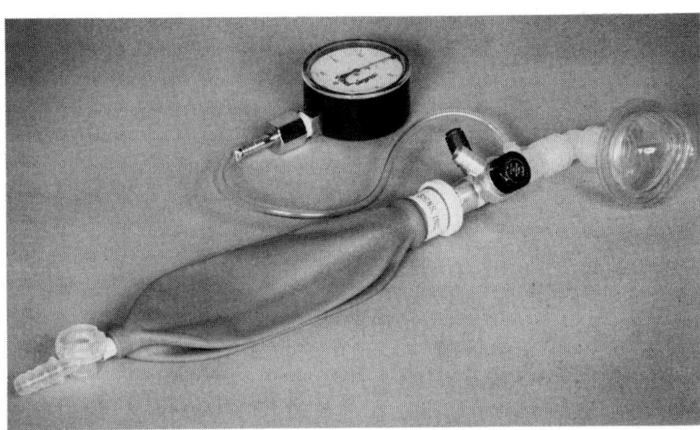

Figure 7-26. Infant resuscitation circuit. (Courtesy of Vital Signs, Totowa, NJ)

TRIGGER. The manual trigger on the device should be positioned so that it can be pressed while using two hands to hold a mask and maintain an open airway. The valve should deliver flow with minimal patient effort.

OPERATOR MANUAL. A detailed operator's manual should be provided that describes use of the unit and sterilization procedures.

CLEANING AND STERILIZATION. The unit should be easy to clean and sterilize using a variety of techniques.

DEADSPACE AND RESISTANCE. The rebreathed volume of the valve should be as small as possible, and the expiratory resistance should be low.

OXYGEN CONNECTIONS. All oxygen connections should be standard Diameter Index Safety System connections. High-pressure connecting hoses should be kinkproof.

CARRYING CASE. Because these devices require a pressurized oxygen source, it is useful for them to be provided with a carrying case for an oxygen cylinder and regulator.

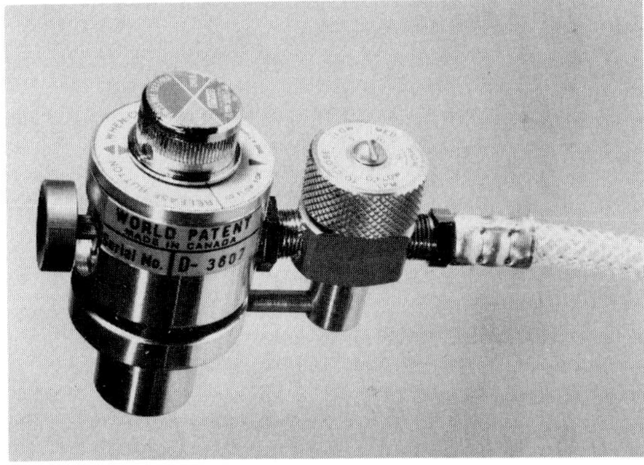

Figure 7-27. Flynn Series III oxygen-powered resuscitator. (Courtesy of O-Two Systems, Buffalo, NY)

COST. The cost should be as low as possible without compromising quality.

AARC Clinical Practice Guideline

Resuscitation in Acute Care Hospitals: Indications, Contraindications, Hazards and Complications

Resuscitation in acute care hospitals for the purpose of this guideline encompasses all care necessary to deal with sudden and often life-threatening events affecting the cardiopulmonary system and involves the identification, assessment, and treatment of patients in danger of or in frank arrest, including the high-risk delivery patient.

- Indications: Cardiac arrest, respiratory arrest, or the presence of conditions that may lead to cardiopulmonary arrest as indicated by rapid deterioration in vital signs, level of consciousness, and blood gas values. Included in those conditions are airway obstruction, acute myocardial infarction, life-threatening dysrhythmias, hypovolvemic shock, severe infections, spinal cord or head injury, drug overdose, pulmonary edema, anaphylaxis, pulmonary embolus, smoke inhalation, and high-risk delivery.
- Contraindications:
  - the patient's desire not to be resuscitated has been clearly expressed and documented in the patient's medical record
  - resuscitation has been determined to be futile because of the patient's underlying condition or disease
- Hazards/Complications:
  - airway: failure to establish a patent airway, failure to intubate the trachea, failure to recognize intubation of the esophagus, upper airway trauma, laryngeal and esophageal damage, aspiration, cervical spine trauma, unrecognized bronchial intubation, eye injury, facial trauma, problems with endotracheal tube cuff, bronchospasm, laryngospasm, dental accidents, dysrhythmias, vagal stimulation, hypertension and tachycardia, inappropriate tube size
  - ventilation: inadequate oxygen delivery, hypo- or hyperventilation, gastric insufflation, barotrauma, hypotension due to high mean airway pressure, vomiting and aspiration, prolonged interruption of ventilation for intubation, failure to establish adequate functional residual capacity in the newborn
  - circulation: ineffective chest compressions, fractured ribs and sternum, laceration of spleen or liver, failure to restore circulation, severe hypovolemia, cardiac tamponade, hemo- or pneumothorax, hypoxia, acidosis, hyperkalemia, massive acute myocardial infarction, hypothermia (in neonates and children), aortic dissection, air embolus, pulmonary embolism

- electrical therapy: failure of defibrillator, shock of team members, inappropriate countershock, induction of malignant dysrhythmias, interference with implanted pacemaker function, fire hazard
- drug administration: inappropriate drug or dose, idiosyncratic or allergic response to drug, endotracheal-tube drug-delivery failure

(Adapted from AARC Clinical Practice Guideline, published in December, 1993, issue of Respiratory Care; see original publication for complete text)

References

1. Guidelines for cardiopulmonary resuscitation and emergency cardiac care. JAMA 1992;268:2171–2302.
2. Emergency Care Research Institute. Manually operated resuscitators. Health Devices 1971;1:13–17.
3. Emergency Care Research Institute. Manual resuscitators. Health Devices 1979;8:133–146.
4. Emergency Care Research Institute. Gas-powered resuscitators. Health Devices 1978;8:24–38.
5. Emergency Care Research Institute. Gas-powered pulmonary resuscitators. Health Devices 1989;18:362–363.
6. Emergency Care Research Institute. Pulmonary resuscitators (gas powered). Health Devices 1988;17:348–354.
7. Emergency Care Research Institute. Exhaled-air pulmonary resuscitators (EAPRs) and disposable manual pulmonary resuscitators (DMPRs). Health Devices 1989;18:333–352.
8. American Society for Testing and Materials. Standard specification for minimum performance and safety requirements for resuscitators intended for use with humans. Designation: F 920-85. Philadelphia: ASTM, 1985.
9. International Organization for Standardization. International Standard ISO 8382:1988 (E): Resuscitators Intended for Use With Humans. New York: American National Standards Institute, 1988.
10. Safer P. Pocket mask for emergency artificial ventilation and oxygen inhalation. Crit Care Med 1974;2:273–276.
11. Stewart RD, Kaplan R, Pennock B, Thompson F. Influence of mask design on bag-mask ventilation. Ann Emerg Med 1985;14:403–406.
12. Palme C, Nystrom B, Tunell R. An evaluation of the efficiency of face masks in the resuscitation of newborn infants. Lancet 1985;1:207–210.
13. Wehrman SF, Radford RR. Evaluation of the effect of lung-system compliance on face mask ventilation (abstract). Respir Care 1986;31:951.
14. Wehrman SF. Effect of mask design on volume delivered during face mask ventilation (abstract). Respir Care 1986;31:950.
15. Anti-infection device for resuscitation (Notes and News). Lancet 1985;2:1255–1256.
16. Hess D, Ness C, Oppel A, Rhoads K. Evaluation of mouth-to-mask devices. Respir Care 1989;34:191–195.
17. Hess D, Kukula C. Evaluation of backleak through mouth-to-mask ventilation devices (abstract). Respir Care 1989;34:1013.
18. Hess D, Fisher D. Evaluation of the filtering ability of the Laerdal Resusci Face Shield (abstract). Respir Care 1993;38:1264.
19. Centers for Disease Control. Recommendations for prevention of HIV transmission in health-care settings. MMWR 1987;36:3S–18S.
20. Healthcare Provider's Manual for Basic Cardiac Life Support. Dallas: American Heart Association, 1988.
21. Melker RJ, Banner MJ. Ventilation during CPR: Two-rescuer standards reappraised. Ann Emerg Med 1985;14:397–402.
22. Admani M, Yeh TF, Jain R, Mora A, Pildes RS. Prevention of gastric insufflation during mask ventilation in newborn infants. Crit Care Med 1985;13:592–593.
23. Salem MR, Wong AY, Mani M, Sellick BA. Efficacy of cricoid pressure in preventing gastric distension during bag-mask ventilation in pediatric patients. Anesthesiology 1974;40:96–98.
24. Johannigman JA, Branson RD, Davis K, Hurst JM. Techniques of emergency ventilation: A model to evaluate tidal volume, airway pressure, and gastric insufflation. J Trauma 1991;31:93–98.
25. Elam JO, Brown ES, Elder JD. Artificial respiration by mouth-to-mask method. N Engl J Med 1954;250:749–754.
26. Harrison RR, Maull KI, Keenan RL, Boyan CP. Mouth-to-mask ventilation: A superior method of rescue breathing. Ann Emerg Med 1982;11:74–76.
27. Elling R, Politis J. An evaluation of emergency medical technicians' ability to use manual ventilation devices. Ann Emerg Med 1983;12:765–768.
28. Sainsbury DA, Davis R, Walker MC. Artificial ventilation for cardiopulmonary resuscitation. Med J Aust 1984;141:509–511.
29. Lawrence PJ, Sivaneswaran N. Ventilation during cardiopulmonary resuscitation: Which method? Med J Aust 1985;143:443–446.
30. Nickalls RWD, Thompson CW. Mouth to mask respiration. Br Med J 1986;292:1350.
31. Hess D, Baran C. Ventilatory volumes using mouth-to-mouth, mouth-to-mask, and bag-valve-mask techniques. Am J Emerg Med 1985;3:292–296.
32. Seidelin PH, Stolarek IH, Littlewood DG. Comparison of six methods of emergency ventilation. Lancet 1986;2:1274–1275.
33. Hess D, Simmons M, Slikkers F, Dickerson R. Resistance to flow through the valves of mouth-to-mask ventilation devices. Respir Care 1993;38:183–188.
34. Fluck RR, Sorbello JG. Comparison of tidal volumes, minute ventilation, and respiratory frequencies delivered by paramedic and respiratory care students with pocket mask versus demand valve. Respir Care 1991;36:1105–1112.
35. Cummins RD, Austin D, Groves JR, Litwin PE, Pierce J. Ventilation skills of emergency medical technicians: A teaching challenge for emergency medicine. Ann Emerg Med 1986;15:1187–1192.
36. Powers WE. Evaluation of a training method that uses volumetric feedback with bag-valve-mask ventilation techniques (abstract). Respir Care 1988;33:942–943.
37. Hess D, Kapp A, Kurtek W. The effect on delivered oxygen concentration of the rescuer's breathing supplemental oxygen during exhaled-gas ventilation. Respir Care 1985;30:631–694.
38. Johannigman JA, Branson RD. Oxygen enrichment of expired gas for mouth-to-mask resuscitation. Respir Care 1991;36:99–103.
39. Barnes TA. Emergency ventilation techniques and related equipment. Respir Care 1992;37:673–694.
40. Redick LF, Dunbar RW, MacDougall DC, Merket TE. An evaluation of hand-operated self-inflating resuscitation equipment. Anesthesia and Analgesia 1970;49:28–32.
41. Carden E, Bernstein M. Investigation of the nine most commonly used resuscitator bags. JAMA 1970;49:28–32.
42. Steinbach RB, Carden E. 1973 assessment of eight adult resuscitator bags. Respir Care 1975;20:69–76.
43. Carden E, Hughes T. An evaluation of manually operated self-inflating resuscitation bags. Anesth Analg 1975;54:133–138.
44. Carden E, Friedman D. Further studies of manually operated self-inflating resuscitation bags. Anesth Analg 1977;56:202–206.
45. LeBouef LL. 1980 assessment of eight adult manual resuscitator. Respir Care 1980;25:1136–1142.
46. Fitzmaurice MW, Barnes TA. Oxygen delivery performance of three adult resuscitation bags. Respir Care 1980;25:928–933.
47. Barnes TA, Watson ME. Oxygen delivery performance of four adult resuscitation bags. Respir Care 1982;27:139–146.
48. Barnes TA, Watson ME. Oxygen delivery performance of old and new designs of the Laerdal, Vitalograph, and Ambu adult manual resuscitators. Respir Care 1983;28:1121–1128.
49. Barnes TA, Potash RJ. Evaluation of five disposable operator-powered adult resuscitators. Respir Care 1989;34:254–261.
50. Hess D, Goff G, Johnson K. The effect of hand size, resuscitator brand, and use of 2 hands on volumes delivered during bag-valve ventilation. Respir Care 1989;34:805–810.
51. Hess D, Goff G. The effects of two-hand versus one-hand ventilation on volumes delivered during bag-valve ventilation at various resistances and compliances. Respir Care 1987;32:1025–1028.
52. Barnes TA, McGarry W. Evaluation of ten disposable manual resuscitators. Respir Care 1990;35:960–968.
53. Barnes TA, Stockwell DL. Evaluation of ten manual resuscita-

tors across an operational temperature range of −18°C to 50°C. Respir Care 1991;36:161–172.

54. Mills PJ, Baptiste J, Preston J, Barnas GM. Manual resuscitators and spontaneous ventilation: An evaluation. Crit Care Med 1991;19:1425—1431.
55. Hess D, Goff G, Johnson K. The effect of hand size, resuscitator brand, and use of two hands on volumes delivered during adult bag-valve ventilation. Respir Care 1989;34:805–810.
56. Hess D, Spahr C. An evaluation of volumes delivered by selected adult disposable resuscitators: The effects of hand size, number of hands used, and use of disposable medical gloves. Respir Care 1990;35:800–805.
57. Hess D, Simmons M. An evaluation of the resistance to flow through the patient valves of twelve adult manual resuscitators. Respir Care 1992;37:432–438.
58. Hess D, Simmons M, Blaukovitch S, Lightner D, Doyle T. An evaluation of the effects of fatigue, impedance, and use of two hands on volumes delivered during bag-valve ventilation. Respir Care 1993;38:271–275.
59. Kissoon N, Connors R, Tiffin N, Frewen TC. An evaluation of the physical and functional characteristics of resuscitators for use in pediatrics. Crit Care Med 1992;20:292–296.
60. Hirsch C, Barker S, Kratohvil J, Hess D, Kacmarek R. Imposed work during spontaneous breathing with adult disposable resuscitators (abstract). Respir Care 1993;38:1282.
61. Jusudian MCS, Harrison R, Keenan RL, Maull KI. Bag-valve-mask ventilation: Two rescuers are better than one: A preliminary report. Crit Care Med 1985:13:122–123.
62. Milner AD, Vyas H, Hopkins IE. Efficiency of facemask resuscitation at birth. Br Med J 1984;289:1563–1565.
63. Kanter RK. Evaluation of mask-bag ventilation in resuscitation of infants. Am J Dis Child 1987;141:761–763.
64. Ornato JP, Bryson BL, Donovan PJ, Farquharson RR, Jaeger C. Measurement of ventilation during cardiopulmonary resuscitation. Crit Care Med 1983;11:79–82.
65. Kravath R, Schonberg SK. Tension-pneumothorax hazard (letter). N Engl J Med 1968;278:1403.
66. Klick JM, Bushnell LS, Bancroft ML. Barotrauma, a potential hazard of manual resuscitators. Anesthesiology 1978;49:3 63–365.
67. Priano LL, Ham J. A simple method to increase the FDO_2 of resuscitator bags. Crit Care Med 1978;6:48–49.
68. Campbell TP, Stewart RD, Kaplan RM, DeMichiei RV, Morton R. Oxygen enrichment of bag-valve-mask units during positive-pressure ventilation: A comparison of various techniques. Ann Emerg Med 1988;17:232–235.
69. Hill SL, Eaton JM. Rebreathing during use of the Air-Viva resuscitation bag: A hazard. Br Med J 1983;287:583–584.
70. Hirschman AM, Kravath RE. Venting vs. ventilating: A danger of resuscitation bags. Chest 1982;82:369–370.
71. Jumper A, Desai S, Liu P, Philip J. Pulmonary barotrauma resulting from a faulty Hope II resuscitation bag. Anesthesiology 1983;58:572–574.
72. Hillman K, Albin M. Pulmonary barotrauma during cardiopulmonary resuscitation. Crit Care Med 1986;14:606–609.
73. Wasserberger J, Ordog GJ, Turner AF, et al. Iatrogenic pulmonary barotrauma accident. Ann Emerg Med 1986;15: 947–951.
74. Marotta J, Greenbaum DM. PEEP attachment for Puritan Manual Resuscitator. Respir Care 1976;21:862–864.
75. Whitley JA. PEEP attachment for resuscitator bags. Respir Care 1977;22:832.
76. Breenbaum DM, Schwarz JO, Goldblatt MB. More on PRM modification for PEEP. Respir Care 1978;23:1137–1140.
77. Perel A, Eimerl D, Grossberg M. A PEEP device for a manual bag ventilator. Anesth Analg 1976;55:745.
78. Lilly JK. An inexpensive portable positive end-expiratory pressure system. Anesth Analg 1979;58:53–55.
79. Page A, Williams A, Spielman FJ, Watson CB. Simple system for portable positive end-expiratory pressure (letter). Anesthesiology 1985;62:698–699.
80. Banner MJ, Lampotang S, Boysen PG, Hurd TE, Desautels DA. Flow resistance of expiratory positive-pressure valve systems. Chest 1986;90:212–217.
81. Pinsky MR, Huhocik D, Culpepper JA, Snyder JV. Flow resistance of expiratory positive-pressure systems. Chest 1988;94: 788–791.
82. Brown SE, Stansbury DW, Merrill EJ, Linden GS, Light RW. Prevention of suctioning-related oxygen desaturation. Chest 1983;83:621–627.
83. Pierce JB, Piazza DE. Differences in postsuctioning arterial blood oxygen concentration values using two postoxygenation methods. Heart Lung 1987;16:34–38.
84. Chulay M, Graeber GM. Efficiency of a hypersufflation and hyperoxygenation suctioning intervention. Heart Lung 1988;17: 15–22.
85. Finer NN, Barrington KJ, Al-Fadley F, Peters KL. Limitations of self-inflating resuscitators. Pediatrics 1986;77:417–420.
86. Kauffman GW, Hess DR. Modification of the infant Laerdal resuscitation bag to monitor airway pressure. Crit Care Med 1982;10:112–113.
87. Bumstead D. A modification of the Laerdal infant resuscitator for the simple and safe delivery of CPAP and PEEP. Respir Care 1984;29:270–272.
88. Gregory GA, Kitterman JA, Phibbs RH, Rooley WH, Hamilton WK. Treatment of the idiopathic respiratory distress syndrome with continuous positive airway pressure. N Engl J Med 1971;284:1333–1340.
89. Arandia HY, Patil VU. PEEP and the Mapleson D Circuit. Anesthesiology 1985;62:846.
90. Paradis IL, Caldwell EJ. Traumatic pneumocephalus: A hazard of resuscitators. J Trauma 1979;19:61–63.
91. Osborn HH, Kayen D, Horne H, Bray W. Excess ventilation with oxygen-powered resuscitators. Am J Emerg Med 1984;2:408–413.
92. Hess D, Simmons M, Ruppert T, McClure S. The effect of inlet pressure on the flow from O_2-powered resuscitators (abstract). Respir Care 1991;36:1288–1289.

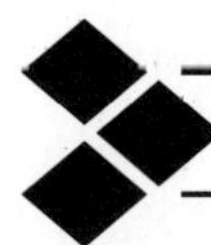
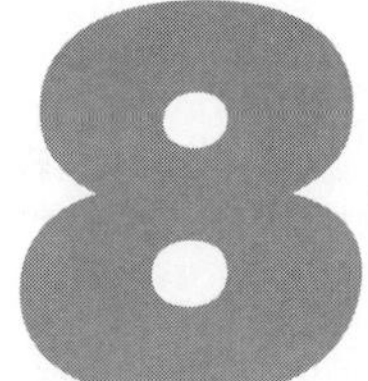

Blood Gases: The Measurement of pH, P_{CO_2}, P_{O_2}, and Related Analytes

Robert F. Moran

Dean R. Hess

OBJECTIVES

1. Compare international and American symbols for blood gases.
2. Explain the relationship between pH and $[H^+]$.
3. Describe the pH, P_{CO_2}, and P_{O_2} measurement systems of blood gas analyzers.
4. Explain the methods of hemoglobin measurement by spectrophotometry and hematocrit measurement by conductivity.
5. Describe the principles of electrode calibration.
6. Discuss the concept of end-point detection.
7. Discuss factors that contribute to analytical sources of error in blood gas analysis.
8. Distinguish between derived and measured blood gas quantities.

(continued)

OBJECTIVES, (continued)

9. Discuss the issues related to temperature adjustment of blood gas values.
10. Distinguish between quality control testing and proficiency testing.
11. Describe the component parts of a blood gas analyzer and a CO-oximeter.
12. Describe the principles of CO-oximetry.
13. Explain the principles of operation of intra-arterial blood gas monitors and mixed venous oxygen saturation monitors.
14. Describe the technique of gastric tonometry.

KEY TERMS

American symbols
base excess
Beer's law
bicarbonate
blood gas measurement
buffer
calibration
carboxyhemoglobin
Clark electrode
CO-oximetry
CO_2 content
conductivity
derived quantity
electrode
end-point detection
fractional oxyhemoglobin
gas tension
gastric tonometry
Henderson-Hasselbach equation
international symbols
methemoglobin
mixed venous blood
optode
oxygen content
oxygen saturation
P_{CO_2} electrode
pH
pH electrode
P_{O_2} electrode
polarographic
proficiency testing
pulmonary artery catheter
quality control
reference electrode
sensor
Severinghaus electrode
spectrophotometry
sulfhemoglobin

Introduction

"Blood gas and pH analysis has more immediacy and potential impact on patient care than any other laboratory determination."[1] In a book on critical care decision making,[2] nearly 70% of the case types described required blood gas analysis at some place in the decision scheme.

The blood gas measurement typically consists of three direct measurements (only two of which are gases), and several calculated or derived values. The measurements are oxygen and carbon dioxide tensions or partial pressures (P_{O_2} and P_{CO_2}, respectively) and hydrogen ion amounts, as pH or as chemical activity. In addition, some analyzers measure total hemoglobin (tHb). Analytical systems are also available that combine blood gas and hemoglobin measurements with measurements of some electrolytes (Na^+, K^+, Ca^{++}, Cl^-), but these are beyond the scope of many respiratory therapy–based blood gas laboratories.

The measurement of blood gases is conceptually simple but requires optimal integration of system and sensor design with operator knowledge and use of the system. A premier consideration in the design is the fact that whole blood is living tissue and as such is a complex milieu that presents unique problems when an attempt is made to assess its physical and chemical properties. For example, it interacts with every surface it contacts and is substantially less stable than serum or plasma when exposed to air. Even in an anaerobic state, it is stable only when iced and then only for a short time. Most measurements in the clinical chemistry laboratory require dilution of the sample by one or more reagents, with subsequent reactions that produce some measurable response. Blood gas analysis relies on sensors in direct contact with the undiluted whole blood specimen. Due to these factors, the operational simplicity of the modern blood gas analyzer (Fig. 8-1) should not mask the underlying complexity

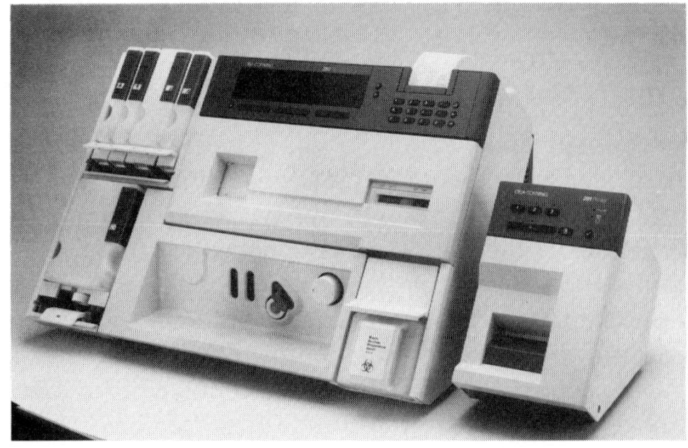

Figure 8-1. Ciba-Corning Model 280 blood gas analyzer. (Courtesy of Ciba-Corning Diagnostics Corp, Medfield, MA)

of this analytical system and the need for the operator to understand not only the *how to* but also the *why* of total system performance.

General Measurement Concepts

International Symbols

Recommendations for symbols and other notations have been made by various national and international standards organizations such as the International Standards Organization (ISO), the International Union of Pure and Applied Chemistry (IUPAC), the International Federation of Clinical Chemistry (IFCC), and the National Committee for Clinical Laboratory Standards—USA (NCCLS). Various documents of these organizations are available, and Sigaard-Andersen's book[3] is also a useful guide.

The kind of quantity is identified by an italicized lower case letter such as "*p*" for partial pressure (tension), "*c*" for concentration, and "*a*" for activity. This is followed by the substance identifier, for example "CO_2" for carbon dioxide (strictly speaking, the "CO_2" should be subscripted to the kind of quantity, but the IFCC has indicated that there is no ambiguity involved by keeping it on the same line). If necessary, the quantity is characterized as a sample source and type in a parenthetical option. The complete symbol then for the partial pressure of carbon dioxide in arterial blood is $p\mathrm{CO_2(aB)}$. If the sample were venous blood or mixed venous blood, the symbols would be, respectively, $p\mathrm{CO_2(vB)}$ and $p\mathrm{CO_2}(\bar{\mathrm{v}}\mathrm{B})$.

If the discussion is generic about the partial pressure of carbon dioxide, or if no ambiguity in the context of the discussion is involved, an abbreviated form is acceptable. The most common application of the abbreviated symbols is for tHb, pH, $p\mathrm{CO_2}$, and $p\mathrm{O_2}$, since it is usually clear from the context or other symbols that blood or alveolar gas in involved. Therefore, the symbol (B) following the substance may be omitted in most circumstances, such as $p\mathrm{CO_2(a)}$ for the partial pressure of carbon dioxide in arterial blood.

American Symbols

Unfortunately, symbols commonly used in the American pulmonary literature do not conform to international standards. Pulmonary literature usually conforms to the standards established for pulmonary terms and symbols by the American College of Chest Physicians and the American Thoracic Society.[4] According to their recommendations, the pressure of a gas is represented by a capital "P," followed by a letter representing the sample source (eg, "a" for arterial, "$\bar{\mathrm{v}}$" for mixed venous). For example, P_{aO_2} is used for the partial pressure of oxygen in arterial blood and P_{aCO_2} is used for the partial pressure of carbon dioxide in arterial blood.

Gas Tension

Gas tension, as measured by the blood gas analyzer, represents the P_{O_2} or P_{CO_2} as dissolved in the blood plasma and in physicochemical equilibrium with the blood cells and their components. The partial pressure of a gas is that fraction of the total gas pressure from that gas alone, as defined by Dalton's law. The total pressure (atmospheric [P_B]) is measured by the height of a column of mercury, which has resulted in the measurement of pressure in millimeters of mercury (see Chapter 1).

The pH Concept

The amount of acid in a system is represented by the hydrogen ion concentration or its activity. In the realm of general chemical applications, the range of hydrogen ion levels is quite wide, extending from as much as 36 mol/L in concentrated sulfuric acid to as little as 0.00000000000001 mol/L in a solution of sodium hydroxide. In the early part of this century, Sorensen,[5] working at the Carlsburg (Brewery) Laboratories in Denmark, initiated the use of a scientific notation that made recording of the hydrogen ion levels more convenient for some chemists.

Sorensen's notation, an extension of the classic scientific notation for very large or very small numbers, is best explained by the following example. If a 0.1 mol/L solution of hydrochloric acid is prepared, its hydrogen ion concentration is 0.1 mol/L or 1×10^{-1} mol/L. If a 0.1 mol/L solution sodium hydroxide (a base) is prepared, its hydrogen ion concentration is 0.00000000000001 or 1×10^{-14} mol/L. If equal amounts of the two are mixed, a neutral solution results. This neutral solution has a hydrogen ion concentration of 0.0000001 mol/L or 1×10^{-7} mol/L.

To avoid the inconvenience of the negative sign and all the zeroes, Sorensen recorded the "power of Hydrogen," or pH; that is, the exponent of the standard scientific notation for large or small numbers. Sorensen's paper in French used the term *puissance Hydrogen*, thus the term *pH*. In the above example, the hydrochloric acid has a pH of 1 and the sodium hydroxide has a pH of 14. For computation purposes (ie, intermediate "concentrations"), the notation is further refined so that pH is defined as the negative base 10 logarithm of the hydrogen ion activity ($\mathrm{pH} = -\log [\mathrm{H^+}]\mathrm{a}$, where "a" signifies activity).

Since it is convenient for general chemical work, this notation (pH) has continued despite some limitations in the biochemical and physiologic disciplines. There is an effort in those disciplines to express the concentra-

TABLE 8-1. Relationship Between pH and [H⁺]

pH	$[H^+]$ (nanomol/L)
7.0	100
7.1	80
7.2	64
7.3	50
7.4	40
7.5	32
7.6	25
7.7	20
7.8	16
8.0	10

tion in different units. Thus, instead of 0.0000001 mol/L, one would use the term 100 nanomol/L (ie, 100 $\times 10^{-9}$ mol/L) to represent pH = 7 (ie, neutral). The relationship between pH and nanomol/L is illustrated in Table 8-1. Note that the relationship between pH and nanomol is inverse. Also, because of the logarithmic relationship, small numeric changes in pH are equivalent to large changes in hydrogen ion concentration and are nonlinear. The advantages and disadvantages of the nanomol/L approach are relative to the interpretation and clinical application of the data. Most blood gas analyzers designed to measure pH can be set up to calibrate, measure, and report hydrogen ions as either pH or nanomol/L. Since the pH notation is most commonly used, we will use that term.

Units

With respect to units of measurement, the metric system (Système International d'Unites [SI]) should be used, with the only major exception being blood gases. This is partially because change in gas tension units from millimeters of mercury (mm Hg) to kilopascals (kPa) offers no clinical advantage. Additionally, no mercury barometers currently manufactured are calibrated in kilopascals. As a result, we will use the conventional units of millimeters of mercury for gas tension and pH for hydrogen ion concentration. To convert to kilopascals for gas tension, multiply the millimeters of mercury by 0.1333 or divide it by 7.5. To understand the numbers, remember that 30, 60, 90, and 120 mm Hg convert to 4, 8, 12, and 16 kPa, respectively.

Sensors and Measurement Concepts

The sensors used in a blood gas analyzer employ two separate principles, electrometric (electrodes) and optical. Of the electrodes, the pH and P_{CO_2} are of the potentiometric type and measure voltage. The P_{O_2} electrode is amperometric and measures current when a constant voltage is applied. The optical system used for measurement of total blood hemoglobin is based on the characteristic absorbance of light by the colored hemoglobin solution. Because of these differences, each sensor presents unique problems with sample handling, calibration, and quality control.

The pH Measurement System

The measurement of pH can be accomplished using a single sensing electrode. However, reliable results for specific pH values require a system composed of a sensor and a reference electrode.

The pH Sensor/Electrode

If two hydrogen ions containing electrolytes are separated by a thin glass membrane of a specific composition (pH glass), a potential (voltage) is produced across the glass membrane. This principle can be used to compare the pH of two solutions. An excellent review of the principles of electrochemistry may be found in the two-volume series on ion-selective electrodes edited by Covington and published by CRC Press.[6] Depending on their pH, a millivoltmeter will show different readings for different solutions on one side of the glass membrane, provided that the pH of the solution on the other side is held constant (Fig. 8-2). The glass pH electrode responds predictably over a wide range of pH. The voltmeter in the circuit is calibrated so that it converts millivolts to pH.

The Reference Electrode

Due to the high impedance of glass, the voltage difference due to differences in pH cannot be measured accurately with the simple system described earlier. Instead, a reference electrode, having a constant reference voltage against which the potential across the pH glass interface can be measured, is necessary for comparison. In a combined pH-reference system, a solu-

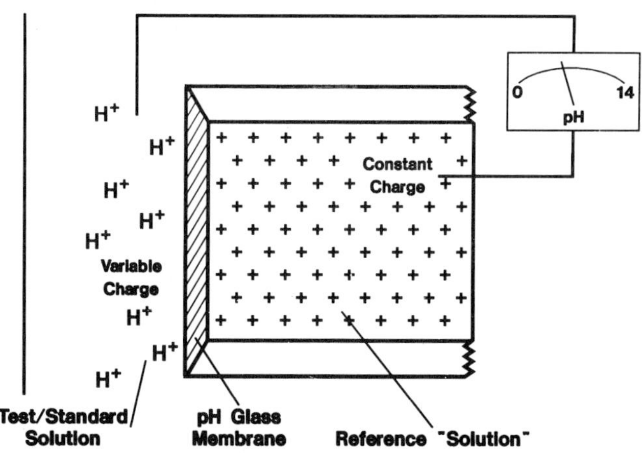

Figure 8-2. Simple glass pH measuring electrode.

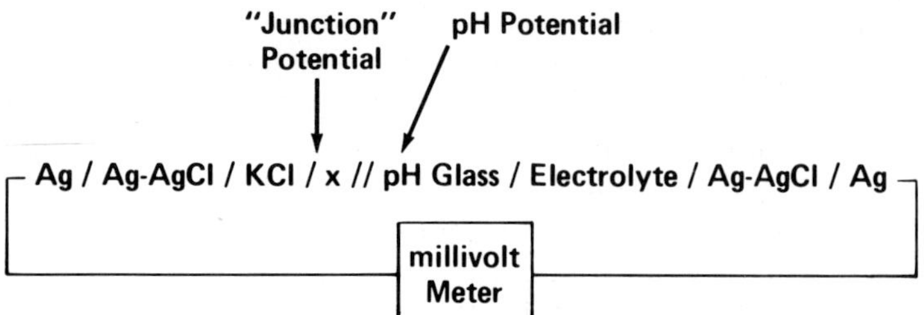

Figure 8-3. Combined pH–reference electrode system; "X" represents solution of unknown pH. Although potentials exist at each junction in the circuit, the only potential that changes is that between the sample and the pH glass.

tion of constant pH is kept sealed on one side of the pH glass membrane while the solution to be measured is on the other side. As illustrated in Figure 8-3, the unknown solution on the left side of the pH-sensitive glass is in electrical contact through a potassium chloride (KCl) salt bridge to either a silver/silver chloride or a calomel reference electrode. A typical pH measurement cell, as found in the blood gas laboratory, is illustrated in Figure 8-4.

Functional Requirements and Characteristics of the pH System

The measured pH of blood is dependent on the temperature of the sample and calibrants as well as on avoidance of contamination of the measuring system with air. For sufficiently accurate results, the temperature of the pH electrode should be maintained at the normal body temperature of 37° ± 0.1°C. Since the blood pH varies by approximately 0.0147 unit/°C, it is also important that blood sample temperature be kept at a constant temperature (usually 37°C) during measurement of pH.

Another consideration in the design of pH electrodes for use with blood samples is the effect of room air contamination on the pH of the blood. Since loss of CO_2 to the air will increase the pH of the sample, blood pH electrodes must be contained in an anaerobic chamber to minimize the possibility of contamination with room air.

To achieve anaerobic and temperature-constant conditions in blood gas analyzers, the pH-sensitive glass may be constructed either as a capillary arrangement or as a dip-type electrode surrounded by temperature-stabilizing materials such as steel, aluminum, electrically conductive (EC) glass, or some combination of these. The use of other materials for maintenance of temperature (eg, water or air circulating in plastic or glass) may be inadequate to quickly heat iced samples to 37°C unless special components such as pre-heaters are used to sufficiently warm and stabilize the blood. Incorporation of an integrated membrane reference electrode into this temperature-controlled module is not essential but minimizes the smaller effects on pH due to temperature fluctuation of the reference system.

In a capillary system (Fig. 8-5), the blood sample is inserted or drawn into the chamber formed by the pH glass capillary. The charge on the inside of the pH glass varies with the pH of the sample. The dip-type pH electrode illustrated in Figure 8-4 acts in the same manner as the capillary electrode except that the outer aspect of pH glass is in contact with the sample. Either solid electrolyte or buffer is used to maintain a constant potential on the one surface of the pH glass. With either system, careful attention to sample chamber geometry and pH glass characteristics is essential to maintain thermostated and anaerobic conditions.

The electrically conducting salt bridge (usually of either saturated or 4 M KCl) is used to complete the

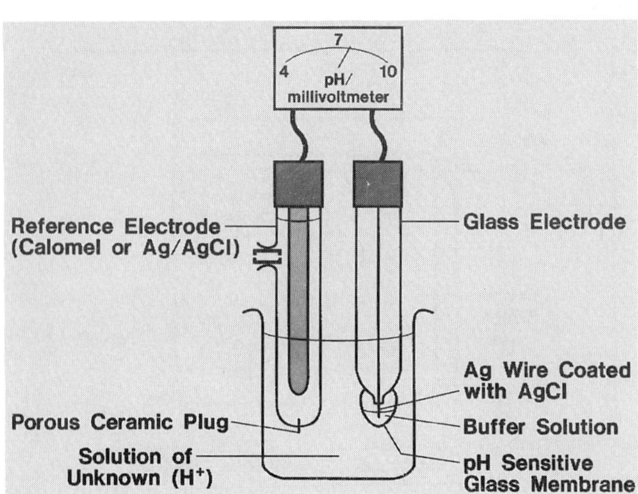

Figure 8-4. Dip-type pH measurement cell.

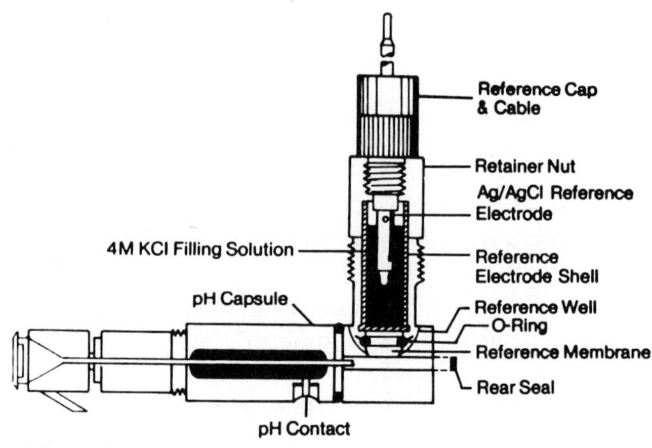

Figure 8-5. Schematic diagram of capillary type pH electrode system.

circuitry between the pH electrode and the external reference half-cell. Near-saturated KCl is chosen since the moderate changes in its concentration that normally result from routine use will not significantly affect the pH and its concentration (4 M) can be well controlled in manufacture and storage.

Although potentials exist at each junction in the circuit (see Fig. 8-3), including the pH glass and buffer or solid electrolyte, the only potential that is allowed to change is that between the sample and the pH glass. Thus, the measured pH changes as a function of the number of free hydrogen ions in the sample. The greater the acidity (hydrogen ion concentration) of the sample, the more positive is the total voltage because an increasing number of hydrogen ions are present.

The reference electrode can be modified to incorporate packed silver chloride granules around the internal wire. This overcomes the drift that often occurs when a new reference electrode is placed into a system by eliminating the porous ceramic plug that has slow diffusion characteristics. A KCl donut can also be added to the reference shell. This helps to maintain a level of about 4 M KCl for much longer periods, while minimizing the build-up of KCl crystals when saturated KCl is used.

The responsiveness of the pH electrode to changes in hydrogen ion levels diminishes with time owing to changes in the pH glass itself. As the electrode is exposed to successive samples, an exchange of hydrogen ions (hydronium, H_3O^-) with the metal ions of the pH glass occurs (Fig. 8-6). Indeed, it is the potential (voltage) between the charge layer at the hydrogen ion–metal ion interface and the reference side of the pH glass that allows pH to be measured. As the depth of this hydrogen ion–metal ion exchange gel layer migrates inward (Fig. 8-7), the pH response time increases. When combined with build-up of protein or other material on the outer glass surface (see Fig. 8-7), a substantially slower or noisier response may occur. Basic maintenance procedures suggested by manufacturers reduce these effects, which include simple cleaning of the glass surface by use of protein digesting enzymes, and in some cases by stripping off layers of glass a few molecules thick with either strong acid or base (see Fig. 8-7). These treatments decrease the distance the sample's hydrogen ions must travel to reach the interface with the metal in the glass matrix.

The Pco_2 Electrode System

The Pco_2 electrode, often called the Severinghaus electrode, was originally developed by Bradley and Severinghaus[7,8] using the principles developed by Stow.[9] The inner chamber of the Pco_2 electrode is similar to the dip-type pH measuring electrode (Fig. 8-8). It consists of a sealed glass cylinder and has a tip of pH-sensitive

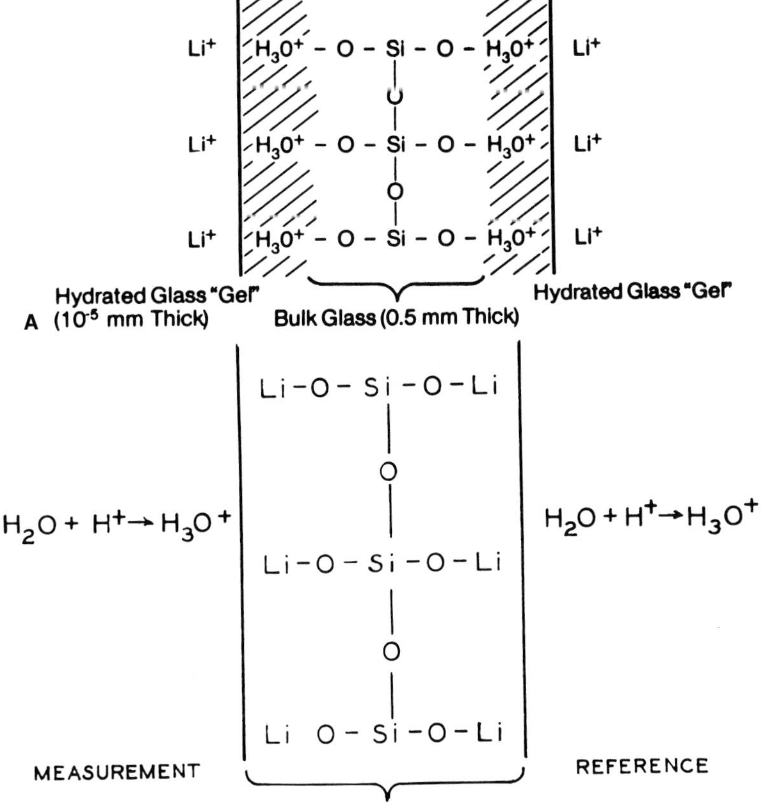

Figure 8-6. New pH glass (A) and normal "hydrated" pH glass (B).

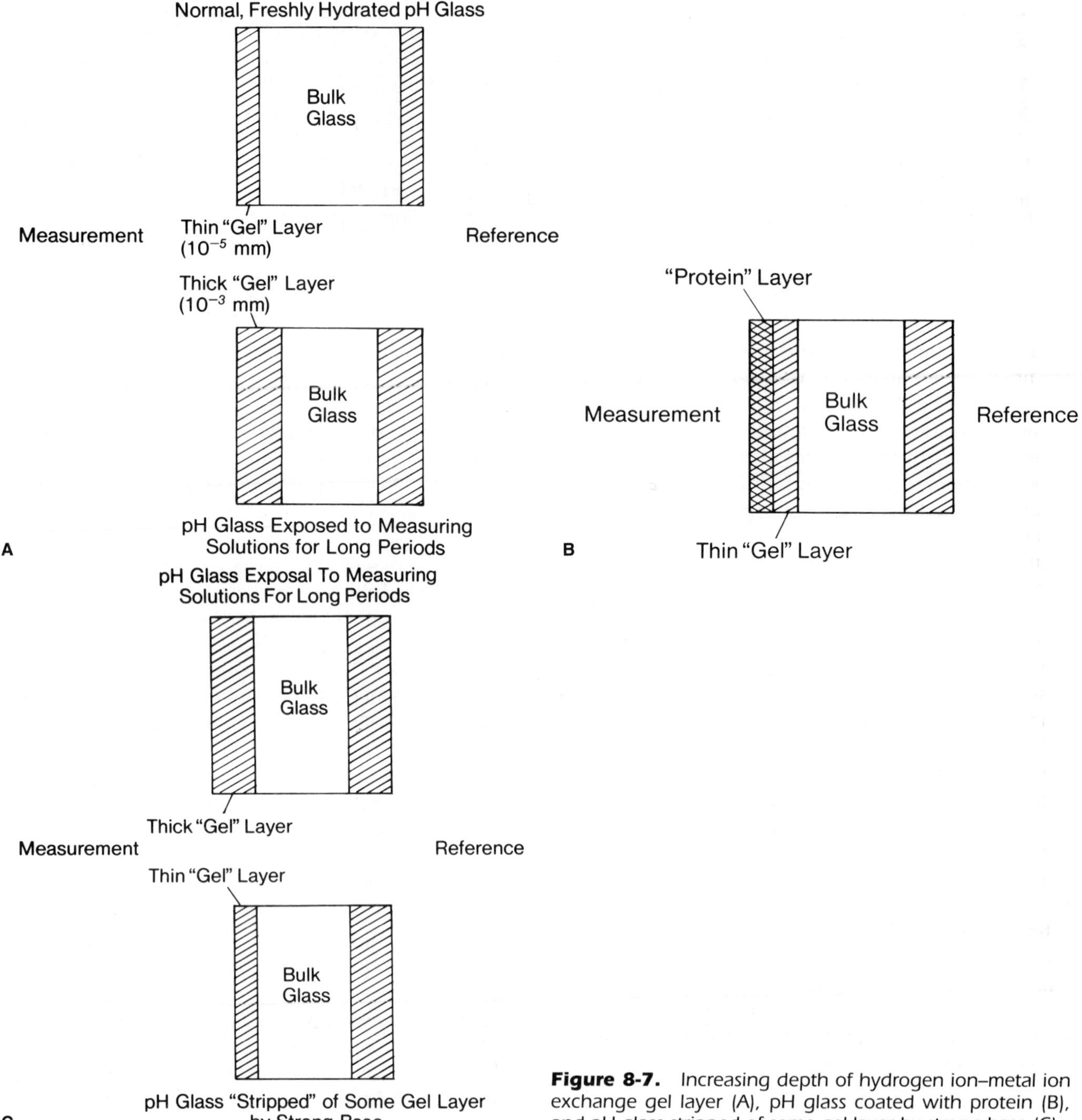

Figure 8-7. Increasing depth of hydrogen ion–metal ion exchange gel layer (A), pH glass coated with protein (B), and pH glass stripped of some gel layer by strong base (C).

glass. A buffer of strong acid solutions is contained inside this glass cylinder. The outer chamber contains a reference half-cell, typically silver/silver chloride and a bicarbonate electrolyte solution. A gas-permeable membrane is placed between the blood sample and the bicarbonate-electrolyte solution. The measurement of P_{CO_2} by this electrode is an adaptation of the pH measurement. CO_2 from the sample chamber diffuses through the gas-permeable membrane, which alters the pH of the bicarbonate solution contained between the membrane and pH-sensitive glass.

Functional Requirements and Characteristics of the P_{CO_2} Electrode

The classic CO_2 membrane material is Silastic (silicone-elastic, General Electric Company), but some electrodes use membranes made of Teflon (DuPont DeNemours Company) or other materials. Different materials can result in different performance characteristics. For example, while Silastic is quite permeable to CO_2, it is not resilient and thus stretches, resulting in the need to change the membrane frequently. Teflon does not stretch but allows CO_2 to diffuse more slowly,

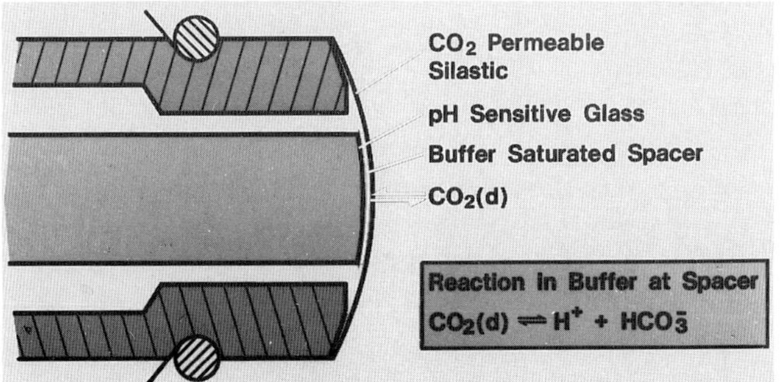

Figure 8-8. Schematic diagram of Pco_2 electrode.

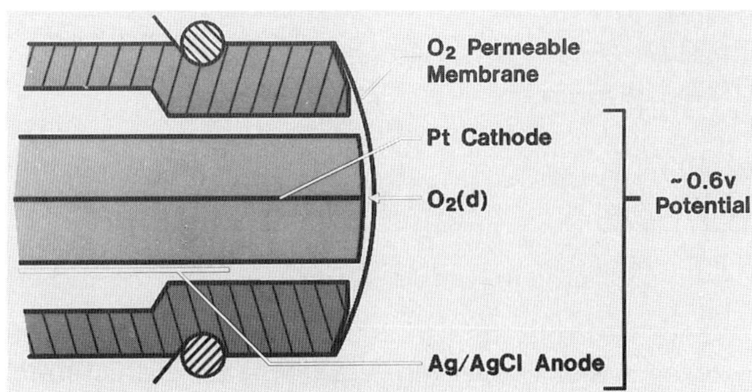

Figure 8-10. Schematic diagram of Po_2 electrode.

resulting in longer response times. The final choice of membrane material by the manufacturer is based on a balance of these factors. The space between the membrane and the pH glass is kept relatively constant by either the interposition of a spacer (eg, nylon, Joseph paper) or by designed-in-engineering (PT = F) features and membrane materials selection.

The chemistry of the CO_2 electrode is illustrated in Figure 8-9. The pH change that results from this reaction is amplified and displayed as Pco_2. Note that the sample cannot produce a direct change in the hydrogen ion concentration of the internal bicarbonate solution because the hydrophobic membrane excludes passage of hydrogen ions. The sample affects the pH of the bicarbonate solution only by the production of H_2CO_3 from the dissolved CO_2.

Changes in CO_2 electrode performance generally occur as a result of stretching of the membrane or protein accumulation on the membrane. Over very long periods (several months), the pH-sensitive glass can also be affected (as noted earlier for the pH electrode). Recently designed electrodes reduce these issues to the extent that some CO_2 electrode–membrane combinations can be used for many months without any maintenance except in situ cleaning. These improvements have resulted from changes in membrane materials, as well as modifications of the internal electrolyte and of system hydraulics.

The Po_2 Electrode System

The O_2 electrode, usually called the Clark electrode[10] for its inventor Leland Clark, differs from the CO_2 electrode and the pH electrode because it is current-generating rather than potential-generating. A small platinum wire inside the electrode is polarized with a specific negative voltage. Oxygen molecules diffuse from the sample through a semi-permeable membrane (PT = F) into the electrode electrolyte and are reduced at the platinum cathode, and the resultant current is measured. This current is proportional to the Po_2 of the sample. The O_2 electrode is often referred to as both polarographic (because the electrode is polarized) and consumptive (because it consumes oxygen that diffuses from the sample).

The Po_2 electrode contains a silver/silver chloride element that acts as the anode and encircles an inner solid glass rod (Fig. 8-10), in which the platinum wire cathode is sealed with its end exposed flush with the glass surface. The semi-permeable membrane covering the tip of the assembly also holds in place an electrolyte solution that serves as the contact medium between an anode and a cathode and into which the oxygen diffuses.

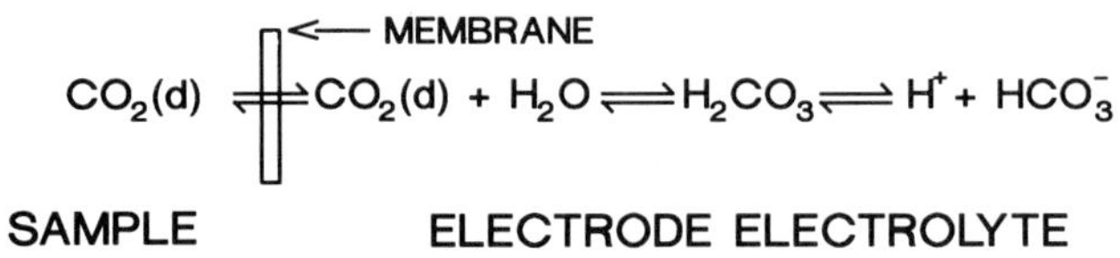

MEMBRANE

$$CO_2(d) \rightleftharpoons CO_2(d) + H_2O \rightleftharpoons H_2CO_3 \rightleftharpoons H^+ + HCO_3^-$$

SAMPLE | ELECTRODE ELECTROLYTE

Figure 8-9. Chemistry of the Pco_2 electrode.

Functional Requirements and Characteristics of the Po_2 Electrode

A constant voltage of 0.6 to 0.7 volt is maintained between the anode and the cathode. The specific voltage chosen for a Po_2 electrode system is dependent on several factors, including the pH of the internal electrolyte. The voltage chosen is kept constant under most internal electrolyte conditions. Generally, voltages above 0.8 volt cause electrolysis of water and as a result are not used in these systems. At the designed voltage for the particular electrode, virtually all oxygen reaching the surface of the cathode will react, leaving none to diffuse back from the cathode surface to the membrane. Thus, the Po_2 at the cathode surface remains zero. Oxygen is reduced at the cathode, as shown in Equation Box 8-1.

Equation Box 8-1:
Reduction of Oxygen in Po_2 Electrode

$$O_2 + 2H_2O + 4e^- \leftrightarrows 4OH^-$$

Equation Box 8-2:
Production of Electrons from Silver Anode in P_{O_2} Electrode

$$4Ag^{\circ} \leftrightarrows 4Ag^{+} + 4e^{-}$$

Four electrons are necessary to reduce each oxygen molecule that comes into contact with the cathode. Under the conditions of the designed voltage and pH, the silver anode (positive electrode) provides the necessary electrons for oxygen reduction as described in Equation Box 8-2. These electrons migrate through the electrolyte to the cathode, where they reduce oxygen. The potential applied between the anode and the cathode provides the driving or polarizing force for the electrons produced at the anode. Thus, there is a continuous flow of electrons between the poles of the electrodes. The electron flow, or current, is proportional to the amount of oxygen that diffuses through the membrane and dissolves in the electrolyte surrounding the cathode tip. The electron flow (current) is measured and displayed as P_{O_2}.

The internal electrolyte composition can affect performance. Oxygen electrodes using a silver chloride (AgCl)–based electrolyte may have deposits form on the cathode tip over time, resulting in a need to change the membrane and clean the cathode tip. Recent design improvements incorporate internal electrolytes having a different silver base and are combined with membranes that are physically more stable than the typical polypropylene membrane. These permit measurement of P_{O_2} over prolonged periods (months) with only minimal in situ maintenance, such as simple cleaning.

Total Hemoglobin Measurement

Hemoglobin, a complex iron-containing protein, is the key blood component that transports oxygen to the tissues. It is found in several forms with differences in both fundamental composition (protein portion) and active group (with respect to oxygen transport). Assessment of the former is beyond the scope of the blood gas laboratory, and the latter is addressed in a later section of this chapter. In situations in which the previous concerns have been addressed, the simple measurement of total hemoglobin may be a useful addition to the analysis of the classic blood gases, since it aids the respiratory care practitioner in assessing oxygen delivery.

Hemoglobin concentration is reliably measured on a well-mixed whole blood sample using the principles of spectrophotometry. According to this principle, if light of a particular wavelength is passed through a light-absorbing material, the absorbance of the light by the material will be proportional to the concentration and length of the light path through that material. This is commonly called Beer's law and is expressed as shown in Equation Box 8-3.

Equation Box 8-3:
Beer's Law

$$A = \epsilon \ell c$$

where A is the absorbance of light, ϵ is a constant (molar extinction coefficient, which is based on the wavelengths of light passing through the solution and the material being tested and is designated by the Greek letter epsilon), ℓ is for the length of the light path, and c is the concentration. Thus, if ϵ for a material such as hemoglobin and the light path ℓ are known, the measurement of the absorbance allows calculation of the concentration.

The fundamental criterion for valid application of this principle is that the material to be measured is the only material present that absorbs light at the chosen wavelength. This is typically controlled by mixing the test solution (blood) with reagents that form a single, stable, colored compound only with the analyte or analytes to be measured. Thus, total hemoglobin, which is composed of several different types of molecules that absorb at different wavelengths, is commonly reacted with a ferricyanide-based reagent to form cyanomethemoglobin, which has a known absorbance spectrum. Combinations of hemoglobin and other reagents that combine ordinary properties with the ability to form a single chromophase with hemoglobin can also be used (Fig. 8-11). The actual wavelength (or narrow band of wavelength) of light chosen for the measuring system typically corresponds to the region of maximum absorbance as seen in Figure 8-10.

The precision of the hemoglobin measurement is determined by many functional considerations, such as completeness of hemolysis, sample mixing, and other preanalytical and analytical factors. Accuracy is a function of the ability to calibrate the system to the reference method established by international convention.[11] A combination of accuracy and precision is paramount if the hemoglobin measured is to be useful in the assessment of oxygen delivery capabilities.

Hematocrit Measurement

Hematocrit, defined as the packed red blood cell volume expressed as a percentage, can also be useful as an index of oxygen delivery. This is due to the strong relationship between the red blood cell volume and

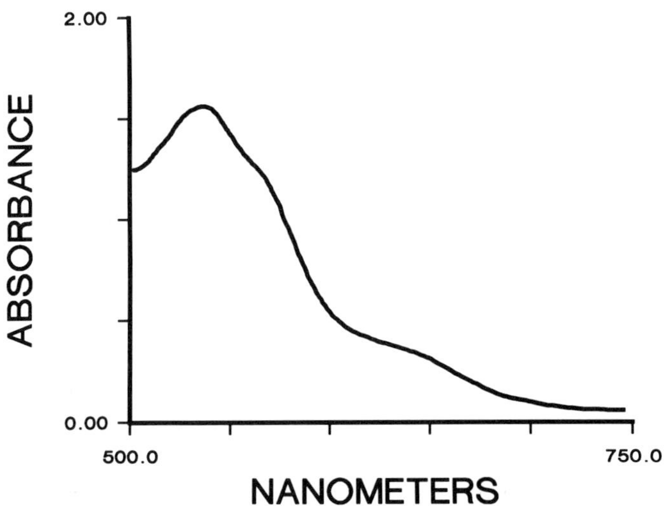

Figure 8-11. Absorbance spectrum for hemoglobin determination, with absorbance as a function of wavelength in nanometers. (Courtesy of Ciba-Corning Diagnostics Corp, Medfield, MA)

the hemoglobin levels. One must be aware, however, that in certain hematologic disorders the quantitative relationship between hemoglobin and hematocrit is not valid.[12] The classic measurement of hematocrit[13] is accomplished by centrifuging a well-mixed sample of whole blood at high speed until the cells are solidly packed. Subsequently, the volume percentage of red blood cells can be measured by use of a template. An alternate method,[14] based on changes in conductivity of the sample with changes in numbers of cells, can be incorporated into a blood gas analyzer.

Since conductivity of whole blood also varies with changes in plasma protein and electrolytes, these must also be taken into account when estimating hematocrit by this method. This is especially important in open-heart surgery and dialysis patients when blood is being diluted by various conductive electrolyte solutions that invalidate the assumptions involved in the hematocrit–hemoglobin relationship.

Calibration Principles

It is important for those who measure pH, blood gases, and hemoglobin to understand the principles of instrument calibration. Only with correct calibration is it possible to relate changes in electrode output to real values of pH, P_{CO_2}, P_{O_2}, and tHb.

Electrode Calibrations

Each electrode (pH, P_{CO_2}, P_{O_2}) has a theoretical slope or change in output as a function of the change in analyte concentration. This should make it possible to set the instrument at a zero response when exposed to a zero level of analyte and then obtain a direct readout of concentration of the analyte exposed to the sensor. In practice, however, the variability in slope of each electrode prevents reliable results from being obtained in this manner.

Because of inaccuracies that result from slope value variability, the electrodes of an instrument must be exposed to two accurately known levels of each analyte. One of these levels will result in a zero value, and the other will result in a slope value. By means of manual or microprocessor adjustment, each level is then set to the appropriately known value. This results in a calibrated or standardized instrument that can be used to measure absolute values of analyte in the sample.

In the case of pH and P_{CO_2}, a setting of zero seems contradictory to practice because a zero pH or P_{CO_2} is not used to calibrate the instrument. In both cases, however, the zero is an electronic zero related to the true characteristics of the standard material used.

For pH, the zero point occurs when buffers on one side of the pH sensitive glass and those on the opposite side (provided by the calibrating buffer solution) result in the same charge on both sides of the glass. Thus, a charge difference of zero and a zero voltage difference exists, which is referred to as the isoelectric (or isopotential) point (Fig. 8-12). After the isopotential pH is set by a potentiometer, another buffer of known pH is introduced and the value of its pH is set by another potentiometer. Isopotential pH is often 7.382, and the other standardization pH is often 6.838.

For P_{CO_2}, most blood gas systems are designed so that a gas that contains 5% CO_2 results in a potential across the pH glass that is approximately zero. Precise adjustment of the appropriate calibration control results in a zero potential at a P_{CO_2} of 35.65 mm Hg (at an atmospheric pressure of 760 mm Hg). The introduction of another gas with a significantly higher P_{CO_2} (often 10%) causes the pH of the bicarbonate to lower

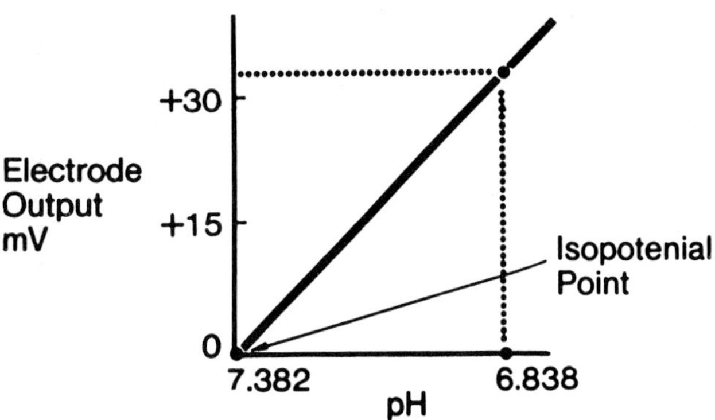

Figure 8-12. Ideal slope of pH measuring system, with isoelectric calibration point.

and the second calibration point is set on the basis of this known P_{CO_2}.

For P_{O_2}, calibration is more straightforward. A gas containing no oxygen is usually used to set zero, although some manufacturers choose to use an electronic zero point. The other non-zero gas used is usually about 12% oxygen, but the specific choice is governed by the manufacturer's designation and has little effect on performance.

As with the electrodes, a number of practical considerations make the routine measurement of hemoglobin concentration easier if the absorbance of a solution with known hemoglobin concentration is measured at the same time as the unknown. By comparison of the two absorbancies, the concentration of the unknown can be determined, as shown in Equation Box 8-4.

These relationships, the basis for many measurements in the clinical laboratory, apply to the blood gas analyzer equipped with a hemoglobin-measuring module (spectrophotometer). However, instead of reading absorbances directly and calculating concentration, the analyzer is set to the known concentration of hemoglobin (or dye equivalent) in the calibration material.

Functional Requirements and Characteristics of Calibration

Some set points for electrodes and optical systems are inherently quite stable and need to be adjusted only occasionally. Because of this stability, it is possible to routinely calibrate or standardize a blood gas analyzer at the less stable points for each parameter and only check the stable set points occasionally. The process of calibrating in this manner is frequently called one-point calibration, and checking both levels is called two-point calibration.

Equation Box 8-4: Comparison of Two Absorbances to Determine the Concentration of an Unknown

$$A_U = \epsilon \ell C_U$$

$$A_S = \epsilon \ell C_S$$

Since the absorbances are proportionate to concentration and the concentration relating to one of the absorbances is known, by canceling the constants and rearranging, the following equation is produced:

$$C_U = \frac{A_U}{A_S} \cdot C_S$$

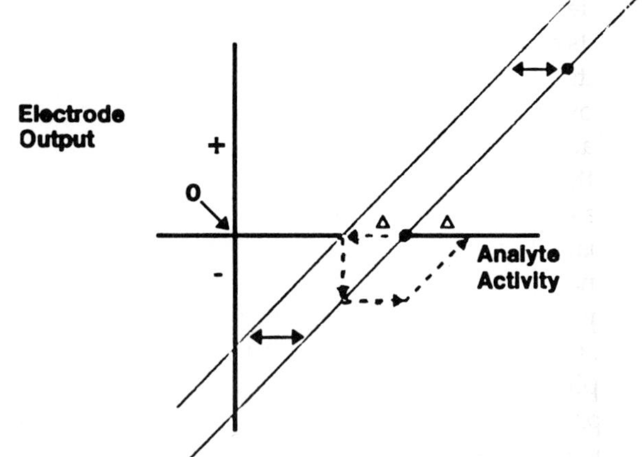

Figure 8-13. Effect of misadjustment of zero point on calibration.

The basic design features of older, manual blood gas analyzers include set points of the nonzero analytes that are dependent on the zero set points. Therefore, in these systems, any two-point calibration must start with the zero output analyte (eg, the isopotential pH buffer, the 5% CO_2, and the 0% O_2). Misadjustment of the zero versus the nonzero level of the analyte can result in significantly different errors in measurement of a sample, dependent on the level of the sample versus the levels of the analyte chosen for standardization. Additionally, the length of time to standardize the analyzer can be significantly prolonged. Misadjustment of the zero point will result in a constant error at all levels (Fig. 8-13). Misadjustment of the nonzero point results in a variable error, with a decrease in error as the sample value approaches the zero point and an increase in error as the sample value deviates from the zero set point (Fig. 8-14).

There are two methods used for calibration. The most common is to pass rehydrated mixtures of CO_2 and O_2 and known buffer solutions for pH across the face of the gas electrodes. Hydration of the gases is required in some systems to minimize cooling of the electrodes by the flowing gas as well as to reduce drying of

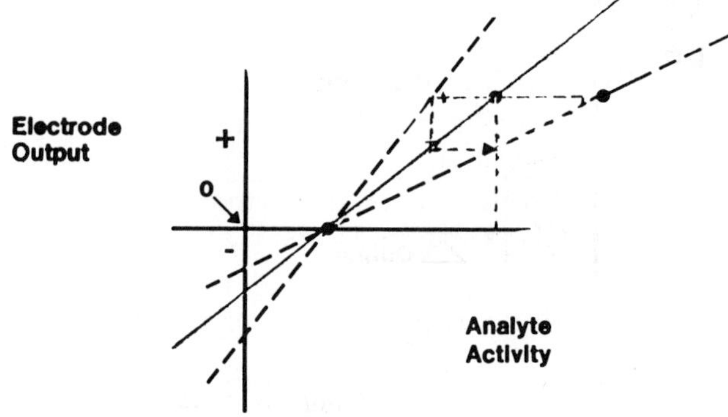

Figure 8-14. Effect of misadjustment of non-zero point on calibration, resulting in constant error.

the measuring chamber, which could cause deposition of salts and contamination of subsequent sample or calibrants. Some Food and Drug Administration (FDA)-approved instruments are designed to take these issues into account without prehydration of the gases. A system that measures hemoglobin would incorporate either a dye or hemoglobin in the buffer or would require a separate hemoglobin calibration sequence.

An alternative approach to calibrating the system is to equilibrate two carefully prepared buffer solutions with two gas mixtures. This choice is made to reduce sample path complexity, since both pH and the gases are present. However, it introduces problems related to the instability of gas-equilibrated aqueous solutions and the aqueous solutions do not behave in the instrument in the same way as whole blood. Despite both theoretical and market arguments to the contrary, either calibration approach seems to be reliable if the system is operated and maintained properly.

Electrode Response and End-Point Detection

Electrodes respond to a sample by changing the signal sent to the analyzing unit and the output display. The initial response is slow, followed by a fast, nearly linear, response and finishing by leveling off to a steady plateau where only minimal changes are seen (Fig. 8-15). The concept of end-point detection is the observation that an electrode's response is no longer changing significantly with respect to time and the electrode has thus reached a plateau.

End-point detection can be determined manually. In this case, the operator accepts a value when an electrode plateau is reached. The major fault with this method is that the criteria used by each operator may vary significantly, which may affect the reported results. Using a microprocessor, a blood gas analyzer can automatically determine electrode end-point. The microprocessor compares the change in electrode output to an internal algorithm and provides a consistent reproducible end-point. Even though an instrument may provide automatic end-point detection, it should also provide the operator with a display of the electrode output during most of the period of response to the sample. This allows the operator to evaluate electrode response for purposes of troubleshooting.

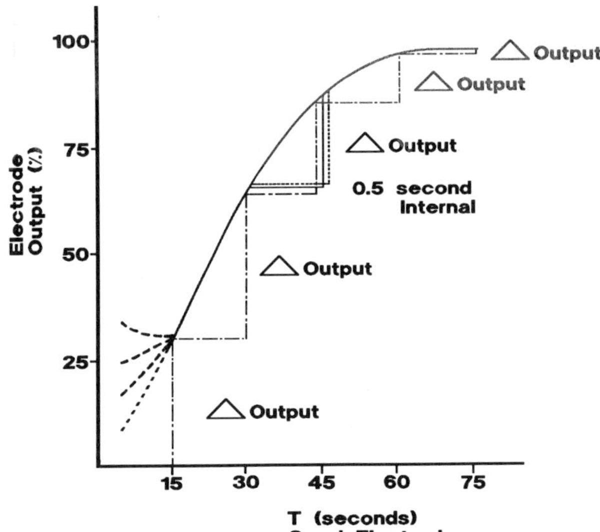

Figure 8-15. Electrode response and end-point detection.

Analytical Sources of Error

Perhaps the most important and unrecognized source of error is the handling of the sample within the analyzer. Blood gases are unlike other blood analytes in that the tubing through which they pass, and even the sensing electrodes, are potential sources of sample contamination. Plastic and rubber materials dissolve both oxygen and CO_2 to varying degrees. For example, silicon and polyurethane have extremely high oxygen and CO_2 solubility coefficients. As a result, their presence in the sample handling path must be minimized. Although there are usually design issues dealt with by the manufacturer, performance problems may result if a user decides to use substitute tubing or other materials for economy or convenience.

The whole blood sample must be moved through the analyzer as rapidly as possible to minimize the above effects, while at the same time ensuring that agitation induced by motion that is too rapid does not cause the formation or entrainment of bubbles that can contaminate the sample. The more automated devices deal with this issue as a fundamental part of design, but older manual analyzers are subject to operator-induced error of this type.

The oxygen measurement presents some interesting characteristics. The slope of the oxyhemoglobin dissociation curve at any point is proportional to the oxygen buffer capacity for the blood at that Po_2. Above a Po_2 of approximately 110 mm Hg, the hemoglobin is nearly saturated and the blood is more easily contaminated with oxygen (ie, the buffer capacity is exhausted). Aqueous materials that do not contain hemoglobin have no oxygen buffer capacity and are easier to contaminate with oxygen. A result of this is that a sample of blood with a Po_2 of 40 mm Hg is difficult to contaminate with oxygen. At a Po_2 of 200 mm Hg, aqueous controls and blood are equally easy to contaminate.

Blood pH is also buffered. However, this buffering action is relatively less constant over the physiologic pH range. The Pco_2 is buffered only in that it is part of the pH/HCO_3 equilibrium. As a result, residual aqueous buffer solutions do not constitute a serious source of contamination for the gases in the blood specimen (except at the high blood oxygen tension levels as noted) but do contribute to an error for pH measurements.

Electrodes have typically been the most common source for instrument performance questions, and these issues are treated as routine by many users. Instrument electronics detects most types of significant electrode irregularities. However, this does not preclude the absolute requirement for the user to perform all of the maintenance procedures according to the operator's and service manuals provided by the manufacturer. Following manufacturer's guidelines, most modern electrodes will operate fault free for extended periods of time. Recently introduced blood gas analyzers, which utilize membranes permanently attached to the electrode, have substantially less frequent electrode maintenance. Coupled with a fixed expiration date or specific, verifiable functional characteristics of each electrode, the net result is good performance and minimized operator interaction.

A frequently misunderstood source of analytical error is the effect of barometric pressure (PB). The tensions of both oxygen and CO_2 depend on their molar percent concentration and on ambient PB. Although optimum accuracy in calibration and patient results requires adjustment of the calibration and patient results requires adjustment of the calibration point with diurnal PB variation, the typical variation is not usually clinically significant. However, PB also depends on altitude. For every 1000 feet of altitude, PB drops about 3%. Depending on the altitude, the effects of this change can be clinically important if not taken into account (Fig. 8-16). Thus, for instruments used at significant altitude, calculation of gas calibration tensions should be based on actual PB taken from a mercury barometer or by setting the instrument barometer to match the mercury barometer reading.

Insidious and difficult to detect are errors resulting from contaminated calibrants, microbial growth within the instrument, small leaks permitting tiny bubbles to enter the sample stream, and inadvertent electrical ground paths created when the instrument is not properly cleaned.

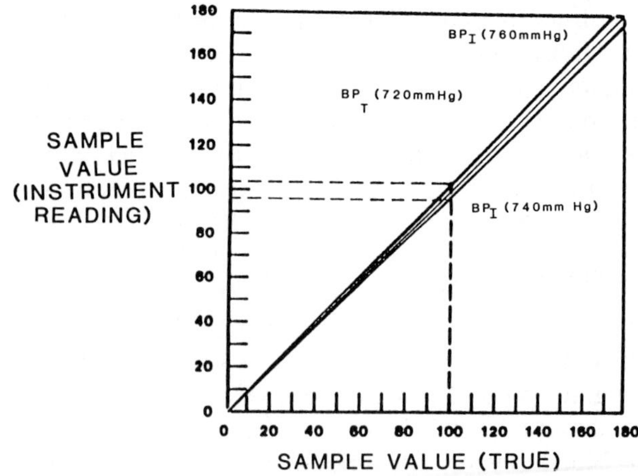

Figure 8-16. Effect of barometric pressure (BP) on accuracy of P_{O_2} measurement. The true P_{O_2} is 100 mm Hg at a BP of 740 mm Hg (center line). If the instrument is incorrectly calibrated to a BP of 760 mm Hg, the instrument reading will be less than the true value. (Courtesy of Ciba-Corning Diagnostics Products, Medfield, MA)

Derived Quantities

The most important measured quantities in blood pH and gas analysis are pH, P_{CO_2}, P_{O_2}, and tHb.[15] Although other quantities may be calculated from these, it should be emphasized that little new information is contained in these derived numbers and that they should be used only if they contribute to the understanding of the acid–base status of the patient. On the other hand, some of these quantities can be measured, either directly or with the incorporation of well-accepted constants. When measured (see section on CO-oximetry), the values do add new and useful information.

Oxygen Saturation of Hemoglobin

Oxygen saturation of hemoglobin, S_{O_2}, is defined as the ratio of oxyhemoglobin, O_2Hb, to the amount of hemoglobin present and capable of binding oxygen. In practice, the terms saturation or oxygen saturation have been used to represent several distinctly different parameters (see later in section on reported values of CO-oximetry). This ambiguous use is sometimes unnoticed, owing to the similarity of the numeric values obtained in some clinical conditions. Other clinical conditions can result in significantly different values, depending on the mode of measurement and reporting.

Calculated Hemoglobin Oxygen Saturation

Although it is possible to measure oxygen saturation (S_{O_2}) directly, it is often estimated from a measured P_{O_2} and calculations based on an empirical equation for the oxyhemoglobin dissociation curve. Such calculations, which may be performed manually using a nomogram or automatically using instrument-resident software, involve several assumptions, and significant systematic errors are possible because the relationship between hemoglobin oxygen saturation and P_{O_2} is a function of several variables. Additionally, the relationship does not take into account the effects of dyshemoglobins such as carboxyhemoglobin, methemoglobin, or sulfhemoglobin. Clinically important errors can result from incorporation of this calculated value infurther calculations, such as shunt fraction, or by assuming that the value obtained is equivalent to oxyhemoglobin fraction.[16] The use of this value is strongly discouraged.

Calculated Oxygen Content

The actual amount of oxygen present in a quantity of blood is called the oxygen content (O_2Ct). The total oxygen content is the sum of oxygen bound to hemoglobin (O_2Hb) and the amount of oxygen dissolved in the blood plasma. The amount of oxyhemoglobin present in the blood sample is a function of the PO_2 and the position and shape of the oxygen dissociation curve. At PO_2 values below 150 mm Hg, not all available hemoglobin is converted to oxyhemoglobin (ie, hemoglobin is not fully saturated with oxygen). The degree of saturation of the available hemoglobin with oxygen is an important factor in the determination of oxygen content, as is the total amount of available hemoglobin. As a result, the reporting of an oxygen content value derived from a calculation of oxygen saturation is totally inappropriate in the clinical setting.

Bicarbonate and CO_2 Content

All modern blood pH and gas analyzers provide a calculation of one or both of these quantities from the measured pH and PCO_2 and applications of the Henderson-Hasselbach equation (Equation Box 8-5).[13] The calculation of bicarbonate (and total CO_2 if the dissolved CO_2 is included) assumes a constant pK′ (usually 6.1). If, as some reports indicate,[17,18] the pK′ is other than this assumed value in critically ill patients, then errors in the bicarbonate and total CO_2 will result. However this issue is resolved, it is still appropriate to remember that no new information is provided by either of these calculated quantities. Most clinicians expect to see one of them on the blood gas report because it helps form a mental picture of the metabolic component of the acid–base abnormality. Therefore, these values will probably continue to be required. The need and extent of therapeutic intervention using various electrolytes may be more easily assessed when the CO_2 content is represented as an electrolyte.

Equation Box 8-5: Henderson-Hasselbach Equation

$$pH = pK' + \log \frac{HCO_3^-}{(0.03 \times PCO_2)}$$

Base Excess

There has been long-term interest in defining a quantity that reflects only the metabolic, and not the respiratory, component of a blood pH alteration. *Base excess* was intended for this purpose, but the term is now ambiguous because it has been defined in two different ways. The classic definition had reference only to the intravascular fluid compartment (ie, whole blood).[15] This has been called base excess (actual), standard base excess, base excess of whole blood, and in vitro base excess.

Others have pointed out that while this quantity has meaning in vitro, it does not reflect the metabolic acid–base status of a patient (in vivo). To reflect this status, one needs a quantity that takes into account the equilibration of CO_2 not only in intravascular fluid but also in interstitial fluid. This calculation can be easily performed on the basis of empirical data. The resultant quantity is usually called extracellular fluid base excess or in-vivo base excess.[15]

Again, it should be emphasized that neither quantity is actually needed, in that no new information is conveyed. However, clinicians who insist on having a calculated base excess should be provided extracellular fluid base excess, not whole blood base excess. Simple algorithms have been published for those whose instruments do not provide this calculation.[15]

Temperature Correction of Blood Gas Values

The values for pH and blood gases vary with respect to temperature. As a result, many laboratories report blood gas values corrected or adjusted to the temperature of the patient. The clinical application of the physiologic facts related to this may not be quite so clear as expected.[19,20] First, there is the issue of reference values for each analyte at each temperature. Although some clinicians may have practical experience and know what to expect at temperatures other than 37°C, there are no widely accepted reference values at different temperatures. Second, there is the issue of how to clinically use the adjusted values. For example, does one adjust the patient's temperature corrected pH and PCO_2 to 7.40 and 40 mm Hg, respectively? Finally, what algorithms does one choose to calculate temperature-adjusted values?

From the perspective of the blood gas laboratory, the first two issues are most reasonably addressed by accepting the recommendations of Ashwood and associates.[19] According to these recommendations, the acid–base values (pH and PCO_2) and calculated quantities such as actual bicarbonate (HCO_3^-) should be reported at the measuring temperature of 37°C. For PCO_2 and PO_2 used in assessing gas exchange and compared with expired gases, temperature-adjusted values should be reported. On a practical basis, this means that the PCO_2 and PO_2 should be reported at both temperatures, while other values should be reported only for 37°C. However, some clinicians may prefer both the adjusted and measured values for each quantity. The blood gas report itself should clearly distinguish between the measured and temperature adjusted values.

The last issue is easiest to address, because the algorithm used for temperature adjustment is that chosen by the manufacturer of the analyzer. NCCLS document C-12T2 provides a recommended algorithm for each temperature correction, and most of the major blood gas manufacturers use the NCCLS criteria.[15] Clinical algorithms for temperature adjustment have also been published.[21]

Quality Control: Initial and Routine Assessment of Analyzer Performance

Because the measurement of pH and blood gases assumes critical importance in the care of seriously ill patients, the quality of results is crucial.[22] Total quality assurance goes beyond the assessment of analyzer performance by considering the multiple factors that affect the quality of the final result (Fig. 8-17). Quality control is a major issue both within and outside the blood gas laboratory. Indeed, some states, as well as the federal government (eg, Clinical Laboratory Improvement Act [CLIA]), have laws and regulations governing general quality control and aspects specific to the blood gases. Whatever the detailed legal requirements, a properly designed laboratory protocol for quality control enables the respiratory care practitioner to determine proper functioning of the analyzer when first introduced into service as well as on a routine, daily, or more often basis. This ensures analytically correct results.

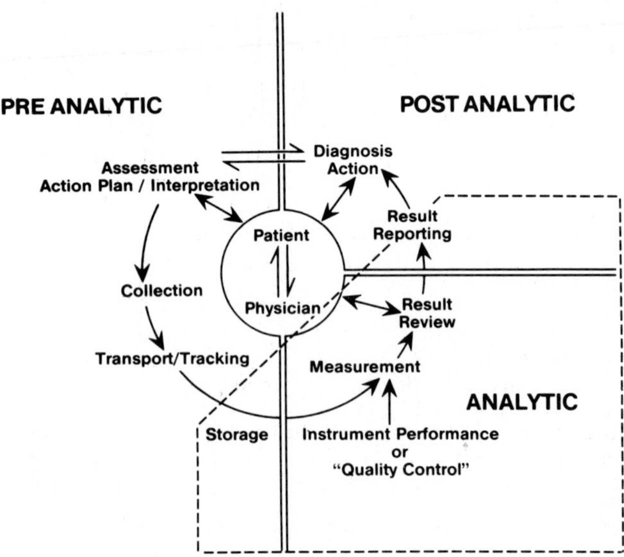

Figure 8-17. The cycle of quality assurance.

The requirements and complications of quality control protocols for a blood gas analyzer are substantially different from other analyses performed in the clinical laboratory environment. This is due not only to the fact that the patient sample is fresh whole blood (ie, living tissue), and thus has characteristics that are not stable, but also to the need to obtain clinical results quickly.

The optimum technique for establishing the extent of inaccuracy and imprecision of an individual blood gas analyzer is the use of whole blood tonometry[1] with samples of fresh anticoagulated whole blood, carefully equilibrated with a known standard mixture of oxygen, CO_2, and nitrogen at 37°C. Properly done, this technique enables determination of the performance of the analyzer when measuring blood at the partial pressures of the tonometry gas mixtures. Tonometry more closely resembles a primary standard in a true sample matrix, not merely an artificial control material. The technical and economic advantages of whole blood tonometry must be balanced by its hazard potential and the labor-intensive nature of the process.

An alternative to whole blood tonometry is the use of commercially available prepackaged materials, with each type having its own advantages and disadvantages. There are currently three major types of commercially available controls used for blood gas quality control, each of which is gas-equilibrated: aqueous buffer solutions, blood-based (hemoglobin-containing) materials, and perfluorocarbon/oil emulsions. The effectiveness of these materials varies and is dependent on the particular analyte and the physical and chemical characteristics of the material itself. The fundamental issue with respect to these controls is that their physical and chemical properties do not, in many respects, match those of whole blood. As a result, they may not detect certain problems or they may signal problems that do not exist. The former situation can result in clinical problems. The latter creates financial issues due to the cost of repeat controls, labor, and unnecessary service calls.

Duplicate analysis of the same blood sample can be a useful quality assurance tool but should not be used as the sole method of assessing instrument performance. Duplicate patient samples measured on two different analyzers are most useful in detecting individual sample errors owing to the improbability of similar errors occurring simultaneously on two different instruments. For example, certain types of pH system malfunction (reference circuit) can only be reliably detected using whole blood. In an emergency situation where analytical reliability and turnaround time are equally important, duplicate analysis may be a requirement. However, it must be recognized that duplicate analysis on the same instrument has marginal usefulness and may provide a false sense of security.

Good laboratory practice as well as some legal and regulatory requirements dictates that a blood gas system be evaluated both before initial use on patient samples as well as periodically during routine use. All of the above approaches can be used as a part of both the initial and routine evaluations of performance.

Initial, pre-use validation should incorporate either primary reference approaches such as whole blood tonometry or traceable reference materials of similar composition to the control materials to verify instrument calibration throughout the reportable range, as well as performance of replicate measurements on the patient's whole blood samples to assess imprecision.

Routine, ongoing evaluation of performance may be less stringent in its technical requirements, since it is primarily addressing the detection of changes from the initial state of either accuracy or precision. However, selection of a particular type of control for routine use must be based on evaluation of its technical and other merits in the context of a complete blood gas quality control program.[1,23] In that context, the prepackaged commercially available controls can serve a primary role in assessing blood gas analyzer performance, while recognizing that a performance issue can (with respect to the reliability of patient results) only be resolved satisfactorily by whole blood tonometry.[1] Whichever materials are chosen to assess performance, the results of the quality control program should be recorded in a manner that allows the operator to easily detect changes in performance of the instrument.[24,25] This is most commonly done by use of Levey-Jennings charts, which are plots of the quality control results over time (Figs. 8-18 and 8-19). Shifts and trends become obvious when results are displayed in this manner. A multiple level quality control program is recommended that uses at least two levels of control for pH, P_{CO_2}, and P_{O_2} on each work shift.

Internal quality control programs are better at estimating the precision of results than they are at estimating the accuracy of results. For this reason, licensed or certified laboratories use external proficiency testing programs. These external proficiency testing programs are available from several sources (such as the College of American Pathologists and the American Thoracic Society). The types of materials used in these programs are the same as those available for routine (internal) programs and thus suffer from the same technical shortfalls. As noted earlier, in those cases, only whole blood tonometry can resolve conflicts involving analyzer performance.

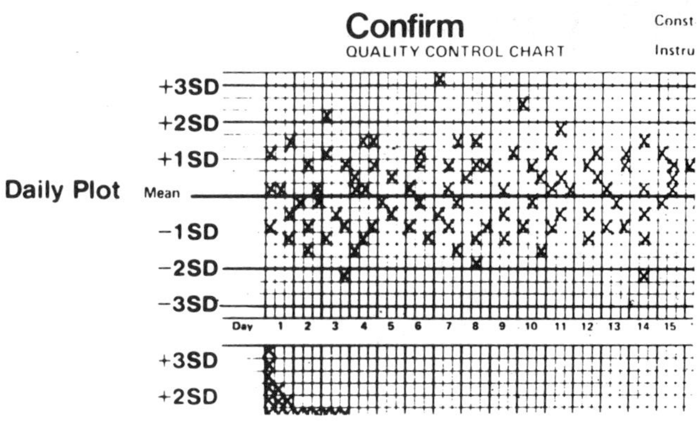

Figure 8-18. Levey-Jennings chart.

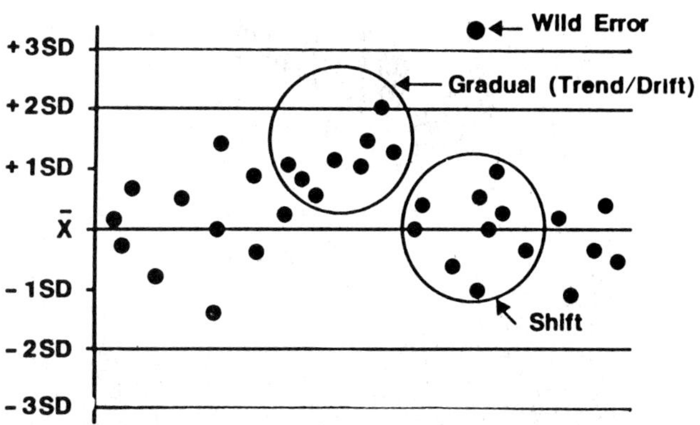

Figure 8-19. Three types of analytical errors identified on Levey-Jennings chart: wild error (outlier), gradual error (trend, drift), and a shift to a new (in this case, lower) mean.

The Modern pH/Blood Gas Analyzer

Although the electrodes or other sensors are essential for the measurement of the blood gases and other analytes such as total hemoglobin, it can be inferred from the earlier portions of this chapter that to effectively combine these sensors in one device requires the balancing of multiple interacting and even opposing factors. For example, reagents typically used for one measurement may interfere with another measurement, response time of one sensor may be substantially different from another, and the costs to produce one type of electrode are offset by the increased useful life.

In the selection, use, maintenance, and troubleshooting of a blood gas analyzer, the user must realize that application of the simple principles described earlier are not necessarily simple in practice. Sensor technology, electronics, chemistry, and fluidics are all combined to obtain the overall performance required. An understanding of the principles of each is only a beginning to the understanding of the whole system.

A complete blood gas analysis system can be conceptually divided into four major modules. However, in practice as well as in effects on overall performance, they are thoroughly integrated. The four major modules are the sensor module, the fluidic control module, the reagents module, and the electronics module.

Sensor modules are generally grouped together according to measuring technology. Therefore, electrodes are generally in close proximity in a temperature-controlled environment. This enables three requirements of analysis to be easily met: thermal stability of 37° ± 0.1°C, sample visibility (to facilitate observation of bubbles or clots in the sample), and the shortest possible sample path. Hemoglobin measurement technology, having different requirements, need not be in the same area as the electrodes. Indeed, during the measurement phase, the hemoglobin measuring chamber cannot be visible since the measurement is affected by ambient light.

The fluidics control module governs the flow of sample reagents, calibrants, and waste. Generally it is physically located central to the system to minimize complexity, tubing length, and so on. The reagents module is designed for easy access to reagents to facilitate replacement. Additional consideration may be given in the placement of this module to aid in observation of fluid levels or, if elevated, to lessen the load on the fluidics module by gravity assistance.

The electronics module, the "brains" of the system, is generally isolated from the wet portion of the system. However, the control panel and display must be easily accessible. Early blood gas electrodes were composed primarily of amplifier circuits and systems to allow manual adjustment of system output (such as calibration). Current models are microprocessor controlled. The electronics not only control operation of the complex components of the system (such as automatically initiating a wash cycle or calibrating the analyzer), but they also enable the operator to set nonstandard calibration frequencies, electrode drift limits, and a myriad of other things. The display and/or printer record instrument performance prompts the operator to take action and even provides a summary of quality control results over a specified time interval.

Although the basic principles of measurement technology used in blood gas analyzers have not changed substantially in many years, refinement of the technology, coupled with creative use of electronics and microprocessors, has made blood gas analyzers relatively simple to use. However, they remain one of the most sophisticated systems used by the respiratory care practitioner.

CO-Oximetry: The Measurement of Oxygen Content, Saturation, and Dyshemoglobins in Blood

Complete laboratory assessment of oxygenation requires measurement not only of gas exchange related variables such as P_{O_2}, but also of quantities that directly relate to oxygen transport and delivery, primarily oxygen content (total oxygen concentration) and oxygen saturation. Additionally, certain clinical situations such as carbon monoxide poisoning or assessment of pulmonary shunting require information that cannot be proved by blood gas and total hemoglobin determinations alone. Rather, the individual oxygen-carrying and non–oxygen-carrying hemoglobin components (oxyhemoglobin, carboxyhemoglobin, and methemoglobin) must be quantified. Although some of these components can be individually measured, the techniques frequently involve a series of time-consuming or technique-dependent steps. As a result,

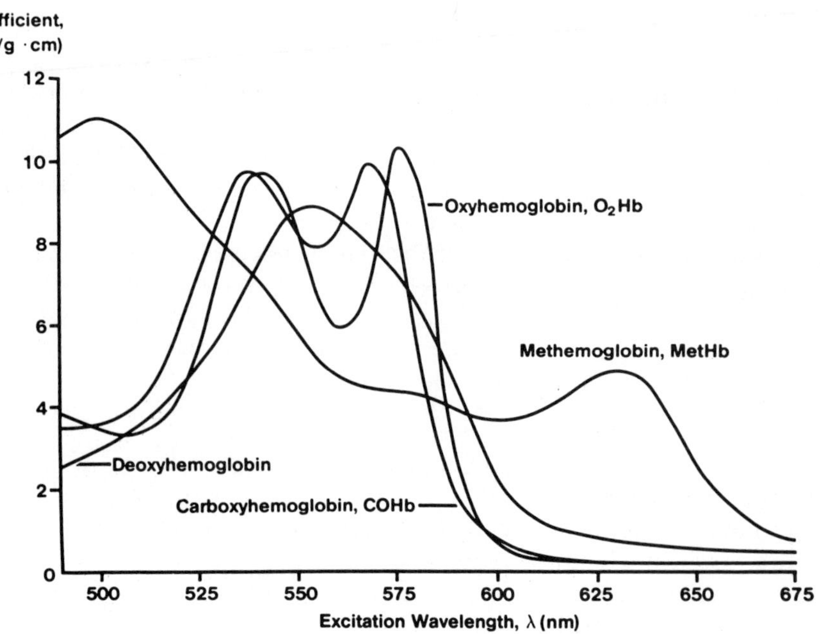

Figure 8-20. Absorption spectra for hemoglobin species.

methods and instruments that allow simultaneous determination of the major component of hemoglobin using the principles of multicomponent spectrophotometry have been developed and standardized working method guidelines have been prepared.[26]

Unlike the situation described earlier in the chapter, when the total hemoglobin combined with a reagent to produce a material with a single absorption spectrum, the measurement of these individual analytes (oxyhemoglobin, deoxyhemoglobin, carboxyhemoglobin, and methemoglobin) requires a spectrophotometer that can differentiate between the four analytes as well as a number of common interferents. This quantitative differentiation is difficult because of smaller and overlapping absorption spectra (Fig. 8-20), the lack of standard solutions for each component, and the complex nature of the whole blood specimen.

The basic procedure relates to the principles of Beer's law discussed earlier in this chapter and extends the principle to multiple absorbing components. It relies on the fact that the absorbance of light at any given wavelength is equal to the sum of the absorption constant/mol (molar extinction constant, absorptivity) of each component (ϵ) times the concentration of that component times the the light path length.

If there are two known components of unknown concentration, measurements of absorbance are made at two wavelengths where the specific absorptivity for each component is known. Because of basic algebraic requirements, two unknowns require two equations. This is expressed in Equation Box 8-6 and Figure 8-21. The math involved becomes very complex if the sample has four components, which is the real life clinical possibility (eg, COHb, O_2Hb, HHb, MetHb). Although possible to perform, the mathematics necessary has precluded the use of a general purpose spectrophotometer for this clinical measurement. The development of CO-oximeters (Fig. 8-22), which are high-quality spectrophotometers designed solely to measure hemoglobin components, enabled the simple routine measurement of the hemoglobin components and, in some cases, interfering compounds. This is based on identical principles to the generic approach described earlier. However, because of its single use design, factors such as light path length, wavelengths selected, and absorption constants are unchanging and thus the computations are designed into the electronics.

Equation Box 8-6: Derivation of Mathematical Relationships Used in CO-oximetry

$$A_1 = [\epsilon_{1d}C_d + \epsilon_{1o}C_o]$$
$$A_2 = [\epsilon_{2d}C_d + \epsilon_{2o}C_o]$$

where the subscripts 1 and 2 refer to the wavelength, o and d refer to oxyhemoglobin and deoxyhemoglobin, A is the absorbance, ϵ the absorption constant/mol, C is the concentration of the designated component, and ℓ is the light path length. To solve these equations, one must either apply standard algebraic substitution and rearrangement techniques or select wavelengths such as one that corresponds to a point where equimolar amounts of oxyhemoglobin and deoxyhemoglobin produce the same absorbance (isosbestic point) and the other corresponds to a maximum absorbance of one component (see Fig. 8-21). The latter aids in the routine measurement and computations, as may be seen below. When an isosbestic wavelength is not chosen, the relationship between C_o/C and A_1/A_2 is nonlinear and the mathematical solutions are more complex. If 2 is an isosbestic wavelength ($\epsilon o_2 = \epsilon d_2$) and if C_d is substituted by the difference ($C - C_o$) between the total concentration (C) of light-absorbing substances and C_o, then the following relationship is obtained:

$$\frac{C_o}{C} = \frac{\epsilon_{2d}A_1}{(\epsilon_{1o} - \epsilon_{1d})A_2} - \frac{\epsilon_{1d}}{\epsilon_{1o} - \epsilon_{1d}}$$

or

$$\frac{C_o}{C} = a \cdot \frac{A_1}{A_2} - b$$

The concentration of a single component expressed as the percentage of the total pigment concentration is thus a linear function of the ratio A_1/A_2. The constants a and b can be calculated from measurements of A_1/A_2 in solutions containing 100% component 1 or 100% component 2. Hence the percentages of the components are calculated as in the second equation above. The experimental determination of a and b produces a calibration curve that is a straight line.

Functional Requirements and Characteristics of CO-Oximeters

The minimum number of wavelengths for a clinically useful CO-oximeter is four, owing to the four components to be measured, which are oxyhemoglobin (O_2Hb), deoxyhemoglobin (HHb), carboxyhemoglobin (COHb), and methemoglobin (MetHb). Additional wavelengths may be used, and the specific wavelengths chosen are manufacturer specific. Different combinations are selected based on type of light source, the hemolysis system (ultrasonic or chemical), if any, the optimization of error detection, and the requirements for detection of interferents such as bilirubin or turbidity or dyes that might be in a blood or medication sample.

Extinction Coefficient, ε (dL/g · cm)
12
10
8
6
4
2
0
B
Oxyhemoglobin
A
Deoxyhemoglobin
500 525 550 575 600 625 650 675
Excitation Wavelength, λ (nm)

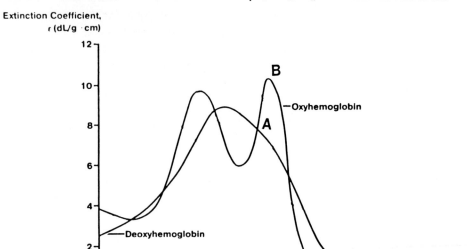

Figure 8-21. Wavelengths at which the isosbestic point occurs (A) and the maximal absorbance of oxyhemoglobin (B).

The operating system of a typical CO-oximeter is illustrated in Figure 8-23. Before the blood enters the sample chamber, it is thoroughly hemolyzed, which ruptures the cell membranes and releases the hemoglobin. A series of monochromatic light beams (either from a thallium hollow cathode lamp or a white light source combined with a stable diffraction grating) are passed through an interference filter, which eliminates extraneous wavelengths of light and passes the selected wavelengths through the sample. During the measurement sequence, the light is split. One portion is passed directly to a reference photodetector. The other is passed through the sample chamber to another photodetector. The photodetectors convert the intensity of the light into an electrical current, which is directly proportional to the intensity of the light and inversely proportional to the amount of light absorbed. Microprocessor-controlled sequencing passes the multiple wavelengths through the sample and measures the (in this example, seven) absorbances at the seven wavelengths. The results for oxyhemoglobin, deoxyhemoglobin, carboxyhemoglobin, and methemoglobin are then calculated from the result of a four by seven set of matrix equations (Equation Box 8-7).

Note that the matrix equations will change depending on the location and number of wavelengths of light passed through the sample, which are manufacturer specific. Potential interfering substances include dyes (eg, indocyanine green, methylene blue), bilirubin, turbidity (lipemia or cell stroma), and sulfhemoglobin. Fetal hemoglobin (HbF) may also produce spectral interference, resulting in an aberrantly high (maximum 6%–7%) carboxyhemoglobin measurement on some CO-oximeters.[27] Others, by judicious selection of wavelengths used, can eliminate HbF as an interferent.

The existence or extent of the interferences is dependent on instrument design, especially with respect to the wavelength chosen. Most interferents can be either identified or quantified by an appropriately designed system, although development cost becomes a factor when that is carried to an extreme (ie, developing an approach to quantify a rare or insignificant interferent).

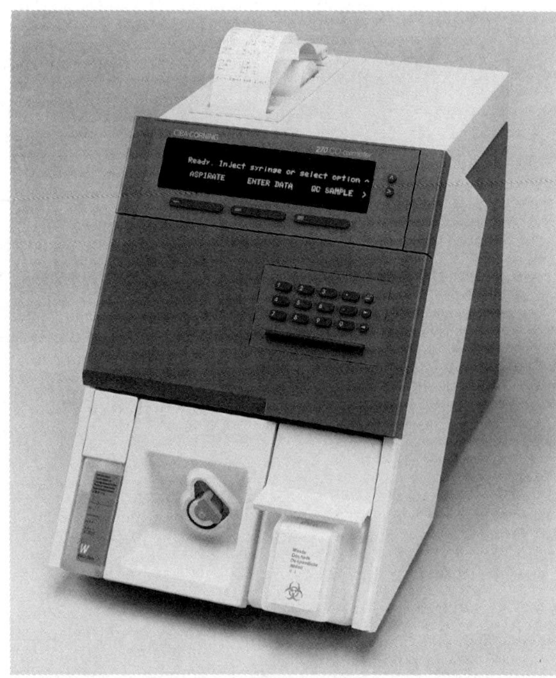

Figure 8-22. Ciba-Corning Model 2500 CO-oximeter. (Courtesy of Ciba-Corning Diagnostics Products, Medfield, MA)

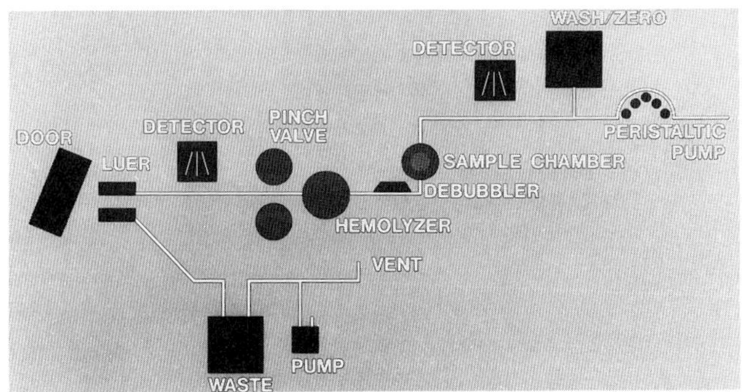

Figure 8-23. Operating system for CO-oximeter. (Courtesy of Ciba-Corning Diagnostics Products, Medfield, MA)

It is important to note that because of the complexity of the matrix equations, an unaccounted interference or any change in one or more of the wavelengths of light used (which may be due to filter delamination, clouded optics, or other conditions) can result in erroneous values for one or all of the components and not just for a component that has similar absorption to the interfering substance. Fortunately, these situations are rare, and in fact some are detected by the analyzer using pattern recognition of the light spectrum detected. Thus, signals from the analyzer are displayed, such as "If blood question data," when a dye-based control is measured or if a real interferent in the blood sample is present.

CO-oximeter Calibration

As with blood gas and pH electrodes, it is important that the CO-oximeter is correctly calibrated and that appropriate quality controls are used. Calibration solutions and quality control materials are usually supplied by the manufacturer of the CO-oximeter, although theoretically calibration solutions may be unnecessary if the right path length variability can be accounted for using other means. Calibration is necessary only for tHb since it is the only analyte whose concentration is measured. Individual fractions are dependent on the proportionate absorbances at the wavelengths tested and thus are determined by inherent absorbance ratios at the predetermined wavelengths. Only changes in absorbing species can cause the hemoglobin fractions to be incorrectly reported.

Equation Box 8-7: Matrix Equations Used by CO-oximeters to Determine O_2Hb, HHb, COHb, and MetHb

$$A_TO_2Hb = a_1A_1 + a_2A_2 + \ldots a_7A_7$$

$$A_THHb = b_1A_1 + b_2A_2 + \ldots b_7A_7$$

$$A_TCOHb = c_1A_1 + c_2A_2 + \ldots c_7A_7$$

$$A_TMetHb = d_1A_1 + d_2A_2 + \ldots d_7A_7$$

where a_1, a_7, b_1, b_7, etc, are coefficients that are analogues of the absorption constant, ϵ, used earlier. These are derived from established reference methods. A_TO_2Hb, A_THHb, etc, are the absorbances of the sample for the particular fraction.

Reported Values

Subsequent to measurement of the hemoglobin fractions, the individual components are reported either as decimal fractions (<1.0) or as a percentage (user choice on some analyzers). In practice, the terms *saturation* or *oxygen saturation* have been used to represent the distinctly different quantities discussed below. This ambiguous use is frequently unnoticed, owing to the similarity in numeric values obtained in some clinical conditions. Other clinical conditions can result in significantly different values, dependent on the mode of measurement and reporting. When reporting or discussing saturation, one must use unambiguous terminology or symbols as described below or both to pre-vent error in clinical management.

Fractional Oxyhemoglobin

Fractional oxyhemoglobin (FO_2Hb) is the amount of oxyhemoglobin in a solution expressed as a fraction of the amount of total hemoglobin as shown in Equation Box 8-8.

Oxygen Saturation of Hemoglobin

Oxygen saturation (of hemoglobin) ($SO_2\%$) is the amount of oxyhemoglobin expressed as a fraction of the total amount of hemoglobin able to bind oxygen (oxyhemoglobin plus deoxyhemoglobin). This is also termed *functional oxygen saturation* or *oxygen saturation of available or active hemoglobin* and is expressed as the percent fraction (Equation Box 8-9). Because available hemoglobin concentration equals the total hemoglobin minus the inactive hemoglobin components, oxygen saturation can also be expressed as shown in Equation Box 8-10. To avoid confusion,

Equation Box 8-8: Fractional Oxyhemoglobin

$$FO_2Hb = \frac{O_2Hb}{O_2Hb + HHb + COHb + MetHb + SulfHb + \ldots}$$

$$= \frac{O_2Hb}{tHb}$$

**Equation Box 8-9:
Functional Oxygen Saturation**

$$SO_2\% = \frac{O_2Hb}{O_2Hb + HHb} \cdot 100\%$$

**Equation Box 8-10:
Oxygen Saturation: Alternate Means to Calculate Functional Saturation**

$$SO_2\% = \frac{O_2Hb}{tHb - (COHb + MetHb + SulfHb + ...)}$$

$$= \frac{O_2Hb}{tHb - Hb}$$

both FO_2Hb and SO_2 should be clearly differentiated when reported.

Oxygen Content

This quantity is formally designated concentration of total oxygen since it is composed of oxygen in various physicochemical states (ie, oxygen dissolved in plasma, oxygen dissolved in intracellular fluid, and oxygen bound to hemoglobin). The more common term, *oxygen content,* which is used here, can legitimately be calculated and reported by the CO-oximeter, from the fractional oxyhemoglobin and tHb as measured, since the major components are measured, not assumed, as with the computation from a blood gas analyzer alone (see Equation Box 8-11).

It is important to understand that an oxygen content calculated in this manner (ie, based on well-defined constants and measured values for O_2Hb, tHb, and PO_2) is a clinically useful value. This is in contrast to an oxygen content calculated from values for saturation derived from a blood gas analyzer alone, as discussed earlier in this chapter.

**Equation Box 8-11:
Oxygen Content**

$$CtO_2 = [FO_2Hb) \cdot (CtHb) \cdot (1.39)] + [(0.0031) \cdot (PO_2)]$$

The value 1.39 is a factor (Hufner's factor) that represents the milliliters of oxygen bound per gram of hemoglobin and is based on the exact chemical structure of adult hemoglobin. In practice, the value may be lower (approximately 1.36), owing to the presence of nonspecific binding of hemoglobin. In the past, a value of 1.34 has also been used. To address this issue, some manufacturers allow the user to select a specific value for this constant. The value 0.00314 represents a combination of the Bunsen solubility coefficient and a unit conversion factor (to give units of mL O_2/100 mL blood/mm Hg PO_2).

Fractional COHb, MetHB, SulfHb

The amount of each entity expressed as a substance fraction of the total hemoglobin is termed the *fractional (prefix) hemoglobin.* The quantitative definition is exactly analogous to that in Equation Box 8-9, except for substitution of the appropriate entity's symbol in the numerator. The value reported may be expressed either as a decimal fraction (<1.0) or, if multiplied by 100, as a percentage.

Intra-arterial Blood Gases and pH

There is much interest in the critical care community for a system to continuously monitor arterial blood gases and pH,[28,29] and several manufacturers now have FDA approval for such systems.[30-33] Current generation in vivo blood gas monitors use optical biosensors called fluorescent optodes. The optode consists of a miniaturized probe containing a fluorescent dye (Fig. 8-24). The

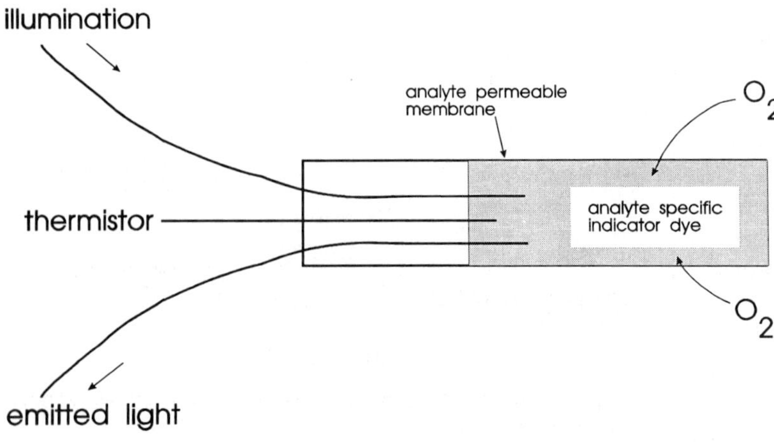

Figure 8-24. A schematic illustration of an optode to measure PO_2. The optode to measure PO_2 is usually bundled with optodes to measure PCO_2 and pH. The entire sensor is miniaturized so that it can fit through an arterial catheter.

dye is capable of absorbing light of a specific wavelength and rapidly re-emitting the light at a longer wavelength (ie, lower energy). Some molecules (eg, O_2, CO_2, H^+) are capable of accepting energy from the fluorescent dye in a process called quenching. This decreases the amount of emitted energy relative to the pH, P_{CO_2}, and P_{O_2}. Photosensors are used to quantify the amount of quenching, and a microprocessor is used to translate the signal into a display of blood gases and pH. The sensor is calibrated before use and can be used for several days before it is replaced.

Minimal requirements for a blood gas monitor in conjunction with an arterial catheter have been suggested by Shapiro (Box 8-1).[28] Several approaches can be used for blood gas monitoring with an arterial catheter. The first uses a probe that passes through an arterial catheter and resides directly within the artery. The second approach connects the optode system to the proximal arterial line but does not pass it through the catheter. With this method, when blood gas and pH values are desired, blood is drawn into a chamber containing the optodes; this is referred to as an "on-demand" system. After analysis, the blood is flushed back into the artery. Thus, frequent, but *not* continuous, blood gas measurements are possible without blood loss.

Box 8-1
Minimal Requirements for Blood Gas Systems Used in Conjunction With Arterial Catheters

- Must accurately measure P_{O_2}, P_{CO_2}, pH, and temperature with a rapid response time
- Must not have any interference from substances normally found in arterial blood
- Must operate with a 20-gauge arterial catheter without affecting continuous blood pressure measurement, obtaining blood samples, or any other functions of the arterial catheter system
- Must be biocompatible and nonthrombogenic
- Must be simple to operate and maintain
- Must be able to withstand the rigors of and abuse of everyday practice within the intensive care unit
- Must be accurate and precise for at least 72 hours
- Must not be adversely affected by reductions in local blood flow or perfusion
- Must not be adversely affected by changes in hemodynamics
- Must be cost effective

Mixed Venous Oxygen Saturation Monitoring

The ability to measure mixed venous oxygen saturation continuously through oximetric methodology became commercially available in the early 1980s.[34] This system uses a microprocessor, an optical module with light sources and photodetectors, and a flow-directed pulmonary artery catheter.[35] By using fiberoptics, wavelengths of light between 650 and 1000 nm are pulsed into the pulmonary artery (Fig. 8-25). The light reflected off red blood cells in the pulmonary artery is returned to the optical module through another fiberoptic bundle. S_{O_2} is the ratio of transmitted and reflected light. Before insertion, the system is calibrated using an in vitro calibration standard, and calibration can be updated periodically by in vivo calibration using a CO-oximetry determined S_{O_2}. Factors that affect the measurement of S_{O_2} using this method include temperature, pH, blood flow velocity, hematocrit, and occlusion of the catheter tip (eg, clot or vessel wall).[34–37] Although lipid emulsion infusions affect CO-oximetry, in vivo venous oximetry appears to be unaffected.[38]

Three systems are commercially available to measure S_{O_2} by oximetry. Each of these uses different methods to deal with interference and drift.[39]

- Edwards Sat-One Catheter: This system uses two reference wavelengths and one detecting fiberoptic filament and allows the user to periodically update the hematocrit to control the effects of hematocrit on S_{O_2} measurements.
- Oximetrix Opticath Catheter: This system uses three reference wavelengths and one detecting filament to improve the accuracy of the system in the presence of physiologic changes such as hematocrit.
- Spectramed Spectracath Catheter: This system uses two reference wavelengths and two detecting filaments. The second detecting filament supposedly

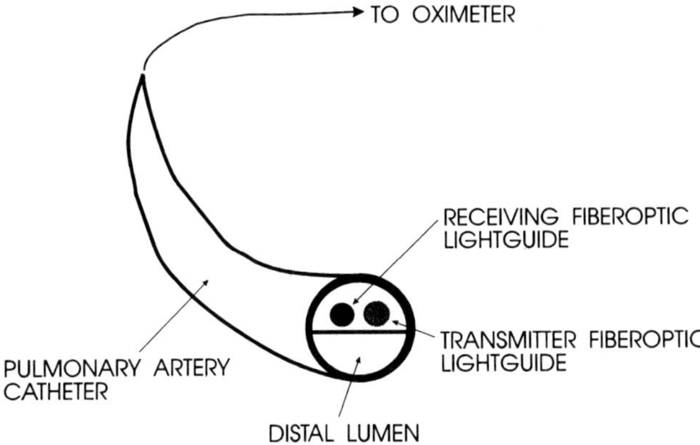

Figure 8-25. Schematic illustration of a mixed venous oximetry catheter.

improves the accuracy of the system when hematocrit changes.

Most studies have found three-wavelength systems to correlate better with CO-oximeter S_{O_2} than two-wavelength systems. It has also been generally found that drift is less with three-wavelength systems. However, if meticulous attention is paid to care of the catheter system (eg, in vivo calibrations, updating the hematocrit setting), either system is probably acceptable.

Gastric Tonometry

Gastric tonometry is a minimally invasive method to assess tissue oxygenation in critically ill patients.[40,41] Perfusion of the gut is affected early in the course of systemic hypoxia. Theoretically, tissue hypoxia should result in a decrease in gastric intramucosal pH (pH_i). Normal pH_i is 7.38 ± 0.03.

The gastric tonometer consists of a nasogastric tube with a distal CO_2-permeable balloon (Fig. 8-26). The balloon is filled with 2.5 to 3 mL of physiologic saline solution. An equilibration time of 1 to 2 hours is allowed for CO_2 in the gastric lumen to equilibrate with the saline inside the balloon. After discarding 1 to 1.5 mL of aspirate from the gastric tube (dead volume), the remaining 1 to 1.5 mL is analyzed for P_{CO_2} using a blood gas analyzer. A simultaneous arterial blood sample is analyzed to determine HCO_3^-. Gastric pH_i is then calculated from the Henderson-Hasselbach equation, using the PCO_2 of the saline from the gastric balloon and the HCO_3^- of arterial blood.

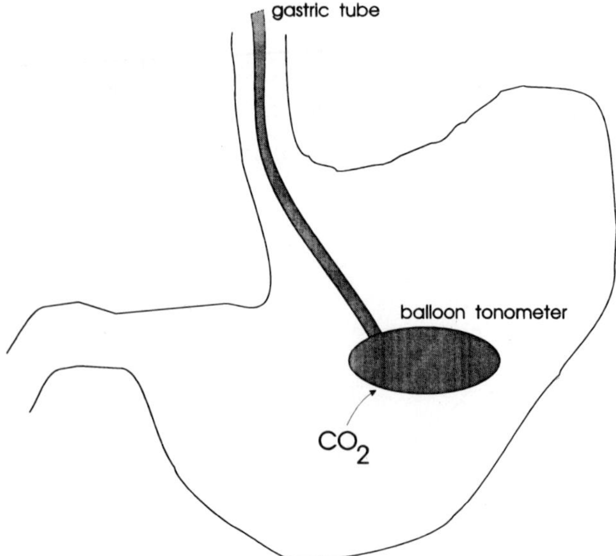

Figure 8-26. Schematic illustration of a gastric tonometer.

AARC Clinical Practice Guideline

Sampling for Arterial Blood Gas Analysis: Indications, Contraindications, Hazards and Complications

Blood is drawn from a peripheral artery, or from an indwelling arterial cannula or catheter for multiple samples.

- Indications:
  - the need to evaluate the adequacy of a patient's ventilatory, acid–base, and/or oxygenation status, and the oxygen-carrying capacity and intrapulmonary shunt.
  - the need to quantitate the response to therapeutic intervention and/or diagnostic evaluation
  - the need to monitor severity and progression of documented disease processes
- Contraindications:
  - negative results of a modified Allen test are indicative of inadequate blood supply to the hand and suggest the need to select another extremity as the site of puncture
  - arterial puncture should not be performed through a lesion or distal to a surgical shunt. If there is evidence of infection or peripheral vascular disease involving the selected limb, an alternate site should be selected
  - agreement is lacking regarding the puncture sites associated with a lesser likelihood of complications. However, because of the need for monitoring the femoral puncture site for an extended period, femoral punctures should not be performed outside the hospital
  - a coagulopathy or medium-to-high-dose anticoagulation therapy may be a relative contraindication for arterial puncture
- Hazards/Complications:
  - hematoma
  - arteriospasm
  - air or clotted-blood emboli
  - anaphylaxis from local anesthetic
  - introduction of contagion at sampling site and consequent infection in patient; introduction of contagion to sample by inadvertent needle stick
  - hemorrhage
  - trauma to the vessel
  - arterial occlusion
  - vasovagal response
  - pain

(Adapted from AARC Clinical Practice Guideline, published in August, 1992, issue of Respiratory Care; see original publication for complete text)

References

1. Eichhorn JH, Cormier AD, Moran RF. Blood Gas Pre-analytical Considerations: Specimen Collection, Calibration and Controls. National Committee for Clinical Laboratory Standards (NCCLS) C-27T, 1988.
2. Don H, ed. Decision Making in Critical Care. St. Louis: CV Mosby, 1985.

3. Siggaard-Andersen O. The Acid–Base Status of Blood, 4th ed. Copenhagen: Munksgaard, 1976.
4. Pulmonary terms and symbols: A report of the absorbancies joint committee on pulmonary nomenclature. Chest 1975;67:583–593.
5. Sorensen SPL. Enzymestudien: II. Uber die Messung und die Bedeutung der wasserstuffionen Konzentration bei enzymatischen Prozessen. Biochem Z 1909;12:131–304.
6. Covington AK, ed. Ion Selective Electrode Methodology, vols I and II. Boca Raton, FL: CRC Press, 1979.
7. Severinghaus JW, Bradley AF. Electrodes for blood P_{O_2} and P_{CO_2} determinations. J Appl Physiol 1958;13:515–520.
8. Bradley AF, Moran RF. Blood gas systems: Major determinants of performance. Lab Med 1981;12:353–358.
9. Stow RW, Baer RF, Randall BF. Rapid measurement of the tension of carbon dioxide in blood. Arch Phys Med Rehabil 1957;38:646–650.
10. Clark LC Jr. Monitor and control of blood and tissue oxygen tensions. Trans Am Soc Artif Intern Organs 1956;2:41–56.
11. Huseby RM, Bacus J, Bull BS, et al: Reference Procedure for the Quantitative Determination of Hemoglobin in Blood. National Committee for Clinical Laboratory Standards (NCCLS) H15-A, 1984.
12. Rice EW. Diagnosing anemia: Blood hemoglobin versus microhematocrit. Am Clin Lab 1988;7(6A):14.
13. Henry JB, ed. Clinical Diagnosis and Management by Laboratory Methods, 17th ed. Philadelphia: WB Saunders, 1984.
14. Kerner JA, Wurzel H, Okada RH. New electronic method for measuring hematocrit: Clinical evaluation. J Lab Clin Med 1961;57:635–641.
15. Eichhorn JH, Barrett RW, Christiansen TF, et al. Standard for Definitions of Quantities and Conventions Related to Blood Gas Analysis. National Committee for Clinical Laboratory Standards (NCCLS) C-12T2, 1989.
16. Hess D, Elser RC, Agarwal N. The effect of measured versus calculated hemoglobin oxygen saturation, carboxyhemoglobin and methemoglobin on the pulmonary shunt calculation. Respir Care 1984;29:1001–1005.
17. Rosan RC, Enlander D, Ellis J. Unpredictable error in calculated bicarbonate homeostasis during pediatric intensive care: The delusion of fixed pK′. Clin Chem 1983;29:69–73.
18. Ream AK, Reitz BA, Silverberg G. Temperature correction of P_{CO_2} and pH in estimating acid–base status: An example of the emperor's new clothes? Anesthesiology 1982;56:41–44.
19. Ashwood ER, Kost G, Kenny M. Temperature correction of blood gas and pH measurements. Clin Chem 1985;29:1877–1885.
20. Delaney KA, Howland MA, Vassallo S, Goldfrank LR. Assessment of acid–base disturbances in hypothermia and their physiologic consequences. Ann Emerg Med 1989;18:72–82.
21. Andritsch RF, Muravchick S, Gold MI. Temperature correction of arterial blood-gas parameters: A comparative methodology. Anesthesiology 1981;55:311–316.
22. Elser RC. Quality control of blood gas analysis: A review. Respir Care 1986;31:807–816.
23. Moran RF, Grenier RE. A simple method of setting reliable target values and limits for blood gas quality control materials. Can J Med Tech 1988;50:95–98.
24. Moran RF, Van Kessell AL. Blood gas quality assurance. NSCPT Analyzer 1981;11:18–26.
25. Moran RF. Assessment of quality control of blood gas/pH analyzer performance. Respir Care 1981;26:538–46.
26. Moran RF, Clausen JL, Feil MC, Ehrmeyer S, Van Kessell Al, Eichhorn JH. The Measurement of Oxygen Content and Saturation in Blood. National Committee for Clinical Laboratory Standards (NCCLS), C-25P, 1984.
27. Zwart A, Buursma A, Oeseburg B, Aijlstra WG. Determination of hemoglobin derivatives with the IL 282 CO-oximeter as compared with a manual spectrophotometric five-wavelength method. Clin Chem 1981;27:1903–1907.
28. Shapiro BA. In-vivo monitoring of arterial blood gases and pH. Respir Care 1992;37:165–169.
29. Hess D, Kacmarek RM. Techniques and devices for monitoring oxygenation. Respir Care 1993;38:646–671.
30. Shapiro BA, Mahutte CK, Cane RD, Gilmour IJ. Clinical performance of a blood gas monitor: A prospective, multicenter trial. Crit Care Med 1993;21:487–492.
31. Zimmerman JL, Dellinger RP. Initial evaluation of a new intraarterial blood gas system in humans. Crit Care Med 1993;21: 495–500.
32. Shapiro BA. Blood gas monitors: Justifiable enthusiasm with a note of caution. Am Rev Respir Dis 1994;149:850–851.
33. Mahutte CK, Holody M, Maxwell TP, Chen PA, Sasse SA. Development of a patient-dedicated, on-demand, blood gas monitor. Am Rev Respir Dis 1994;149:852–859.
34. Schweiss JF. Mixed venous hemoglobin saturation: Theory and application. Int Anesthesiol Clin 1987;25(3):113–136.
35. Paulus DA. Invasive monitoring of respiratory gas exchange: Continuous measurement of mixed venous oxygen saturation. Respir Care 1987;32:535–543.
36. Rahey PJ, Harris K, Vanderwarf C. Clinical experience with continuous monitoring of mixed venous oxygen saturation in respiratory failure. Chest 1984;86:748–752.
37. Baraka A, Baroody M, Haroun S, et al. Continuous venous oximetry during cardiopulmonary bypass: Influence of temperature changes, perfusion flow, and hematocrit levels. J Cardiothorac Anesth 1990;4:35–38.
38. Howdieshell TR, Sussman A, Dipiro J, McCarten M, Mansberger A. Reliability of in vivo mixed venous oximetry during experimental hypertriglyceridemia. Crit Care Med 1992;20: 999–1004.
39. Rouby JJ, Poete R, Bodin L, Bourgeois J, Arthaud M, Viars P. Three mixed venous saturation catheters in patients with circulatory shock and respiratory failure. Chest 1990;98:954–958.
40. Gutierrez G, Bismar H, Danzker DR, Silva N. Comparison of gastric intramucosal pH with measures of oxygen transport and consumption in critically ill patients. Crit Care Med 1992;20: 451–457.
41. Gutierrez G, Palizas F, Doglio G, et al. Gastric intramucosal pH as a therapeutic index of tissue oxygenation in critically ill patients. Lancet 1992;339:195–199.

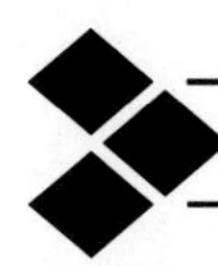

9

Noninvasive Respiratory Monitoring Equipment

Dean R. Hess
Richard D. Branson

OBJECTIVES

1. Compare the following principles of oxygen analysis: polarographic, galvanic cell, paramagnetic, wheatstone bridge, and the zirconium analyzer.
2. Describe the use of transcutaneous monitors and conjunctival oxygen monitors.
3. Describe the principle of operation of a pulse oximeter, and list factors that affect the accuracy of pulse oximetry.
4. Distinguish between capnometry and capnography and compare mainstream and sidestream capnometers.
5. List advantages and disadvantages of transcutaneous monitors, conjunctival monitors, pulse oximeters, and capnometers.
6. Describe the principle of operation of mass spectroscopy.
7. Compare open-circuit and closed-circuit indirect calorimeters.
8. List advantages and disadvantages of open-circuit and closed-circuit calorimeters.
9. Describe the use of mechanics and waveforms during mechanical ventilation.

KEY TERMS

Braschi valve	infrared absorption spectroscopy	pulse oximeter
calorimetry	mainstream monitor	sidestream monitor
capnography	mass spectroscopy	silica gel crystals
capnometry	noninvasive respiratory monitoring	spectrophotometry
closed-circuit calorimetry	open-circuit calorimetry	thermoconductivity
collision broadening effect	oxygen analyzer	transcutaneous monitor
conjunctival oxygen monitor	paramagnetic	variable orifice pneumotachometer
direct calorimetry	Pauling principle	Weir method
esophageal pressure	plethysmography	wheatstone bridge
galvanic cell	polarographic	zirconium analyzer
indirect calorimetry		

Introduction

Respiratory care practitioners are often responsible for noninvasive respiratory monitoring. This monitoring is frequently used with critically ill patients and provides important information in the care of these patients. To derive valid information, respiratory care practitioners must understand the correct operation of this equipment. In this chapter we describe oxygen analyzers, transcutaneous monitors, conjunctival monitors, pulse oximetry, capnography and capnometry, mass spectroscopy, raman spectroscopy, calorimetry, and waveforms during mechanical ventilation.

Oxygen Analysis

Respiratory care practitioners commonly use an oxygen analyzer to measure the concentrations of oxygen administered to patients. The four principal types of oxygen analyzers are the polarographic, galvanic cell, paramagnetic, and wheatstone bridge.[1,2] Of these, the galvanic cell and the polarographic electrode are most commonly used. Characteristics of the ideal oxygen analyzer are listed in Box 9-1. For clinical use, it should be recognized that oxygen analyzers are constructed as much for ruggedness as they are for accuracy. The accuracy of the oxygen analyzers that are commonly used clinically is ± 2%.

Box 9-1
Properties of the "Ideal" Oxygen Analyzer

- Accurate at a variety of conditions of temperature, pressure, humidity, and altitude
- Quick response
- Rugged
- Inexpensive
- Easy to calibrate
- Alarms
- Minimal easy-to-perform maintenance

Polarographic Analyzers

Polarographic analyzers are electrochemical and use a Clark electrode to measure oxygen. The Clark electrode is adapted for use in a gas environment. Although it actually measures PO_2, it usually displays $\%O_2$. The $\%O_2$ is calculated from the PO_2 and the barometric pressure

$$\%O_2 = \frac{PO_2}{\text{barometric pressure}} \cdot 100\%$$

Polarographic analyzers are accurate at any altitude, provided that the instrument is calibrated at that altitude. Calibration is usually accomplished by exposing the electrode to room air (21% oxygen) or 100% oxygen. Because this analyzer actually measures PO_2, it is affected by changes in pressure, as might occur in a ventilator circuit (particularly if positive end-expiratory pressure [PEEP] is added).

Because these analyzers use a Clark electrode, an external power source is required. The power is usually provided by a battery, which makes these analyzers portable. The electrode has a finite life. Inability to calibrate each analyzer usually means that the electrolyte in the electrode needs to be changed. Many of these electrodes are disposable, so that the entire electrode is replaced. Older polarographic analyzers require replacement of the electrolyte solution within the electrode.

Polarographic analyzers can be used for continuous measurement of gas samples. Many of these analyzers are designed for continuous use and have alarms for high and low oxygen concentrations. Polarographic analyzers are affected by temperature and must be temperature compensated for their normal operating range of temperatures. They may also be affected by humidity. Condensation of water on the surface of the membrane may decrease diffusion of oxygen into the electrode, with a resultant inaccurately low $\%O_2$ displayed. Because of the effects of water vapor pressure on oxygen concentration and PO_2, the accuracy of these analyzers will be affected if they are calibrated with a dry gas and then used with a humidified gas sample.

There are many commercially available polarographic oxygen analyzers. These include the IL, IMI, Ohio, Critikon, and Hudson-Ventronics (Fig. 9-1).

Galvanic Cell Analyzers

The galvanic cell analyzers, like the polarographic analyzers, use an electrochemical principle. Oxygen is reduced in the electrode, which produces a current flow proportional to the PO_2. Although the electrode responds to changes in PO_2, the analyzer usually displays $\%O_2$. The analyzer is calibrated with either room air (21% oxygen) or 100% oxygen. Because it can be calibrated, it can be used at any altitude. It is affected by pressure and humidity in a manner similar to that of polarographic analyzers. Like polarographic analyzers, galvanic cell analyzers can be used with continuous sampling and often include alarms.

Unlike polarographic analyzers, galvanic cell analyzers do not require an external power source. Although the response time of the galvanic cell tends to be slower than that of the polarographic analyzer, the life of the galvanic cell tends to be longer than that of the polarographic electrode. The life expectancy of either cell depends on the oxygen concentrations to which the cell is exposed (higher oxygen concentrations reduce the life of the cell).

Galvanic cell analyzers are commonly used in respiratory care. Commercially available examples include the BioMarine, Hudson, MiniOx, Teledyne, Ohmeda, and Harlake (Fig. 9-2).

Paramagnetic Oxygen Analyzers

These analyzers use the Pauling principle, which is based on the fact that oxygen is a paramagnetic gas.

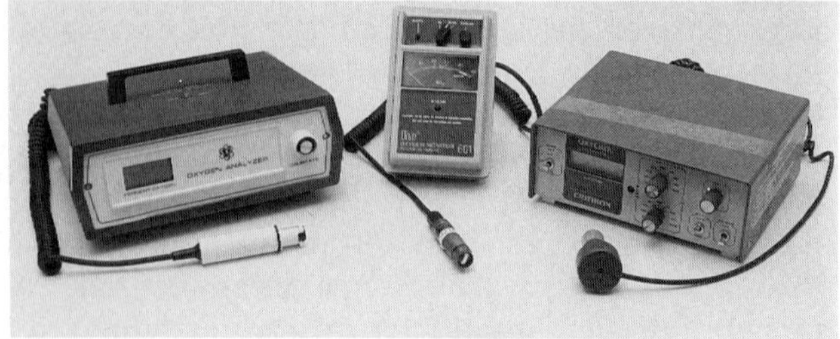

Figure 9-1. Polarographic oxygen analyzers.

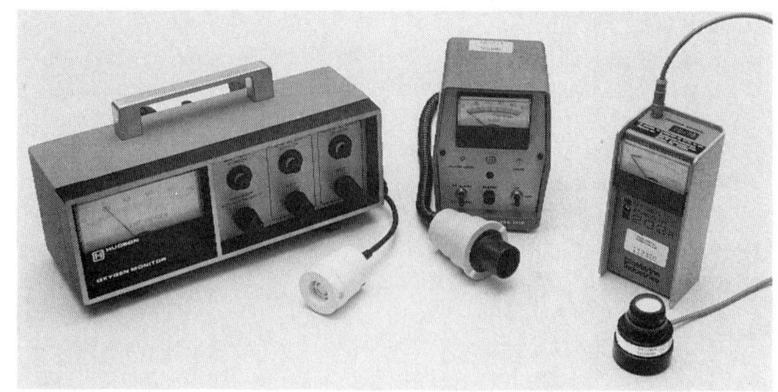

Figure 9-2. Galvanic cell oxygen analyzers.

Other gases such as nitrogen and carbon dioxide are diamagnetic. Unlike a diamagnetic gas, oxygen is attracted to a magnetic field.

The paramagnetic oxygen analyzer is illustrated in Figure 9-3. Two hollow glass spheres are attached together in the shape of a dumbbell and suspended by a quartz fiber between two static magnets. The glass spheres contain nitrogen (a diamagnetic gas). The dumbbell and the magnetic field are enclosed within an airtight sample chamber. When oxygen is introduced into the sample chamber, it is attracted to the magnetic field, displacing the nitrogen and causing the dumbbell to rotate. A mirror is attached to the quartz fiber, which directs a beam of light onto a translucent scale. The light beam thus translates the rotation of the dumbbell into a display of oxygen concentration. Although the paramagnetic principle does not require an electric power source per se, battery power is needed to produce the beam of light.

When 100% oxygen is introduced to the sample chamber, the dumbbell is displaced so that the light beam moves to 100% (760 mm Hg) on the translucent scale. When the sample chamber is flushed with room air, the torque on the quartz fiber causes the dumbbell to rotate so that the light beam falls at 21% (159 mm Hg) on the translucent scale. The paramagnetic oxygen analyzer is calibrated at sea level conditions and cannot be user-calibrated. As a result, the $\%O_2$ scale is inaccurately low at barometric pressures less than 760 mm Hg. However, the mm Hg scale is accurate at any ambient pressure. Thus, the oxygen concentration can be correctly calculated by dividing the readout in millimeters of mercury by the ambient barometric pressure. Conversion charts for use at high altitude are also available from the manufacturer.

The displacement of the dumbbell is determined by the number of oxygen molecules in the sample. Because the number of oxygen molecules depends on the PO_2 of the sample, the paramagnetic analyzer responds directly to PO_2, not $\%O_2$. Because the analyzer is calibrated with dry gas, the sample must be dried before it enters the sample chamber. This is accomplished by

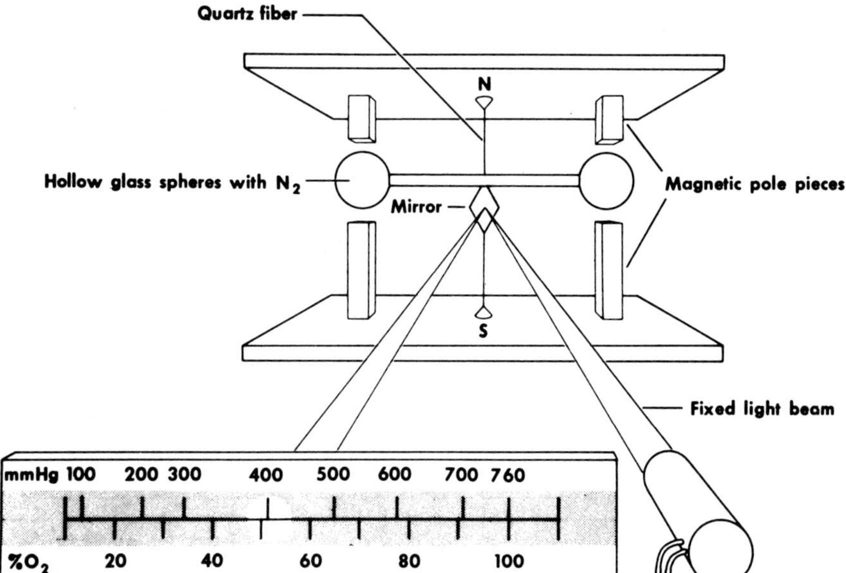

Figure 9-3. Paramagnetic oxygen analyzer. (From Bagent RA. Oxygen analyzers. Respir Care 1976;21:410–416)

drawing the sample through a drying chamber containing dry silica gel crystals. The silica gel contains anhydrous cobaltous chloride. Because cobaltous chloride is blue when it is dry and pink when it is saturated with water, this color change (blue to pink) indicates that the silica gel crystals must be replaced.

The paramagnetic analyzer will not allow a continuous flow of oxygen through the sample chamber. Thus, this method of oxygen analysis can be used only with static samples and cannot be used for continuous gas sampling. These analyzers do not consume oxygen, and they are safe for use with flammable gases. An analyzer using this principle is the Beckman Model D2 (Fig. 9-4).

Wheatstone Bridge Analyzers

A wheatstone bridge is an electrical circuit (Fig. 9-5) consisting of four resistors. The circuit is constructed so that two of the resistors are parallel to the other two. A galvanometer compares the resistances to electrical flow through the two sides of the wheatstone bridge. One of the resistors, Rv, is variable and used to calibrate (or balance) the wheatstone bridge. Another resistor, Rx, varies with the measurement being made (in this case, oxygen concentration). In the wheatstone bridge oxygen analyzers, the resistors are platinum.

The wheatstone bridge oxygen analyzers use the principle of thermoconductivity, which states that the resistance to electrical flow varies with temperature. The higher the temperature of a resistor, the greater is its resistance to electrical flow. Nitrogen and oxygen differ in their abilities to cool an electrical resistor. Oxygen, being of higher molecular weight, cools the wire more than nitrogen. The wheatstone bridge prin-

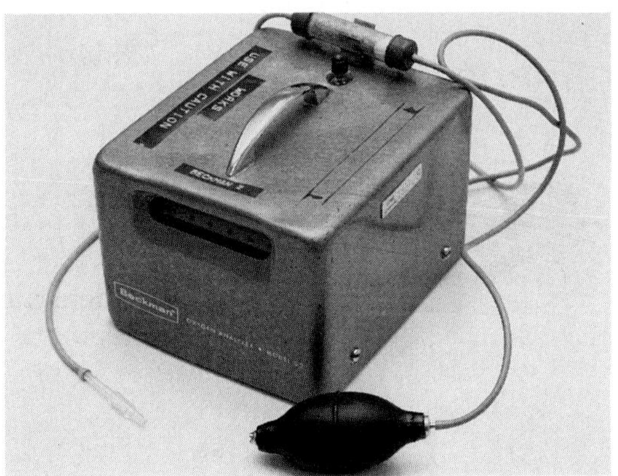

Figure 9-4. Beckman Model D2 oxygen analyzer.

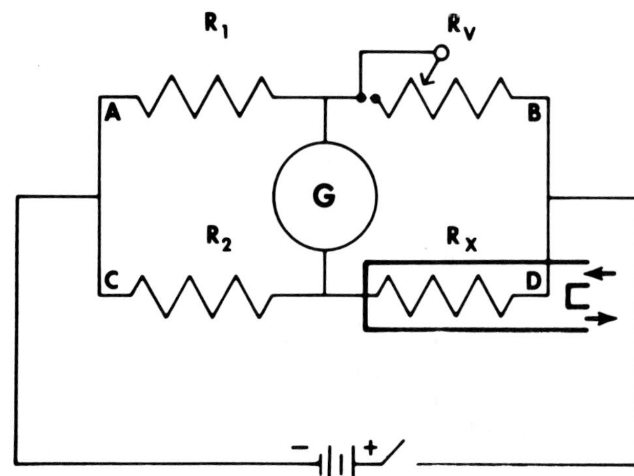

Figure 9-5. Wheatstone bridge used in an oxygen analyzer. (From Bagent RA. Oxygen analyzers. Respir Care 1976; 21:410–416)

ciple of oxygen analysis depends on the ability of oxygen to cool the resistor Rx.

When room air is drawn into a sample chamber around Rx, the electrical resistance at Rv is adjusted so that the resistance through both sides of the wheatstone bridge is equal, and the galvanometer displays 21% oxygen. In this manner, the oxygen analyzer is calibrated. If higher concentrations of oxygen are placed into the sample chamber (Rx), the wheatstone bridge will be unbalanced relative to the oxygen concentration, with a resultant change in $\%O_2$ displayed on the galvanometer.

The wheatstone bridge actually compares the oxygen concentration in an unknown sample with the oxygen concentration of room air. Thus, it compares a known O_2/N_2 mixture (room air) to an unknown O_2/N_2 mixture. Because thermoconductivity is a physical property of all gases, mixtures containing gases other than nitrogen and oxygen will cause these analyzers to be inaccurate. The principle of thermoconductivity can be adapted for use in the measurement of gases other than oxygen. For example, the catharometer found in pulmonary function laboratories uses thermoconductivity to measure helium concentrations.

Because these oxygen analyzers use hot wires, they cannot be used with flammable gases. These analyzers can be used only for static gas samples, because a continuous flow through the sample chamber would cool Rx and result in inaccuracies. Because they compare the oxygen concentration of an unknown sample to the oxygen concentration of air, they can be used at any altitude. For the same reason, they respond to changes in $\%O_2$ rather than PO_2 per se.

Two examples of wheatstone bridge oxygen analyzers are the Mira (Fig. 9-6) and the OEM. The Mira requires that the gas sample is completely saturated with water vapor and thus uses pink silica gel crystals. The OEM requires the gas sample to be dry, and thus uses blue silica gel crystals.

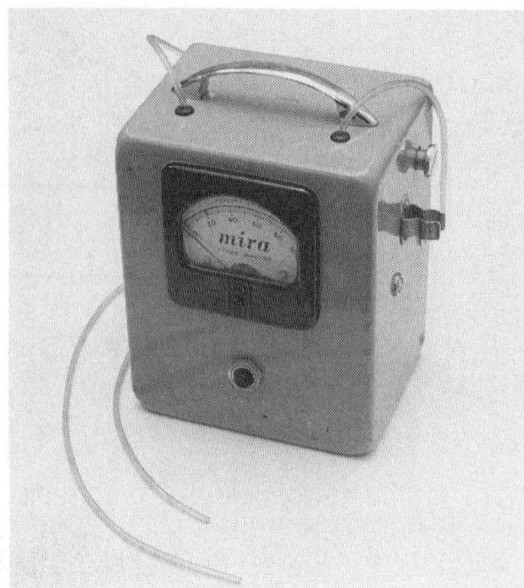

Figure 9-6. Mira oxygen analyzer.

Zirconium Analyzers

The zirconium analyzer is a very accurate oxygen cell with a rapid response time.[3] In this analyzer, an electric potential is developed across heated zirconium oxide (Fig. 9-7). The potential is proportional to the PO_2. These cells are used in applications such as indirect calorimetry in which accuracy and rapid response are important. The cell must be heated to 700°C to 800°C, which requires substantial time for thermal stabilization, as well as considerable thermal insulation.

Transcutaneous PO_2 and PCO_2

Transcutaneous monitors (Fig. 9-8) use an electrode placed directly on the skin to measure skin PO_2 and PCO_2.[4-6] Although both transcutaneous PO_2 ($PtcO_2$) (Fig. 9-9) and transcutaneous PCO_2 ($PtcCO_2$) electrode systems are available, most currently used transcutaneous monitoring systems have the PO_2 electrode and PCO_2 electrode built into a common electrode body (Fig. 9-10). Transcutaneous PO_2 is measured with a miniaturized Clark electrode, and transcutaneous PCO_2 is measured with a miniaturized Severinghaus electrode.

Measurement of transcutaneous PO_2 and PCO_2 is dependent on diffusion of oxygen and carbon dioxide from the circulation through the skin to the transcutaneous electrode that rests on the skin. Human skin is

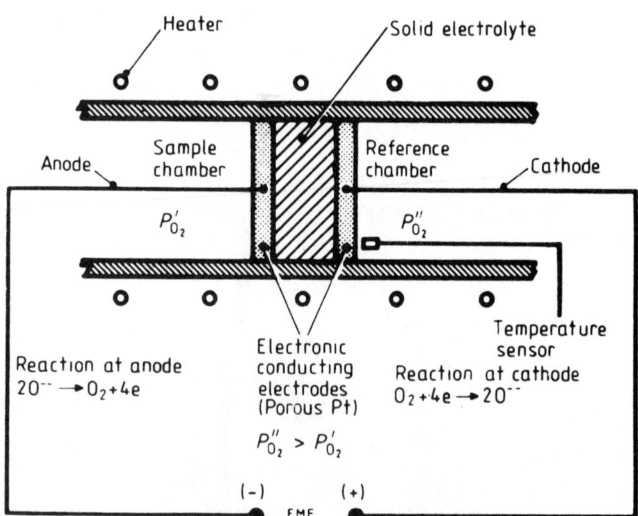

Figure 9-7. Zirconium oxygen analyzer. This analyzer uses a solid electrolyte of yttrium zirconium that conducts oxygen ions, flanked by two platinum-conducting electrodes. A reference cell and a measurement cell are located on either side of the solid electrolyte. The difference in the partial pressures of oxygen on either side of the electrolyte causes an electrical potential to develop. If the partial pressure of oxygen in the reference side (air) is known, then the partial pressure of oxygen in the sample chamber can be determined. (Courtesy of Sensormedics)

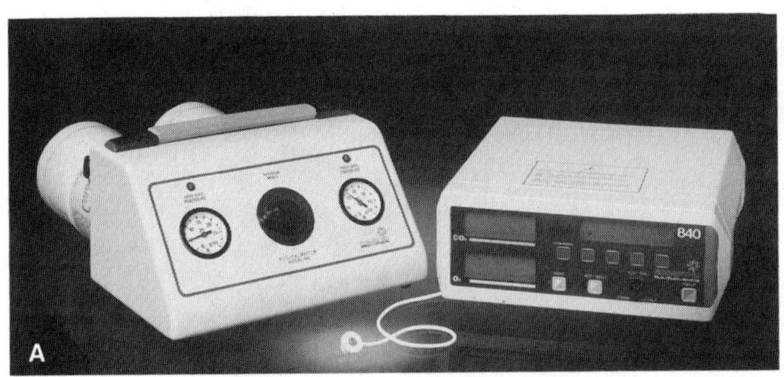

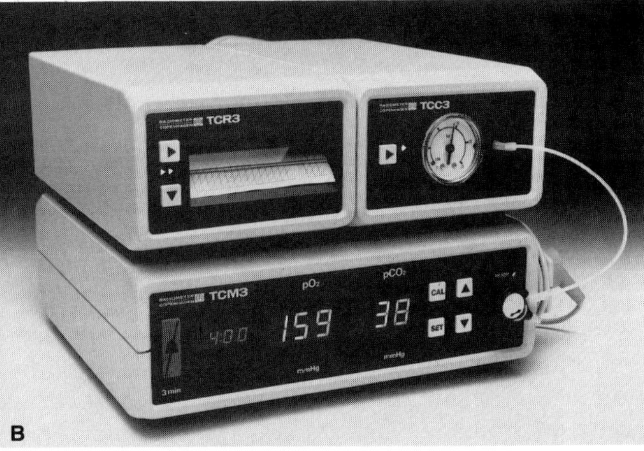

Figure 9-8. (A.) Novametrix transcutaneous blood gas monitoring system with autocalibrator and combined Po_2/Pco_2 electrode. (B.) Radiometer transcutaneous blood gas monitoring system. (A, courtesy of Novametrix; B, courtesy of Radiometer)

relatively impermeable to oxygen and carbon dioxide and poses a formidable barrier to the diffusion of blood gases. Although this is particularly true for the skin of adults, the skin of neonates may be more permeable to oxygen and carbon dioxide. To overcome this permeability obstacle, the transcutaneous electrode is heated. A principle unique to transcutaneous blood gas monitors is that the electrode is heated to some temperature greater than body temperature.[7,8]

Transcutaneous monitors measure the Po_2 and Pco_2 of the skin. It is important to recognize that transcutaneous Po_2 and Pco_2 are not the same as arterial blood gases.[5-9] A number of factors affect the relationship between arterial blood gas levels and the transcutaneous blood gas. First, there is consumption of oxygen by the skin between the vascular bed and the transcutaneous electrode, which tends to decrease the $Ptco_2$ and increase the $Ptcco_2$. Second, the electrode heats the underlying skin. This tends to increase the $Ptco_2$ and the $Ptcco_2$.

For $Ptco_2$, the skin consumption and heating effects nearly cancel one another so the $Ptco_2$ is similar to Pao_2. This is particularly true in neonates, which has created the illusion that $Ptco_2$ should be the same as arterial Po_2. However, it is only coincidental (and artifact) that $Ptco_2$ is often similar to the arterial Po_2. For $Ptcco_2$, the skin consumption and heating effects are additive. The $Ptcco_2$ should thus be higher than the arterial Pco_2, and some manufacturers incorporate a correction factor to account for this effect.

A number of technical considerations must be observed to obtain reliable data from transcutaneous blood gas monitors. The electrode must be maintained according to the manufacturer's specifications. This involves proper preparation of the membrane (eg, cleaning, replacing electrolyte) and proper placement of the electrode membrane. The electrode also needs

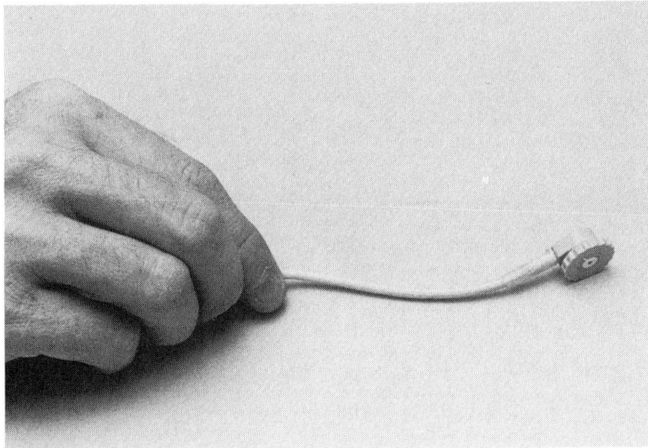

Figure 9-9. Transcutaneous Po_2 electrode.

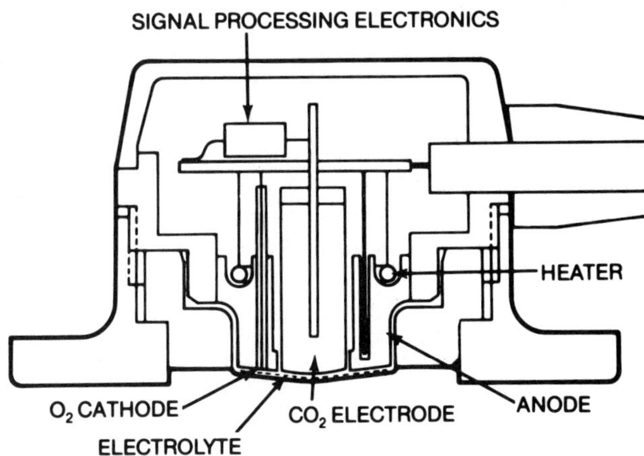

Figure 9-10. Combination electrode for transcutaneous oxygen and carbon dioxide. (From Mahutte CK, Michiels TM, Hassell KT, et al. Evaluation of a single transcutaneous Po_2-Pco_2- sensor in adult patients. Crit Care Med 1984;12: 1063–1066)

to be properly calibrated. Transcutaneous electrodes are usually calibrated with 0% and 12% O_2 and 5% and 10% CO_2. Many transcutaneous monitors feature automatic or semiautomatic calibration.

Proper preparation of the skin and correct attachment of the electrode is most important for obtaining useful transcutaneous P_{O_2} and P_{CO_2} data.[10] The skin should be cleaned and degreased with soap and water, then wiped with an alcohol swab. The skin should be shaved if there is hair on the intended site. A monitoring site should be chosen that has good capillary blood flow, and sites with large fat deposits or bony prominences should be avoided. The sites most commonly used are the anterior chest and abdomen. It is also important to choose a site where an airtight seal between the electrode and the skin can be maintained. Contact gel should also be placed between the electrode and the skin.

For best results, an electrode temperature of 44°C should be used with transcutaneous monitors in neonates,[10] and electrode temperatures of 44°C to 45°C should be used in adults. For P_{tcCO_2} monitoring (without P_{tcO_2}), cooler temperature settings can be used. To avoid skin burns, the electrode site must be changed at least every 2 hours in neonates and every 2 to 4 hours in adults. Each time the electrode site is changed, an equilibration time of at least 10 to 20 minutes is required before stable readings are obtained.

Transcutaneous monitors are usually equipped with a number of alarms. These include alarms for high P_{O_2}, high P_{CO_2}, low P_{O_2}, low P_{CO_2}, and high temperature. There may also be alarms to indicate that it is time to change the electrode site.

Some transcutaneous monitors provide an indication of heating power (ie, the amount of energy needed to maintain the temperature of the electrode). Theoretically, this should provide a noninvasive measure of tissue perfusion. If blood flow under the electrode increases, then more power should be required to maintain the temperature of the electrode (because blood temperature is less than the electrode temperature). Conversely, a decrease in blood flow under the electrode should result in less power required to maintain the electrode temperature. Although this concept is potentially useful to monitor tissue perfusion, it has not been found to very useful in the clinical setting.

Many studies have evaluated the relationship between arterial blood gases and the corresponding transcutaneous values.[5–13] Correlation between arterial blood gases and corresponding transcutaneous values is better in neonates than adults and in hemodynamically stable patients. For adults, P_{tcCO_2} is more reliable than P_{tcO_2}. The P_{tcO_2} tends to be lower than the arterial P_{O_2}, and the P_{tcCO_2} tends to be higher than the arterial P_{CO_2}.

It is important to recognize the effect of perfusion (cardiac output) on the transcutaneous P_{O_2} and P_{CO_2}.[14,15] With a decrease in cardiac output, the P_{tcO_2} decreases and the P_{tcCO_2} increases, even with no change in arterial P_{O_2} or P_{CO_2}. Thus, the ratio of transcutaneous P_{O_2} to arterial P_{O_2} and the ratio of transcutaneous P_{CO_2} to arterial P_{O_2} may be good indicators of cardiac output. A decrease in P_{tcO_2} might be due to a decrease in arterial P_{O_2} or a decrease in cardiac output. Hence, the P_{tcO_2} is an indicator of tissue oxygen delivery (arterial oxygenation and cardiac output). P_{tcO_2} is not an indicator of arterial P_{O_2} per se, which is particularly true in hemodynamically unstable patients in whom the P_{tcO_2} might be an indicator of cardiac output. Similarly, an increase in P_{tcCO_2} might be due to an increase in arterial P_{CO_2} or a decrease in cardiac output. Like P_{tcO_2}, P_{tcCO_2} is not an indicator of arterial P_{CO_2} per se. Although transcutaneous monitoring is continuous and noninvasive, the relationship of transcutaneous P_{O_2} and P_{CO_2} with arterial blood gases must be understood if these data are to be clinically useful.

Conjunctival Oxygen Monitoring

The conjunctival oxygen monitor uses a miniaturized Clark electrode to measure the oxygen tension of the palpebral conjunctiva.[16] The palpebral conjunctiva is the capillary bed that supplies oxygen to the cornea when the eyelid is closed. The eyelid sensor consists of a Clark electrode mounted on a hollow acrylic oval conformer (Fig. 9-11). Right-eye and left-eye conformers are available. The sensor fits into the conjunctival fornices and does not come into contact with the cornea (Fig. 9-12). The system provides a continuous digital display of conjunctival P_{O_2}. A thermistor incorporated in the electrode provides information on eye-

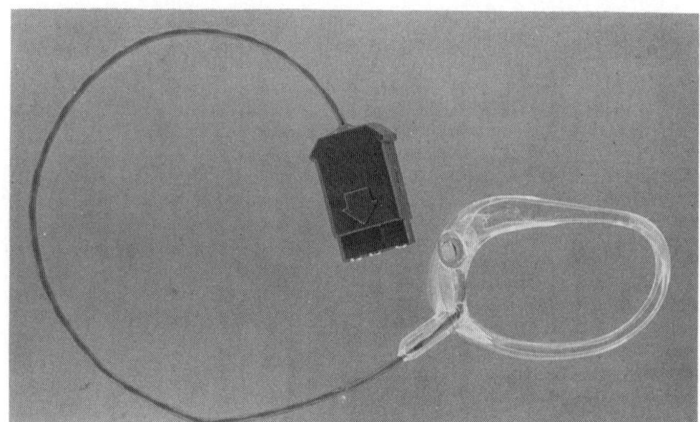

Figure 9-11. Conjunctival P_{O_2} electrode mounted on oval conformer. (From Hess D, Evans C, Thomas K, Eitel D, Kochansky M. The relationship between conjunctival P_{O_2} and arterial P_{O_2} in 16 normal persons. Respir Care 1986;31:191–198)

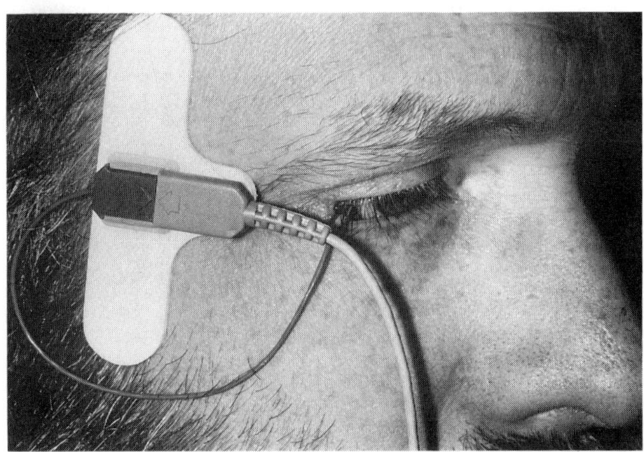

Figure 9-12. Conjunctival P_{O_2} electrode in place. (From Hess D, Evans C, Thomas K, Eitel D, Kochansky M. The relationship between conjunctival P_{O_2} and arterial P_{O_2} in 16 normal persons. Respir Care 1986;31:191–198)

lid temperature and allows temperature compensation of the conjunctival P_{O_2} reading. The electrode is calibrated with room air and to zero using a zeroing solution. High and low alarms can be set on the monitor to signal extreme changes in conjunctival P_{O_2}.

Conjunctival P_{O_2} evaluates tissue P_{O_2}, which is always less than arterial P_{O_2}. The conjunctival P_{O_2} is normally 60% to 70% of the arterial P_{O_2}. It has been suggested that conjunctival P_{O_2} may be useful in tracking changes in arterial P_{O_2}.[16] However, variability in the relationship between the conjunctival and the arterial P_{O_2} may make it difficult to adequately predict arterial P_{O_2} from conjunctival P_{O_2}.[17]

A low cardiac output due to hemorrhage or cardiac arrest[18–20] has been shown to result in a drop in conjunctival P_{O_2}. A decrease in conjunctival P_{O_2} may indicate a decrease in tissue oxygen delivery, which may be due to a drop in arterial P_{O_2} or a drop in cardiac output. Although the conjunctival P_{O_2} may be useful in the evaluation of gross hemorrhage (greater than 15% of blood volume), it is probably insensitive to small amounts of blood loss.[21] The conjunctival P_{O_2} may also be of limited usefulness during cardiopulmonary resuscitation because of the effect of epinephrine on blood flow to the conjunctiva.[22] Although it has been suggested that the conjunctival P_{O_2} may be a useful index of cerebral perfusion during hemorrhage and cardiac arrest,[23] this has yet to be proven.

Pulse Oximetry

Pulse oximeters (Fig. 9-13) provide continuous and noninvasive monitoring of hemoglobin oxygen saturation (Sp_{O_2}). The pulse oximeter combines the principles of spectrophotometric oximetry and plethysmography.[24–27] Although pulse oximeters traditionally use transmission spectrophotometry, some have been developed that use reflectance spectrophotometry.[28,29] The absorption of selected wavelengths of light that passes through (or is reflected from) a living tissue sample are measured. Unlike CO-oximetry, pulse oximetry only uses two wavelengths of light. Also, pulse oximetry is an in vivo measurement, whereas CO-oximetry is an in vitro measurement. Pulse oximeters are unique as monitoring devices in that they do not require user calibration.

The absorption spectra of oxyhemoglobin and deoxyhemoglobin are shown in Figure 9-14. Oxyhemoglobin and deoxyhemoglobin exhibit different absorption characteristics at the wavelengths of red light (660 nm) and infrared light (940 nm). With pulse oximetry, the principal problem is differentiation between the absorption due to oxyhemoglobin and deoxyhemoglobin and the absorptions due to all other tissue constituents.

When light is transmitted through a tissue, some of that light is absorbed by each constituent of the tissue (Fig. 9-15). However, the only variable absorption is due to arterial pulsations. This varying absorption due to arterial pulsation is translated into a plethysmographic waveform at both the red and infrared wavelengths. The ratio between the amplitude of these two plethysmographic waveforms can then be converted to oxygen saturation. For example, it can be seen in Figures 9-16 and 9-17 that equal plethysmographic amplitudes at 660 nm and 940 nm result in an arterial oxygen saturation of 85%.

The pulse oximeter uses a probe that passes light through a pulsating tissue bed (Figure 9-18). The probe consists of two light sources (light-emitting diodes) and a photodetector (photodiode). To obtain correct data, the probe must be correctly positioned so that the two light sources and the photodetector are directly opposite one another across the arteriolar bed. The probe may be incorrectly placed so that light passes from the light source to the photodetector without passing through the pulsating tissue bed. This effect, called optical shunting, results in errors in the saturation measurement. The probe must be placed to avoid ambient light coming into contact with the photodetector, and care must be taken to avoid placement of opaque material (such as artificial finger nails) between the light source and the photodetector.

To facilitate proper placement, a number of probes have been developed. These include finger probes, toe probes, ear probes, nasal probes, and foot probes. The probes are available in adult, pediatric, and neonatal sizes. Either single-patient-use disposable or reusable permanent probes can be used. To obtain valid data, manufacturer's instructions must be followed regarding proper placement of the probe. To prevent pressure necrosis, care must also be taken to

(text continues on page 194)

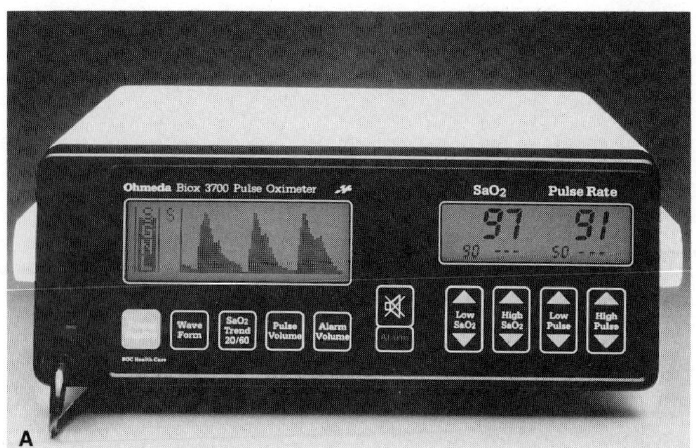

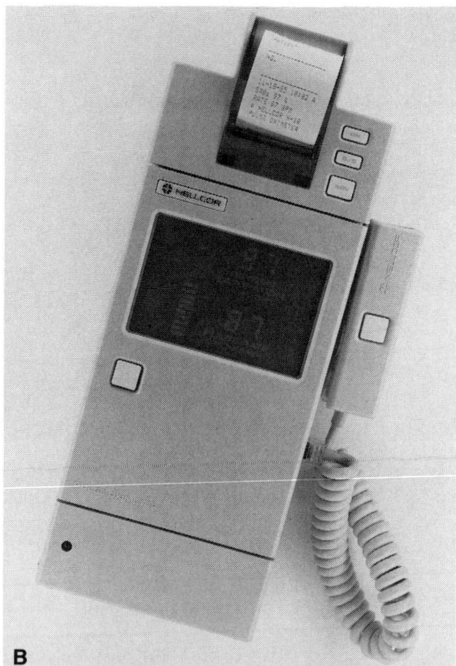

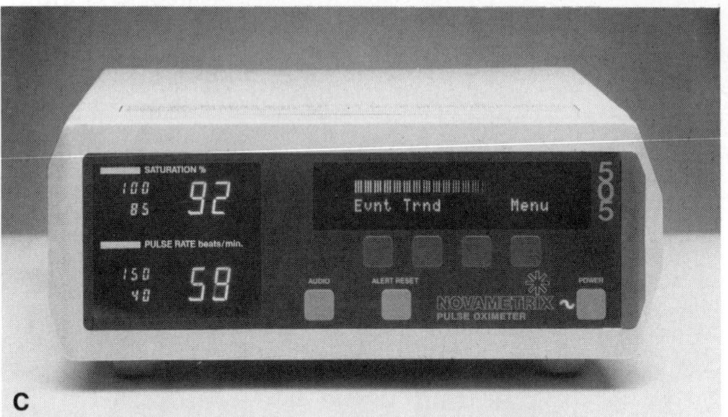

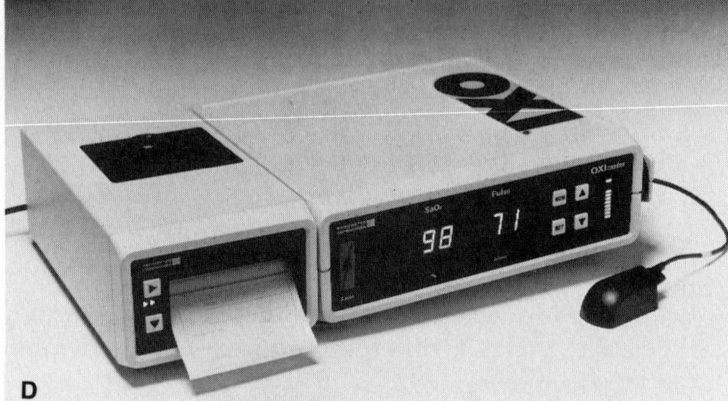

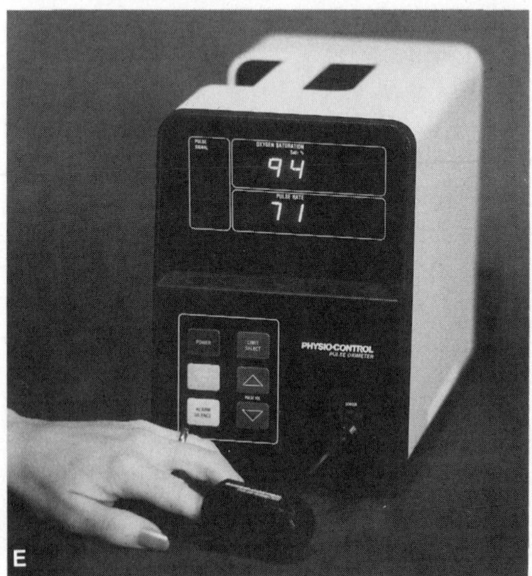

Figure 9-13. (A.) Ohmeda 3700 pulse oximeter. Note plethysmographic waveform. (Courtesy of Ohmeda Inc., Madison, WI). (B.) Nellcor N-10 pulse oximeter. (C.) Novametrix 505 pulse oximeter. (Courtesy of Novametrix Medical Systems, Wallingford, CT). (D.) Radiometer Oximeter pulse oximeter. (Courtesy of Radiometer America, Westlake, OH). (E.) Physio-Control pulse oximeter (Courtesy of Physio-Control, Redland, WA).

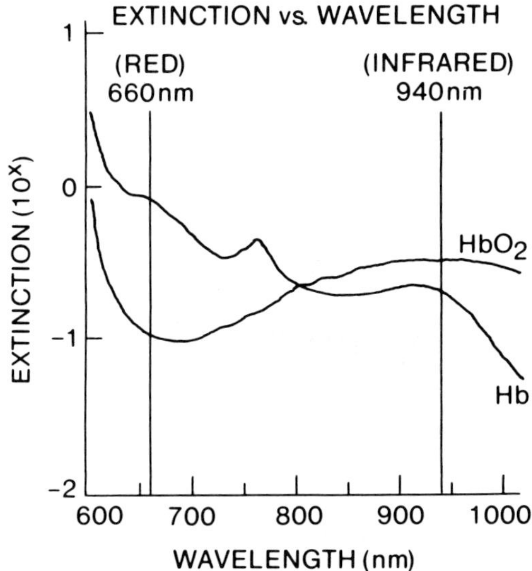

Figure 9-14. Absorption spectra of oxyhemoglobin and deoxyhemoglobin. Pulse oximeters use red (660 nm) and infrared (940 nm) light. (Courtesy of Ohmeda Inc., Madison, WI)

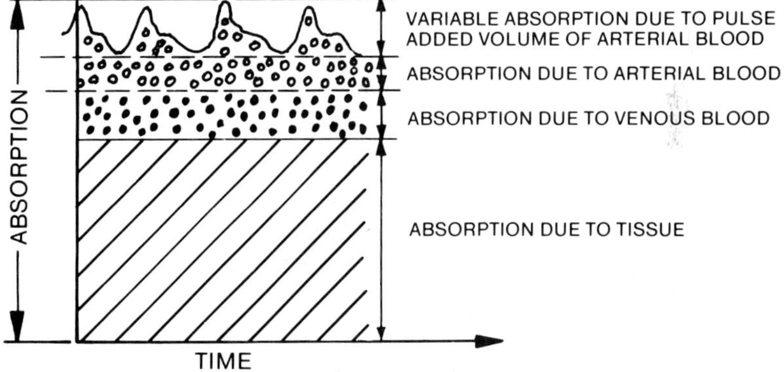

Figure 9-15. When light is passed through tissue, some of that light is absorbed by each constituent of the tissue, but the only variable light absorption is due to arterial blood. (Courtesy of Ohmeda Inc., Madison, WI)

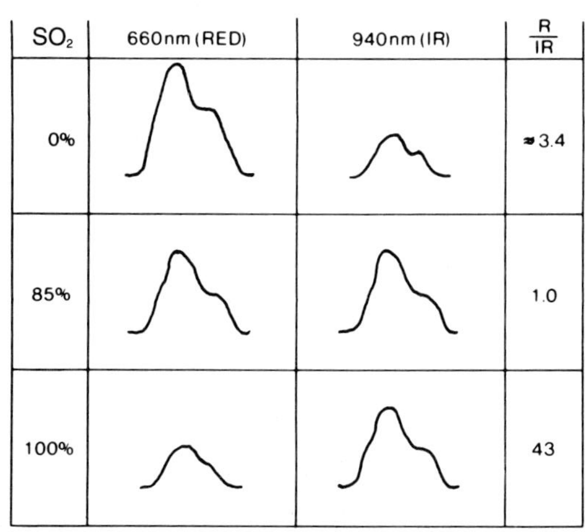

RELATIVE PLETHYSMOGRAPHIC SIGNAL AMPLITUDES ASSUMING THE TRANSMISSION INTENSITIES ARE EQUAL.

Figure 9-16. The ratio between the amplitude of the red and infrared wavelength is used to determine oxygen saturation by the pulse oximeter. (Courtesy of Ohmeda Inc., Madison, WI)

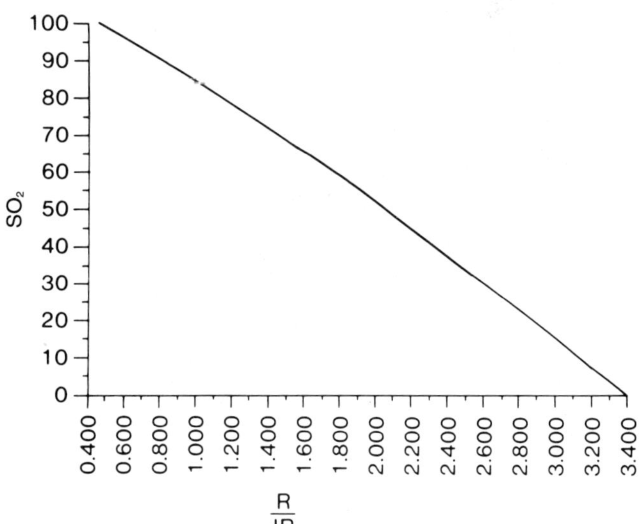

Figure 9-17. With pulse oximetry, oxygen saturation is determined by the ratio of the red light absorbed to that of the infrared light absorbed. (Courtesy of Ohmeda Inc., Madison, WI)

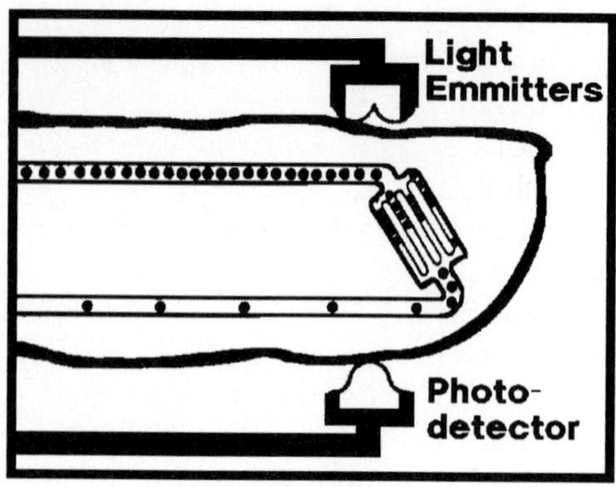

Figure 9-18. The pulse oximeter sensor passes light through a pulsating tissue bed. (Courtesy of Nellcor, Pleasanton, CA)

avoid excessive pressure when pulse oximeter probes are attached.[30]

Because it uses plethysmographic information to determine arterial oxygen saturation, the pulse oximeter must be able to adequately detect an arterial waveform. If perfusion is poor, the pulse oximeter may not be able to adequately differentiate between arterial pulsations and background noise. Most pulse oximeters provide a visual indication of pulse amplitude. If pulse amplitude is poor, the user may elect to choose an alternate site or sensor. Some pulse oximeters display the plethysmographic waveform, which provides a visual indication of the adequacy of perfusion. In an attempt to improve the validity of results in conditions of poor perfusion, some manufacturers have synchronized pulse oximeter measurements with the R wave of the electrocardiogram and others have increased the intensity of the light source.

Pulse oximeters are subject to motion artifact. Movement of the sensor makes it difficult for the oximeter to differentiate motion from arterial pulsations, with a resultant inaccuracy in the oxygen saturation displayed. Motion artifact can be reduced by use of low mass and snugly fitting sensors. Adjusting the oximeter for a longer signal averaging time may also reduce the effects of motion artifact, and electrocardiographic synchronization may be useful in reducing the deleterious effects of motion artifact.

Because pulse oximeters use two-wavelength spectrophotometry, they are susceptible to inaccuracies in the presence of dysfunctional hemoglobins.[31–35] Due to the absorption spectra of carboxyhemoglobin and methemoglobin relative to those of oxyhemoglobin and deoxyhemoglobin (Fig. 9-19), the effects of these dysfunctional hemoglobins are different. In the presence of carboxyhemoglobin, the pulse oximeters overestimate the true oxygen saturation by an amount roughly equal to the carboxyhemoglobin level. In the presence of methemoglobin, the pulse oximeter reading of oxygen saturation shifts toward 85%, thus causing the pulse oximeter to read inaccurately low when the oxygen saturation is high and inaccurately high when the saturation is low. Pulse oximetry is accurate in the presence of fetal hemoglobin.[36,37] As seen in Figure 9-20, the absorption spectra of adult hemoglobin and fetal hemoglobin are similar.

The accuracy of pulse oximetry may be affected by venous pulsation. Because pulse oximetry evaluates the light absorption of hemoglobin, its accuracy may also be affected by severe anemia or hemodilution. High-intensity external light can also affect the accuracy of pulse oximetry. Because pulse oximetry is dependent on a pulsating arteriolar vascular bed, it does not function well under pulseless conditions such as cardiac arrest or poor peripheral perfusion.[38] The accuracy of pulse oximetry is not affected by high bilirubin levels[39] but is affected by intravascular dyes[40] and an

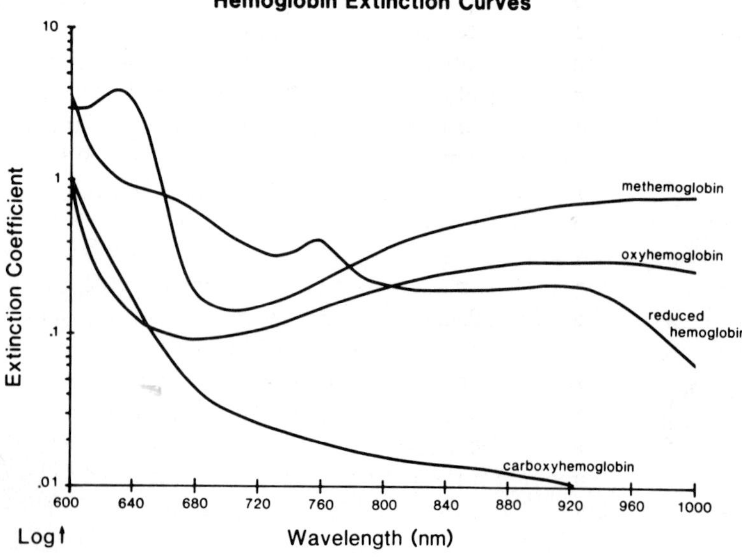

Figure 9-19. Absorption spectra of oxyhemoglobin, deoxyhemoglobin, carboxyhemoglobin, and methemoglobin in the range of wavelengths used with pulse oximetry. (From Tremper KK, Nickerson BG. Oximeters [letter]. Chest 1988;94: 1110–1113)

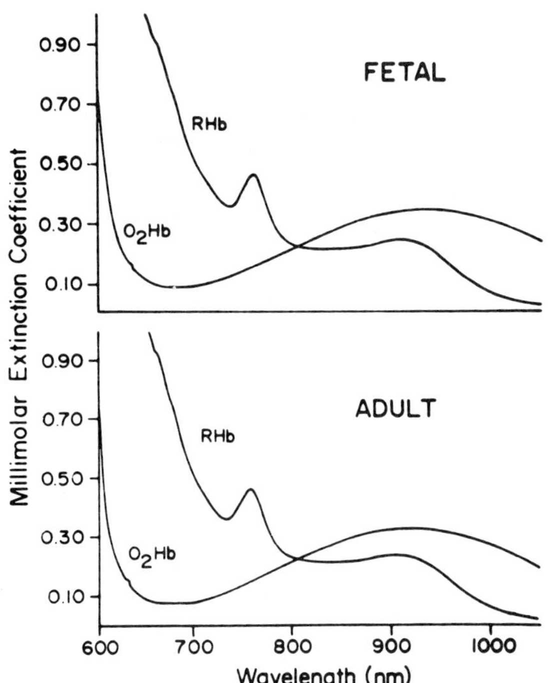

Figure 9-20. Absorption spectra of adult hemoglobin and fetal hemoglobin. (From Harris AP, Sendak MJ, Donham RT, Thomas M, Duncan D. Absorption characteristics of human fetal hemoglobin at wavelengths used in pulse oximetry. J Clin Monit 1988;4:175–177)

impedance by an intra-arterial catheter.[41] To avoid spectral interference, nail polish should be removed if the pulse oximeter probe is placed on the finger.[42] The accuracy and reliability of pulse oximetry is less in individuals with deeply pigmented skin.[43]

To fully appreciate the use of pulse oximetry, one must understand the relationship between Spo_2 and arterial Po_2. If the oxyhemoglobin dissociation curve shifts, Spo_2 can change without any change in arterial Po_2.[44,45] Or, if the oxyhemoglobin dissociation curve shifts concurrently with a change in Po_2, there may be no change in Spo_2. Also, at a high Spo_2, there can be little change in Spo_2 with a large change in arterial Po_2. However, at a low Spo_2, a small change in Po_2 may result in a relatively large change in Spo_2. Because of this relationship between Spo_2 and Po_2, it may not be advisable to predict arterial Po_2 from Spo_2.

The accuracy of many commercially available pulse oximeters is $\pm$ 5%.[25-27,46-50] Because of the sigmoid shape of the oxyhemoglobin dissociation curve, the implications of this accuracy depends on the Spo_2. When the Spo_2 is greater than 90%, this accuracy represents a relatively wide range of Po_2 values. When the Spo_2 is lower, however, this accuracy represents a smaller range of Po_2 values. For quality control purposes, pulse oximeter Spo_2 should be compared periodically with a concurrent Spo_2 determined by CO-oximetry. It should also be recognized that pulse oximetry provides no indication of ventilation or acid–base status, which requires periodic arterial blood gas analysis. The limitations of pulse oximetry should be appreciated by all clinicians who use this technology.[51]

Because pulse oximeters use plethysmography as well as spectrophotometry, they can measure heart rate as well as Spo_2. If the heart rate displayed by the pulse oximeter differs significantly from the patient's actual heart rate, then the pulse oximeter results should be questioned. However, it should be recognized that agreement between the pulse oximeter heart rate and the patient's actual heart rate does not necessarily imply that the saturation displayed is accurate. Many pulse oximeters also feature alarms for high saturation, low saturation, high heart rate, and low heart rate. Pulse oximeters may be combined with other monitoring equipment such as capnographs, intensive care bedside monitors, mechanical ventilators, and transcutaneous monitors.

Capnometry and Capnography

Capnometry is the measurement of carbon dioxide concentration (usually Pco_2) at the patient's airway during the ventilatory cycle. The capnometer provides a numerical measurement of inspired and end-tidal CO_2 ($Petco_2$). Capnography is the graphic waveform display of carbon dioxide as a function of time. When the waveform is displayed, capnography includes capnometry.[52-55]

Carbon dioxide analysis of respiratory gas is measured using mass spectroscopy, infrared absorption spectroscopy, or raman spectroscopy. Because of the expense and nonportability of mass spectrometers, most capnometers used in critical care units by respiratory care practitioners use infrared absorption. The absorption peak used in capnometry is 4.26 μm (Fig. 9-21). The capnometer compares the amount of infrared light absorbed in a sample cell to the amount of infrared light absorbed in a carbon dioxide–free reference cell. For correct results, the accuracy of infrared capnometry must be confirmed using a gas of known carbon dioxide concentration (usually 5% CO_2).

Capnometers can be either sidestream or mainstream monitors (Fig. 9-22). With the sidestream monitor, gas samples at the airway are aspirated through a fine-bore tubing to the sample measurement chamber of the capnometer. Most sidestream capnometers use a flow of 150 to 250 mL/min to aspirate gas from the airway. With this system, the measurement chamber is not attached directly to the patient's airway. With the mainstream monitor, the sample measurement chamber is placed directly at the airway. With the sidestream method, respiratory gas is lost from the ventilation cir-

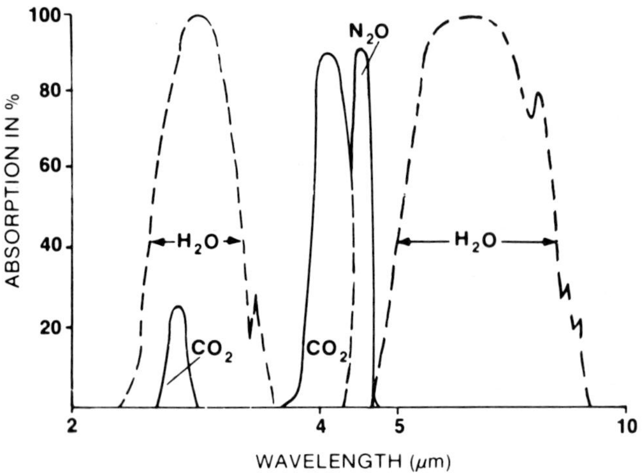

Figure 9-21. Absorption spectra for CO_2, N_2O, and H_2O. (From Carbon dioxide monitors. Health Devices 1986;15: 255–285)

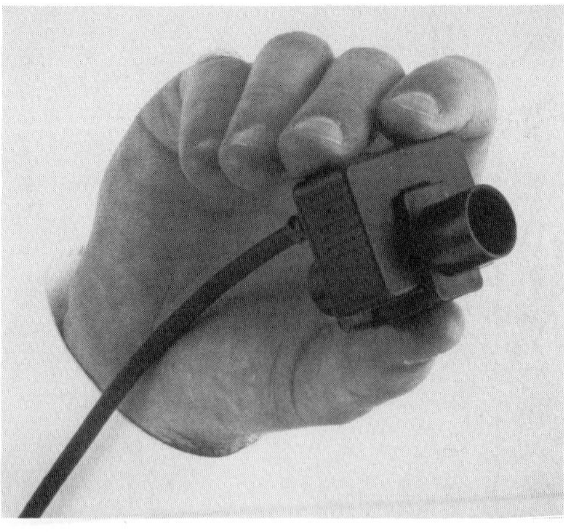

Figure 9-23. Sample measurement chamber for the Novametrix mainstream monitor.

cuit due to sampling, which might compromise ventilation if low tidal volumes are used. The mainstream system may produce a faster response and less damping of the waveform because no sampling system is required, but it has a larger deadspace (undesirable with low tidal volumes) and adds weight to the airway (which could result in inadvertent extubation). Although many commercially available capnometers are sidestream monitors, low-deadspace low-weight mainstream capnometers are available (Fig. 9-23).

A typical nondispersive double-beam positive-filter capnometer is illustrated in Figure 9-24.[55] The detector is filled with carbon dioxide. Radiation that comes through the reference and sample cells affects the absorption by carbon dioxide in the detection chamber. Carbon dioxide in the sample cell decreases the radiation transmitted to the detector. The increased radiation transmitted from the reference cell (relative to that from the sample cell) produces movement of a diaphragm, which is translated to a display of the amount of carbon dioxide present in the sample cell. Interference from nitrous oxide is removed by a filter that absorbs the radiation from the nitrous oxide absorption band. A chopper periodically permits measurement of reference signal, sample signal, and dark signal (neither reference or sample signals).

A double-beam negative-filter capnometer can be applied to mainstream capnometers (Fig. 9-25).[55] The infrared signal is directed through the sample cell to the detector. However, to reach the detector, the signal must also pass through the cell in a chopper wheel. Two cells are present on the chopper wheel; one contains carbon dioxide and the other contains nitrogen. Thus, two signals are generated, and the ratio of these signals is used to determine the carbon dioxide concentration.

With the mainstream capnometer, the sample chamber on the airway can serve as the reference cell during inhalation.[55] This device assumes that the inspired P_{CO_2} is zero (Fig. 9-26), and will not function correctly if there is carbon dioxide in the inspired gas.

A chopper is used in most capnometers[55] and is important for several reasons. First, it allows a common source and detector to be used with the double beam capnometer. Second, it provides an alternating signal from the reference and sample cells. Third, it produces a null signal (ie, no signal from either sample or reference cell), which helps to eliminate drift and interference.

To provide accurate measurements, capnometers must be calibrated at regular intervals. This involves

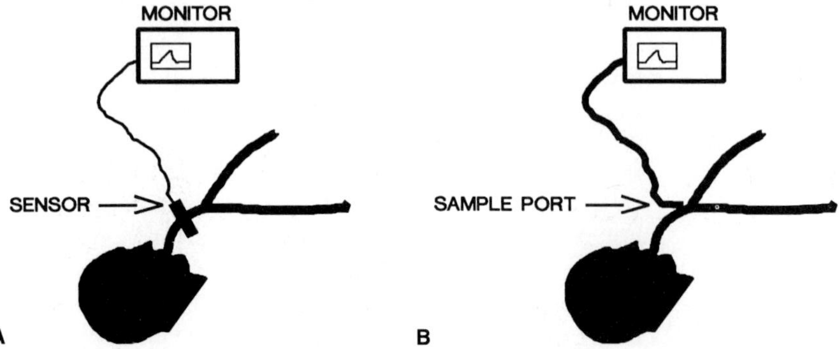

Figure 9-22. Sidestream and mainstream capnographs.

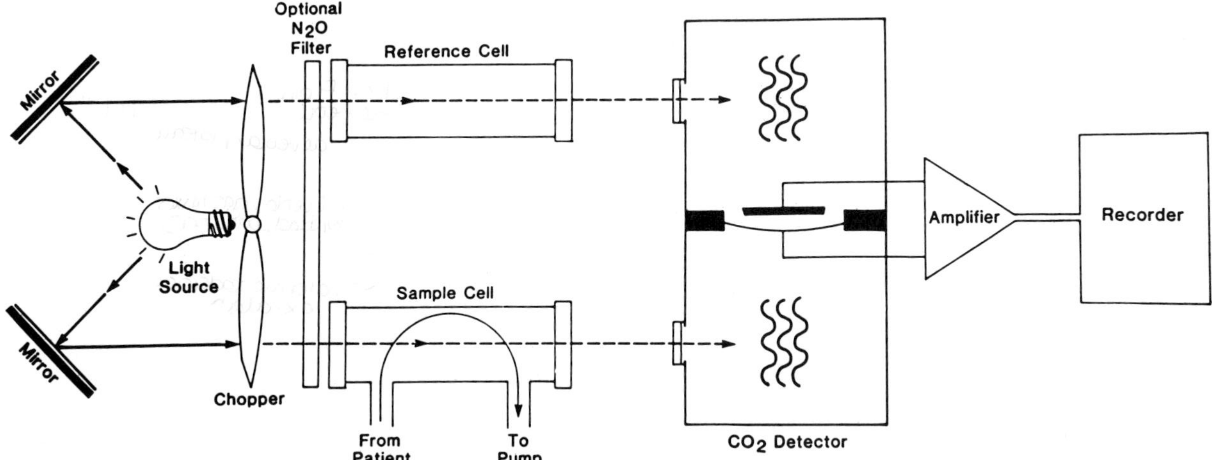

Figure 9-24. A nondispersive double-beam positive-filter capnometer.

occasional use of a 5% carbon dioxide gas mixture and more frequent zero calibration with room air. The accuracy of a capnometer should be ± 10% or ± 3 mm Hg, whichever is larger.[52]

Capnometry is usually used with intubated patients. However, it can be used with nonintubated patients using a tight-fitting face mask, nasal catheter, nasal cannula, or mouthpiece. Particularly with nonintubated patients, it is important that the exhaled gas sample is not contaminated with room air, which will invalidate the P_{ETCO_2}. A sidestream monitor usually performs better than a mainstream monitor for nonintubated patients.

There are several technical difficulties with the use of capnometry. The greatest of these is water condensation within the sidestream system, which results in instrument failure. Manufacturers of capnometers have incorporated numerous designs into the construction of the device to deal with this problem. These include use of nafion tubing (which allows water vapor to diffuse through the tubing wall), condensation water traps, and moisture-absorbent filters. With the sidestream monitor, the sampling tube can become obstructed with water or secretions, which may be recognized by the monitor and purged from the line. With the mainstream sensor, water can condense on the windows of the sensor cell, resulting in inaccurate measurements. To avoid this problem, the mainstream sensor is often heated. Another technical problem is that of increased mechanical deadspace in the respiratory circuitry, which is particularly a problem with low tidal volume ventilation and with the use of mainstream sensors. The sidestream capnometer results in a loss of tidal volume due to aspiration of gas samples from the airway, which can be a problem with low tidal volume ventilation such as in pediatric or neonatal applications.

If nitrous oxide is present in the gas mixture analyzed, it will produce a "collision broadening effect," which will affect the accuracy of the capnometer. Due to this effect, the absorption band for carbon dioxide is affected by the presence of other constituents in the gas mixture. Correction factors to adjust for the effects of pressure broadening are known and can be used to correct for the presence of gases other than carbon dioxide in the mixture being analyzed.

The normal capnogram is illustrated in Figure 9-27. During inspiration, the P_{CO_2} is zero. At the beginning of exhalation, P_{CO_2} remains zero as anatomic deadspace gas exits the airway (A). The curve then rises sharply as alveolar gas mixes with deadspace gas (B). The curve then levels off and forms a plateau during most of exhalation (C), which represents gas flow from alveoli. This plateau is called the " alveolar plateau,"and the P_{CO_2} at the end of the alveolar plateau (ie, end-exhalation) is the P_{ETCO_2}. A characteristic of obstructive lung disease is

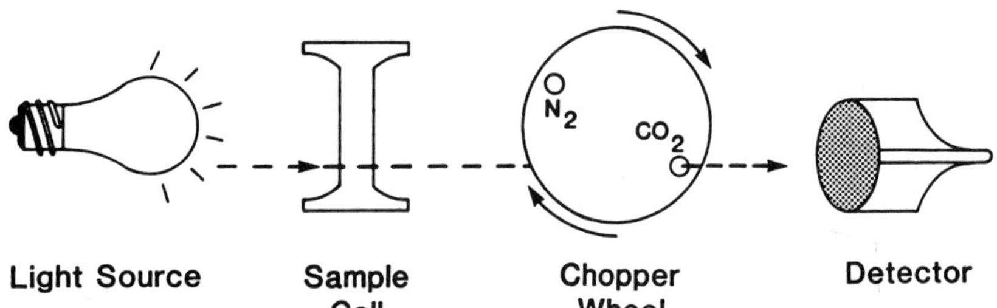

Figure 9-25. A double-beam negative-filter capnometer applied to a mainstream capnometer.

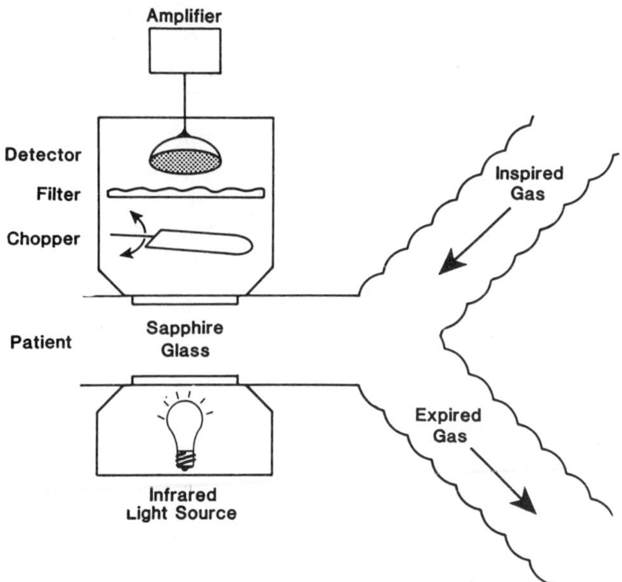

Figure 9-26. A sample chamber on the airway that serves as the reference cell during inhalation.

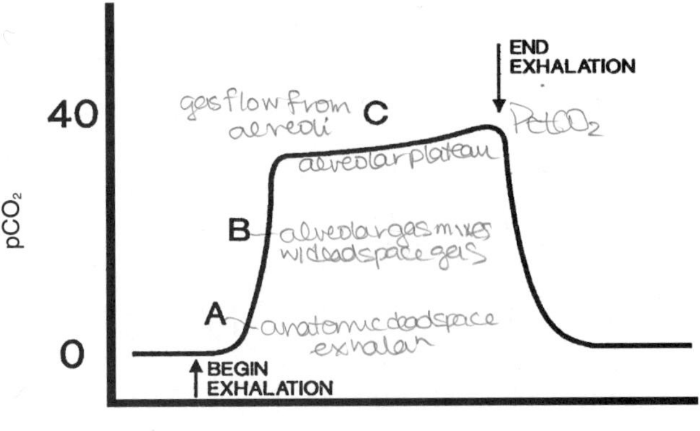

Figure 9-27. The normal capnogram.

an increased slope of the alveolar plateau, so that a true plateau is not reached. The capnogram may be displayed in fast speed (Fig. 9-28) or slow speed (Fig. 9-29). The fast speed recording allows evaluation of the fine detail of each breath, whereas the slow speed allows evaluation of trends.

With normal lung function, the $P_{ET}CO_2$ is within ± 5 mm Hg of arterial PCO_2. However, with pulmonary or cardiac disease, the $P_{ET}CO_2$ may be significantly different than the arterial PCO_2.[56–70] An arterial PCO_2 much greater than $P_{ET}CO_2$ indicates deadspace ventilation, which can be due to maldistribution of ventilation within the lung or poor pulmonary blood flow (pulmonary embolus, low cardiac output, cardiac arrest). It is also possible for the $P_{ET}CO_2$ to be greater than the arterial PCO_2 with ventilation–perfusion mismatch. Theoretically, the $P_{ET}CO_2$ could be as great as the mixed venous PCO_2 or as low as the inspired PCO_2. Under normal conditions, the $P_{ET}CO_2$ will correlate well with changes in arterial PCO_2. However, in patients with heart or lung disease, the $P_{ET}CO_2$ may not correlate well with arterial PCO_2. To adequately assess the $P_{ET}CO_2$, the arterial PCO_2 must be known. Thus, capnometry may not necessarily reduce the need for arterial PCO_2 measurements. Also, a large gradient between arterial PCO_2 and $P_{ET}CO_2$ is relatively nonspecific, with a variety of potential etiologies. Capnography may be useful in the detection of changes in the patient's condition, thus alerting the respiratory care practitioner of the need for further assessment. Capnography may be as useful in the evaluation of the waveform produced as it is in the determination of $P_{ET}CO_2$. It has been suggested that capnography should be viewed as a qualitative rather than a quantitative technique.[71]

Capnometry may be useful in the detection of equipment failures. A ventilator disconnect should result in a $P_{ET}CO_2$ of zero.[72] An esophageal intubation will also result in a $P_{ET}CO_2$ of zero.[73,74] Inspired PCO_2 should be zero, and an increase in inspired PCO_2 indicates rebreathing. With cardiac arrest, PCO_2 will drop to zero, and failure of $P_{ET}CO_2$ to increase during resuscitation is an ominous sign.[68]

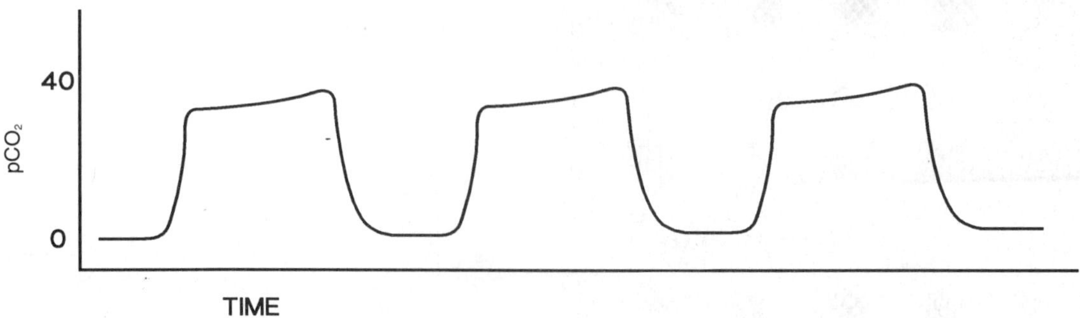

Figure 9-28. Capnogram recorded in fast speed.

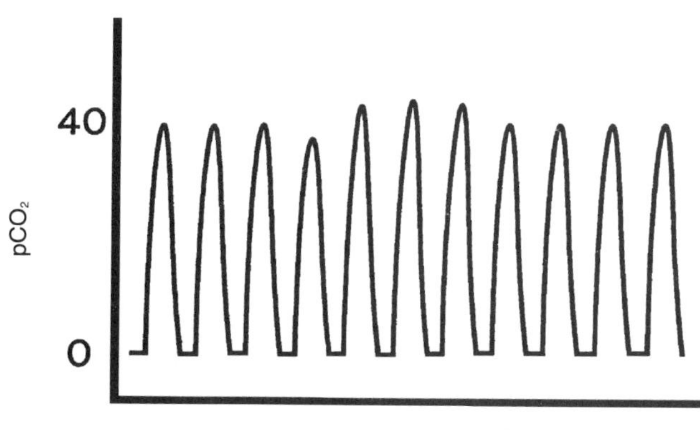

Figure 9-29. Capnogram recorded in slow speed.

Several manufacturers now market monitors that combine pulse oximetry and capnography (Fig. 9-30). These monitors allow continuous noninvasive monitoring of oxygenation and ventilation. Some of these monitors also measure nitrous oxide and F_{IO_2}, and all are equipped with numerous alarms.

A disposable device, the Nellcor EasyCap, is available to verify tracheal intubation. It produces a color change due to carbon dioxide in the exhaled gas. Absence of carbon dioxide (<4 mm Hg) produces a purple color, more than 2% of carbon dioxide (15–38 mm Hg) produces a yellow color, and 0.5% to 2% (4–15 mm Hg) produces an intermediate color. The color of the indicator is compared with a reference color on the dome of the device (Fig. 9-31). Because there is very little carbon dioxide in the stomach, esophageal intubation results in no color change. The device is generally reliable but may not produce a color change with a correctly placed endotracheal tube (ie, in the trachea) if pulmonary blood flow is very low (eg, cardiac arrest).[75]

Mass Spectroscopy

The mass spectrometer is used for respiratory gas analysis.[76–79] It is very accurate, has a rapid response time, and can be used for breath-to-breath analysis of inspired and expired gases. The mass spectrometer can be used to measure the concentrations of oxygen, nitrogen, carbon dioxide, and anesthetic gases. A multiplex system can be used to monitor several patients simultaneously in the intensive care unit or operating room. The principal disadvantage of the mass spectrometer is its high initial cost.

A schematic diagram of the mass spectrometer is shown in Figure 9-32. The gas to be analyzed is drawn

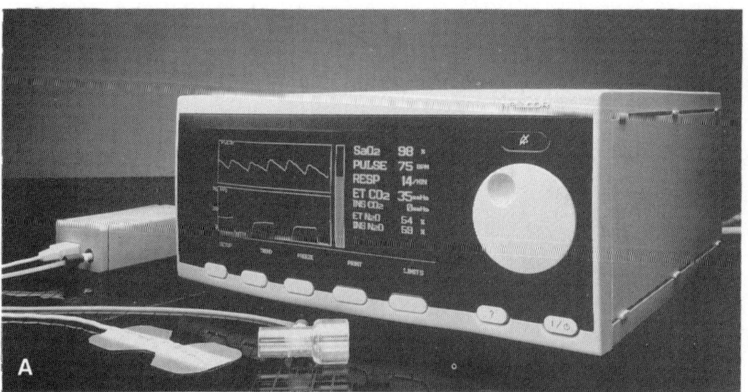

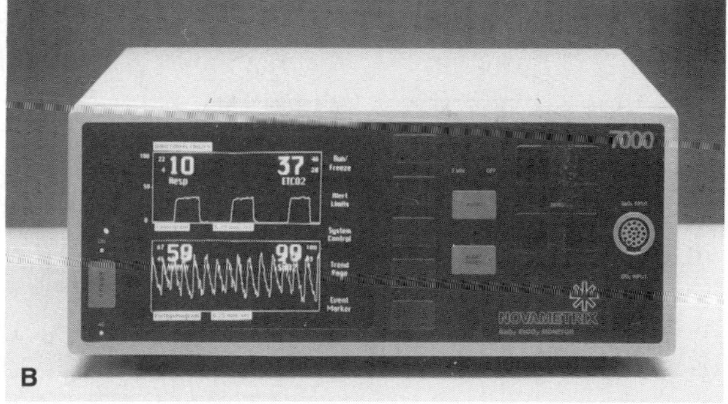

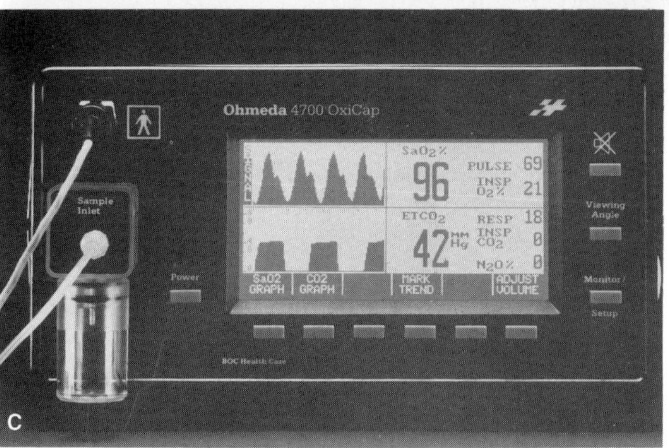

Figure 9-30. (A.) Nellcor N-1000 combined pulse oximeter/capnograph. (B.) Novametrix 7000 combined pulse oximeter/capnograph. (C.) Ohmeda 4700 OxiCap combined pulse oximeter/capnograph.

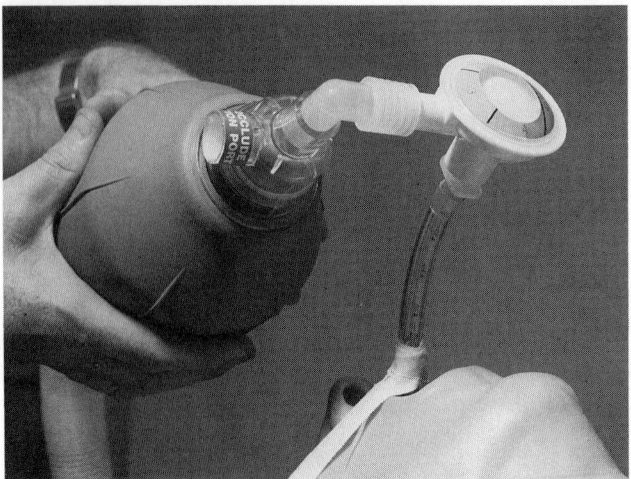

Figure 9-31. End-tidal CO_2 detector used to detect tracheal versus esophageal intubation.

into the system by a vacuum pump. The gas molecules are then ionized by bombarding them with an electron beam. The ionized gases (which are primarily cations) are then projected into the analyzer. By application of a magnetic field, the gases are separated onto collector plates in the analyzer according to their mass-to-charge ratios. The heavier the ionized particle, the less it curves. When the ionized gases strike the collector plates, they produce an electric charge. These electric charges are then quantified, which allows the mass spectrometer to determine the concentration of each gas present.

Raman Spectroscopy

When light collides with gas molecules, the photon loses energy to the gas molecule, resulting in a longer wavelength (lower frequency). This can be used to measure gas concentrations by isolating the specific raman wavelengths for each gas using multiple optical wavelength filters.[80] Because the magnitude of the raman signal is small, high-intensity light sources such as lasers are used. Because raman scattering takes place almost instantaneously, breath-by-breath measurements are possible. This method can be used to measure anesthetic gas concentrations. In respiratory care, this technique can be used in sidestream capnometers.[81]

Calorimetry

Calorimetry is the technique by which energy expenditure of a human or an animal is measured. In clinical practice, the measurement of energy expenditure can be useful in the care of malnourished patients, as well as in those unable to eat (such as mechanically ventilated patients) requiring enteral or parenteral nutri-

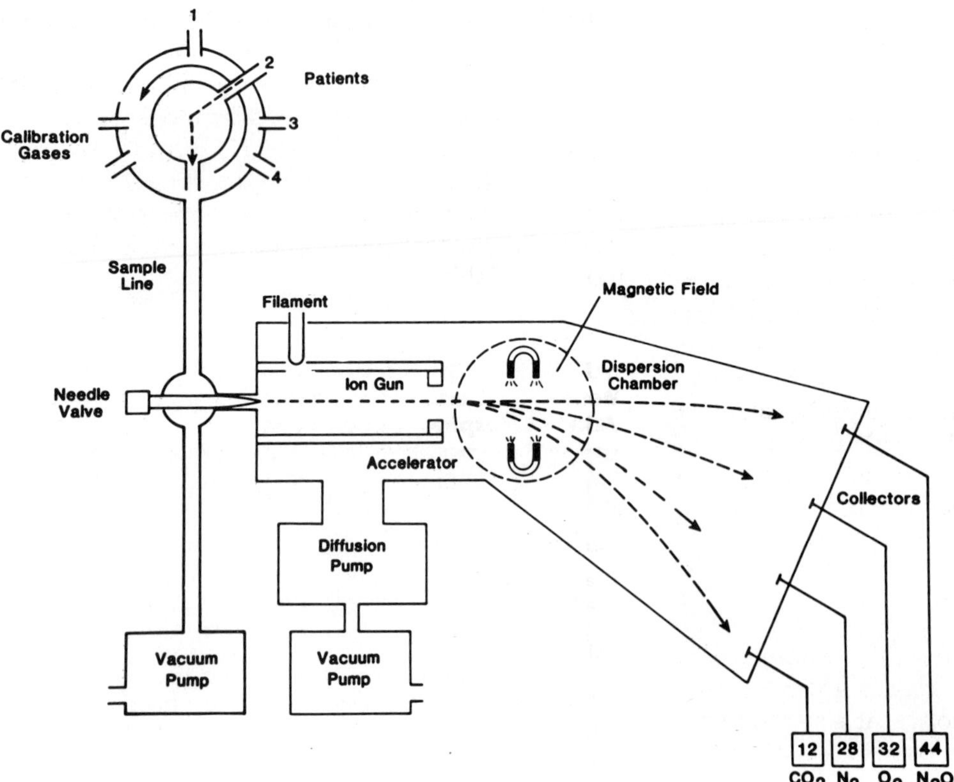

Figure 9-32. Mass spectrometer.

Equation Box 9-1: Weir Equation

$$\text{Energy} = [(\dot{V}O_2)(3.941) + (\dot{V}CO_2)(1.11)] \cdot 1440$$

tion. Respiratory function and nutritional status are closely related.[82] Both malnutrition and excessive nutrition have been shown to adversely effect weaning from mechanical ventilation.[83–85] Until the late 1970s the technology to measure energy expenditure in mechanically ventilated patients was unavailable. Improved sensor design and microprocessor technology, however, have made these measurements feasible in all but the most severe cases.[86] The components of systems used to measure energy expenditure are familiar to respiratory therapists and are described below.

Direct Calorimetry

Direct calorimetry is the determination of energy expenditure by measuring heat production. This technique confines the subject to a relatively small chamber for long periods of time. Direct calorimetry is impractical for use on patients who require constant care (such as critically ill patients). The primary use of direct calorimetry has been in the study of animals, where understanding the process of converting food to animal products improves the yield of milk, meat, or eggs.

Indirect Calorimetry

Indirect calorimetry is the calculation of energy expenditure by the measurement of oxygen consumption ($\dot{V}O_2$) and carbon dioxide production ($\dot{V}CO_2$). These measurements are converted to energy expenditure (kilocalories per day) by the Weir method (Equation Box 9-1).[87] Another important determination from indirect calorimetry data is the respiratory quotient (RQ). RQ is the relationship of $\dot{V}CO_2/\dot{V}O_2$. Normal RQ is 0.8 to 0.85 with variations according to the type of substrate being used (Table 9-1). The RQ also serves as a quality control of the measurement since RQ cannot be less than 0.67 or greater than 1.3. Although many systems have been devised, all indirect calorimeters work by one of two methods, the open-circuit method or the closed-circuit method.

Open-Circuit Method

The open-circuit method measures the concentrations and volumes of inspired and expired gases to determine $\dot{V}O_2$ and $\dot{V}CO_2$. The equations that are used to calculate these variables are shown in Equation Box 9-2. The key components of an open-circuit calorimeter are the analyzers (O_2 and CO_2), a volume measuring device, and mixing chamber. The analyzers must be capable of measuring small changes in gas concentrations (0.001%) in room air and oxygen-enriched environments. The volume measuring device may be a turbine spirometer or pneumotachometer and must be capable of accurately measuring volumes from 0.05 to 1 L. Another important component is a pressure transducer. Since most oxygen analyzers in indirect calorimeters use the polarographic principle, changes in pressure (such as those that occur during mechanical ventilation) will effect the measurement of FIO_2.[88] The pressure transducer corrects the analyzers for periodic changes in partial pressure.

The open-circuit method can be used to measure energy expenditure in spontaneously breathing subjects and those requiring mechanical ventilation (Fig. 9-33). Figure 9-34 illustrates the movement of gas into the components of an open-circuit indirect calorimeter. Expired gas from the patient is directed into the mixing chamber, where baffles interrupt flow and prevent streaming of gases and uneven gas concentrations. At the end of the mixing chamber a vacuum pump withdraws a small sample of mixed expired gas for measurement by the oxygen and carbon dioxide analyzers. The pressure transducer is also within this circuit to ensure pressure-compensated gas measurements. This sample of gas is returned to the mixing chamber after analysis. At preselected intervals, the analyzers also measure the inspired gas concentration for determination of inspired/expired differences. The entire volume of gas then exits through a volume transducer for measurement of minute ventilation. A thermistor is used for correction of volumes to BTPS (Body Temperature Pressure Saturated 37°C at 1 atmosphere saturated with water). A microprocessor system controls the calorimeter functions, writes the data to the memory, and performs the necessary calculations. A printed copy of the information is also commonly available.

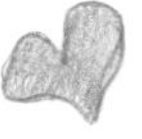

TABLE 9-1. The Effect of Substrate Metabolized and Other Factors on the Value of Respiratory Quotient

	Respiratory Quotient
Substrate	
Carbohydrate	1.0
Protein	0.8–0.85
Lipids	0.7
Alcohol	0.67
Other Factors	
Hyperventilation	>1.0
Lipogenesis	>1.0

Equation Box 9-2: Calculations of Oxygen Consumption and Carbon Dioxide Production

Oxygen consumption is measured by the relationship:

$$\dot{V}O_2 = (\dot{V}I)(FIO_2) - (\dot{V}E)(FEO_2)$$

Carbon dioxide production is measured by the relationship:

$$\dot{V}CO_2 = (\dot{V}E)(FECO_2) - (\dot{V}I)(FICO_2)$$

$(\dot{V}I)(FICO_2)$ is often deleted, since $FICO_2$ is less than 0.03% when breathing room air and in a ventilator circuit should equal 0%. Of the two measurements, oxygen consumption represents the greatest technical challenge. One of the difficulties is encountered in measuring $\dot{V}I$. Since $\dot{V}E$ is commonly measured, however, $\dot{V}I$ can be calculated using the Haldane transformation. If $\dot{V}I$ is assumed to equal $\dot{V}E$, an error between 15% and 20% in $\dot{V}O_2$ may result (at a normal $\dot{V}O_2$ of 250 mL and RQ of 0.8), depending on patient tidal volume and respiratory frequency. The Haldane transformation[88] measures nitrogen (an insoluble gas) in inspired and expired gas to calculate $\dot{V}I$ in the following manner:

$$\dot{V}I = \frac{FEN_2}{FIN_2} \cdot \dot{V}E$$

Oxygen consumption can be rewritten as

$$\dot{V}O_2 = \left[\left(\frac{FEN_2}{FIN_2} \cdot FIO_2\right) - FEO_2\right] \cdot \dot{V}E$$

The nitrogen content is not measured but is determined by measurement of the other gases in the sample:

$$FIN_2 = 1 - (FIO_2 - FICO_2)$$
$$FEN_2 = 1 - (FEO_2 - FECO_2)$$

The resulting final equation is

$$\dot{V}O_2 = \left[\frac{(1 - FEO_2 - FECO_2) \cdot FIO_2}{(1 - FIO_2)} - FEO_2\right] \cdot \dot{V}E$$

Most manufacturers use this calculation to measure $\dot{V}O_2$ when only $\dot{V}E$ is measured. In some systems, $\dot{V}I$ is measured by pneumotachometry at the airway, but build-up of water droplets or secretions in the device generally makes this technique undesirable.

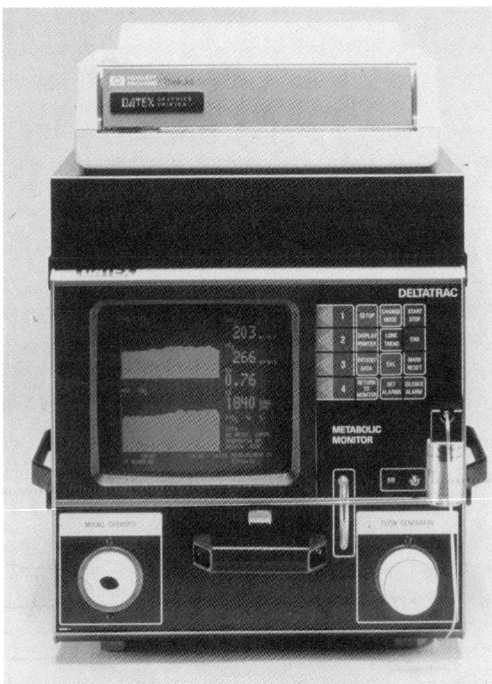

Figure 9-33. Commercially available open-circuit calorimeter.

For the open-circuit technique to work properly, the following points must be observed.[89] First, the FIO_2 must be stable (± 0.005%). In most cases, an air–oxygen blender should be used to prevent the fluctuations caused by changes in air–oxygen line pressure and instability of the mixing systems in mechanical ventilators, which tend to drift with changes in patient demand.[90] Second, the entire system must be leak free. Loss of gas from the system does not allow for complete gas collection, and addition of gas from the atmosphere causes dilution of gas concentrations. Clinically, patients with uncuffed endotracheal or tracheostomy tubes and those with bronchopleural air leaks cannot be accurately measured. Third, inspired and expired gases must be completely separated. This is especially true in continuous-flow systems.

Closed-Circuit Method

The closed-circuit method differs from the open-circuit method only in the measurement of $\dot{V}O_2$. The $\dot{V}CO_2$ measurement and calculation of energy expenditure are identical.

The key components of a closed-circuit calorimeter are a volumetric spirometer (often a rolling seal), mixing chamber, carbon dioxide analyzer, and carbon dioxide absorber. The measurement of $\dot{V}O_2$ is accomplished by filling the spirometer with a known volume of oxygen and connecting it to the

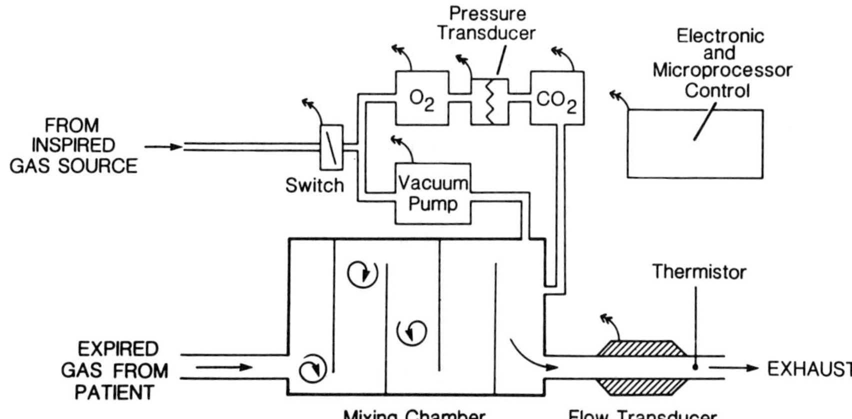

Figure 9-34. Open-circuit indirect calorimeter.

patient by mask, mouthpiece, or endotracheal tube. As the patient breathes from the spirometer, oxygen is consumed and carbon dioxide is produced. The carbon dioxide is scrubbed out of the system by a carbon dioxide absorber before the gas returns to the spirometer. The decrease in volume over time equals $\dot{V}O_2$.

Figure 9-35 depicts the movement of gases in a closed-circuit indirect calorimeter. Gas from the patient flows into the mixing chamber where gases are baffled to ensure homogeneity. A small sample of gas is withdrawn for analysis of $FECO_2$. From the mixing chamber, gas flows through a carbon dioxide scrubber and into the spirometer. Spirometer movement is electronically monitored to allow measurement of tidal volume. The difference between end-expiratory volumes is calculated at preselected intervals by the microprocessor for determination of $\dot{V}O_2$ (volume change in milliliters divided by time in seconds). During inspiration, the patient rebreathes from the spirometer. If mechanical ventilation is necessary, a bag-in-the-box system is an integral part of the inspiratory limb of the calorimeter. A bellows containing the gas to be respired is pressurized by the ventilator. The compression of the bellows results in ventilation of the patient. A series of one-way valves controls gas flow appropriately. Measurement time is limited by FIO_2 and the total volume of the spirometer. As the volume of the spirometer decreases to a critical point, the measurement must be interrupted until the spirometer is refilled with oxygen.

Critical to the accurate measurement of $\dot{V}O_2$ by the closed-circuit technique is prevention of leaks. Leaks out of the system will result in erroneously high $\dot{V}O_2$ measurements. Since the system is closed and usually pressurized, leaks into the system rarely occur. Another potential problem with the closed-circuit technique is related to ventilatory support. Since the calorimeter is placed between the patient and ventilator, compressible volume is increased and sensitivity (for triggering assisted breaths) is decreased. Depending on peak airway pressure, ventilator volume may have to be increased by 50% to 75% to ensure adequate ventilation of the patient. Generally, the closed-circuit system should not be used when patients are on low-rate intermittent mandatory ventilation or continuous-flow systems.

The major advantage of the closed-circuit technique is the ability to make measurements without being concerned about FIO_2 stability or high FIO_2 (up to 1.0).

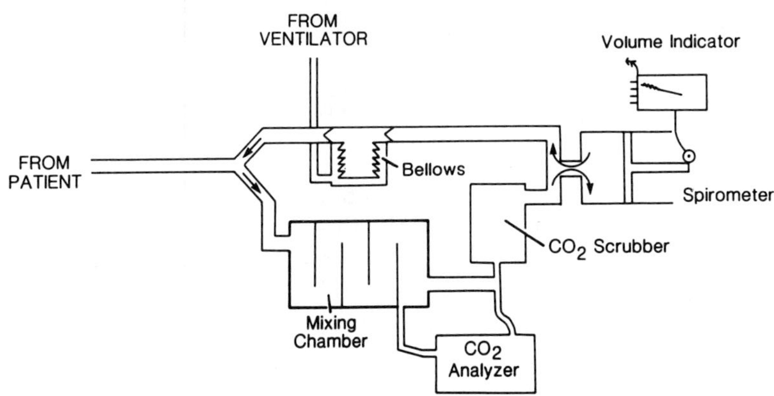

Figure 9-35. Closed-circuit indirect calorimeter.

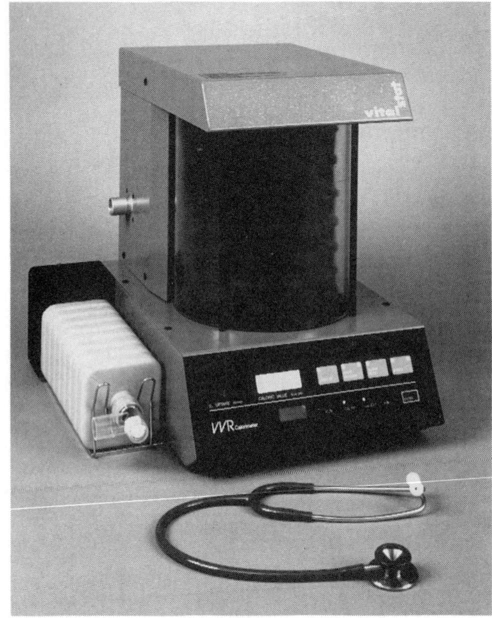

Figure 9-36. Vital Stat VVR calorimeter. (Courtesy of Vital Signs, Totowa, NJ)

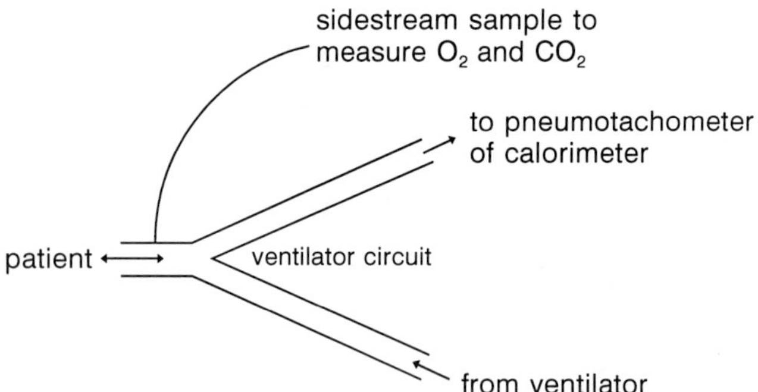

Figure 9-38. Breath-by-breath calorimeter.

Closed-Circuit Replenishment Technique

A modified version of the closed-circuit method for measuring $\dot{V}O_2$ is known as the replenishment technique.[91] Rather than measuring the volume of oxygen consumed from a spirometer, this technique determines the amount of oxygen necessary to maintain the volume of the spirometer constant. This eliminates the need for a large bulky spirometer and the need to interrupt measurements to refill the spirometer.

The Vital Stat VVR Calorimeter (Fig. 9-36) is a $\dot{V}O_2$ meter (technically it is not a calorimeter since $\dot{V}CO_2$ is not measured) specifically designed for use with mechanically ventilated patients that uses the replenishment technique. A diagram of the VVR is shown in Figure 9-37. The major components are a bellows spirometer, carbon dioxide absorber, and an ultrasonic sensor. Before testing, the system is primed with oxygen and the position of the bellows measured by the ultrasonic sensor. The patient is connected to the system and rebreathes from the bellows while carbon dioxide is removed by the carbon dioxide absorber. After a programmed number of breaths, the ultrasonic sensor determines the new position of the bellows. Since oxygen is consumed, the end-expiratory level of the bellows is raised. Calibrated pulses of oxygen, from a cylinder or bulk oxygen system, are returned to the bellows until the original level, as measured by the ultrasonic sensors, is reached. The number of pulses multiplied by the pulse volume equals $\dot{V}O_2$.

The problems with this system are the same as with the other closed-circuit systems. Also, since the bellows is contained in a rigid canister, mechanical ventilation is accomplished with the same bag-in-the-box technique.

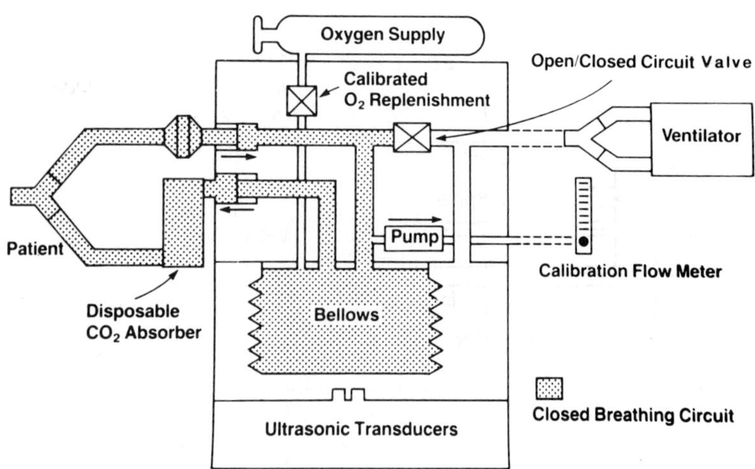

Figure 9-37. Vital Stat VVR calorimeter.

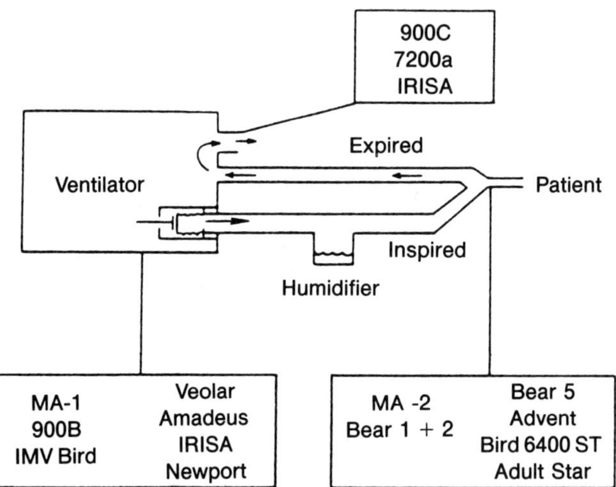

Figure 9-39. Sites where pressure is monitored in mechanical ventilator systems. (From Branson RD. Enhanced capabilities of current ICU ventilators: Do they really benefit patients? Respir Care 1991;36:362–376)

Breath-by-Breath Technique

As its name implies, the breath-by-breath technique measures $\dot{V}O_2$ and $\dot{V}CO_2$ on a breath-by-breath basis. Gases are sampled directly at the airway using a sidestream technique, and the volume of exhaled gas is measured using a pneumotachometer (Fig. 9-38). Generally, this technique is similar to the open-circuit method. It can be used with mechanically ventilated patients and with spontaneously breathing patients using a mouthpiece or canopy.

Waveforms and Mechanics During Mechanical Ventilation

In recent years, it has become possible to evaluate waveforms of pressure, flow, and volume at the bedside of mechanically ventilated patients. From these primary measurements, derived values of resistance, compliance, and work can be calculated. This technology is incorporated into the design of most current-generation microprocessor ventilators. There are also commercially available systems designed solely to monitor waveforms and mechanics during mechanical ventilation.

Site of Measurement

Pressure can be measured at a number of sites in the patient-ventilator system (Fig. 9-39).[92] Ventilator systems measure pressure in the inspiratory limb of the ventilator, in the expiratory limb of the ventilator, or at the proximal airway. Of these three sites, pressure should ideally be measured at the proximal airway. However, many ventilator systems do not measure pressure at this site due to technical limitations. Some current-generation ventilators measure pressure on the expiratory limb of the ventilator during inspiration and on the inspiratory limb during exhalation. This approximates proximal airway pressure, provided that the ventilator circuit is patent.

Most ventilator systems do not measure volume directly. They measure flow and integrate the flow signal to calculate volume. Flow monitoring sites in ventilator systems are shown in Figure 9-40.[92] Inspiratory flow and volume are measured on the inspiratory limb of the ventilator system, and expiratory flow and volume are measured on the expiratory limb of the ventilator system. One ventilator system (Hamilton) measures flow directly at the patient's airway.

Pressure can be monitored in the trachea,[93] but this is not commonly done, owing to technical limitations. The potential advantage of measuring airway pressure in the trachea is that this bypasses the high resistance (and associated pressure drop) across the endotracheal tube.

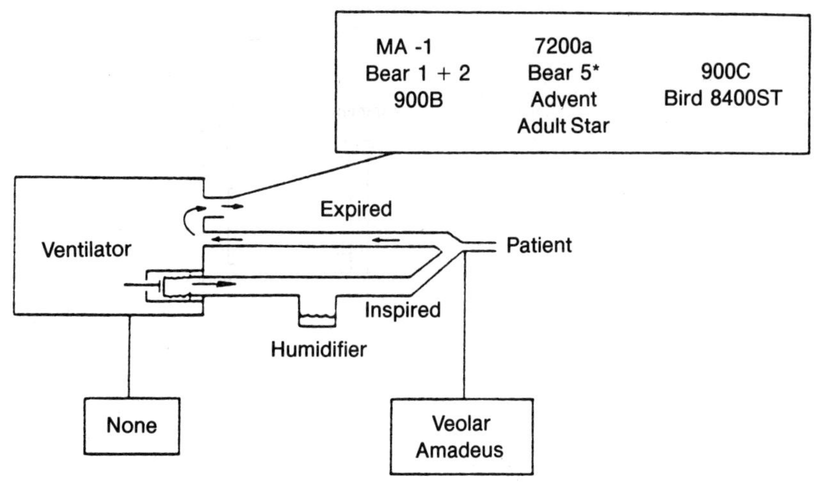

Figure 9-40. Sites where flow is monitored in mechanical ventilator systems. (From Branson RD. Enhanced capabilities of current ICU ventilators: Do they really benefit patients? Respir Care 1991;36:362–376)

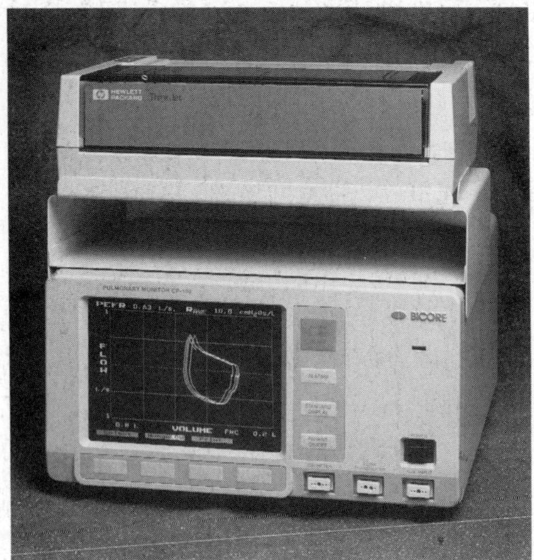

Figure 9-41. Bicore monitoring system. (Courtesy of Bicore Monitoring Systems, Irvine, CA)

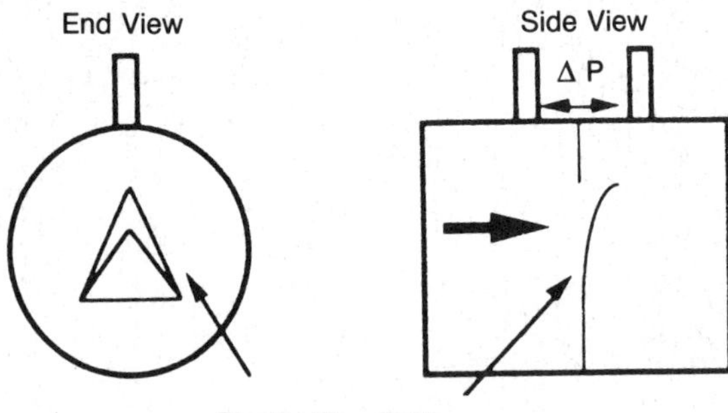

Figure 9-43. Variable orifice pneumotachometer, such as that used with the Bicore and VenTrak systems. (From East TD. What makes noninvasive monitoring tick? A review of basic engineering principles. Respir Care 1990;35:500–519)

Pressure can also be monitored in the esophagus.[94] Esophageal pressure is a reflection of intrapleural pressure. It is measured from an air-filled balloon placed in the lower third of the esophagus. The catheter is inserted into the stomach where positive pressure is measured during inspiration, then slowly withdrawn until negative pressure is measured during inspiration. The balloon is initially inflated with 6 to 10 mL of air to expand it completely, after which all of the air except 0.5 to 1.5 mL is removed. In the spontaneously breathing patient, proper placement can be assessed by having the patient breathe against an occluded airway, which should result in equal changes in airway and esophageal pressures. Gastric tubes are commercially available with a built-in esophageal balloon, which allows esophageal pressure monitoring during enteral feeding.

Several commercially available systems are available to monitor waveforms and mechanics of mechanically ventilated patients (Bicore and VenTrak) (Figs. 9-41 and 9-42). These systems measure pressure and flow at the proximal airway and are also capable of measuring esophageal pressure. They use a variable orifice pneumotachometer to measure flow (Fig. 9-43)[80] and an electronic transducer to measure pressure (see Chapter 11).

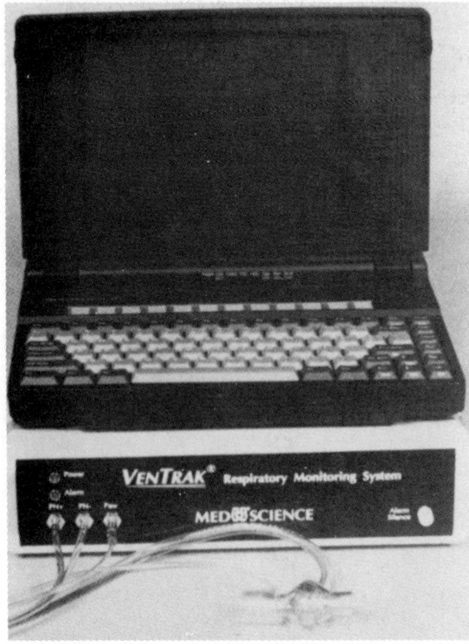

Figure 9-42. VenTrak monitoring system. (Courtesy of Novametrix Medical Systems, Wallingford, CT)

Pressure Monitoring

A typical proximal airway pressure waveform during volume ventilation is shown in Figure 9-44. The pressure during exhalation is the PEEP level. During inspiration, pressure rises to the peak pressure (Pmax).

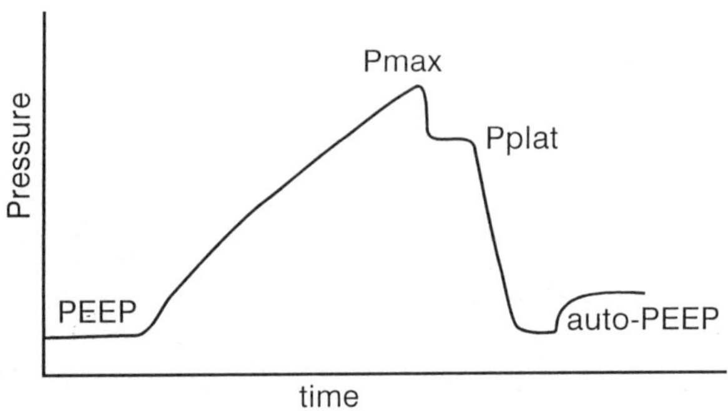

Figure 9-44. Proximal airway pressure waveform, with an end-inspiratory hold and an end-expiratory hold.

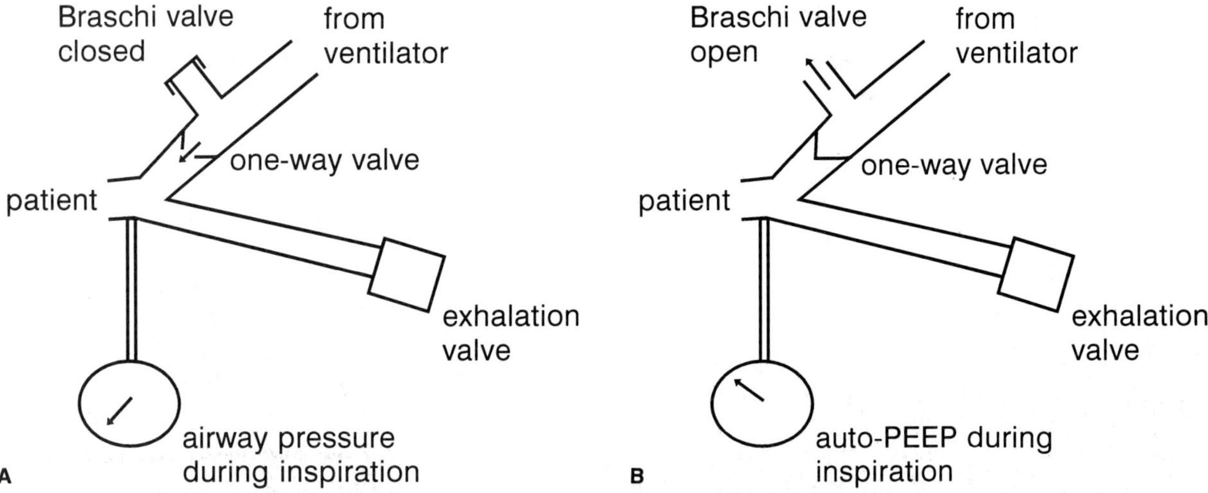

Figure 9-45. Braschi valve. (A.) When the valve is closed to the atmosphere, the ventilator operates normally and proximal airway pressure reflexes the pressure delivered during inspiration and the set PEEP level during exhalation. (B.) When the valve is opened to atmosphere during exhalation, the next breath is dumped to the atmosphere and the pressure at the proximal airway rises to the auto-PEEP level.

Pmax is determined by tidal volume, inspiratory flow, airway resistance, and lung/thorax compliance. Additional information related to airway pressure can be obtained by applying an end-inspiratory and end-expiratory hold. With an end-inspiratory hold of 0.5 to 1.5 seconds, pressure at the proximal airway equilibrates with the peak alveolar pressure, and this is commonly called plateau pressure (Pplat). With an end-expiratory hold, proximal airway pressure equilibrates with the auto-PEEP level. Most ventilator systems are capable of producing an end-inspiratory hold, and some can provide an end-expiratory hold. For those ventilators that do not provide and end-expiratory hold, a Braschi valve can be used (Fig. 9-45*A*, *B*).[94]

With pressure-targeted ventilation, the inspiratory pressure waveform approximates a square wave and end-inspiratory proximal airway pressure is virtually equivalent to peak alveolar pressure. However, due to characteristics of the ventilator system and the patient's lungs, the proximal airway pressure may not be a perfect square wave (Fig. 9-46).[95]

Monitoring tracheal pressure can be used to determine the appropriate level of pressure support to virtually eliminate the imposed work of breathing due to the endotracheal tube (Fig. 9-47).[96] Tracheal pressure measurements can also be used to trigger the ventilator. From a practical standpoint, tracheal pressure measurements are difficult and are not commonly performed.

Esophageal pressure can be used to compute chest wall compliance during controlled mechanical ventilation.[97] During spontaneous breathing, esophageal pressure monitoring allows calculation of resistance, compliance, work of breathing, and auto-PEEP. Esophageal pressure monitoring also allows patient effort during spontaneous breathing modes, such as pressure sup-

Ventilator Type	Respiratory Parameters*	Load Effect	Desired Waveform	Actual Waveform
Pressure-Controller	↑ C, ↓ R	large		
	↑ C, ↑ R	medium		
	↓ C, ↓ R	medium		
	↓ C, ↑ R	small		
Flow-Controller	↑ C, ↓ R	small		
	↑ C, ↑ R	medium		
	↓ C, ↓ R	medium		
	↓ C, ↑ R	large		

* ↑ = high; ↓ = low; C = compliance; R = resistance.

Figure 9-46. The effect of load on waveform for constant pressure and constant flow ventilators. (From Chatburn RL. A new system for understanding mechanical ventilators. Respir Care 1991;36:1123–1155)

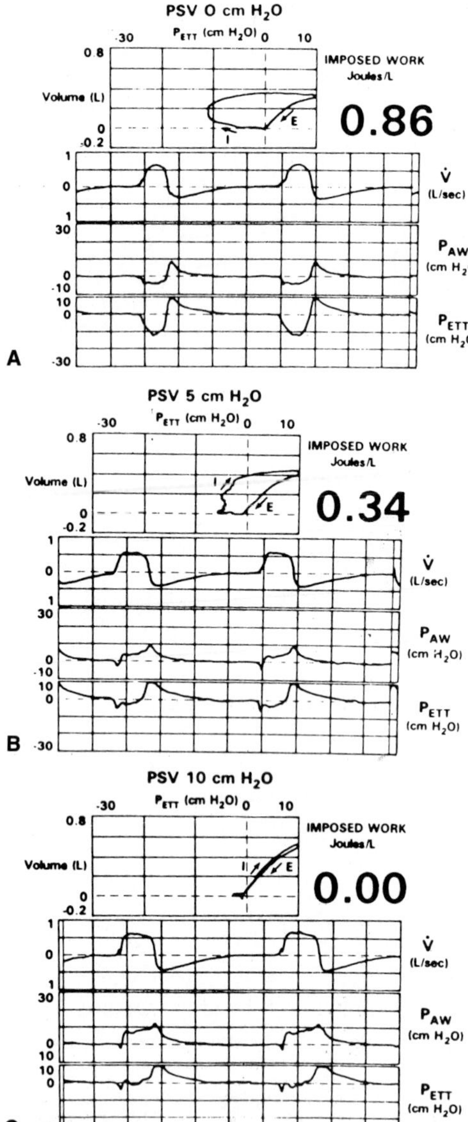

Figure 9-47. Imposed work of breathing evaluated by monitoring tracheal pressure during pressure support ventilation. Note the elimination of tracheal pressure drop during inhalation with the addition of pressure support ventilation. (From Banner MJ, Kirby RR, Blanch PB, Layon AJ. Decreasing imposed work of the breathing apparatus to zero using pressure-support ventilation. Crit Care Med 1993;21:1333–1338)

port to be evaluated (Fig. 9-48). Esophageal pressure monitoring is not commonly performed, owing to its semi-invasive nature and technical difficulties with proper placement of the esophageal balloon. Newer monitors such as the Bicore and the VenTrak, used with a gastric tube fitted with an esophageal balloon, have made these measurements easier and more reliable in the critical care unit.

Flow Monitoring

A typical flow waveform during volume-targeted ventilation is shown in Figure 9-49. During inspiration, the flow is determined by the flow setting of the ventilator (eg, square wave, sine wave, decelerating). With pressure-targeted ventilation, the inspiratory flow tapers and a period of zero flow may occur with a long inspiratory time (Fig. 9-50). Expiratory flow is determined by the characteristics of the patient's lungs and is reduced with obstructive lung disease. If auto-PEEP is present, flow will be present at end-exhalation; this method allows the detection of auto-PEEP but does not allow its measurement.

Volume Monitoring

A typical volume waveform during volume-targeted ventilation is shown in Figure 9-51. If there is a leak in the system, the volume waveform does not return to zero during exhalation. This may be particularly useful in neonatal and pediatric patients who are intubated with uncuffed airways and can be used to quantify the amount of leak around the tube (Fig. 9-52). With constant-flow ventilation, the volume increases linearly during inhalation. With constant-pressure ventilation, the volume is delivered early during inspiration.

Flow–Volume Loops

Flow can be plotted as a function of volume to produce a flow–volume loop (Fig. 9-53). The inspiratory part of the flow–volume loop is determined by the ventilator settings, and the expiratory part of the flow–volume loop is determined by the characteristics of the patient's lungs. The flow–volume loop is characteristically abnormal in patients with obstructive lung disease (Fig. 9-54). The flow–volume loop can be used to assess the response to inhaled bronchodilators (Fig. 9-55).

Volume–Pressure Loops

Volume can be plotted as a function of pressure to produce a volume–pressure loop (Fig. 9-56). The slope of the volume–pressure loop is the dynamic compliance. During constant-flow ventilation, the volume–pressure loop can be used to detect overinflation, indicating that the tidal volume should be decreased (Fig. 9-57).

Airway Resistance

Several methods can be used to estimate airway resistance during mechanical ventilation. During con-

(text continues on page 214)

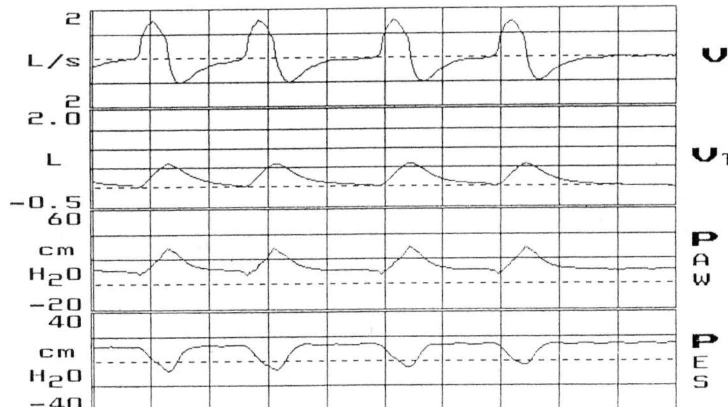

Figure 9-48. Esophageal pressure (bottom tracing) of a patient on pressure support ventilation. The large fluctuations in esophageal pressure indicate that the pressure support level is too low.

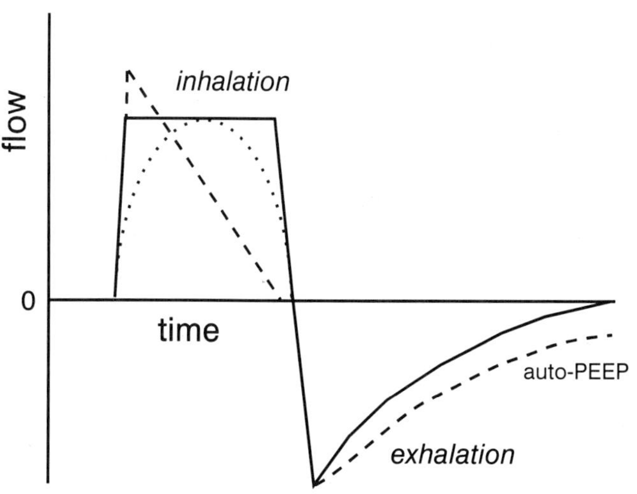

Figure 9-49. Flow waveform during mechanical ventilation. The flow above baseline occurs during inspiration and is determined by the flow setting on the ventilator. The flow below baseline is the expiratory flow.

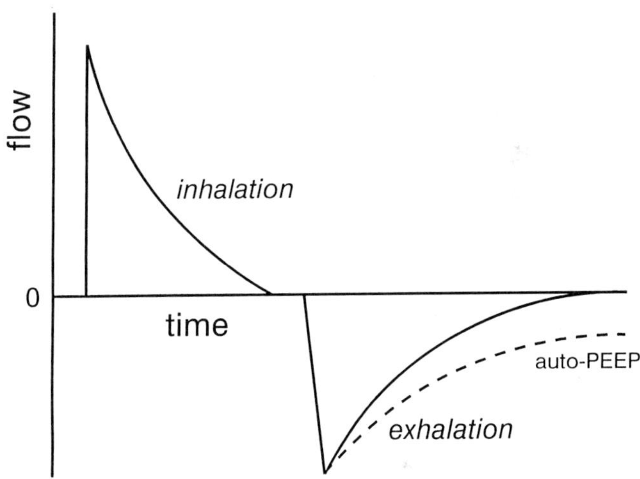

Figure 9-50. Typical flow waveforms during pressure-targeted ventilation.

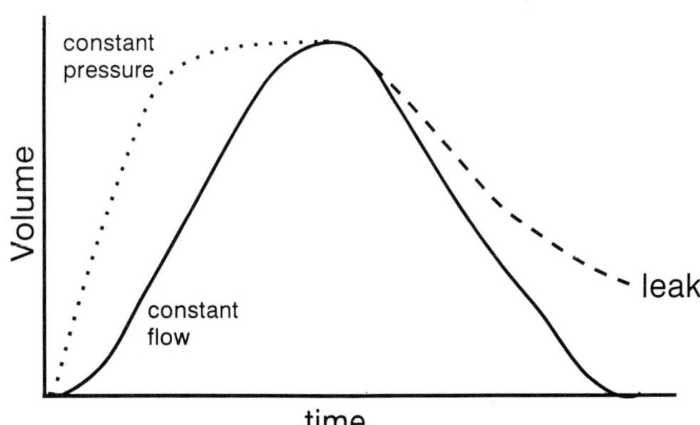

Figure 9-51. Volume waveform during mechanical ventilation. With constant pressure ventilation, the volume is delivered earlier in the inspiratory phase.

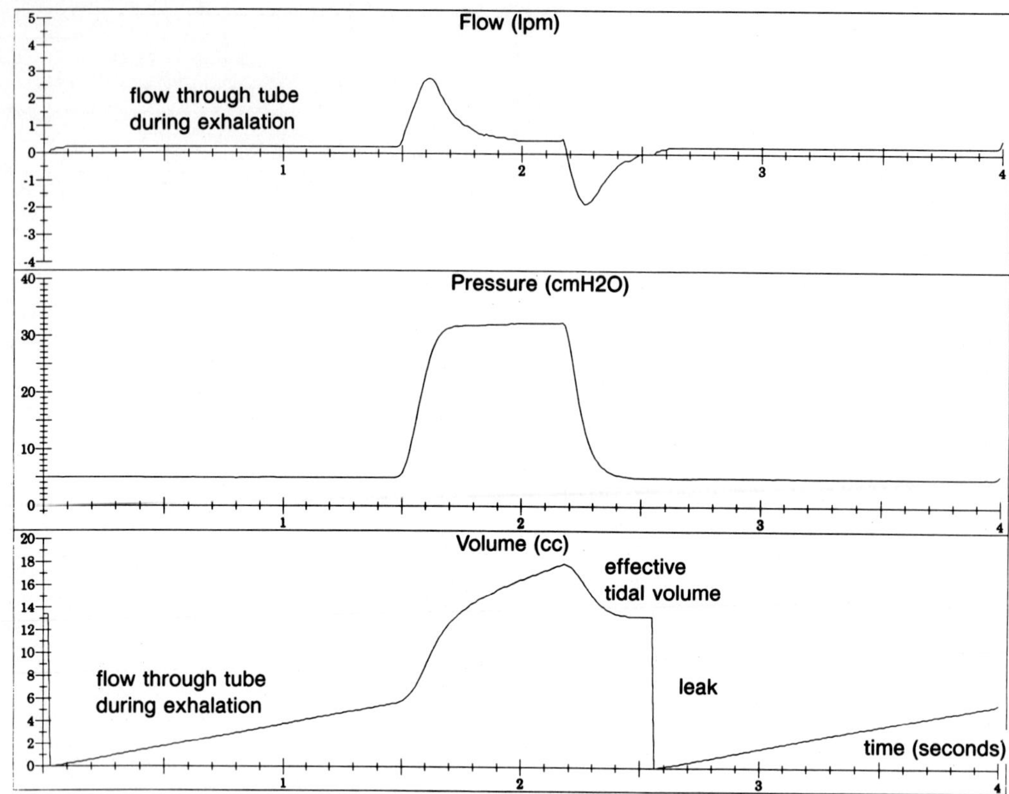

Figure 9-52. Flow, pressure, and volume waveforms of a neonatal patient with a leak around the endotracheal tube.

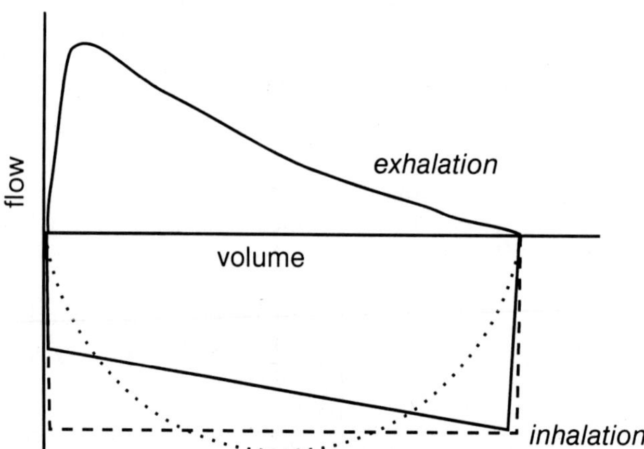

Figure 9-53. Flow–volume loop. In this example, expiratory flow is above baseline and inspiratory flow (determined by the ventilator) is below baseline.

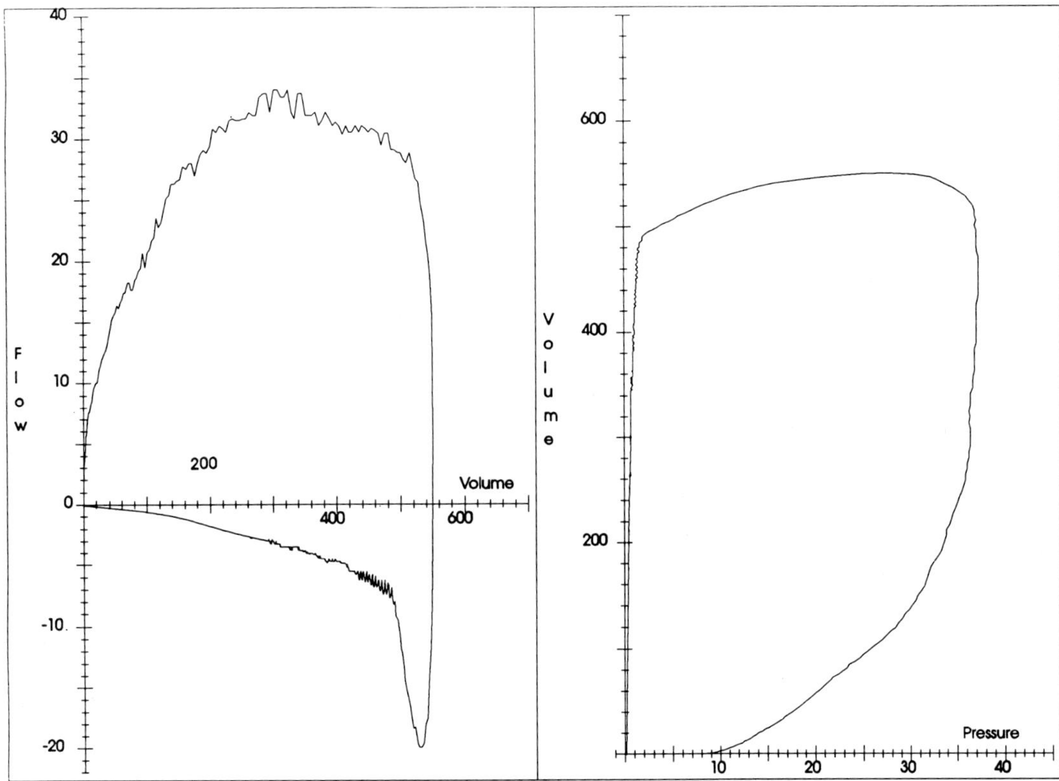

Figure 9-54. Flow—volume and volume–pressure loops of a patient with severe chronic obstructive lung disease. In this case, inspiratory flow is above baseline and expiratory flow is below baseline.

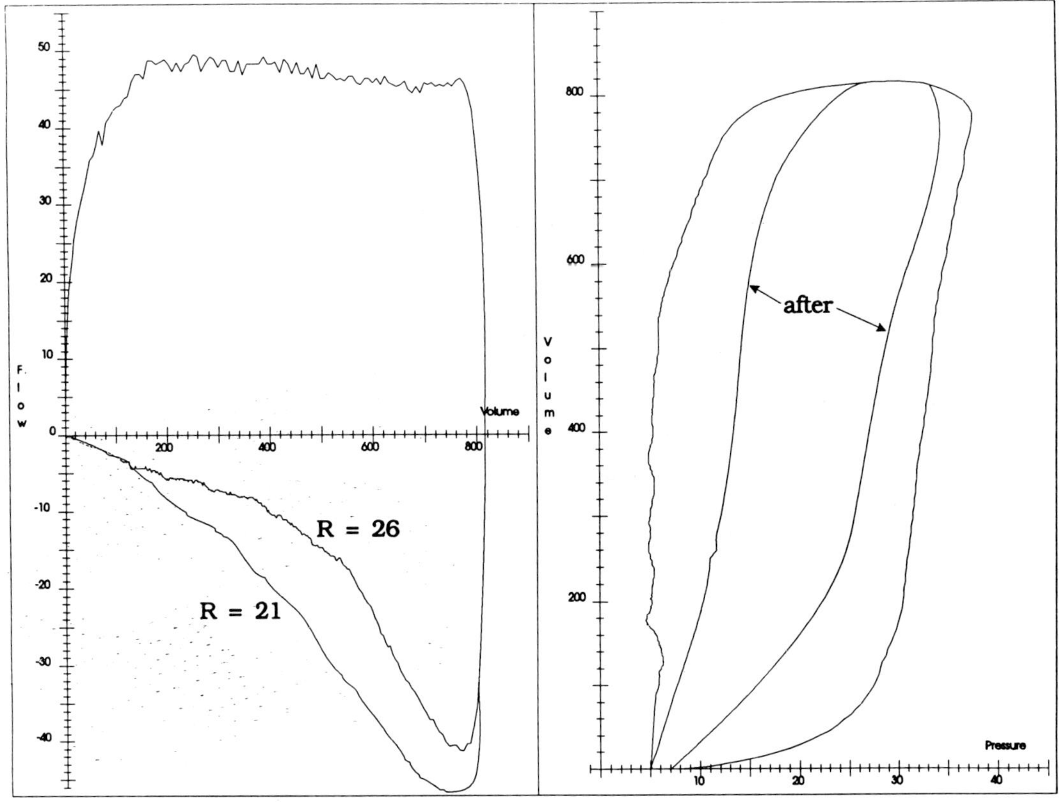

Figure 9-55. Flow-volume and volume-pressure loops of an asthmatic patient before and after administration of an inhaled bronchodilator. Expiratory flow is below baseline.

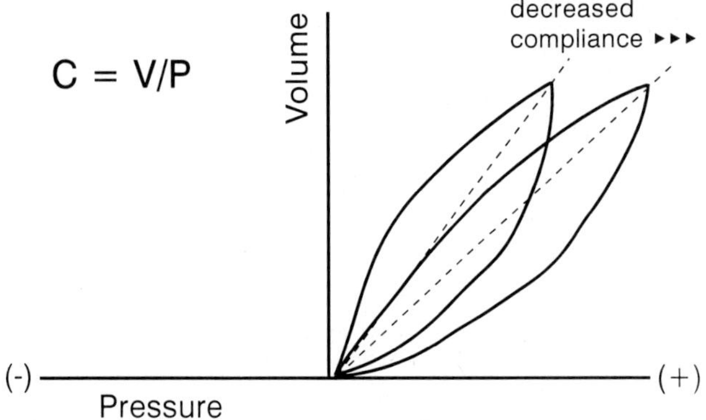

Figure 9-56. Volume–pressure loop during constant flow ventilation, with compliance line indicated.

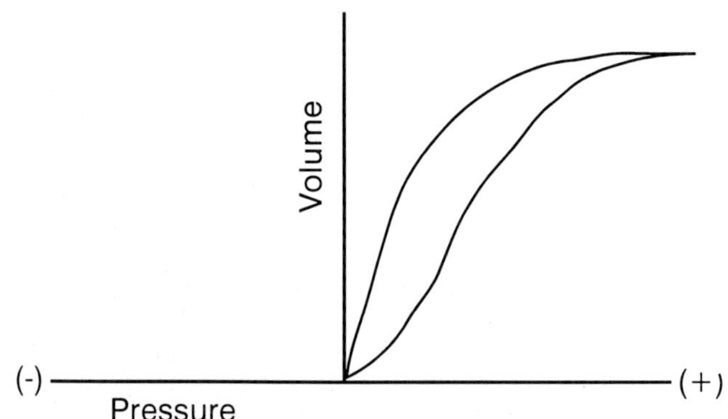

Figure 9-57. Volume–pressure loop during constant flow ventilation, with tidal volume set too high

Resistance — Jonson Method

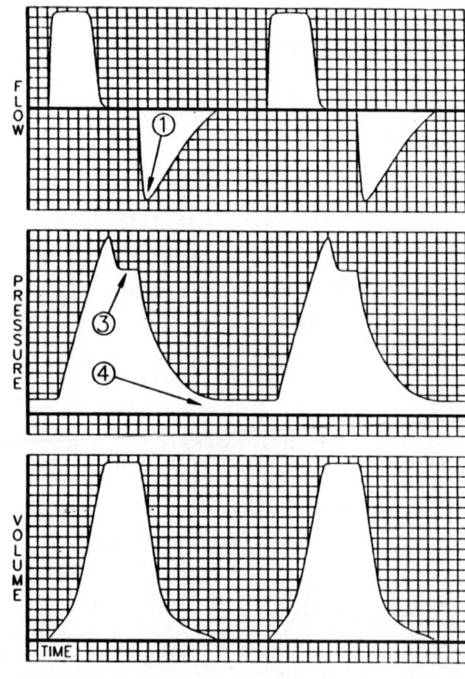

① Measure and record peak expiratory flow.

② Convert flow in step 1 from L/min to L/sec:

$$\text{Flow (L/sec)} = \frac{\text{Peak exp flow in L/min}}{60}$$

③ Measure and record plateau pressure

④ Calculate expiratory pressure drop:

Press drop = (plateau press) − (PEEP)

⑤ Calculate resistance:

$$R = \frac{\text{Pressure drop in step 4}}{\text{Peak exp flow in step 2}}$$

Figure 9-58. (A.) Technique for calculation of expiratory resistance during mechanical ventilation using the Jonson method. (B.) Technique for calculation of expiratory resistance during mechanical ventilation using the Comroe method. (C.) Technique for calculation of expiratory resistance during mechanical ventilation using the time constant method.

Resistance – Comroe Method

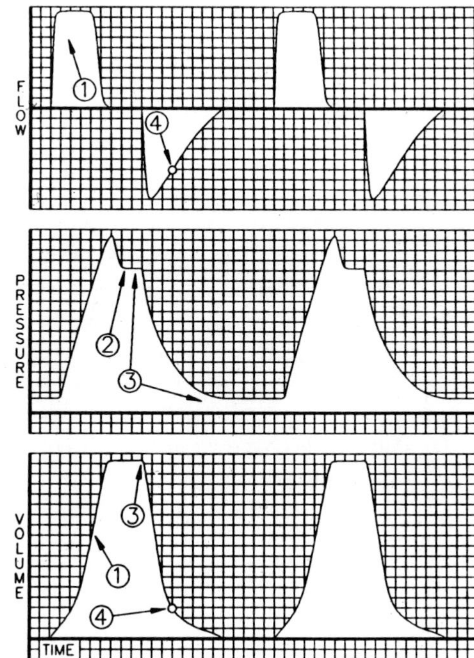

B

(1) Integrate inspiratory flow into volume through the inspiratory phase. Record volume value.

(2) Measure and record plateau pressure.

(3) Calculate compliance:

$$C = \frac{\text{Volume (step 1)}}{\text{Plateau pressure} - \text{PEEP}}$$

(4) Integrate expiratory flow until flowrate drops to 0.5 L/sec.

(5) Calculate portion of peak volume remaining in lung at 0.5 L/sec:

$$V = (\text{Vol step 1}) - (\text{Vol step 4})$$

(6) Calculate resistance for breath:

$$R = \frac{V / C}{0.5\ \text{L/sec}}$$

Where: R = Expiratory resistance
V = Volume step 5
C = Compliance step 3

Resistance – Time Constant Method

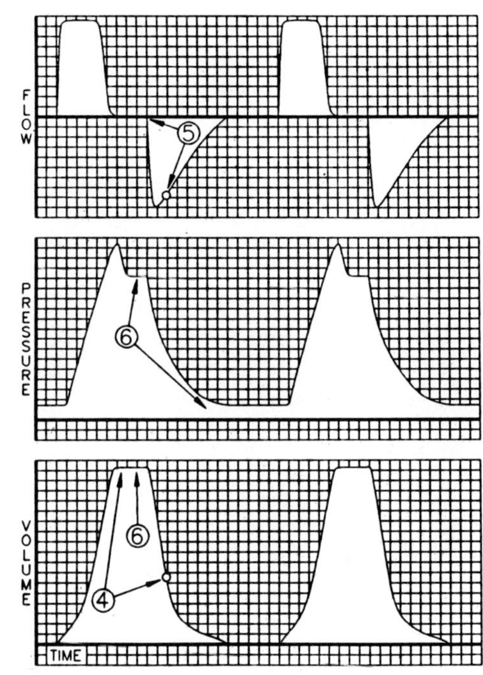

C

(1) Formula: Tau = (R)(C)

Where: Tau = 1 time constant
R = resistance
C = compliance

(2) Definition: 63% of expiratory tidal volume takes place during 1 time constant.

(3) Definition: At the end of 1 expiratory time constant, 37% of the expiratory tidal volume remains in the lung.

(4) Calculate tidal volume remaining in lung after 1 time constant:

$$\text{Vol rem} = (\text{Peak volume})(0.37)$$

(5) Measure and record time from begin expiration until exp volume in step 4.

(6) Calculate compliance:

$$C = \frac{\text{Peak volume}}{\text{Plateau pressure} - \text{PEEP}}$$

(7) Convert compliance from cc/cm to L/cm:

$$C \text{ in L/cm} = \frac{C \text{ in cc/cm}}{1000}$$

(8) Calculate resistance:

$$R = \frac{\text{Time Step 5}}{\text{Compliance step 7}}$$

Figure 9-58. continued

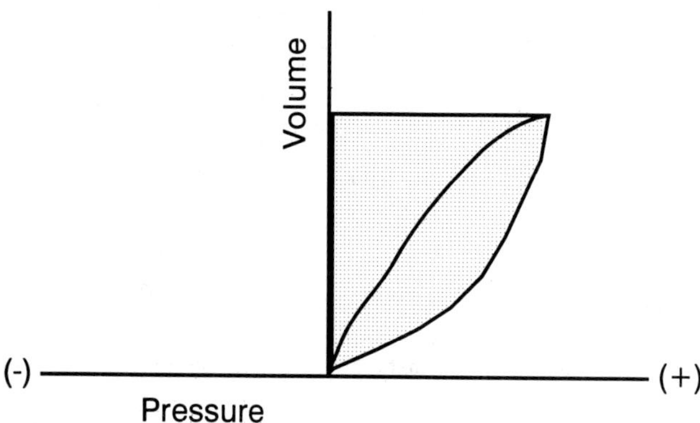

Figure 9-59. Work of breathing, as determined from the volume–pressure loop. The shaded area represents the work of breathing.

stant-flow ventilation, inspiratory resistance can be estimated as

$$Ri = \frac{Pmax - Pplat}{\dot{V}}$$

where $\dot{V}$ is the inspiratory flow. Inspiratory resistance usually significantly underestimates expiratory resistance. Expiratory resistance can be calculated as shown in Figure 9-58. Clinically, expiratory resistance is often more useful than inspiratory resistance.[98] Resistance is increased with bronchospasm, secretions, and small endotracheal tubes.

Compliance

During mechanical ventilation, static compliance can be calculated as

$$C = \frac{V_T}{Pplat - PEEP}$$

where V_T is tidal volume and PEEP is the total PEEP level (including auto-PEEP). Dynamic compliance can also be calculated as the slope of the volume–pressure curve, which is the slope of the line connecting the point of zero flow and end-inhalation and end-exhalation (see Fig. 9-56). Normal compliance during mechanical ventilation is 50 to 100 mL/cm H_2O. Disorders that can decrease compliance during mechanical ventilation include tension pneumothorax, mainstem intubation, congestive heart failure, adult respiratory distress syndrome, pleural effusion, atelectasis, consolidation, hyperinflation, fibrosis, and abdominal distention.

Work of Breathing

Work of breathing during mechanical ventilation can be calculated as the area under the volume–pressure curve (Fig. 9-59). Calculation of work of breathing is clinically difficult, unless a computerized system is used. Work of breathing is increased with an increase in resistance, a decrease in compliance, or an increase in minute ventilation. Normal work of breathing is 0.5 J/L or 0.05 kg-m/L.

AARC Clinical Practice Guideline

Pulse Oximetry: Indications, Contraindications, Hazards and Complications

Pulse oximetry provides estimates of arterial oxyhemoglobin saturation by utilizing selected wavelengths of light to noninvasively determine the saturation of oxyhemoglobin.

- Indications:
  - the need to monitor the adequacy of arterial oxyhemoglobin saturation
  - the need to quantitate the response of arterial oxyhemoglobin saturation to therapeutic intervention, or to a diagnostic procedure
  - the need to comply with mandated regulations or recommendations by authoritative groups
- Contraindications: the presence of an ongoing need for measurement of pH, PCO_2, total hemoglobin, and abnormal hemoglobin may be a relative contraindication to pulse oximetry.
- Hazards/Complications: Pulse oximetry is considered a safe procedure, but because of device limitations, false negative results for hypoxemia and/or false positive results for normoxemia or hyperoxemia may lead to inappropriate treatment of the patient. In addition, tissue injury may occur at the measuring site as a result of probe misuse.

(Adapted from AARC Clinical Practice Guideline, published in December, 1993, issue of Respiratory Care; see original publication for complete text)

References

1. Bagent RA. Oxygen analyzers. Respir Care 1976;21:410–416.
2. Wilson RS, Laver MB. Oxygen analysis: Advances in methodology. Anesthesiology 1972;37:112–126.
3. Sodal IE, Bowman RR, Filley GF. A fast-response oxygen analyzer with high accuracy for respiratory gas measurement. J Appl Physiol 1968;25:181–183.
4. Dubbers DW. Theory and development of transcutaneous oxygen pressure measurement. Int Anesthesiol Clin 1987;26 (Fall):31–65.
5. Martin R. Transcutaneous monitoring: Instrumentation and clinical applications. Respir Care 1990;35:577–583.
6. Koff PB, Hess D. Transcutaneous oxygen and carbon dioxide measurements. In: Kacmarek RM, Hess D, Stoller JK, eds. Monitoring in Respiratory Care. St. Louis, Mosby–Year Book, 1993.
7. Mahutte CK, Michiels TM, Hassell KT, et al. Evaluation of a single transcutaneous PO_2-PCO_2 sensor in adult patients. Crit Care Med 1984;12:1063–1066.

8. Severinghaus JW. Transcutaneous blood gas analysis. Respir Care 1982;27:152–159.
9. Tremper KK, Barker SJ. Transcutaneous oxygen measurement: Experimental studies and adult applications. Int Anesthesiol Clin 1987;26(Fall):67–96.
10. Rooth G, Huch A, Huch R. Transcutaneous oxygen monitors are reliable indicators of arterial oxygenation (if used correctly). Pediatrics 1987;79:283–286.
11. Cassady G. Transcutaneous monitoring in the newborn infant. J Pediatrics 1983;103:837–848.
12. Palmisano BW, Severinhaus JW. Transcutaneous PCO_2 and PO_2: A multicenter study of accuracy. J Clin Monit 1990;6:189–195.
13. Lanigan C, Ponte J, Moxham J. Performance of transcutaneous PO_2 and PCO_2 dual electrodes in adults. Br J Anaesth 1988;60: 736–742.
14. Tremper KK, Waxman K, Shoemaker WC. Effects of hypoxemia and shock on transcutaneous PO_2 values in dogs. Crit Care Med 1979;7:526–531.
15. Tremper KK, Mentelos RA, Shoemaker WC. Effect of hypercarbia and shock on transcutaneous carbon dioxide at different electrode temperature. Crit Care Med 1980;8:608–612.
16. Abraham E. Conjunctival oxygen tension monitoring. Int Anesthesiol Clin 1987:(Fall):97–112.
17. Hess D, Evans C, Thomas K, Eitel D, Kochansky M. The relationship between conjunctival PO_2 and arterial PO_2 in 16 normal persons. Respir Care 1986;31:191–198.
18. Smith M, Abraham E. Conjunctival oxygen tension monitoring during hemorrhage. J Trauma 1986;26:217–224.
19. Rutherford WF, Albertson TE, Panacek EA, Mogannam J, Fisher CJ. Deterioration of conjunctival PO_2 after CPR. Ann Emerg Med 1987;16:894–897.
20. Abraham E, Fink S. Conjunctival oxygen tension monitoring in emergency department patients. Am J Emerg Med 1988;6: 549–554.
21. Klein M, Hess D, Eitel D, Bauernshub D, Sabulsky N. Conjunctival oxygen tension monitoring during a controlled phlebotomy. Am J Emerg Med 1988;6:11–13.
22. Guerci AD, Thomas K, Hess D, et al. Correlation of transconjunctival PO_2 with cerebral oxygen delivery during cardiopulmonary resuscitation in dogs. Crit Care Med 1988;16:612–614.
23. Abraham E, Fink S. Conjunctival oxygen tension monitoring in emergency department patients. Am J Emerg Med 1988;6: 549–554.
24. Pologe JA. Pulse oximetry. Technical aspects of machine design. International Anesthesiology Clinics 1987;26(Fall):137–153.
25. Welsh JP, DeCesare R, Hess D. Pulse oximetry: Instrumentation and clinical applications. Respir Care 1990;35:584–601.
26. Kelleher JF. Pulse oximetry. J Clin Monit 1989;5:37–62.
27. Severinghaus JW, Kelleher JF. Recent developments in pulse oximetry. Anesthesiology 1992;76:1018–1038.
28. Mendelson Y, Kent JC, Yocum BL, Birle MJ. Design and evaluation of a new reflectance pulse oximeter sensor. Med Instrument 1988;22:167–173.
29. Cheng EY, Hopwood MB, Kay J. Forehead pulse oximetry compared with finger pulse oximetry and arterial blood gas measurements. J Clin Monit 1988;4:223–226.
30. Berge KH, Lanier WL, Scanlon PD. Ischemic digital skin necrosis: A complication of the reusable Nellcor Pulse Oximeter probe. Anesth Analg 1988;67:712–713.
31. Barker SJ, Tremper KK. Pulse oximetry: Applications and limitations. Int Anesthesiol Clin 1987;26(Fall):155–176.
32. Barker SJ, Tremper KK. The effect of carbon monoxide inhalation on pulse oximetry and transcutaneous PO_2. Anesthesiology 1987;66:677–679.
33. Harris K. Noninvasive monitoring of gas exchange. Respir Care 1987;32:544–557.
34. Barker SJ, Tremper KK, Hyatt J, Zaccari J. Effects of methemoglobinemia on pulse oximetry and mixed venous oximetry. Anesthesiology 1987;67:A170.
35. Tremper KK, Nickerson BG. Oximeters (letter). Chest 1988;94: 1110–1113.
36. Fanconi S, Doherty P, Edmonds JF, Barker GA, Bohn DJ. Pulse oximetry in pediatric intensive care: Comparison with measured saturations and transcutaneous oxygen tension. J Pediatr 1985;107:362–366.
37. Harris AP, Sendak MJ, Donham RT, Thomas M, Duncan D. Absorption characteristics of human fetal hemoglobin at wavelengths used in pulse oximetry. J Clin Monit 1988;4:175–177.
38. New W. Pulse oximetry. J Clin Monit 1985;1:126–129.
39. Veyckemans F, Baele P, Guillaume JE, Willems E, Robert A, Clerbaux T. Hyperbilirubinemia does not interfere with hemoglobin saturation measured by pulse oximetry. Anesthesiology 1989;70: 118–122.
40. Scheller MS, Unger RJ, Kelner MJ. Effects of intravenously administered dyes on pulse oximetry readings. Anesthesiology 1986;65:550–552.
41. Kurki TS, Sanford TJ, Smith NT, Dec-Silver H, Head N. Effects of radial artery cannulation on the function of finger blood pressure and pulse oximeter monitors. Anesthesiology 1988;69: 778–782.
42. Cote CJ, Goldstein A, Fuchsman WH, Hoaglin DC. The effect of nail polish on pulse oximetry. Anesth Analg 1988;67:683–686.
43. Jubran A, Tobin MJ. Reliability of pulse oximetry in titrating supplemental oxygen in ventilator-dependent patients. Chest 1990;97:1420–1425.
44. Kochansky M. Oximetry, technology, and the Medicare Guidelines. Respir Care 1986;31:1185–1187.
45. Carlin BW, Clausen JL, Ries AL. The use of cutaneous oximetry in the prescription of long-term oxygen. Chest 1988;94:239–241.
46. Hess D, Kochansky M, Hassett L, Frick R, Rexrode WO. An evaluation of the Nellcor N-10 Portable Pulse Oximeter. Respir Care 1986;31:796–802.
47. Hess D, Mohlman A, Kochansky M, Kriss T. An evaluation of the accuracy of the Physio-Control Lifestat 1600 pulse oximeter in measuring arterial oxygen saturation. Respir Care 1987;32: 19–23.
48. Chapman KR, D'Urzo A, Rebuck AS. The accuracy and response characteristics of a simplified ear oximeter. Chest 1983; 83:86–864.
49. Severinghaus JW, Naifeh KH. Accuracy of response of six pulse oximeters to profound hypoxia. Anesthesiology 1987;67:551–558.
50. Yelderman M, New W. Evaluation of pulse oximetry. Anesthesiology 1983;59:349–352.
51. Hess D, Kacmarek RM. Techniques and devices for monitoring oxygenation. Respir Care 1993;38:646–671.
52. Carbon dioxide monitors. Health Devices 1986;15:255–285.
53. Paloheimo MPJ. A carbon dioxide monitor that does not show the waveform has value. J Clin Monit 1988;4:210–212; Block FE. A carbon dioxide monitor that does not show the waveform is worthless. J Clin Monit 1988;4:213–214.
54. Hess D. Capnometry and capnography: Technical aspects, physiologic aspects, and clinical applications. Respir Care 1990;35: 557–576.
55. Gravenstein JS, Paulus DA, Hayes TJ. Capnography in Clinical Practice. Butterworths, Boston, 1989.
56. Raemer DB, Francis D, Philip JH, Gabel RA. Variation in PCO_2 between arterial blood and peak expired gas during anesthesia. Anesth Analg 1983;62:1065–1069.
57. Whitesell R, Asiddao C, Gollman D, Jablonski J. Relationship between arterial and peak expired carbon dioxide pressure during anesthesia and factor influencing the difference. Anesth Analg 1981;60:508–512.
58. Lindahl SGE, Yates AP, Hatch DJ. Relationship between invasive and noninvasive measurements of gas exchange in anesthetized infants and children. Anesthesiology 1987;66:168–175.
59. Phan CQ, Tremper KK, Lee SE, Barker SJ. Noninvasive monitoring of carbon dioxide: A comparison of the partial pressure of transcutaneous and end-tidal carbon dioxide with the partial pressure of arterial carbon dioxide. J Clin Monit 1987;3:149–154.
60. Jones NL, Robertson DG, Kane JW. Difference between end-tidal and arterial PCO_2 in exercise. J Appl Physiol 1979;47:954–960.
61. Moorthy SS, Losasso M, Wilcox J. End-tidal PCO_2 greater than $PaCO_2$. Crit Care Med 1984;12:534–535.
62. Hoffman RA, Kreiger BP, Kramer MR, et al. End-tidal carbon dioxide in critically ill patients during changes in mechanical ventilation. Am Rev Respir Dis 1989;140:1265–1268.
63. Hess D, Schlottag A, Levin B, Mathai J, Rexrode WO. An evaluation of the usefulness of end-tidal PCO_2 to aid weaning from mechanical ventilation following cardiac surgery. Respir Care 1991; 36:837–843.

64. Graybeal JM, Russell GB. Capnometry in the surgical ICU: An analysis of the arterial-to-end-tidal carbon dioxide difference. Respir Care 1993;38:923–928.
65. Yamanaka MK, Sue DY. Comparison of arterial-end-tidal P_{CO_2} difference and dead space/tidal volume ratio in respiratory failure. Chest 1987;92:832–835.
66. Hatle L, Rokseth R. The arterial to end-expiratory carbon dioxide tension gradient in acute pulmonary embolism and other cardiopulmonary disease. Chest 1974;66:352–357.
67. Weil MH, Bisera J, Trevino RP, Rackow EC. Cardiac output and end-tidal carbon dioxide. Crit Care Med 1985;13:907–909.
68. Sanders AB, Ewy GA, Bragg S, Atlas M, Kern KB. Expired P_{CO_2} as a prognostic indicator of successful resuscitation from cardiac arrest. Ann Emerg Med 1985;14:948–952.
69. Trevino RP, Bisera J, Weil MW, Rackow EC, Grundler WG. End-tidal CO_2 as a guide to successful cardiopulmonary resuscitation: A preliminary report. Crit Care Med 1985;13:910–911.
70. Falk JL, Rackow EC, Weil MH. End-tidal carbon dioxide concentration during cardiopulmonary resuscitation. N Engl J Med 1988;318:607–611.
71. Carlon GC, Ray C, Miodownik S, Kopec I, Groeger JS. Capnography in mechanically ventilated patients. Crit Care Med 1988;16:550–556.
72. Swedlow DB. Capnometry and capnography: The anesthesia disaster early warning system. Semin Anesth 1986;5:194–205.
73. Owen RL, Cheney FW. Use of an apnea monitor to verify endotracheal intubation. Respir Care 1985;30:974–976.
74. Murray IP, Modell JH. Early detection of endotracheal tube accidents by monitoring carbon dioxide concentration in respiratory gas. Anesthesiology 1983;59:344–346.
75. Hess D, Eitel D. Monitoring during resuscitation. Respir Care 1992;37:739–768.
76. Lichtiger M. Recent advances in clinical monitoring: Mass spectrometry. Curr Rev Clin Anesth 1985;5:115–119.
77. Riker JB, Haberman B. Expired gas monitoring by mass spectrometry in a respiratory intensive care unit. Crit Care Med 1976;4:223–229.
78. Ayres SM. Use of mass spectrometry for evaluation of respiratory function in the critically ill patient. Crit Care Med 1976;4: 219–222.
79. Yukulis R, Snyder JV, Powner D, Fusco D, Grenvik A. Mass spectrometry monitoring of respiratory variables in an intensive care unit. Respir Care 1978;23:671–679.
80. East TD. What makes noninvasive monitoring tick? A review of basic engineering principles. Respir Care 1990;35:500–519.
81. Graybeal JM, Russell GB. Relative agreement between raman and mass spectroscopy for measuring end-tidal carbon dioxide. Respir Care 1994;39:190–194.
82. Branson RD, Hurst JM. Nutrition and respiratory function: Food for thought. Respir Care 1988;33:89–92.
83. Askanazi J, Elwyn DH, Silverberg PA, Rosenbaum SH, Kinney JM. Respiratory distress secondary to a high carbohydrate load: A case report. Surgery 1980;87:596–598.
84. Covelli HD, Black JW, Olsen MW, Beckman JF. Respiratory failure precipitated by high carbohydrate loads. Ann Intern Med 1981;95:579–581.
85. Dark DS, Pingleton SK, Kerby GR. Hypercapnia during weaning: A complication of nutritional support. Chest 1985;88: 141–143.
86. Damask MC, Schwarz Y, Weissman C. Energy measurements and requirements of critically ill patients. Crit Care Clin 1987;3: 71–96.
87. Weir JB. New method for calculating metabolic rate with special reference to protein metabolism. J Physiol 1949;109:1–9.
88. Ultman JS, Burszstein S. Analyses error in the determination of respiratory gas exchange at varying F_{IO_2}. J Appl Physiol 1981;50: 210–216.
89. Branson RD. The measurement of energy expenditure: Instrumentation, practical considerations, and clinical application. Respir Care 1990;35:640–659.
90. Browning JA, Lindberg SE, Turney SF, et al. The effects of fluctuating F_{IO_2} on metabolic measurements in mechanically ventilated patients. Crit Care Med 1982;10:82–85.
91. Branson RD, Hurst JM, Davis K, Pulsfort R. A laboratory evaluation of the Biergy VVR calorimeter. Respir Care 1988;33: 341–347.
92. Branson RD. Enhanced capabilities of current ICU ventilators: Do they really benefit patients? Respir Care 1991;36:362–376.
93. Banner MJ, Kirby RR, Blanch PB, Layon AJ. Decreasing imposed work of the breathing apparatus to zero using pressure-support ventilation. Crit Care Med 1993;21:1333–1338.
94. Kacmarek RM, Hess D. Airway pressure, flow, and volume waveforms, and lung mechanics during mechanical ventilation. In: Kacmarek RM, Hess D, Stoller JK. Monitoring in Respiratory Care. St. Louis, Mosby–Year Book, 1993.
95. Chatburn RL. A new system for understanding mechanical ventilators. Respir Care 1991;36:1123–1155.
96. Banner MJ, Blanch PB, Kirby RR. Imposed work of breathing and methods of triggering a demand-flow continuous positive airway pressure system. Crit Care Med 1993;21:183–190.
97. Banner MJ, Jaeger MJ, Kirby RR. Components of the work of breathing and implications for monitoring ventilator-dependent patients. Crit Care Med 1994;22:515–523.
98. Hess D, Tabor T. Comparison of six methods to calculate airway resistance during mechanical ventilation in adults. J Clin Monit 1993;9:275–282.

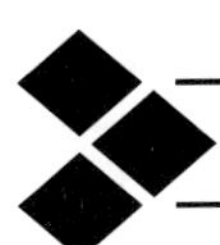

10

Flow and Volume Measuring Devices

F. Herbert Douce

OBJECTIVES

1. Explain the characteristics of volume and flow measuring devices including accuracy, precision, and linearity.
2. Describe the operation and limitations of volume displacement spirometers.
3. Describe the operation and limitations of flow measuring devices.
4. Describe the operation and limitations of thermistors, turbinometers, and sonic flow measuring devices.
5. Describe the operation and limitations of body and respiratory inductive plethysmography.

KEY TERMS

accuracy
ATPS
ATS
bellows spirometer
body plethysmography
calibration
capacity
dry rolling seal spirometer
error
inertia
linearity
peak flowmeter
plethysmography
pneumotachograph
pneumotachometer
potentiometer
precision
respiratory inductive plethysmography
respirometer
spirometer
spirometry
turbinometer
volume
volume displacement spirometer
water-sealed spirometer
WEDGE spirometer

Introduction

Measuring respiratory volumes and flow rates for patient monitoring, pulmonary function screening, and diagnostic testing can be accomplished by a wide variety of instruments and principles of measurement. These instruments are commonly divided into two broad categories: (1) devices that directly measure gas volumes and (2) devices that directly measure gas flow rates. In this chapter the discussion focuses on describing the general characteristics of volume and flow measuring devices, various principles of measurement used by these instruments, and the clinical application of the principles. Specific examples of volume and flow measuring devices and the professional standards applied to diagnostic spirometers are also included. Many diagnostic pulmonary function testing systems are computerized, as described in Chapter 21.

General Characteristics of Volume and Flow Measuring Devices

Regardless of the general type of device and the specific principle of measurement, there are several characteristics that are common to all volume and flow measuring devices. Every measuring instrument has the characteristics of capacity, accuracy, error, precision, linearity, durability, simplicity of operation, maintenance of asepsis, output, and cost.[1-3]

The *capacity* of an instrument refers to how much it can measure; capacity is also referred to as the range or limits of measurement. The capacity of a volume measuring device is how small as well as how large a volume it can measure; the capacity of a flow measuring device is how slow and fast a flow rate it can measure. Both of these devices also have a time capacity—how long the device will measure volume or flow during any specific test or measurement.

The *accuracy* of a measuring instrument is how well it measures a known reference value. A volume or flow measuring device is perfectly accurate if it indicates values identical to reference values for volume or flow. For volume measurements, standard reference values are provided by a graduated 3-L calibration syringe.[4] When 3 L is injected into a volume or flow measuring device and the device indicates 3 L, then the device is perfectly accurate for volume. For flow measurements, known reference values can be provided by constant-flow precision rotometers, by dynamic-flow forced vital capacity simulators, and by Hankinson's system of computerized forced vital capacity waveforms.[5] However, no measuring instrument is perfect, and there is usually an arithmetic difference between known reference values and measured reference values; this difference is called *error*. Accuracy and error are opposite and complementary terms; the greater the accuracy, the smaller the error. The sum of the percent accuracy and percent error always equals 100%. To determine percent accuracy and percent error (see Equation Box 10-1), measure several known reference values, compute the mean of the measured reference values, and compare the mean measured value to the known reference value.

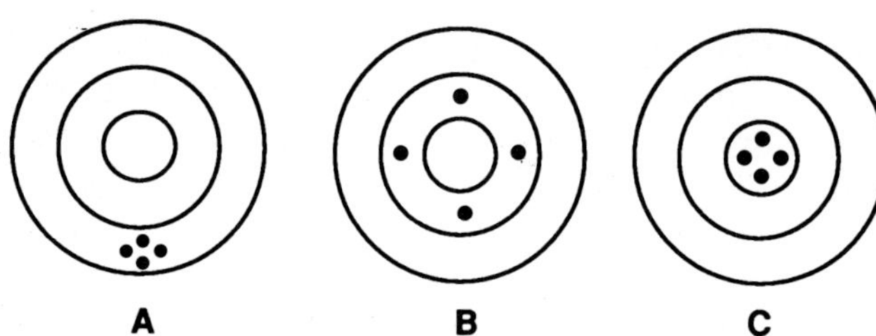

Figure 10-1. Target analogy for accuracy. In target A, the measurements are precise but not certain. In target B, the measurements are near the center but scattered; there is certainty but little precision. In target C, the measurements are accurate; they have certainty and precision.

Precision is synonymous with reproducibility and is a measure of the reliability of measurements. The standard deviation of the mean measured reference values is the statistic that indicates the relative precision of an instrument. The classic target analogy depicts the concepts of precision, certainty, and accuracy (Fig. 10-1). When the measurements of reference values cluster together the instrument is precise. When the measurements of reference values are close to the known reference value but not clustered, the instrument has certainty. Only when the measurements of reference values are certain and precise is the instrument accurate.[6]

Linearity refers to the accuracy of the instrument over its entire range of measurement or its capacity.

Equation Box 10-1: Accuracy and Error

To determine percent accuracy and percent error, measure several known reference values, compute the mean of the measured reference values, and compare the mean measured value to the known reference value.

$$\%\ \text{Accuracy} = \frac{\text{Mean measured reference value}}{\text{Mean known reference value}} \cdot 100$$

$$\%\ \text{error} = \frac{\text{Mean known reference value} - \text{mean measured reference value}}{\text{Mean known reference value}} \cdot 100$$

Some devices may accurately measure large volumes or high flow rates but may be less accurate when measuring small volumes or low flow rates. To determine linearity, one must calculate accuracy and precision at different points over the entire range or capacity of the device and plot measured reference values against known reference values on a graph. On the graph, a linear instrument has a slope of 1.0 and a y-intercept of 0.0 (Fig. 10-2).

Durability is an important characteristic of any medical instrument. Most clinical volume and flow measuring devices are frequently used by many practitioners and patients. Under the stress of high utilization these instruments must be durable to remain accurate and precise. An accurate, precise, and linear device is worthless if it is always broken. *Simplicity of operation* and *maintaining asepsis* are also important practical characteristics. Consider warm-up time, calibration procedures, the number and sequence of buttons, and the ability to clean and disinfect the device. Some excellent devices are complex and require extensive operator training and frequent calibration.[1]

The characteristic of *output* includes the form of the output and the content of the output. Every measuring instrument communicates or "outputs" its measurements. The form of the communication may be an indicating needle on a dial, a digital display, a graph with volume and time axis, or a graph with flow and volume axis; or there may be a RS-232 computer connection and interface, and a computer will calculate, display and print the measurements (see Chapter 21). Some instruments have more than one method of output. The content of the output includes the specific measurements made or computed by the instrument and the conditions of measurement. Some volume and flow measuring devices measure the forced vital capacity and forced expiratory volume in 1 second (FEV_1); others may also calculate a variety of forced expiratory flow rates, while some measure tidal volume and minute ventilation. Some devices report measurements at ambient temperature (ATPS); others output at body temperature (BTPS) conditions. The performance of each volume and flow measuring device compared with national standards for diagnostic spirometers and the specific output of the device determines its appropriate clinical application.

National Performance Standards and Clinical Applications

In 1978, the American Thoracic Society (ATS) adopted standards for diagnostic spirometers for the characteristics of capacity, accuracy, error, linearity, and graphic recordings.[7] These standards, which were updated in 1987 and include a detailed methodology of evaluating spirometers, have been adopted by other medical organizations and government agencies, including the National Institute of Occupational Safety and Health (NIOSH) and the Social Security Administration (Table 10-1).[4] Spirometer sales literature often indicates that ATS standards are met or exceeded. Some spirometers have been independently evaluated against the ATS standards or compared with instruments that meet those standards.[8–20]

According to the ATS standards, when measuring the vital capacity and forced expiratory flow rate in 1 second, a diagnostic spirometer should have a capacity of at least 7 L, measure flow rates between 0 and 12 L/s, and have less than 3% error or measure within 50 mL of a reference value, whichever is greater. When measuring a slow vital capacity, the spirometer should be able to measure for up to 30 seconds, and for the forced vital capacity the time capacity should be at least 15 seconds. A diagnostic spirometer that measures flow should be at least 95% accurate (or within 0.2 L/s, whichever is greater) over the entire 0 to 12 L/s range of gas flow. A summary of the recommen-

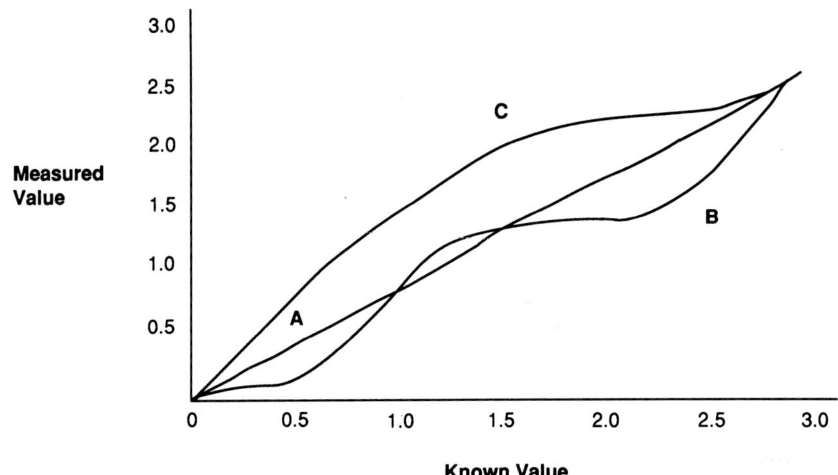

Figure 10-2. Linearity. Line A indicates a linear measuring device. Lines B and C indicate nonlinear devices that are accurate at specific points.

TABLE 10-1. Minimal Spirometry Standards Summary

Test	Range/Accuracy BTPS (L)	Flow Range (L/s)	Time (s)	Resistance and Back-Pressure	Test Signal
VC	7 L ± 3% of reading or ± 0.05 L, whichever is greater	0 to 12	30		3-L calibrating syringe
FVC	7 L ± 3% of reading or ± 0.05 L, whichever is greater	0 to 12	15		24 standard waveforms
FEV_1	7 L ± 3% of reading or ± 0.05 L, whichever is greater	0 to 12	1	Less than 1.5 cm H_2O/L/s, from 0 to 12 L/s	24 standard waveforms
Time zero	The time point from which all FEV_1 measurements are taken			Determined by back extrapolation	
FEF 25–75	7 L ± 5% of reading or ± 0.200 L/s, whichever is greater	0 to 12	15	Same as FEV_1	24 standard waveforms
$\dot{V}$	12 L/s ± 5% of reading or ± 0.200 L/s, whichever is greater	0 to 12	15	Same as FEV_1	Manufacturer proof
MVV	Sine wave 250 L/min at V_T of 2 L within ±5% of reading	0 to 12 ±5%	12 to 15 ±3%	Pressure less than ± 10 cm H_2O at 2-L V_T 2.0 Hz	Sine wave pump 0 to 4 Hz ± 10% at ± 12 L/s

dations is provided in Tables 10-1 and 10-2. Diagnostic spirometers that meet the ATS standards must provide a graphic recording of sufficient size for hand measurements and analysis.

Diagnostic spirometers usually measure and calculate vital capacity, forced vital capacity, forced expiratory flow rate in 1 second, peak expiratory flow rate, and forced expiratory flow rates, and some measure and calculate maximum voluntary ventilation and inspiratory volumes and flow rates. Some of these instruments may be a component of a laboratory system to provide the volume or flow measuring capability for other diagnostic tests of pulmonary function. For example, they are used with gas analyzers or a body plethysmograph to measure thoracic gas volume, functional residual capacity, and total lung capacity, or to measure the inspiratory vital capacity during the single-breath diffusing capacity (D_LCO_{SB}).

TABLE 10-2. Minimum Required Scale Factors for Volume, Flow, and Time Graphics for Diagnostic Spirometric Measurements

Variable	Resolution Required	Scale Factor
Volume	0.050 L	5 mm/L
Flow	0.20 L/s	2.5 mm/L/s
Time	20 ms	1 cm/s

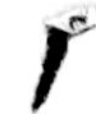

The 1978 ATS standards had a significant impact on the quality of instrumentation available. In response to these standards, some manufacturers produced more accurate, precise, and linear devices with larger capacities while others redefined their market to nondiagnostic spirometry and bedside respiratory assessments. The 1987 ATS standards for diagnostic spirometers expand the application of the standards to include clinical and epidemiologic purposes as well as cardiopulmonary diagnostic testing.[4] With the updated standards there may no longer be an appropriate utilization of volume and flow measuring devices that fail to meet or exceed the ATS Standards. The newer standards recommend at least 15 seconds for measuring the forced vital capacity, whereas the original standard indicated only 10 seconds. As a result, some devices that met the 1978 standards may not meet the 1987 updated standards. In Tables 10-3 through 10-8 of this chapter, appropriate clinical applications of devices that substantially comply with the ATS standards are "diagnostic spirometry" and "diagnostic spirometry and pulmonary function testing" when the measuring device may be incorporated in a laboratory system. "Nondiagnostic spirometry" is listed for those devices that do not substantially comply with the standards.

The ATS standards do not apply to those devices that measure tidal volume and minute ventilation and count frequency; these devices are suited for measuring spontaneous ventilatory parameters and for checking tidal volumes and minute ventilation during continuous mechanical ventilation. The devices that are not adversely affected by water vapor and condensation are appropriate and well suited for continuous or long-term monitoring of spontaneous or mechanically assisted ventilation. Some ventilators have a volume or flow measuring device built in or as a monitoring option.

Volume Measuring Devices

Volume measuring devices are also called volume displacement spirometers or volume collecting devices. In general, these instruments tend to mechanically collect an expired volume of gas into a leakproof and expandable container; the expansion of the container is designed to be linear, and the container is calibrated for volume. These devices are inherently simple, accurate for measuring volumes, and dependable. Because mechanical parts must move as the container expands, the forces of inertia, friction, and momentum and the effect of gravity need to be minimized in the design of these instruments to measure volumes and calculate flow rates accurately and precisely.

The measurements made by volume displacement devices can be recorded directly on moving graph paper, or their expandable component can be fitted with a potentiometer that provides an electrical output signal for a digital readout or computer interface. Volume displacement devices often incorporate an electronic circuit called an analogue differentiator that integrates the volume signal with time to calculate and indicate flow rates. Having a direct, real-time mechanical recording as well as an electrical output for a computer interface is a distinct advantage of most volume displacement spirometers because there is not a total dependence on computer-generated data.

Volume displacement spirometers linearly expand with expiration and contract with inspiration, but the exhaled or inhaled gas volumes and the volume actually measured by these spirometers are not identical. The temperature of gas that occupies the lungs is body temperature (37°C) and fully saturated with water vapor. As gas is exhaled, it tends to cool to ambient temperature; and according to Charles' law, as the temperature decreases the volume also decreases. As the gas cools some of the water vapor condenses and forms water droplets, which causes an additional volume loss. For measurements of inspired gases the opposite mechanisms occur; gas volume expands when heated and humidified by the body.

Corrections from the measuring conditions to body conditions are necessary for accurate measurements of gas volumes and flow rates by volume displacement spirometers, although the validity of the correction for some spirometers has been questioned.[8,21,22] All recorded volumes are routinely converted from ambient temperature and saturated (ATPS) conditions to body temperature and saturated (BTPS) conditions so that the actual volume exhaled or inhaled by the subject can be calculated.[4] Ambient temperature is measured by a mercury, alcohol, or electronic thermometer that is placed within most volume displacement spirometers, or a constant value such as 25°C is assumed.[23] Computerized spirometers often automatically convert output signals to BTPS conditions; otherwise, conversion tables or slide rules facilitate the conversion.

Volume displacement spirometers are more commonly found in pulmonary function laboratories than at the bedside or in intensive care units. These devices are often the gas volume and flow rate measuring component of a complete pulmonary function testing system and provide the volume and flow rate measuring capability for all pulmonary function tests. There are three distinctly different types of volume collecting containers, including water-sealed spirometers, bellows spirometers, and dry rolling seal spirometers; and within each general type of volume measuring device, the configuration and characteristics can also vary. These three types of spirometers and their different configurations are described in this section, and specific examples are listed in Table 10-3.

Water-Sealed Spirometers

The first type of volume displacement device is also the oldest. In 1846, John Hutchinson used a water-sealed bell to measure the vital capacity.[24,25] A "bell" is actually a cylinder with one open end and one closed end; this cylinder is submerged in water, which creates a leakproof seal and provides minimal resistance to movement. Water-sealed bell spirometers are accurate, precise, and linear as long as the bell shape remains cylindrical and there are no leaks in the bell or tubing. Water-sealed bells are generally less portable than other devices because of the weight of the water and the splashing that can occur. Water also provides the opportunity for corrosion and bacterial growth within the instrument, although using "soft" or distilled water and weekly draining and replacing the water can minimize these potential problems. Cleaning the water cavity can also be difficult, but the risks of cross-infection between subjects are considered minimal.

To obtain a direct volume output from a water-sealed, bell-type spirometer that is not equipped to provide electrical output or digital readouts, the recording of bell movement can be seen on graph paper graduated for volume, or the recording pen's vertical movement can be measured in millimeters

TABLE 10-3. Examples of Volume Displacement Spirometers and Clinical Applications

Classification	Manufacturer/Model	Applications
Water Sealed	Warren E. Collins 9.0 & 13.5 L Respirometer	Nondiagnostic spirometry Parameters of ventilation
	Warren E. Collins Stead-Wells Survey Spirometer, Eagle and APEX systems	Diagnostic spirometry and pulmonary function testing
	Sensormedics 2400 (formerly Godart)	Diagnostic spirometry and pulmonary function testing
	S & M Instrument Co. Pyramid II	Diagnostic spirometry and pulmonary function testing
Bellows		
Horizontal	Jones Medical Instrument Co. Pulmonor II and Pulmonaire 10	Diagnostic spirometry and pulmonary function testing
Vertical	Puritan-Bennett Monitoring Spirometer	Continuous ventilation monitoring of tidal volume
	Puritan-Bennett PS 600	Diagnostic spirometry
Diagonal	American Electromedics Corp. Airomax 629V	Diagnostic spirometry
	Cybermedic CM-110	Diagnostic spirometry and pulmonary function testing
	Med-Science 570 WEDGE Spirometer	Diagnostic spirometry and pulmonary function testing
	Vitalograph Spirometer and S-Model Spirometer	Diagnostic spirometry
Dry Rolling Seal		
Horizontal	Cardio-Pulmonary Instr. Corp. Model 220	Diagnostic spirometry and pulmonary function testing
	Ohio Medical Products Model 822 Spirometer	Diagnostic spirometry and pulmonary function testing
	Sensormedics 922 (formerly Ohio Medical)	Diagnostic spirometry and pulmonary function testing
	Spirotech S400 and S500	Diagnostic spirometry and pulmonary function testing
	Vacumed UCI-500 & PC Spiropak	Diagnostic spirometry and pulmonary function testing
Vertical	S & M Instr Co. VSR 2000 and Vacumed Vicatest-3	Diagnostic spirometry
	Sensormedics Pulmograph & 2450 (formerly CPI)	Diagnostic spirometry and pulmonary function testing

and multiplied by the "bell factor." Bell factors are used to convert vertical distances measured in millimeters on graph paper to volume in millimeters. Examples of bell factors are 20.45 mL/mm for a 10.0-L bell to 41.73 mL/mm for a 13.5-L bell. Each size bell has its own bell factor, which is equivalent to the volume contained in a cross-section of 1 mL of cylinder height. It is dependent on the cross-sectional area of the bell, which is a function of the radius of the bell. The recording system of a water-sealed bell spirometer is known as a kymograph, and there are often several controlled speeds of paper movement. Common kymograph speeds are 1920 mm/min (or 32 mm/s) for recording the forced vital capacity; 160 mm/min (or 32 mm/12 s) for recording the maximum voluntary ventilation or the single breath diffusing capacity, and 32 mm/min for recording minute ventilation and oxygen consumption. There are two configurations of water-sealed bell spirometers.

Chain-Compensated Spirometers

The original water-sealed bell is also called a chain-compensated spirometer (Fig. 10-3). This spirometer incorporates a metal bell with a capacity of 9 or 13.5 L. Because of the weight of the bell, the bell is counterbalanced by a chain and pulley system. A counterweight equal to the weight of the bell is designed to minimize the force of gravity, but the additional mass of the counterweight increases the inertia and momentum of the system. This configuration produces a recording that is inverted because when the bell rises during an exhalation the pen attached to the counterweight falls, and when the bell falls during an inspiration the pen rises. The pulley can be fitted with a rotary potentiometer for electrical output signals to provide a computer interface.

The chain-compensated spirometer with metal bell is excellent for recording quiet breathing, minute ventilation, and oxygen consumption. With the addition of nitrogen, helium, and carbon monoxide analyzers, it can also be used to measure lung volumes and diffusing capacity. Because of the inertia and momentum of the metal bell and counterweight, these spirometers do not meet the criteria for diagnostic measurements of forced expiratory volumes and maximal voluntary ventilation.[11] Replacing the metal bell with a plastic one and reducing the counterweight enhances the performance of these spirometers for measuring pulmonary mechanics.

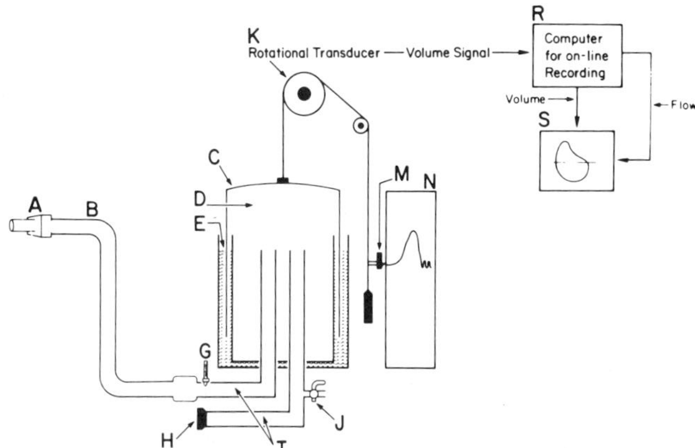

Figure 10-3. Chain-compensated, water-sealed, volume-displacement spirometer. This spirometer uses a metal or lightweight plastic bell (C) placed over a hollow cylinder (D). The patient forcefully exhales through large-bore tubing (B) into the bell. As the bell rises, the pen (M) traces a curve representing the exhaled volume on the paper attached to the rotating drum (N). A stopcock (J) on one of the inlet tubes allows filling with special gas mixtures when necessary (ie, helium and oxygen mixture). A thermometer (G) is placed in the inlet for ambient air recording. The output voltage from the rotational potentiometer (K) may be used as volume input to a computer (R) for on-line recording and calculation. The computer may be used to derive a flow signal, which may then be sent out along with the volume signal to an X-Y recorder (S). A, mouthpiece and valve; E, water seal; H, stopper; I, spirometer tubes. (From Miller WF, Scacci R, Gast LR. Laboratory Evaluation of Pulmonary Function. Philadelphia: JB Lippincott, 1987)

Stead-Wells Spirometer

The second type of water-sealed bell spirometer was created because of the weight of the metal bell and problems with bell movement during rapid breathing maneuvers such as forced vital capacity and maximum voluntary ventilation. Stead and Wells[26] redesigned the water-sealed spirometer specifically for rapid breathing tests. Their design incorporates a 7-, 10-, or 14-L lightweight plastic bell that eliminates the need for counterbalancing (Fig. 10-4). The graph recorded by a Stead-Wells spirometer is direct: when the bell rises with an exhalation, the recording pen rises; and when the bell falls with an inspiration, the pen falls. The Stead-Wells spirometer can be fitted with a linear potentiometer to provide an electrical output signal. The Stead-Wells spirometer meets all of the criteria for diagnostic spirometry and is often considered the standard on which other volume displacement instruments are compared.[11,12,18,19,23]

Bellows Spirometer

The second general type of volume displacement device is the bellows spirometer. These instruments expand and contract like an accordion with one fixed and one movable plate, and there are several configurations of bellows movement. The Jones 10-L bellows spirometer unfolds horizontally; as gas enters the bellows, it expands in a horizontal direction or motion. Another configuration of bellows movement is vertical, and some bellows expand in a diagonal motion using a hinge on one end to connect the plates. One of the bellows spirometers that expands diagonally and horizontally is also known as the WEDGE spirometer. WEDGE is an acronym for Waterless, Effortless, Data-Generating, Electro-mechanical spirometer.[27] Other hinged bellows spirometers are sometimes called wedge bellows because of their shape when partially inflated (Fig. 10-5).

Some of the configurations that have a vertical movement or a diagonal-vertical movement can be affected by gravity and significantly underestimate volumes and flow rates; some vertical bellows spirometers, such as the Puritan-Bennett Monitoring Spirometer, are used only for tidal volume monitoring during volume-oriented intermittent positive pres-

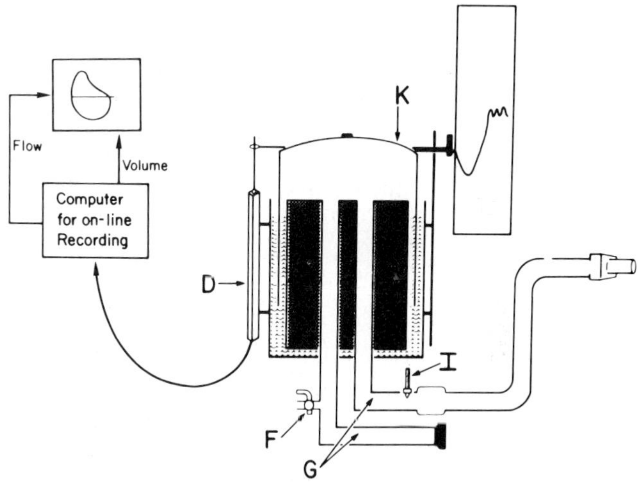

Figure 10-4. Stead-Wells water-sealed volume-displacement spirometer. The Stead-Wells spirometers use a lightweight plastic bell (K) and a water seal to contain the exhaled air. A pen is attached directly to the spirometer bell and produces a volume-time tracing upside down from that produced by the chain-compensated spirometer. A stopcock is available for adding special gases (F), and a thermometer (I) is placed in an inlet for ambient temperature recording. A linear potentiometer (D) is attached to the spirometer bell and produces a voltage output proportional to volume as the bell moves up and down. This voltage output may be used by a computer for automatic processing of test results. The computer can integrate the volume signal to obtain flow, and these outputs may be sent to an X-Y recorder for display. G indicates the spirometers tube, one of which is stoppered. (From Miller WF, Scacci R, Gast LR. Laboratory Evaluation of Pulmonary Function. Philadelphia: JB Lippincott, 1987)

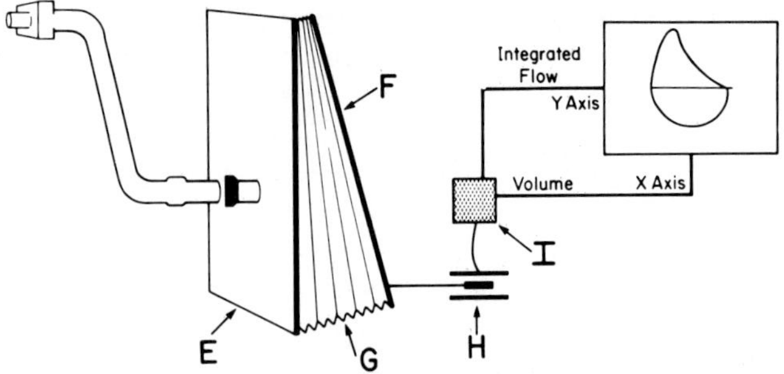

Figure 10-5. Typical bellows or WEDGE spirometer. This spirometer uses an accordian-type folding bellows (G) to attach a lightweight movable bellows plate (F) to a fixed front plate (E). As gas enters the spirometers, the bellows unfolds and the bellows plate moves outward. A rod attached to the bellows plate is attached to a linear potentiometer (H), which provides an output voltage to the spirometer electronics (I) that is proportional to volume. This spirometer also contains differentiating circuitry that provides for direct recording of computer processing. Internal electronic calibration signals are available for standardizing external displays, and adjustments for changing output signals from ATPS to BTPS are also contained in this spirometer.

sure breathing or continuous mechanical ventilation. Some manufacturers, such as Vitalograph and Puritan-Bennett in their model PS 600, have compensated for their vertical movement against gravity with springs and gears, and these devices are used for diagnostic spirometry.

The bellows are commonly composed of a soft and compliant silicone rubber or polyvinylchloride (PVC) material that is important for minimizing the inertia and friction of bellows movement and expansion. The compliance of a bellows spirometer can be temperature dependent; cold environments can decrease the compliance, and warm environments can increase the compliance. When measuring volumes in ambient temperature that deviate from normal room temperature of 22°C to 25°C, changes in bellows compliance can affect accuracy and precision.[8] The bellows of all newer Vitalograph spirometers are composed of polythene, which is less susceptible to temperature variations.[21]

With multiple exhalations into a bellows spirometer, the folds of the bellows may become wet and stick and not open in a uniform manner, which may create nonlinearity. Aged bellows may tear and leak along the folds, which may not be identified by an accuracy check with a 3-L syringe.[28] These potential problems may be minimized by periodically fully expanding the bellows to dry it and performing leak tests for at least 15 seconds.[28] Some bellows spirometers can require up to 30 mL of exhaled gas to inflate the bellows before any expansion and recording pen movement occurs, which may affect accuracy for measuring small volumes.[23]

The movable plate can have a pen attached to mechanically record bellows expansion or a potentiometer for providing an electrical output signal or both.

Dry Rolling Seal Spirometer

The third general type of volume displacement spirometer incorporates a movable piston attached to a cylinder by a soft, flexible rolling seal (Fig. 10-6). The piston is usually lightweight aluminum, which minimizes the effects of inertia and momentum. The piston moves in a horizontal direction, which minimizes the effect of gravity, or in a vertical direction. The size of the cylinder is usually 8 to 12 L with a large diameter, so a large volume change occurs with a small movement of the piston. With the rolling seal of silicone rubber or plastic, the short piston movements offer minimal friction or resistance. Although a pen can be attached to the piston rod to record volume on graduated graph paper, a rotary potentiometer can also be attached to the piston rod for electrical output signals of volume and flow rates.

Similar to the bellows spirometers, failure to clean and dry the piston and rolling seal can cause the piston to stick and hesitate during breathing maneuvers. Hesitations of piston movement could affect accuracy of flow rate as well as volume measurements. Dry rolling seal spirometers are often used in diagnostic spirometry and pulmonary function testing.

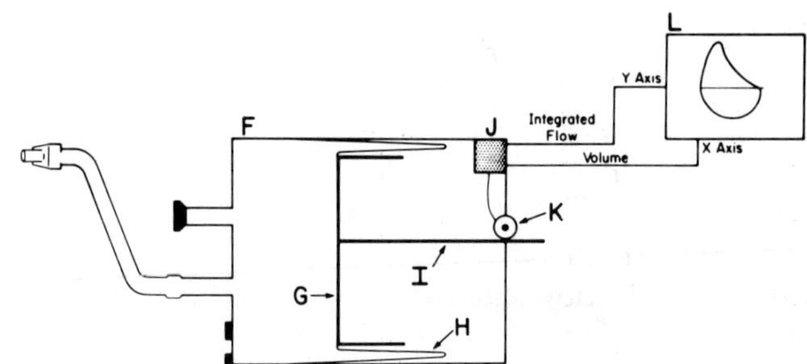

Figure 10-6. Typical rolling-seal spirometer. This spirometer (F) uses a lightweight aluminum piston (G) attached to the inside of a cylinder by a soft, flexible seal (H). As the patient forcefully exhales, the seal rolls between the piston and the sides of the cylinder. A rod (I) attached to the piston causes the voltage on a rotational potentiometer to change, producing a voltage output proportional to the volume change in the spirometer. The volume signal is also differentiated electronically (J) and made available as a flow signal. Thus, both a flow and volume signal are available as outputs from this spirometer. One or both of these signals may be displayed on an X-Y recorder (L) or input into a computer for automatic processing. These spirometers also have a built-in electronic calibration signal for external display devices as well as electronics that adjusts the spirometer output signal from ATPS to BTPS. (From Miller WF, Scacci R, Gast LR. Laboratory Evaluation of Pulmonary Function. Philadelphia, JB Lippincott, 1987)

Flow Measuring Devices

The second general category of instruments directly measures gas flow rates and electronically integrates flow rate to provide a calculated measurement of volume. Flow measuring devices are also called pneumotachometers, although some practitioners reserve the name pneumotachometer for devices that use the gas flow measuring device originally designed by Fleisch.[6,29] Flow measuring devices are generally smaller, lighter, and more portable; many are more dependent on electronics and less mechanical than volume displacement devices. Because airflow is the primary measurement, factors that can affect flow, such as gas density and viscosity, can affect the accuracy and precision of some of these instruments. In other instruments, humidity can be an important variable.

There are four distinctly different devices for measuring gas flow rates, including pneumotachometers, thermistors, turbinometers, and sonic devices. Peak flowmeters comprise a fifth group of devices. Within each of these five broad classifications there are a variety of instruments with important distinctions.

Pneumotachometers

The original flow measuring device was described by Fleisch in 1925, and since then there have been several modifications in an attempt to improve the original design. All of these devices measure a pressure created by breathing through a very low resistance. The newer modifications have been in structure and in materials used to create the resistance. This principle of measurement is based on Poiseuille's law of laminar flow and on the definition of airflow resistance (see Chapter 1). If the resistance is constant, known, and low enough so that flow is not limited by that resistance, during expiration against the resistance there is a small but measurable increase in pressure. During inspiration there is a small decrease in pressure on the proximal side of the resistance. A differential pressure transducer is used to measure the change in pressure across the resistance, and flow rates are calculated by dividing the pressures by the value of the resistance (Fig. 10-7). The remaining variables of Poiseuille's law (viscosity, radius, and length) are additional factors that can affect the accuracy and precision of pneumotachometers.[30] All three factors can affect the resistance, but only viscosity of the gases being measured is a factor that can vary in clinical use. As a result, pneumotachometers should be calibrated with gas of a viscosity similar to the gas that is to be measured. Since temperature affects viscosity, the temperature of the calibrating gas should also be similar to that being measured.[31]

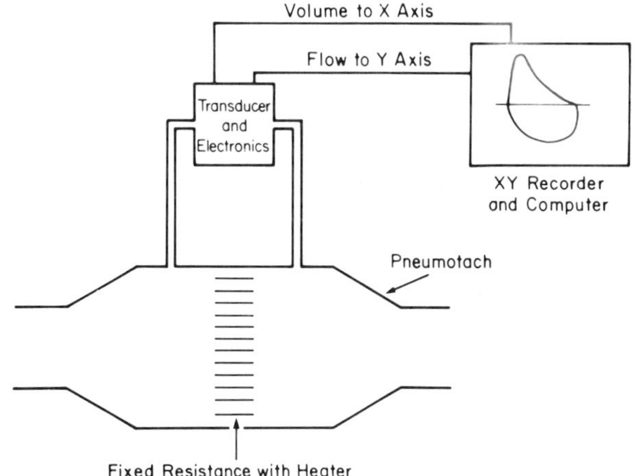

Figure 10-7. The Fleisch-type pneumotachometer. (From Miller WF, Scacci R, Gast LR. Laboratory Evaluation of Pulmonary Function. Philadelphia, JB Lippincott, 1987)

Inspiratory and expiratory gases differ in composition and temperature. Room air has a viscosity of approximately 184 poise. The viscosity of oxygen is 206 poise, the viscosity of carbon dioxide is 149 poise, and viscosity of water vapor is only 120 poise. The proportions of these gases differ between inhalations and exhalations with more carbon dioxide and water vapor and less oxygen in exhaled air. Therefore, exhaled air should have a lower viscosity than inhaled air. Temperature also affects viscosity. An increase in temperature increases viscosity. At least for room air, the differences in gas composition and temperature for inhaled air and exhaled air tend to cancel out their effects on viscosity. When gas mixtures other than room air are being measured, such as a mixture of 80% helium/20% oxygen, a bag-in-box system may be needed to ensure accurate measurements.[30,32]

The pneumotachometer principle of measurement is valid for measuring laminar flow, but the presence of turbulent flow creates unpredictably high pressures and inaccurately high measurements. Therefore, these instruments have been designed to minimize turbulence. Using a cone-shaped adapter to connect smoothbore tubing to a large-diameter resistance element are common strategies to minimize turbulence. Electronic linearizers that reduce the gain from the pressure transducer at high flow rates are also used to compensate for the presence of turbulence.

Fleisch Pneumotachometer

The Fleisch pneumotachometer is the standard to which all other flow measuring devices are compared.[3,9,33,34] Several companies manufacturer Fleisch pneumotachometers, and specific examples are listed in Table 10-4. The resistance of the Fleisch pneumotachometer is created by breathing through a bundle of

TABLE 10-4. Examples of Fleisch-type Pneumotachometers and Clinical Applications

Manufacturer/Model	Applications
American Electromedics Corp. SPIROcomp	Diagnostic spirometry
Brentwood Instruments, Inc. Sprioscan 1000 & 2000	Diagnostic spirometry
Cavitron SC-20	Diagnostic spirometry
CDX Corp. Spiro 110	Diagnostic spirometry
Cybermedic Medistor II	Diagnostic spirometry
Cybermedic CM-160	Diagnostic spirometry and pulmonary function testing
Erich Jaeger Inc. Pneumotac	Diagnostic spirometry and pulmonary function testing
Fukuda Sangyo Model ST-100/ST-200	Diagnostic spirometry
Hewlett Packard 47402A	Diagnostic spirometry and pulmonary function testing
Med-Science Model 4000	Diagnostic spirometry
Medical Equipment Design, Inc. MultkSPIRO SA/100	Diagnostic spirometry
MAS Inc. PEDS	Continuous ventilation monitoring and mechanics of breathing
Puritan-Bennett REMAC	Diagnostic spirometry and lung volumes
Spirometrics Flowmate	Diagnostic spirometry and pulmonary function testing

brass capillary tubes, and a differential pressure transducer provides for both inspiratory and expiratory pressure and flow measurements. Fleisch pneumotachometers are available in several different sizes and resistances for different ranges of flow rate measurements. In the original Fleisch design, the capillary tubes are heated to approximately 37°C in an attempt to prevent condensation within the capillary tubes and to ensure that measurements are being made under BTPS conditions. If condensation occurs and some of the capillary tubes became clogged with water droplets, the resistance of the device will increase to an unknown value, and all volume and flow rate measurements will be falsely increased.[31] In Fleisch pneumotachometers that are not heated above room temperature, a BTPS correction factor is applied to the measurements, and some caution is recommended for developing condensation. Miller suggests that the optimal temperature of a Fleisch pneumotachometer may be 30°C because he found no condensation and the highest degree of accuracy and linearity at 30°C, as compared with room temperature or 37°C.[31]

Fleisch pneumotachometers are commonly used as the flow measuring device in body plethysmographs, indirect calorimeters, and diagnostic spirometers. Even when heated and accompanied with water/mucus traps, Fleisch pneumotachometers often become occluded when used for continuous monitoring during mechanical ventilation.

Metal Screen Pneumotachometer

There have been several modifications of the original Fleisch design, and specific examples are listed in Table 10-5. The first modification of the Fleisch pneumotachometer replaced the brass capillary tubes with one or three stainless-steel heated screens. These devices are known as metal screen, triple screen, Silverman's, or Rudolph pneumotachometers (Fig. 10-8). The middle screen provides the resistance; the outer screens tend to prevent particulate matter of other objects from reaching the middle screen, and to some limited extent the outer screens tend to laminarize the airflow. Although the screens are heated to 37°C, there is little heat transfer to the gases because the surface area of the screens is minimal. The heating prevents condensation on the screens but does not always ensure that gases are measured at body temperature. A measurement of gas temperature or an assumed gas temperature is needed to correct the gas volumes to BTPS conditions. Frequent cleaning of the outer screens may be necessary, and cleaning can be accomplished by soaking the device in a mild detergent and brushing the screens with a soft bristle brush.

The triple-screen Hans Rudolph Linear Pneumotachometer is used in the Sensormedic body plethysmograph, for diagnostic spirometry, and in pulmonary function testing. Seimens uses a single metal screen pneumotachometer in their 900 series ventilators to control and monitor tidal volumes and minute ventilation.

Fiber Screen Pneumotachometer

The metal screen pneumotachometer was further modified by replacing the metal screens with a single layer of fibrous material, such as filter paper, fabric, nylon, or styrofoam. These devices are called fiber screen pneumotachometers and are designed to measure only exhaled air (Fig. 10-9). The fibrous resistance and mouthpiece are one unit and are disposable, which eliminates cleaning but creates potential variability in the resistance between mouthpiece units. These devices are not heated, and some of the fibrous materials absorb water vapor, which affects the resistance of the material and the accuracy of the measurements. As a result, these mouthpiece units should be limited to only a few exhalations before disposing. Fiber screen pneumotachometers are commonly used for nondiagnostic spirometry and bedside respiratory assessments.[9,14,16]

TABLE 10-5. Examples of Modified Fleisch-type Pneumotachometers and Clinical Applications

Classification	Model/Manufacturer	Applications
Metal screen	Hans Rudolph Linear Pneumotachometer	Diagnostic spirometry and pulmonary function testing
Fiber screen	Chesebrough-Ponds Respiradyne	Nondiagnostic spirometry
	Life Support Equipment Corp. Vanguard	Nondiagnostic spirometry
	Sherwood Medical Respiradyne II	Nondiagnostic spirometry, parameters of ventilation, and inspiratory force
	Puritan-Bennett PB 900 and 900L	Diagnostic spirometry
	Timeter L.A.P. Spirometer	Diagnostic spirometry
Ceramic	Biotrine, Inc. Flo-Cor	Diagnostic spirometry
	CDX Corp. 121	Diagnostic spirometry
	Medical Equipment Designs MultiSPIRO-PC	Diagnostic spirometry
Variable orifice	Critikon	Continuous ventilation monitoring
	Hamilton Veolar	Continuous ventilation monitoring
	McGaw VR-1/Accutach	Continuous ventilation monitoring
Fixed orifice	Monaghan RVM 761	Continuous ventilation monitoring

Ceramic Pneumotachometer

In another modification, the brass capillary tubes have been replaced by a ceramic resistance element, and these devices are called ceramic pneumotachometers. The advantages of using ceramics include excellent heat conduction to the gases, which ensures measurements at BTPS conditions and the capacity to absorb water vapor. Ceramic materials are porous, and water tends to be absorbed into the material instead of clogging the capillary tubes. Ceramic pneumotachometers are somewhat larger and heavier than Fleisch pneumotachometers and are unwieldy at the mouth. A length of tubing usually connects the mouthpiece to the ceramic resistance, and these devices are used for diagnostic spirometry.

Orifice Pneumotachometer

The need to continuously monitor tidal volume, minute ventilation, and frequency during mechanical ven-

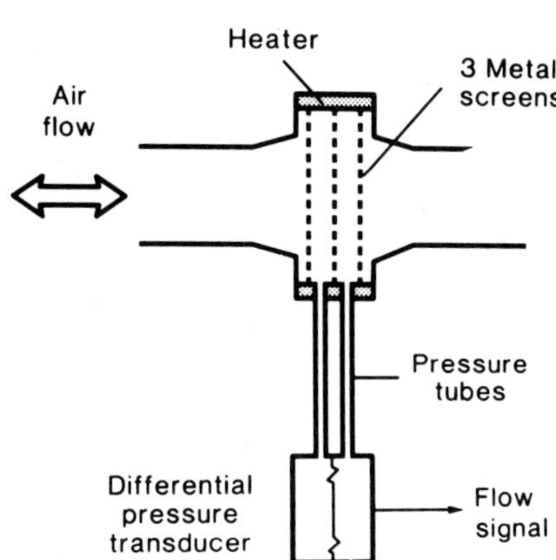

Figure 10-8. Rudolph pneumotachometer. (From Sullivan WJ, Peters GM, Enright PL. Pneumotachometers: Theory and clinical application. Respir Care 1984;29:736–749)

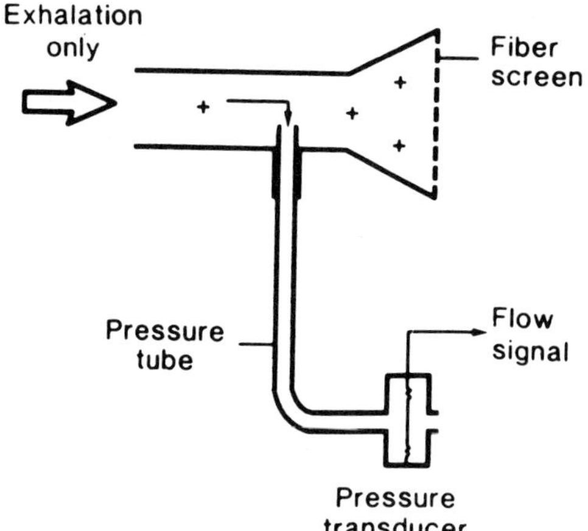

Figure 10-9. Fiber screen pneumotachometer. (From Sullivan WJ, Peters GM, Enright PL. Pneumotachometers: Theory and clinical application. Respir Care 1984;29:736–749)

tilation and the condensation problems associated with the pneumotachometers led to further modifications of the Fleisch pneumotachometer. Elliot[33] removed the resistance element, replaced it with a small chamber, and measured pressures proximally and distally to the chamber. The chamber created turbulent flow, and the flow rate calculations were linearized electronically to compensate for the presence of turbulence. The turbulent flowmeter led to the development of the orifice pneumotachometers.

There are two types of orifice pneumotachometers: fixed and variable (Fig. 10-10). The size of the fixed orifice is large enough so water droplets are less likely to accumulate and change its resistance but small enough to produce measurable increases in pressure. Saklad and associates[34] reported no effect of humidity or temperature and minimal effect of varying oxygen concentrations on the accuracy of the fixed orifice pneumotachometer. Because gas passing through an orifice creates turbulence and turbulence creates nonlinearity in pneumotachometers, fixed orifice pneumotachometers have the electronic circuits that reduce the gain from the pressure transducer at high flow rates to compensate for the presence of turbulence. The variable orifice pneumotachometer incorporates a single flap or fish-mouth type valve that covers the orifice. At higher flow rates when turbulence is more likely to occur, the valve opens and turbulence is decreased. Osborn[35] reported that the resistance of the variable orifice (V-0) pneumotachometer remains constant for flow rates between 0.1 and 2.5 L/s.

Both fixed and variable orifice pneumotachometers are used for tidal volume and ventilation monitoring during spontaneous breathing and mechanical ventilation because they are less susceptible to water effecting the resistance. The Hamilton mechanical ventilators and the Bicore and VenTrak monitors use a variable orifice pneumotachometer. The Monaghan Rate Volume Monitor uses small fixed orifices for monitoring ventilation.

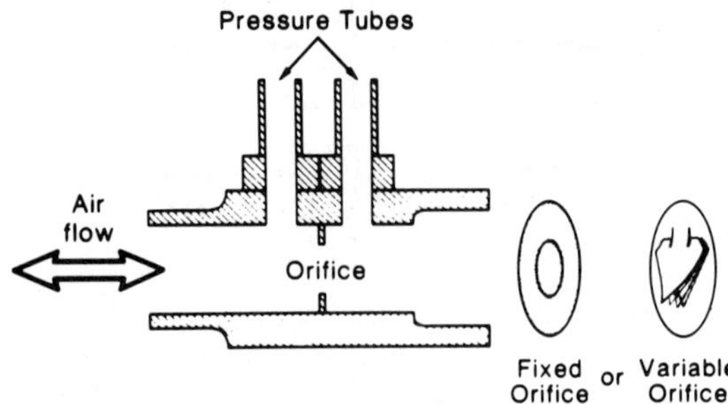

Figure 10-10. Orifice pneumotachometers. (From Sullivan WJ, Peters GM, Enright PL. Pneumotachometers: Theory and clinical application. Respir Care 1984;29:736–749)

Thermistors

The second general principle to measure airflow uses thermal convection or heat transfer from a hot object to the gas flow. The devices that use this principle are called thermistors, hot wire systems, or mass flow anemometers. Specific examples of devices that use heat transfer are listed in Table 10-6. Some of these were independently evaluated before the ATS standards were adopted.[19,36,37] In these devices there are one or two thin metal wires, a bead, or film that is heated and maintained at a constant temperature as high as 400°C (Fig. 10-11). Gas flow removes heat from the hot object; the higher the flow rate the greater the heat transfer. The amount of electrical current needed to maintain the constant temperature of the hot object is proportional to the rate of airflow. Because the relationships between electrical current, electrical resistance of the wire, airflow, and thermal convection are not linear, an electronic linearizer circuit is necessary, and the electronic sophistication of these circuits varies among manufacturers. The Puritan-Bennett 7200 has a temperature-compensated hot-film anemometer to monitor exhaled volumes during continuous mechanical ventilation, and Monaghan M-700 ventilation monitor can be used with spontaneously breathing patients as well as those being mechanically ventilated.[38]

Thermistors perform best when measuring laminar flow because heat transfer is more linear and predictable. Turbulent flow is minimized by placing the flow sensor away from the mouth and connected to the mouthpiece by several feet of smooth, large-diameter tubing. By placing the hot wire away from the mouth, protective screens, which can cause high resistance to airflow, can also be eliminated and there is less effect of the temperature of the gas being measured.[36] This type of device can measure either inspiratory or expiratory airflow but cannot distinguish the direction of flow. A low-resistance one-way valve can separate inspiratory from expiratory flow rates.

Some manufacturers use two hot wires in their sensors. Sensormedics use the second hot wire in their mass flow anemometer to correct for the temperature of the airflow in devices requiring accuracy and precision for diagnostic spirometry, and Bear Medical uses a shielded second hot wire to separate measurements of inspired and expired flows in their infant ventilation monitor.

Turbinometers

The third general principle for measuring airflow uses a windmill effect. Similar to wind turning a windmill, airflow through a sensor causes a turbine, blades, vanes, or cogs to oscillate or spin; the faster the airflow, the faster the oscillations or spinning

TABLE 10-6. Examples of Thermistors and Clinical Applications

Manufacturer/Model	Applications
Bear Medical Neonatal Volume Monitor	Continuous ventilation monitoring
Cavitron DONTI PA 70	Nondiagnostic spirometry Pulmonary performance analyzer
Cavitron RM-73 Respiratory Monitor	Parameters of ventilation and continuous ventilation monitoring
Hospal Medical Corp. Calculair	Nondiagnostic spirometry and incentive spirometry
Marion Laboratories Spirocare	Incentive spirometry
Monaghan Pulmonary Function Analyzer M-402 and M-403	Nondiagnostic spirometry
Monaghan M-700 Ventilation Monitor	Parameters of ventilation and continuous ventilation monitoring
RICO Medical and Scientific Spiromate AS=500 and AS=600	Diagnostic spirometry
Sensormedics Mass Flow Anemometer (formerly SRL, Gould, Spectromed)	Diagnostic spirometry and pulmonary function testing

(Fig. 10-12). Because of the moving component, inertia, friction, and momentum are factors that must be minimized in these instruments. In an effort to reduce these factors, lightweight spinning elements and lubricants are used, but the result is sometimes inaccurately high measurements due to too much momentum, which causes the turbine to continue to spin after exhalation is completed. In general, turbinometers are not designed to meet the accuracy and precision standards of rapid breathing maneuvers for diagnostic spirometry. These devices work best when airflow is relatively constant or when the direction of flow changes rapidly, as in exercise testing. Many of these devices are suitable for nondiagnostic spirometry, for measurements of ventilation, or in incentive spirometers.

Turbinometers are not affected by turbulence, gas composition, temperature, or water vapor, but all turbinometers have airflow measuring limits or thresholds. A minimal airflow is necessary to initiate spinning, and a maximal airflow should not be exceeded because the spinning element cannot turn fast enough, may be damaged, and will indicate inaccurate measurements. Because of the flow rate limit, some turbinometers are not suitable for diagnostic spirometry, including forced vital capacity and peak expiratory flow rate.[12,13,39,40]

Turbinometers can be electronic or mechanical; some specific examples are listed in Table 10-7. In electronic turbinometers, each rotation or oscillation of the turbine or blades interrupts or reflects a light beam focused on a photocell. Each interruption or reflection creates a pulse of electricity, which is counted by a digital circuit, and each pulse of current represents a volume of gas. The Ohmeda 5410 and P. K. Morgan spirometers use a spinning vane, while the Ohio Vortex uses an oscillating vane. Electronic turbinometers provide a digital display of their measurements.

In mechanical turbinometers, the spinning vanes or cogs are connected through gears to one or more needles on an indicating dial for volumes or flow rate. The Wright Respirometers, Ohio Haloscale Respirometers, and Wright Peak Flow Meter are examples of mechanical turbinometers that use spinning vanes. Wright respirometers have flow rate limits of 3 and 300 L/min, whereas the Boehringer Adult spirometer

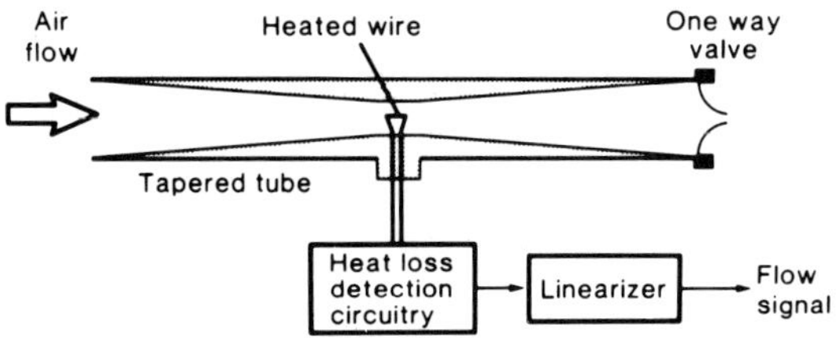

Figure 10-11. Thermistor. (From Sullivan WJ, Peters GM, Enright PL. Pneumotachometers: Theory and clinical application. Respir Care 1984;29:736–749)

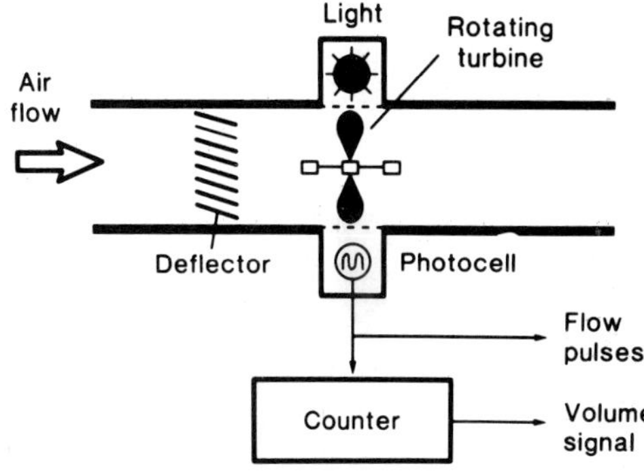

Figure 10-12. Turbinometer. (From Sullivan WJ, Peters GM, Enright PL. Pneumotachometers: Theory and clinical application. Respir Care 1984;29:736–749.

TABLE 10-7. Examples of Turbinometers and Clinical Applications

Classification	Model/Manufacturer	Applications
Electronic	Ferraris Medical, Inc. Magtrac II/III	Parameters of ventilation and continuous ventilation monitoring
	Kintex Pulmometer	Nondiagnostic spirometry
	Ohio Medical Products Vortex Respiration Monitor	Parameters of ventilation
	Ohmeda 5410 Spirometer	Nondiagnostic spirometry and parameters of ventilation
	P.K. Morgan Pocket Spirometer	Nondiagnostic spirometry
	Scitec Spirometer 4800	Diagnostic spirometry and recorder
	Sensormedics Digital Volume Transducer	Exercise testing
	Vacumed Pneumoscan S-310	Diagnostic spirometry and recorder
Mechanical	Wright's Pattern Respirometers	Parameters of ventilation
	Wright Peak Flow Meter	Nondiagnostic peak flow
	Boehringer Adult and "Mini" Spirometers	Parameters of ventilation

has only a 200 L/min high flow rate limit. The Wright Peak Flow Meter is designed to only measure peak expiratory flow rate; both adult and pediatric sizes are available.[41] The Boehringer Adult and "Mini" spirometers have interchangeable turbines, while the Dragger Volumeter uses a pair of rotating wooden cogs that must be periodically dried.

Sonic Devices

There are two principles of airflow measurement that are related to the production and transmission of sound waves: the vortex principle and the ultrasonic principle. Specific examples are listed in Table 10-8. Although ultrasonic sound is common to both, each principle uses sound uniquely. The sonic principles are not affected by humidity, temperature, gas composition, or viscosity and are ideally suited for monitoring tidal volumes and minute ventilation during continuous mechanical ventilation.

The vortex principle gets its name from the swirling action that results when a flowing fluid encounters an obstruction; a vortex is an individual swirl of turbulent flow. In the vortex airflow sensor (Fig. 10-13) there is a partial obstruction called a strut; and when airflow encounters this strut, turbulence is created and vortices are formed. The faster the airflow, the greater the turbulence and the more vortices are produced. Downstream to the strut is an ultrasonic transmitter and receiver. When there is no flow through the sensor, the ultrasonic beam is uninterrupted; when there is airflow, the sound beam is interrupted by the vortices. Each vortex represents a specific volume of air, and each interruption of the ultrasonic beam creates an electrical pulse. The pulses are counted and volumes are calculated. Because of an upper flow rate limit of 250 L/min, the vortex principle is not suited for measuring the forced vital capacity. This principle is applied in the Bear Medical LS-75 and LS-80 ventilation monitors for bedside measurements of the parameters of ventilation and in Bear Adult Volume Ventilators to measure inspiratory and expiratory volumes.[42]

The ultrasonic principle differs from the vortex

TABLE 10-8. Examples of Sonic Devices and Clinical Applications

Classification	Model/Manufacturer	Applications
Vortex	Bourns LS 75 and LS 80	Parameters of ventilation and continuous ventilation monitoring
	Medical Equipment Designs Microspiro-SDS and Autospiro SD-System	Diagnostic spirometry
Ultrasonic	Perkin-Elmer Ultraflow 3	Diagnostic spirometry and pulmonary function testing

principle because there are no struts in the airflow sensor and no vortices are produced. In the ultrasonic airflow sensor, there is an ultrasonic transmitter at one end and a receiver at the other end (Fig. 10-14). The speed of the sound transmission is measured because airflow predictably affects the speed of the ultrasonic wave from transmitter to receiver; ultrasound transit time is decreased with gas flow and increased against flow.[43] The ultrasonic principle is applied in the Perkin-Elmer ventilation monitor.

Peak Flowmeters

The need for an inexpensive instrument for monitoring peak expiratory flow rate at home by asthmatics and at the bedside after bronchodilator administration has resulted in the development of several mechanical peak flow measuring devices. Some of these devices are functionally similar to Thorpe tubes or rotameters. When one exhales forcibly into the device, the pressure created by exhaling through an orifice results in a steel ball rising against gravity. The greater the forced expiratory flow rate, the higher the ball will rise, indicating a higher flow rate. HealthScan's ASSESS has two scales and an end-cap that provides a second orifice, and it can measure flows between 120 and 480 L/min. Although the steel ball can stick with frequent use due to condensation, these rotameter-like devices have been shown to meet the ATS Standards for flow accuracy when used in a vertical position and have compared favorably with the Wright Peak Flow Meter.[10,44]

Exhaling into the second type of peak flowmeter results in a disk expanding a spring. The greater the expiratory flow, the farther the disk will be moved against the tension of the spring. The accuracy of these devices is dependent on maintaining a horizontal position and the length–tension relationship of the spring. Variability in the length–tension relationship due to age may account for less accuracy and precision of these devices as compared with the rotameter type and the Wright Peak Flow Meter.[45] These devices, which are designed to measure only peak expiratory flow rate, have a resetable indicator that rests at the maximum flow rate. The Flo-scope Peak Flow Meter has four different fixed orifices and corresponding scales to provide measurements from 50 to 900 L/min. The "mini-Wright" and the Vitalograph Pulmonary Monitor have been independently evaluated and found suitable for patient self-assessment, although precision was decreased with age of the spring.[46,47,48]

Body Plethysmography

The body plethysmograph is used to measure thoracic gas volume and airway resistance.[49] In normal persons, the thoracic gas volume is similar to functional residual capacity, as measured by open-circuit (nitrogen washout) and closed-circuit (helium dilution) techniques. However, in patients with air trapping, such as those with chronic airflow obstruction, the thoracic gas volume can significantly exceed the functional residual capacity measured by these methods.

The body plethysmograph, commonly called a body box, is a large airtight box in which the subject is seated. As the subject breathes in and out, the volume of gas in the box changes. This change in volume within the box can be measured one of three ways: direct volume measurement, pressure measurement, or flow integration (Fig. 10-15).[50] Of these three methods, pressure measurement is the most commonly used.

When the body plethysmograph is used to measure thoracic gas volume, the subject breaths through a special mouthpiece that is equipped with a shutter and pressure transducer (Fig. 10-16). At end-expiration, the shutter is closed and the subject is instructed

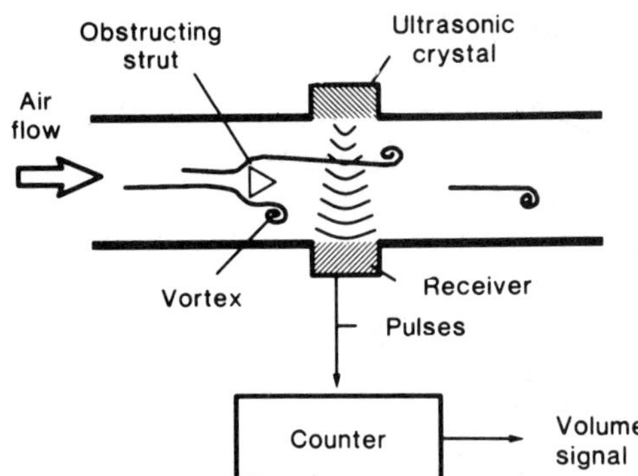

Figure 10-13. Vortex device. (From Sullivan WJ, Peters GM, Enright PL. Pneumotachometers: Theory and clinical application. Respir Care 1984;29:736–749.

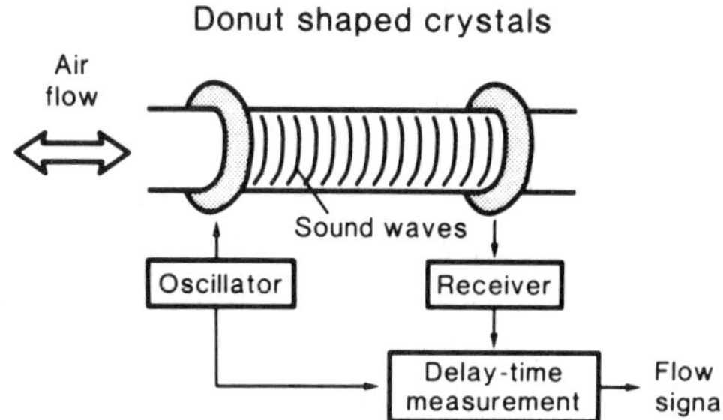

Figure 10-14. Ultrasonic device. (From Sullivan WJ, Peters GM, Enright PL. Pneumotachometers: Theory and clinical application. Respir Care 1984;29:736–749)

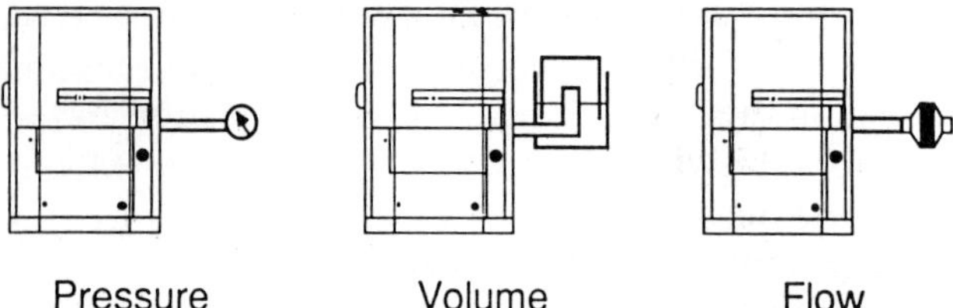

Figure 10-15. Three types of body plethysmography: pressure, volume, and flow. (From Snow MG. Determination fo functional residual capacity. Respir Care 1989;34: 586–596)

to pant. Pressure is measured at the mouth, which is equal to alveolar pressure because there is no airflow. Pressure in the plethysmograph is measured simultaneously, which is a reflection of changes in thoracic gas volume. The relationship between the pressure change in the plethysmograph and the corresponding volume change is determined by adding a known volume of gas to the box and noting the resultant change in pressure. Thoracic gas volume is calculated by application of Boyle's law (Equation Box 10-2).

The body plethysmograph can also be used to measure airway resistance. For this application, a pneumotachometer is added to measure airflow at the mouth. As with the thoracic gas volume measurement, the subject pants against a closed airway and changes in alveolar pressure and changes in plethysmograph pressure are measured. The shutter is then released, and flow from the airway (as measured by the pneumotachometer) is measured as well as changes in box (plethysmograph) pressure. Airway resistance is then calculated (Equation Box 10-3).

Body plethysmography is not commonly used for several reasons. First, the equipment is very expensive. Second, the techniques used for measurement of thoracic gas volume and airway resistance are technically difficult. Finally, measurement of thoracic gas volume and airway resistance (in addition to the measurement of spirometry and lung volumes) has limited clinical usefulness in everyday clinical respiratory care.

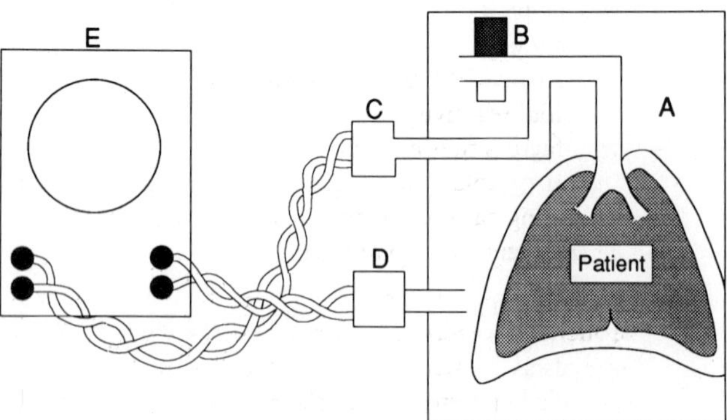

Figure 10-16. Body plethysmograph used to measure thoracic gas volume. A, airtight box; B, electronic shutter; C, pressure transducer to measure mouth (alveolar) pressure; D, transducer to measure pressure in the plethysmograph; E, oscilloscope to display data

Equation Box 10-2: Use of Boyle's Law to Calculate TGV by Body Plethysmography

$$TGV = \frac{(P)\,(\Delta V)}{\Delta P}$$

where P is the barometric pressure, ΔV is the change in the volume of the plethysmograph, and ΔP is the change in alveolar pressure while panting against the closed shutter. In practice, the measurement of ΔV and ΔP is facilitated by the use of an oscilloscopic display.

Respiratory Inductive Plethysmography

Respiratory inductive plethysmography is a relatively new method for semi-quantitative measurement of respiratory rate, tidal volume, chest–abdomen synchrony, and end-expiratory thoracic gas volume (auto-PEEP).[51] Respiratory inductive plethysmography consists of two coils of insulated Teflon wire, which are sewn onto elastic cloth bands in a sinusoidal fashion. In practice, two bands are used. One band encircles the abdomen (AB), and the second encircles the rib cage (RC). Changes in the cross-sectional area of the bands, as occurs with breathing, alter the self-inductance of the wire coils. On commercially available systems such as the Respitrace and Respigraph, the RC and AB waveforms are usually displayed (Fig. 10-17).

Equation Box 10-3: Calculation of Airway Resistance by Body Plethysmography

$$R = \frac{\dfrac{\Delta P_A}{\Delta P_B}}{\dfrac{\dot{V}}{\Delta P_B}} = \frac{\Delta P_A}{\dot{V}}$$

where ΔP_A is the change in alveolar pressure, ΔP_B is the change in box (plethysmograph) pressure, and $\dot{V}$ is flow.

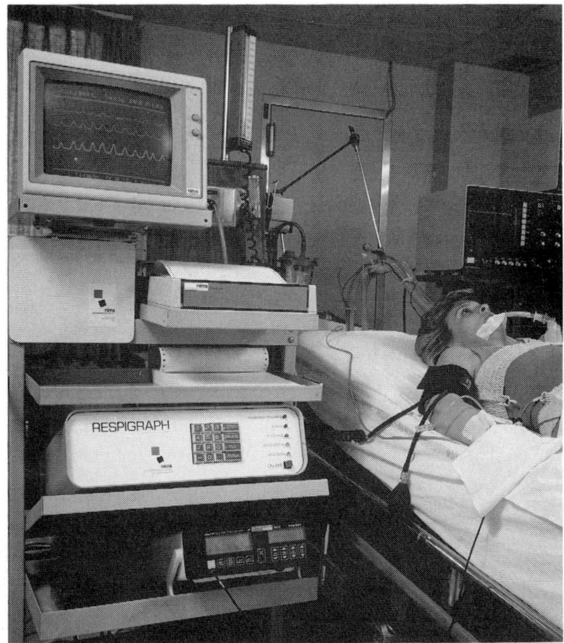

Figure 10-17. Respigraph RIP system. (From Kreiger BP. Respirative inductive plethysmography. In: Hicks GH, ed. Applied Noninvasive Respiratory Monitoring. Philadelphia: JB Lippincott, 1989;156–175)

By use of calibrating methods, the output of respiratory inductive plethysmography can be used to approximate tidal volume. By calibrating the gains of the RC and AB signals, their sum (TC + AB) can be made equivalent to a tidal volume simultaneously measured by spirometry (Fig. 10-18). The accuracy of respiratory inductive plethysmography is ± 10% if there is no change in the patient's body position after calibration and is ± 20% with changes in body position or end-expiratory lung volume.

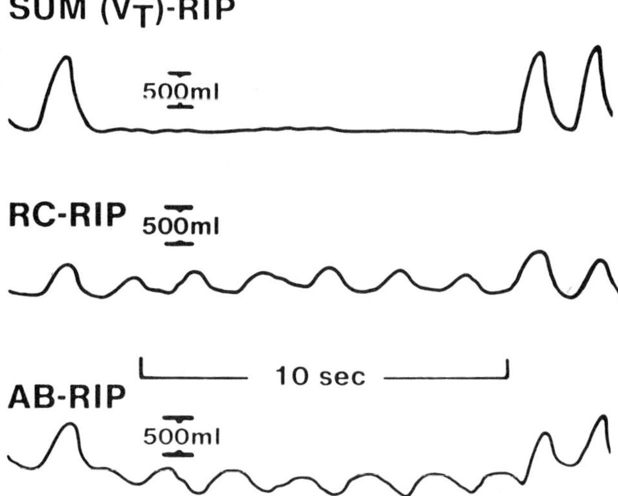

Figure 10-18. RIP tracing performed on a trained subject. Volume is shifted between the RC to the AB while the glottis is closed. This results in a flat (apneic) sum (tidal volume) signal during paradoxical RC and AB movements. (From Kreiger BP. Respirative inductive plethysmography. In: Hicks GH, ed. Applied Noninvasive Respiratory Monitoring. Philadelphia: JB Lippincott, 1989:156–175

Respiratory inductive plethysmography can be used in critical care units, intermediate care units, sleep laboratories, and pulmonary function laboratories. It can be used for continuous monitoring of a wide variety of patients in a variety of clinical situations.

AARC Clinical Practice Guideline

Bronchial Provocation: Indications, Contraindications, Hazards and Complications

Bronchial provocation testing identifies and characterizes hyperresponsive airways by having the patient inhale an aerosolized bronchospastic agent.

- Indications:
  - the need to diagnose or to confirm a diagnosis of airway hyperreactivity
  - the need to follow changes in hyperresponsiveness
  - the need to document the severity of hyperresponsiveness
  - the need to determine who is at risk in the military or workplace
  - the need to establish a control or baseline prior to a series of environmental or occupational exposures
- Contraindications:
  - existence of ventilatory impairment at the time of the proposed challenge
  - significant response to the diluent
  - upper or lower respiratory tract infection within previous six weeks
  - specific antigen exposure within previous one week
  - exposure to high atmospheric pollution with previous one week
  - pregnancy
  - failure to withhold medications that may affect the bronchial reactivity test
  - other factors that may confound the test including ingestion of cola drinks, chocolate, and other agents containing caffeine or theobromides; smoking; occupational exposure to antigens
- Hazards/Complications:
  - bronchoconstriction, hyperinflation, severe coughing
  - hazards associated with spirometry
  - systemic hypotension and flushing from histamine
  - possible exposure of technologists to provocating substances

(Adapted from AARC Clinical Practice Guideline, published in Respiratory Care, August, 1992; see original publication for complete text)

AARC Clinical Practice Guideline

Single-Breath Carbon Monoxide Diffusing Capacity: Indications, Contraindications, Hazards and Complications

Diffusing capacity is a test in which the subject inspires a gas containing carbon monoxide and one or more tracer gases in order to determine the gas exchange capacity of the lungs.

- Indications:
  - evaluation and follow-up of parenchymal lung diseases associated with dusts or drug reactions, or related to sarcoidosis
  - evaluation and follow-up of emphysema and cystic fibrosis
  - differentiating among chronic bronchitis, emphysema, and asthma in patients with obstructive patterns
  - evaluation of pulmonary involvement in systemic diseases
  - evaluation of cardiovascular diseases
  - prediction of arterial desaturation during exercise in chronic obstructive pulmonary disease
  - evaluation and quantification of disability associated with interstitial lung disease
  - evaluation of the effects of chemotherapy agents, or other drugs known to induce pulmonary dysfunction
  - evaluation of hemorrhagic disorders
- Contraindications:
  - mental confusion or muscular incoordination preventing the subject from adequately performing the maneuver
  - a large meal or vigorous exercise immediately before the test
  - smoking within 24 hours of test administration—smoking may have a direct effect on diffusing capacity independent of the effect of carboxyhemoglobin
- Hazards/Complications:
  - single breath diffusing capacity requires breath holding at total lung capacity; some patients may perform either a Valsalva or a Müeller maneuver. Either of these can result in alteration of venous return to the heart.
  - transmission of infection is possible via improperly cleaned mouthpieces or as a consequence of the inadvertent spread of droplet nuclei of body fluids (to patient or technologist).

(Adapted from AARC Clinical Practice Guideline, published in May, 1993, issue of Respiratory Care; see original publication for complete text)

AARC Clinical Practice Guideline

Spirometry: Indications, Contraindications, Hazards and Complications

The objective of spirometry is to assess ventilatory function. Spirometry includes but is not limited to the measurement of forced vital capacity (FVC), the forced expiratory volume in the first second (FEV_1), and other forced expiratory flow measurements.

- Indications:
  - detecting the presence or absence of lung dysfunction suggested by history or physical indicators (eg, smoking history, family history of lung disease, cough) and/or the presence of other abnormal diagnostic tests (eg, chest x-ray, arterial blood gases)
  - quantifying the severity of known lung disease
  - assessing the change in lung function over time or following administration of or change of therapy
  - assessing the potential effects or response to environmental or occupational exposure
  - assessing the risk for surgical procedures known to affect lung function
- Contraindications: relative contraindications to performing spirometry are
  - hemoptysis of unknown origin
  - untreated pneumothorax
  - unstable cardiovascular status
  - thoracic, abdominal, or cerebral aneurysms
  - recent eye surgery (e.g., cataract)
  - presence of an acute disease process that might interfere with test performance
- Hazards/Complications:
  - pneumothorax
  - increased intracranial pressure
  - syncope, dizziness, light-headedness
  - chest pain
  - paroxysmal coughing
  - contraction of nosocomial infections
  - oxygen desaturation due to interruption of oxygen therapy
  - bronchospasm

(Adapted from AARC Clincal Practice Guideline, published in December, 1991, issue of Respiratory Care; see original publication for complete text)

References

1. Shigeoka JW. Calibration and quality control of spirometer systems. Respir Care 1983;28:747–753.
2. Norton A. Accuracy in pulmonary measurements. Respir Care 1979;24:131–137.
3. Clausen JL, Tisi GM, Moser KM. Methods of evaluation of accuracy of spirometers and pneumotachographs (abstract). Med Instrum 1974;8:117.
4. Gardner RM, Hankinson JL, Clausen JL, Crapo RO, Johnson RL, Epler GR. Standardization of spirometry: 1987 update. Respir Care 1987;32:1039–1061.
5. Hankinson JS, Gardner RM. Standard wave forms for spirometry testing. Am Rev Respir Dis 1982;126:363–364.
6. Sullivan WJ, Peters GM, Enright PL. Pneumotachographs: Theory and clinical application. Respir Care 1984;29:736–749.
7. Gardner RM (chairman). ATS Statement I, Snowbird Workshop on Standardization of Spirometry. Am Rev Respir Dis 1978;119: 831–838.
8. Cramer D, Peacock A, Denison D. Temperature correction in routine spirometry. Thorax 1984;39:771–774.
9. Clayton J, Morgan WJ, Taussig LM. Spirometric variables measured by a new hand-held digital device (DS) correlate well with results from a #3 Fleish pneumotachograph (PT) (abstract). Am Rev Respir Dis 1986;133:A336.

10. Eichenhorn MS, Beauchamp RK, Harper PA, Ward JC. An assessment of three portable peak flow meters. Chest 1982;82: 306–309.
11. Gardner RM, Hankinson JL, West RF. Evaluating commercially available spirometers. Am Rev Respir Dis 1980;121:73–82.
12. Hess D, Kacer K, Beener C. An evaluation of the accuracy of the Ohmeda 5410 spirometer. Respir Care 1988;33:21–26.
13. Hess D, Lehman E, Troup J, Smoker J. An evaluation of the P.K. Morgan spirometer. Respir Care 1986;31:786–791.
14. Hess D, Chieppor P, Johnson K. An evaluation of the Respiradyne II spirometer. Respir Care 1987;32:1123–1130.
15. Hudson LD, Petty TL, Baldwan B, Stark K. Clinical evaluation of a new office spirometer. JAMA 1978;240:2754–2755.
16. Jenkins SC, Barnes NC, Moxham J. The Respiradyne: A pocket-size pulmonary function monitor (abstract). Thorax 1986;41:243.
17. Kraman SS. The pulmometer: A compact, self-contained spirometer. Am Rev Diagnostics 1983;4:108–111.
18. Rode A, Shephard RJ. Accuracy of an electronic spirometer—a field test. Respiration 1986;50:66–69.
19. Shanks DE, Morris JF. Clinical comparison of two electronic spirometers with a water-sealed spirometer. Chest 1976;69: 461–466.
20. Zimnicki GL, Kline JL, MacDonell RF. Evaluation of the Respiradyne pulmonary function monitor. Respir Care 1987;69:461–466.
21. Forche G, Harnoncourt K, Stadlober E, Zenker G. BTPS correction with dynamic spirometers. Respiration 1986;49:274–279.
22. Perks WH, Sopwith T, Brown D. The effect of temperature on the Vitalograph spirometer (abstract). Am Rev Respir Dis 1981; 123:124.
23. Glindmeyer HW, Anderson ST, Diem JE, Weill H. A comparison of the Jones and Stead-Wells spirometers. Chest 1978;73: 596–602.
24. Hutchinson J. On the capacity of the lungs and on the respiratory functions, with a view of establishing a precise and easy method of detecting disease by the spirometer. Trans Med Chir Soc Lond 1846;29:137–252.
25. Spriggs EA. John Hutchinson, the inventor of the spirometer—His north country background, life in London, and scientific achievements. Med Hist 1977;21:357–364.
26. Wells HS, Stead WW, Rossing TD, Ognanovich J. Accuracy of an improved spirometer for recording of fast breathing. J Appl Physiol 1959;14:451–454.
27. Med-Science. Silver anniversary of the WEDGE. Med Sci Inspir 1986;1:1.
28. Townsend MC. The effects of leaks in spirometers on measurements of pulmonary function. J Occup Med 1984;26:835–841.
29. Fleisch A. Pneumotachograph: Apparatus for recording respiratory flow. Arch Gen Physiol 1925;209:713–722.
30. Gelfand R, Lambertsen CJ, Peterson RE, Slater A. Pneumotachograph for low and volume measurement in normal and dense atmospheres. J Appl Physiol 1976;41:120–124.
31. Miller MR, Pincock AC. Linearity and temperature control on the Fleisch pneumotachograph. J Appl Physiol 1986;60:710–715.
32. Muller NL, Zamel N. Pneumotachograph calibration for inspiratory and expiratory flows during HeO_2 breathing. J Appl Physiol 1981;51:1038–1041.
33. Elliot SE. A turbulent flowmeter. J Appl Physiol 1977;42:456–459.
34. Saklad M, Sullivan M, Paliotta J, Lipsky M. Pneumotachography: A new low-dead-space, humidity-independent device. Anesthesiology 1979;51:149–153.
35. Osborn JJ. Flowmeter for respiratory monitoring. Crit Care Med 1978;6:349–351.
36. Fitzgerald MX, Smith AA, Gaensler EA. Evaluation of "electronic" spirometers. N Engl J Med 1973;289:1283–1288.
37. Cox P, Miller L, Petty TL. Clinical evaluation of a new electronic spirometer. Chest 1973;63:517–520.
38. Sutton FD, Nett LM, Petty TL. A new ventilation monitor for the intensive respiratory care unit. Respir Care 1974;19:196.
39. Chowienczyk PJ, Lawson CP. Pocket-sized device for measuring forced expiratory volume in one second and forced vital capacity. Br Med J 1982;285:15–17.
40. Wernerus H, Silve G, Wanner A. Accuracy of Drager and Wright ventilation meters. Respir Care 1978;23:856–859.
41. Wright BM, McKerrow CB. Maximum forced expiratory flow rate as a measure of ventilatory capacity. Br Med J 1959;2:1041–1044.
42. Westenskow DR, Tucker SM. Evaluation of a ventilation monitor. Crit Care Med 1981;9:64–66.
43. Blumenfeld W, Turney SZ, Denman RS. A coaxial ultrasonic pneumotachometer. Med Biol Eng 1975;13:855–860.
44. Darden MD, Sly RM. Evaluation of Healthscan ASSESS peak flow meters. Ann Allergy 1985;54:486–488.
45. Morrill CG, Dickey DW, Weiser PC, Kinsman RA, Chai H, Spector SL. Calibration and stability of standard and mini-Wright peak flow meters. Ann Allergy 1979;43:246–249.
46. Burns KL. An evaluation of two instruments for assessing airway flow. Ann Allergy 1979;43:246–249.
47. Perks WH, Cole M. Steventon RD, et al. An evaluation of the Vitalgraph pulmonary monitor. Br J Dis Chest 1981;75:161–164.
48. Wright BM. A miniature Wright peak flowmeter. Br Med J 1978;2: 1627–1628.
49. Miller WF, Scacci R, Gast TR. Laboratory Evaluation of Pulmonary Function. Philadelphia: JB Lippincott, 1987:110–128, 214–221.
50. Snow MG. Determination of functional residual capacity. Respir Care 1989;34:586–596.
51. Kreiger BP. Respiratory inductive plethysmography. In: Hicks GH, ed. Applied Noninvasive Respiratory Monitoring. Philadelphia: JB Lippincott, 1989:156–175.

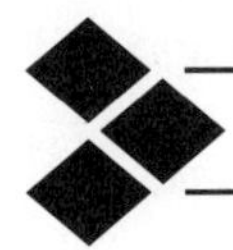

11 Airway Pressure Monitoring Devices

Richard D. Branson

OBJECTIVES

1. Explain how pressure measurements are made.
2. Compare the advantages and disadvantages of pressure monitoring devices.
3. Describe the proper use of a disconnect alarm.
4. Describe the measurement of mean airway pressure.
5. Determine the factors associated with inadvertent disconnection from the ventilator.
6. Describe methods to prevent accidental disconnections.

KEY TERMS

electromechanical pressure transducers
gravity-dependent manometer
mean airway pressure
mechanical aneroid manometers
pressure disconnect alarm

Introduction

Airway pressure monitoring is one of the most common measurements performed by respiratory care practitioners. Accurate measurement of airway pressure is equally important in the pulmonary function laboratory and the intensive care unit. In this chapter the principles of pressure measurement are reviewed and commercially available airway pressure monitors and disconnect alarms are described.

Pressure Measurement Devices

Pressure is, by definition, force per unit area. Atmospheric pressure is the force exerted by the atmosphere. Gauge pressure is the pressure measured relative to atmospheric pressure (positive or negative). Absolute pressure is the total force per unit area and is equal to atmospheric pressure plus gauge pressure. All of these pressure measurements are of importance to the respiratory care practitioner.

Devices used to measure pressure can be classified into three categories: gravity-dependent fluid manometers, mechanical aneroid manometers, and electromechanical transducers.[1] Each will be considered with respect to principle of operation, limitations, and clinical uses.

Gravity-Dependent Fluid Manometers

Gravity-dependent fluid manometers are the simplest devices used to monitor pressure. A classic example of a gravity-dependent device is the mercury barometer, used to measure atmospheric pressure. Invented in 1643, by Evangelista Torricelli, the mercury barometer equilibrates atmospheric pressure with the weight of a column of mercury. This device consists of an evacuated glass tube or column, a scale to measure height, and a mercury reservoir. The glass tube is inverted, with its open end into the mercury reservoir. The atmospheric pressure exerts a force on the surface of the mercury reservoir that equilibrates with the weight of the mercury in the column (Fig. 11-1). The resulting height of the mercury column is equivalent to the barometric pressure in millimeters (mm Hg) or centimeters of mercury (cm Hg).

The use of mercury is for practical purposes. Mercury is a dense liquid that at normal atmospheric pressure stands at a height that is conveniently measured. A water barometer could likewise be constructed but owing to the density of water (13.6 times less than that of mercury) it would have to be 34 feet in height.

The mercury barometer is used for measuring atmospheric pressure in the hospital to allow accurate calibration of blood gas and flow and volume monitoring devices.

Another type of gravity-dependent device is the U-tube manometer. The U-tube manometer is, as its name suggests, a U-shaped tube filled with a fluid, typically water or mercury (Fig. 11-2). The pressure on one leg of the tube is open to atmospheric pressure (Patm), and the pressure to be measured is applied to the other leg. The resulting shift of the liquid between the two legs is proportional to the pressure applied.

The U-tube manometer is suitable for monitoring static pressures but is unreliable in monitoring dynamic pressures. This device is most often used to create a known pressure against which other pressure monitoring devices can be calibrated.

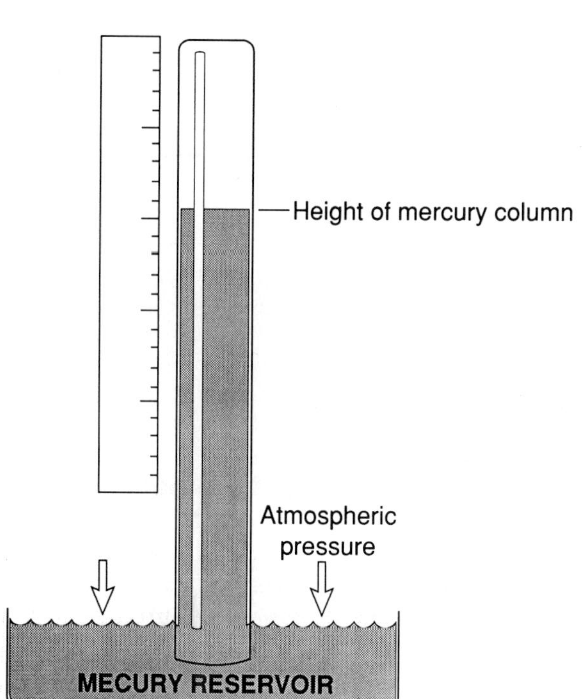

Figure 11-1. Gravity-dependent mercury barometer used for measuring atmospheric pressure.

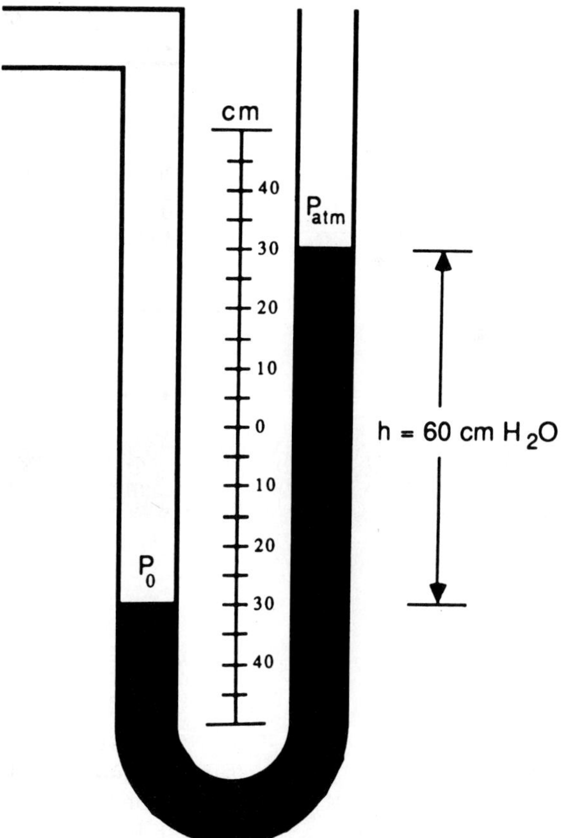

Figure 11-2. U-tube manometer. The height (h) of the column of liquid indicates a pressure of 60 cm H_2O is being measured.

Mechanical Aneroid Manometers

These devices are the most frequently used devices for monitoring pressure in respiratory care. They can be found as integral parts of ventilators and as stand-alone devices for measuring a wide range of clinical indices (Fig. 11-3).

The majority of mechanical manometers are modified Bourdon tube gauges (Figs. 11-4 and 11-5). An expandable metal or plastic bellows is connected to the pressure source to be measured. As pressure is exerted, the bellows expands, causing a gear mechanism to rotate a needle across a calibrated dial. A restrictive orifice is often included in these devices to prevent damage to the manometer during high and/or rapidly changing pressures. Excessive pressures will cause the spring to become stretched or dislodged, rendering the device useless.

These devices can measure static and dynamic pressures and are often used in ventilators, disconnect alarms, and along with resuscitation equipment to monitor airway pressures. However, the reliability of these devices at rapidly changing pressures is suspect. The restrictor causes a dampening of applied pressure, which causes peak pressure to be underestimated and baseline pressure to be overestimated.

Mechanical manometers are also sensitive to humidity and are easily broken if dropped. This necessitates both protection from moisture and encasement of stand-alone devices in rubber or foam padding.

Although these devices are extremely popular, they should not be considered alternatives to electromechanical devices.

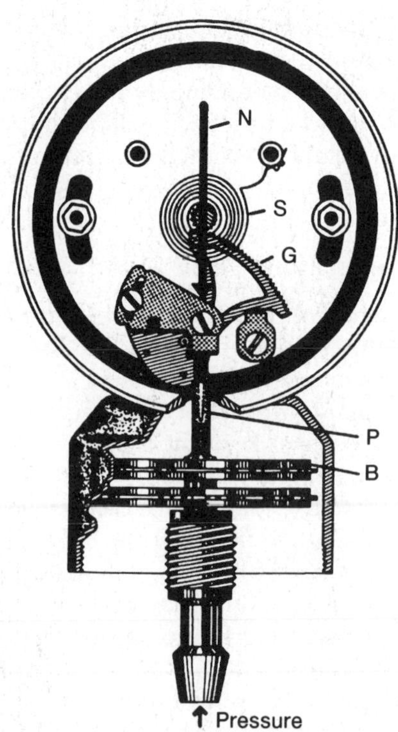

Figure 11-4. Aneroid manometer. Variations in pressure within the bellows (B) activate a pin (P), which sets the gear (G) in motion. The gear, in turn, operates the spring (S), which causes the needle (N) to rotate across the face of a calibrated dial. (From Wilkins R, Hicks GH. Gas volume, flow, pressure, and temperature monitoring. Prob Respir Care 1989;2:126–155)

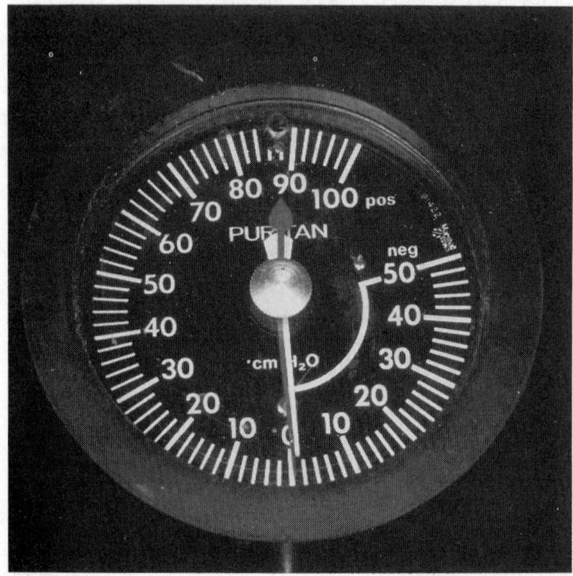

Figure 11-3. Typical aneroid pressure gauge used for monitoring pressure during manual ventilation with a non–self-inflating resuscitation bag.

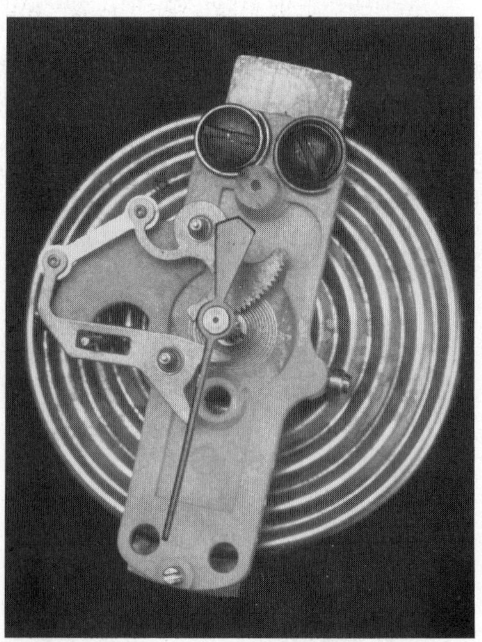

Figure 11-5. Internal components of an aneroid pressure gauge. The bellow is copper, and its expansion causes the gears to move the needle.

Electromechanical Transducers

There are a wide variety of electromechanical transducers used to monitor pressure. Those used in respiratory care are typically strain gauge transducers. A strain gauge transducer relies on measuring the change in electrical resistance created when a fine wire (25 µm in diameter) is stretched.[2] Typically, strain gauges use wire made from chromium, copper, germanium, nickel, platinum, and silicone or a combination of these materials.[3] When used to monitor airway pressure, the strain gauge is attached to a diaphragm, one side of which is open to atmosphere and the other side open to the desired site of pressure measurement (Fig. 11-6). As airway pressure rises, the diaphragm moves, stretching the wires in the strain gauge. The change in diameter and length of the wire causes its resistance to change. Resistance changes are most conveniently measured with a wheatstone bridge circuit (Fig. 11-7). The wheatstone bridge is extremely sensitive in detecting resistance changes and can compensate for changes in temperature.

A wheatstone bridge circuit uses a reference circuit and a measurement circuit. The change in output of the wheatstone bridge when pressure is applied to the measurement circuit (causing the bridge to be unbalanced) is proportional to the change in resistance. The change in resistance is proportional to the pressure applied, which can then be digitally or graphically displayed.

Piezoelectric Pressure Measuring Devices

Many of the new disposable pressure transducers used for monitoring vascular pressures are solid-state piezoelectric devices. Similar to the strain gauge in principle, the piezoelectric crystal creates a change in voltage when strained (Fig. 11-8). The crystal is asymmetric; and when pressure is applied its shape is distorted, causing a reorientation of charges within the crystal. When this distortion occurs the positive and negative charges that produce surface changes in opposite polarity on opposite sides of the crystal are displaced. The resulting voltage (v) is calculated as shown in Equation Box 11-1.

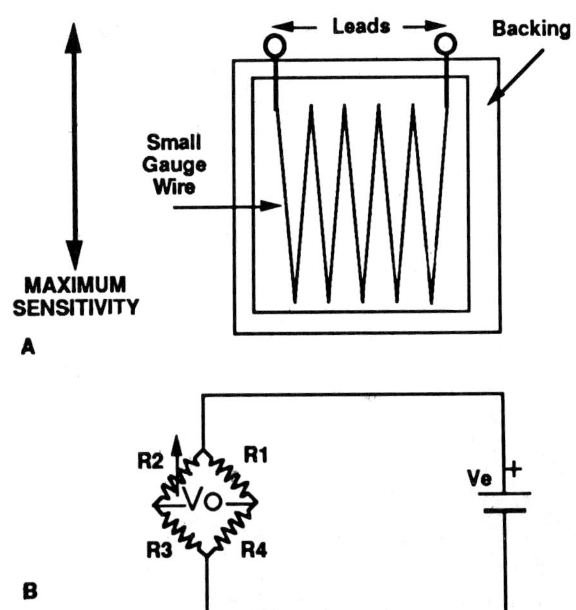

Figure 11-7. Strain gauge pressure transducers: A. Diagram of a strain gauge pressure transducer. B. Wheatstone bridge used to measure the resistance of the strain gauge.

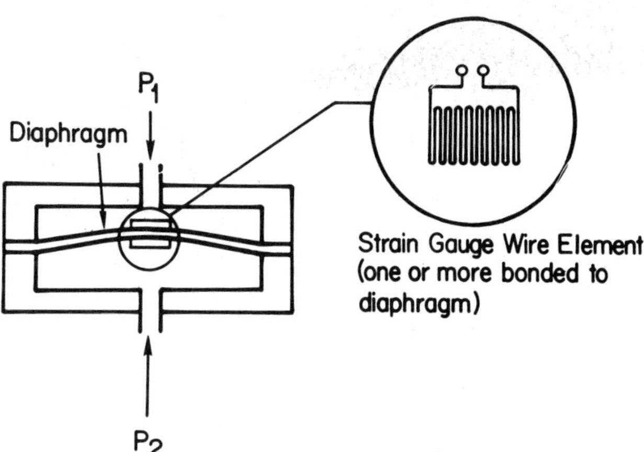

Figure 11-6. Attachment of a strain gauge wire to the diaphragm of a pressure transducer. P_1, reference pressure, P_2, measured pressure. (From Chatburn RL, Craig KC. Fundamentals of Respiratory Care Research. Norwalk, CT: Appleton & Lange, 1988:288)

Disconnect Alarms

Unrecognized disconnection of the patient from a mechanical ventilator is a life-threatening event and has

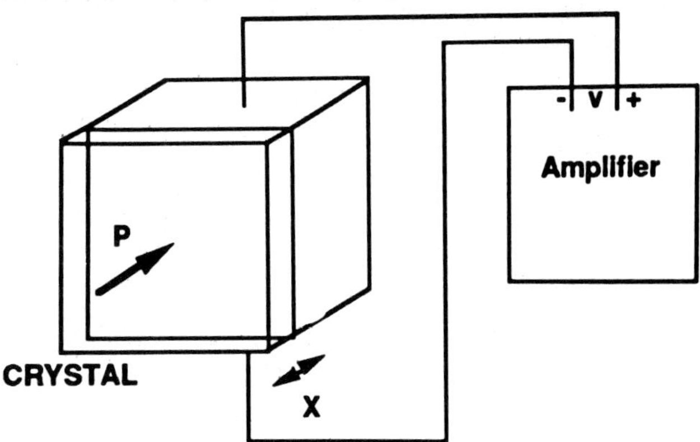

Figure 11-8. Functional diagram of a piezoelectric pressure transducer. (From East TD. What makes non-invasive monitoring tick? A review of basic engineering principles. Respir Care 1990;35:500-519.

Equation Box 11-1: Voltage Output of a Piezoelectric Crystal

$$v = \frac{k \times f}{c}$$

where k is the piezoelectric constant, f is the force applied, and c is the capacitance. If the area of the crystal that is exposed to the desired pressure remains constant, then the output of the device is proportional to the applied pressure (pressure = force ÷ area).

been implicated in a number of anesthetic mishaps.[4–13] Pressure monitoring systems and disconnect alarms have been developed to combat this problem.

A disconnect alarm is the simplest of these devices. Disconnect alarms may or may not measure pressure and may or may not display airway pressure. Effective use of a disconnect alarm requires proper set up by the practitioner, proper placement of the pressure monitoring site, and understanding of the device's principle of operation.

A low-pressure or disconnect alarm should be set to signal at a value ± 10% or ± 5 cm H_2O, whichever is greater, of the desired pressure. That is, if the pressure being monitored is 20 cm H_2O, then the disconnect alarm should be set to sound at a pressure below 15 cm H_2O. If the low-pressure setting is set improperly, for example, at 5 cm H_2O, the alarm may fail to sound (Fig. 11-9). This is most often due to resistance to gas flow caused by a humidifier or by the ventilator circuit being trapped in the bed sheets, preventing pressure from falling below this level.[14]

A typical disconnect alarm has a calibrated setting for the pressure below which the alarm sounds, a time delay for the low-pressure alarm, and a temporary alarm silence button.

The low-pressure setting is set as previously described. The time delay is set according to the set ventilator rate. If the set rate is 10 breaths per minute, which allows 6 seconds per ventilatory cycle, and inspiratory time is 1 second, then expiratory time will be 5 seconds. The time delay should be set to 6 seconds. That is, if the following breath is not detected, then 1 second after it should have been delivered the alarm will sound. This delay is clinically adjustable, and longer delays may be indicated depending on the situation. The temporary alarm silence button is used to disable the alarm during times when the patient is purposely taken off the ventilator (ie, for suctioning) as a convenience for practitioners. The alarm silence should automatically reactivate at a period of 30 to 60 seconds after its inactivation.

Many new disconnect alarms have other safety functions. The first is the absence of an on/off switch. When the device is plugged in or connected to battery

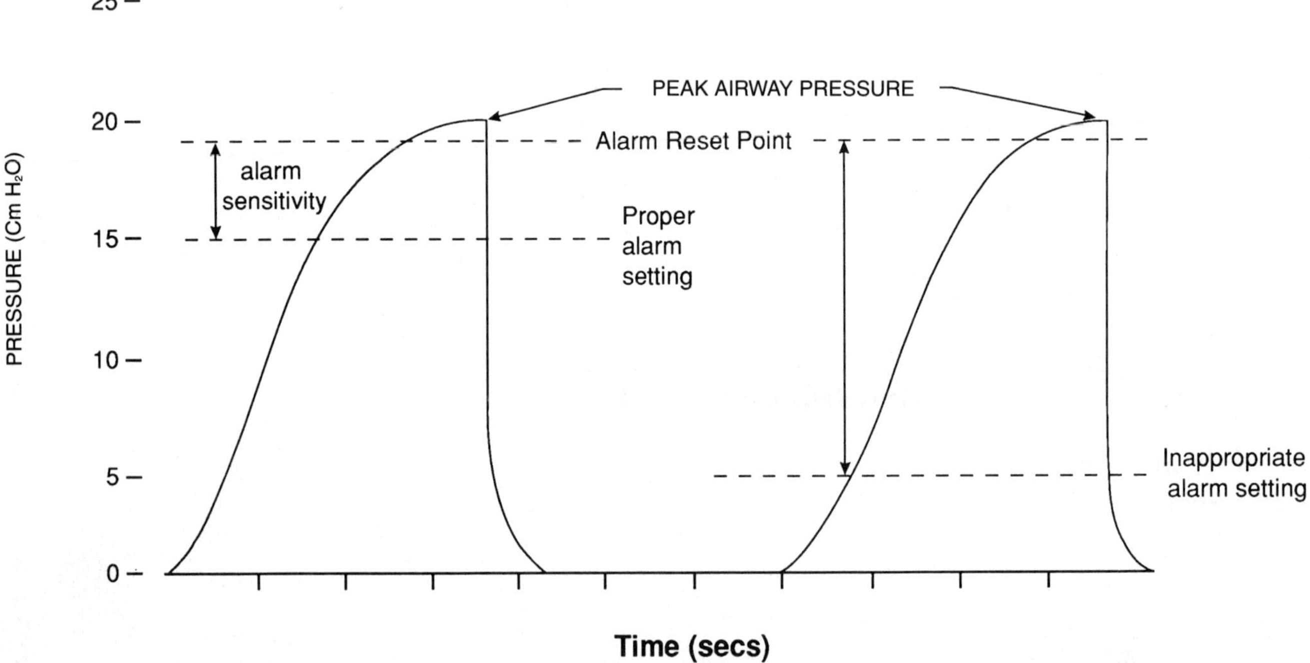

Figure 11-9. Airway pressure during two mechanical breaths. The dotted lines represent the appropriate (left) and inappropriate (right) low-pressure alarm settings.

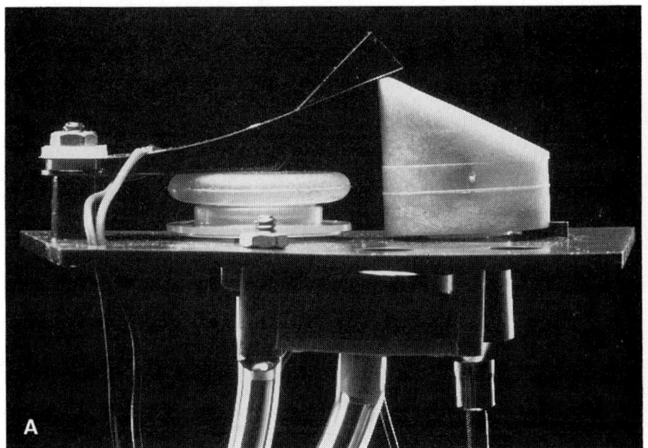

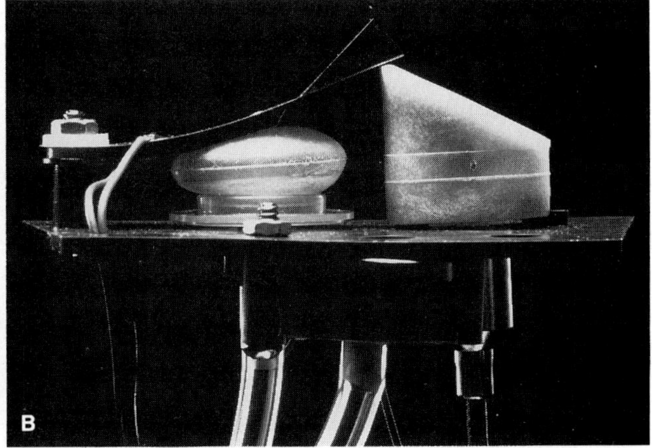

Figure 11-10. (A.) Position of diaphragm and contact plates during the absence of pressure in the circuit. (B.) Position of diaphragm (inflated) and contact plates (touching) during the presence of pressure in the circuit.

power, it is always on. This prevents the clinician from forgetting to turn the alarm on after prolonged patient disconnection and from accidentally turning the alarm off.

The second is used in devices with an on/off switch. These devices emit a continuous alarm if they sense pressure, with the alarm turned off. Both these methods are useful and necessary to prevent catastrophe.

The simplest disconnect alarms use pressure-activated switch contacts to generate the alarm (Fig. 11-10). The relative position of the contact plates to each other is controlled by the low-pressure alarm setting. The closer the plates, the lower the pressure has to be in the diaphragm to allow the plates to touch. In Figure 11-10*A* the diaphragm is deflated and there is space between the contact plates. If after the set time delay the diaphragm does not inflate causing the plates to touch, the alarm will sound. In Figure 11-10*B*, the diaphragm is inflated, causing the contact plates to touch, resetting the alarm. A schematic of a similar low-pressure alarm is shown in Figure 11-11,[15] and a typical low-pressure alarm is shown in Figure 11-12.

Airway Pressure Monitoring Devices

Airway pressure monitoring devices act as low- and high-pressure alarms as well as monitors, digitally displaying values for peak inspiratory pressure (PIP), positive end-expiratory pressure (PEEP) or continuous positive airway pressure (CPAP), mean airway pressure ($\bar{P}$aw), respiratory frequency (f), inspiratory time (TI), and the ratio of inspiratory to expiratory time (I:E). These devices use an electromechanical pressure transducer and process the measurements using an on-board microprocessor to allow for automatic or clinician adjustable alarm settings.

Most airway pressure monitors are used in conjunction with neonatal or pediatric ventilators that do not have the sophisticated monitoring of adult ventilators.

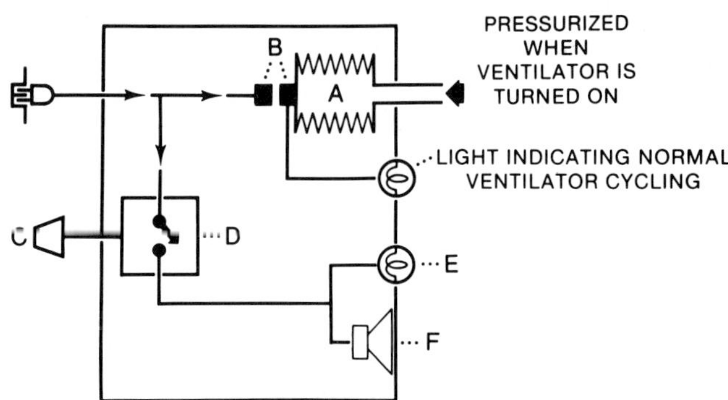

Figure 11-11. Single-channel low-pressure monitor. When the ventilator fires to the inspiratory phase, diaphragm A is compressed, engaging the two contact points B (these complete the circuit), resulting in a discharge of current that turns on a light indicating that the ventilator is cycling normally. If the ventilator becomes disconnected, pressure is lost and the circuit is broken. For example, if the IMV rate is set at 4 breaths per minute, the ventilator is activated every 15 seconds, and the delay timer control C is set for a 20-second delay. If the ventilator is then disconnected, no pressure will be detected at the 15-second interval. Since switch B cannot become activated under this condition, current discharge is impossible by this route, and current can only flow through resistor switch D after the previously set 20-second delay has elapsed. Discharge of current through D activates another light (E) and the low-pressure audible alarm (F), signifying that the ventilator is not working. This is usually caused by a leak in the ventilator circuit or disconnection from the patient. (From Hudson-Civetta J, Banner M. Nursing assessment of intermittent mandatory ventilation. Int Anesthesiol Clin 1980;18:143–177)

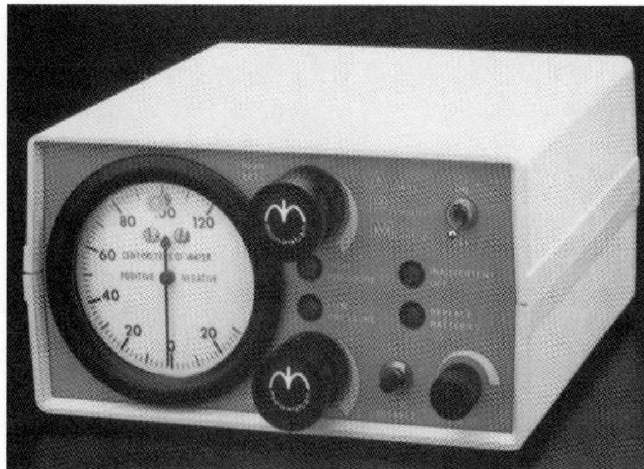

Figure 11-12. A typical disconnect alarm.

Mean airway pressure has been shown to be an important determinant of oxygenation and hemodynamic embarrassment and is frequently measured.[16–19] Typically, an airway pressure monitor will sample pressure 100 times per second and update the display on a breath-to-breath or gliding-average basis. See Equation Box 11-2.[20–23]

Commercially available airway pressure monitors can monitor and alert health care personnel with high and low alarms for a variety of pressures as well as respiratory frequency, inspiratory and expiratory times, and I:E ratio. Table 11-1 compares the commercially available monitors. These range from hand-held devices (Fig. 11-13) to devices mounted on the ventilator (Figs. 11-14 through 11-16).

Equation Box 11-2: Calculation of Mean Airway Pressure

Mean airway pressure may be calculated as the arithmetic mean using the following equation:

$$\overline{Paw} = \frac{\sum_{X_1}^{X_n} P}{N}$$

where $\overline{Paw}$ is mean airway pressure in cm H_2O, X_n is the last pressure measurement, X_1 is the first pressure measurement, and N is the number of pressure measurements made. Mean airway pressure can also be calculated using the following formula:

$$\overline{Paw} = K[(PIP - PEEP) \times (T_I/T_{TOT})] + PEEP$$

where K is the empirical flow waveform constant (constant or square flow waveform = 1.0, decelerating flow waveform = 0.5, and sine wave flow form = $2/\pi$. PIP = peak inspiratory pressure (cm H_2O), PEEP = positive end-expiratory pressure (cm H_2O), T_I = inspiratory time (seconds), and T_{TOT} = total cycle time (seconds).

The relative accuracy of this formula depends on the ability of the ventilator to deliver the specified waveform despite changes in respiratory system impedance and the absolute values for T_I, frequency, and PIP.[20–23]

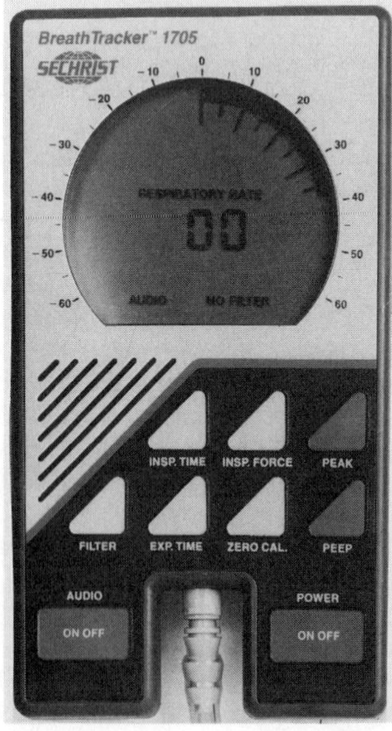

Figure 11-13. The Sechrist 1705 Breath Tracker is a hand-held device that uses an electromechanical transducer to measure airway pressures. (Courtesy of Sechrist Industries, Anaheim, CA)

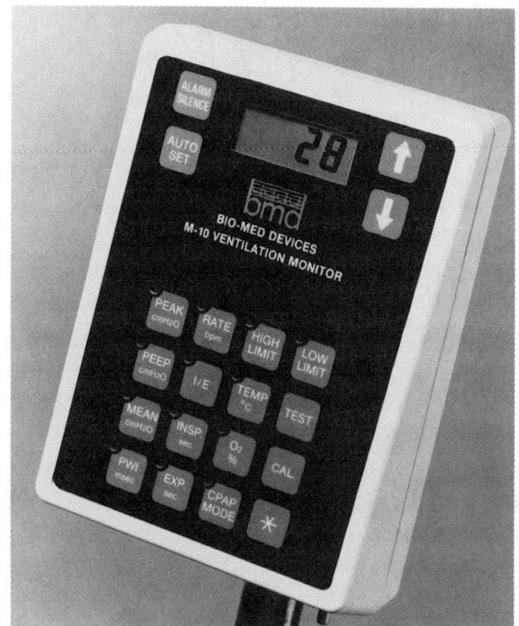

Figure 11-14. The Bio-Med Devices M-10 ventilation monitor. (Courtesy of Bio-Med Devices, Madison, CT)

TABLE 11-1. Commercially Available Airway Pressure Monitors

Variables	Device					
	Bio-Med M-10	Bunnell	Nova Metrix	Sechrist 1705	Sechrist 400	Sechrist 600*
Peak inspiratory pressure	A⁺, D	A⁺, D	A, D	D	D, A	D, A⁺
Positive end-expiratory pressure	A⁺, D	A⁺, D	A, D	D	D	D
Mean airway pressure	A, D	A⁺, D	A, D	NA	D, A	D
Frequency	A⁺, D	D	D	NA	D	D
Inspiratory time	D	D	D	D	D	D
Expiratory time	D	NA	NA	D	NA	D
I:E ratio	A, D	D	D	NA	NA	D
Maximum inspiratory pressure	NA	NA	NA	D	NA	NA

*Graphic display of pressure waveform.
A, alarmed; A⁺, automatic alarm setting; D, displayed; NA, not available.

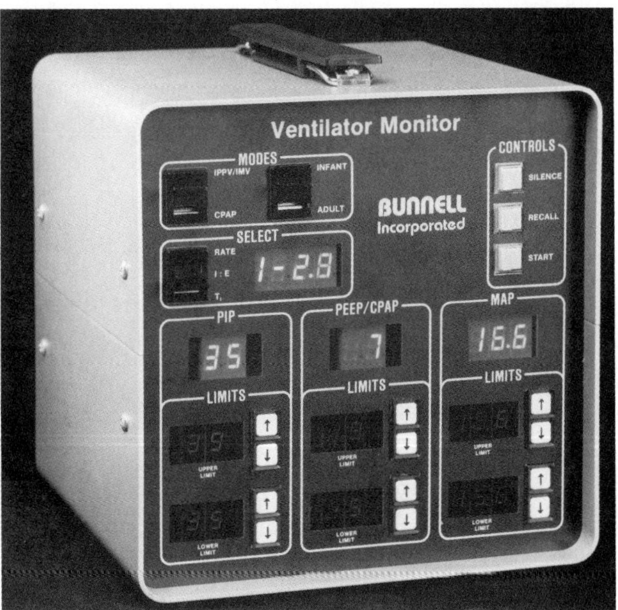

Figure 11-15. The Bunnell ventilator monitor.

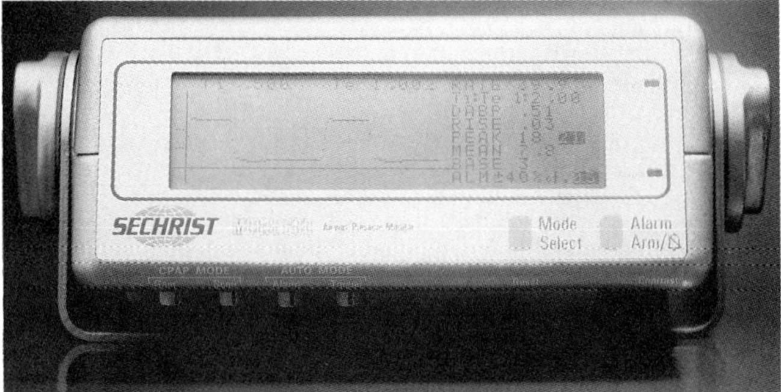

Figure 11-16. The Sechrist 600 airway pressure monitor. This device provides a graphic display of airway pressure. (Courtesy of Sechrist Industries, Anaheim, CA)

Despite the use of disconnect alarms and airway pressure monitors, inadvertent disconnection of the mechanically ventilated patient can be disastrous. Alarms will not function under all conditions.[24,25] Boxes 11-1 and 11-2 list the causes of accidental disconnections and the reasons why detection can be elusive. Precautions in preventing ventilator disconnection have been published by the Food and Drug Administration (Fig. 11-17) and respiratory care practitioners should be familiar with these techniques.[26]

Box 11-1
Reasons for Accidental Breathing Circuit Disconnections

- Incompatible components due to
  - Nonstandard dimensions
  - Dissimilar or inappropriate materials
  - Effects of reuse
- Inadequate connection force
- Intentional loose assembly
  - To facilitate required disconnections
  - To use connection as "circuit breaker"
- High pressure within circuit
- Tension on tubing
- Environmental changes affecting connector performance
  - Humidity
  - Temperature
- Patient movement
- Deliberate disconnection by patient

Box 11-2
Reasons Why Accidental Disconnections May Elude Detection

- Complacency due to reliance on alarms
- Desensitization due to frequent false alarms
- Inappropriate alarm settings
- Inappropriate sensor location
- Inadequate understanding of monitor/alarm function
- Misinterpretation of alarms
- Incompatible combination of monitors/alarms
- Disabled alarms
- Inaudible alarms
- Malfunctioning alarms

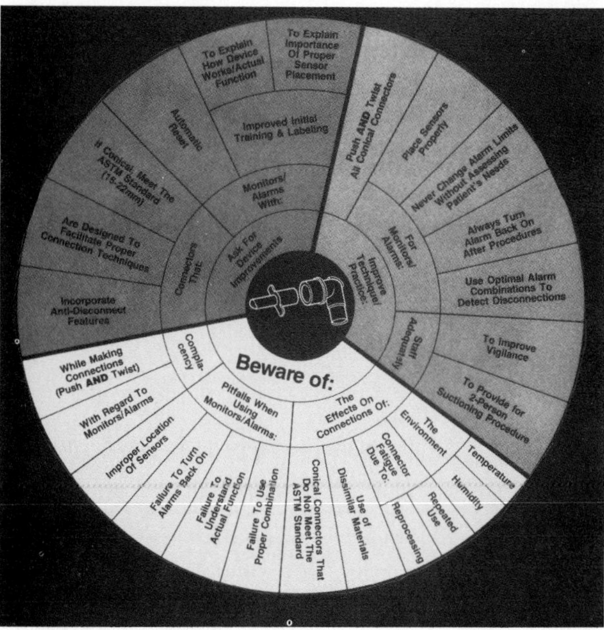

Figure 11-17. Chart describing methods to avoid and prevent accidental ventilator disconnections in the critical care setting.

References

1. Wilkins R, Hicks GH. Gas volume, flow, pressure, and temperature monitoring. Probl Respir Care 1989;2:126–155.
2. Peura RA, Webster JG. Basic transducers and principles. In: Webster JG, ed. Medical Instrumentation. Boston: Houghton Mifflin, 1978:511–557.
3. East TD. What makes noninvasive monitoring tick? A review of basic engineering principles. Respir Care 1990;35:500–519.
4. Cooper JB, Newbower RS, Long DC, McPeek M. Preventable anesthesia mishaps: A study of human factors. Anesthesiology 1978;49:399–406.
5. Stirt JA, Lewenstein LN. Circle system failure induced by gastric suction. Anaesth Intensive Care 1981;9:161–162.
6. Patel KD, Dalal FY. A potential hazard of the Drager scavenging interface system for wall suction. Anesth Analg 1979;58:327–328.
7. Ghanooni S, Wilks DH, Finestone SC. A case report of an unusual disconnection. Anesth Analg 1983;62:696–697.
8. Morrison AB. Failure to detect anesthetic circuit disconnections. Medical Devices Alert, Health and Welfare, Canada, Health Protection Branch, January 15, 1981.
9. McEwen JA, Small CF, Saunders BA, Jenkins LC. Hazards associated with the use of disconnect monitors. Anesthesiology 1980;53:S391.
10. Reynolds AC. Disconnect alarm failure. Anesthesiology 1983; 58:488.
11. Sarnquist FH, Demas K. The silent ventilator. Anesth Analg 1982;61:713–714.
12. Heard SO, Munson ES. Ventilator alarm nonfunction associated with a scavenging system for waste gases. Anesth Analg 1983; 62:230–232.
13. Craig J, Wilson ME. A survey of anaesthetic misadventures. Anaesthesia 1981;36:933–936.
14. Slee TA, Paulin EG. Failure of low pressure alarm associated with the use of a humidifier. Anesthesiology 1988;69:791–793.
15. Hudson-Civetta J, Banner M. Nursing assessment of intermittent mandatory ventilation. Int Anesthesiol Clin 1980;18:143–177.
16. Boros SJ. Variations in inspiratory:expiratory ratio and airway pressure waveform during mechanical ventilation: The significance of mean airway pressure. J Pediatr 1979;94:114–118.
17. Boros SJ, Matalon SV, Ewald R, et al. The effect of independent variations in inspiratory-expiratory ratio and end-expiratory pressure during mechanical ventilation in hyaline membrane disease. J Pediatr 1977;91:794–797.
18. Banner MJ, Gallagher TJ, Bluth LI. A new microprocessor device for mean airway pressure measurement. Crit Care Med 1981;9: 51–53.
19. Dillard R. Mean airway pressure calculation. J Pediatr 1980;97: 506–507.
20. Primiano FP, Chatburn RL, Lough MD. Mean airway pressure: Theoretical considerations. Crit Care Med 1982;10:378–383.
21. Glenski JA, Marsh HM, Hall RT. Calculation of mean airway pressure during mechanical ventilation in neonates. Crit Care Med 1984;12:642–644.
22. Marini JJ, Crooke P, Truwit J. Determinants and limits of pressure preset ventilation: A mathematical model of pressure control. J Appl Physiol 1989;67:1081–1092.
23. Berman L, Downs JB, Van Eeden A, Delhagen D. Inspiration:expiration ratio: Is mean airway pressure the difference? Crit Care Med 1981;9:775–777.
24. Myerson KR, Ilsley AH, Runciman WB. An evaluation of ventilator monitoring alarms. Anaesth Intens Care 1986;14:174–185.
25. Raphael DT, Weller RS, Doran DJ. A response algorithm for the low pressure alarm condition. Anesth Analg 1988;67:876–883.
26. Accidental breathing circuit disconnections in the critical care setting. HHS publication No. FDA 90-4233. (1991). Rockville, MD: US Department of Health and Human Services.

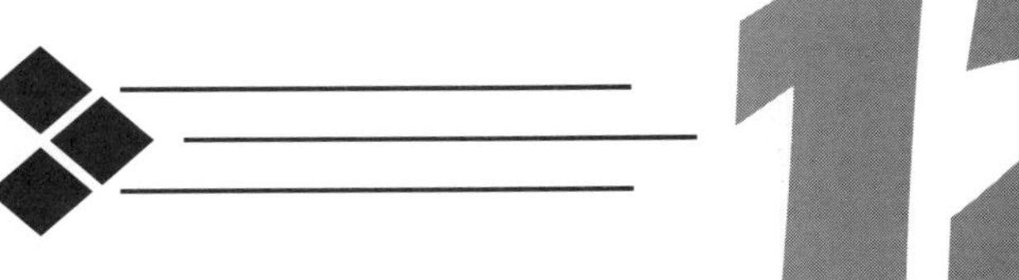

Devices for Chest Physiotherapy, Incentive Spirometry, and Intermittent Positive-Pressure Breathing

Dean R. Hess
Richard D. Branson

OBJECTIVES

1. Explain the difference between manual devices, electrically powered devices, and pneumatically powered devices to perform chest percussion and vibration.
2. Compare the principle of operation of volume-oriented and flow-oriented incentive spirometers.
3. Compare the Bird and Bennett IPPB devices.
4. Describe the Percussionaire Intrapulmonary Percussive Ventilator.
5. Describe the principle of operation of a positive expiratory pressure device.

KEY TERMS

chest percussor
chest vibrator
electrically powered percussor
flow-oriented incentive spirometer
incentive spirometer
intermittent positive-pressure breathing (IPPB)
manual percussor
mechanical chest percussor
pneumatically powered percussor
positive expiratory pressure (PEP)
volume-oriented incentive spirometer

Chest Percussors and Vibrators

Chest physiotherapy is commonly performed to assist in the removal of secretions from the respiratory tract.[1-4] This therapy has been traditionally performed manually, with the respiratory care practitioner clapping or vibrating the chest wall with the hands. Manual percussion is effective and allows the practitioner to assess the chest by palpation. However, it is also fatiguing and is quite variable from one practitioner to another. For these reasons, mechanical chest percussors have become available. Chest percussors and vibrators can be categorized as manual devices, electrically powered devices, or pneumatically powered devices.

Manual Devices

Manual percussors are used to replace the cupping action of the practitioner's hands. The practitioner manually operates the device, but the percussor produces the cupping. These devices are designed to increase patient comfort, improve practitioner efficiency, reduce practitioner fatigue, and increase uniformity of percussion between practitioners. The DHD Palm Cups (Fig. 12-1) are molded from soft vinyl. The Palm Cups are available in four sizes—neonatal, pediatric, medium, and large. The Ballard neonatal percussor (Fig. 12-2) features an absorbent percussor head and is designed to be used with neonates.

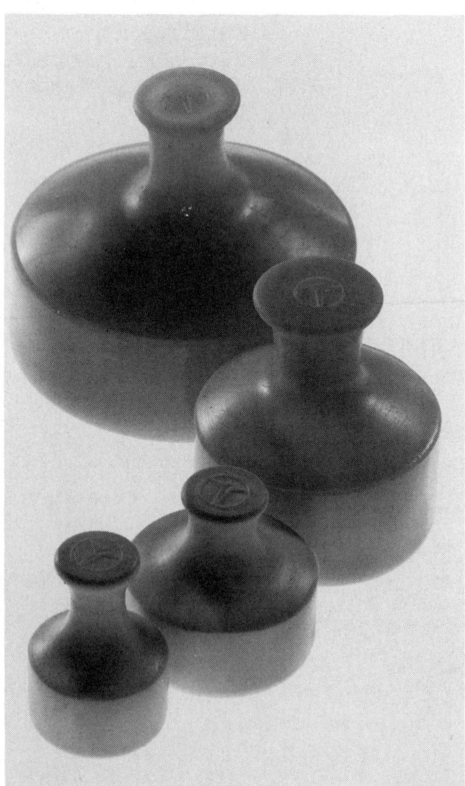

Figure 12-1. DHD palm cups: adult, pediatric, and neonatal sizes. (Courtesy of DHD Medical Products, Canastota, NY)

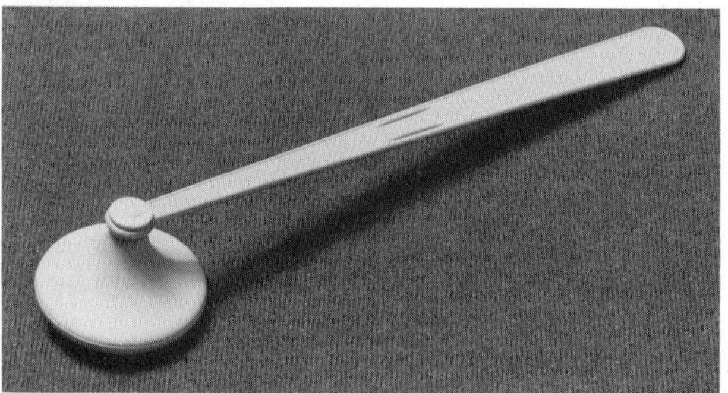

Figure 12-2. Ballard neonatal percussor. (Courtesy of Ballard, Medvale, UT)

Electrically Powered Devices

These devices are powered by 110 volts AC or they are battery operated. They are available in adult and pediatric sizes.

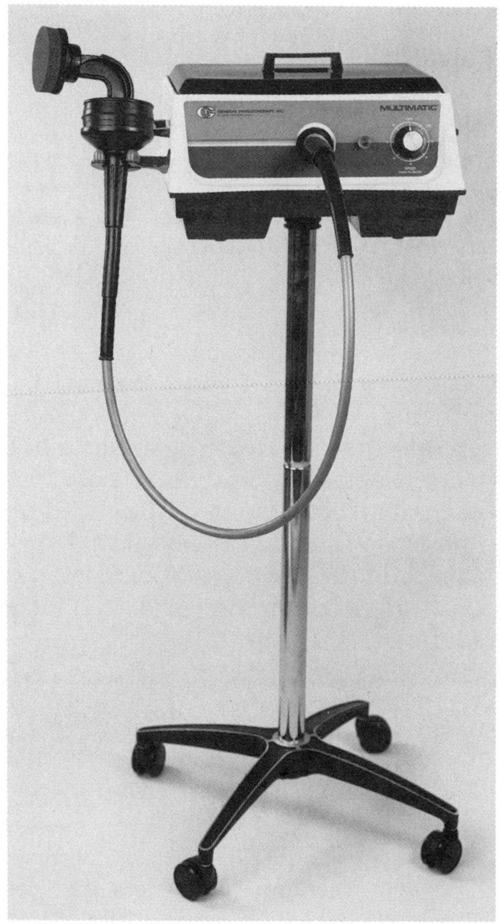

Figure 12-3. General Physiotherapy Vibramatic/Multimatic. (Courtesy of General Physiotherapy St. Louis, MO)

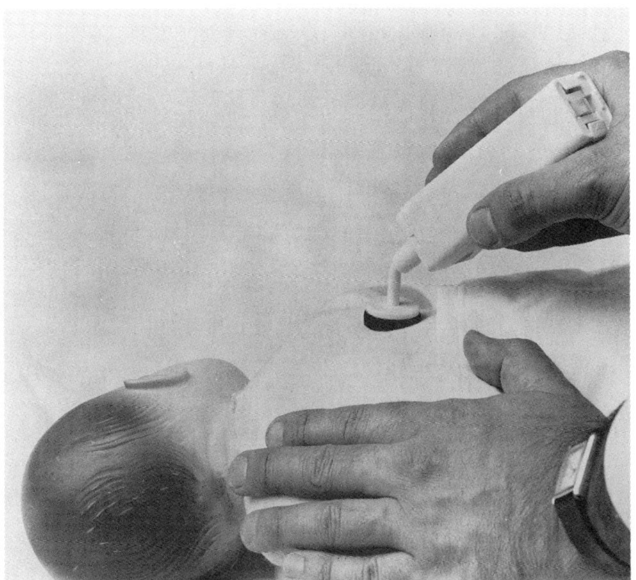

Figure 12-4. General Physiotherapy Neo-Cussor. (Courtesy of General Physiotherapy, St. Louis, MO)

A variety of electrically powered chest physiotherapy devices are available from General Physiotherapy. These devices feature a percussive directional stroking action. This rotational direction stroke has two force components. According to the manufacturer, a force component perpendicular to the body helps to loosen mucus, and a force component parallel to the body helps move mucus in the direction selected by the practitioner. The Vibramatic/Multimatic (Fig. 12-3) is designed for use in the hospital or clinic and has a variable-speed output, a speed indicator gauge, and a timer with automatic shutoff. The Flimm Fighter is designed for home care, and both variable-speed and single-speed versions are available. The Flimm Fighter uses a foam pad and Velcro belt to allow self-application of the device. The Vibracare can be used on children and adults and is of a smaller size to allow it to be more portable. The Neo-Cussor is a pocket-sized, battery-operated percussor for neonates that uses a disposable applicator (Fig. 12-4).

Electrically powered percussors are also available from Strom and Puritan-Bennett. The Strom percussor (Fig. 12-5) features a variable-speed, 3/4-inch stroke, and suction cup covered with leather. The Strom percussor can be used for either percussion or vibration. The Puritan-Bennett Vibrator/Percussor (Fig. 12-6) independently controls stroke intensity and frequency.

Pneumatically Powered Devices

Pneumatically powered percussors and vibrators are available from several manufacturers. The principal advantage of these devices is that they do not require an electrical power source. They do, however, require a pressurized gas source, which will usually be 50 psig air or oxygen.

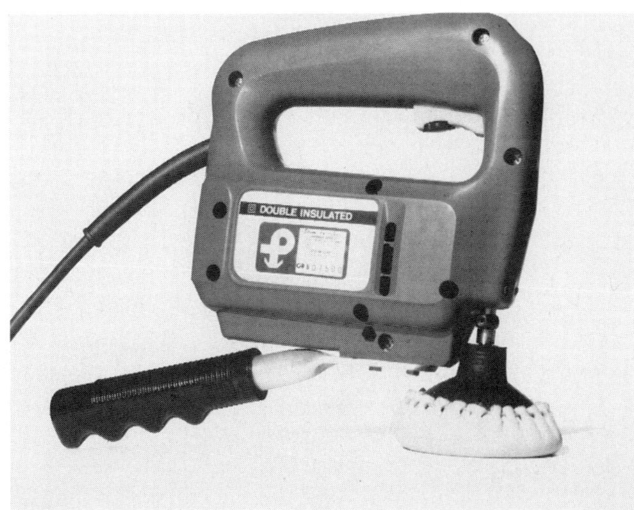

Figure 12-5. Strom electronic percussor. (Courtesy of Strom, Lewisville, TX)

The Strom PPS 3 (Fig. 12-7) is a pneumatically powered sonic percussor that can be used with neonates or adults. The PPS 3 has an adjustable speed control to produce low clapping or mid/high vibration. The bellows-shaped cup of the PPS 3 is shock absorbing and is intended to produce percussion with little trauma to the patient. The Fluid Flo Percussor is a pneumatically powered adult percussor with a variable-speed control (Fig. 12-8). The Mercury MJ Percussor is pneumatically powered, available in adult and child sizes, and has a variable speed control (Fig. 12-9).

Incentive Spirometers

Incentive spirometers are used to encourage deep breathing, and thus prevent atelectasis, in postopera-

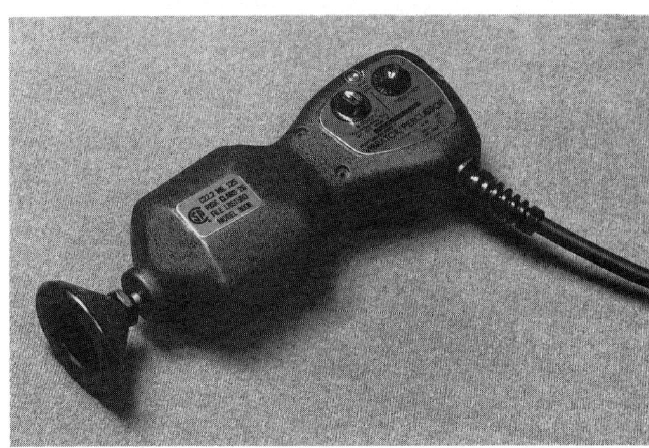

Figure 12-6. Puritan-Bennett Vibrator/Percussor. (Courtesy of Puritan-Bennett Corporation Lenexa KS)

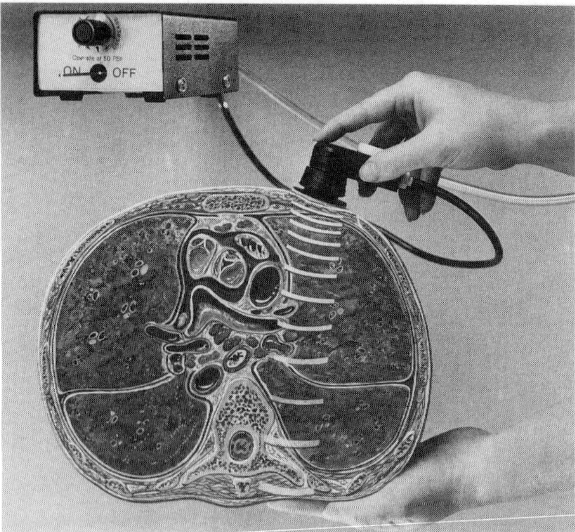

Figure 12-7. Strom PPS 3 sonic percussor. (Courtesy of Strom, Lewisville, TX)

tive patients. Incentive spirometry may be the most commonly used respiratory therapy in postoperative patients. Incentive spirometers are of two primary types, volume-oriented devices and flow-oriented devices. Although there may be differences in the performance of various incentive spirometers available on the market, differences among devices may be negligible in terms of clinical outcome. Theoretically, volume-oriented devices are superior to flow-oriented devices, but the use of volume-oriented devices rather than flow-oriented devices may make little difference clinically.[5–10]

Volume-Oriented Incentive Spirometers

The first commercially available incentive spirometer was the Bartlett-Edwards (Fig. 12-10), which is no longer commercially available. It is a lightweight, portable, battery-operated device that consists of a piston in a cylinder. When the patient inhales from the device, the piston rises and activates a light when the prescribed inhaled volume is reached. Because of a fixed leak in the piston, the patient needs to continue active inhalation after the signal light comes on to keep it lit for a few seconds. A digital indicator automatically records the number of inspirations that meet the volume goal set on the device.

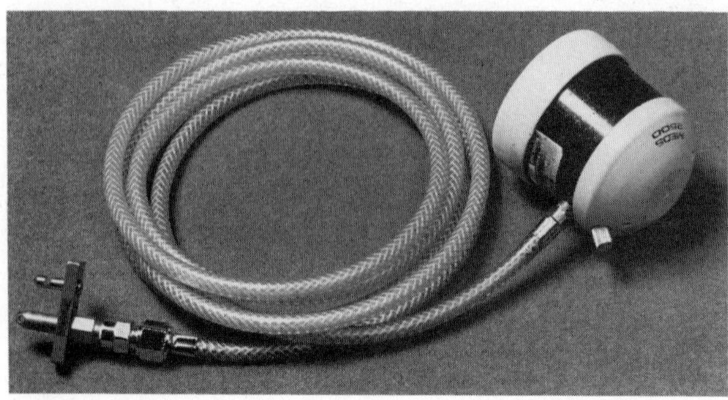

Figure 12-8. Fluid Flo Percussor.

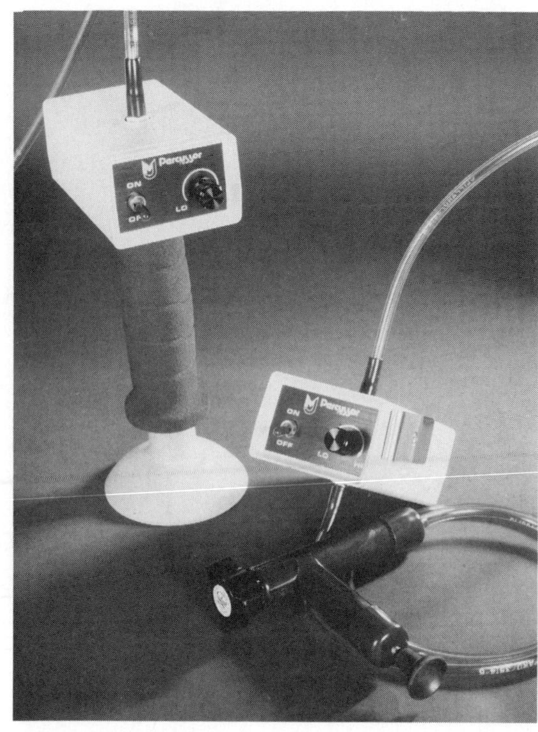

Figure 12-9. Mercury MJ percussor. (Courtesy of Mercury Medical, Clearwater, FL)

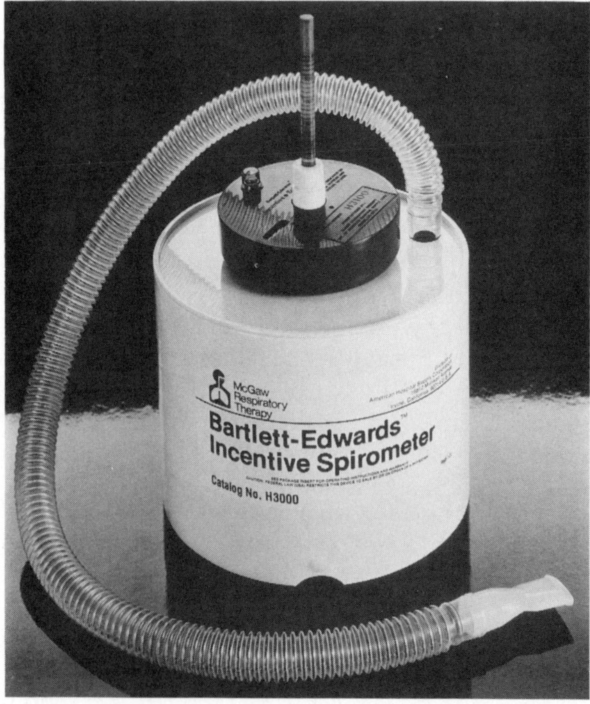

Figure 12-10. Bartlett-Edwards incentive spirometer.

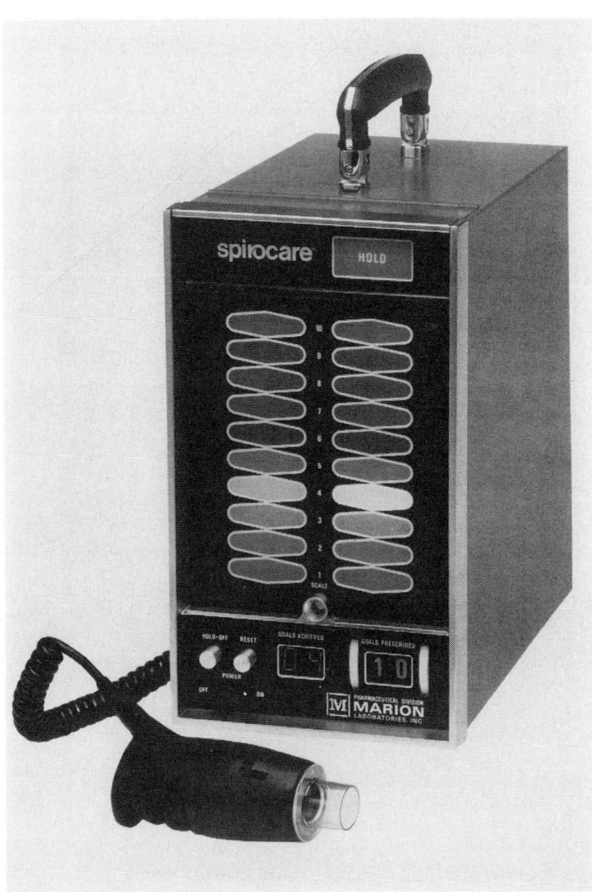

Figure 12-11. Spirocare incentive spirometer.

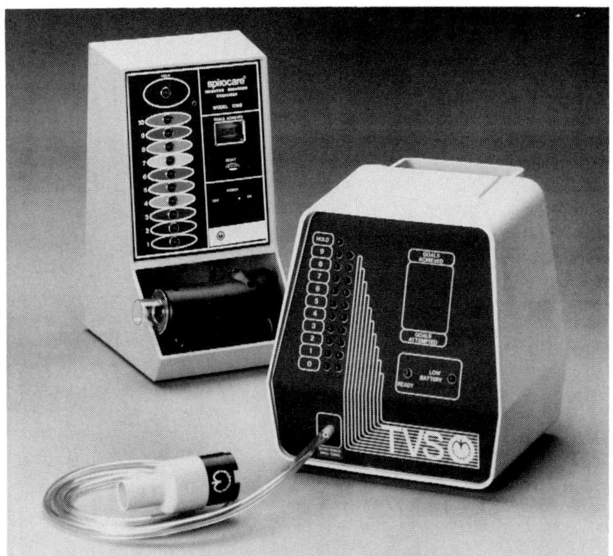

Figure 12-12. Battery-operated Spirocare (left) and TVS incentive spirometer (right).

The Spirocare is available in two versions, one that is powered by 110 volts AC (Fig. 12-11) and one that is battery operated (Fig. 12-12). Both of these use a disposable mouthpiece/flow tube, which contains a turbine that spins as the patient inhales. A light signal is interrupted as the patient breathes through the flow tube, and this is translated into an inspired volume display. The patient's inspired volume is indicated by 10 goal lights. Volume ranges of 250 to 1375 mL, 500 to 2750 mL, and 1000 to 5500 mL can be selected by the respiratory care practitioner. A hold light is activated and remains lit for 2.5 seconds when the patient reaches the inspiratory goal. The number of goals achieved is digitally indicated. The TVS is similar to the Spirocare in that it is also electrically powered (see Fig. 12-12).

The Volurex is a disposable incentive spirometer with a 4000-mL capacity (Fig. 12-13). The bottom edge of the bellows serves as the inspired volume indicator. After each breath, a reset button is depressed to return the bellows to the bottom of the unit. A one-way valve prevents the patient from rebreathing. This device requires assembly by the respiratory care practitioner before use.

Several incentive spirometers are available from DHD Medical Products that consist of a piston in a cylinder configuration. The DHD Coach (Fig. 12-14) has a compact size, a 4000-mL capacity, a one-way valve to prevent exhaling into the unit, and an inspiratory flow guide to coach the patient to inhale slowly. The DHD Coach 2500 is similar to the DHD Coach except that it has a 2500-mL capacity. Both the DHD Coach and DHD Coach 2500 have a sliding pointer to indicate the prescribed inspired volume. The DHD Coach Jr has a 2000-mL capacity for use with children, has colorful packaging to hold the child's interest, and a bubble gum fragrance for the child's added enjoyment.

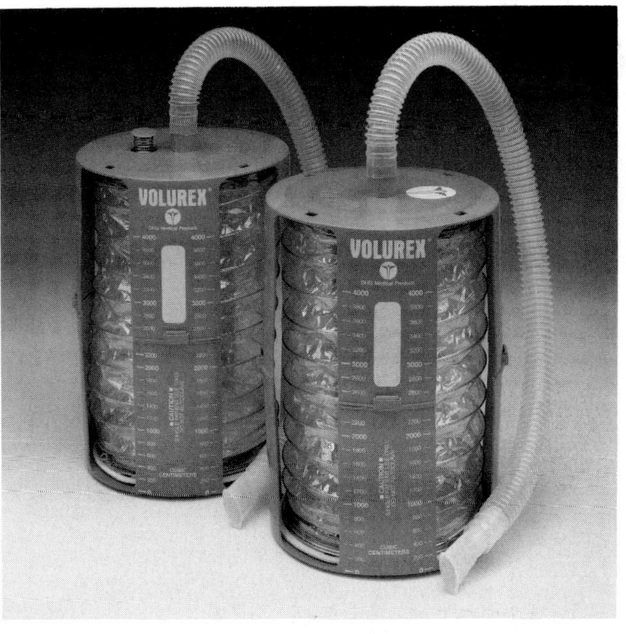

Figure 12-13. DHD Volurex incentive spirometer. (Courtesy of DHD Medical Products, Canastota, NY)

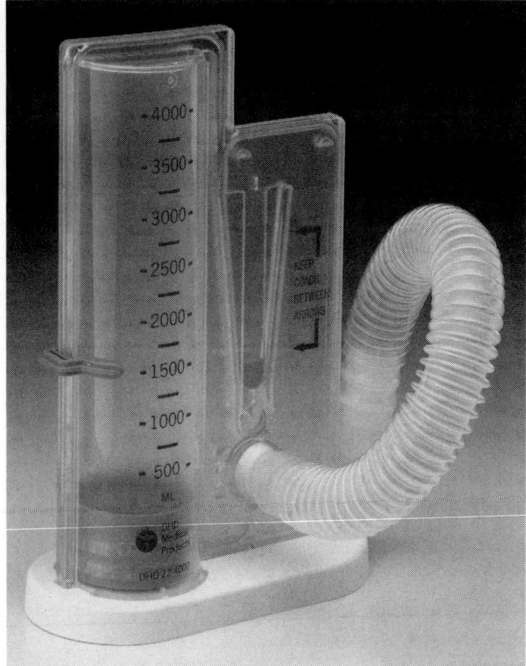

Figure 12-14. DHD Coach incentive spirometer. (Courtesy of DHD Medical Products, Canastota, NY)

The Voldyne volumetric exerciser has a capacity of 4000 mL and is a piston in a cylinder similar to the DHD Coach (Fig. 12-15). A sliding indicator is used to indicate the prescribed inspiratory volume, and a flow indicator encourages the patient to inspire slowly.

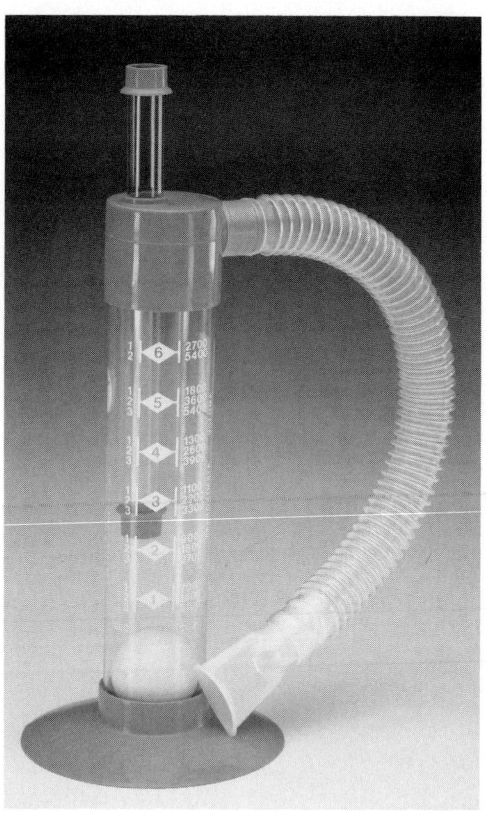

Figure 12-16. DHD Respirex incentive spirometer. (Courtesy of DHD Medical Products, Canastota, NY)

Flow-Oriented Incentive Spirometers

The DHD Respirex incentive spirometer has an adjustable inspiratory volume indicator (Fig. 12-16).

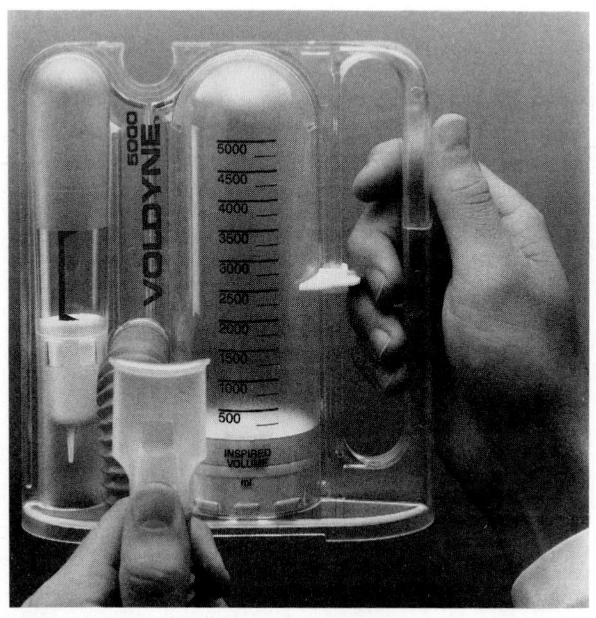

Figure 12-15. Voldyne incentive spirometer. (Courtesy of Sherwood Medical, St. Louis, MO)

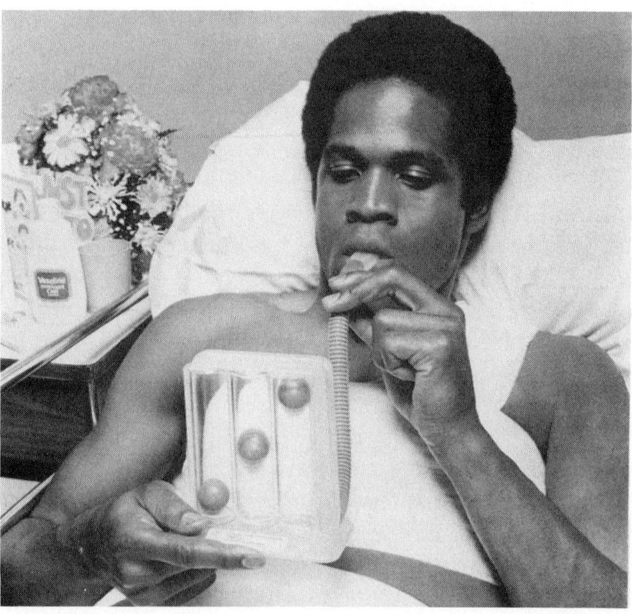

Figure 12-17. Triflow incentive spirometer. (Courtesy of Sherwood Medical, St. Louis, MO)

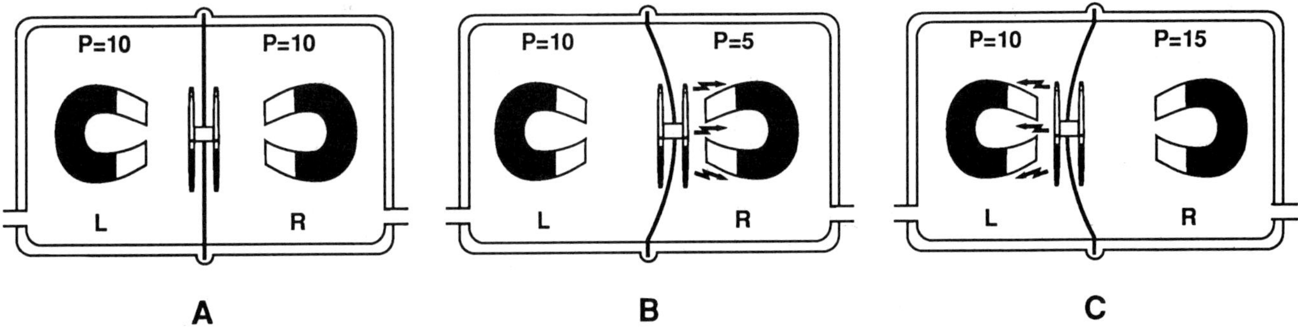

Figure 12-21. Conceptual drawing demonstrating the use of pressure gradients and magnetism as seen with the Bird respirators. (Courtesy of Bird Corporation, Palm Springs, CA)

The Mark 7 uses pressure gradients and magnetism to control inspiration and expiration. A simplified drawing of this concept is shown in Figure 12-21. The drawing depicts two chambers separated by a flexible diaphragm. Note that both chambers communicate with ambient pressure. Attached to the diaphragm are two metal plates (one on each side of the diaphragm). Each chamber contains a magnet. When pressure in the two chambers and magnetic attraction of the plates by the magnets are equal, the diaphragm remains in a neutral position (A). When the right chamber has a reduction in its pressure (as would occur clinically with a spontaneous inspiration), the diaphragm shifts to the right. This causes the metal plate to contact the right magnet (B). As pressure increases in the right chamber (it must increase greater than atmospheric pressure to overcome force of the magnetic attraction), the diaphragm is shifted back to the left, where the left magnet holds the metal plate (C). In actual operation of the Mark series of ventilators, the position of the diaphragm shown in A does not occur. The attraction of the magnets and the pressure changes in the chambers or both serve to hold the diaphragm to the left (expiration) or to the right (inspiration).

A functional schematic of the Mark 7 is shown in Figure 12-22. Depicted is the position of the components during expiration and at the start of inspiration. During the expiratory phase, the ceramic switch that is attached to the metal clutch plates is moved toward the ambient compartment. This occurs when the ambient magnet is in contact with the ambient clutch plate, preventing flow from entering the patient circuit. When the ventilator is triggered on, the pressure magnet holds the pressure clutch plate, sliding the ceramic switch to the right. This allows gas flow from the flow control to travel through an opening in the ceramic switch and begin inspiration. Gas from the ceramic switch travels to the air/mix control. The air/mix control (Fig. 12-23) is a plunger mechanism that controls F_{IO_2} by allowing or preventing gas flow to a venturi. When the air/mix control is pushed in, O-rings on the plunger prevent gas from traveling to the venturi. In this instance, gas flow to the patient comes from the nebulizer output and through the bleed hole in the metal center body of the Mark 7. When the air/mix control is pulled out, gas flow is directed to the venturi. The venturi entrains gas from the ambient compartment for delivery to the pressure compartment and finally to the patient. During operation of the venturi, gas delivered to the patient comes from the nebulizer output and the venturi output. Because entrainment of room air is dependent on back-pressure, the F_{IO_2} delivered with the air/mix control open fluctuates throughout the ventilatory cycle. A gate placed on the venturi outlet is actually a spring-loaded

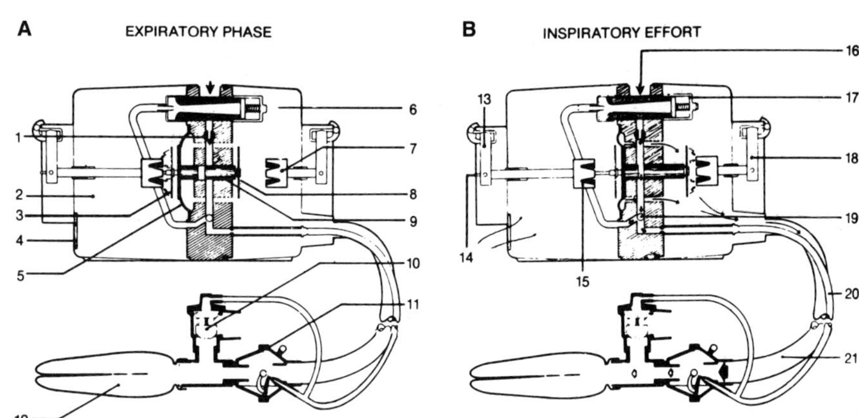

Figure 12-22. Internal schematic of the Bird Mark 7 with breathing circuit: 1, flow rate control; 2, ambient compartment; 3, ambient clutch plate; 4, air inlet filter; 5, diaphragm; 6, pressure compartment; 7, pressure magnet; 8, pressure clutch plate; 9, ceramic switch; 10, exhalation valve; 11, micro nebulizer; 12, test lung, 13, sensitivity arm; 14, hand timer rod; 15, ambient magnet; 16, source gas inlet; 17, venturi; 18, pressure limit arm; 19, air/mix plunger; 20, inspiratory drive line; 21, mainstream line. (Courtesy of Bird Corporation, Palm Springs, CA)

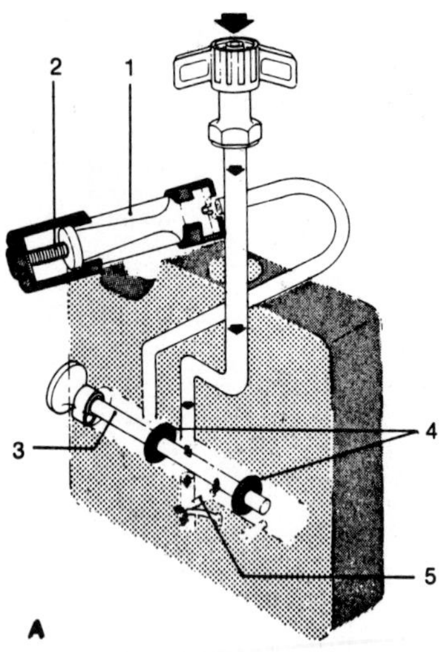

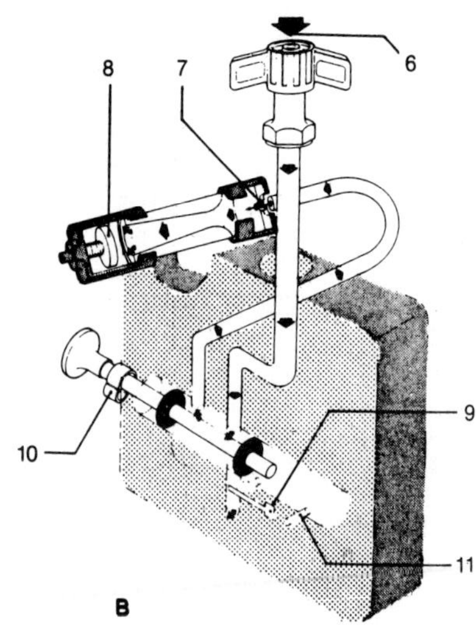

Figure 12-23. Air/mix control of the Bird Mark 7. Air/mix control is pulled out (right) allowing flow to the venturi. Air/mix control pushed in prevents flow from entering the venturi (left) causing 100% source gas to be delivered to the patient. (Courtesy of Bird Corporation, Palm Springs, CA)

valve that requires 2 cm H_2O to open. The gate's purpose is to prevent gas from the ambient compartment from entering the pressure compartment during a patient's spontaneous inspiration. If the gate was not present, the small flow of gas through the venturi could prevent pressure in the pressure compartment from falling to a level sufficient to trigger inspiration during the patient's inspiratory effort. Operating of the air/mix control also effects the Mark 7's output waveform. At the 100% F_{IO_2} setting, the Mark 7 produces a rectangular flow waveform and ascending ramp pressure waveform. When the venturi is activated, a descending flow waveform is produced and an irregular pressure waveform ranging from nearly a rectangular waveform to an ascending waveform occurs, depending on the patient's compliance and resistance. Inspiration can be triggered manually by pushing the hand timer rod, which pushes the ceramic switch/clutch plate assembly into the inspiratory position. It may also be triggered by the patient, when an inspiratory effort causes pressure in the pressure compartment to fall below pressure in the ambient compartment. Pressure triggering is controlled by the sensitivity arm. Time triggering is also available by use of the expiratory timer (Fig. 12-24). The expiratory timing mechanism consists of a cartridge containing a diaphragm, spring, timer arm, and a needle valve. When the expiratory time control is off (needle valve is closed) during inspiration (A) and expiration (B), the cartridge remains pressurized and no movement of the arm takes place. As the expiratory time control is opened, gas passes by the needle valve and into the pressure compartment. During inspiration (C), the cartridge remains pressurized, but when the ceramic switch returns to the expiratory position (D), gas exits through the needle valve through a bleed hole. As the cartridge loses pressure, the diaphragm and spring move to the right, causing the timer arm to push the ambient clutch plate into the inspiratory position. The faster gas is released from the cartridge (by opening the needle valve), the shorter expiratory time becomes. During IPPB, the expiratory timer is turned off.

Normal operation of the Bird Mark 7 allows the operator to set sensitivity, peak pressure limit, flow rate, and F_{IO_2}. Sensitivity is controlled by positioning the ambient pressure magnet closer (less sensitive) or farther away (more sensitive) from the ambient clutch plate. With the sensitivity arm, pressure limit is set by positioning the pressure magnet closer (higher pressure) or farther away (lower pressure) from the pressure clutch plate with the pressure limit arm. The flow rate control is a simple needle valve that has an uncal-

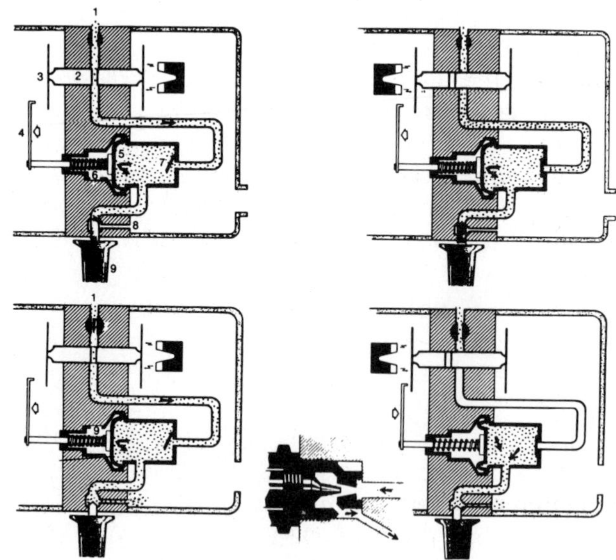

Figure 12-24. Operation of the expiratory timer cartridge: 1, source gas inlet; 2, ceramic switch; 3, ambient clutch plate; 4, expiratory timer arm; 5, diaphragm; 6, spring; 7, check valve; 8, drain hole; 9, expiratory timer control. (Courtesy of Bird Corporation, Palm Springs, CA)

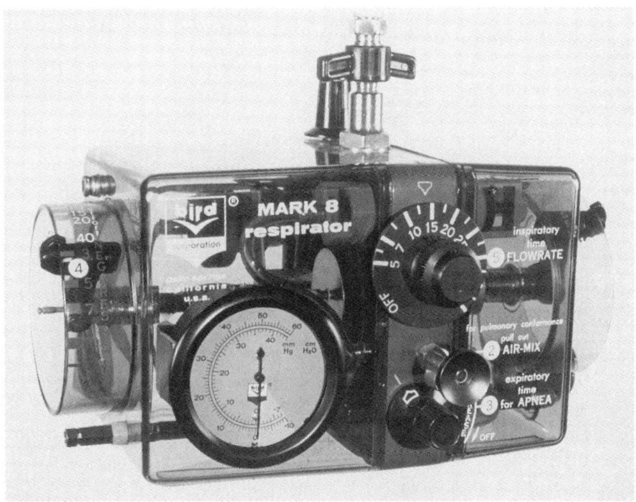

Figure 12-25. Bird Mark 8 ventilator. (Courtesy of Bird Corporation, Palm Springs, CA)

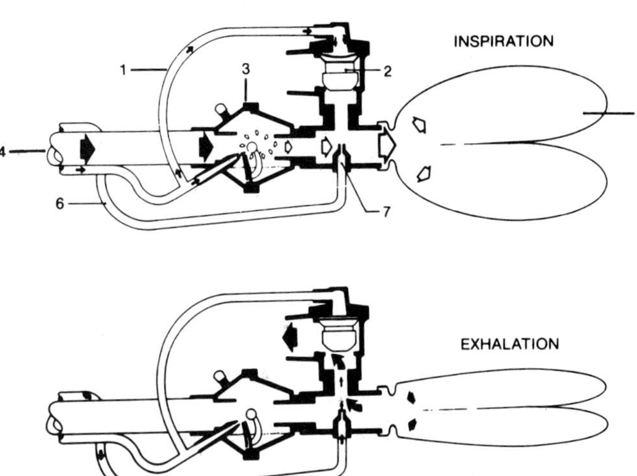

Figure 12-26. Breathing assembly for the Bird Mark 8 ventilator: 1, inspiratory drive line; 2, exhalation valve; 3, micronebulizer; 4, mainstream line; 5, test lung; 6, expiratory drive line; 7, negative venturi. (Courtesy of Bird Corporation, Palm Springs, CA)

ibrated control knob. Placing the air/mix control in either the in or out position allows delivery of gas at either 100% source gas or a level less than that, as previously described.

An integral aneroid pressure gauge measures pressure in the pressure compartment over a range of −10 to 60 cm H_2O.

Bird Mark 8

The Bird Mark 8 ventilator (Fig. 12-25) is identical to the Mark 7 except that a system for generating a constant flow during the expiratory phase is present. The knob for adjusting this flow is located on the top of the ventilator and consists of a needle valve and a "negative interrupter" cartridge. Activation of the needle valve allows a flow of gas to travel to a venturi in the breathing circuit (Fig. 12-26). During expiration, gas flowing through the venturi entrains expired gas from the circuit and patient and directs it out the exhalation valve. This system was used to create negative end-expiratory pressure (NEEP), which was thought to help alleviate air trapping. In clinical use, the use of NEEP proved to be of little benefit and may actually have exacerbated air trapping. The use of NEEP has since been abandoned.

Bird Mark 9

The Bird Mark 9 ventilator (Fig. 12-27) is a modified Mark 8 that was primarily intended for veterinary use. Differences between the Mark 9 and Mark 8 include (1) a larger pressure magnet to allow for higher pressure limit settings, (2) an aneroid pressure gauge calibrated over a range of −30 to 200 mm Hg, and (3) replacement of the air/mix control with a dual flow range control. When the dual flow control is "in," only a single venturi is operational (peak flow = 200 L/min) while when the control is pulled "out," two venturis were activated (peak flow 270 L/min).

Bird Mark 10

The Bird Mark 10 (Fig. 12-28) is similar to the Mark 7 with two major differences. First, there is not an air/mix control on the Mark 10, which means it always operates in the air dilution mode. Second, the Mark 10 has an additional control known as inspiratory flow acceleration. This control allows for an automatic increase in flow at the end of inspiration based on the control setting. The purpose of the inspiratory flow acceleration is to compensate for leaks in the system.

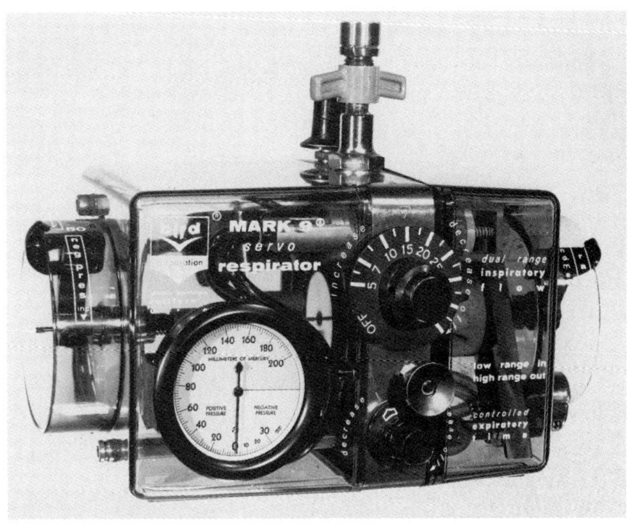

Figure 12-27. Bird Mark 9. (Courtesy of Bird Corporation, Palm Springs, CA)

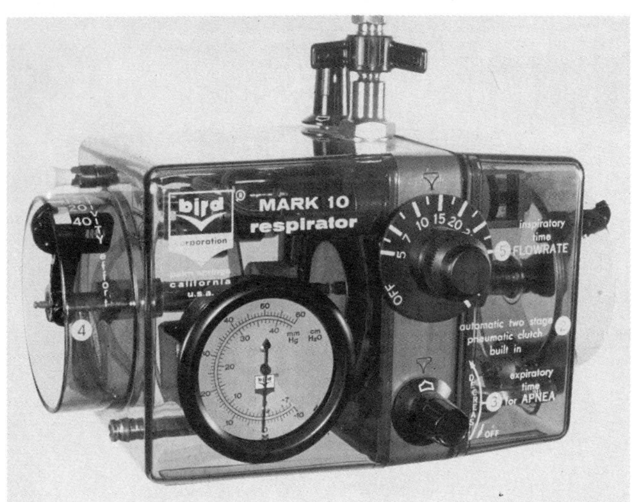

Figure 12-28. Bird Mark 10. (Courtesy of Bird Corporation, Palm Springs, CA)

Bird Mark 14

The Bird Mark 14 (Fig. 12-29) is essentially a Mark 10 with a Mark 9 pressure magnet that allows peak pressures of approximately 200 cm H_2O. The Mark 14 has an integral aneroid pressure gauge with a range of −30 to 200 mm Hg. Additionally, the Mark 14 has an improved sensitivity control known as a vernier.

Puritan-Bennett IPPB Units

Puritan-Bennett PR-2

The Puritan-Bennett PR-2 (Fig. 12-30) is a pressure controller that may be time or pressure triggered and is pressure limited and flow or time cycled. Like the Bird Mark series of ventilators, the PR-2 is pneumatically powered and controlled and, although capable of providing mechanical ventilation, is normally used to deliver IPPB therapy.

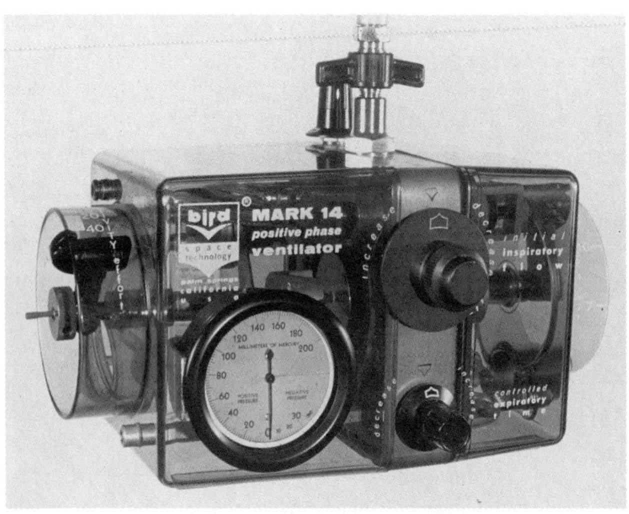

Figure 12-29. Bird Mark 14. (Courtesy of Bird Corporation, Palm Springs, CA)

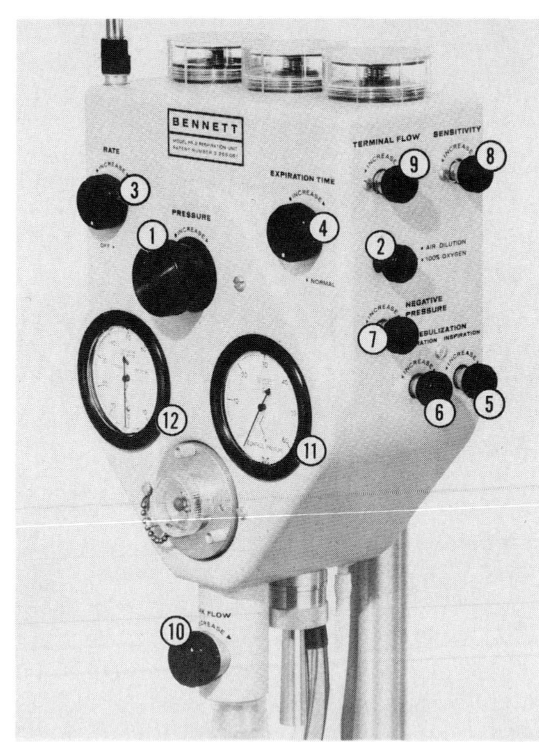

Figure 12-30. The Puritan-Bennett PR-2: 1, peak pressure control (0 to 50 cm H_2O); 2, air/mix control; 3, respiratory rate control; 4, expiratory time control; 5, inspiratory nebulization; 6, expiratory nebulization; 7, negative expiratory pressure control (0 to -6 cm H_2O); 8, sensitivity control; 9, terminal flow control; 10, peak flow control; 11, control pressure gauge; 12, system pressure gauge. (Courtesy of Puritan-Bennett Corporation, Kansas City, MO)

A schematic of the PR-2 is shown in Figure 12-31. Gas at 50 psig enters the ventilator through a brass filter and is delivered to the control pressure regulator, the low-pressure regulator, and the nebulizer pressure switch. Gas entering the control pressure regulator is reduced to the pressure set by the pressure control knob in the center of the face panel. Adjustment of the control knob simply works to increase or decrease spring tension on a diaphragm. Within the control pressure regulator is a venturi, which may be activated by the air-dilution control. This allows the PR-2 to deliver either 100% source gas or an FIO_2 of 0.40 to 0.60, depending on back-pressure. Gas from the control pressure regulator is delivered to the Bennett valve, which controls gas delivery to the patient. The Bennett valve was developed by V. Ray Bennett in 1944 to provide oxygen to pilots flying in unpressurized aircraft at high altitudes. It consists of a hollow cylinder that is closed at either end with two rectangular openings on its opposite sides (Fig. 12-32). Attached externally to the cylinder is a drum vane and within the cylinder is a counterweight. Dur-

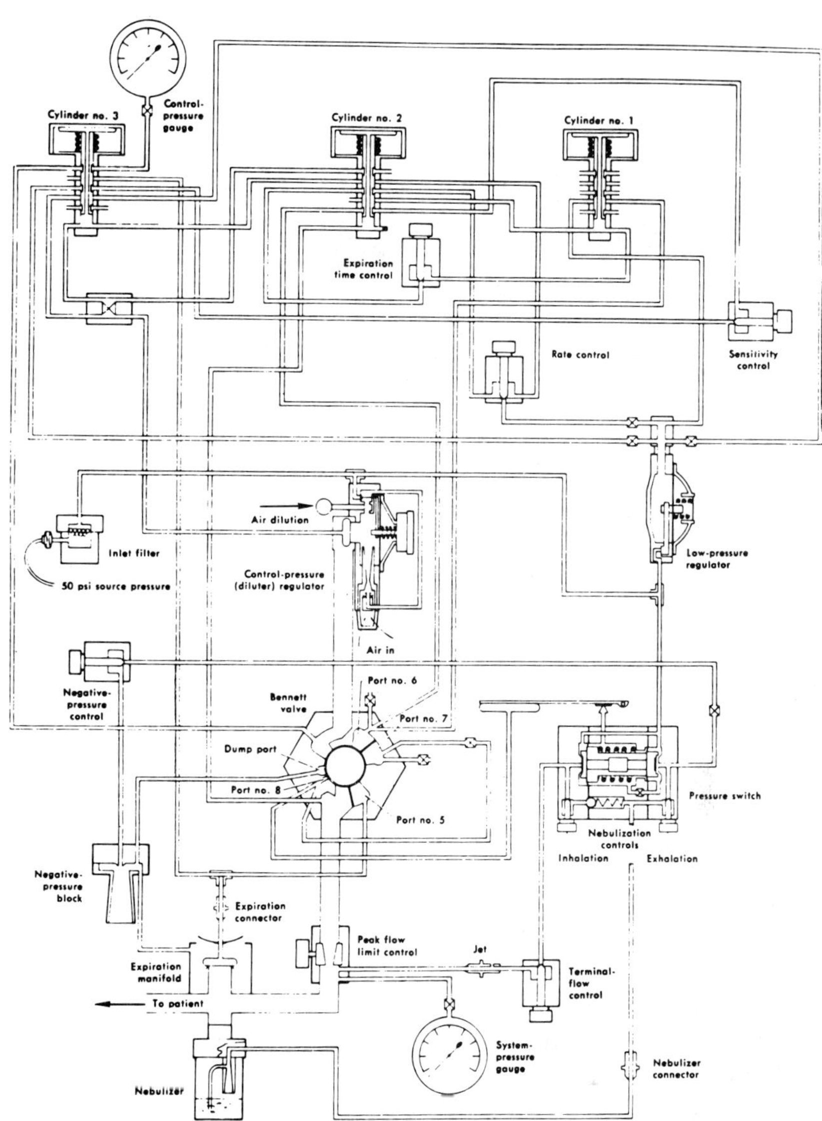

Figure 12-31. Pneumatic components of the PR-2. (Courtesy of Puritan-Bennett Corporation, Kansas City, MO)

ing expiration the counterweight keeps the drum rotated such that gas from the pressure control regulator is blocked and allows the exhalation valve to communicate with the atmosphere through the dump port. When the drum rotates counterclockwise into the inspiratory position, the upper and lower windows allow gas from the pressure control regulator to flow through the valve to the peak flow control and on to the patient. In the inspiratory position, gas is also directed to the exhalation valve and system pressure gauge. As pressure in the system builds, the difference between the set pressure (controlled by the regulator) and circuit pressure diminishes and the flow across the valve falls. When flow reaches a level, less than 1 to 3 L/min, the counterweight overcomes the effects of gas flow on the drum vane and inspiration ends. The peak flow control is simply a needle valve and allows flow to be adjusted from 15 to 80 L/min.

Gas that was directed to the nebulizer pressure switch controls gas flow to the inspiratory and expiratory nebulizer controls and the terminal flow control. Depending on the position of the Bennett valve, the nebulizer pressure switch will allow gas flow to the nebulizer as selected by the operator. The terminal flow control allows gas to enter a venturi and deliver a flow of up to 15 L/min into the patient circuit. This flow is delivered below the peak flow control to increase system pressure and facilitate closure of the Bennett valve when leaks are present. Because gas flow to the nebulizer switch is source gas (it has not passed through the air-dilution system), if air-dilution is operable, use of the terminal flow control will increase delivered F_{IO_2}. Gas from the nebulizer pressure switch is also used to power an optional negative pressure control. Gas flow from the negative pressure control operates a venturi, which allows the application of NEEP from 0 to −6 cm H_2O.

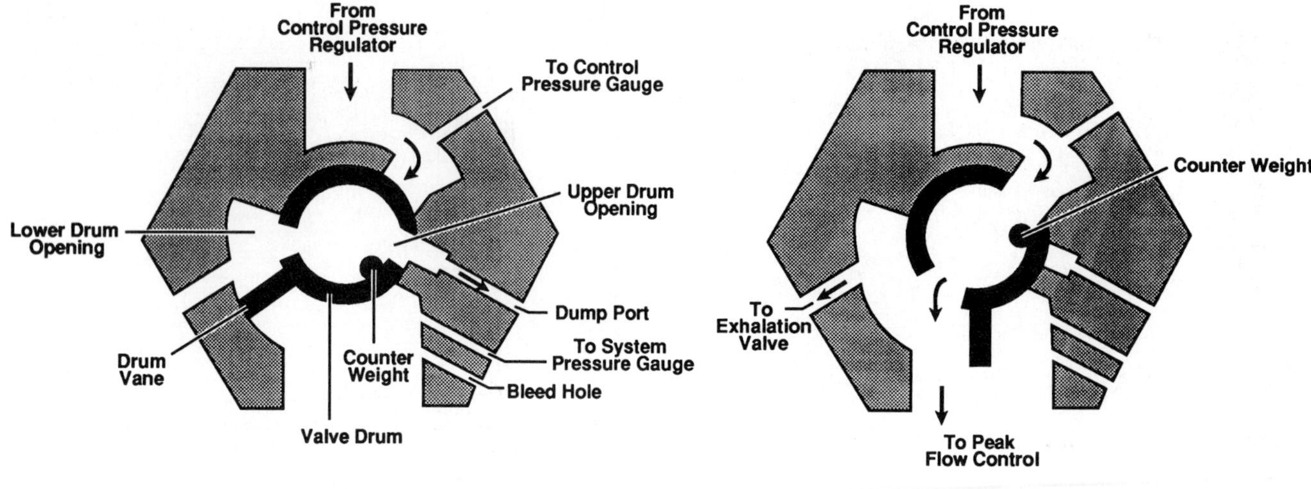

Figure 12-32. The Bennett valve. During expiration, the counterweight maintains the valve in the off position. When inspiration begins (either by creation of a negative inspiratory effort by the patient or time-triggered by the ventilator), the drum rotates to allow gas flow through the drum openings and on to the peak flow control and patient. (Note: The Bennett valve used in the PR-2 utilizes two vanes on the drum.) (Courtesy of Puritan-Bennett Corporation, Kansas City, MO)

Gas that was directed to the low-pressure regulator is reduced to a pressure of 60 cm H_2O and used to control ventilator rate, expiratory time, and sensitivity. Since ventilator rate and expiratory time are normally not used during IPPB therapy, only the sensitivity control is discussed here. When the sensitivity control is functional, it allows gas from the low-pressure regulator to flow to the Bennett valve to a port above the upper drum vane. This flow tends to rotate the drum clockwise toward inspiration. This biasing of the drum allows the patient to trigger inspiration with less effort. During inspiration, flow to the sensitivity control is terminated.

Puritan-Bennett AP-5

The Puritan-Bennett AP-5 (Fig. 12-33) is an electronically powered, pneumatically controlled, pressure

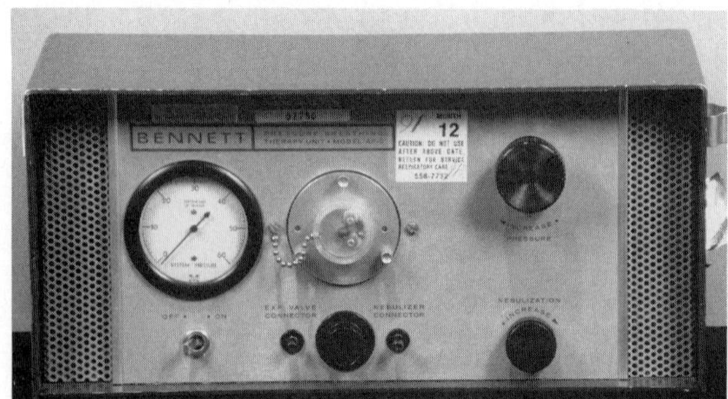

Figure 12-33. The Puritan-Bennett AP-5. (Courtesy of Puritan-Bennett Corporation, Kansas City, MO)

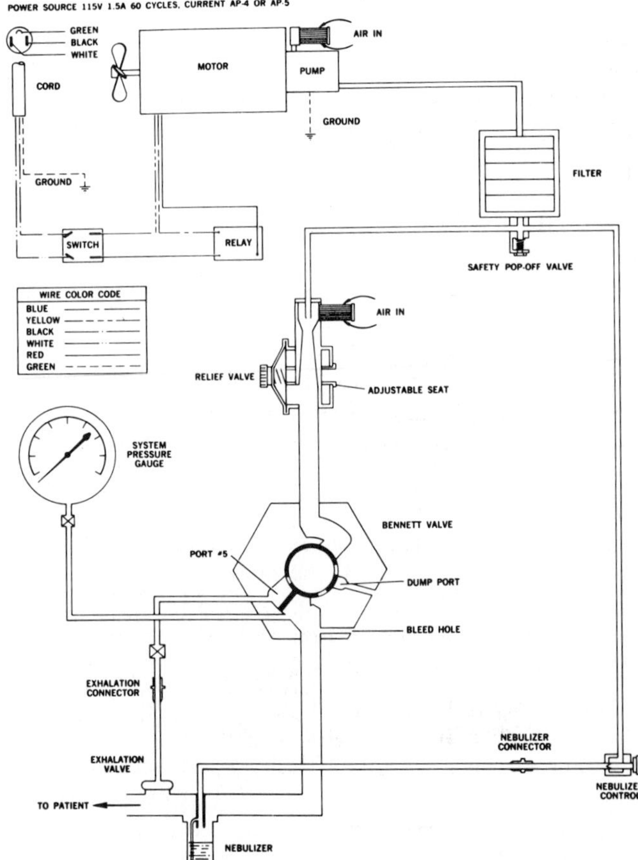

Figure 12-34. Internal components of the AP-5. (Courtesy of Puritan-Bennett Corporation, Kansas City, MO)

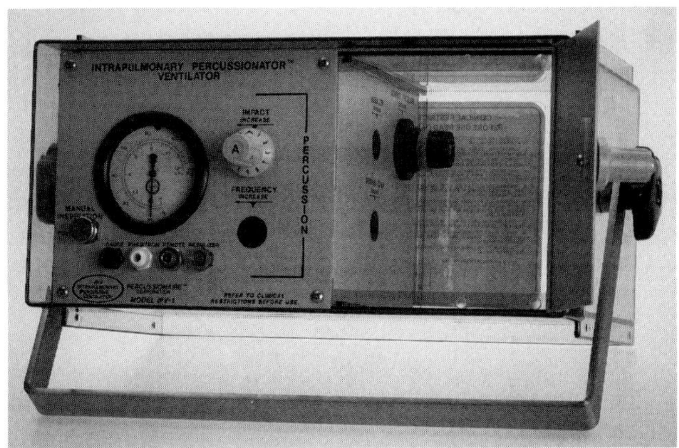

Figure 12-35. The IPV-1. (Courtesy of Percussionaire, Sandpoint, ID)

controller that can be pressure triggered, pressure limited, and flow cycled. The AP-5 is only used for the delivery of IPPB therapy and is most commonly used in the home.

A schematic of the AP-5 is shown in Figure 12-34. Gas supplied by a compressor passes through a filter and is directed to either the pressure control or nebulizer control. A safety pressure pop-off valve is located at the filter outlet to vent excessive pressure. Gas flows to the pressure relief valve (in place of the pressure control regulator of the PR-2) by means of a venturi. The pressure relief valve is a simple spring-disk system that allows excess pressure to vent to ambient. Adjustment of the pressure control knob adjusts spring tension on the disk and thus peak pressure

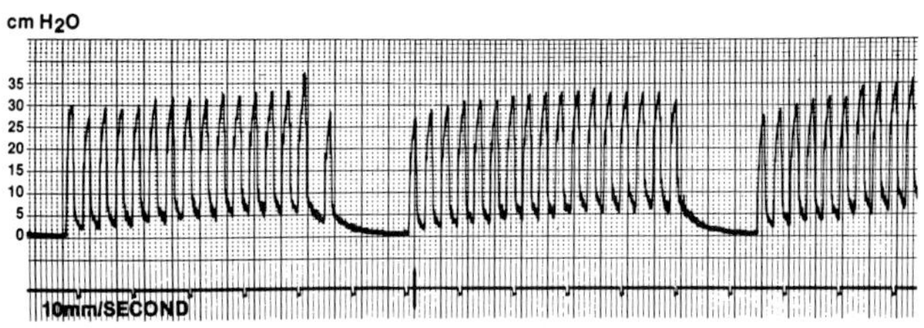

Figure 12-36. Airway pressure pattern seen during IPV therapy. (Courtesy of Percussionaire, Sandpoint, ID)

(0–30 cm H_2O). From the pressure relief valve gas flows to the Bennett valve, which operates as previously described. Gas from the compressor also travels to the nebulizer control, which is a simple needle valve. Opening the nebulizer control allows more flow to travel to the nebulizer.

Percussionaire Intrapulmonary Percussive Ventilator-1 (IPV-1)

The IPV-1 (Fig. 12-35) is a recently developed method of providing IPPB in a unique fashion. Rather than trigger on a positive-pressure breath, the IPV-1 allows the patient to manually trigger a group of high-frequency or "percussive" breaths. This method of gas delivery increases lung volume to a selected pressure, and the percussive breaths are continuously supplied as a method to increase secretion mobilization (Fig. 12-36).

The IPV-1 has only two controls: the operational pressure (20 to 50 psig) and the "impact" or peak pressure. An internal schematic is shown in Figure 12-37. Gas at 50 psig enters a filter and travels to a pressure

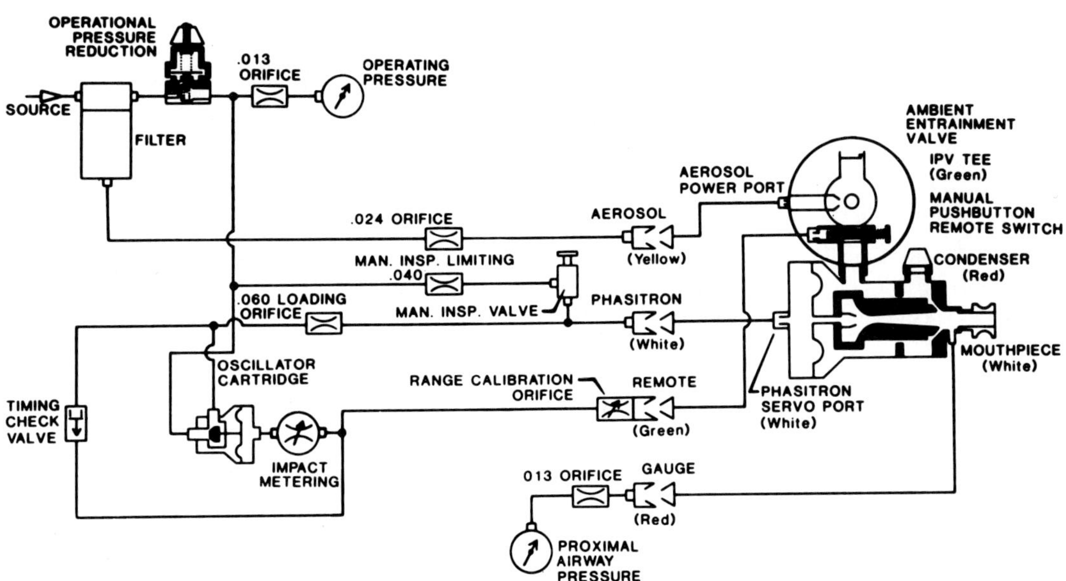

Figure 12-37. Internal schematic of the IPV-1. (Courtesy of Percussionaire, Sandpoint, ID)

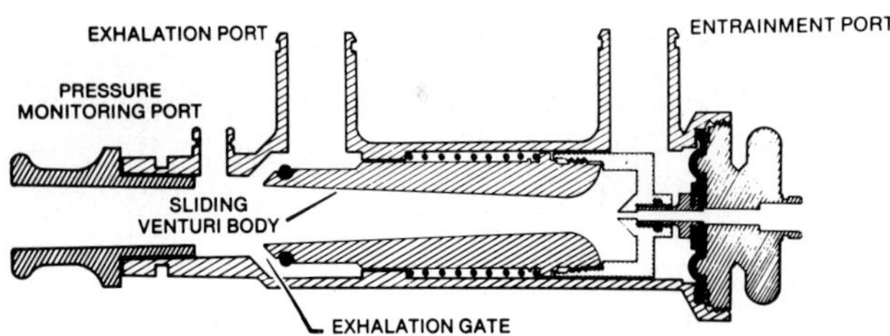

Figure 12-38. The phasitron is a sliding venturi that directs both inspiratory and expiratory gases at the airway. The expiratory phase is depicted here. (Courtesy of Percussionaire, Sandpoint, ID)

regulator, where pressure is set at the desired level (psig). Gas pressure is displayed by an aneroid gauge on top of the unit (0 to 100 psig). From the pressure regulator, gas travels to the nebulizer output, remote output, and phasitron output. Prior to the phasitron output is an oscillator cartridge that creates the percussive breaths. The pressure or impact control acts to adjust pressure in the oscillator cartridge, which increases or decreases airway pressure.

Gas exits the IPV-1 through the phasitron and remote or nebulizer sockets. Gas from the nebulizer socket travels through small-bore tubing to the nebulizer. Gas from the phasitron socket travels through small-bore tubing to the "phasitron" or sliding venturi (Fig. 12-38). This is the gas flow that creates the percussive action. The venturi body slides back and forth within the outer body as gas is delivered to the venturi jet. The entrainment port of the venturi is connected by large-bore aerosol tubing to the nebulizer (Fig. 12-39). This allows entrainment of aerosolized medications for delivery to the patient. Inspiration may be triggered by the manual push button on the nebulizer (by the patient) or by the manual inspiration button on the control panel. Airway pressure is displayed on an aneroid gauge located on the control panel.

The IPV-1 is not intended for mechanical ventilation. It can be classified as a manually triggered, flow or pressure limited, manually cycled, pressure controller. Experience with IPV-1 units in patients with chronic sputum production has been promising.

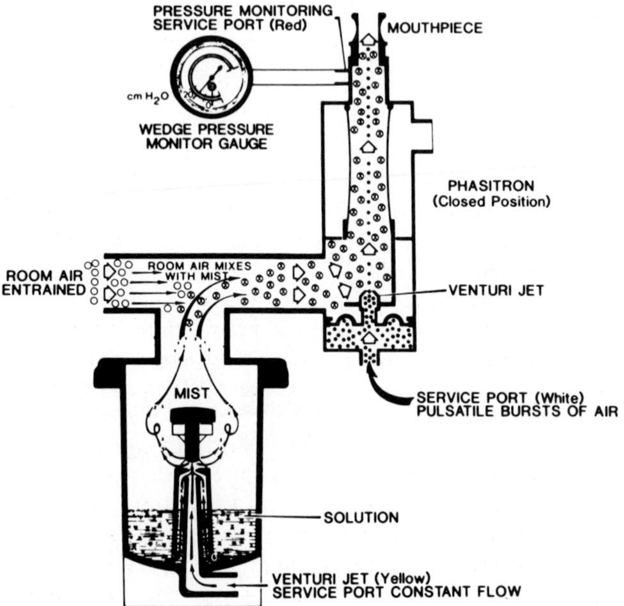

Figure 12-39. Gas from the nebulizer socket aerosolizes medication in the nebulizer, which along with room air is entrained by the venturi for delivery to the patient. (Courtesy of Percussionaire, Sandpoint, ID)

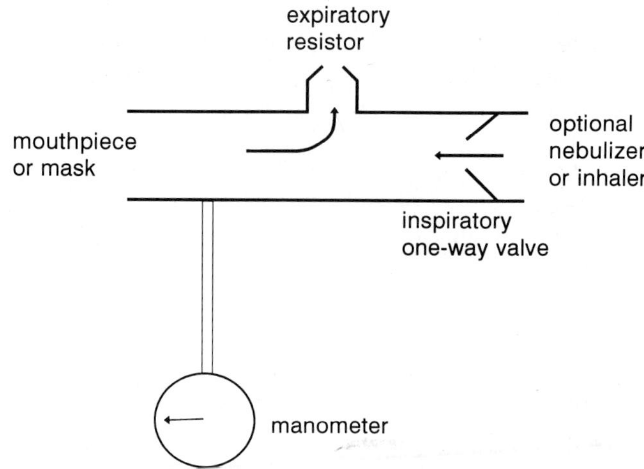

Figure 12-40. Diagram of PEP device.

Positive Expiratory Pressure Devices

Positive expiratory pressure (PEP) is a bronchial hygiene therapy used in the management of airway secretions and postoperative atelectasis. It was originally introduced in Europe for the treatment of patients with cystic fibrosis. It has since gained acceptance in the United States, and its use has been expanded to include patients with chronic bronchitis and in patients after upper abdominal surgery. Although PEP devices were originally homemade, commercially available units have been introduced.

Equipment required for PEP therapy includes a mask (or mouthpiece), T-piece, one-way valve, adjustable fixed-orifice resistor, and manometer (Fig. 12-40). A threshold resistor can be substituted for the fixed orifice, but this increases the cost of the device. The patient is instructed to inhale a volume of air larger than a normal tidal volume through the one-way valve. The patient then exhales actively, but not forcibly, through the fixed orifice to a normal level of exhalation. The size of the fixed orifice is chosen to achieve a PEP of 10 to 20 cm H_2O during exhalation. The desired inspiratory:expiratory ratio is 1:3 to 1:4.

Flow resistors of 2.5 to 4.0 mm are usually appropriate. The patient performs a series of 10 to 20 breaths using the PEP device, followed by several huff coughs; this is repeated four to six times per treatment session.[11]

PEP therapy can be combined with aerosol bronchodilator therapy. For this, a nebulizer or inhaler is attached to the inspiratory one-way valve of the PEP device.

AARC Clinical Practice Guideline

Use of Positive Airway Pressure Adjuncts to Bronchial Hygiene Therapy: Indications, Contraindications, Hazards and Complications

Positive airway pressure adjuncts are used to mobilize secretions and treat atelectasis and include continuous positive airway pressure (CPAP), positive expiratory pressure (PEP), and expiratory positive airway pressure (EPAP).

- Indications:
  - to reduce air trapping in asthma and COPD
  - to aid in mobilization of retained secretions (in cystic fibrosis and chronic bronchitis)
  - to prevent or reverse atelectasis
  - to optimize delivery of bronchodilators in patients receiving bronchial hygiene therapy
- Contraindications:
  - patients unable to tolerate the increased work of breathing (acute asthma, COPD)
  - intracranial pressure greater than 20 mm Hg
  - hemodynamic instability
  - recent facial, oral, or skull surgery or trauma
  - acute sinusitis
  - epistaxis
  - esophageal surgery
  - active hemoptysis
  - nausea
  - known or suspected tympanic membrane rupture or other middle ear pathology
  - untreated pneumothorax
- Hazards/Complications:
  - increased work of breathing that may lead to hypoventilation and hypercarbia
  - increased intracranial pressure
  - cardiovascular compromise (myocardial ischemia, decreased venous return)
  - air swallowing, with increased likelihood of vomiting and aspiration
  - claustrophobia
  - skin breakdown and discomfort from mask
  - pulmonary barotrauma

(Adapted from AARC Clinical Practice Guideline, published in May, 1993, issue of Respiratory Care; see original publication for complete text)

AARC Clinical Practice Guideline

Postural Drainage Therapy: Indications, Contraindications, Hazards and Complications

Postural drainage therapy is designed to improve the mobilization of bronchial secretions, and the matching of ventilation and perfusion, and to normalize functional residual capacity based upon the effects of gravity and external manipulation of the thorax. This includes turning, postural drainage, percussion, vibration, and cough. This procedure has been commonly referred to as chest physiotherapy, chest physical therapy, postural drainage and percussion, and percussion and vibration.

- Indications:
  - Postural drainage: evidence or suggestion of difficulty clearing secretions with expectorated sputum production greater than 25–30 mL/day, evidence or suggestion of retained secretions in the presence of an artificial airway, presence of atelectasis caused by or suspected of being caused by mucus plugging, diagnosis of certain diseases (such as cystic fibrosis, bronchiectasis, or cavitating lung disease, presence of foreign body in the airway).
  - External manipulation of the thorax: sputum volume or consistency suggesting a need for additional manipulation to assist movement of secretions by gravity, in a patient receiving postural drainage.
- Contraindications:
  - All positions are contraindicated for intracranial pressure greater than 20 mm Hg, head and neck injury until stabilized, active hemorrhage with hemodynamic instability, recent spinal injury, acute spinal injury or active hemoptysis, empyema, bronchopleural fistula, pulmonary edema associated with congestive heart failure, larger pleural effusions, pulmonary embolism, patients who do not tolerate position changes, rib fracture, surgical wound or healing tissue.
  - Trendelenburg position is contraindicated for intracranial pressure greater than 20 mm Hg, patients in whom increased intracranial pressure is to be avoided, uncontrolled hypertension, distended abdomen, esophageal surgery, recent gross hemoptysis, uncontrolled airway at risk for aspiration.
  - Reverse Trendelenburg is contraindicated in the presence of hypotension or vasoactive medication.
  - External manipulation of the thorax is contraindicated for subcutaneous emphysema, recent epidural spinal infusion or spinal anesthesia, recent skin grafts of the thorax, burns or open wounds or skin infections of the thorax, recently placed transvenous pacemaker or subcutaneous pacemaker, suspected pulmonary tuberculosis, lung contusion, bronchospasm, osteomyelitis of the ribs, osteoporosis, coagulopathy, complaint of chest wall pain.
- Hazards/Complications:
  - hypoxemia
  - increased intracranial pressure

- acute hypotension during procedure
- pulmonary hemorrhage
- pain or injury to muscles, ribs, or spine
- vomiting and aspiration
- bronchospasm
- dysrhythmias

(Adapted from AARC Clinical Practice Guideline, published in December, 1991, issue of Respiratory Care; see original publication for complete text)

AARC Clinical Practice Guideline

Intermittent Positive Pressure Breathing: Indications, Contraindications, Hazards and Complications

IPPB is a technique used to provide short-term or intermittent mechanical ventilation for the purpose of augmenting lung expansion, delivering aerosol medication, or assisting ventilation.

- Indications:
  - the need to improve lung expansion when other forms of therapy have been unsuccessful
  - the need for short-term ventilator support for patients who are hypoventilating as an alternative to tracheal intubation and continuous ventilatory support
  - the need to deliver aerosol medication
- Contraindications:
  - intracranial pressure greater than 15 mm Hg
  - hemodynamic instability
  - recent facial, oral, or skull surgery
  - tracheoesophageal fistula
  - recent esophageal surgery
  - active hemoptysis
  - nausea
  - air swallowing
  - active untreated tuberculosis
  - radiographic evidence of bleb
  - singultation
- Hazards/Complications:
  - increased airway resistance
  - barotrauma, pneumothorax
  - nosocomial infection
  - hypocarbia
  - hemoptysis
  - hyperoxia when oxygen is the gas source
  - gastric distention
  - impaction of secretions
  - psychological dependence
  - impedance of venous return
  - exacerbation of hypoxemia
  - hypoventilation
  - increased mismatch of ventilation and perfusion
  - air trapping, auto-PEEP, overdistended alveoli

Adapted from AARC Clinical Practice Guideline, published in December, 1993, issue of Respiratory Care; see original publication for complete text)

AARC Clinical Practice Guideline

Incentive Spirometry: Indications, Contraindications, Hazards and Complications

Incentive spirometry is designed to mimic natural sighing or yawning by encouraging the patient to take long, slow, deep breaths. This is accomplished by using a device that provides patients with visual or other positive feedback when they inhale at a predetermined flow rate or volume and sustain the inflation for a minimum of 3 seconds.

- Indications:
  - presence of conditions predisposing to the development of pulmonary atelectasis
  - presence of pulmonary atelectasis
  - presence of a restrictive lung defect associated with quadriplegia and/or dysfunctional diaphragm
- Contraindications:
  - Patient cannot be instructed or supervised to ensure appropriate use of the device.
  - Patient cooperation is absent or patient is unable to understand or demonstrate proper use of the device.
  - Incentive spirometry is contraindicated in patient unable to deep breathe effectively.
  - The presence of an open tracheal stoma is not a contraindication but requires adaptation of the spirometer.
- Hazards/Complications:
  - ineffective unless closely supervised or performed as ordered
  - inappropriate as sole treatment for major lung collapse or consolidation
  - hyperventilation
  - barotrauma
  - discomfort due to inadequate pain control
  - hypoxia secondary to interruption of prescribed oxygen therapy if face mask is being used
  - exacerbation of bronchospasm
  - fatigue

(Adapted from AARC Clinical Practice Guideline, published in December, 1991, issue of Respiratory Care; see original publication for complete text)

References

1. Zidulka A, Chrome JF, Wright DW, Burnett S, Bonnier L, Fraser R. Clapping or percussion causes atelectasis in dogs and influences gas exchange. J Appl Physiol 1989;66:2833–2838.
2. Holody B, Goldberg HS. The effect of mechanical vibration physiotherapy on arterial oxygenation in acutely ill patients with atelectasis or pneumonia. Am Rev Respir Dis 1981;124:372–375.
3. MacKenzie CE, Shiner B. Cardiorespiratory function before and after chest physiotherapy in mechanically ventilated patients with post-traumatic respiratory failure. Crit Care Med 1985;13: 483–486.
4. Radford RR, Barutt J, Billingsley JG, Hill WH, Lawson WH, Willick WA. Rational basis for percussion-augmented mucociliary clearance. Respir Care 1982;27:556–563.
5. Bartlett RH, Gazzaniga AB, Geraghty TR. Respiratory maneuvers to prevent postoperative pulmonary complications: A critical review. JAMA 1973;224:1017–1021.

6. Bakow ED. Sustained maximal inspiration: A rationale for its use. Respir Care 1977;22:379–382.
7. Lederer DH, Van deWater J, Indech RB. Which deep breathing device should the postoperative patient use? Chest 1980;77:610–613.
8. Krastins IRB, Corey ML, McLeod A, Edmonds J, Levison H, Moes F. An evaluation of incentive spirometry in the management of pulmonary complications after cardiac surgery in a pediatric population. Crit Care Med 1982;10:525–528.
9. Mang H, Obermayer A. Imposed work of breathing during sustained maximal inspiration: Comparison of six incentive spirometers. Respir Care 1989;34:1122–1128.
10. Scuderi J, Olsen GN. Respiratory therapy in the management of postoperative complications. Respir Care 1989;34:281–291.
11. Mahlmeister MJ, Fink JB, Hoffman GI, Fifer LF. Positive-expiratory mask therapy: Theoretical and practical considerations and a review of the literature. Respir Care 1991;36:1218–1229.

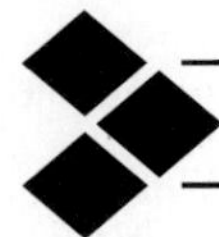

13

Classification of Mechanical Ventilators

Robert L. Chatburn

OBJECTIVES

1. Write the general outline for classification of ventilators.
2. Describe the major drive mechanisms and output control valves of mechanical ventilators.
3. Describe the equation of motion and how it relates to ventilator classification.
4. Compare open- and closed-loop control of mechanical ventilators.
5. Discuss the differences between pressure, volume, and flow control.
6. Define control variables, phase variables, and conditional variables.

(continued)

OBJECTIVES, (continued)

7. Draw the pressure, volume, and flow curves for:
   a. Rectangular and exponential pressure output
   b. Ramp and sinusoidal volume output
   c. Rectangular, ramp, and sinusoidal flow output
8. Describe the major modes of ventilation in terms of the control and phase variables for mandatory and spontaneous breaths.
9. Define mandatory and spontaneous breaths.
10. Describe the effects of patient circuit compliance and resistance on ventilator output.

KEY TERMS

active expiration
alarm event
assisted expiration
assisted inspiration
assisted ventilation
closed-loop control
compressor
constant airway pressure (CAP)
control circuit
control variable
cycle
demand valve
end-expiratory pressure (EEP)
event
external compressor
expiratory phase (expiration)
expiratory time
gauge pressure
inspiratory phase (inspiration)
inspiratory time
internal compressor
limit
mandatory breath
mean airway pressure
open-loop control
passive expiration
phase
phase variable
phase variable value
spontaneous breath
transient expiratory assist pressure (TEAP)
transrespiratory pressure
trigger
ventilatory period

Introduction*

Over the past few years, ventilators have evolved into highly complex, microprocessor-controlled devices with a wide range of operating characteristics. Unfortunately, our language and conceptual models, which we use to understand how ventilators work, have not kept pace with the technologic development. Most authors use some version of Mushin's classic text,[1] based on ventilators common in the 1960s. This chapter presents an updated classification scheme that has been accepted by leading members of the pulmonary medicine community.[2-4]

Basic Concepts

A ventilator is simply a machine—a system of related elements designed to alter, transmit, and direct applied energy in a predetermined manner to perform useful work.[5] We put energy into the ventilator in the form of electricity (energy = volts × amperes × time) or compressed gas (energy = pressure × volume). That energy is transmitted or transformed (by the ventilator's drive mechanism) in a predetermined manner (by the control circuit) to augment or replace the patient's muscles in performing the work of breathing (the desired output). Therefore, to understand mechanical ventilators in general, we must first understand their basic functions of

- Power input
- Power transmission or conversion
- Control scheme
- Output (pressure, volume, and flow waveforms)

This simple outline format can be expanded to add as much detail about a given ventilator as desired (Box 13-1).

Input Power

All ventilators require a source of power that can be used to perform the work of ventilating the respiratory system. In effect, they convert input power in a readily available form to a form that is more convenient for the delicate and exacting task of supporting ventilation. The most common forms of input power for ventilators are electric and pneumatic. Input power should not be confused with the power for the control circuit. For

*Much of this chapter appeared in Respir Care 1991;36:1123-1155.

Box 13-1
Outline of Ventilator Classification System

- I. Input
  - A. Electric
    - 1. AC
    - 2. DC (battery)
  - B. Pneumatic
- II. Power Conversion and Transmission (drive mechanism)
  - A. Compressor
    - 1. External
    - 2. Internal
  - B. Motor and linkage
    - 1. Electric motor/rotating crank and piston rod
    - 2. Electric motor/rack and pinion
    - 3. Electric motor/direct
    - 4. Compressed gas/direct
  - C. Output control valves
    - 1. Electromagnetic poppet valve
    - 2. Pneumatic poppet valve
    - 3. Electromagnetic proportional valve
    - 4. Pneumatic diaphragm
- III. Control Scheme
  - A. Control circuit
    - 1. Mechanical
    - 2. Pneumatic
    - 3. Fluidic
    - 4. Electric
    - 5. Electronic
  - B. Control variables and waveforms
    - 1. Pressure
    - 2. Volume
    - 3. Flow
    - 4. Time
  - C. Phase variables
    - 1. Trigger variable
    - 2. Limit variable
    - 3. Cycle variable
    - 4. Baseline variable
  - D. Modes of ventilation and conditional variables
- IV. Output
  - A. Pressure
    - 1. Rectangular
    - 2. Exponential
    - 3. Sinusoidal
    - 4. Oscillating
  - B. Volume
    - 1. Ramp
    - 2. Sinusoidal
  - C. Flow
    - 1. Rectangular
    - 2. Ramp
      - a) ascending ramp
      - b) descending ramp
    - 3. Sinusoidal
  - D. Effects of the patient circuit
- V. Alarm Systems
  - A. Input power alarms
    - 1. Loss of electric power
    - 2. Loss of pneumatic power
  - B. Control circuit alarms
    - 1. General systems failure (ventilator inoperative)
    - 2. Incompatible ventilator settings
    - 3. Inverse I:E ratio
  - C. Output alarms
    - 1. Pressure
    - 2. Volume
    - 3. Flow
    - 4. Time
      - a) high/low ventilatory frequency
      - b) high/low inspiratory time
      - c) high/low expiratory time (high expiratory time = apnea)
    - 5. Inspired Gas
      - a) high/low inspired gas temperature
      - b) high/low FIO_2

example, many ventilators use pneumatic input power to drive inspiration but electric power for the control circuit.

Electric

Most American ventilators use 110 to 115 volts AC (60 Hz) from common electrical outlets to power drive mechanisms. The AC voltage is also reduced and converted to DC to power electronic control circuits. Some current ventilators, notably infant and transport ventilators, are designed to use rechargeable batteries as alternative sources of power when the usual AC current is not available. This capability makes them useful for transferring ventilator-dependent patients from one place to another within the hospital as well as for external transport. In the home care setting, a battery backup can be a lifesaving feature in the event of a power outage. Common ventilator batteries are the lead-acid type, which supply about 2.5 amp-hours of energy. This will usually power a ventilator for up to 1 hour. This type of battery normally requires 8 to 12 hours to recharge.

Pneumatic

Because compressed air and oxygen are in abundant supply in most hospital intensive care units, many ventilators are designed to use the energy stored in pressurized gas. We usually think of pressure as a force per unit area, but it can be shown that pressure also has the units of energy density. Thus, the more pressure available, the more useful work that can be generated. Besides being used to inflate the lungs, the input pressure is often used as the source of power for the control circuit, as in the case of fluidic logic circuits. Ventilators operated by pressurized gas typically have internal reducing regulators, so that the normal operating pressure is lower than the source pressure. This allows uninterrupted operation from piped gas sources in hospitals, which are usually regulated to 50 psi but are subject to periodic fluctuations. The use of compressed gas as a power source makes a ventilator useful in environments where no electrical power is available, such as during transports, or where it is undesirable, such as near magnetic resonance imaging (MRI) equipment.

Power Transmission and Conversion

The power transmission and conversion system, sometimes referred to as the drive mechanism, generates the force necessary to deliver gas to the patient. In general terms, this system is composed of either a compressor external to the ventilator in conjunction with a regulator inside the ventilator or else an internal compressor linked to a motor. A complete description of all possible systems is beyond the scope of this chapter but may be found elsewhere.[6]

Compressor

A compressor is a device whose internal volume can be changed to increase the pressure of the gas it contains. Large, water-cooled, piston-type compressors are often used to supply gas under pressure to outlets near patient beds in hospitals. When a ventilator uses compressed gas from wall outlets as its only source of power to drive inspiration, the ventilator is considered to have an external compressor. Alternatively, a small compressor designed for use with a single ventilator may be employed. There are four types of compressors commonly used inside ventilators:

- Piston and cylinder (eg, Emerson IMV)
- Diaphragm (eg, Engstrom Erica)
- Bellows (eg, Siemens Servo 900C)
- Rotating vane (eg, Bear 2)

Motor and Linkage

A motor is anything that produces motion. As it relates to a mechanical ventilator, the motor is the device used to drive the compressor. For those ventilators with internal compressors, the characteristics of interest are the type of motor and the linkage between the compressor and motor, since these influence the waveforms the ventilator can produce.

Electric Motor/Rotating Crank and Piston Rod

This is sometimes referred to as an "eccentric wheel" (Fig. 13-1). It produces a quasi-sinusoidal motion at the distal end of the piston rod (eg, Emerson IMV). A true sinusoidal motion is generated only by a rotating crank in combination with a Scotch yoke.[7]

Electric Motor/Rack and Pinion

This produces a linear motion of the rack, driving the piston forward at either a constant rate (eg, Bourns LS 104-150) or a variable rate, depending on the control circuit (Fig. 13-2).

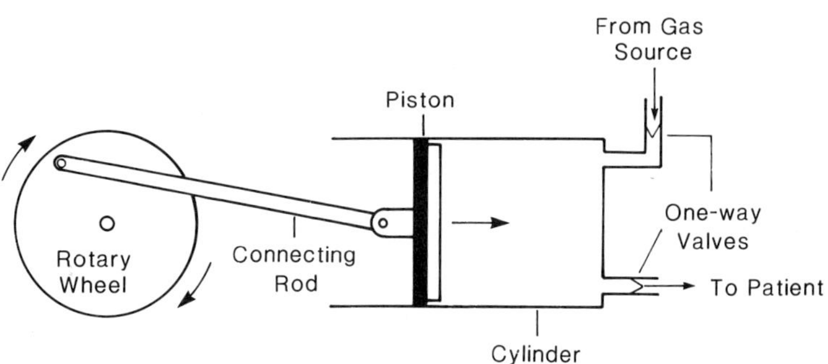

Figure 13-1. Drive mechanism consisting of eccentric wheel, piston rod, and piston.

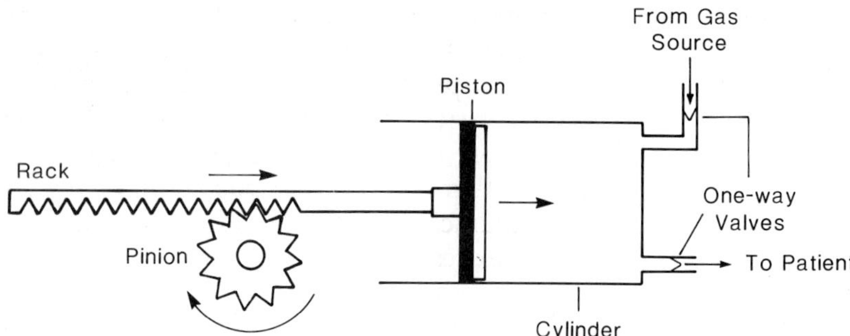

Figure 13-2. Drive mechanism consisting of a rack and pinion, piston rod, and piston.

Electric Motor/Direct

This can either produce a rotary motion of the output shaft such as on a rotating vane air compressor (eg, Bear 2) or a linear motion as in the case of a linear drive motor (eg, Mira Hummingbird). The linear drive motor is particularly versatile because it can produce a wide variety of easily controllable output waveforms.

Compressed Gas Regulator/Direct

When compressed gas is used as the motor, its force is often adjusted by a pressure regulator (pressure reducing valve). The compressed gas either directly inflates the lungs (eg, Bennett 7200), displaces a diaphragm that forces gas into the patient (eg, Engstrom Erica), or stores energy in a weight or spring (eg, Siemens Servo 900C, mechanism shown in Figure 13-3).

Output Control Valve

This valve is used to regulate the flow of gas to the patient. It may be a simple on/off valve (also called an exhalation valve) as in the Puritan-Bennett MA-1, or it may be used to shape the output waveform as in the Siemens Servo 900C. The most commonly used types are discussed below.

Electromagnetic Poppet Valve

This type of device uses magnetic force caused by an electric current to allow a small voltage to control a large pneumatic pressure in an on/off fashion. Examples include the electronic interface valve (eg, Infrasonics Infant Star, which uses a set of valves to approximate various pressure or flow waveforms), the plunger (eg, Bear Cub), and the pinch valve (eg, Bunnell Life Pulse Jet Ventilator).

Pneumatic Poppet Valve

This type of valve is similar to a solenoid valve except that it uses a small pneumatic pressure (eg, a fluidic signal) to control a larger pneumatic pressure. They are particularly useful when electronic signals are inconvenient or hazardous.

Proportional Valve

Also known in industrial settings as a mass flow control valve, this device is similar to the solenoid valve in that it is operated by an electromagnet, perhaps in the form of a stepper motor (ie, an electric motor whose rotation can be controlled in discrete arcs or "steps"). The major difference is that rather than simply turning flow on and off, this type of valve can shape the flow waveform during inspiration by changing the diameter of its outflow port and can be used to create a variety of waveforms. Proportional valves are used in the Bennett 7200 and the Hamilton Veolar ventilators and in the form of scissors valves in the Siemens Servo 900C or stepper motors in the Bear 5.

Pneumatic Diaphragm

Usually an on/off type of valve, this device uses a flexible diaphragm or membrane (eg, a "mushroom" valve) to divert gas from one pathway to another. These are commonly referred to as "exhalation valves," which is a misnomer because they are primarily responsible for diverting gas into the patient's lungs during inspiration. However, they may also be responsible for slowing exhalation ("expiratory retard") and maintaining positive end-expiratory pressure (PEEP). Pneumatic di-

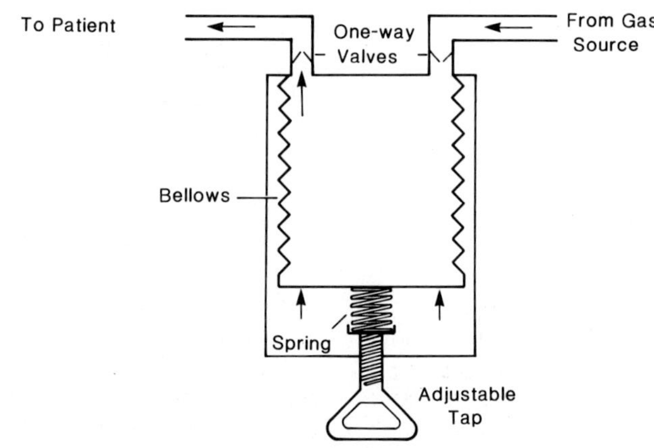

Figure 13-3. Drive mechanism consisting of a bellows under spring tension.

aphragms are used on many ventilators, such as the Bear 5 and the Sechrist IV-100B.

Many ventilators use more than one output control valve. In particular, one valve is often used to direct flow into the patient's airway (eg, a mushroom valve) while another may be used to shape the waveform (eg, a proportional valve).

Control Scheme

To understand how a machine can be controlled to replace or supplement the natural function of breathing, we need to understand something about the mechanics of breathing. The study of mechanics deals with forces, displacements, and the rate of change of displacement. In physiology, force is measured as pressure (pressure = force ÷ area), displacement is measured as volume (volume = area × displacement), and the relevant rate of change is measured as flow (eg, average flow = Δvolume ÷ Δtime; instantaneous flow = dv/dt, the derivative of volume with respect to time). Specifically, we are interested in the *pressure* necessary to cause a *flow* of gas to enter the airway and increase the *volume* of the lungs.

The study of respiratory mechanics is essentially the search for simple but useful models of respiratory system mechanical behavior. Conceptually, the relatively complex respiratory system can be represented by a simple graphic model (eg, a straw connected to a balloon). The simple graphic model is analogous to simple electrical circuits in which compliance is analogous to capacitance, flow resistance is analogous to electrical resistance, and pressure is analogous to a voltage source. The similarity of the physical and electrical model makes it possible to borrow mathematical models from electrical engineering, substituting pressure, volume, and flow for voltage, charge, and current, respectively (Fig. 13-4). The result is known as the equation of motion for the respiratory system (a simplified version)[8,9]:

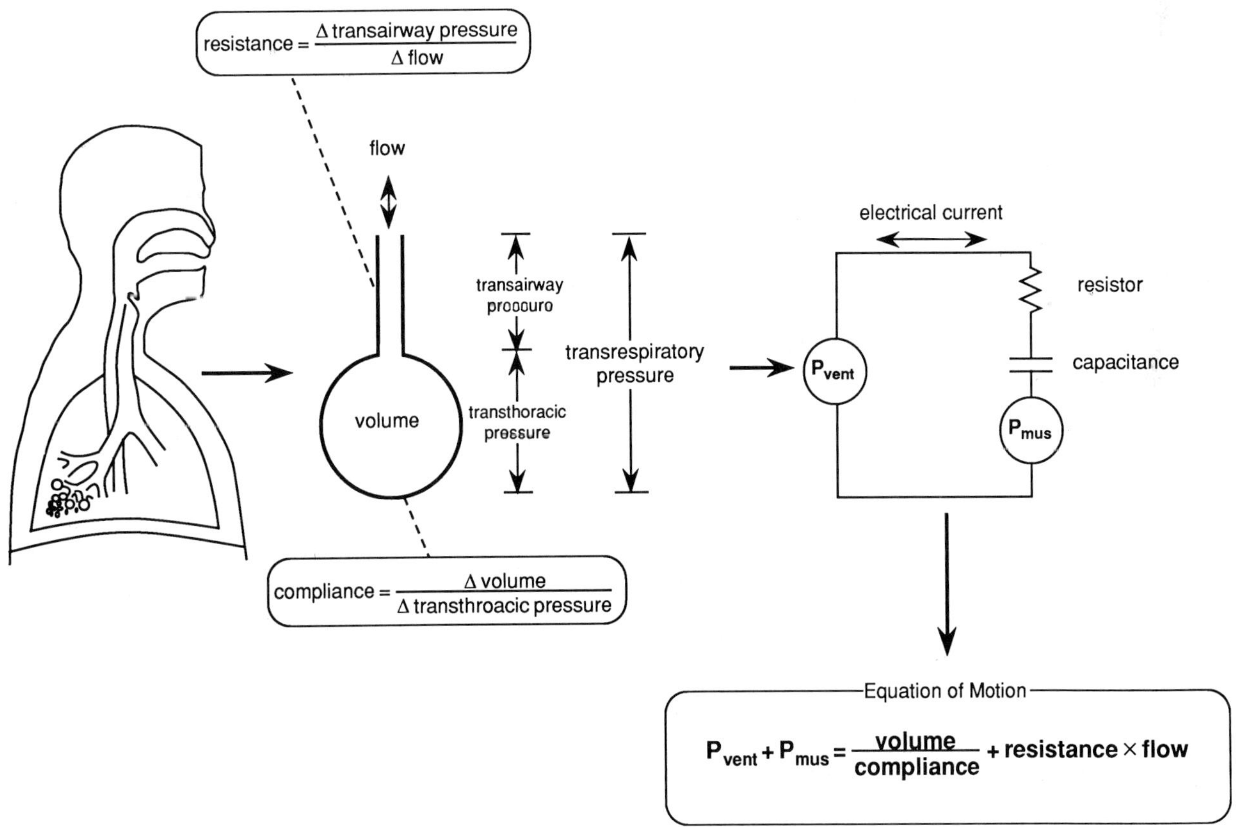

Figure 13-4. The study of respiratory system mechanics is based on graphical and mathematical models. The respiratory system can be modeled as a single-flow conducting tube connected to a single elastic compartment. This physical model is analogous to a simple electrical circuit consisting of a resistor and a capacitor. Two voltage sources in the circuit represent pressures generated by the muscles and the ventilator; electrical current represents airflow. The electrical circuit can be modeled by a mathematical model called the equation of motion for the respiratory system. In this model, pressure, volume, and flow are variables (ie, functions of time) while resistance ana compliance are constants.

(1) Muscle pressure + ventilator pressure

$$= \frac{\text{volume}}{\text{compliance}} + \text{resistance} \times \text{flow}$$

(2) Muscle pressure + ventilator pressure

= elastic load + resistive load

In this simplified form,* muscle pressure is the imaginary transrespiratory pressure (ie, airway pressure minus body surface pressure) generated by the ventilatory muscles to expand the thoracic cage and lungs. Muscle pressure is said to be imaginary because it is not directly measurable. Ventilator pressure is the transrespiratory pressure generated by the ventilator during inspiration. The combined muscle and ventilator pressure causes volume and flow to be delivered to the patient. Pressure, volume, and flow change with time and hence are *variables*. Compliance and resistance are assumed to remain constant and are called *parameters,* and their combined effect constitute the *load* experienced by the ventilator and ventilatory muscles. The elastic load is the pressure necessary to overcome the elastance (or compliance) of the respiratory system, and the resistive load is the pressure necessary to overcome the flow resistance of the airways (including endotracheal tube) along with lung and chest wall tissue resistance. The term *parameter* may also refer to a particular aspect of a variable such as the peak or mean value.

Note that pressure, volume, and flow are all measured relative to their baseline values (ie, their values at end-expiration). This means that the pressure to cause inspiration is measured as the change in airway pressure† above PEEP. This is the reason, for example, that pressure support levels are measured relative to PEEP. Thinking of ventilator pressure as simply airway pressure (ie, pressure measured at one point in space, the airway) limits our understanding of the mechanics involved in breathing. Volume is measured as the change in lung volume above functional residual capacity, and the change in lung volume during the inspiratory period is defined as the tidal volume. Flow is measured relative to its end-expiratory value (usually zero). When pressure, volume, and flow are plotted as functions of time, characteristic waveforms for volume-controlled ventilation and pressure-controlled ventilation are produced (Fig. 13-5).

*This is not an algebraic equation but rather a differential equation. Specifically, it is a linear differential equation with constant coefficients that must be solved using calculus to get any of the three variables as functions of the other variables and time. Volume and flow are inverse functions (ie, volume is the integral of flow with respect to time and flow is the derivative of volume with respect to time).

†Airway pressure measured by a ventilator at the patient's airway opening is actually transrespiratory pressure. This is true because the ventilator's manometer measures gauge pressure (ie, pressure measured relative to atmospheric or body surface pressure).

Notice that if the patient's ventilatory muscles are not functioning, muscle pressure = 0 and the ventilator must generate all of the pressure required to deliver the tidal volume and inspiratory flow. On the other hand, if ventilator pressure = 0 (ie, airway pressure does not rise above baseline during inspiration), there will be no ventilatory support. In between these two extremes there are an infinite variety of combinations of muscle pressure (ie, patient effort) and ventilator support that are theoretically possible for partial ventilatory support.

Analysis of ventilator–patient interaction based on a mathematical model suggests the proper use of the word "assist," which is another frequently confused concept. *Webster's Dictionary* defines assist as "to help; to aid; to give support." From the perspective of the equation of motion, whenever airway pressure (ie, ventilator pressure) rises above baseline during inspiration, the ventilator does work on the patient.‡ Thus, the breath is said to be *assisted,* independent of other breath parameters (ie, whether the breath is classified as spontaneous or mandatory). Do not confuse this meaning of the word "assist" with specific names of modes of ventilation (eg, ASSIST/CONTROL). Ventilator manufacturers often coin terms for modes without regard to consistency or theoretical relevance.

In the equation of motion, the form of any one of the three variables (ie, pressure, volume, or flow expressed as functions of time) can be predetermined, making it the independent variable and making the other two dependent variables. This is precisely analogous to the way ventilators operate. Thus, during pressure-controlled ventilation, pressure is the independent variable and the shape of the volume and flow waveforms depends on the shape of the pressure waveform and also on the resistance and compliance of the respiratory system. On the other hand, during flow-controlled ventilation, we can specify the shape of the flow waveform. This makes flow the independent variable and the shape of the volume waveform depends on the shape of the flow waveform. The shape of the pressure waveform depends on the flow waveform as well as on resistance and compliance.

We now have a theoretical basis for classifying ventilators as either pressure, volume, or flow controllers. The necessary and sufficient criteria for determining which variable is controlled (ie, which variable is the independent variable) are illustrated in Figure 13-6. Note that if the waveforms for all three variables are not predetermined (ie, none of the variables can be considered independent), then the ventilator is considered to control only the timing of the inspiratory and expiratory phase and is called a time controller.

‡Work is the integral of pressure with respect to volume, that is, the area under the pressure–volume curve.

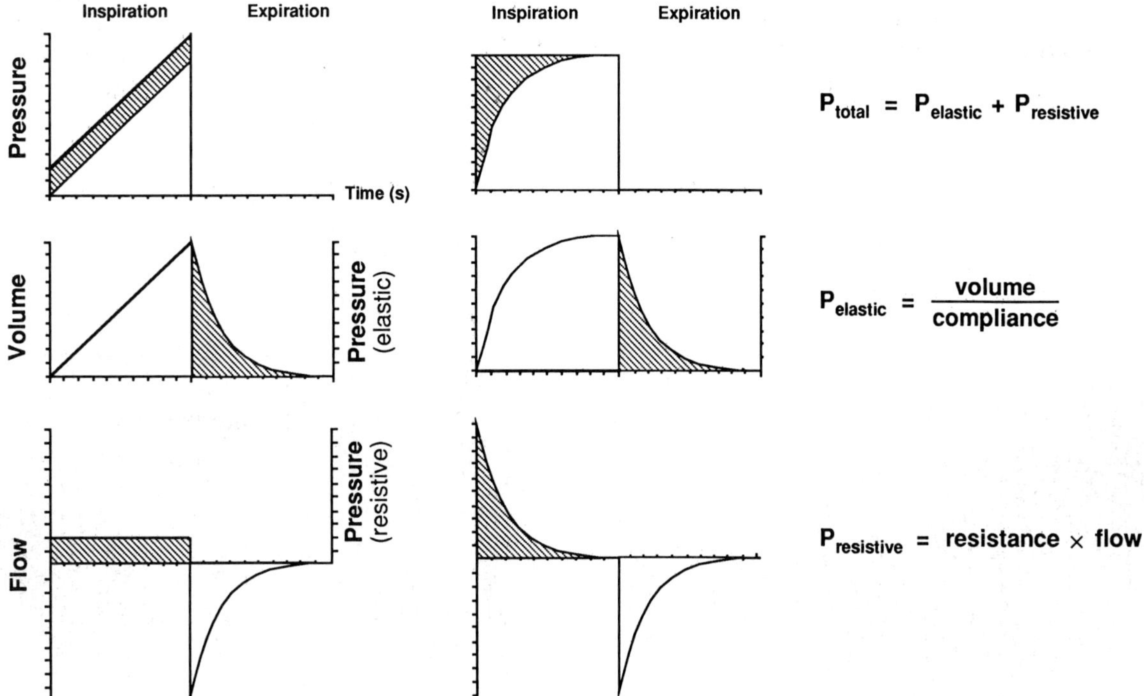

Figure 13-5. This figure illustrates some conventions for the presentation of graphical data. It shows the theoretical output waveforms for flow-controlled inspiration with a rectangular (ie, pulse) flow waveform on the left compared with pressure-controlled inspiration with a rectangular pressure waveform. The order of presentation is pressure, volume, and flow, according to the order specified by the equation of motion. Note that the volume waveform has the same shape as the transthoracic or lung pressure waveform (ie, pressure due to elastic recoil). The flow waveform has the same shape as the transairway pressure waveform (ie, pressure due to airway resistance). If all the pressure scales are the same, then the height of the airway pressure waveform at any instant is the sum of the heights of the other two waveforms. The origin of the airway pressure waveform is the end-expiratory pressure; the origins of the volume and flow waveforms are both zero. The shaded areas represent pressures due to flow resistance; the open areas represent pressure due to elastic recoil.

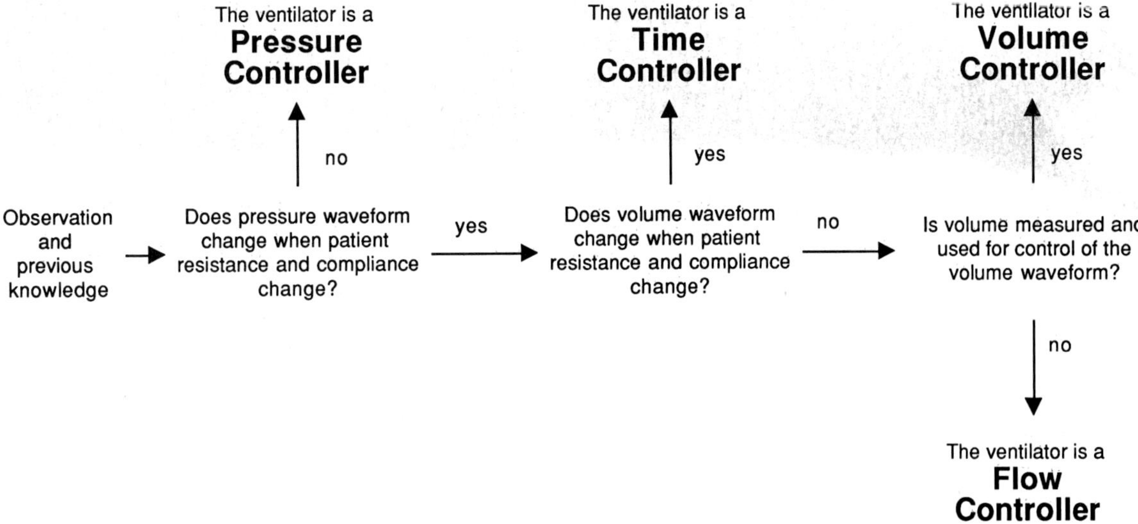

Figure 13-6. Criteria for determining the control variable during a ventilator-assisted inspiration.

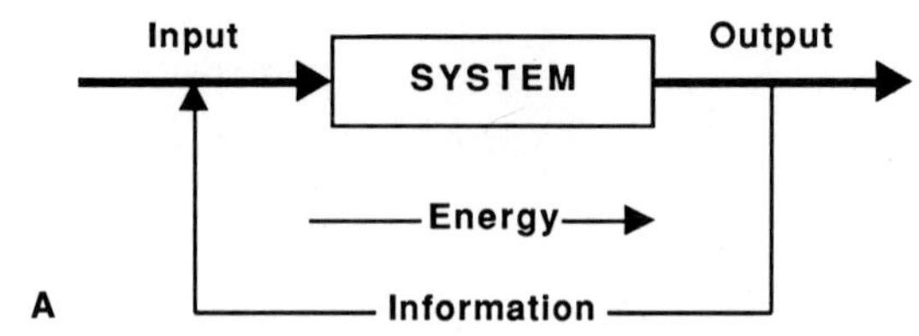

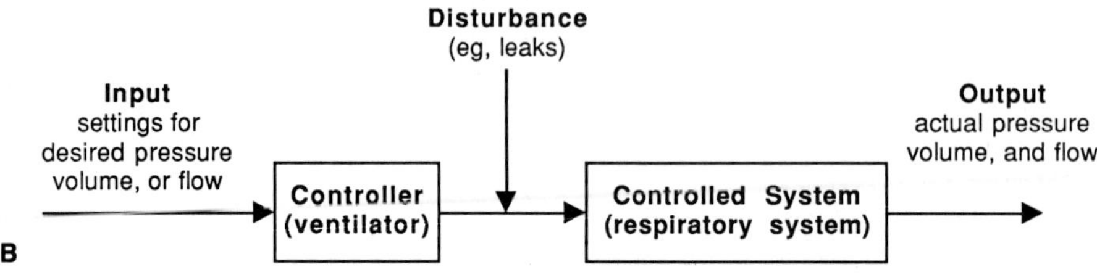

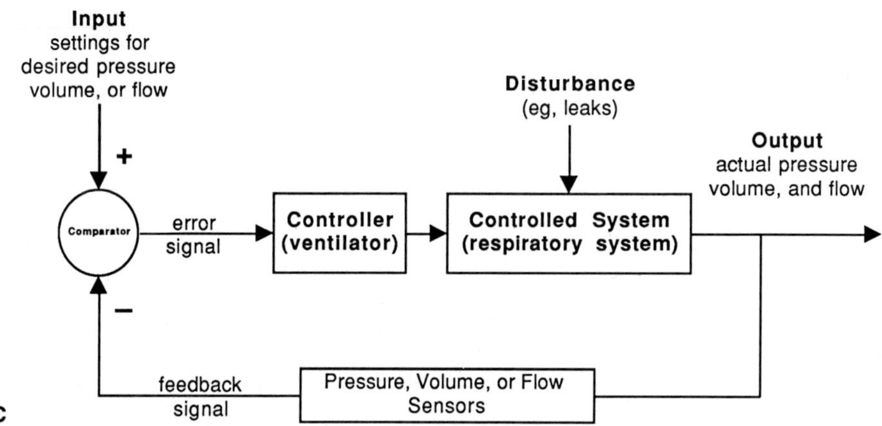

Figure 13-7. A. A simple block diagram of an unspecified system having one input and one output. Energy flows from input to output, and information flows from output to input. B. Block diagram for a ventilator using open-loop control. For example, the Newport Breeze ventilator controls airway pressure using open-loop control. C. Block diagram for a ventilator using closed-loop control. This is also called feedback or servo control. For example, the Infrasonics Infant Star ventilator uses closed-loop control of airway pressure.

The most significant revelation provided by the equation of motion, however, is that *any conceivable ventilator can directly control only one variable at a time: pressure, volume, or flow.* Therefore, we can think of a ventilator as simply a machine that controls either the airway pressure waveform, the inspired volume waveform, or the inspiratory flow waveform. Thus, pressure, volume, and flow are referred to in this context as *control variables.** Time is a variable that is implicit in the equation of motion. We will see below that in some cases, time is viewed as a control variable.

*If the ventilator directly controls the flow waveform, it indirectly controls the volume waveform (and vice versa) independent of the resistance and compliance.

Having said *what* is controlled, we can now explore *how* it is controlled. In discussing respiratory mechanics, we have used the term *system* without definition. Formally, a system is defined as a collection of elements that interact according to some particular process or function. A model is a simplified version of a real world system used to help us understand the relationships between system elements (eg, the equation of motion is a model of the respiratory system). Specifically, we are interested in understanding the relation between the input and the output of the system (ie, we need to create a model). This understanding may then help us to control the system behavior.

A system can be controlled in two different ways to achieve the desired output[10]:

1. Select an input and wait for an output with no interference during the waiting period.
2. Select an input, observe the trend in the output, and modify the input accordingly to get as close as possible to the desired output.

For example, when a helmsman steers a boat toward the dock, he may do it in one of the two ways described earlier:

1. Point the boat in the direction of the dock and retire to his cabin.
2. Continuously steer the boat toward the dock, by observing the direction of the dock, observing the direction the boat is moving, and making adjustments as necessary.

In this example, the system is the boat (motor, propeller, steering mechanism, etc.), the input is the position of the boat's steering wheel, and the output is the direction of the boat's motion. In both cases a change in the input causes a change in the output. But in the first case there is no flow of information from the output to generate a new input to "close the loop." Hence, this type of control scheme is called *open-loop control.* In the second case, the helmsman uses information about the output to modify the input, which in turn, improves the output. This control scheme is called *closed-loop control* or *feedback control.* Feedback control is also called *servo control.* Figure 13-7 illustrates block diagrams (ie, models) of open- and closed-loop control systems.

To perform closed-loop control, the output must be measured and compared with a reference value. In the above example, a human performed the measuring and comparing functions. But in ventilators, a transducer and electronic circuitry are necessary to perform automatic closed-loop control. Closed-loop control provides the advantage of a more consistent output in the presence of unanticipated disturbances. In the previous example, disturbances that affect the direction of the boat might include wind and water currents. In the case of ventilators, disturbances that might affect the delivery of pressure, volume, and flow include pooled condensation or leaks in the patient circuit, endotracheal tube obstructions, and changes in respiratory system resistance and compliance.

Control Circuit

The control circuit is the subsystem responsible for controlling the drive mechanism and/or the output control valve. A ventilator may have more than one control circuit, which may be of several types.

Mechanical

Mechanical control circuits use levers, pulleys, cams, and so on. These types of circuits were used in the early manually operated ventilators illustrated in history books.[11]

Pneumatic

Pneumatic control circuits use gas pressure to operate diaphragms, jet entrainment devices, pistons, and so on. The original Bird and Bennett PR series ventilators used pneumatic control. A simple ventilator can be constructed with just two poppet valves and three flow resistors (Fig. 13-8).

Fluidic

Fluidic circuits are analogs of electronic logic circuits (Fig. 13-9).[12] They use minute gas flows to generate signals that operate timing systems and pressure switches. This makes them immune to failure from electromagnetic interference (such as around magnetic resonance imaging equipment). Fluidic circuits can be constructed with discrete components like comparators and flip-

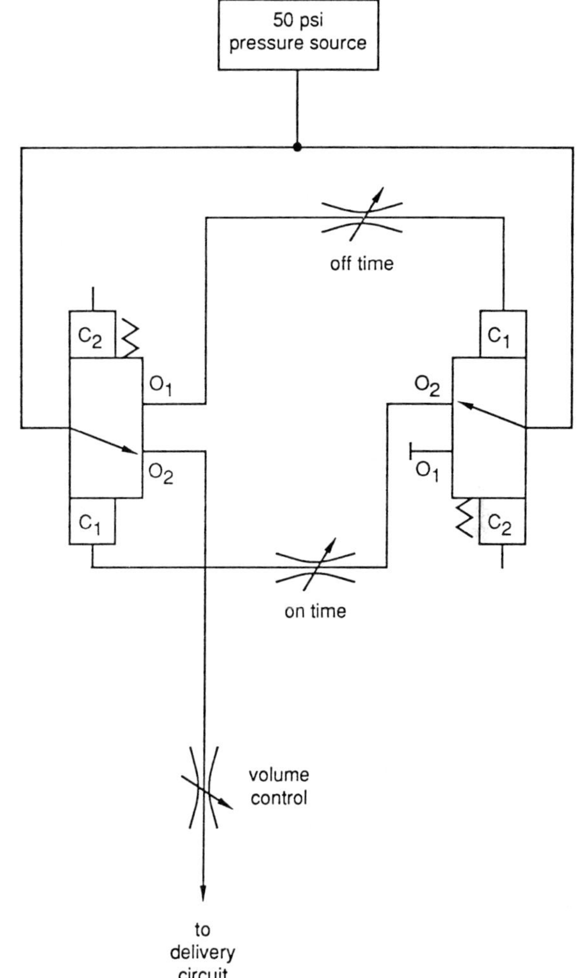

Figure 13-8. A simple ventilator control circuit composed of pneumatic components. Two poppet valves are connected to form a simple oscillator circuit. The on and off times (ie, inspiratory and expiratory times) are controlled by two flow resistors. O_1 and O_2 are pneumatic signal outputs. C_1 ports are pneumatic signal inputs. The C_2 ports are spring loaded.

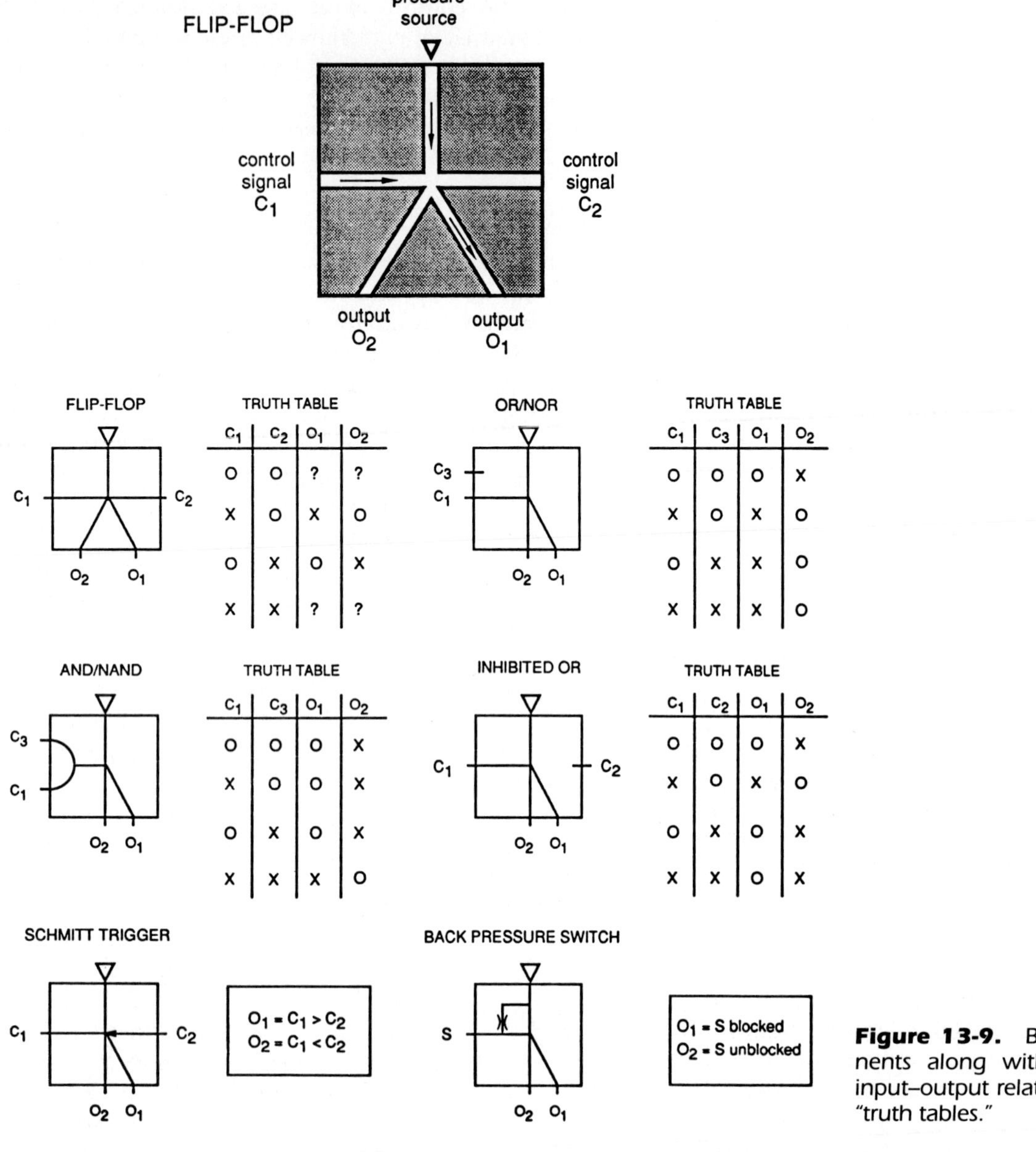

Flip-flop truth table:

C_1	C_2	O_1	O_2
O	O	?	?
X	O	X	O
O	X	O	X
X	X	?	?

OR/NOR truth table:

C_1	C_3	O_1	O_2
O	O	O	X
X	O	X	O
O	X	X	O
X	X	X	O

AND/NAND truth table:

C_1	C_3	O_1	O_2
O	O	O	X
X	O	O	X
O	X	O	X
X	X	X	O

Inhibited OR truth table:

C_1	C_2	O_1	O_2
O	O	O	X
X	O	X	O
O	X	O	X
X	X	O	X

Figure 13-9. Basic fluidic components along with their associated input–output relations in the form of "truth tables."

flops, or they can be combined in the form of integrated circuits, analogous to electronic integrated circuits. Examples of ventilators using fluidic logic control circuits are the Sechrist IV-100B and the Bio-Med MVP-10. A simple fluidic ventilator is shown in Figure 13-10.

Electric

Electric control circuits use only simple switches, rheostats (or potentiometers), and magnets to control ventilator operation. One example of a completely electrically controlled ventilator would be the Emerson Iron Lung.

Electronic

Electronic control circuits use devices such as resistors, capacitors, diodes, and transistors as well as combinations of these components in the form of integrated circuits. Integrated circuits can range in complexity from simple logic gates and operational amplifiers to microprocessors.

Control Variables and Waveforms

A ventilator may be classified as either a *pressure, volume,* or *flow controller* and may be further characterized in terms of the types of waveforms it can generate. In some cases, it is logical to classify a ventilator as a *time controller* (ie, it controls only inspiratory and expiratory times).

Ventilators can combine control schemes to create complex modes. For example, the Puritan-Bennett 7200a ventilator can mix flow-controlled breaths with pres-

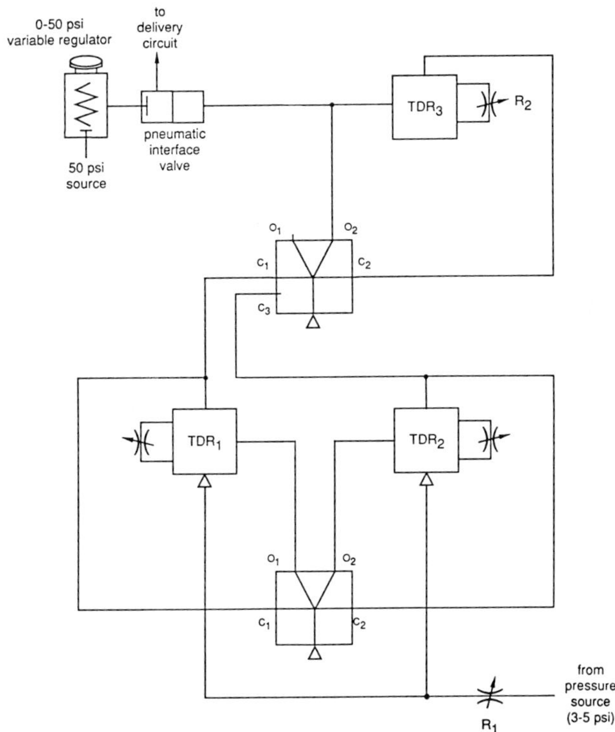

Figure 13-10. A simple ventilator control circuit composed of fluidic logic components. This circuit is an improvement over the one shown in Figure 13-8 in that it allows independent control of frequency (R_1) and % inspiration (R_2). TDR stands for time delay relay, which is a device that delays the signal introduced to its input by a time period determined by the setting of the variable resistor (ie, a needle valve).

sure-controlled breaths in the SIMV + PRESSURE SUPPORT mode. The Bear 1000 can mix pressure control with flow control within a single breath in its PRESSURE AUGMENT mode. The Siemens Servo 300 can adjust the level of pressure control automatically to achieve a pre-set target volume. The great flexibility of today's ventilators is achieved at the expense of added complexity. Thus, when evaluating ventilator performance it is important to have simple and unambiguous criteria for deciding which control variables are in effect.

Pressure

The equation of motion tells us that if the ventilator is an ideal *pressure controller,* then the left side of the equation (ie, ventilator pressure as a function of time) will be determined by the ventilator settings and will be unaffected by changes in parameter values on the right side (ie, compliance and resistance).

If the control variable is pressure, the ventilator can control either the airway pressure (causing it to rise above body surface pressure for inspiration) or the pressure on the body surface (causing it to fall below airway opening pressure for inspiration). This is the basis for classifying ventilators as being either positive or negative pressure types.* For example, the Newport Wave ventilator would be classified as a positive-pressure controller that generates a rectangular pressure waveform, and the Emerson Iron Lung is a negative-pressure controller that produces a quasi-sinusoidal pressure waveform.

Volume

If the pressure waveform varies as the load imposed by the patient's respiratory system changes, we then examine the volume waveform. However, the observation that the volume waveform remains unchanged is a necessary but not a sufficient condition to warrant the classification of volume controller, because the same holds true for a flow controller. The reason is that once the volume waveform is specified, the flow waveform is determined, since they are functions of each other (ie, volume is the integral of flow and flow is the derivative of volume). Therefore, if changes in compliance and resistance do not change the volume waveform, they will not affect the flow waveform and vice versa.

To qualify as a *volume controller* a ventilator must (1) maintain a consistent volume waveform in the presence of a varying load and (2) measure volume and use the signal to control the volume waveform. Volume can be measured directly only by the displacement of a piston or bellows or similar device. With a piston or bellows, controlling the excursion of the device automatically controls the volume waveform. Alternatively, a volume signal could be derived by integrating a flow signal. Note that although some ventilators like the Siemens Servo 900C, the Puritan-Bennett 7200, the Bear 5, and the Hamilton Veolar display volume readings, they all actually measure and control flow and calculate volume for displays. Thus, they are all flow controllers unless they are operated in a pressure-controlled mode (eg, during pressure support ventilation). An examination of a ventilator's schematic diagrams and operator's manual should provide the information necessary to decide whether volume or flow is being measured.

Flow

If the volume change (ie, tidal volume) remains consistent when compliance and resistance are varied, and if volume change is not measured and used for

*The terms *positive-pressure ventilator* and *negative-pressure ventilator* obscure the fact that both devices generate a positive transrespiratory pressure. Positive-pressure ventilators cause airway pressure to rise above atmospheric pressure (resulting in positive gauge pressure), while negative-pressure ventilators cause body surface pressure to fall below atmospheric pressure (resulting in negative gauge pressure). *Gauge pressure* is defined as pressure measured relative to atmospheric pressure.

control, the ventilator is classified as a *flow controller.* The simplest example of open loop flow control in a ventilator consists of a pressure regulator supplying gas to a flowmeter, such as found in infant ventilators. An infant ventilator becomes a flow controller rather than a pressure controller if the airway pressure does not reach the set pressure limit.[13] (However, the flowmeter is usually not back-pressure compensated and will vary its output slightly in the presence of a changing load.) In contrast, the Siemens Servo 900C (so-called because it uses servo control) measures flow and adjusts the output control valve (ie, the inspiratory scissors valve) accordingly. It can maintain a more consistent inspiratory flow waveform as the load changes.

Time

Suppose that both pressure and volume are affected substantially by changes in lung mechanics. Then the only form of control is that of defining the ventilatory cycle, or alternating between inspiration and expiration. Therefore, the only variables being controlled are the inspiratory and expiratory times. This situation arises in some forms of high-frequency ventilation when even the designation of an inspiratory and expiratory phase becomes somewhat obscure.

Phase Variables

Once the control variables and the associated waveforms are identified, more detail can be obtained by examining the events that take place during a ventilatory cycle, that is, the period of time between the beginning of one breath and the beginning of the next. Mushin and colleagues[14] proposed that this time span be divided into four phases: (1) the change from expiration to inspiration, (2) inspiration, (3) the change from inspiration to expiration, and (4) expiration. This convention is useful for examining how a ventilator starts, sustains, and stops an inspiration and what it does between inspirations. In each phase, a particular variable is measured and used to *start, sustain, and end* the phase. In this context, pressure, volume, flow, and time are referred to as *phase variables.*[15] The criteria for determining phase variables are defined in Figure 13-11.

Trigger

All ventilators measure one or more of the variables associated with the equation of motion (ie, pressure, volume, flow, or time). Inspiration is started when one of these variables reaches a pre-set value. Thus, the variable of interest is considered an initiating or *trigger variable.* The most common trigger variables are time (ie, the ventilator initiates a breath according

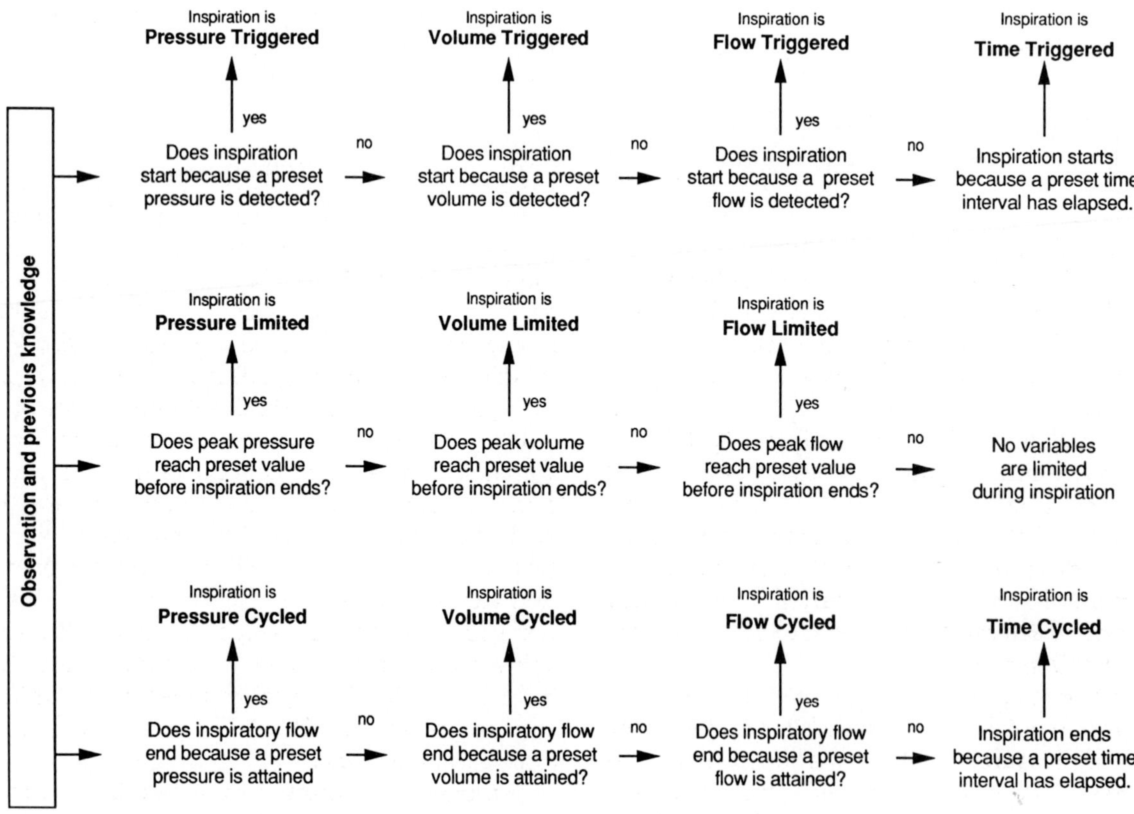

Figure 13-11. Criteria for determining the phase variables during a ventilator-assisted breath.

to a set frequency, independent of the patient's spontaneous efforts) and pressure (ie, the ventilator senses the patients's inspiratory effort in the form of a drop in baseline pressure and starts inspiration independent of the set frequency). Any variable that can be measured can potentially be used to trigger inspiration (eg, the Infrasonics Star Sync module allows triggering of the Infant Star ventilator by chest wall movement). Of course it may be possible to *manually trigger* inspiration.

It is feasible for a ventilator to measure volume and flow changes caused by the patient's inspiratory efforts and use them to trigger inspiration, but the technology is more complex and is not commonly used. Triggering on flow has been shown to be more sensitive than triggering on pressure (at least with conventional patient circuits); hence the patient has to do less work on the ventilator to obtain a breath.[16] Newer ventilators such as the Puritan-Bennett 7200a and the Bird V.I.P. may be flow triggered and the Dräger Babylog may be volume triggered.

The patient effort required to trigger inspiration is determined by the ventilator's sensitivity. Sensitivity is adjusted by changing the pre-set value of the trigger variable. For example, to make a pressure-triggered ventilator more sensitive, the trigger pressure might be adjusted from 5 to 1 cm H_2O below the baseline pressure.

Limit

Inspiratory time is defined as the time interval from the start of inspiratory flow to the start of expiratory flow. During inspiration, pressure, volume, and flow increase above their end expiratory values. If one (or more) of these variables rises no higher than some pre-set value, we will refer to the variable as a *limit variable*. But we must distinguish the limit variable from the variable that is used to end inspiration (called a *cycle variable*). Therefore, we impose the additional criterion that *inspiration is not terminated because a variable has met its pre-set limit value.* In other words, a variable is "limited" if it increases to a pre-set value before inspiration ends. These criteria are illustrated in Figure 13-12.

Clinicians commonly misuse the terms *limit* and *cycle* by using them interchangeably. This is encouraged by some ventilator manufacturers who use the term *limit* to describe what happens when a pressure alarm threshold is met (ie, inspiration is terminated and an alarm is activated). The term *cycle* is more appropriate in this situation.

Another potentially confusing issue is that, by convention, peak inspiratory pressure (PIP) and baseline pressure are measured relative to atmospheric pressure whereas the pressure limit is sometimes measured relative to baseline pressure (eg, Siemens Servo 900C) and sometimes relative to atmospheric pressure

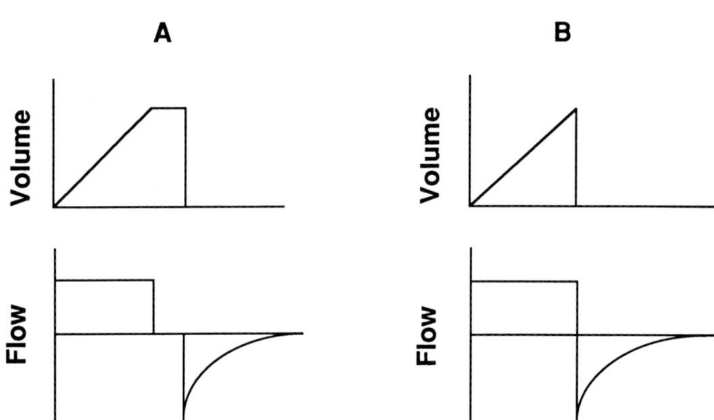

Figure 13-12. This figure illustrates the importance of distinguishing between the terms limit and cycle. In A, both volume and flow are limited (because they reach pre-set values before end inspiration) and inspiration is time cycled (after the pre-set inspiratory pause time). In B, flow is limited but volume is not and inspiration is volume cycled.

(eg, Bird V.I.P.). On the Bird V.I.P., the high pressure limit control sets the PIP limit (above ambient pressure) during pressure-controlled ventilation but cycles the breath off and activates a high-pressure alarm during volume-controlled ventilation. Hence the term *pressure limit* in common usage can indicate several different clinically significant situations depending on both the mode of ventilation and the manufacturer! Clearly, the lack of standardization among ventilator manufacturers makes it especially important that clinicians understand what they say and say what they mean.

Cycle

Inspiration always ends (ie, is cycled off) because some variable has reached a pre-set value. The variable that is measured and used to terminate inspiration is called the *cycle variable.* Deciding which variable is used to cycle off inspiration for a given ventilator can be confusing. For a variable to be used as a feedback signal (in this case a cycling signal) it must first be measured. Most third-generation adult ventilators allow the operator to set a tidal volume and inspiratory flow rate, which would lead one to believe that the ventilator could be volume cycled. However, closer inspection reveals that these ventilators do not measure volume (which is consistent with the fact that all third-generation ventilators are flow controllers). Rather, they set the inspiratory time necessary to achieve the set tidal volume with the set inspiratory flow rate, making them time cycled. The tidal volume dial can be thought of as an inspiratory time dial calibrated in units of volume rather than time.

Some persons think that a ventilator can have "mixed" cycling, which is contrary to the idea presented here that a ventilator can only control one variable at a time. The most common example given by these authors is a ventilator drive mechanism composed of a piston connected to a rod and a rotating crank. It is argued that one cannot distinguish time (ie, inspiratory time set by the frequency at which the crank rotates) or volume (ie, the stroke volume of the piston) as the cycling variable. However, if the inspiratory time is set low enough and the volume and patient load are high enough, a point will be reached when a piston-driven ventilator will "sacrifice" (ie, extend) the set inspiratory time to deliver the volume, thus unmasking its true volume-cycled nature.

Baseline

The variable that is controlled during the expiratory time is the *baseline variable.* Note that in the equation of motion, pressure, volume, and flow are measured relative to end-expiratory or baseline values and are thus initially all zero. Although the baseline value of any of these variables could theoretically be controlled, pressure control is the most practical and is implemented by all commonly used ventilators.

There is another interpretation of baseline pressure: during high-frequency oscillatory ventilation, airway pressure takes on both positive and negative values relative to the mean airway pressure. In this context, the baseline pressure is the mean airway pressure.

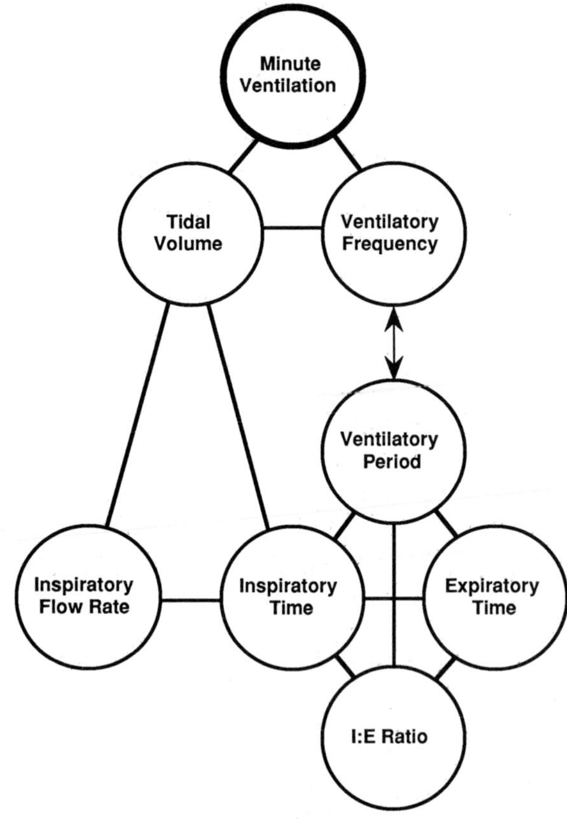

Figure 13-13. Influence diagram for volume-controlled ventilation. Variables are connected by straight lines such that if any two are known, the third can be calculated using standard equations.[21] The double arrow line indicates that ventilatory period is the reciprocal of ventilatory frequency. (Adapted from Perry DG. A simplified diagram for understanding the operation of volume-preset ventilators. Respir Care 1977; 22:42–49)

Modes of Ventilation and Conditional Variables

There are two general approaches to supporting the patient's inspiration: volume/flow control and pressure control. Figure 13-13 is a simplified influence diagram[17,18] that illustrates the important variables for ventilators that are either volume or flow controllers. Figure 13-14 is the influence diagram for ventilators that are pressure controllers. The equations relating these variables for inspiration are given in Table 13-1.[21]

Beyond these two general approaches to ventilatory support, it is possible to create a variety of breathing patterns or "modes" of ventilation. A mode of ventilation represents a specific set of characteristics that are of particular importance to the clinician. Specifically, *a mode of ventilation is defined as a particular set of control variables, phase variables, and conditional variables (explained later).* Using this approach, modes are conveniently defined in tabular form as shown in Table 13-2.

Figure 13-15 illustrates that for each breath, the ventilator creates a specific pattern of control and phase variables. The ventilator either may keep this pattern constant for each breath or it may introduce other patterns (eg, one for mandatory and one for spontaneous breaths). In essence, the ventilator must decide which pattern of control and phase variables to implement before each breath, depending on the value of some pre-set *conditional variables.* Conditional variables can be thought of as initiating conditional logic in the form of "if-then" statements. That is, *if* the value of a conditional variable reaches some pre-set threshold, *then* some action occurs to change the ventilatory pattern.

A simple example would be the Puritan-Bennett MA-1 in the control mode. Each breath is time triggered, flow limited, and volume cycled. The trigger, limit, and cycle variables have pre-set values (eg, trigger at frequency = 20 cycles/min, limit inspiratory flow at 60 L/min, and cycle at tidal volume = 750 mL). However, every few minutes a sigh breath is introduced that has a different set of phase variable values (eg, trigger at frequency = two sighs every 15 minutes; cycle at tidal volume = 1500 mL). How did the ventilator know to do this? Conceptually, we can say that before each breath pattern is selected, the ventilator examines the value of some conditional variable to see if it has reached a pre-set threshold value. If the threshold has been met, one pattern is selected, if not, another pattern is selected. In the case of the Puritan-

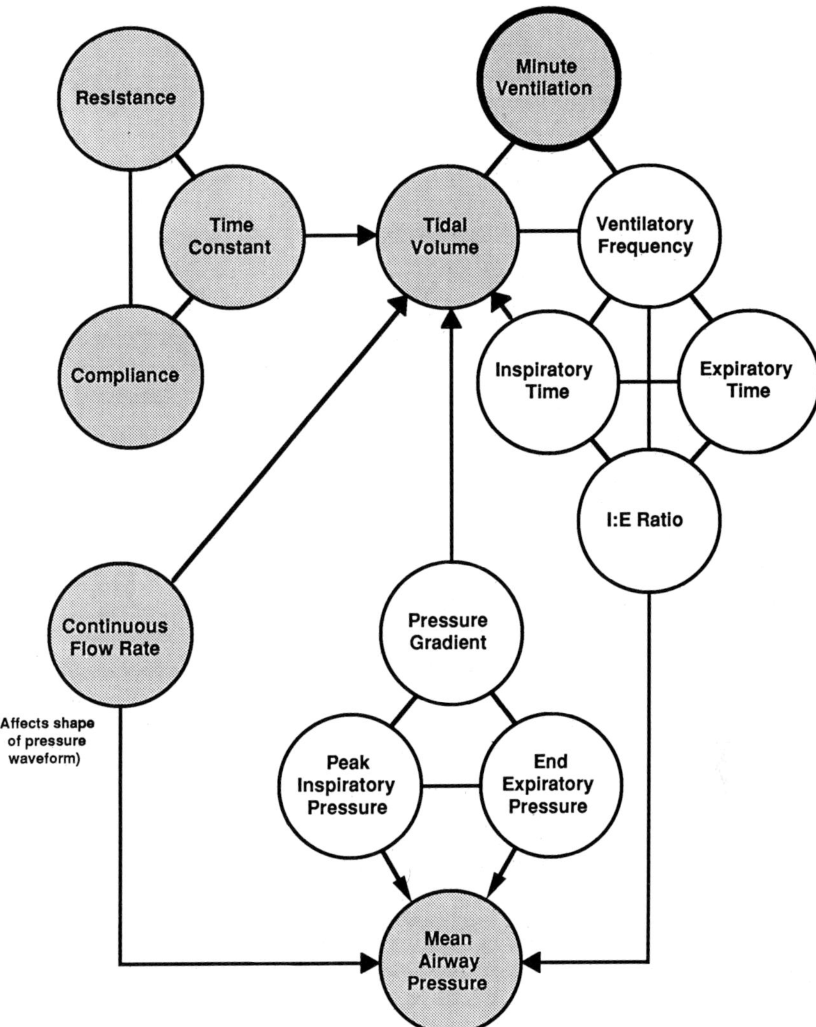

Figure 13-14. Influence diagram for pressure-controlled ventilation. Variables are connected by straight lines such that if any two are known, the third can be calculated using standard equations.[21] Arrows represent relations that are either more complex or less predictable. Open circles represent variables that can be directly controlled by the ventilator; shaded circles are controlled indirectly. (Adapted from Chatburn RL, Lough MD. Mechancal ventilation. In: Lough MD, Doershuk CF, Stern RC., eds. Pediatric respiratory therapy. Chicago: Year Book Medical Publishers, 1985: (148–191)

Bennett MA-1, the conditional variable was time—*if* a pre-set time interval has elapsed (ie, the sigh interval), *then* the ventilator switches to the sigh pattern. Other examples include switching from patient-triggered to machine-triggered breaths in the SIMV and mandatory minute ventilation (MMV) modes.

So far in this discussion we have used the terms *mandatory* and *spontaneous* without explanation. Clinicians have an intuitive understanding of the meanings of these terms. But because they play a central role in defining and understanding modes of ventilation, formal definitions must be provided. *Spontaneous* breaths are those that are *both* initiated *and* terminated by the patient. If the ventilator determines either the start or end of inspiration, then the breath is considered to be *mandatory*. Figure 13-16 illustrates these definitions with an algorithm. Note that if the ventilator either time or volume cycles an inspiration, the breath is considered mandatory because it is terminated by the ventilator. If, however, the ventilator flow cycles as in the pressure support mode, the inspiration is not considered mandatory. The rate of decay of inspiratory flow is determined by the patient's lung mechanics and ventilatory muscle activity. Hence, during the PRESSURE SUPPORT mode, pressure-limiting inspiration does not constrain inspiratory flow rate, and flow cycling does not necessarily dictate either the inspiratory time or the tidal volume if the ventilatory muscles are active. In other words, the ventilator attempts to match the patient's inspiratory demand and it is really the patient who terminates the breath. What is confusing to some clinicians is that if a breath is assisted, as in pressure support ventilation, it somehow seems to them to be mandatory rather than spontaneous. The advantages of separating the definitions of "mandatory" versus "spontaneous" from the definitions of "assisted" versus "unassisted" should now be clear.

Examination of Table 13-2 reveals an interesting fact: the commonly used mode names are not very specific in describing a given pattern of ventilation. For example, assist/control can mean that inspiration is pressure triggered, flow limited, and volume cycled, or volume triggered, flow limited, and time cycled, or pressure triggered, volume limited, and time cycled,

(Text continues on page 282)

TABLE 13-1. Pressure, Volume, and Flow as Functions of Time Related to Ventilator Settings and Respiratory System Parameters

Volume/Flow-Controlled Inspiration		Any mode	
$V = \int \dot{V}_I dt$	$\dot{V}_E = (V_T)(f)$	$\overline{P}aw = (K)(PIP - PEEP)\left(\frac{I}{I + E}\right) + PEEP$	
$V = (\dot{V}_I)(t)$ (for constant flow)			
$Paw = \frac{V}{C} + (R)(\dot{V})$	$\text{Period} = \frac{f}{60} = T_I + T_E$	$T_I = \frac{(I)(60)}{(I + E)(f)}$	$T_E = \frac{(E)(60)}{(I + E)(f)}$
Pressure-Controlled Inspiration			
$V = (\Delta Paw)(C)(1 - e^{-t/\tau})$			$I{:}E = \frac{T_I}{T_E}$
	$V = (\Delta Paw)(C)(e^{-t/\tau})$ (expiration)		
$\dot{V} = \left(\frac{\Delta Paw}{R}\right)(e^{-t/\tau})$			
$\tau = (R)(C)$	$\dot{V} = -\left(\frac{\Delta Paw}{R}\right)(e^{-t/\tau})$ (expiration)		

where
- Paw = airway pressure
- $\overline{P}aw$ = mean airway pressure
- V = lung volume
- $\dot{V}$ = flow
- $\dot{V}_I$ = inspiratory flow
- $\dot{V}_E$ = exhaled minute ventilation
- K = waveform constant, ranging from 0.5 for triangular pressure waveform to 1.0 for rectangular waveform
- R = respiratory system resistance
- C = respiratory system compliance
- t = time from begining of inspiration
- τ = time constant of respiratory system
- f = ventilatory frequency (cycles/min)
- T_I = inspiratory time
- T_E = expiratory time
- I = numerator of I:E ratio
- E = denominator of I:E ratio
- PIP = peak inspiratory pressure
- PEEP = positive end expiratory pressure

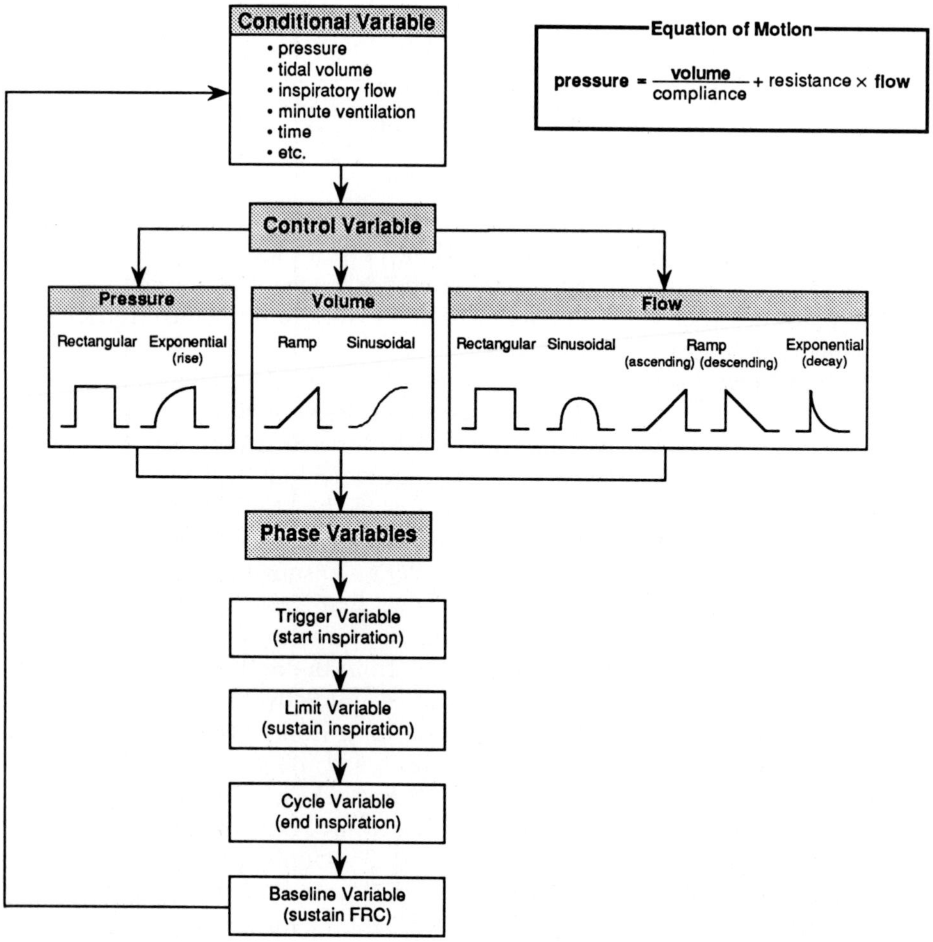

Figure 13-15. This figure illustrates a ventilator classification scheme based on a mathematical model known as the "equation of motion" for the respiratory system. This model indicates that during inspiration the ventilator is able to directly control one and only one variable at at time (ie, pressure, volume, or flow). Some common waveforms provided by current ventilators are shown for each control variable. Pressure, volume, flow, and time are also used as phase variables that determine the parameters of each ventilatory cycle (eg, trigger sensitivity, peak inspiratory flow rate or pressure, inspiratory time, and baseline pressure).

TABLE 13-2. Suggested Terminology for Operational Modes, Their Classification, and Relationship to Old Terminology

	Mandatory				Spontaneous				Control Logic			
Mode	Control	Trigger	Limit	Cycle	Control	Trigger	Limit	Cycle	Assisted?	Conditional Variable	Action	Prior Terms
Constant airway pressure (CAP)	—	—	—	—	Pressure	Pressure, volume, or flow	Pressure	Pressure	No	—	—	CPAP
Continuous spontaneous ventilation (CSV)	—	—	—	—	Pressure	Pressure, volume, or flow	Pressure	Volume	Yes	—	—	PSV
Continuous mandatory ventilation (CMV)	Pressure	Pressure, volume, flow, or time	Pressure	Time	—	—	—	—	—	Time or patient effort	Machine-to-patient trigger	PC-CMV, PCIRV, PC-A/C
	Volume/flow	Pressure, volume, flow, or time	Volume/flow	Volume, flow, or time	—	—	—	—	—	Time or patient effort	Machine-to-patient trigger	CMV, A/C
Intermittent mandatory ventilation (IMV)	Pressure	Pressure, volume, flow, or time	Pressure	Time	Pressure	Pressure, volume, or flow	Pressure	Pressure	No	Time or patient effort	Machine-to-patient trigger	PC-IMV, APRV, BiPAP, PC-SIMV
	Volume/flow	Pressure, volume, flow, or time	Volume or flow	Volume, flow, or time	Pressure	Pressure, volume, or flow	Pressure	Pressure	No	Time or patient effort	Machine-to-patient trigger	IMV, SIMV
Mandatory minute ventilation (MMV)	Volume/flow	Time	Volume or flow	Volume, flow, or time	Pressure	Pressure, volume, or flow	Pressure	Pressure	Yes*	Minute volume or time	Spontaneous-to-mandatory breath	MMV, EMMV

*Optional

CMV, continuous mandatory ventilation; A/C, assist/control; AMV, assisted mechanical ventilation; IMV, intermittent mandatory ventilation; SIMV, synchronized mandatory ventilation; CPAP, continuous positive airway pressure; PCV, pressure-controlled ventilation; PC-IMV, pressure-controlled IMV; PCIRV, PC inverse-ratio ventilation; APRV, airway pressure release ventilation; PSV, pressure support ventilation; MMV, mandatory minute ventilation; BiPAP, bilevel positive airway pressure.

From Branson RD, Chatburn RL. Technical description and classification of modes of ventilator operation. Respir Care 1992;37:1026–1044.

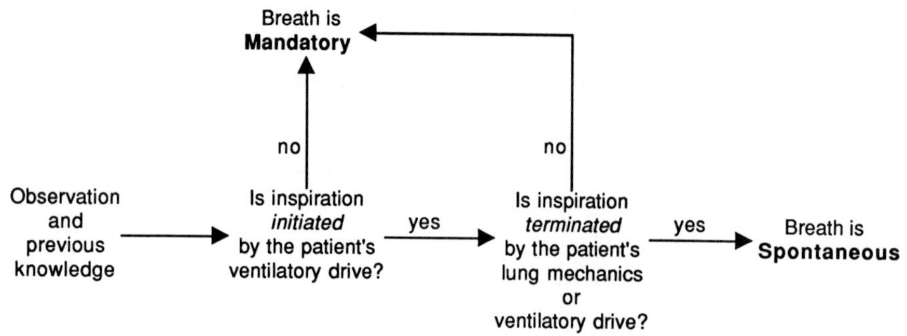

Figure 13-16. Algorithm defining spontaneous and mandatory breaths. In terms of current technology, if the breath is triggered according to a pre-set frequency or minimum minute ventilation or cycled according to a pre-set frequency or tidal volume, the breath is mandatory. All other breaths are spontaneous.

and so on. But it was not always this way. Back when the Puritan-Bennett MA-1 was the most commonly used ventilator, ASSIST/CONTROL was understood by everyone to mean simply that the tidal volume was pre-set and inspiration was pressure triggered on every breath (ie, the breath was either pressure or time triggered, flow limited, and volume cycled). Our traditional concepts do not fit today's more flexible technology. And the situation promises to get worse with future ventilators.

One way to simplify the naming and hierarchical organization of ventilator modes is illustrated in Figure 13-17.[4] There are three parent modes: pressure control (PC), volume/flow control (VC), and time control (TC). For each of these, there are three (daughter) breath patterns: continuous mandatory ventilation (CMV), intermittent mandatory ventilation (IMV), and continuous spontaneous ventilation (CSV). IMV is a daughter of both VC and PC because mandatory breaths can be either volume or pressure controlled. Further hierarchical categories are derived by examining the trigger pattern (ie, patient triggered, machine triggered, or combined triggering) and whether spontaneous breaths are assisted (eg, pressure support versus constant airway pressure).

The way a person describes a ventilator depends on how the information will be used. An administrator may need to know only where and for what type of patient the ventilator can be used (making the input power and control variables important). In addition to this information, the clinician would want to know how the ventilator is operated (making phase variables and output characteristics of interest). The student, educator, or researcher may need to understand the internal workings of the ventilator (requiring the knowledge of drive mechanism, compressor motor/linkage, output control valves, and control variables/waveforms). Certainly, the manufacturer's representatives should be conversant with all of this information and be able to provide it to interested parties. The classification system presented here was designed to meet these needs in a logical, consistent, and unambiguous manner. Let us explore some ways that it could be used to communicate ideas in "ventilator lingo."

The average clinician needs to describe very little about a ventilator during the course of the daily routine. Hence, the terms *volume ventilator* and *pressure ventilator* are often heard, referring to ventilators that allow a pre-set inspiratory pressure or tidal volume, respectively. Confusion quickly arises, however, when one attempts to describe how a ventilator operates, especially when speaking to someone who has little experience with the subject. Terms such as *pressure generator* or *flow generator* are often used but may be ambiguous because all ventilators generate pressure, volume, and flow all at once. The idea one would like to convey is that a ventilator controls a particular variable; hence the terms *pressure controller, volume controller,* and *flow controller* are more specific.

The outline approach to classification lends itself to varying degrees of detail. For example, a simple description of an Emerson Iron Lung would be that it is an electrically powered, negative pressure controller that produces a sinusoidal pressure waveform. A more detailed description would add that it is time triggered, is time cycled, provides no baseline pressure control, and uses an electrically controlled drive mechanism consisting of a diaphragm, rotating crank, and connecting rod driven by an electric motor. It operates in the continuous mandatory ventilation mode only and has no alarms.

A simple description of a more complex ventilator like the Bennett 7200 would be that it is an electrically powered, pressure or flow controller. A more detailed description would include that it is time, pressure, flow, or manually triggered; is pressure or volume limited; is time, or flow cycled; controls baseline pressure (PEEP/CPAP); and uses an electronic (microprocessor) control circuit and a drive mechanism/output control valve consisting of a pressure regulator and proportional valve with a pneumatic diaphragm exhalation manifold valve. One could go on and list the multitude of operating modes and alarms. The more complicated the ventilator, the more involved the description will be.

Perhaps more commonly, clinicians need to refer to a mode of ventilation rather than to a specific ventilator per se. The most general terms seem to be *volume-controlled* versus *pressure-controlled* ventilation. The term *pressure-controlled ventilation* should cause no problems but the use of *volume-controlled ventilation* may be confusing. A strict interpretation of the classification system presented in this discussion would require a distinction between volume-controlled and flow-controlled modes. However, in the interest of convenience, the term *volume controlled* should be acceptable for both. Any breath that is directly flow controlled is indirectly volume controlled and vice versa. (But when describing a ventilator rather than a mode of ventilation, you should make the distinction between volume and flow control.) More information about the mode of ventilation can be conveyed by stating the breath and trigger patterns and whether spontaneous breaths are assisted (see Fig. 13-17). For example, a neonatal ventilator is typically operated in the pressure-controlled IMV mode in which mandatory breaths are time triggered and spontaneous breaths are unassisted.

A complete description of a mode must specify the control and phase variables for mandatory and spontaneous breaths, as illustrated in Table 13-2. But you can communicate most of the important information by just specifying the phase variables for the mandatory and spontaneous breaths. For example, a description of volume-controlled SIMV with pressure support might be "mandatory breaths are pressure triggered, flow limited, and time cycled; spontaneous breaths are pressure triggered, pressure limited, and flow cycled."

Use of this system may seem uncomfortable at first, especially to those who are already familiar with some other system. Yet if the basic ideas are learned, the rest is easy. It is similar to the way that the game of checkers has only a few simple rules but leads to an almost infinite variety of playing strategies and tactics. However, if two persons playing the game do not know and use the same set of rules, confusion and conflict result. To carry the analogy further, the person who sees the similarity of positional patterns is much more likely to be successful at the game than the player who sees each position as different and unique. In the same way, the clinician who sees the similarity of design features and applies the same operational definitions to all ventilators more easily understands ventilators

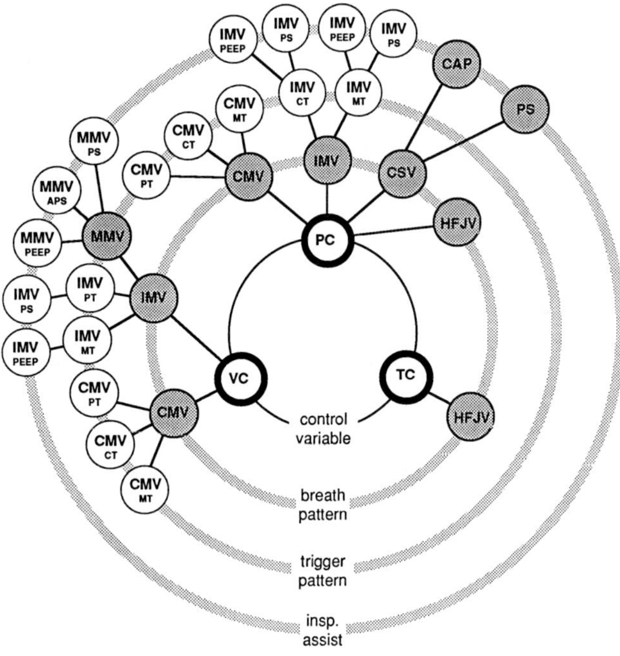

Figure 13-17. The constellation of ventilator modes. The parent mode is determined by the control variable (inner ring). The second generation is derived on the basis of the mandatory versus spontaneous breath pattern. The third generation is based on the trigger pattern. The fourth generation distinguishes between spontaneous breaths that are assisted (eg, pressure support mode) or unassisted (eg, continuous airway pressure or CAP, also known as CPAP).

Purpose

1. Illustrates all distinguishable modes currently described
2. Groups modes according to progressively more complex characteristics
3. Suggests possible modes not yet described

Explanation of Chart Organization

Generation	Distinguishing Characteristic
1	Root control variable pattern (pressure, volume/flow, time)
2	Mandatory breath pattern (continuous, intermittent, absent, or superimposed on spontaneous breaths)
3	Trigger variable pattern (mandatory breaths)
4	Spontaneous breath assist (yes, no)
5	Expiratory assist (yes, no)

* shaded circles represent primary set of mode names

Definitions

CAP = constant airway pressure
CMV = continuous mandatory ventilation
CSV = continuous spontaneous ventilation
CT = combined triggering
HFJV = high frequency jet ventilation
IMV = intermittent mandatory ventilation
MMV = mandatory minute ventilation
MT = machine triggered
PC = pressure control
PEEP = positive end expiratory pressure
PS = pressure support
PT = patient triggered
TC = time control
VC = volume/flow control

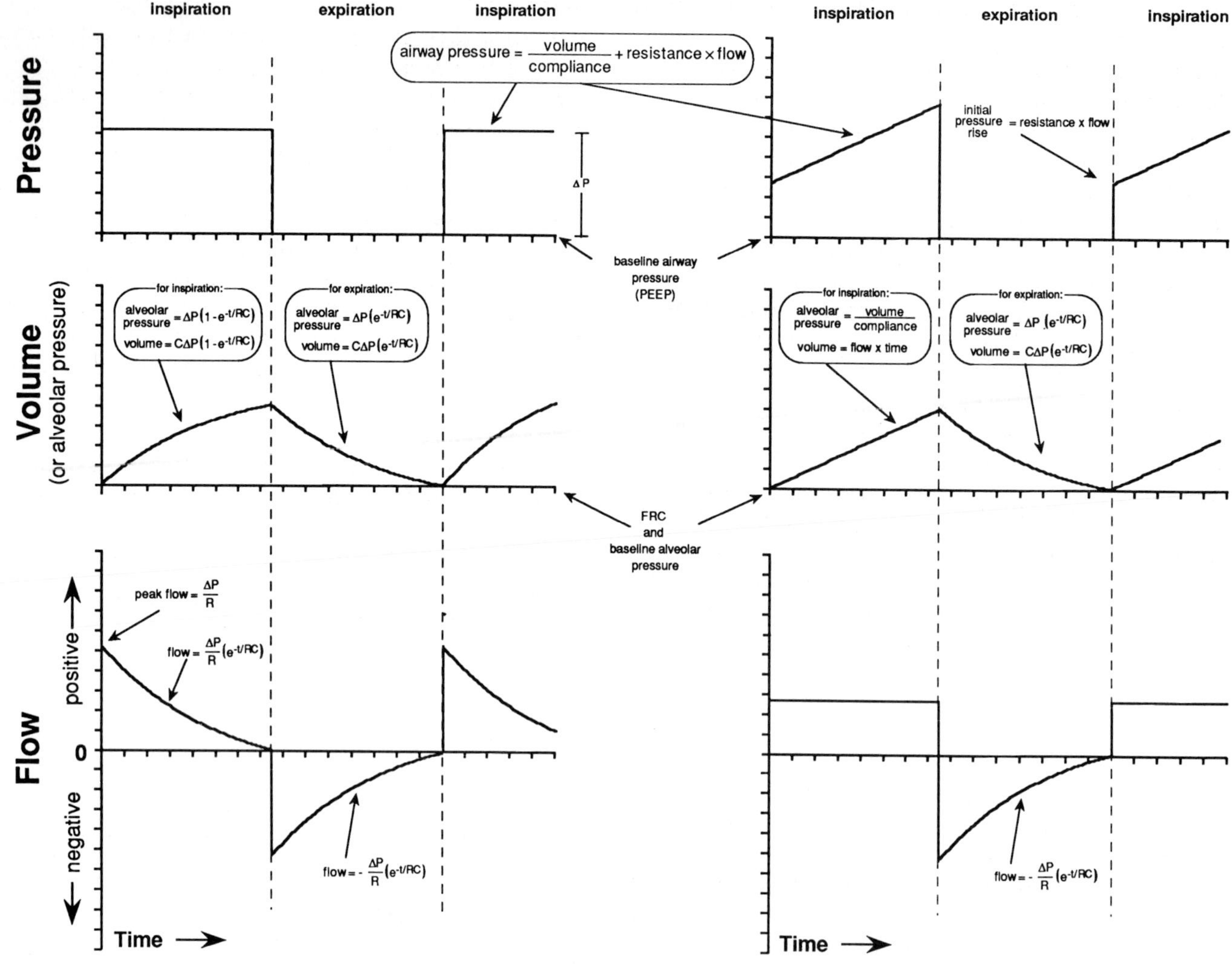

Figure 13-18. Typical pressure, volume, and flow waveforms for pressure-controlled (rectangular pressure waveform) and volume-controlled (rectangular flow waveform) ventilation. The curves show pressure, volume, and flow as functions of time in accordance with the equation of motion (where muscle pressure is zero). Note that all variables are measured relative to their baseline, or end-expiratory, values. ΔP, change in airway pressure; R, resistance, C, compliance; t, time; e, base of natural logarithm (≈ 2. 72); FRC, functional residual lung capacity.

and modes of ventilation than the clinician who tries to memorize endless lists of different features.

Output

Just as the study of heart physiology involves the study of electrocardiograms and blood pressure waveforms, the study of ventilator operation requires the examination of output waveforms. The waveforms of interest, of course, are the pressure, volume, and flow waveforms we have used throughout this discussion.

For each control variable, there are a limited number of waveforms that are commonly used by current ventilators. These waveforms can be idealized as shown in Figure 13-15 and have been grouped into four basic categories; pulse (rectangular), exponential, ramp, and sinusoidal. (Note that a rectangular volume waveform is theoretically impossible because volume cannot change instantaneously from zero to some pre-set value as pressure and flow can.)

Output waveforms are graphed in groups of three (Fig. 13-18).* The horizontal axes of all graphs are the same and have the units of time. The vertical axes are in units of the measured variables (eg, cm H_2O for pressure). For the purpose of identifying output wave-

*The conventional order of presentation is pressure, volume, and flow, respectively, from top to bottom. This order is based on the mathematical convention used for the form of the equation of motion, which is a specific example of a general class of expressions called first-order linear differential equations. Convention also dictates that positive flow values (above the horizontal axis) correspond to inspiration and negative flow values (below the horizontal axis) correspond to expiration.

forms, the specific baseline values of each variable are irrelevant. Therefore, the origin of the vertical axis is labeled zero. What is important is the relative magnitude of each of the variables and how the value of one affects or is affected by the value of the others.

Characteristic ventilator output waveforms are shown in Figs. 13-19 through 13-25. They are idealized. That is, they are precisely defined by mathematical equations and are meant to characterize the operation of the ventilator's control system. As such, they do not show the minor deviations or "noise" often seen in waveforms recorded during actual ventilator use. These waveform imperfections can be caused by a variety of extraneous variables such as vibration and turbulence, and the appearance of the waveform will be affected by the scaling of the time axis. The waveforms also do not show the effects of the resistance of the expiratory side of the patient circuit, since this will vary depending on the ventilator and type of circuit.

No ventilator is an ideal controller and ventilators are designed to only approximate a particular waveform. Idealized or standard waveforms are nevertheless helpful because they are common in other fields (eg, electrical engineering), which makes it possible to use mathematical procedures and terminology that have already been developed. For example, a standard mathematical equation is used to describe the most common waveforms for each control variable. This known equation may be substituted into the equation of motion, which is then solved to get the equations of the other two variables. Once the equations for pressure, volume, and flow are known, they are easily graphed. This is the process used to generate the graphs in Figures 13-19 through 13-25.

As mentioned previously, most ventilator waveforms can be classified as one of four general types: rectangular, exponential, ramp, or sinusoidal (including sigmoidal and oscillating). Although a variety of subtypes is possible, only the most common will be described here. Waveforms are listed according to the shape of the control variable waveform. Any new waveforms produced by future ventilators can easily be accommodated by this system.

Pressure

Rectangular

Mathematically, a rectangular waveform is referred to as a step or instantaneous change in transrespiratory pressure from one constant value to another (see Fig. 13-19). In response, volume rises exponentially from zero to a steady-state value equal to compliance times the change in airway pressure (ie, PIP − PEEP). Inspiratory flow falls exponentially from a peak value (at the start of inspiration) equal to (PIP − PEEP) ÷ resistance.

Exponential

Exponential pressure waveforms are most commonly used during neonatal ventilation (see Fig. 13-20). Ventilators such as the Bear Cub are designed to deliver a modified rectangular waveform that typically results in a gradual rather than an instantaneous change in pressure at the start of inspiration. Thus, depending on the specific ventilator settings (eg, short inspiratory time, low flow rate, and high PIP), the pressure waveform may never attain a constant value and resembles an exponential curve instead. In response, the volume and flow waveforms are also exponential but their peak values are less than with a rectangular pressure waveform.

Sinusoidal

A sinusoidal pressure waveform can be created by attaching a piston to either a rotating crank or to a lin-

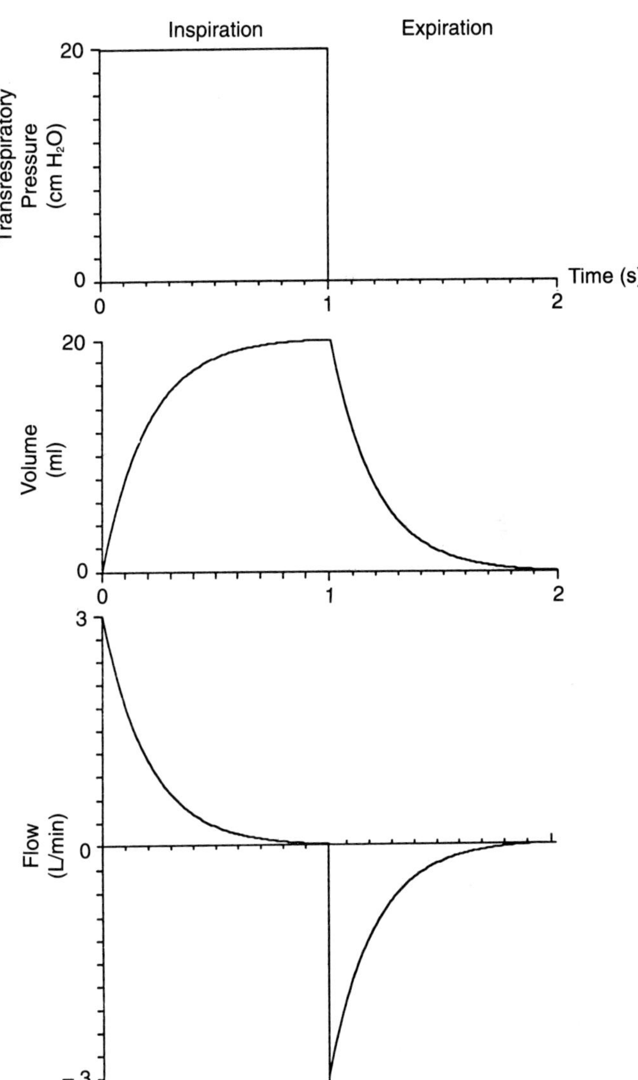

Figure 13-19. Characteristic waveforms for pressure-controlled ventilation with a rectangular pressure waveform. C = 0.001 L/cm H_2O; R = 200 cm H_2O/L/s.

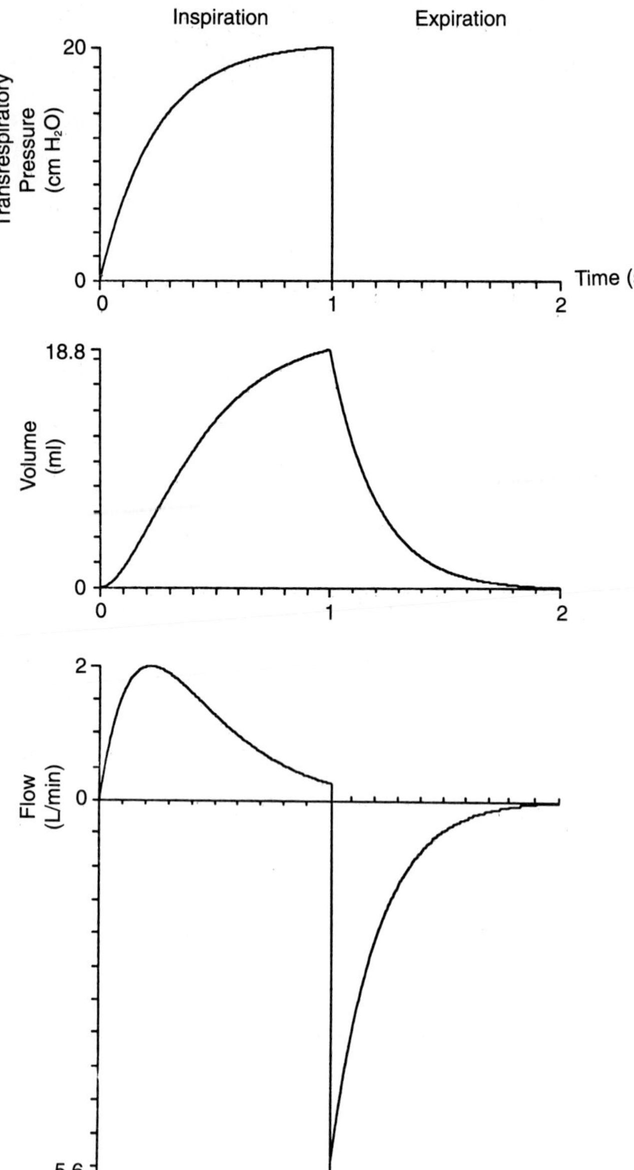

Figure 13-20. Characteristic waveforms for pressure-controlled ventilation with an exponential pressure waveform. C = 0.001 L/cm H_2O; R = 200 cm H_2O/L/s.

ear drive motor driven by an oscillating signal generator (see Fig. 13-21). In response, the volume and flow waveforms are also sinusoidal but they attain their peak values at different times.

Oscillating

Oscillating pressure waveforms can take on a variety of shapes from sinusoidal (eg, Mira Hummingbird) to ramp (eg, SensorMedics 3100 oscillator) to roughly triangular (eg, Infrasonics Star Oscillator). The distinguishing feature of a ventilator classified as an oscillator is that it can generate negative transrespiratory pressure. That is, if the mean airway pressure is set equal to atmospheric pressure, then the airway pressure waveform oscillates above and below zero. If the pressure waveform is sinusoidal, volume and flow will also be sinusoidal but out of phase with each other (ie, their peak values occur at different times).

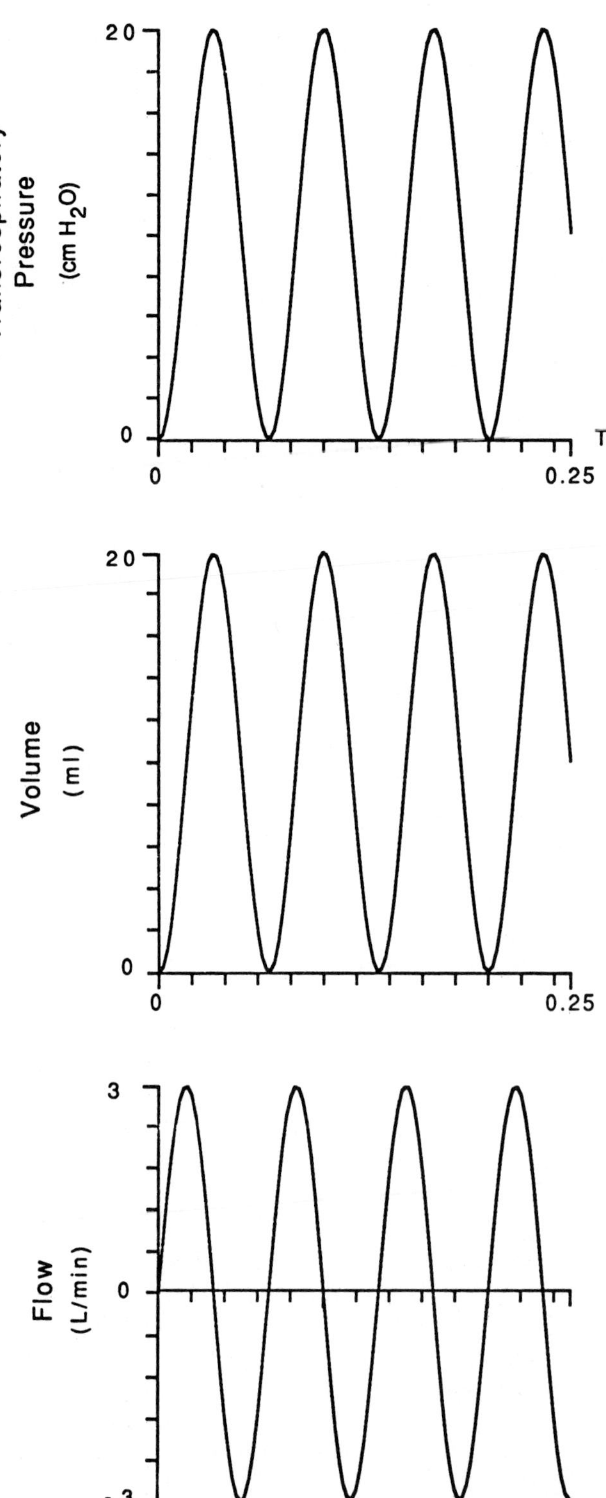

Figure 13-21. Characteristic waveforms for pressure-controlled ventilation with a sinusoidal pressure waveform. C = 0.001 L/cm H_2O; R = 200 cm H_2O/L/s.

Other waveforms produce more complex volume and flow waveforms.

Volume

Ramp

Volume controllers that produce an ascending ramp waveform (eg, the Bennett MA-1) produce a linear rise in volume from zero at the start of inspiration to the peak value (ie, the set tidal volume) at end inspiration (see Fig. 13-22). In response, the flow waveform is rectangular. The pressure waveform rises instantaneously from zero to a value equal to resistance × flow at the start of inspiration. From here it rises linearly to its peak value (ie, PIP) equal to (tidal volume/compliance) + (flow × resistance).

Sinusoidal

This waveform is most often produced by ventilators whose drive mechanism is a piston attached to a rotating crank (eg, Engstrom and Emerson ventilators). The output waveform of this type of ventilator can be approximated by the first half of a cosine curve, whose shape in this case is sometimes referred to as a sigmoidal curve (see Fig. 13-23). Because volume is sinusoidal during inspiration, pressure and flow are also sinusoidal.

Flow

Rectangular

A rectangular flow waveform is perhaps the most common output (see Fig. 13-22). When the flow waveform is rectangular, volume is a ramp waveform and pressure is a step followed by a ramp as described for the ramp volume waveform.

Ramp

The ramp waveform is what many respiratory care practitioners (and ventilator manufacturers) call an "accelerating" or "decelerating" flow waveform. The term *ramp* is borrowed from electronic engineering and is preferred for three reasons. First, the name "ramp" gives a more obvious visual image of actual shape of the waveform. Second, the term *ramp* has been described mathematically and used universally for much longer than mechanical ventilators have been in existence. Third, the analogy of something accelerating or decelerating is misapplied. For example, when a car is moving we say it has a certain speed (ie, speed = Δdistance/Δtime). If the speed increases with time we say that the car accelerates (ie, acceleration = Δspeed/Δtime) not that the speed accelerates. The speed of moving gas is expressed as a flow rate (ie, flow rate = area of tube × Δdistance/Δtime). If the flow rate increases, we would properly say that the gas accelerates (ie, acceleration = Δflow rate/Δtime) not that the flow accelerates. In scientific terms: the acceleration of a particle is the rate of change of its velocity with time.[22]

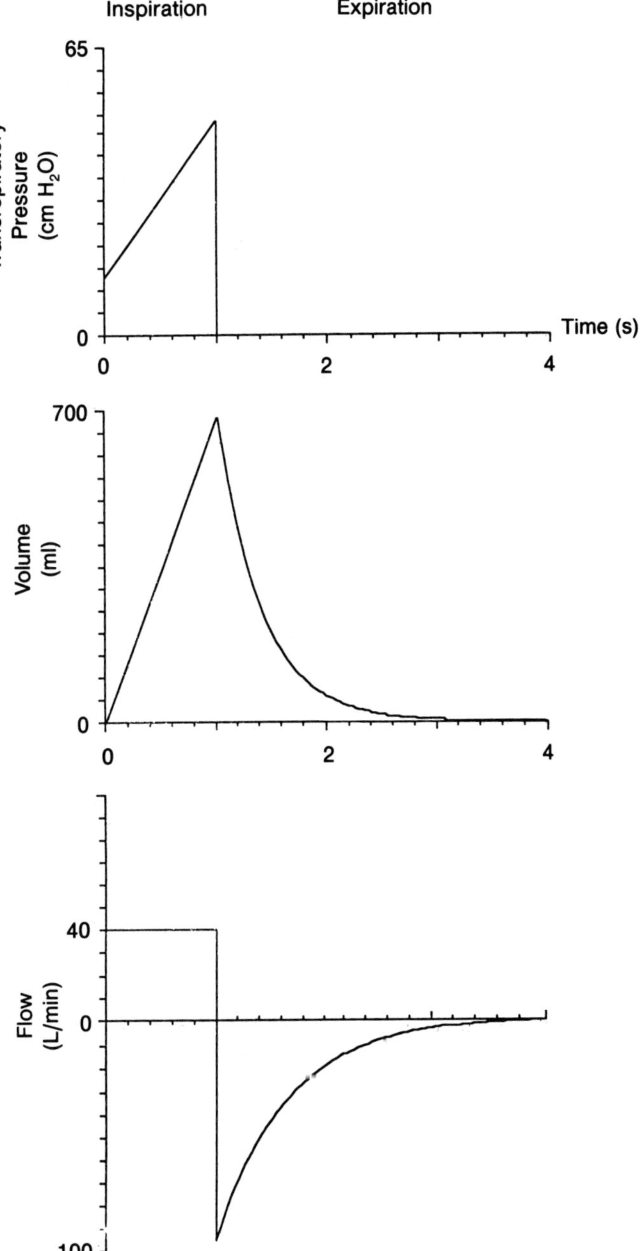

Figure 13-22. Characteristic waveforms for volume-controlled ventilation with an ascending ramp volume waveform. Identical to flow-controlled ventilation with a rectangular flow waveform. C = 0.02 L/cm H_2O; R = 20 cm H_2O/L/s.

ASCENDING RAMP. A true ascending ramp waveform starts at zero and increases linearly to the peak value (see Fig. 13-24). Ventilator flow waveforms are sometimes truncated; inspiration starts with an initial instantaneous flow (eg, the Bear 5 ventilator starts

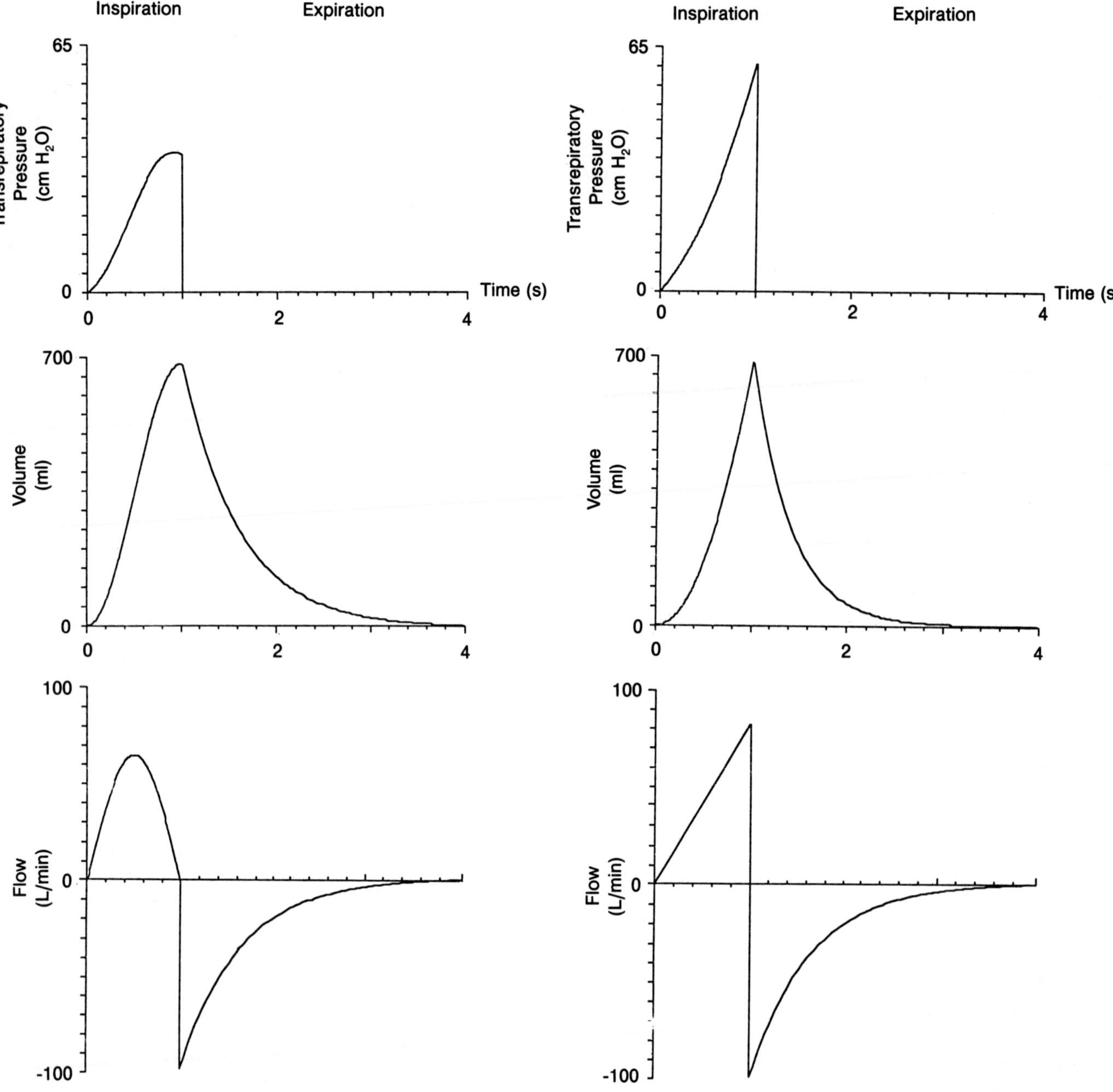

Figure 13-23. Characteristic waveforms for volume-controlled ventilation with a sinusoidal volume waveform. Identical to flow-controlled ventilation with a sinusoidal flow waveform. C = 0.02 L/cm H_2O; R = 20 cm H_2O/L/s.

Figure 13-24. Characteristic waveforms for volume-controlled ventilation with an ascending ramp flow waveform. C =0.02 L/cm H_2O; R = 20 cm H_2O/L/s.

inspiration at 50% of the set peak flow). Flow then increases linearly to the set peak flow rate. In response to an ascending ramp flow waveform, the pressure and volume waveforms are exponential with a concave upward shape.

DESCENDING RAMP. A true descending ramp waveform starts at the peak value and decreases linearly to zero (see Fig. 13-25). Ventilator flow waveforms are sometimes truncated; inspiratory flow rate decreases linearly from the set peak flow until it reaches some arbitrary threshold where flow drops immediately to zero (eg, the Bennett 7200a ends inspiration when the flow rate drops to 5 L/min). In response to a descending ramp flow waveform, the pressure and volume waveforms are exponential with a concave downward shape.

Sinusoidal

Some ventilators offer a mode in which the inspiratory flow waveform approximates the shape of the first half of a sine wave (see Fig. 13-23). As with the ramp waveform, ventilators often truncate the sine wave-

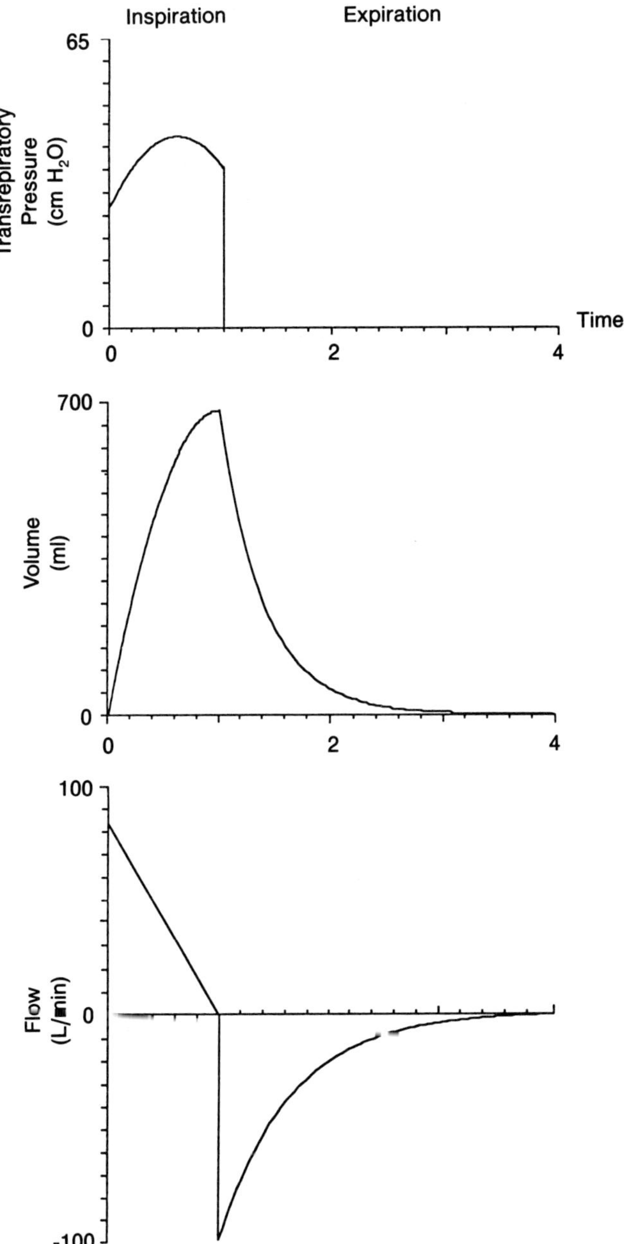

Figure 13-25. Characteristic waveforms for volume-controlled ventilation with a descending ramp flow waveform. C = 0.02 L/cm H_2O; R = 20 cm H_2O/L/s.

form by starting and ending flow at some percentage of the set peak flow rather than start and end at zero flow. In response to a sinusoidal flow waveform, the pressure and volume waveforms will also be sinusoidal but out of phase with each other.

Effects of the Patient Circuit

So far in this discussion we have implied that what comes out of the ventilator is the same as what goes into the patient. However, pressure, volume, and flow measured inside the ventilator are never the same as pressure, volume, and flow measured at the patient's airway opening. The reason, of course, is because the patient circuit has its own compliance (actually, the compliance of the tubing material plus the compressibility of the inspired gas) and resistance. Therefore, the pressure measured inside the ventilator on the inspiratory side (eg, on a Puritan-Bennett MA-1) will always be higher than the pressure at the airway opening owing to the elastic and flow resistive pressure drops created by the patient circuit. Volume and flow coming out of the ventilator will always be more than that delivered to the patient because of the effective compliance of the patient circuit. Patient circuit compliance includes not only the compliance of the material the circuit is made from but also the compressibility of the gas within the circuit. This compliance effect absorbs both volume and flow.

It can be shown by analogy to electrical circuits that the compliance of the delivery circuit is connected in parallel with the compliance of the respiratory system. That is, pneumatic compliance is analogous to electrical capacitance and pneumatic resistance is analogous to electrical resistance.[9] Therefore, the total compliance of the ventilator–patient system is simply the sum of the two compliances. In a similar manner, the resistance of the delivery circuit is shown to be connected in series with the respiratory system resistance so that the total resistance is the sum of the two. From these assumptions, it can be shown that the relation between the volume input to the patient (at the point of connection to the patient's airway opening) and the volume output from the ventilator (at the point of connection to the patient circuit) is described by:

$$\text{(3) Volume input to patient} = \left(\frac{1}{1 + \frac{C_{PC}}{C_{RS}}}\right) \times \text{volume output from ventilator}$$

where C_{PC} is the compliance of the patient circuit and C_{RS} is the total compliance of the patient's respiratory system. The equation shows that the larger the patient circuit compliance is compared with the patient's respiratory system, the larger the denominator on the right hand side of the equation and hence the smaller the delivered tidal volume will be compared with the volume coming out of the ventilator's drive mechanism.

Assuming that the volume exiting the ventilator is the set tidal volume, the patient circuit compliance is calculated as:

$$\text{(4)} \qquad C_{PC} = \frac{\text{Set tidal volume}}{\text{Pplt} - \text{EEP}}$$

where Pplt is the pressure measured during an inspiratory hold maneuver with the wye adapter of the patient circuit occluded (patient is not connected) and EEP is end-expiratory pressure (ie, baseline pressure). Most authors recommend the use of peak inspiratory pressure, PIP, for Pplt in the above equation. This is acceptable, but it may lead to a slight underestimation of patient circuit compliance. Pplt is slightly lower than PIP because of the flow resistive pressure drop of the patient circuit if pressure is not measured at the wye adapter. This difference will be greatest in small-bore, corrugated patient circuit tubing but is probably insignificant.

The effects of patient circuit compliance are most troublesome during volume-controlled ventilation. For example, when ventilating neonates, the patient circuit compliance can be as much as three times that of the respiratory system, even with small-bore tubing and a small-volume humidifier. Thus, when trying to deliver a pre-set tidal volume, the volume delivered to the patient may be as little as 25% of that coming from the ventilator, while 75% is compressed in the patient circuit. An example using adult values is shown in Figure 13-26.

Another area in which patient circuit compliance causes trouble is in the determination of auto-PEEP. The patient's airway opening is occluded at end-expiration until static conditions prevail throughout the lungs. The pressure at this time is auto-PEEP (PEEPA) and is an index of the volume of gas trapped in the lungs:

$$(5) \qquad \text{True PEEP}_A = \frac{V_{RS}}{C_{RS}}$$

where V_{RS} is the volume of the respiratory system at end-expiration and C_{RS} is respiratory system compliance.

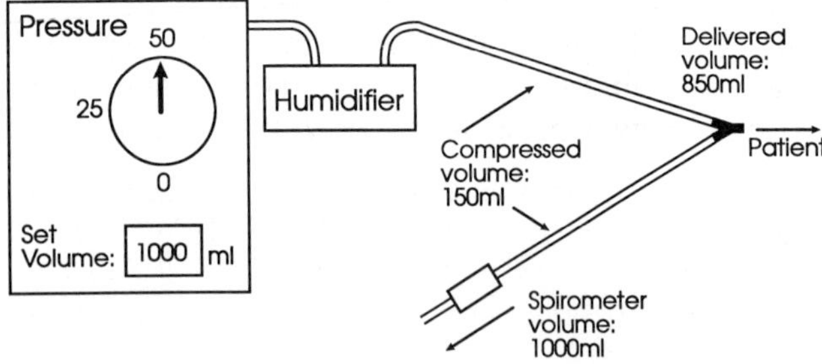

Figure 13-26. Illustration of the concept of compressible volume. The ventilator is set to deliver 1000 mL to the patient. If the tubing compliance is 3 mL/cm H_2O and plateau pressure is 50 cm H_2O, then compressible volume is (3 mL/cm H_2O) ÷ 50 cm H_2O = 150 mL. Actual volume delivered to the patient is 1000 mL − 150 mL = 850 mL. If the ventilator measures volume distal to the exhalation valve, tidal volume will equal set volume but will not reflect the actual tidal volume delivered to the patient.

Some ventilators (eg, Siemens Servo 900C) allow the clinician to perform the maneuver without disconnecting the patient from the ventilator. In this case, however, the end-expiratory respiratory system volume is distributed between the lungs and the patient circuit. Thus, the auto-PEEP measured under these conditions will underestimate the true auto-PEEP because the patient circuit compliance is added in parallel with the compliance of the respiratory system:

$$(6) \qquad \text{Estimated PEEP}_A = \frac{V_{RS}}{C_{RS} + C_{PC}}$$

The relation between true and estimated auto-PEEP is derived by solving equation for volume and substituting it into equation:

$$(7) \ \text{True PEEP}_A = \left(\frac{C_{RS} + C_{PC}}{C_{RS}}\right) \cdot \text{estimated PEEP}_A$$

Thus, true auto-PEEP may be calculated from the estimated auto-PEEP by multiplying by an error factor that is a function of the patient circuit compliance. This error can be substantial for small patients with stiff lungs.

You can see that the patient circuit has the same magnitude of effect on mean inspiratory flow rate by dividing both sides of equation 3 by inspiratory time. The discrepancy between the set and delivered tidal volume and flow must be taken into account when using most ventilators. However, some ventilators, such as the Puritan-Bennett 7200 series, make the appropriate calculations and adjustments automatically.

During pressure-controlled ventilation, the compliance of the patient circuit has the effect of rounding the leading edge of a rectangular pressure waveform, which could possibly reduce the volume delivered to the patient. This effect is avoided if the pressure limit is maintained for at least five time constants (ie, time constants of the respiratory system). The *time constant* is a measure of the time required for the passive respiratory system to respond to abrupt changes in ventilatory pressure. It is measured in units of seconds and is calculated as resistance times compliance.[9,21]

For both pressure- and volume-controlled ventilation, the patient circuit compliance increases the expiratory time constant. Thus, a large circuit compliance coupled with a short expiratory time can lead to inadvertent end-expiratory pressure.

In general, the "set" values for pressure, volume, and flow may be different from the "output (from ventilator)" values owing to calibration errors and different from the "input (to the patient)" owing to the effects of the patient circuit. Thus there are two general sources of error that cause discrepancies between the desired and actual patient values.

Ventilator Alarm Systems

The ventilator classification scheme described previously centers on the basic functions of input, control, and output. If any of these functions fails, a life-threatening situation may result. Thus, ventilators are equipped with various types of alarms, which may be classified in the same manner as the other major ventilator characteristics.

Day and MacIntyre[23,24] have stressed that the goal of ventilator alarms is to warn of *events*. They define an "event" as any condition or occurrence that requires clinician awareness or action. *Technical events* are those involving an inadvertent change in the ventilator's performance; *patient events* are those involving a change in the patient's clinical status that can be detected by the ventilator.[23] A ventilator may be equipped with any conceivable vital sign monitor, but we will limit the scope here to include the ventilator's mechanical/electronic operation and those variables associated with the mechanics of breathing (ie, pressure, volume, flow, and time). Because the ventilator is in intimate contact with exhaled gas, we will also include the analysis of exhaled oxygen and carbon dioxide concentrations as possible variables to monitor.

Alarms may be audible, visual, or both, depending on the seriousness of the alarm condition. Visual alarms may be as simple as colored lights or may be as complex as alphanumeric messages to the operator indicating the exact nature of the fault condition. Specifications for an alarm event should include (1) conditions that trigger the alarm, (2) the alarm response in the form of audible and/or visual messages, (3) any associated ventilator response such as termination of inspiration or failure to operate, and (4) whether the alarm must be manually reset or resets itself when the alarm condition is rectified. Table 13-3 outlines the various levels of alarm priority along with alarm characteristics and appropriate alarm categories. Alarm categories are based on the ventilator classification scheme and are detailed below.

Input Power Alarms

Loss of Electric Power

Most ventilators have some sort of battery backup in the case of electrical power failure, even if the batteries only power alarms. Ventilators typically have alarms that are activated if the electrical power is cut off while the machine is still switched on (eg, if the power cord is accidentally pulled out of the wall socket).

If the ventilator is designed to operate on battery power (eg, transport ventilators), there is usually an alarm to warn of a low-battery condition.

Loss of Pneumatic Power

Ventilators that use pneumatic power have alarms that are activated if either the oxygen or air supply is cut off or reduced below some specified driving pressure. In some cases, the alarm is activated by an electronic pressure switch (eg, Puritan-Bennett 7200), but in others the alarm is pneumatically operated as a part of the blender (eg, Siemens Servo 900C).

Control Circuit Alarms

Control circuit alarms are those that either warn the operator that the set control variable parameters are incompatible (eg, inverse I:E ratio) or indicate that some aspect of a ventilator self-test has failed. In the latter case, there may be something wrong with the ventilator control circuitry itself (eg, a microprocessor failure) and the ventilator generally responds with some generic message like "Ventilator Inoperative."

Output Alarms

Output alarms are those that are triggered by an unacceptable state of the ventilator's output. More specifically, an output alarm is activated when the value of a control variable (pressure, volume, flow, or time) falls outside an expected range. Some possibilities include the following.

Pressure

Pressure alarms may be available for the following conditions.

HIGH AND LOW PEAK AIRWAY PRESSURE. These alarms occur when there is a possible endotracheal tube obstruction or leak in the patient circuit, respectively.

HIGH AND LOW MEAN AIRWAY PRESSURE. These alarms indicate a possible leak in the patient circuit or a change in ventilatory pattern that might lead to a change in the patient's oxygenation status (ie, within reasonable limits, oxygenation is roughly proportional to mean airway pressure).

HIGH AND LOW BASELINE PRESSURE. These alarms indicate a possible patient circuit or exhalation manifold obstruction (or inadvertent PEEP) and disconnection of the patient from the patient circuit, respectively.

FAILURE TO RETURN TO BASELINE. Failure of airway pressure to return to baseline within a specified period indicates a possible patient circuit obstruction or exhalation manifold malfunction.

Volume

HIGH AND LOW EXPIRED VOLUME. These alarms indicate changes in respiratory system time constant

TABLE 13-3. Classification of Ventilator Alarms

	Priority			
	Level 1	Level 2	Level 3	Level 4
Event	critical* ventilator malfunction	noncritical† ventilator malfunction	patient status change‡	operator alert§
Alarm characteristics				
Mandatory	Yes	Yes	No	Yes
Redundant‖	Yes	No	No	No
Noncancelling¶	Yes	No	No	Yes
Audible	Yes	Yes	Yes	No
Visual	Yes	Yes	Yes	Yes
Automatice backup response#	Yes	No	No	No
Automatic reset				
Audible	Yes	Yes	Yes	—
Visual	No	Yes	Yes	Yes
Applicable Alarm Categories				
Input				
Electric power	Yes	No	No	No
Pneumatic power	Yes	No	No	No
Control circuit				
Inverse I:E ratio	No	Yes	No	Yes
Incompatible settings	No	No	No	Yes
Mechanical/electronic fault	Yes	No	No	No
Output				
Pressure**	Yes	Yes	Yes	Yes
Volume††	Yes	Yes	Yes	Yes
Flow‡‡	Yes	Yes	Yes	Yes
Minute ventilation	Yes	Yes	Yes	Yes
Time§§	Yes	Yes	Yes	Yes
Inspired gas (F_{IO_2}, temp)‖‖	Yes	Yes	No	Yes
Expired gas (F_{EO_2}, F_{ECO_2})‖‖	No	No	Yes	No

*Immediately life threatening.

†Not immediately life threatening.

‡Change in neurologic ventilatory drive, respiratory system mechanics, hemodynamic or metabolic status, etc.

§Ventilator warns of potential danger (eg, control variable settings unusually high or low; alarm thresholds inappropriately set).

‖Specific alarm mechanisms designed in duplicate or backed up by related alarm mechanisms.

¶Operator cannot reset the alarm until the alarm condition has been corrected.

#Backup ventilator mode or patient circuit opens to atmosphere.

**High/low peak, mean, and baseline pressure.

††High/low inhaled and exhaled tidal volume. May also include alarm for leak (inhaled volume minus exhaled volume expressed as a percent of inhaled volume).

‡‡Alarm triggered if expiratory flow rate does not fall below set threshold. Warns of alveolar gas trapping.

§§Warns that inspiratory or expiratory times are too long/short.

‖‖Analysis of inspired and expired gas may include other tracer gases that enable calculation of functional residual capacity.

during pressure-controlled ventilation, leaks around the endotracheal tube or from the lungs, or possible disconnection of the patient from the patient circuit.

Flow

HIGH AND LOW EXPIRED MINUTE VENTILATION. These alarms indicate hyperventilation (or possible machine self-triggering) and possible apnea or disconnection of the patient from the patient circuit, respectively.

Time

HIGH OR LOW VENTILATORY FREQUENCY. When these alarms occur, hyperventilation (or possible machine self-triggering) and possible apnea, respectively, may be happening.

INAPPROPRIATE INSPIRATORY TIME. Inspiratory time too long indicates a possible patient circuit obstruction or exhalation manifold malfunction. Inspiratory time too short indicates that adequate tidal volume may not be delivered (in a pressure-controlled mode) or that gas distribution in the lungs may not be optimal.

INAPPROPRIATE EXPIRATORY TIME. Expiratory time too long may indicate apnea. Expiratory time too short may warn of alveolar gas trapping (ie, expiratory time should be greater than or equal to five time constants of the respiratory system.

Inspired Gas

Inspired gas conditions have been standard alarm parameters for some time.

- High/low inspired gas temperature
- High/low FIO_2

Expired Gas

Because ventilators are designed to control the mechanical results of exhalation, they may be easily adapted to the analysis of exhaled gas composition and alarms may be set for specific parameters.

EXHALED CARBON DIOXIDE TENSION. End-tidal carbon dioxide monitoring may reflect arterial carbon dioxide tension and thus indicate the level of ventilation. Calculation of mean expired carbon dioxide tension along with minute ventilation measurements could provide information about carbon dioxide production and contribute to the calculation of the respiratory exchange ratio and the tidal volume/dead space ratio.

EXHALED OXYGEN TENSION.[25] Analysis of end-tidal and mean expired oxygen tension may provide information about gas exchange and could be used along with carbon dioxide data to calculate the respiratory exchange ratio.

References

1. Mushin M, Rendell-Baker W, Thompson PW, Mapelson WW. Automatic Ventilation of the Lungs. Oxford: Blackwell Scientific Publications, 1980:62–166.
2. Consensus statement on the essentials of mechanical ventilators—1992. Respir Care 1992;37:1000–1008.
3. Chatburn RL. Classification of mechanical ventilators. Respir Care 1992;37:1009–1025.
4. Branson RD, Chatburn RL. Technical description and classification of modes of ventilator operation. Respir Care 1992;37: 1026–1044.
5. Morris W. The American Heritage Dictionary of the English Language. Boston: American Heritage Publishing Co. and Houghton Mifflin, 1975:780.
6. Dupuis YG. Ventilators: Theory and Application. St. Louis: CV Mosby, 1986.
7. Beckwith TG, Buck NL, Marangoni RD. Mechanical Measurements, 3rd ed. Reading, MA: Addison-Wesley, 1982:25.
8. Otis AB, McKerrow CB, Bartlett RA, et al. Mechanical factors in distribution of pulmonary ventilation. J Appl Physiol 1956;8: 427–443.
9. Chatburn RL, Primiano FP Jr. Mathematical models of respiratory mechanics. In: Chatburn RL, Craig KC, eds. Fundamentals of Respiratory Care Research. Norwalk, CT: Appleton & Lange, 1988.
10. Rubinstein MF. Patterns of Problem Solving. Englewood Cliffs, NJ: Prentice-Hall, 1975:409–473.
11. Morch ET. History of mechanical ventilation. In: Kirby RR, Smith RA, Desautels DA, eds. Mechanical Ventilation. New York: Churchill Livingstone, 1985:1–58.
12. Russell DF, Ross DG, Manson HJ. Fluidic cycling devices for inspiratory and expiratory timing in automatic ventilators. J Biomed Eng 1983;5:227–234.
13. Hess D, Lind L. Nomograms for the application of the Bourns Model BP200 as a volume-constant ventilator. Respir Care 1980;25:248–250.
14. Mushin WW, Rendell-Baker L, Thompson PW, Mapleson WW. Automatic Ventilation of the Lungs, 3rd ed. Oxford: Blackwell Scientific Publications, 1980:62–131.
15. Desautels DA. Ventilator performance evaluation. In: Kirby RR, Smith RA, Desautels DA. Mechanical ventilation. New York: Churchill Livingstone, 1985;120.
16. Sassoon CSH, Giron AE, Ely EA, Light RW. Inspiratory work of breathing on flow-by and demand-flow continuous positive airway pressure. Crit Care Med 1989;17:1108–1114.
17. Shachter RD. Evaluating influence diagrams. Operations Res 1986;34:871–882.
18. Seiver A, Holtzman S. Decision analysis: A framework for critical care decision assistance. Int J Clin Monit Comput 1989;6:137–156.
19. Perry DG. A simplified diagram for understanding the operation of volume-preset ventilators. Respir Care 1977;22:42–49.
20. Chatburn RL, Lough MD. Mechanical ventilation. In: Lough MD, Doershuk CF, Stern RC, eds. Pediatric Respiratory Therapy. Chicago: Year Book Medical Publishers, 1985:148–191.
21. Chatburn RL, Lough MD, Primiano FP Jr. Mechanical ventilation. In: Chatburn RL, Lough MD, eds. Handbook of Respiratory Care, 2nd ed. Chicago: Year Book Medical Publishers, 1990:159–223.
22. Halliday D, Resnick R. Fundamentals of Physics, 2nd ed. New York: John Wiley & Sons, 1981:29.
23. Day S, MacIntyre NR. Ventilator alarm systems. Probl Respir Care 1991;4:118–126.
24. MacIntyre NR, Day S. Essentials for ventilator-alarm systems. Respir Care 1992;37:1108–1112.
25. Weingarten M. Respiratory monitoring of carbon dioxide and oxygen: A ten-year perspective. J Clin Monit 1990;6:217–225.

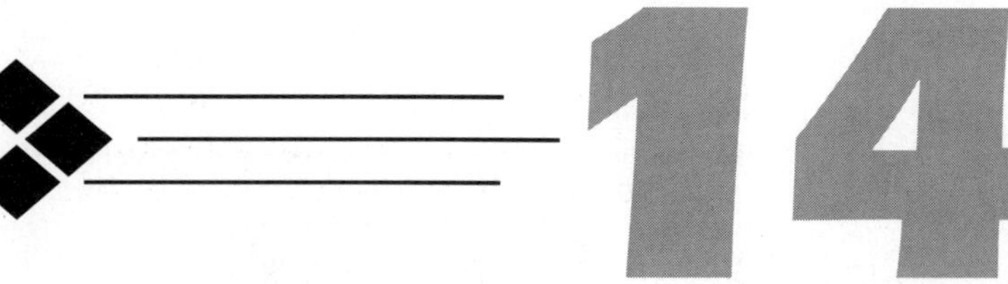

Mechanical Ventilators

Robert L. Chatburn
Richard D. Branson

OBJECTIVES

1. Classify adult and pediatric ventilators using the scheme in Chapter 13.
2. Describe the pneumatic circuitry of adult and pediatric ventilators.
3. List the modes available on adult and pediatric ventilators.
4. Describe the inspiratory waveforms available on adult and pediatric ventilators.
5. Describe the phase variables available on adult and pediatric ventilators.
6. Describe the drive mechanisms of adult and pediatric ventilators.
7. List the alarms available on pediatric and adult ventilators.
8. List the specific operator selections available on the control panel of adult and pediatric ventilators.

Introduction

In this chapter our focus is on describing a representative group of ventilators used in the United States. We have not divided this information into that for adult and pediatric ventilators or used any other arbitrary system. We believe that a critical care ventilator can be described by the classification system in Chapter 13 regardless of the intended patient population.

We did not attempt to describe every ventilator because of space limitations. Likewise, we did not attempt to describe devices only used outside the United States with which we were not familiar. This would have been a disservice to the manufacturers as well as the readers.

Table 14-1 provides a comparison of the devices discussed.

(Text continues on page 298)

TABLE 14-1. Comparison of Characteristics of Ventilators

	Bear 1	Bear 2	Bear 5	Bear 1000	Bear Cub	Bird 8400ST	Bird V.I.P.	Emerson 3MV	Hamilton Veolar	Infant Star Infrasonics	Adult Star Infrasonics	Newport Breeze	Newport E100i	Newport Wave	Puritan-Bennett MA-1	Puritan-Bennett 7200	PPG IRISA	Sechrist IV-100B	Sechrist 2200B	Siemens 900C	Siemens 300
Drive Power*																					
Pneumatic	•	•	•	•	•	•	•		•	•	•	•	•	•	•	•	•	•		•	•
Electric								•											•		
Drive Mechanism																					
Compressor																					
External			•	•	•	•	•		•	•	•	•	•	•		•	•	•		•	•
Internal	•	•						•							•				•		
Motor and linkage																					
Compressed gas/direct	•	•	•	•	•	•	•		•	•	•	•	•	•	•	•	•	•		•	•
Electric motor/crank								•													
Electric motor/threaded rod																			•		
Output control valves																					
Pneumatic diaphragm	•	•	•	•	•			•		•	•	•	•	•	•	•	•	•	•		
Pneumatic poppet valve											•	•	•								
Electric poppet valve	•	•		•	•					•		•	•	•		•	•	•	•		
Electric proportional valve			•	•		•	•		•		•			•		•	•		•	•	•
Control Scheme																					
Control circuit																					
Mechanical								•							•						
Pneumatic	•	•	•	•	•					•	•	•	•	•	•	•	•	•	•		
Fluidic																		•			
Electronic	•	•	•	•	•	•	•		•	•	•	•	•	•	•	•	•		•	•	•
Control variables																					
Pressure	•	•	•	•	•	•	•		•	•	•	•	•	•		•	•	•	•	•	•
Volume	•	•		•				•							•				•		
Flow			•		•	•	•		•	•	•	•	•	•		•	•	•		•	•
Phase variables																					
Trigger																					
Pressure	•	•	•	•		•	•		•		•	•	•	•	•	•	•		•	•	•
Volume Flow	•	•				•	5									•					•
Time	•	•	•	•	•	•	•	•	•	•	•	•	•	•	•	•	•	•	•	•	•
Manual	•	•	•	•	•	•	•	•	•	•	•	•	•	•	•	•	•	•	•	•	•
Optional External Source										•											
Limit variable																					
Pressure	•	•	•	•	•	•	•	•	•	•	•	•	•	•		•	•	•	•	•	•
Volume	•	•	•	•		•			•		•				•	•	•		•	•	•
Flow	•	•	•	•	•	•	•		•	•	•	•	•	•	•	•	•	•	•	•	•
Cycle variable																					
Pressure	•	•	•	•		•	•		•	•	•	•	•	•	•	•	•		•	•	•
Volume	•	•		•			•	•							•				•		
Flow			•	•		•	•		•		•			•		•	•		•	•	•
Time	•	•	•	•	•	•	•	•	•	•	•	•	•	•	•	•	•	•	•	•	•

(continued)

TABLE 14-1. Continued

	Bear 1	Bear 2	Bear 5	Bear 1000	Bear Cub	Bird 8400ST	Bird V.I.P.	Emerson 3MV	Hamilton Veolar	Infant Star Infrasonics	Adult Star Infrasonics	Newport Breeze	Newport E100i	Newport Wave	Puritan-Bennett MA-1	Puritan-Bennett 7200	PPG IRISA	Sechrist IV-100B	Sechrist 2200B	Siemens 900C	Siemens 300
Output																					
Pressure Rectangular			•	•		•	•	•	•	•	•	•	•	•		•	•	•	•	•	•
Exponential				•	•												•	•			•
Adjustable				•	3					3		3	3	3			•	3			
Volume Ascending ramp				•											4						
Sinusoidal									•												
Flow Rectangular	•	•	•	•	•	•	•		•	•	•	•	•	•			•	•	•	•	•
Ascending ramp			•						•		•								•		
Descending ramp	•	•	•	•		•			•		•					•			•		
Sinusoidal			•	•					•		•					•			•	•	
Adjustable	•																				
Alarms																					
Input power alarms Loss of electric power	•	•	•	•	•	•	•	•	•	•	•	•	•	•	•	•	•	•	•	•	•
Loss of pneumatic power	•	•	•	•	•	•	•	•	•	•	•	•	•	•	•	•	•	•	•	•	•
Control circuit alarms General systems failure	•	•	•	•	•	•	•	•	•	•	•			•		•	•		•		•
Incompatible settings				•	•				•	•	•			•							
Inverse I:E ratio	•	•	•	•	•	•					•		•	•	•	•					
Output alarms Pressure High peak	•	•	•	•		•	•	5	•	•	•	•	•	•	•		•		•	•	•
Low peak	•	•	•	•	•	•	•	5		•	•	•	•	•		•	•	•	•		
High baseline			•	•						•	•										
Low baseline	•	•	•	•	•	•	•		•	•	•					•					
High/low mean			•																		
Volume Low tidal volume	•	•	•								•					•			•		
Flow High minute ventilation			•	•					•					•			•		•	•	•
Low minute ventilation			•	•		•	5		•		•			•		•	•		•	•	•
Time High/low ventilatory rate		•	•	•		•	5		•		•					•	•		•		
Apnea	•	•				•	•		•			•	•			•	•			•	•
Inspired gas High/low F_{IO_2}								5	•								•		•	•	•
Mode Types																					
Volume-controlled CMV	•	•	•	1		•	•		•		•	•	•	•	•	•	•		•	•	•
Volume-controlled IMV/SIMV	•	•	•	1	•	•	•	•	•	•	•	•	•	•		•	•	•	•	•	•

(continued)

TABLE 14-1. Continued

	Bear 1	Bear 2	Bear 5	Bear 1000	Bear Cub	Bird 8400ST	Bird V.I.P.	Emerson 3MV	Hamilton Veolar	Infant Star Infrasonics	Adult Star Infrasonics	Newport Breeze	Newport E100i	Newport Wave	Puritan-Bennett MA-1	Puritan-Bennett 7200	PPG IRISA	Sechrist IV-100B	Sechrist 2200B	Siemens 900C	Siemens 300
Mode Types (cont)																					
Pressure-controlled CMV				•								•	•	•		•	•		•	•	6
Pressure-controlled IMV/SIMV			•	•	•		•	•		•		•	•	•		•	•	•	•		•
Pressure Support			•	2		•	•		•		•			•		•	•		•	•	6
Constant airway pressure	•	•	•	•	•	•	•		•	•	•	•	•	•		•	•	•	•		•
Mandatory minute ventilation			•	•					•								•		•		
Sigh	•	•	•	•		•					•	•			•	•			•	•	
Apnea backup ventilation																•					
Mode Descriptions																					
Mandatory Breaths																					
Control variable: Pressure			•	•	•		•	•		•		•	•	•		•	•	•	•	•	•
Volume	•	•						•							•				•		
Flow			•	•	•	•	•		•	•	•	•	•	•		•	•	•		•	•
Phase variable: Trigger: Pressure			•	•		•	•		•		•	•	•	•	•	•	•		•	•	•
Volume																					
Flow	•	•				•	5									•					•
Time	•	•	•	•	•	•	•	•	•	•	•	•	•	•	•	•	•	•	•	•	•
Manual	•	•	•	•	•	•	•	•	•	•	•	•	•	•	•	•	•	•	•	•	•
Option external source										•											
Limit variable: Pressure				•	•	•	•	•		•		•	•	•		•	•	•	•	•	•
Volume	•	•		•		•			•						•	•	•		•	•	•
Flow	•	•		•	•	•	•		•	•	•	•	•	•	•	•	•	•	•	•	•
Cycle variable: Pressure	•	•	•	•		•	•		•		•	•	•	•	•	•	•		•	•	•
Volume	•	•		•			•	•							•	•			•		
Flow				•															•		•
Time	•	•	•	•	•	•	•	•	•	•	•	•	•	•	•	•	•	•	•	•	•
Spontaneous Breaths																					
Control variable: Pressure	•	•	•	•	•	•	•	•	•	•	•	•	•	•		•	•	•	•	•	•
Phase variable: Trigger: Pressure	•	•	•	•		•	•		•		•			•		•	•		•	•	•
Volume																					
Flow						•	5									•					•
Limit variable: Pressure (to baseline only)	•	•			•			•		•		•	•					•			
Pressure (to baseline and above)			•	•		•	•		•		•			•		•	•		•	•	•

(continued)

TABLE 14-1. Continued

	Bear 1	Bear 2	Bear 5	Bear 1000	Bear Cub	Bird 8400ST	Bird V.I.P.	Emerson 3MV	Hamilton Veolar	Infant Star Infrasonics	Adult Star Infrasonics	Newport Breeze	Newport E100i	Newport Wave	Puritan-Bennett MA-1	Puritan-Bennett 7200	PPG IRISA	Sechrist IV-100B	Sechrist 2200B	Siemens 900C	Siemens 300
Spontaneous Breaths (cont)																					
Cycle variable																					
• Pressure	•	•				•	•									•	•		•		
• Flow			•	•		•	•		•					•		•	•		•	•	
Time						•	•														
• Bias flow				•	•		•	•		•	•	•	•	•		•		•			
Conditional variables																					
• Pressure			•	•		•	•		•		•	•	•	•	•	•	•		•	•	
• Tidal volume			•	•					•								•				
Minute volume			•	•					•								•				
• Flow	•	•				•	5									•					
• Time	•	•	•	•		•	•		•		•	•	•	•	•	•	•		•	•	

* Power source for generating breath; electricity is usually required for control system.

1 Patient will receive flow and volume beyond set values in response to increased demand.

2 Ventilator will switch to flow control during breath if tidal volume not delivered.

3 Pressure waveform adjustable as a function of pressure and flow settings.

4 Under heavy patient load, flow waveform degenerates to an exponential form.

5 Requires optional monitor.

6 Pressure limit adjusts automatically to achieve set tidal volume.

Types of Ventilators

BEAR 1

The Bear 1 ventilator (Bear Medical Corporation, Riverside, CA) (Fig. 14-1) is a pressure or flow controller that is triggered by a combination of pressure and flow or may be triggered manually. It may be volume or flow limited and pressure or time cycled. It has an integral compressor, air–oxygen blender, and a gas outlet port that will power a nebulizer during inspiration.

Input Variables

The Bear 1 uses 115 volts AC at 60 Hz to power the control circuitry. The main electrical power switch is located on the front panel. The pneumatic circuit, which includes an integral air–oxygen blender, operates on external compressed gas sources (ie, air and oxygen) at 25 to 100 psig. It has an internal compressor that will supply air at 9.5 psig if an external source is not available.

The front panel of the Bear 1 is illustrated in Figure 14-2 The operator may select the mode of ventilation, pressure-triggering and pressure-cycling thresholds, PEEP/CPAP, tidal volume, sigh volume, peak inspiratory flow rate, flow waveform, ventilatory frequency, inspiratory pause time, and F_{IO_2}.

Control Variables

The Bear 1 controls either inspiratory pressure or flow. It controls pressure in the CPAP mode and flow in the CONTROL and ASSIST/CONTROL modes. It switches between pressure control (for spontaneous breaths) and volume control (for mandatory breaths) in the SIMV mode.

INSPIRATORY WAVEFORMS. The Bear 1 offers a continuously adjustable inspiratory flow waveform by means of the WAVEFORM knob. The two extremes of

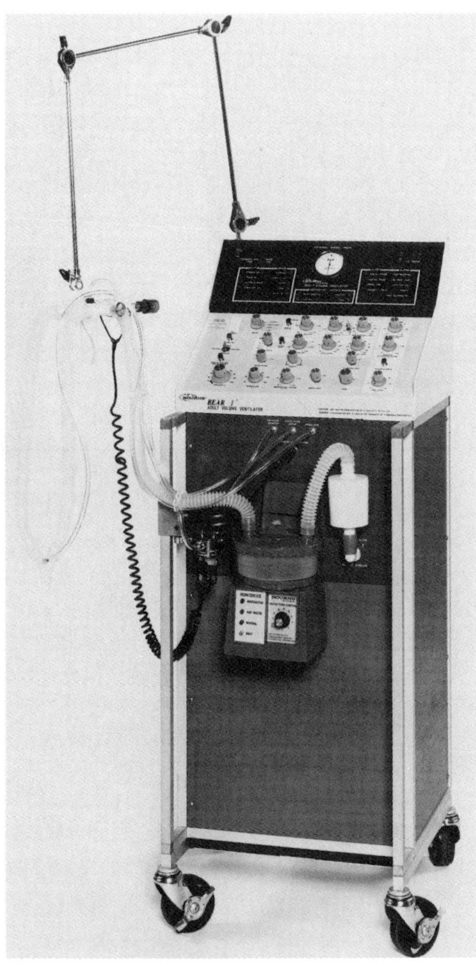

Figure 14-1. The Bear 1 ventilator. (Courtesy of Bear Medical Corporation, Riverside, CA)

the adjustable range yield rectangular and descending ramp waveforms. When the rectangular waveform is selected, the driving pressure to the peak flow valve (see Output Control Valves later) is set at 3.2 psig (225 cm H_2O), which is sufficient to maintain a nearly constant inspiratory flow rate even at high airway pressures. The rectangular waveform results in the shortest inspiratory time for a given tidal volume. When the descending ramp waveform (actually a truncated exponential decay waveform) is selected, the driving pressure is set at 1.8 psig (125 H_2O). Because this is not much higher than airway pressures commonly encountered with diseased lungs, inspiratory flow rate decays as tidal volume accumulates in the lungs and the airway pressure increases. A reduction in peak flow by a much as 50% may be obtained.

PHASE VARIABLES. Inspiration is pressure triggered when the patient receives all inspiratory flow from the demand valve (see Control Circuit later) during spontaneous breaths in the SIMV and CPAP modes. Inspiration is flow triggered when the patient inspires from the demand valve fast enough to cross the triggering threshold (see Control Circuit later). Triggering sensitivity is set with the ASSIST knob, although it is calibrated only as "less" or "more" sensitive. Time triggering is a function of the ventilator frequency, which is set with the NORMAL RATE knob over two ranges: 0.5 to 6 breaths per minute or 5 to 60 breaths per hour, depending on the setting of a "÷10" switch. Time triggering is also in effect when using the SIGH RATE and MULTIPLE dials. The SIGH RATE works only in the CONTROL and ASSIST/CONTROL modes and offers a range of 2 to 60 sighs per hour. The MULTIPLE switch allows two or three sighs to be delivered in a row, with each set delivered at the frequency set by the SIGH RATE knob. The Bear 1 may be manually triggered using either the SINGLE BREATH or the SINGLE SIGH pushbutton.

Inspiration is pressure limited during spontaneous breaths in both the SIMV and the CPAP modes. A demand valve controls inspiratory pressure (ie, attempts to maintain the set PEEP level) and may deliver an inspiratory flow rate of up to 100 L/min. Inspiration is volume limited whenever the inspiratory pause time is greater than zero. INSPIRATORY PAUSE may be adjusted from 0 to 2 seconds. Inspiration is flow limited for volume-controlled breaths. Peak inspiratory flow rate can be set over a range of 20 to 120 L/min.

Inspiration is terminated when one of three variables reaches a pre-set threshold. Inspiration may be pressure cycled using either the NORMAL PRESSURE LIMIT or the SIGH PRESSURE LIMIT knobs. Both may be set over a range of 0 to 100 cm H_2O. Active inspiratory flow from the demand valve is also pressure cycled for spontaneous breaths in the SIMV and CPAP modes. Inspiration is volume cycled because the Bear 1 measures instantaneous volume by integrating the signal from the flow transducer at the main flow control valve outlet. Tidal volume may be set from 100 to 2000 mL and sigh volume from 150 to 3000 mL. Inspiration is time cycled for volume-controlled breaths whenever the inspiratory pause time is set above zero. Inspiratory pause time is adjustable from 0 to 2.0 seconds. Inspiration is also time cycled if the I:E ratio exceeds 1:1 while the I:E RATIO LIMIT is on.

Baseline pressure may be adjusted from 0 to 30 cm H_2O using the PEEP/CPAP knob.

Control Subsystems

CONTROL CIRCUIT. The Bear 1 uses pneumatic, mechanical, and electronic control components (Fig. 14-3). In the SIMV and CPAP modes, a mechanical demand valve delivers flow to accommodate the patient's spontaneous inspiratory effort. If the patient withdraws enough volume from the circuit to drop

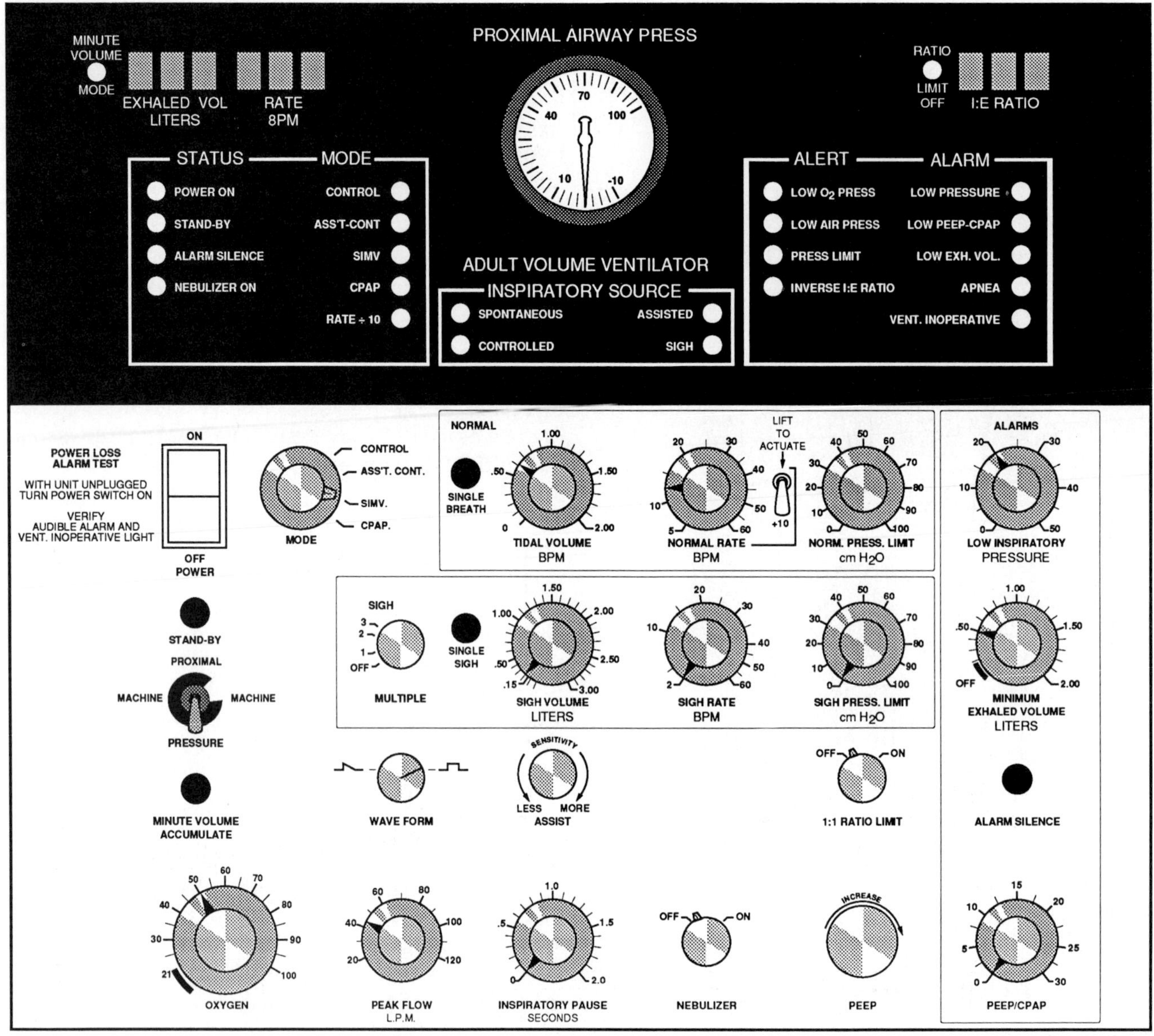

Figure 14-2. Control panel of the Bear 1 ventilator.

the pressure in the valve to a pre-set (and unchangeable) threshold of 1 cm H_2O below the baseline pressure (ie, PEEP), the valve opens and flow begins. Flow stops if the pressure rises above the threshold. Thus, flow rates of up to 100 L/min will be delivered to maintain the airway pressure at the desired baseline level.

The demand valve also plays a role in delivering mandatory breaths in the ASSIST/CONTROL and SIMV modes. A flow transducer (thermistor) measures the rate of change of inspiratory flow from the demand valve. If it senses a rate of sufficient magnitude as the patient begins to inspire, it provides a feedback signal to the main solenoid valve (see Output Control Valves later) that triggers the delivery of a pre-set tidal (or sigh) volume. The magnitude of flow change necessary to trigger inspiration (ie, the sensitivity) is adjusted by the ASSIST knob. If the patient inspires slowly enough, or if the sensor is not calibrated correctly, patient-initiated inspirations may not be triggered in the ASSIST/CONTROL mode or synchronized in the SIMV mode.

In the CONTROL mode, a "lockout solenoid" prevents gas from entering the demand valve, thus inactivating it.

Inspiratory flow rate is measured by a vortex-type flow transducer located between the peak flow control system and the patient circuit output port. During inspiration, the flow signal from the sensor is integrated to obtain a volume signal, which is compared with the tidal volume or sigh volume setting. When the desired volume is delivered, inspiration is terminated.

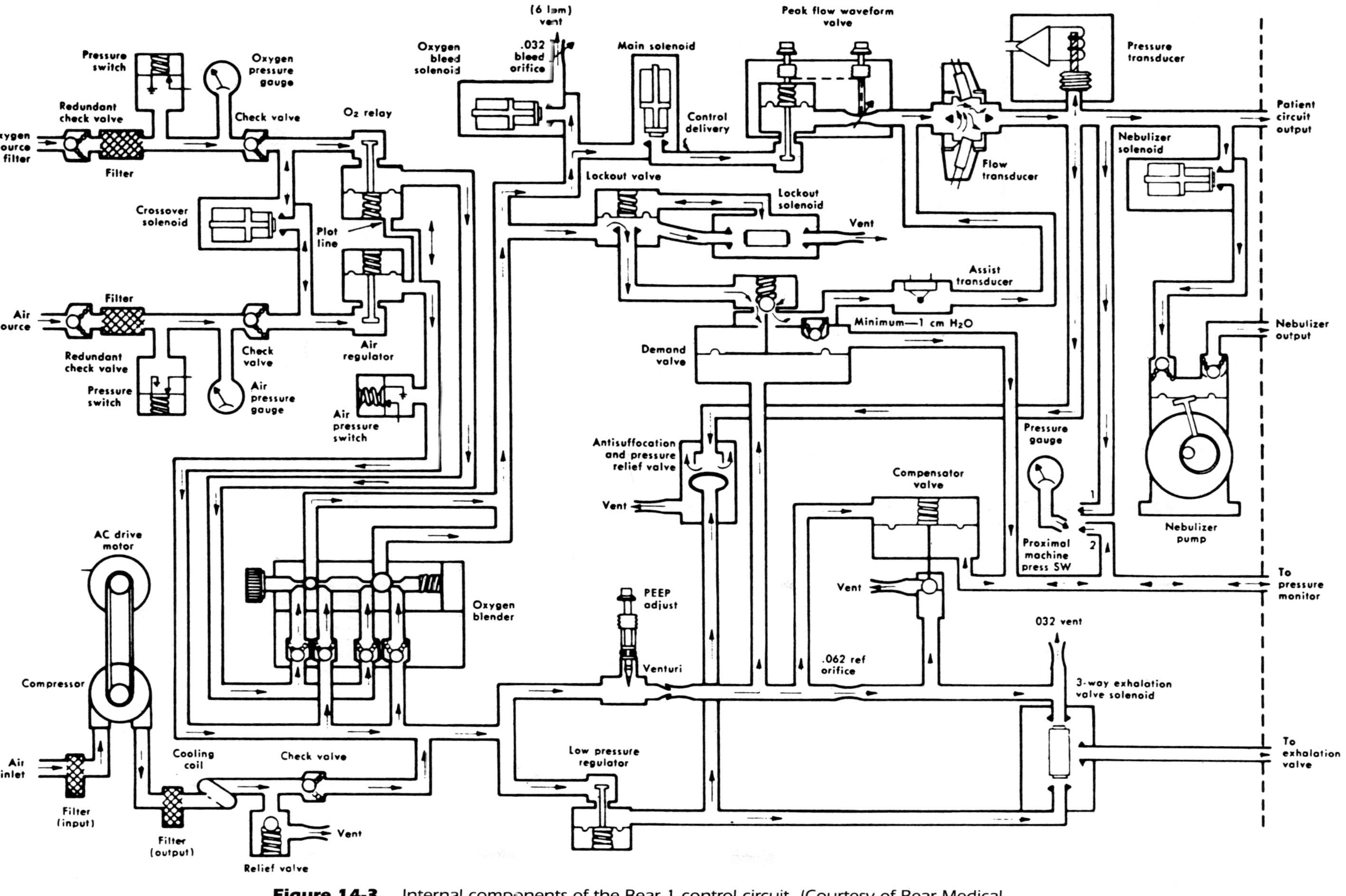

Figure 14-3. Internal components of the Bear 1 control circuit. (Courtesy of Bear Medical Corporation, Riverside CA)

A pressure transducer is located between the vortex flow transducer and the patient circuit output port. If the inspiratory pressure at that point exceeds the thresholds set by the NORMAL PRESSURE LIMIT or the SIGH PRESSURE LIMIT, inspiration is terminated. This transducer also provides the signal that operates the pressure alarms.

A pneumatic signal from a venturi device is directed to the exhalation manifold to control PEEP.

DRIVE MECHANISM. The Bear 1 uses either external compressed gas (for air and oxygen) or an electric motor and rotary vane-type compressor (for air) in conjunction with a pressure regulator. Gas pressure is initially reduced to about 10 psig before reaching the air–oxygen blender mechanism. The pressure is further reduced, after it leaves the blender, by the inspiratory flow waveform control system. The inspiratory flow waveform is adjusted by varying the driving pressure supplied to the PEAK FLOW valve. Driving pressure is controlled from 1.8 to 3.2 psig with a variable pressure regulator connected to the WAVE FORM knob. The effects of loading on this type of drive mechanism are similar to those described for the Puritan-Bennett MA-1 (see later). Gas from the blender also powers the demand valve.

OUTPUT CONTROL VALVES. There are several output control valves that work together to shape the inspiratory flow waveform. A main solenoid valve controls flow to the WAVEFORM and PEAK FLOW controls. At the same time that the main solenoid valve turns flow on, a three-way exhalation valve solenoid (inside the ventilator) sends a pneumatic signal to a mushroom-valve type exhalation manifold (outside the ventilator) that blocks gas from leaving the exhalation side of the patient circuit, thus forcing gas into the patient's lungs. Inspiratory flow rate is adjusted mechanically by a variable-orifice restrictor valve connected to the PEAK FLOW knob.

During expiration, the main solenoid valve is off and the three-way exhalation valve solenoid directs a pressure signal (adjusted by the PEEP knob) to the exhalation manifold to maintain baseline pressure.

Output Displays

Digital displays include exhaled tidal volume or minute volume, ventilatory frequency, and I:E ratio. An analog meter displays ventilating pressures. There are many LEDs that indicate ventilator status and operating and alarm conditions.

Modes of Operation

The following modes are those named on the mode selector switch of the Bear 1:

CONTROL. Inspiration is volume controlled, time triggered (according to the frequency set on the NORMAL RATE knob), may be volume limited (when using an inspiratory pause), is flow limited, and volume cycled.

ASSIST/CONTROL. The same as CONTROL except that inspiration may be flow triggered between time-triggered breaths, depending on the presence of spontaneous breathing efforts and the ASSIST sensitivity setting.

SIMV. Mandatory breaths are volume controlled, flow triggered (depending on the presence of spontaneous breathing efforts and the sensitivity setting) or time triggered (according to the frequency setting), and volume cycled. Spontaneous inspirations between mandatory breaths are pressure controlled (ie, inspiratory flow varies to maintain the set PEEP value), pressure triggered, and pressure cycled.

A mandatory breath is flow triggered the first time a spontaneous breathing effort is detected during each ventilatory period (the time equal to the reciprocal of the SIGH RATE). Subsequent breathing efforts during the same period will not trigger another mandatory breath. If a breathing effort is not detected during a given ventilatory period, a mandatory breath will be delivered at the beginning of the next period. The ventilator will continue to deliver mandatory breaths according to the SIGH RATE setting until a spontaneous breath is detected, and the sequence of events repeats itself.

CPAP. Spontaneous inspirations are pressure controlled (ie, inspiratory flow varies to maintain the set CPAP value), pressure triggered, and pressure cycled.

Alarms

INPUT POWER ALARMS. Visual and audible alarms are activated if the electrical or either pneumatic power supplies are interrupted. Separate visual and audible alarms are provided for the air and oxygen sources.

CONTROL VARIABLE ALARMS. Visual and audible alarms are activated if the peak inspiratory pressure (PIP) exceeds the NORMAL PRESSURE LIMIT setting (adjustable from 0 to 100 cm H_2O), if it fails to exceed the LOW INSPIRATORY PRESSURE setting (adjustable from 0 to 50 cm H_2O), or if end-expiratory pressure falls below the LOW PEEP/CPAP setting (adjustable from 0 to 30 cm H_2O).

Visual and audible alarms are activated if the exhaled tidal volume does not exceed the MINIMUM EXHALED VOLUME setting for three consecutive breaths (an external vortex-type flow sensor must be attached to the exhalation manifold). Alarm settings are adjustable from 0 to 2 L/min.

Visual and audible (APNEA) alarms activate if spontaneous or assisted breaths are more than 20 seconds apart.

CONTROL CIRCUIT ALARMS. Visual and audible alarms indicate either a flow sensor malfunction, that the I:E ratio is greater than 1:1, or that inspiratory flow above 20 L/min continues for more than 9 to 12 seconds. The digital I:E RATIO display will flash if the I:E ratio is less than 1:10.

BEAR 2

The Bear 2 ventilator (Bear Medical Corporation, Riverside, CA) (Fig. 14-4) is a pressure or volume controller that is triggered by a combination of pressure and flow or may be triggered manually. It may be volume or flow limited and pressure, volume, or time cycled. It has an integral compressor, air–oxygen blender, and a gas outlet port that will power a nebulizer during inspiration.

Input Variables

The Bear 2 uses 115 volts AC at 60 Hz to power the control circuitry. The main electrical power switch is located on the front panel. The pneumatic circuit, which includes an integral air–oxygen blender, operates on external compressed gas sources (ie, air and oxygen) at 25 to 100 psig. It has an internal compressor that will supply air at 9.5 psig if an external source is not available.

The front panel of the Bear 2 is illustrated in Figure 14-5. The operator may select the mode of ventilation, pressure-triggering and pressure-cycling thresholds, PEEP/CPAP, tidal volume, sigh volume, peak inspiratory flow rate, flow waveform, ventilatory frequency, inspiratory pause time, and F_{IO_2}.

Control Variables

The Bear 2 controls either inspiratory pressure or flow. It controls pressure in the CPAP mode and flow in the CONTROL and ASSIST/CONTROL modes. It switches between pressure control (for spontaneous breaths) and volume control (for mandatory breaths) in the SIMV mode.

INSPIRATORY WAVEFORMS. The Bear 2 offers an adjustable inspiratory flow waveform by means of the WAVEFORM switch. The two settings of the switch yield rectangular and descending ramp waveforms. When the rectangular waveform is selected, airway pressure is directed to the waveform regulator in a manner that provides positive feedback. That is, as airway pressure increases during inspiration, it augments the force of the regulator's spring, thus increasing the driving pressure and maintaining a constant inspiratory flow rate. The rectangular waveform results in the shortest inspiratory time for a given tidal volume. When the descending ramp waveform (actually a truncated exponential decay waveform) is selected, the waveform regulator is shut off from airway pressure and the driving pressure is determined solely by the regulator's spring tension. Because this force is not much higher than airway pressures commonly en-

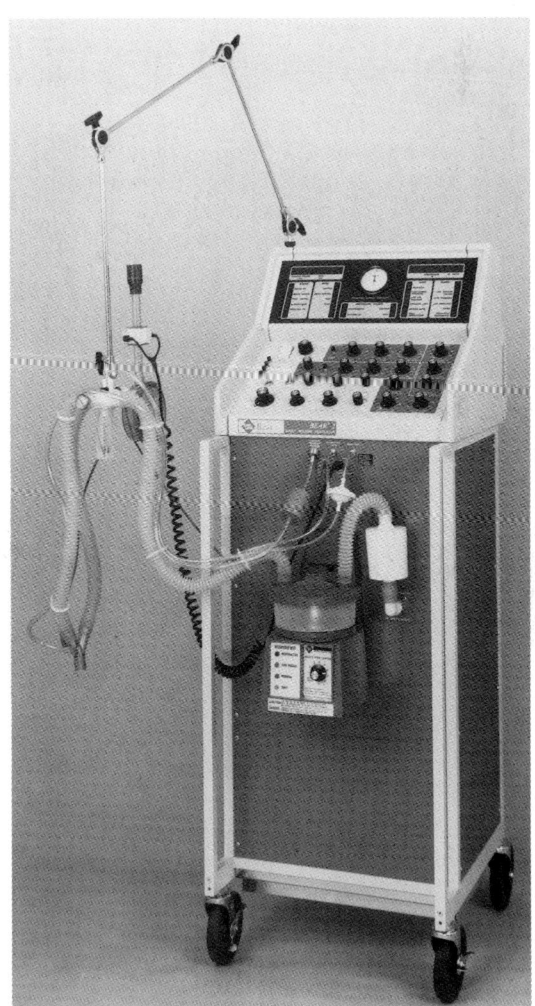

Figure 14-4. The Bear 2 ventilator. (Courtesy of Bear Medical Corporation, Riverside, CA)

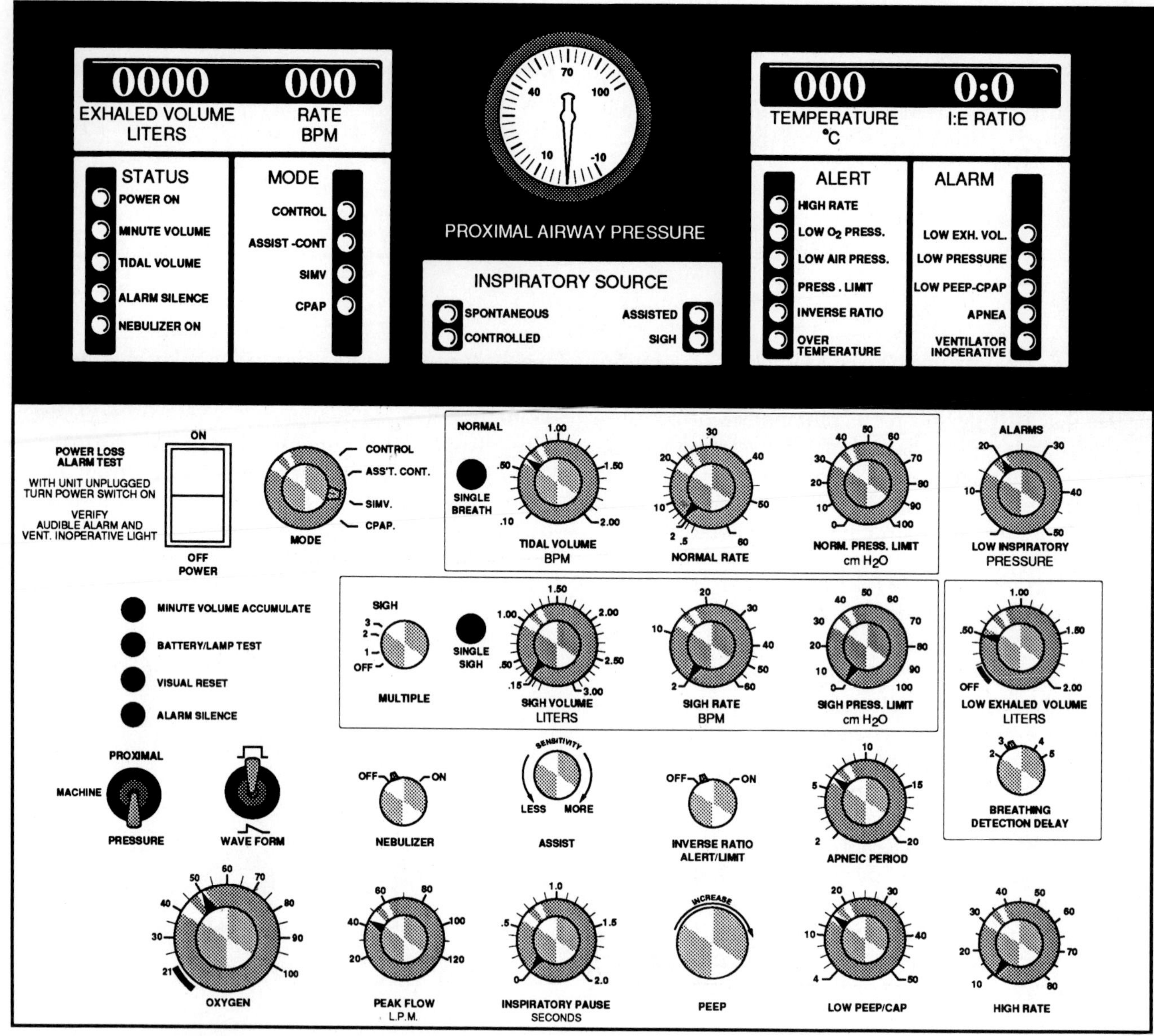

Figure 14-5. Control panel of the Bear 2 ventilator.

countered with diseased lungs, inspiratory flow rate decays as tidal volume accumulates in the lungs and the airway pressure increases. A reduction in peak flow by a much as 50% may be obtained, but flow rate will not drop below 10 L/min. If PEAK FLOW is set at 20 L/min, the waveform control system is bypassed and a rectangular waveform is delivered.

PHASE VARIABLES. Inspiration is pressure triggered when the patient receives all inspiratory flow from the demand valve (see Control Circuit later) during spontaneous breaths in the SIMV and CPAP modes. Inspiration is flow triggered when the patient inspires from the demand valve fast enough to cross the triggering threshold (see Control Circuit later). Triggering sensitivity is set with the ASSIST knob, although it is calibrated only as "less" or "more" sensitive. Time triggering is a function of the ventilator frequency, which is set with the NORMAL RATE knob from 0.5 to 60 breaths per minute. Time triggering is also in effect when using the SIGH RATE and MULTIPLE dials. The SIGH RATE works only in the CONTROL and ASSIST/CONTROL modes and offers a range of 2 to 60 sighs per minute. The MULTIPLE switch allows two or three sighs to be delivered in a row, with each set delivered at the frequency set by the SIGH RATE knob. The Bear 2 may be manually triggered using either the SINGLE BREATH or the SINGLE SIGH pushbutton.

Inspiration is pressure limited during spontaneous breaths in both the SIMV and the CPAP modes. A demand valve controls inspiratory pressure (ie, attempts to maintain the set PEEP level) and may deliver an inspiratory flow rate of up to 100 L/min. Inspiration is volume limited whenever the inspiratory pause time is greater than zero. INSPIRATORY PAUSE may be adjusted from 0 to 2 seconds. Inspiration is flow limited for volume-controlled breaths. Peak inspiratory flow rate can be set over a range of 20 to 120 L/min.

Inspiration is terminated when one of three variables reaches a pre-set threshold. Inspiration may be pressure cycled using either the NORMAL PRESSURE LIMIT or the SIGH PRESSURE LIMIT knobs. Both may be set over a range of 0 to 120 cm H_2O. Active inspiratory flow from the demand valve is also pressure cycled for spontaneous breaths in the SIMV and CPAP modes. Inspiration is volume cycled because the Bear 2 measures instantaneous volume by integrating the signal from the flow transducer at the main flow control valve outlet. Tidal volume may be set from 100 to 2000 mL and sigh volume from 150 to 3000 mL. Inspiration is time cycled when the inspiratory pause time is set above zero. Inspiratory pause time is adjustable from 0 to 2.0 seconds. Inspiration is also time cycled if the I:E ratio exceeds 1:1 while the I:E RATIO LIMIT is on.

Baseline pressure may be adjusted from 0 to 50 cm H_2O using the PEEP/CPAP knob.

Control Subsystems

CONTROL CIRCUIT. The Bear 2 uses pneumatic, mechanical, and electronic control components (Fig. 14-6). In the SIMV and CPAP modes, a mechanical demand valve delivers flow to accommodate the patient's spontaneous inspiratory effort. If the patient withdraws enough volume from the circuit to drop the pressure in the valve to a pre-set (and unchangeable) threshold of 1 cm H_2O below the baseline pressure (ie, PEEP), the valve opens and flow begins. Flow stops if the pressure rises above the threshold. Thus, flow rates of up to 100 L/min will be delivered to maintain the airway pressure at the desired baseline level.

The demand valve also plays a role in delivering mandatory breaths in the ASSIST/CONTROL and SIMV modes. A flow transducer (thermistor) measures the rate of change of inspiratory flow from the demand valve. If it senses a rate of sufficient magnitude as the patient begins to inspire, it provides a feedback signal to the main solenoid valve (see Output Control Valves later) that triggers the delivery of a pre-set tidal (or sigh) volume. The magnitude of flow change necessary to trigger inspiration (ie, the sensitivity) is adjusted by the ASSIST knob. If the patient inspires slowly enough, or if the sensor is not calibrated correctly, patient-initiated inspirations may not be triggered in the ASSIST/CONTROL mode or synchronized in the SIMV mode.

In the CONTROL mode, a "lockout solenoid" prevents gas from entering the demand valve, thus inactivating it.

Inspiratory flow rate is measured by a vortex-type flow transducer located between the peak flow control

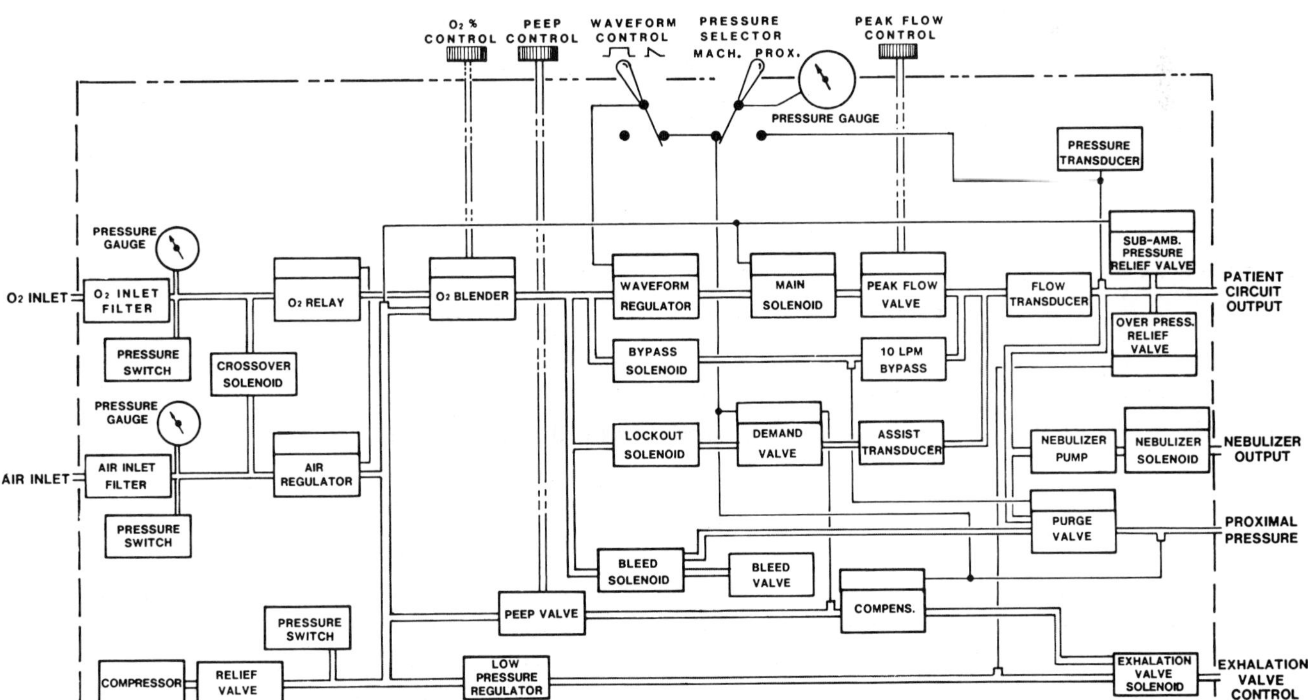

Figure 14-6. Internal components of the Bear 2 ventilator control circuit. (Courtesy of Bear Medical Corporation, Riverside, CA)

system and the patient circuit output port. During inspiration, the flow signal from the sensor is integrated to obtain a volume signal, which is compared with the tidal volume or sigh volume setting. When the desired volume is delivered, inspiration is terminated.

A pressure transducer is located between the vortex flow transducer and the patient circuit output port. If the inspiratory pressure at that point exceeds the thresholds set by the NORMAL PRESSURE LIMIT or the SIGH PRESSURE LIMIT, inspiration is terminated. This transducer also provides the signal that operates the pressure alarms.

A pneumatic signal from a venturi device is directed to the exhalation manifold to control PEEP.

DRIVE MECHANISM. The Bear 2 uses either external compressed gas (for air and oxygen) or an electric motor and rotary vane-type compressor (for air) in conjunction with a pressure regulator. Gas pressure is initially reduced to about 10 psig before reaching the air–oxygen blender mechanism. The pressure is further reduced, after it leaves the blender, by the inspiratory flow waveform control system. The inspiratory flow waveform is adjusted by varying the driving pressure supplied to the PEAK FLOW valve. Driving pressure is controlled from 1.8 to 3.2 psig with a variable pressure regulator connected to the WAVE FORM knob. The effects of loading on this type of drive mechanism are similar to those described for the Bennett MA-1 (see later). Gas from the blender also powers the demand valve.

OUTPUT CONTROL VALVES. There are several output control valves that work together to shape the inspiratory flow waveform. A main solenoid valve controls flow to the WAVEFORM and PEAK FLOW controls. At the same time that the main solenoid valve turns flow on, a three-way exhalation valve solenoid (inside the ventilator) sends a pneumatic signal to a mushroom-valve type exhalation manifold (outside the ventilator) that blocks gas from leaving the exhalation side of the patient circuit, thus forcing gas into the patient's lungs. Inspiratory flow rate is adjusted mechanically by a variable-orifice restrictor valve connected to the PEAK FLOW knob.

During expiration, the main solenoid valve is off and the three-way exhalation valve solenoid directs a pressure signal (adjusted by the PEEP knob) to the exhalation manifold to maintain baseline pressure.

Output Displays

Digital displays include exhaled tidal volume or minute volume, ventilatory frequency, and I:E ratio. An analog meter displays ventilating pressures. There are many LEDs that indicate ventilator status and operating and alarm conditions.

Modes of Operation

The following modes are those named on the mode selector switch of the Bear 2:

CONTROL. Inspiration is volume controlled, is time triggered (according to the frequency set on the NORMAL RATE knob), may be volume limited (when using an inspiratory pause), is flow limited, and volume cycled. Tidal volume remains relatively constant from breath to breath as determined by the TIDAL VOLUME and SIGH VOLUME settings.

ASSIST/CONTROL. This mode is the same as CONTROL except that inspiration may be flow triggered between time-triggered breaths, depending on the presence of spontaneous breathing efforts and the ASSIST sensitivity setting.

SIMV. Mandatory breaths are volume controlled, flow triggered (depending on the presence of spontaneous breathing efforts and the sensitivity setting) or time triggered (according to the frequency setting), and volume cycled. Spontaneous inspirations between mandatory breaths are pressure controlled (ie, inspiratory flow varies to maintain the set PEEP value), pressure triggered, and pressure cycled.

A mandatory breath is flow triggered the first time a spontaneous breathing effort is detected during each ventilatory period (the time equal to the reciprocal of the SIGH RATE). Subsequent breathing efforts during the same period will not trigger another mandatory breath. If a breathing effort is not detected during a given ventilatory period, a mandatory breath will be delivered at the beginning of the next period. The ventilator will continue to deliver mandatory breaths according to the SIGH RATE setting until a spontaneous breath is detected and the sequence of events repeats itself.

CPAP. Spontaneous inspirations are pressure controlled (ie, inspiratory flow varies to maintain the set CPAP value), pressure triggered, and pressure cycled.

Alarms

INPUT POWER ALARMS. Visual and audible alarms are activated if the electrical or both pneumatic power supplies are interrupted. Separate visual and audible alarms are provided for the air and oxygen sources.

CONTROL VARIABLE ALARMS. Visual and audible alarms are activated if the PIP exceeds the NORMAL PRESSURE LIMIT setting (adjustable from 0 to 120 cm H_2O), if it fails to exceed the LOW INSPIRATORY PRESSURE setting (adjustable from 3 to 75 cm H_2O) during inspiration or drops below it during expiration, or if end-expiratory pressure falls below the LOW PEEP/CPAP setting (adjustable from off to 50 cm H_2O). The LOW PEEP/CPAP alarms will also be activated if the internal flow transducer detects flow in excess of 25 L/min for 7 to 9 seconds.

Visual and audible alarms are activated if the exhaled tidal volume does not exceed the LOW EXHALED VOLUME setting for the number of breaths selected by the DETECTION DELAY knob (an external vortex-type flow sensor must be attached to the exhalation manifold). Alarm settings are adjustable from off/0 to 2 L/min.

Visual and audible alarms are activated if the total respiratory frequency exceeds the HIGH RATE setting, which is adjustable from 10 to 80 breaths per minute.

Visual and audible (APNEA) alarms activate if the interval between spontaneous or assisted breaths exceeds the APNEIC PERIOD setting.

CONTROL CIRCUIT ALARMS. Visual and audible alarms indicate either a flow sensor malfunction, that the I:E ratio is greater than 1:1, or that inspiratory flow above 20 L/min continues for more than 9 to 12 seconds. The digital I:E RATIO display will flash if the I:E ratio is less than 1:10 or if the inspiratory time exceeds 6 seconds.

BEAR 5

The Bear 5 ventilator (Bear Medical Corporation, Riverside, CA) (Fig. 14-7) is a pressure or flow controller that may be pressure, time, or manually triggered; pressure, volume, or flow limited; and pressure, flow, or time cycled. It has an optional compressor, an integral air–oxygen blender, and a gas outlet port that will power a nebulizer during inspiration.

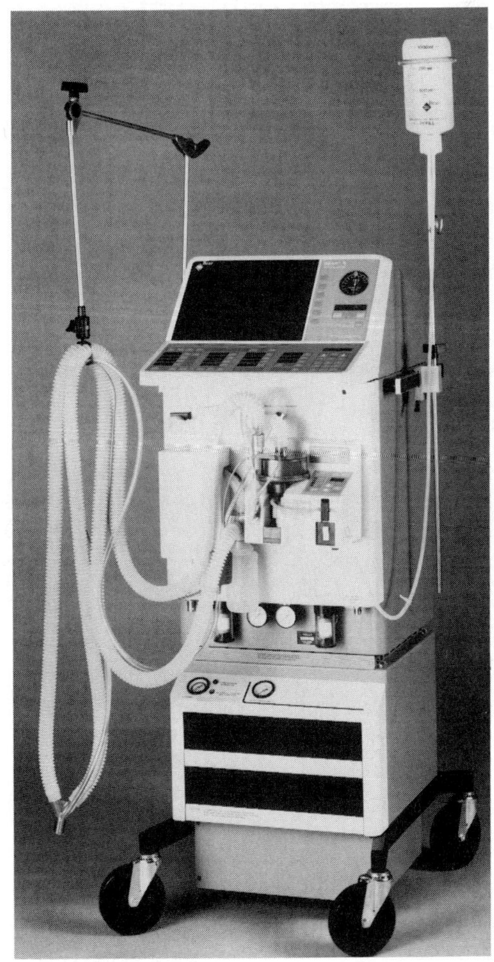

Figure 14-7. The Bear 5 ventilator. (Courtesy of Bear Medical Corporation, Riverside, CA)

Input Variables

The Bear 5 uses 115 volts AC at 60 Hz to power the control circuitry. The pneumatic circuit, which includes an integral air–oxygen blender, operates on external compressed gas sources (ie, air and oxygen) at 30 to 100 psig.

The front panel of the Bear 5 is illustrated in Figure 14-8 The operator may select the mode of ventilation; pressure-triggering, pressure-limiting, and pressure-cycling thresholds; PEEP/CPAP; tidal volume; sigh volume; peak inspiratory flow rate; flow waveform; ventilatory frequency; inspiratory pause time; and F_{IO_2}. Settings are selected using a keypad in conjunction with a CRT display.

Control Variables

The Bear 5 controls either inspiratory pressure or flow. It controls inspiratory pressure in the TIME CYCLE, PRESSURE SUPPORT, and CPAP modes, and flow in the CONTROL, ASSIST/CONTROL, and AUGMENTED MINUTE VOLUME modes. It switches between pressure control (for spontaneous breaths) and

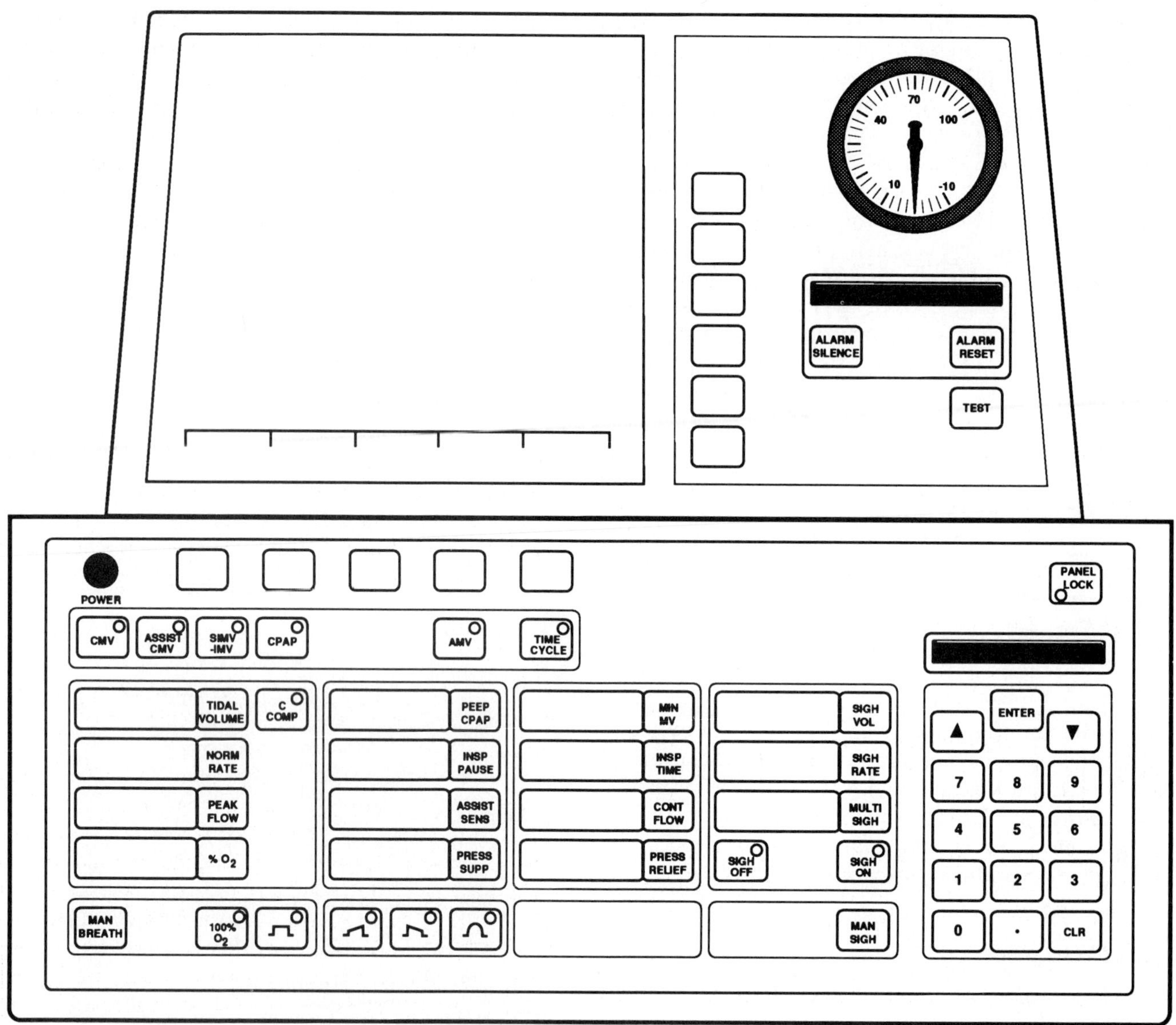

Figure 14-8. Control panel of the Bear 5 ventilator.

flow control (for mandatory breaths) in the IMV and SIMV modes.

INSPIRATORY WAVEFORMS. The Bear 5 offers one inspiratory pressure and four inspiratory flow waveforms. A rectangular pressure waveform can be achieved in the time-cycled or pressure-support modes. Flow waveforms include square (rectangular), accelerating (ascending ramp), decelerating (descending ramp), and sine. Gas delivery with the rectangular waveform is relatively constant at the peak flow setting. With the ascending ramp waveform, inspiratory flow begins at 50% of peak flow setting and increases linearly to peak flow. Conversely, it begins at the peak flow value with the descending ramp waveform and decreases linearly to 50% of peak flow by end-inspiration. When the sine waveform is selected, inspiratory flow goes from zero to peak flow and back to zero in a sinusoidal fashion.

PHASE VARIABLES. Inspiration is pressure triggered when a spontaneous ventilatory effort removes enough gas from the patient circuit to drop the pressure below the assist sensitivity threshold. The threshold for triggering a mandatory breath is adjustable from 0.5 to 5.0 cm H_2O below the baseline pressure. Sensitivity for spontaneous breathing from the demand valve is pre-set and nonadjustable at 0.5 H_2O below the baseline pressure. Inspiration is time triggered as a function of the ventilator frequency or normal rate, which is adjustable from 0 to 150 cycles/min. Time triggering is also in effect when using the sigh rate and multiple sigh functions. The sigh rate works in all modes except time cycle and is adjustable from 2 to 60 sighs per minute. The multiple sigh function allows two or three sighs to be delivered in a row, with each set delivered at the frequency set by the sigh rate. The Bear 5 may also be manually triggered.

Inspiration is pressure limited during spontaneous breaths in the PRESSURE SUPPORT, TIME CYCLE, and the PEEP/CPAP modes. A demand valve controls inspiratory pressure by attempting to maintain the set PEEP/CPAP level, which is adjustable from 0 to 50 cm H_2O, if pressure support is not used. If pressure support is used, the pressure limit may be set from 0 to 72 cm H_2O above the PEEP/CPAP level. Inspiration is volume limited whenever the inspiratory pause time is greater than zero. Inspiration is flow limited for flow-controlled breaths. Peak inspiratory flow rate can be pre-set over a range of 5 to 150 L/min, although peak flow for a spontaneous breath can be as high as 170 L/min. Inspiration will also be flow limited at the continuous-flow setting in the TIME CYCLE mode if inspiration ends before the airway pressure reaches the pressure relief threshold. The continuous flow rate can be adjusted from 5 to 40 L/min, although flow of up to 170 L/min is available if the patient tries to inspire at a flow rate higher than the pre-set value.

Inspiration is terminated when one of three variables reaches a pre-set threshold. Inspiration may be pressure cycled when either the high peak normal pressure limit or the high peak sigh pressure limit thresholds are violated. Both may be set over a range of 0 to 140 cm H_2O (0 to 80 cm H_2O in the TIME CYCLE mode). Active inspiratory flow is also pressure cycled for spontaneous breaths when pressure support is not used (when expiration causes airway pressure to rise above the PEEP setting). Inspiration cannot be volume cycled because the Bear 5 does not measure instantaneous volume. However, when inspiration is flow controlled, tidal volume may be set from 50 to 2000 mL and sigh volume from 65 to 3000 mL. Inspiration is flow cycled in the PRESSURE SUPPORT mode when inspiratory flow rate decays to 25% of the set peak flow rate. Inspiration is time cycled for flow-controlled breaths whenever the inspiratory time reaches the value determined by the volume and flow rate settings. Inspiration is time cycled when the inspiratory pause time is set above zero. Inspiratory pause time is adjustable from 0 to 2.0 seconds. Inspiration is also time cycled according to the inspiratory time setting (adjustable from 0.1 to 3.0 seconds) in the time cycle mode.

Baseline pressure may be adjusted from 0 to 50 cm H_2O using the PEEP/CPAP function.

Control Subsystems

CONTROL CIRCUIT. The Bear 5 uses pneumatic and electronic control components (Fig. 14-9). A Motorola MC 68000 16-bit microprocessor accepts input signals from a pressure transducer (which measures pressure at the airway opening), an internal (vortex-type) flow transducer, and the control variable settings and outputs control signals to the output control valves. Feedback from the airway pressure transducer is used to provide triggering, cycling, and alarm signals and to control the airway pressure waveform during pressure-controlled breaths. A pneumatic signal from a venturi device is directed to the exhalation manifold to control inspiratory pressure and PEEP.

Flow is delivered to the patient circuit whenever the following holds true:

$$\text{Pre-set baseline pressure} - \text{airway opening pressure} - 0.5 = \text{a positive number}$$

A positive number may result from a leak in the patient circuit or when the patient tries to inspire at a flow rate greater than the peak flow setting. Flow ceases when the equation evaluates to a negative number.

A second pressure transducer monitors the primary pressure transducer. If the two signals do not agree within ± 6 cm H_2O, a ventilator inoperative condition is created.

Information from the flow transducer provides the feedback for shaping the inspiratory flow waveform and for calculating delivered volume. A temperature sensor (thermistor) is located downstream of the the flow transducer. It generates a signal used by the microprocessor to convert gas delivery to the BTPS (body temperature, pressure, saturated) standard. In addition, the operator has the ability to input the value of the patient circuit compliance and the ventilator will automatically adjust the delivered volume to compensate for the volume normally compressed in the patient circuit. Under these conditions, the inspiratory time (determined by the tidal volume and peak flow settings) is held constant and the ventilator adds volume by increasing the inspiratory flow rate by an amount determined by the patient circuit compliance (ie, flow added = [compliance factor × end-inspiratory pressure of previous breath ÷ inspiratory time). In this way, both the pre-set tidal volume and peak flow rate are delivered to the airway opening, assuming that the compliance factor is accurate.

An external vortex-type flow transducer is used to measure exhaled volumes for display and alarm functions. When compliance compensation is used, the added volume is automatically subtracted from the exhaled volume measurement. Because exhaled volume is used in the calculation of respiratory mechanics, the displayed value for static compliance is for the respiratory system only and does not include the ventilator system compliance.

The inspired oxygen concentration is also controlled by the microprocessor by means of a stepper motor that adjusts a pneumatic blender. The expected error in oxygen concentration within a breath is about ± 0.2% (1% worst case) while the overall error of the

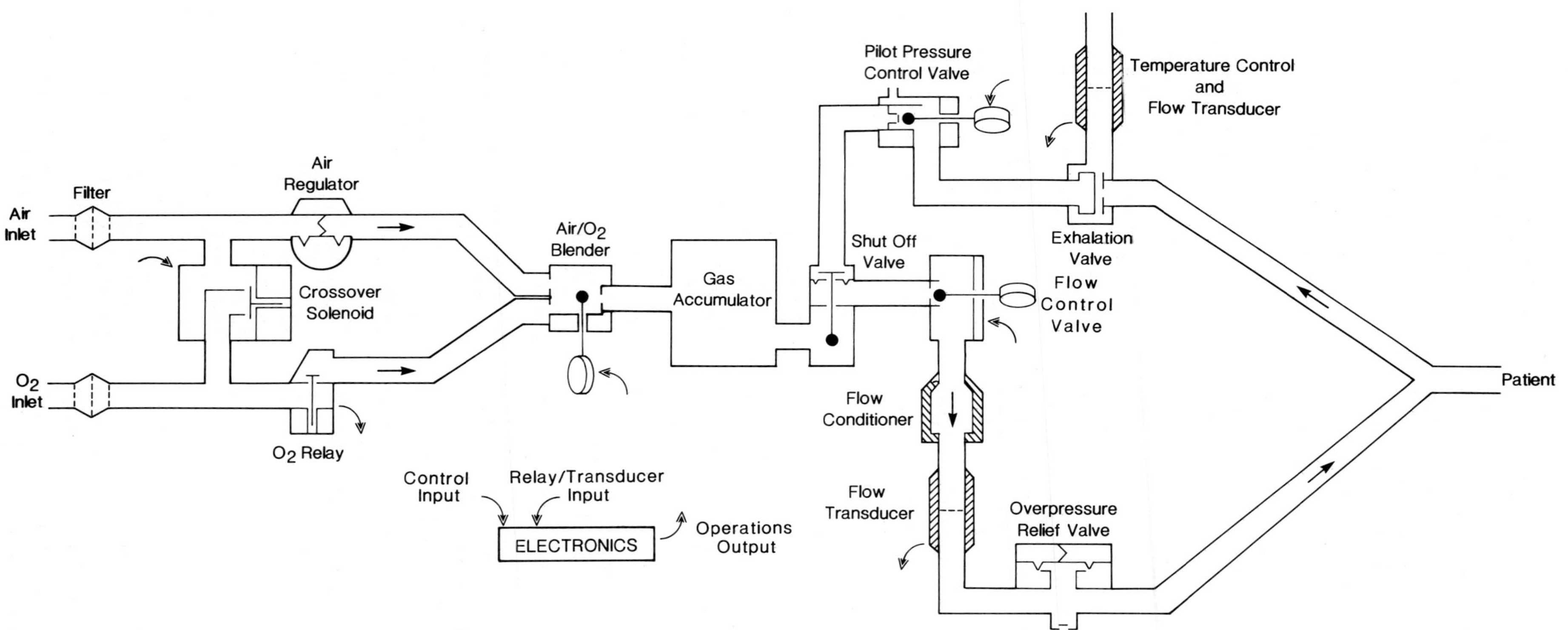

Figure 14-9. Internal components of the Bear 5 ventilator control circuit.

blending system over the range of 21% to 100% is about ± 3%.

DRIVE MECHANISM. The Bear 5 uses either external compressed gas (for air and oxygen) or an electric motor and rotary vane–type compressor (for air) in conjunction with a pressure regulator. Gas pressure is initially regulated to about 18 psig before reaching the air–oxygen blender mechanism. Mixed gas leaves the blender and enters a rigid-walled vessel (the "accumulator") with an internal volume of about 3.6 L. The flow control system is driven by the pressure from the accumulator. The pressure inside the accumulator varies from 10 to 18 psig, representing a stored (ie, compressed) gas volume of 6 to 8 L. During a flow demand, the volume stored in the accumulator is exhausted quickly, reducing the instantaneous flow demand required of the blending system and upstream pressure regulating system. This action allows a wide range of peak flow settings, reduces the flow required of the compressed gas supply, and improves response time. The accumulator also acts as a mixing chamber, which helps to stabilize the delivered oxygen concentration within a given breath.

OUTPUT CONTROL VALVES. All gas flow to the patient is regulated by the main flow control valve, which is a pneumatic valve connected to a stepper motor. Another stepper motor is connected to the pilot pressure control valve that supplies a pneumatic signal to the exhalation valve. The microprocessor coordinates the activity of both valves such that the exhalation valve closes as the flow control valve begins to deliver flow to the patient circuit.

The flow control system is capable of delivering calibrated peak flow up to 150 L/min and demand flow (in response to spontaneous inspiratory efforts) up to 170 L/min. In all modes, there is a continuous background or bias flow of 5 L/min through the patient circuit. This improves the accuracy of the the oxygen blending system at low flows, enhances the response time of the demand system, and improves the accuracy of volume measurement.

There is a 90 to 140 mL/min bleed flow of blended gas directed through the proximal airway pressure line. This discourages the accumulation of condensation in the line that might interfere with pressure measurement.

Output Displays

In addition to the various control settings, the CRT displays include inspiratory source indicators (ie, whether a breath was controlled, assisted, spontaneous, etc.); mandatory and spontaneous tidal volumes; minute volume; peak, mean, and baseline airway pressures; and a wide variety of alarm and special operational help messages. An analog pressure gauge provides redundant airway pressure measurement over the range of −10 to 150 cm H_2O.

Exhaled volumes are displayed after being measured by an external flow transducer. All volume measurements are converted to BTPS and corrected for the volume of gas compressed in the patient circuit during inspiration (ie, to provide an accurate estimate of true exhaled volumes). The Bear 5 also calculates and displays static compliance and resistance, which requires the use of an inspiratory pause. Real-time display of pressure, volume, and flow waveforms can be viewed on the CRT. Analog and digital signals of the measured and calculated data may be output from the back of the ventilator.

Modes of Operation

The following modes are those named on the control panel of the Bear 5:

CMV. During continuous mechanical ventilation, inspiration is flow controlled, is time triggered (according to the normal rate setting), may be volume limited (when using an inspiratory pause), is flow limited, and time cycled. Tidal volume remains relatively constant from breath to breath as determined by the tidal volume and sigh volume settings.

ASSIST CMV. This is the same as CMV except that inspiration may be pressure triggered between time-triggered breaths, depending on the presence of spontaneous breathing efforts and the assist sensitivity setting.

SIMV/IMV. In SIMV, mandatory breaths are flow controlled, pressure triggered (depending on the presence of spontaneous breathing efforts and the sensitivity setting) or time triggered (according to the frequency setting), and time cycled.

Spontaneous inspirations between mandatory breaths are pressure controlled (ie, inspiratory flow varies to maintain the set PEEP value), pressure triggered, and either pressure or flow cycled, depending on whether the pressure support function is used.

A mandatory breath is pressure triggered the first time a spontaneous breathing effort is detected during each ventilatory period (the time equal to the reciprocal of the normal rate). Subsequent breathing efforts during the same period will not trigger another mandatory breath. If a breathing effort is not detected during a given ventilatory period, a mandatory breath will be delivered at the beginning of the next period. The ventilator will continue to deliver mandatory breaths according to the normal rate setting until a spontaneous breath is detected, and the sequence of events repeats itself.

If the continuous flow function is used, the ventilator will deliver a fixed number of mandatory breaths according to the normal rate setting with a continuous bias flow delivered through the patient circuit. Mandatory breaths will not be synchronized with the patient's inspiratory efforts.

CPAP. Spontaneous inspirations are pressure controlled (ie, inspiratory flow varies to maintain either the set CPAP or pressure support value), pressure triggered, and pressure or flow cycled, depending on whether pressure support is activated.

AMV. Augmented minute ventilation (AMV) is identical to SIMV except that the average exhaled minute volume must exceed the threshold determined by the minimum minute volume setting. If it does not, a new backup rate (greater than the normal rate) is established according to the equation:

$$\frac{\text{Backup rate}}{\text{(cycles/min)}} = \frac{\text{Minimum minute volume setting (L/min)}}{\text{Tidal volume setting (L/cycle)}}$$

The ventilator will resume operation at the normal rate when the average exhaled minute volume exceeds the threshold by 1 L or 10%, whichever is less.

TIME CYCLE. Inspiration is usually pressure controlled, time triggered (according to the the normal rate setting), pressure limited (at the pressure relief setting), and time cycled according to the inspiratory time setting. The continuous-flow function is used to provide for spontaneous breathing between time-triggered breaths. By definition, inspiration is flow controlled if it ends before the pressure relief threshold is met.

PRESSURE SUPPORT. Unlike some other ventilators, the Bear 5 does not treat PRESSURE SUPPORT as a separate mode of ventilation. Rather, it is used to assist spontaneous breaths in the SIMV, AMV, and CPAP modes. If a spontaneous effort drops the airway opening pressure below the assist sensitivity threshold, then inspiration is pressure limited to the PRESSURE SUPPORT setting and flow cycled when the inspiratory flow rate decays to 25% of the peak flow setting.

Alarms

INPUT POWER ALARMS. Visual and audible alarms are activated if the electrical or pneumatic power supplies drop below pre-set levels (102 volts and 27 psig, respectively). Separate visual and audible alarms are provided for the air and oxygen sources.

CONTROL VARIABLE ALARMS. There are seven visual and audible alarms associated with ventilating pressures. These include low (0 to 50 cm H_2O) and high (0 to 55 cm H_2O) PEEP/CPAP, low and high mean airway pressure (both 0 to 75 cm H_2O), low inspiratory pressure, high peak normal pressure, and high peak sigh pressure (all 0 to 140 cm H_2O; high peak normal pressure in TIME CYCLE mode is 0 to 80 cm H_2O).

There are four visual and audible alarms associated with exhaled volumes. Three consecutive mechanical breaths below the threshold setting activate the low mandatory volume alarm (0 to 3000 mL). Three consecutive spontaneous breaths below the alarm setting activate the low spontaneous volume alarm (0 to 3000 mL). There are also low (0.3 to 40 L/min) and high (1.0 to 80 L/min) exhaled minute volume alarms.

There are visual and audible alarms for low (3 to 155 cycles/min) and high (3 to 155 cycles/min) breath rate. Low (0.05 to 3.00 seconds) and high (0.10 to 3.20 seconds) inspiratory time alarms are available in the TIME CYCLE mode.

Alarm thresholds may be set either manually or by allowing the ventilator to provide automatic ranging for the variables specific to the given mode of ventilation.

CONTROL CIRCUIT ALARMS. Visual and audible alarms indicate flow sensor malfunction, prolonged high airway pressure, and airway pressure reaching the maximum working pressure (150 cm H_2O or 90 cm H_2O in TIME CYCLE mode). All of these alarms will be indicated by name on the CRT display and will be accompanied by a ventilator-inoperative message. A visual alert is activated if the temperature control chamber door is left open. This may progress to a low temperature alert and, if uncorrected, will progress to a ventilator-inoperative condition.

There are two visual and audible alarms associated with the I:E ratio. If the I:E ratio limit function is enabled, the alarms will be activated if the tidal volume, normal rate, and peak flow settings result in an I:E ratio greater than 1:1. If the I:E ratio limit function is overridden, the maximum allowable I:E ratio is 3:1. Tidal volume, normal rate, and peak flow settings that would result in I:E ratios greater than 3:1 activate the alarms, and the actual I:E ratio is limited to 3:1.

BEAR 1000

The Bear 1000 ventilator (Bear Medical Corporation, Riverside, CA) (Fig. 14-10) is a pressure or volume controller that may be pressure, time, or manually triggered; pressure, volume, or flow limited; and pressure, volume, flow, or time cycled. It can also combine pressure and flow control within a single breath (see discussion of pressure augmentation in section on Modes of Operation). The Bear 1000 has an optional compressor, an integral air–oxygen blender, and a gas outlet port that will power a nebulizer during inspiration.

Input Variables

The Bear 1000 uses 115 volts AC at 60 Hz to power the control circuitry. The pneumatic circuit operates on external compressed gas sources (ie, air and oxygen) at 27.5 psig.

The front panel of the Bear 1000 is illustrated in Figure 14-11. The design of the panel incorporates flat panel touch keys (with associated digital displays) to select variables and a single control knob to set the selected variable. Each touch key is labeled and has an LED that lights if that variable is available in the selected mode. The front panel is divided into three groups of displays: one for controls, one for monitors, and one for alarms.

On the control panel, the operator may select the mode of ventilation, pressure-triggering and pressure-limiting thresholds, pressure slope (see Waveforms), tidal volume, compliance compensation factor (adds to set tidal volume to compensate for patient circuit compliance), inspiratory flow rate, inspiratory flow waveform, minimum minute volume (MMV), ventilatory frequency, inspiratory time, inspiratory pause time, and F_{IO_2}. PEEP/CPAP is controlled by a separate knob located under the aneroid pressure gauge.

Control Variables

The Bear 1000 controls either inspiratory pressure or volume. It controls inspiratory pressure in the CPAP and PRESSURE CONTROL modes, and volume in the ASSIST CMV, SIMV, and MMV modes. It switches between pressure control (for spontaneous breaths) and volume control (for mandatory breaths) in the SIMV (PSV) and MMV modes. It switches between pressure control and volume control within a breath when PRESSURE AUGMENT is activated in the ASSIST CMV and SIMV modes. The ventilator will switch from volume control to pressure control within a breath if the patient demands more flow than is set and drops airway pressure below the set PEEP. In this case, the ventilator will increase flow to maintain the PEEP level.

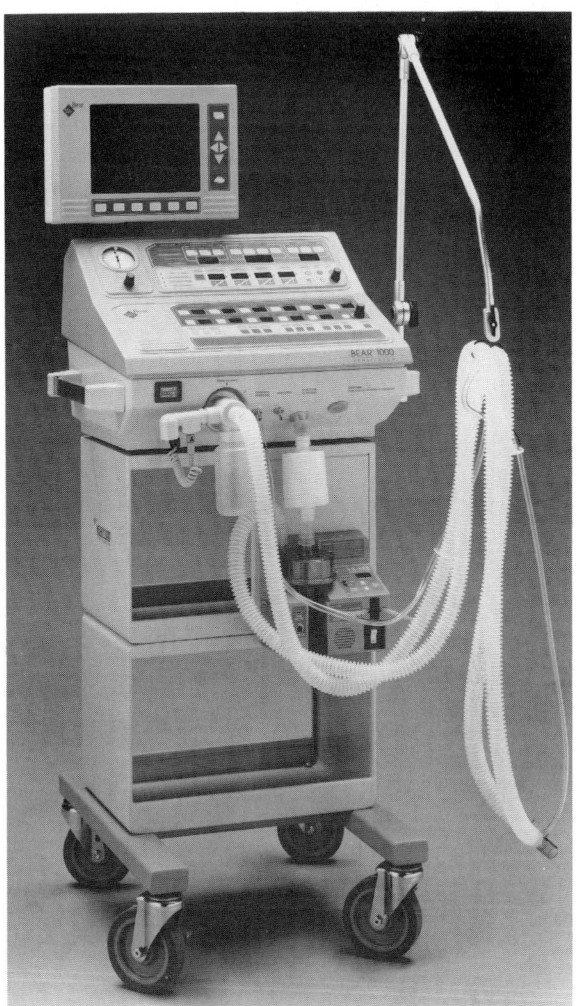

Figure 14-10. The Bear 1000 ventilator. (Courtesy of Bear Medical Corporation, Riverside, CA)

INSPIRATORY WAVEFORMS. The Bear 1000 offers a variable inspiratory pressure and three inspiratory flow waveforms. A rectangular pressure waveform can be achieved in the PRESSURE CONTROL mode and when pressure support is used to assist spontaneous breaths. A PRESSURE SLOPE control permits the adjustment of the pressure–time relation for pressure-limited breaths. That is, the pressure can be made to rise slowly or quickly to the limit, whichever is required by patient demand and patient circuit mechanics. Flow waveforms include SQUARE (rectangular), DECELERATING (descending ramp), and SINE. Gas delivery with the rectangular waveform is relatively constant at the PEAK FLOW setting. For the descending ramp waveform, flow begins at the PEAK FLOW value and decreases linearly to 50% of peak flow by end-inspiration. When the SINE waveform is selected,

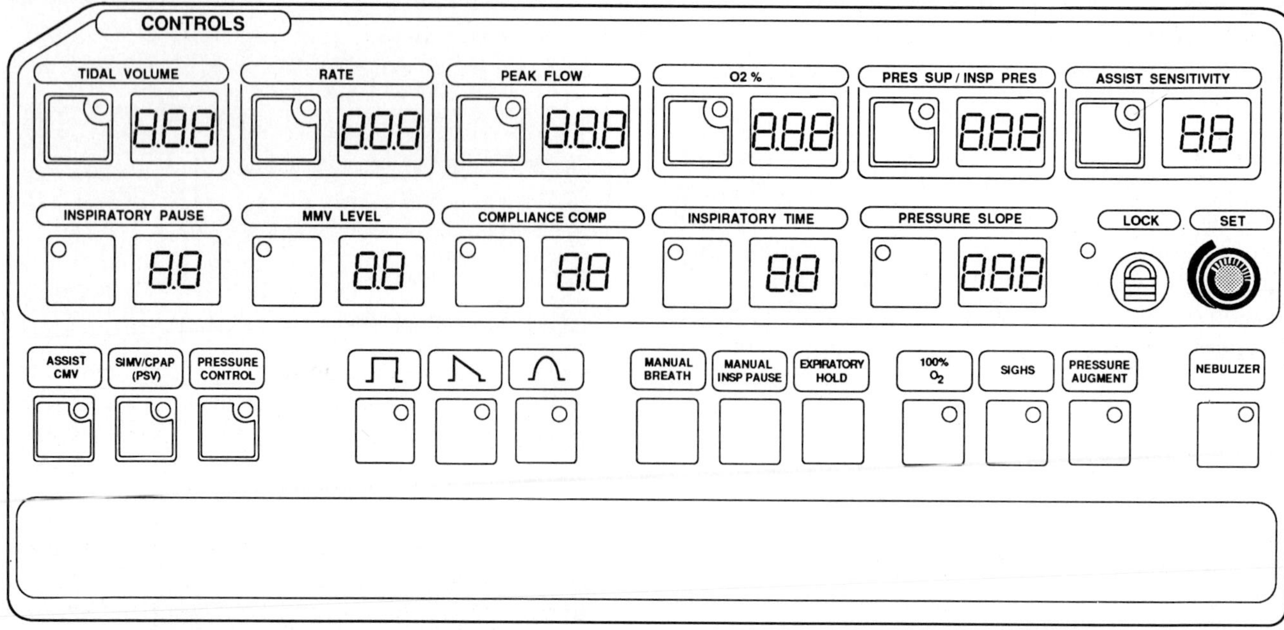

Figure 14-11. Control panel of the Bear 1000 ventilator. (Courtesy of Bear Medical Corporation, Riverside, CA)

inspiratory flow goes from zero to peak flow and back to zero in a sinusoidal fashion.

PHASE VARIABLES. Inspiration is pressure triggered when a spontaneous ventilatory effort removes enough gas from the patient circuit to drop the pressure below the ASSIST SENSITIVITY threshold. The threshold for triggering all assisted breaths is adjustable from 0.2 to 5.0 cm H_2O below the baseline pressure. Unassisted breaths can access demand flow with as little as 0.1 cm H_2O pressure drop. Inspiration is time triggered as a function of the ventilator frequency, or RATE, which is adjustable from 0 to 120 cycles/min. Time triggering is also in effect when using SIGH. When SIGH is activated, a single sigh breath is automatically delivered as the one hundredth mandatory breath. The Bear 1000 may also be manually triggered. Time and pressure triggering can be manually overridden using the EXPIRATORY HOLD key.

Inspiration is pressure limited for mandatory breaths in the PRESSURE CONTROL mode and for all spontaneous breaths. A demand valve controls inspiratory pressure by attempting to maintain the set PEEP/CPAP level, which is adjustable from 0 to 50 cm H_2O. If PRES SUP/INSP PRES is set above zero (range, 0–65 H_2O above baseline), spontaneous breaths will be pressure supported. (Note that there is no explicit mode selection for pressure support). If PRES SUP/INSP PRES is set above zero and PRESSURE AUGMENT is activated, some portion of volume-controlled breaths will be pressure limited (see Modes of Operation). If a patient demand causes airway pressure to drop below the set PEEP level during a volume-controlled breath (because the set inspiratory flow is too low), the ventilator will switch to pressure control, increasing flow to maintain the PEEP level. Inspiration is volume limited whenever the inspiratory pause time is greater than zero. Inspiration is flow limited for volume-controlled breaths. Peak inspiratory flow rate can be pre-set over a range of 10 to 150 L/min, although peak flow for a mandatory pressure-controlled or spontaneous breath can be as high as 200 L/min. Flow limitation may be overridden for some portion inspiration if PRESSURE AUGMENT is activated.

Inspiration is terminated when one of four variables reaches a pre-set threshold. Inspiration may be pressure cycled when the high PEAK INSPIRATORY PRESSURE alarm threshold is violated. Inspiration is also pressure cycled for spontaneous breaths when PRES SUP/INSP PRES (pressure support) is not used (when expiration causes airway pressure to rise above the PEEP setting). Inspiration is volume cycled in the ASSIST CMV and SIMV modes. Although volume is not directly measured, the microprocessor uses feedback information from the flow control valve to end-inspiration when the TIDAL VOLUME and optional COMPLIANCE COMP volume have been delivered. Tidal volume may be set from 100 to 2000 mL and is corrected to STPD. Sigh volume is automatically set at 150% of the set tidal volume. Volume cycling may be overridden if PRESSURE AUGMENT is active and the patient demands more than the set tidal volume. Inspiration is flow cycled for PRES SUP/INSP PRES (pressure supported) spontaneous breaths when inspiratory flow rate decays to 30% of the peak inspiratory flow rate. Flow cycling also occurs when PRESSURE AUGMENT is activated and a patient effort prolongs inspiration beyond the pre-set tidal volume in the ASSIST CMV and SIMV modes. Inspiration is time cycled for mandatory breaths in the PRESSURE CONTROL mode. The INSPIRATORY TIME may be set from 0.1 to 5.0 seconds. Inspiration is time cycled when the INSPIRATORY PAUSE time is set above zero (adjustable from 0 to 2.0 seconds). Inspiration is also time cycled when the TIME/I:E LIMIT alarm is activated.

Baseline pressure may be adjusted from 0 to 50 cm H_2O using the PEEP/CPAP knob.

Control Subsystems

CONTROL CIRCUIT. The Bear 1000 uses pneumatic and electronic control signals (Fig. 14-12). A microprocessor accepts input from six pressure transducers (proximal airway pressure, machine pressure, proximal/PEEP differential pressure, flow control valve pressure, air, and oxygen supply pressures). Input signals also come from a temperature sensor and the external flow sensor to measure delivered gas temperature and exhaled flow. Output control signals go to the air-oxygen blender, flow control valve, nebulizer solenoid valve, exhalation solenoid valve, and others. The exhalation solenoid valve outputs pneumatic signals to the exhalation valve that allow control of peak inspiratory and baseline pressures.

DRIVE MECHANISM. The Bear 1000 uses either external compressed gas (for air and oxygen) or an electric motor and compressor (for air) in conjunction with a pressure regulator. Gas pressure is initially regulated to about 18 psig before reaching the air–oxygen blender mechanism. Mixed gas leaves the blender and enters a rigid-walled vessel (the "accumulator") with an internal volume of about 3.5 L. The flow control system is driven by the pressure from the accumulator. The pressure inside the accumulator varies from 10 to 18 psig, representing a stored (ie, compressed) gas volume of 6 to 8 L. During a flow demand, the volume stored in the accumulator is exhausted quickly, reducing the instantaneous flow demand required of the blending system and upstream pressure regulating system. This action allows a wide range of PEAK FLOW settings, reduces the flow required of the compressed gas supply, and improves response time. The accumulator also acts as a mixing chamber, which helps to stabilize the delivered oxygen concentration within a given breath.

OUTPUT CONTROL VALVES. All gas flow to the patient is regulated by the main flow control valve, which is a pneumatic valve connected to a stepper motor. An electromagnetic poppet valve switches between two sources of a pneumatic signal to the exhalation valve. One source is a 2-psig pressure regulator that keeps a diaphragm-type exhalation manifold closed during assisted breaths. The other source is a jet venturi that generates an adjustable pressure signal to control baseline pressure (ie, PEEP/CPAP). The microprocessor coordinates the activity of both valves such that the exhalation valve closes as the flow control valve begins to deliver flow to the patient circuit.

Output Displays

As mentioned earlier, the front panel is divided into three groups of displays: controls, monitors, and alarms. There is also an aneroid pressure gauge. The control panel is discussed earlier under Input Variables. The monitors panel contains indicator lights for:

- Controlled breath (lit whenever a mandatory breath is delivered)
- Sigh breath (lit whenever a sigh breath is delivered)
- Patient effort (lit whenever the patient inspiratory effort causes a pressure drop greater than the set ASSIST SENSITIVITY)
- MMV active (lit when the MMV backup rate is activated)

A set of three keypads controlling one digital readout is used to display peak, mean, and plateau pressures. Baseline pressure (ie, PEEP/CPAP) is read from an aneroid pressure gauge.

A set of three keypads and one digital readout are used to display exhaled tidal volume, total minute ventilation, and spontaneous minute ventilation. All exhaled readings are corrected to STPD (standard temperature 77°F [25°C], set ambient barometric pressure, dry) to be consistent with the set tidal volume readout.

A set of four keypads with one digital readout are used to display total ventilatory rate, spontaneous ventilatory rate, I:E ratio, and MMV% (the percentage of time during the last half hour that the MMV backup rate has been used rather than the normal breath RATE control).

Modes of Operation

The following modes are those named on the control panel of the Bear 1000:

ASSIST CMV. Inspiration is volume controlled, is pressure triggered (depending on the presence of spontaneous breathing efforts and the ASSIST SENSITIVITY setting) or time triggered (according to the RATE setting), may be volume limited (when INSPIRATORY PAUSE is set above zero), is flow limited, and volume cycled (according to the TIDAL VOLUME setting) or time cycled (when INSPIRATORY PAUSE is set above zero).

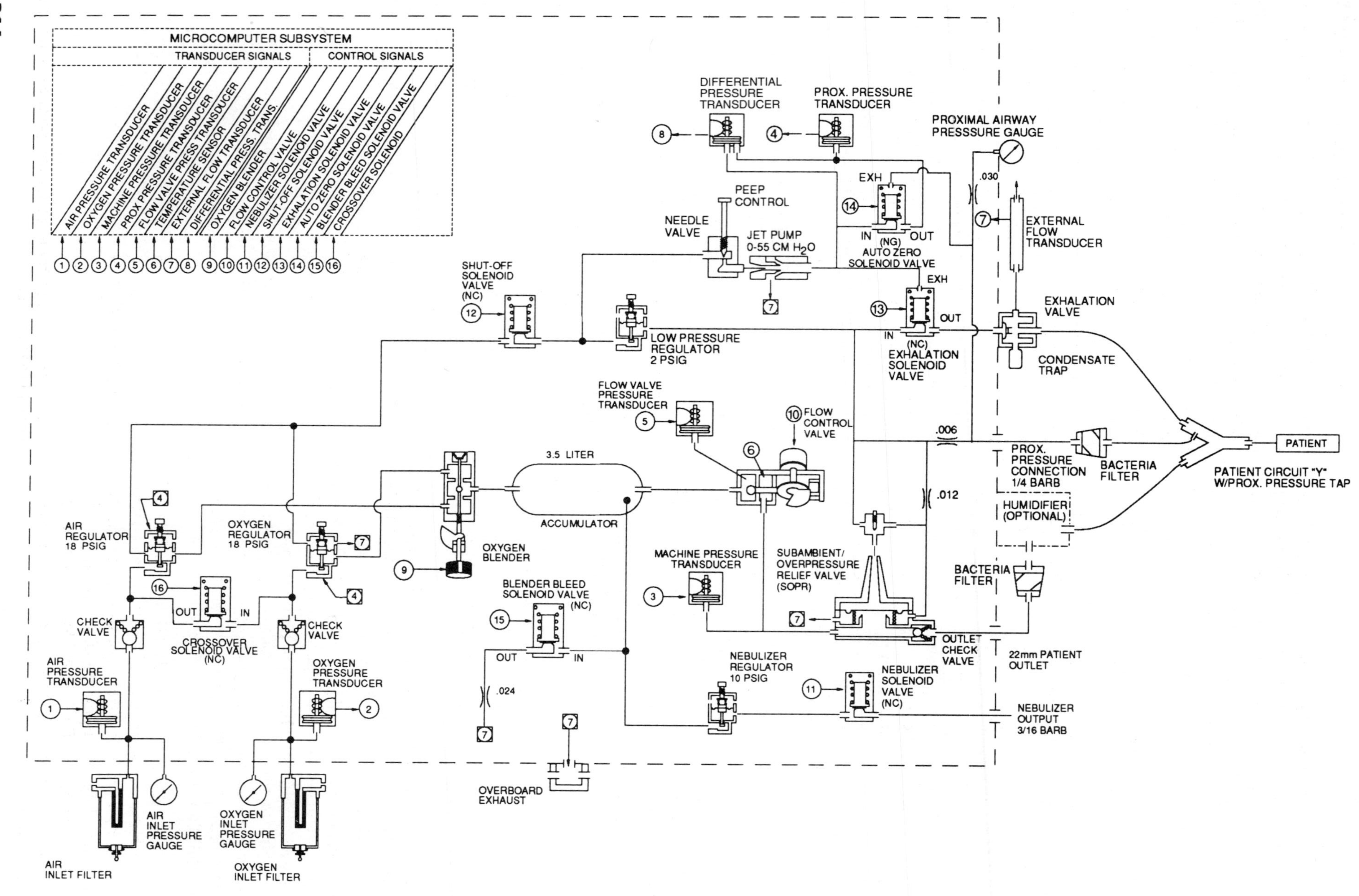

Figure 14-12. Internal components of the Bear 1000 ventilator control circuit. (Courtesy of Bear Medical Corporation, Riverside, CA)

SIMV/CPAP (PSV). In SIMV, mandatory breaths are volume controlled, are pressure triggered (depending on the presence of spontaneous breathing efforts and the ASSIST SENSITIVITY setting) or time triggered (according to the RATE setting), may be volume limited (when INSPIRATORY PAUSE is set above zero), flow limited, and volume cycled (according to the TIDAL VOLUME setting) or time cycled (when INSPIRATORY PAUSE is set above zero). CPAP is instituted if the RATE and PRES SUP/INSP PRES settings are zero. Spontaneous breaths may be pressure supported during CPAP by setting PRES SUP/INSP PRES above zero.

A mandatory breath is pressure triggered the first time a spontaneous breathing effort is detected during each ventilatory period (the time equal to the reciprocal of the RATE). Subsequent breathing efforts during the same period will not trigger another mandatory breath. If a breathing effort is not detected during a given ventilatory period, a mandatory breath will be delivered at the beginning of the next period. The ventilator will continue to deliver mandatory breaths according to the RATE setting until a spontaneous breath is detected and the sequence of events repeats itself.

Spontaneous inspirations between mandatory breaths are pressure limited (ie, inspiratory flow varies to maintain the set PEEP value), pressure triggered, and pressure cycled. They are flow cycled and assisted by pressure support if PRES SUP/INSP PRES is set above zero.

MMV. Minimum minute volume (MMV) is identical to SIMV except that the average exhaled minute volume must exceed the threshold determined by the MMV LEVEL setting. If it does not, a new backup rate (greater than the RATE setting) is established according to the equation:

$$\text{Backup rate (cycles/min)} = \frac{\text{MMV level (L/min)}}{\text{Tidal volume (L/cycle)}}$$

The ventilator will resume operation at the RATE setting when the average exhaled minute volume meets or exceeds the MMV LEVEL setting.

PRESSURE CONTROL. Mandatory breaths are pressure controlled, pressure triggered (depending on the presence of spontaneous breathing efforts and the ASSIST SENSITIVITY setting) or time triggered (according to the RATE setting), pressure limited (determined by PRES SUP/INSP PRES setting), and time cycled (by the INSPIRATORY TIME setting).

PRESSURE AUGMENT. The PRESSURE AUGMENT mode combines pressure control and volume control within one breath. This is thought to benefit the patient by providing the superior assist synchrony effect of pressure control (ie, flow more closely matches patient demand) with the volume "guarantee" effect of volume control.

When the PRESSURE AUGMENT button is activated, inspiration begins under pressure control with the pressure limit determined by the PRES SUP/INSP PRES setting (pressure rise time may be adjusted using the PRESSURE SLOPE function). Inspiratory flow decays from its initial peak value (which is determined by the PRES SUP/INSP PRES setting and the resistance of the patient's respiratory system). If the set tidal volume is achieved, pressure control continues until flow decays to 30% of the initial peak value, when inspiration is cycled off. If the tidal volume is not achieved, flow decays to the PEAK FLOW setting. At this point, the breath continues under volume control at the set flow rate until the tidal volume is delivered and inspiration is cycled off. Inspiration may switch from volume control back to pressure control if the patient's inspiratory effort drops patient circuit pressure below the PRES SUP/INSP PRES setting. The control logic for PRESSURE AUGMENT is illustrated in Figure 14-13. The pressure, volume, and flow curves during PRESSURE AUGMENT may vary con-

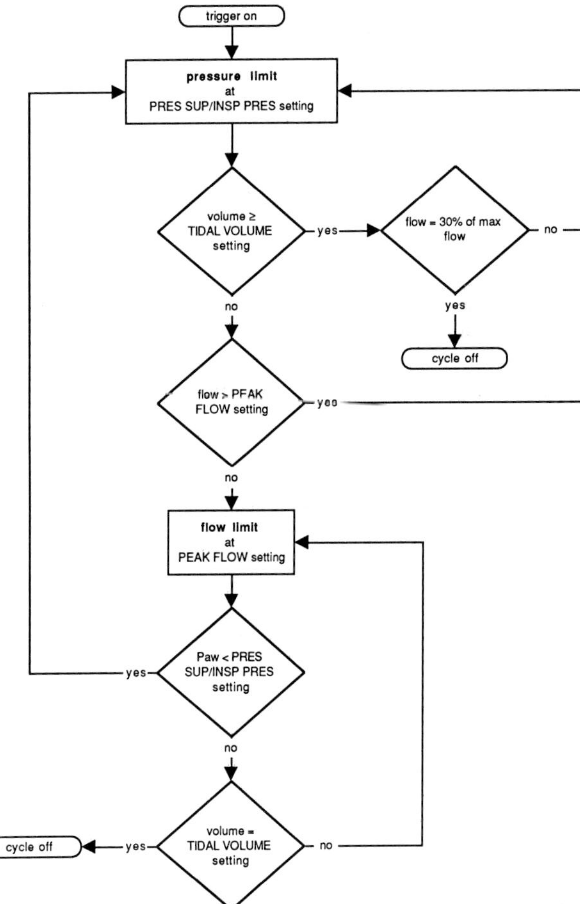

Figure 14-13. Control logic for the pressure augment mode of the Bear 1000.

siderably depending on pressure and volume settings and patient demand.

Alarms

INPUT POWER ALARMS. Visual and audible alarms are activated if there is an electrical power failure or if the pneumatic power supply drops below 27.5 psig.

CONTROL VARIABLE ALARMS. Low (3–99 cm H_2O) and high (0–120 cm H_2O) alarm thresholds can be set for PIP. Activation of the high pressure alarm terminates inspiration. Low (0–50 cm H_2O) and high (0–55 cm H_2O) alarm thresholds can be set for baseline pressure. A proximal disconnect alarm is activated ("Pro" is displayed in the PEAK INSP PRESSURE readout) when proximal pressure measures less than 3 cm H_2O while machine pressure measures greater than the high PEAK INSP PRESSURE setting plus 10 cm H_2O.

There are alarms for low (0–50 L) and high (0–80 L) total minute volume, as well as low (3–99 breaths per minute) and high (0–55 breaths per minute) total breath rate.

CONTROL CIRCUIT ALARMS. Visual and audible alarms are activated if the ventilator fails due to an internal or external condition. "Failure to cycle" means the ventilator is not providing any mechanical breaths or demand flow and PEEP is not maintained.

Visual and audible alarms are activated and inspiration is cycled off if the inspiratory time exceeds the sum of 5 seconds plus the INSPIRATORY PAUSE setting or if the I:E ratio reaches the set limit for a mandatory breath. The set limit is normally 1:1. However, the clinician can override this default value by activating the I:E OVERRIDE button. Once activated, a new default I:E of 4:1 is imposed.

BEAR CUB (BP 2001)

The Bear Cub (Bear Medical Corporation, Riverside, CA) (Fig. 14-14) is a pressure or flow controller that is time or manually triggered and time cycled. It has an integral air–oxygen blender.

Input Variables

The Bear Cub requires 117 volts AC at 60 Hz to power the control circuitry. The ventilator also requires pneumatic power and operates on external compressed gas sources: air at 15 to 75 psig and oxygen at 30 to 75 psig. The Bear Cub has no internal compressor.

The front panel of the Bear Cub is illustrated in Figure 14-15. The operator may select mode of ventilation, desired pressure limit (PIP), desired baseline pressure (PEEP), ventilatory frequency, inspiratory time, and flow rate.

Control Variables

The Bear Cub is normally set to control inspiratory pressure. However, as with most infant ventilators, the Bear Cub is designed more to limit rather than truly control inspiratory pressure. In the first place, the PRESSURE LIMIT control knob is uncalibrated. But more to the point, the peak inspiratory flow rate is always limited to the value set on the flowmeter. For a given inspiratory time, this flow rate may not be sufficient to achieve the set inspiratory pressure limit in the allotted inspiratory time (depending also on the compliance and resistance of the patient's respiratory system). Thus, in this situation, the Bear Cub becomes a flow controller by default.

INSPIRATORY WAVEFORMS. The Bear Cub is capable of producing either a rectangular (approximately rectangular, it is usually rounded early in the inspiratory phase) pressure or a flow waveform. It is most often operated with a semi-rectangular pressure waveform in a pressure-controlled (ie, pressure-limited) mode. A rectangular flow waveform results from setting the

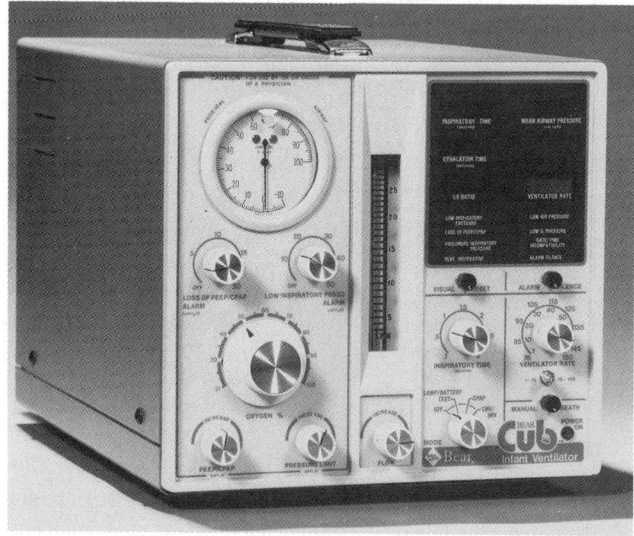

Figure 14-14. The Bear Cub ventilator. (Courtesy of Bear Medical Corporation, Riverside, CA)

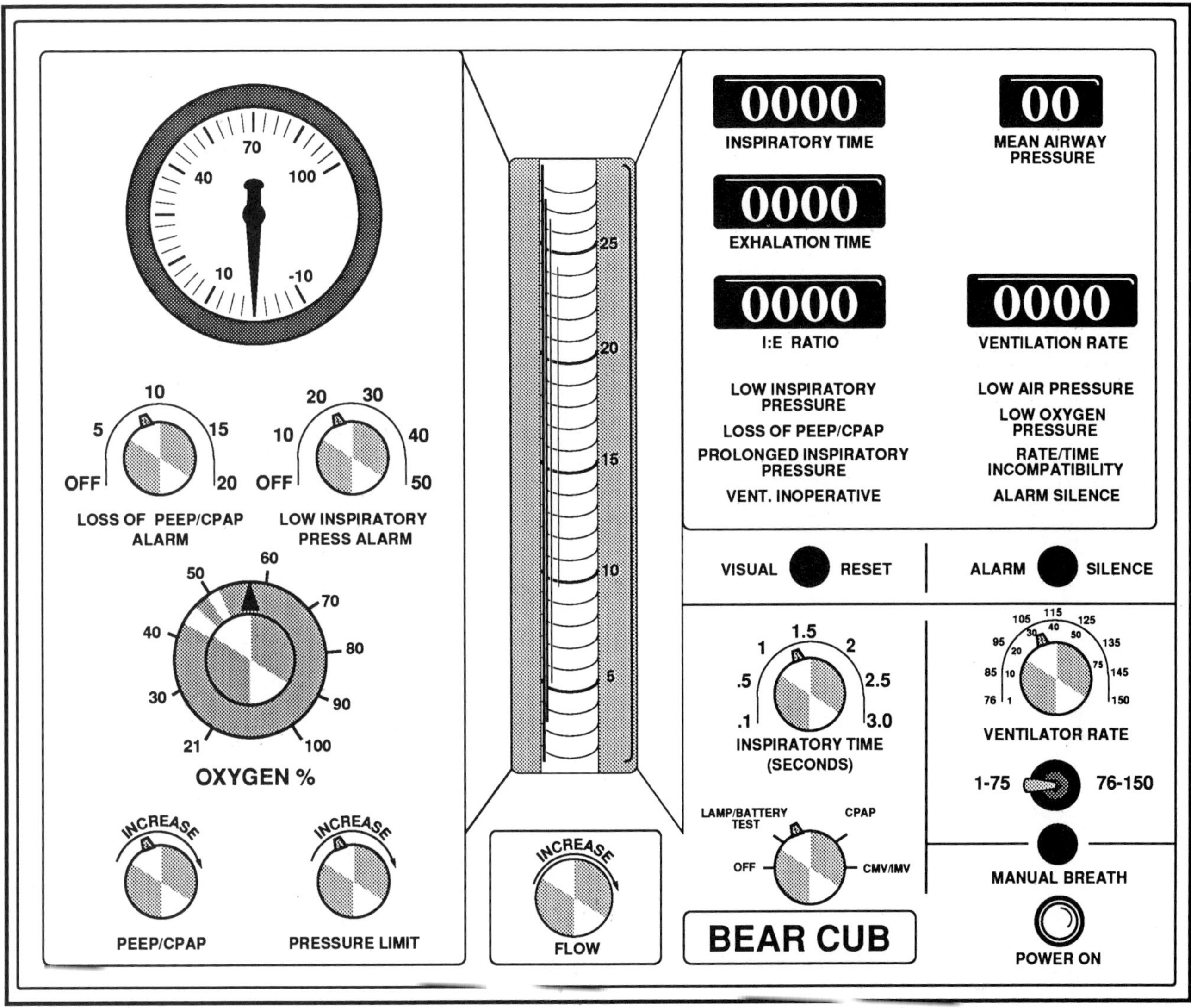

Figure 14-15. Control panel of the Bear Cub ventilator.

PIP limit high enough to achieve flow control (mentioned earlier).

PHASE VARIABLES. Inspiration is time triggered and is a function of the set ventilator frequency, adjustable from 1 to 150 cycles/min. Inspiration may also be manually triggered.

Inspiration may be pressure limited from 0 to 72 cm H_2O. If inspiration is not pressure limited, it is flow limited. The continuous flow rate may be adjusted from 3 to 30 L/min. When inspiration is pressure limited, tidal volume is a function of inspiratory time for a given respiratory system resistance, compliance, and a given inspiratory pressure waveform. When inspiration is flow limited, tidal volume is estimated by calculating the product of the set flow rate and the inspiratory time and subtracting the compressed gas volume.

Inspiration is time cycled as a result of the inspiratory time setting (adjustable from 0.1 to 3.0 seconds).

Baseline pressure may be adjusted over the range of 0 to 20 cm H_2O using the (uncalibrated) CPAP/PEEP control knob.

Control Subsystems

CONTROL CIRCUIT. The Bear Cub is electronically controlled and pneumatically powered (Fig. 14-16). The control circuit is based on a timer that sends inspiratory and expiratory timing signals to the three-way solenoid. The solenoid switches the source of exhalation manifold's pneumatic signal from either the pressure limit control valve or the PEEP control valve. A pneumatic signal from the airway opening pressure sensing line is feedback to the pressure limit control system. This feedback mechanism not only helps control the inspiratory pressure but also results in an exponential pressure waveform.

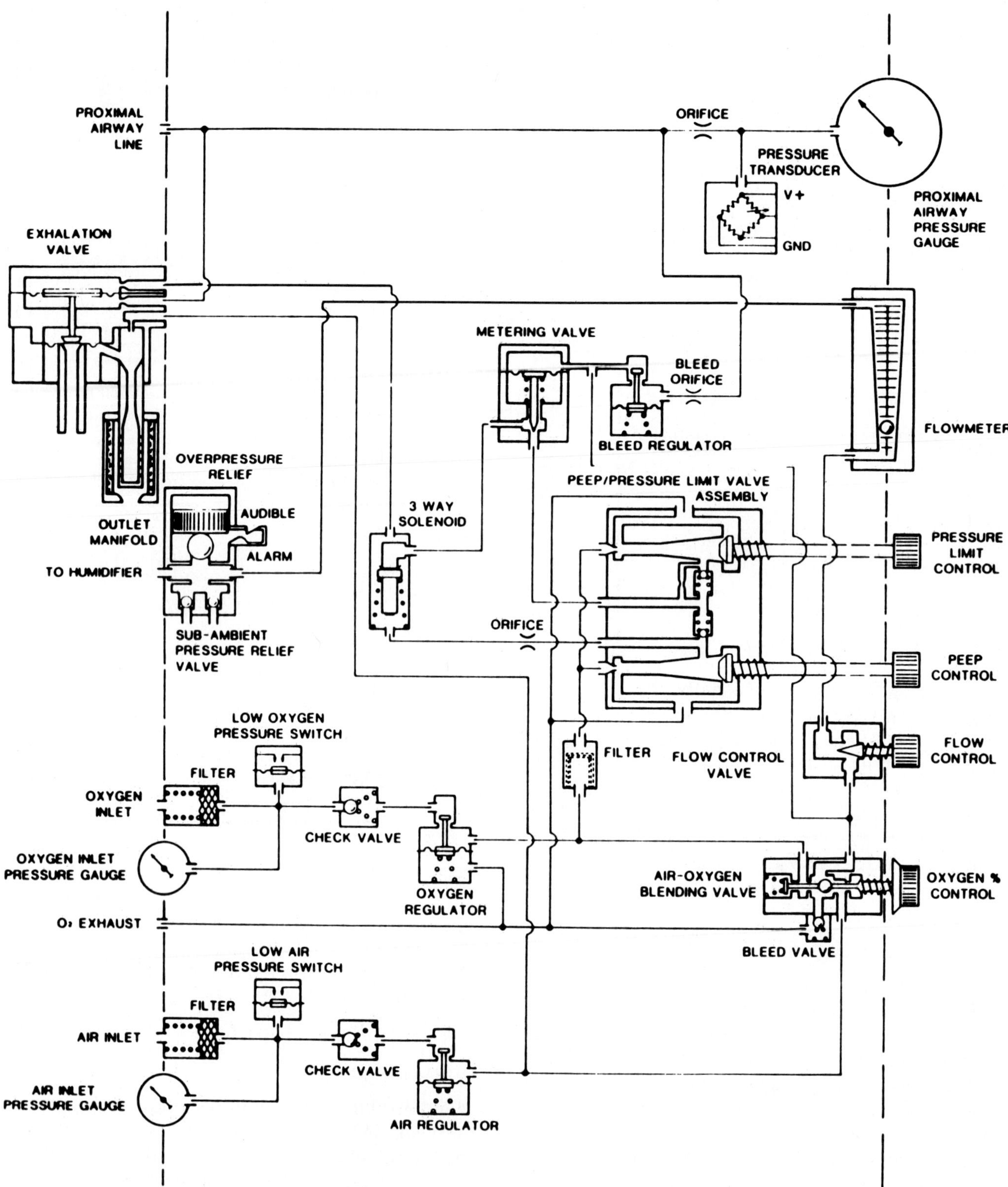

Figure 14-16. Internal components of the Bear Cub ventilator control circuit. (Courtesy of Bear Medical Corporation, Riverside, CA)

DRIVE MECHANISM. The Bear Cub requires an external pneumatic source to power the internal blender. This blender delivers pressurized gas to a flowmeter, which then routes a continuous flow of gas to the patient circuit.

OUTPUT CONTROL VALVES. The ventilatory cycle is controlled by six valves: the flow control valve, the PEEP and inspiratory pressure limit valves, the metering valve, the three-way solenoid valve, and the exhalation valve. The flow control valve in conjunction with the flowmeter sets the rate of continuous gas flow through the patient circuit. The PEEP and inspiratory pressure limit valves are both devices designed to generate reference pressures using jet venturies. The venturies are driven by the oxygen pressure source. As the control knob is rotated clockwise, a plunger occludes the output of the jet venturi, which increases the reference pressure inside the venturi tube. Two check valves between the pressure limit control valve and the PEEP control valve, which prevent the PEEP level from being set above the inspiratory pressure limit.

The exhalation valve has two chambers separated by a flexible diaphragm connected to a plunger. The upper chamber is connected to the reference pressure signal, and the lower chamber is connected to the airway pressure signal.

During the expiratory phase, the three-way solenoid valve directs the PEEP/CPAP reference pressure to the upper chamber of the exhalation valve. This drives the plunger downward to partially occlude the expiratory limb of the patient circuit. The back-pressure caused by this resistance and the continuous flow through from the flow-control valve is the PEEP. Gas from the expiratory limb exits through the outlet manifold, which is configured as a venturi tube. The venturi is driven by flow from the air source and is intended to overcome the resistive pressure drop (ie, inadvertent PEEP) across the expiratory portion of the patient circuit.

During the inspiratory phase, the three-way solenoid directs the inspiratory reference pressure through the metering valve to the upper chamber of the exhalation manifold. The plunger occludes the expiratory limb of the patient circuit causing the airway pressure to rise as the lungs are inflated. When the airway pressure approaches the reference pressure, the forces across the diaphragm in the exhalation manifold equilibrate, the plunger unseats, the continuous flow of gas from the flow control valve is vented to the atmosphere, and airway pressure remains constant at the set inspiratory pressure limit until inspiration is cycled off.

If the airway pressure sensing line becomes disconnected or blocked, the airway pressure will rise uncontrolled until it reaches the limit set by the internal pressure relief valve (87 ± 4 cm H_2O). For this reason, most Bear Cubs have been retrofitted with an external adjustable pressure pop-off valve located on the back panel of the Bear Cub in the inspiratory limb of the patient circuit. In practice, the pressure limit determined by this valve is set above the normal inspiratory pressure limit set on the front of the machine.

The metering valve is a type of needle valve flow controller that is designed to shape the inspiratory pressure waveform. It controls the flow of gas from the inspiratory reference pressure mechanism to the upper chamber of the exhalation manifold and hence controls the rate at which the pressure in the chamber equilibrates with the reference pressure. The flow rate through the metering valve is determined by a pressure signal from a point in the pneumatic circuit just before the flow control valve. At low patient circuit flow rates, the flow control valve is nearly closed and creates a relatively high back-pressure. This pressure causes a low flow rate through the metering valve, a gradual pressure rise in the upper chamber of the exhalation manifold, and, ultimately, an exponential airway pressure waveform. At high flow rates through the patient circuit, the situation is reversed and the airway pressure waveform assumes a more rectangular waveform.

Output Displays

Peak airway pressure and baseline pressure are displayed by an aneroid pressure gauge. Mean airway pressure is digitally displayed along with inspiratory time, expiratory time, I:E ratio, and ventilatory frequency. There are also indicators for power on and various alarms. Flow is indicated on a Thorpe tube flowmeter.

Modes of Operation

The following modes are those named on the control panel of the Bear Cub:

CMV/IMV. Inspiration is normally pressure limited, time triggered (based on the set ventilator rate), and time cycled (based on the inspiratory time). There is a continuous flow of gas from the ventilator at the rate set on the FLOW CONTROL knob to allow for spontaneous breathing between mandatory breaths. If inspiration is not pressure limited (due to insufficient flow or inspiratory time), it is flow limited, time triggered, and time cycled.

If, during spontaneous breaths, the patient's inspiratory flow rate exceeds that delivered by the ventilator such that negative airway pressure is generated below the baseline pressure, the Bear Cub is incapable of varying flow rate to meet the patient's demand. It is therefore important that the operator have the continuous flow rate set sufficiently high to meet all the patient's demands.

CPAP. Inspiration is not controlled in the CPAP mode. The patient breathes the continuous flow of gas from the flowmeter. The pressure at the airway opening during inspiration fluctuates as a function of the fixed resistance through the exhalation manifold (determined mainly by the PEEP/CPAP setting) and the surplus inspiratory flow. Surplus inspiratory flow is the difference between the flow rate set on the flowmeter and the patient's instantaneous inspiratory flow rate.

Alarms

INPUT POWER ALARMS. Audible and visual alarms are activated when the external electrical power supply to the Bear Cub is interrupted or if the source gas pressures drop below 22.5 ± 2.5 psig.

CONTROL VARIABLE ALARMS. There are three audible and visual pressure alarms. The low inspiratory pressure alarm is activated if the inspiratory pressure fails to exceed the set threshold (adjustable from off to 50 cm H_2O). The loss of PEEP/CPAP alarm light is activated when the PEEP level falls below the set threshold value (adjustable from off to 20 cm H_2O). The prolonged inspiratory pressure indicator will light if the proximal airway pressure remains above the threshold value for more than 3.5 seconds. The threshold value is automatically set by the ventilator at 10 cm H_2O above the setting of loss of PEEP/CPAP alarm.

Control Circuit Alarms

If the ventilator is operated so that the I:E ratio is greater than 3:1, the I:E ratio light will flash and an audible alarm will sound.

The rate/time incompatibility indicator lights when the ventilator rate and inspiratory time controls are set at a combination such that expiratory time would be less than 0.25 second. The flashing of the light indicates that an internal timer is preventing the exhalation time from being any shorter than this. In this case, the ventilating frequency is held constant and the inspiratory time is shortened. The digitally displayed inspiratory time will reflect the shortened value.

The ventilator inoperative alarm detects six different alarm conditions, including (1) fail to cycle, (2) electrical power failure, (3) control panel malfunction, (4) prolonged solenoid "on" time, (5) inspiratory time variation by more than ± 24% of setting, and (6) timing circuit failure.

BIRD 8400ST

The Bird 8400ST ventilator (Bird Products Corporation, Palm Springs, CA) (Fig. 14-17) is a pressure or flow controller that may be pressure, flow, or time triggered, pressure or flow limited, and pressure, flow, or time cycled. A software upgrade is available to provide flow triggering. It has an integral gas outlet port that will power a nebulizer during inspiration. This ventilator requires an external air–oxygen blender.

Input Variables

The Bird 8400ST uses 120 volts AC at 60 Hz (or optional European voltages) to power the control circuitry. The pneumatic circuit, which requires an external air–oxygen blender (eg, Bird 3800 MicroBlender), operates on external compressed gas sources (ie, air and oxygen) at 30 to 70 psig.

The front panel of the Bird 8400ST is illustrated in Figure 14-18. The operator may select the mode of ventilation; pressure-triggering, pressure-limiting, and pressure-cycling thresholds; PEEP/CPAP; tidal volume; peak inspiratory flow rate; flow waveform; flow triggering threshold (optional); and ventilatory frequency. Settings are selected using dials in conjunction with LED displays. Control settings, alarm settings, and output displays are conveniently grouped into three separate panels.

Control Variables

The Bird 8400ST controls either inspiratory pressure or flow. It controls inspiratory pressure in the CPAP mode. It controls flow in the ASSIST/CONTROL mode and switches between pressure control (for spontaneous breaths) and flow control (for mandatory breaths) in the SIMV mode.

INSPIRATORY WAVEFORMS. The Bird 8400ST offers one inspiratory pressure and two inspiratory flow waveforms. A rectangular pressure waveform can be achieved in the SIMV or CPAP modes when PRESSURE SUPPORT is activated. Flow waveforms include

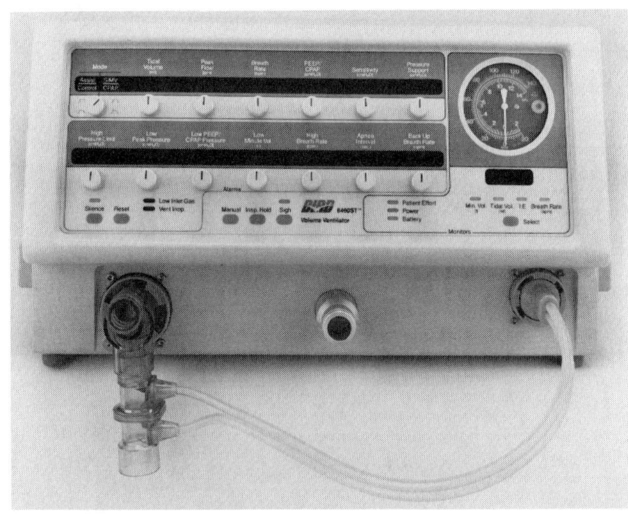

Figure 14-17. The Bird 8400ST ventilator. (Courtesy of Bird Products Corporation, Palm Springs, CA)

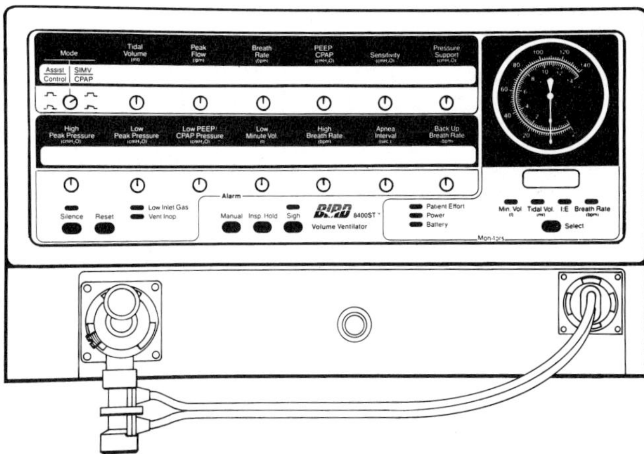

Figure 14-18. Control panel of the Bird 8400ST ventilator. (Courtesy of Bird Products Corporation, Palm Springs, CA)

rectangular and descending ramps. Gas delivery with the rectangular waveform is relatively constant, and peak inspiratory flow rate is operator selectable. When the descending ramp waveform is selected, flow is initially delivered at the peak flow setting and then decreases to 50% of this value at end-inspiration.

PHASE VARIABLES. Inspiration is pressure triggered when a spontaneous ventilatory effort removes enough gas from the patient circuit to drop the pressure below the SENSITIVITY setting. The threshold for triggering a mandatory breath is adjustable from 1.0 to 20.0 cm H_2O below the baseline pressure and may be turned off. When flow triggering is activated, the SENSITIVITY window will display Fxx, where "F" indicates activation of the flow trigger option and "xx" indicates the flow trigger level in L/min (range, 1 to 10 L/min). Inspiration is time triggered as a function of the BREATH RATE setting, which is adjustable from 0 to 80 cycles/min. A BACK UP BREATH RATE is activated if the apnea alarm is triggered (cannot be set less than BREATH RATE setting). The Bird 8400ST may also be manually triggered.

Inspiration is pressure limited during spontaneous breaths in the SIMV or CPAP modes. A demand flow system controls inspiratory pressure by attempting to maintain the set PEEP/CPAP level, which is adjustable from 0 to 30 cm H_2O if PRESSURE SUPPORT is not used. If PRESSURE SUPPORT is used, the pressure limit may be set from 0 to 50 cm H_2O above the PEEP/CPAP level. Inspiration can be manually volume limited by pressing the INSPIRATORY HOLD button. Inspiration is flow limited for mandatory breaths. Peak flow is adjustable from 10 to 120 L/min.

Inspiration is terminated when one of three variables reaches a pre-set threshold. Inspiration may be pressure cycled when the maximum inspiratory pressure threshold is violated. It may be set over a range of 0 to 140 cm H_2O. Inspiration is also pressure cycled for spontaneous breaths when PRESSURE SUPPORT is not used (when expiration causes airway pressure to rise above the PEEP setting). Inspiration cannot be volume cycled because the 8400ST does not measure inspired volume. However, for mandatory breaths, tidal volume may be set from 50 to 2000 mL. When SIGH is activated, a volume equal to 150% of the set tidal volume (available range is 75 to 3000 mL) will be delivered once every 100 breaths (the pressure alarm setting is automatically adjusted to 150% of the set value for the sigh breath). Inspiration is flow cycled when using PRESSURE SUPPORT as soon as the inspiratory flow rate decays to 25% of the PEAK FLOW setting. Inspiration is also flow cycled in the CPAP mode when the FLOW SUPPORT option is activated. Inspiration is time cycled for mandatory breaths whenever the inspiratory time reaches the value determined by the tidal volume and flow rate settings. Pressure-supported spontaneous breaths will be time cycled if inspiratory flow fails to reach 25% of the peak value within 3 seconds.

Baseline pressure may be adjusted from 0 to 30 cm H_2O using the PEEP/CPAP function.

Control Subsystems

CONTROL CIRCUIT The Bird 8400ST uses only electronic control components, although there is a pneumatically driven safety valve that allows the patient to inspire room air in the event of an electrical power failure or a ventilator-inoperative state (Fig. 14-19). A microprocessor accepts input signals relating to airway pressure and control variable settings and outputs control signals to the output control valves.

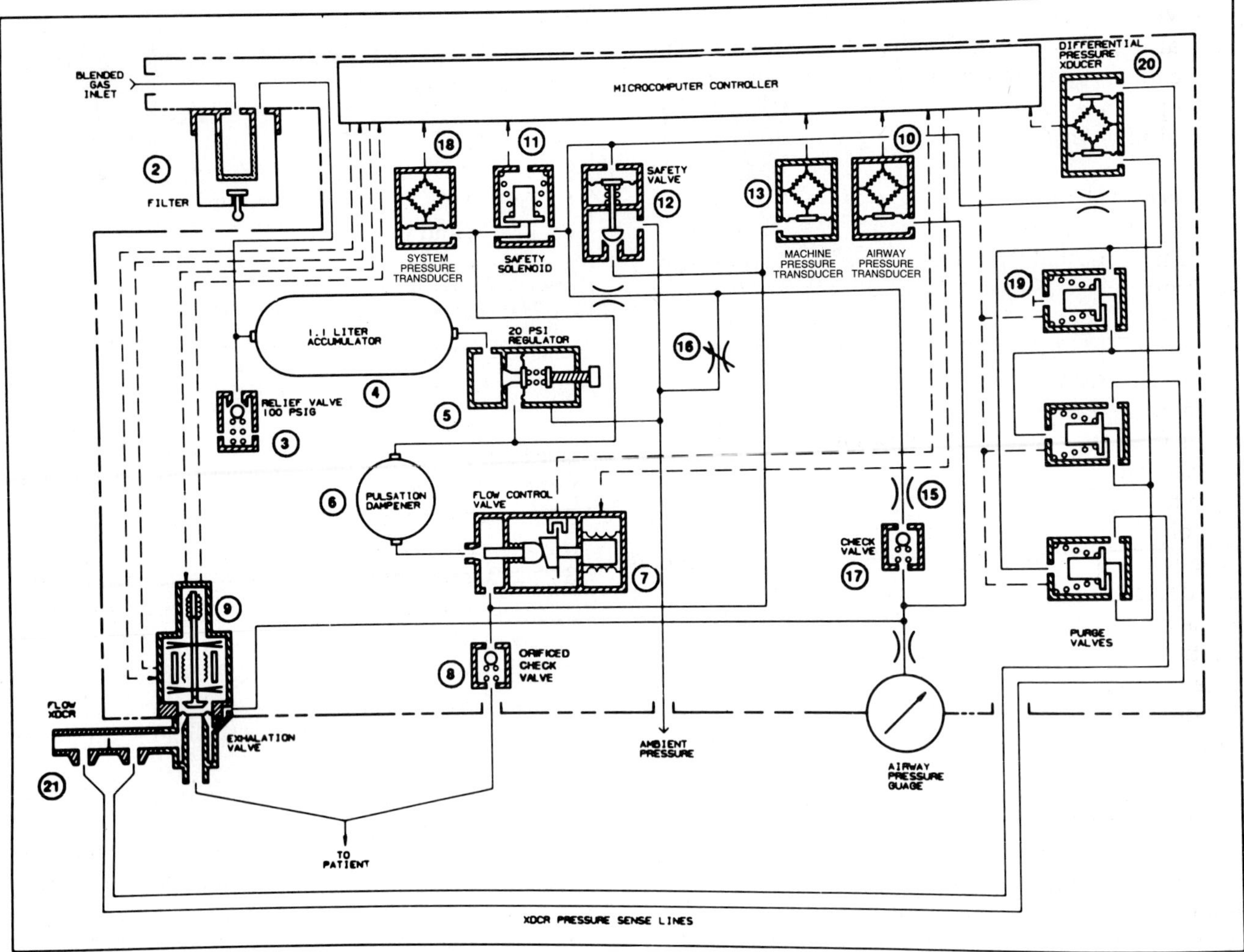

Figure 14-19. Internal components of the Bird 8400ST ventilator control circuit. (Courtesy of Bird Products Corporation, Palm Springs, CA)

Airway pressure is measured both at the airway opening and inside the ventilator. Feedback from the airway pressure transducer is used to provide triggering, cycling, and alarm signals and to control the airway pressure waveform during pressure-controlled breaths. The internal pressure signal is used to detect the CIRC fault (see Alarms).

Flow information is obtained by sensing the position of the stepper motor inside the flow control valve (see Output Control Valves). Signals from the flow control valve are used for shaping the inspiratory flow waveform and for adjusting volume. A flow transducer connected to the exhalation valve measures exhaled tidal volume and minute volume.

When the FLOW SUPPORT option is activated, there is a constant bias flow of 10 L/min through the patient circuit. The patient's flow (inspiratory and expiratory) is determined by comparing the flow leaving the flow control valve with the flow measured at the exhalation manifold, according to the equation:

$$F(pt) = F(vlv) - F(trn)$$

where F(pt) is the patient flow, F(vlv) is the flow leaving the main flow control valve, and F(trn) is the flow measured by the transducer at the exhalation manifold. At end-expiration, F(vlv) is pre-set to 10 L/min baseline flow so F(trn) is also 10 L/min and F(pt) = 0 L/min. When the patient inspires, F(trn) falls below 10 L/min and F(pt) is greater than 0. The exhalation manifold closes and the flow valve opens to provide additional flow equal to the patient demand in an attempt to bring F(tm) back to 10. For example, if the patient's inspiratory flow is 20 L/min, the flow control valve opens to 30 L/min (20 L/min to meet the patient's demand + 10 L/min of baseline flow). As the patient demand decreases near end-inspiration, F(vlv) approaches the value of F(trn). When F(vlv) = F(trn), F(pt) = 0 and the ventilator cycles from inspiration to expiration (ie, the exhalation manifold is opened).

DRIVE MECHANISM. The Bird 8400ST uses either external compressed gas (for air and oxygen) or an electric motor and compressor (for air) in conjunction with a pressure regulator. Compressed gas from the external blender (a Bird 3800 MicroBlender) passes into a 1.1-L rigid chamber accumulator. The purpose of the accumulator is to store pressurized gas for augmenting the blender flow during high inspiratory flow demands. The blender is capable of delivering approximately 75 L/min with inlet and outlet pressures of 50 and 35 psig, respectively, while the accumulator allows the ventilator to deliver up to 120 L/min. This extra flow capacity is provided from gas stored in the accumulator during the expiratory phase.

Gas from the accumulator flows through a regulator that sets the driving pressure of the flow control valve to 20 psig. Between the regulator and the flow control valve is another accumulator, referred to as a pulsation dampener, with a volume of about 200 mL. This device compensates for transient pressure fluctuations caused by the regulator's slow response time (relative to flow rate changes during a ventilatory cycle) and thus helps to maintain a constant driving pressure to the flow control valve. A constant pressure is necessary to maintain the accuracy of the delivered flow rates and tidal volumes.

OUTPUT CONTROL VALVES. Gas flow to the patient is regulated by two electromechanical valves, each consisting of a stepper motor connected to a piston. Rotary motion of the stepper motor is transformed to linear motion required for controlling flow through a variable poppet type orifice. One valve controls the instantaneous flow rate of gas during inspiration. This valve is designed and calibrated to obtain a known relationship between position and orifice opening. With the system pressure at 20 psig, flow through the variable orifice is unaffected by downstream patient circuit pressures up to 210 cm H_2O. The range of the valve is 0 to 120 L/min, with an approximate resolution of 1 L/min/step. An optical sensor detects the zero flow position.

The second output control valve is used to occlude the expiratory path during inspiration and to control the baseline pressure (ie, PEEP/CPAP). The microprocessor coordinates the activity of both valves such that the exhalation valve closes as the flow control valves begin to deliver flow to the patient circuit.

Output Displays

In addition to the various control settings, the front panel displays include total (spontaneous and mandatory) frequency, exhaled tidal volume and minute volume, and I:E ratio. Airway pressures are displayed on an aneroid pressure gauge.

Modes of Operation

The following modes are those named on the control panel of the Bird 8400ST:

CONTROL. In the CONTROL mode, inspiration is flow controlled, is time triggered (according to the BREATH RATE setting; sensitivity is turned off), is flow limited, and time cycled.

ASSIST/CONTROL. ASSIST/CONTROL is the same as control except that the SENSITIVITY is set such that the patient's inspiratory efforts trigger each breath.

SIMV. In SIMV, mandatory breaths are flow controlled, pressure triggered (depending on the presence of spontaneous breathing efforts and the SENSITIVITY setting), flow triggered (with FLOW SUPPORT option) or time triggered (according to the BREATH RATE setting), and time cycled.

Spontaneous inspirations between mandatory breaths are pressure controlled (ie, inspiratory flow varies to maintain the set PEEP value), pressure triggered or flow triggered (with FLOW SUPPORT option), and normally pressure cycled. Inspiration is flow cycled at 25% of peak flow when the PRESSURE SUPPORT setting is above zero.

A mandatory breath is pressure triggered the first time a spontaneous breathing effort is detected during each ventilatory period (the time equal to the reciprocal of the BREATH RATE setting). Subsequent breathing efforts during the same period will not trigger another mandatory breath. If a breathing effort is not detected during a given ventilatory period, a mandatory breath will be delivered at the beginning of the next period. The ventilator will then deliver another mandatory breath the first time a spontaneous inspiratory effort is detected at which time the sequence of events repeats itself.

CPAP All inspirations are pressure controlled (ie, inspiratory flow varies to maintain either the set CPAP value or the PRESSURE SUPPORT value if this option is used), pressure triggered, or flow triggered (with FLOW SUPPORT option) and normally pressure cycled. Inspiration is flow cycled when using PRESSURE SUPPORT.

SIGH. When activated, the SIGH mode delivers a time-triggered, flow-limited, time-cycled breath once every 100 breaths. The volume of the sigh breath is 150% of the set tidal volume, which is delivered at the set peak flow rate.

Alarms

All alarms are visual and audible.

INPUT POWER ALARMS. Audible and visual alarms are activated if the AC power supply fails or if the compressed gas supply drops below 17 psig.

CONTROL VARIABLE ALARMS. There are three alarms associated with ventilating pressures. One is a LOW PEEP/CPAP alarm, which is adjustable from − 20 to + 30 cm H_2O. This alarm can be set below zero baseline to detect return of ventilatory drive of a patient previously being controlled. A high inspiratory pressure alarm is adjustable from 1 to 140 cm H_2O. A low inspiratory pressure alarm (active for mandatory breaths) is triggered if the airway pressure fails to exceed the alarm setting during inspiration (adjustable from 2 to 140 cm H_2O and may be turned off).

There is a LOW MINUTE VOLUME alarm that is triggered whenever the minute volume measured by the transducer at the exhalation valve does not exceed the alarm setting. It is adjustable from 0 to 99.9 L.

A HIGH BREATH RATE alarm is activated if the total breath rate (spontaneous plus mandatory) exceeds the alarm setting. The range is 3 to 150 breaths per minute.

An APNEA INTERVAL alarm is triggered if no breaths (mandatory or spontaneous) are sensed within the selected time interval (10 to 60 seconds). Audible and visual alarms are activated and APNEA BACKUP VENTILATION is initiated. The ventilator will revert automatically to the ASSIST/CONTROL mode of ventilation and begin to deliver breaths as determined by the settings on the TIDAL VOLUME, PEAK FLOW, WAVEFORM, PEEP, and BACK UP RATE controls. APNEA BACKUP VENTILATION will be reset to normal ventilation if (1) the patient initiates two consecutive breaths and exhales at least 50% of the set tidal volume or (2) the operator depresses the ALARM RESET button.

If the flow transducer assembly is disconnected during operation of the ventilator, audible and visual alarms will be activated.

CONTROL CIRCUIT ALARMS. When inspiratory time exceeds expiratory time, the I:E light on the front panel display will flash.

A VENTILATOR INOPERATIVE alarm is activated if any of the following conditions occur:

- Loss of electrical power
- Extended low ventilator inlet gas pressure, less than 16 psig or greater than 24 psig for 1 second
- An electrical or mechanical system failure is detected by the ventilator control system

A CIRC alarm detects possible patient circuit or pressure transducer faults by comparing pressure measurements from the airway pressure transducer and the machine pressure transducer. If a pressure mismatch occurs, a "CIRC" message will be visually displayed in the monitor's display window along with an audible alarm. Once activated, inspiration is terminated. The following conditions can cause this alarm to be activated:

- Blocked airway pressure sensing port
- Occluded or kinked inspiratory or expiratory limb of breathing circuit
- Pressure transducer failure

If a pressure support breath is time cycled, the digital display will flash.

BIRD V.I.P. INFANT PEDIATRIC VENTILATOR

The Bird V.I.P. ventilator (Bird Products Corporation, Palm Springs, CA) (Fig. 14-20) is a pressure or flow controller that may be pressure, time, or manually triggered; pressure or flow limited; and pressure, volume, or time cycled. Optional flow triggering is accomplished with the addition of the Bird Partner volume monitor. It has an auxiliary blender output port that can be used to attach a flowmeter to power a nebulizer.

Input Variables

The Bird V.I.P. uses 115 volts AC at 60 Hz (or optional European voltages) to power the control circuitry. The pneumatic circuit operates on external compressed gas sources (ie, air and oxygen) at 40 to 75 psig.

The front panel of the Bird V.I.P. is illustrated in Figure 14-21. The operator may select the mode of ventilation; pressure-triggering, pressure-limiting, and pressure-cycling thresholds; PEEP/CPAP; tidal volume; inspiratory flow rate; and ventilatory frequency. Flow-cycling thresholds may be set if the optional Bird Partner volume monitor is used. Settings are selected using dials in conjunction with LED displays.

Control Variables

The Bird V.I.P. controls either inspiratory pressure or flow. It controls inspiratory pressure in the TIME CYCLED (S)IMV/CPAP and ASSIST/CONTROL modes. It controls flow in the VOLUME CYCLED ASSIST/CONTROL and SIMV/CPAP modes and

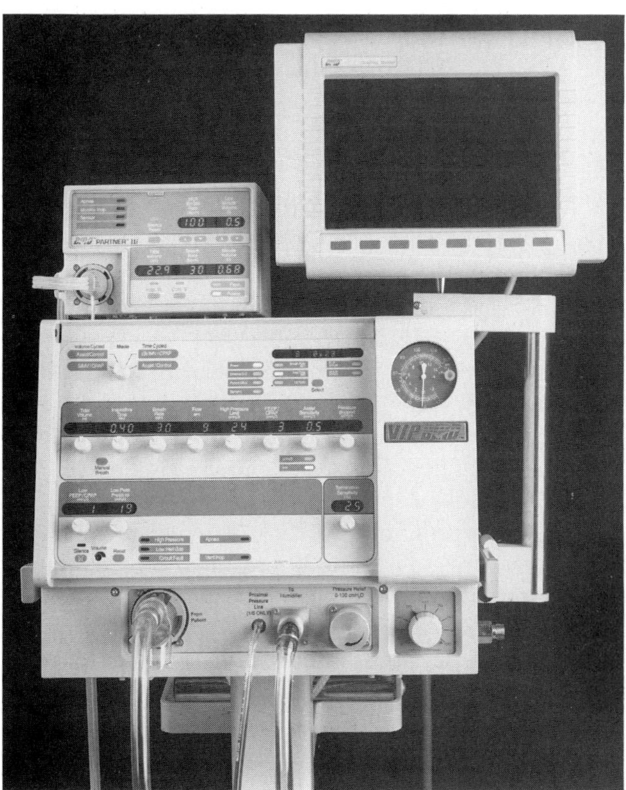

Figure 14-20. The Bird V.I.P. ventilator. (Courtesy of Bird Products Corporation, Palm Springs, CA)

switches between pressure control (for spontaneous breaths) and flow control (for mandatory breaths) in the VOLUME CYCLED SIMV mode.

INSPIRATORY WAVEFORMS. The Bird V.I.P. offers one inspiratory pressure and one inspiratory flow waveform. A rectangular pressure waveform can be achieved in the TIME CYCLED modes and in the VOLUME CYCLED SIMV/CPAP mode when PRESSURE SUPPORT is activated. A rectangular flow waveform can be achieved in the VOLUME CYCLED modes.

PHASE VARIABLES. Inspiration is pressure triggered when a spontaneous ventilatory effort removes enough gas from the patient circuit to drop the pressure below the SENSITIVITY setting. The threshold for triggering a mandatory breath is adjustable from 1.0 to 20.0 cm H_2O below the baseline pressure and may be turned off. Sensitivity is pre-set at 1.0 cm H_2O in the TIME CYCLED IMV mode. With the flow synchronization upgrade (ie, using the Bird Partner volume monitor), two indicators are added below the ASSIST SENSITIVITY control. These indicators identify the trigger source and the calibration of the control. In the VOLUME CYCLED modes, the "H_2O" indicator will illuminate and the control is adjustable from 1.0 to 20.0 cm H_2O. In the TIME CYCLED modes, the "lpm" indicator will illuminate and the control is adjustable from 0.2 to 5.0 L/min in 0.1 L/min increments up to 2.0 L/min and 0.2 L/min increments above 2.0 L/min. In the (S)IMV/CPAP mode, if the breath rate is set to zero, the display will dim indicating that it is not functional. Inspiration is time triggered as a function of the ventilator frequency which is adjustable from 0 to 150 cycles/min. The Bird V.I.P. may also be manually triggered.

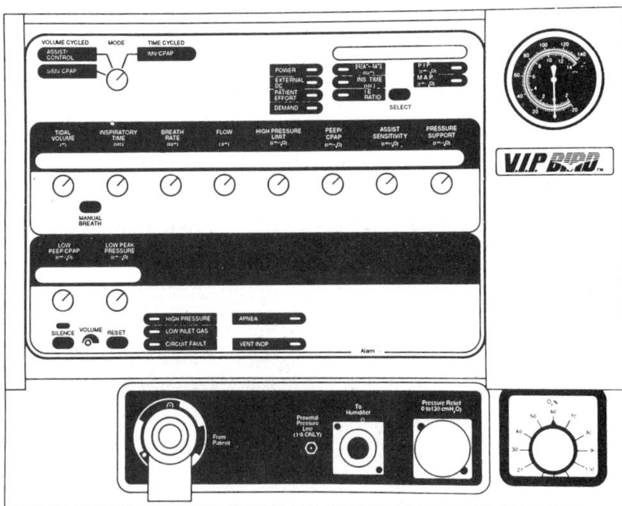

Figure 14-21. Control panel of the Bird V.I.P. ventilator. (Courtesy of Bird Products Corporation, Palm Springs, CA)

Inspiration is pressure limited during spontaneous breaths in all modes. A demand flow system controls inspiratory pressure by attempting to maintain the set PEEP/CPAP level, which is adjustable from 0 to 24 cm H_2O. If PRESSURE SUPPORT is used, the pressure limit may be set from 0 to 50 cm H_2O above the PEEP/CPAP level. In the TIME CYCLED modes, inspiratory pressure may be limited at 3 to 80 cm H_2O. There is a mechanical pressure relief control that may be set from 0 to 130 H_2O in any mode. Inspiration cannot be volume limited as there is no provision for an inspiratory hold. Inspiration is flow limited in the VOLUME CYCLED modes. Peak inspiratory flow rate (in this case the same as mean inspiratory flow rate) is adjustable from 3 to 100 L/min. Demand flow during spontaneous breaths is not affected by the flow control setting and may be as high as 120 L/min. In the TIME CYCLED modes, the flow control setting limits the maximum inspiratory flow rate and the baseline to which flow returns during the expiratory phase. Note that in the TIME CYCLED modes, the actual inspiratory flow rate after the pressure limit is reached is a function of the pressure settings (ie, peak and baseline pressures), respiratory system resistance and compliance, and time.

Inspiration is terminated when one of four variables reaches a pre-set threshold. Inspiration may be pressure cycled in the VOLUME CYCLED modes when the maximum inspiratory pressure threshold is violated during mandatory breaths. It may be set over a range of 3 to 120 cm H_2O. Spontaneous breaths are pressure cycled (factory pre-set threshold above PEEP) when PRESSURE SUPPORT is not used. The manufacturer claims that the Bird V.I.P. is volume cycled. However, there is no direct measurement of volume as a control signal. The microprocessor uses time measurements and the known relationship between flow control valve position and flow rate to move the valve in a predetermined sequence to satisfy the tidal volume and peak flow settings. Thus, it may be argued that the Bird V.I.P. is actually time cycled in the VOLUME CYCLED modes. But to avoid confusion, we will assume that the manufacturer's nomenclature is correct. Tidal volume may be set from 20 to 995 mL. The set tidal volume is equal to the volume delivered to the patient circuit corrected to body temperature (37°C). Inspiration is flow cycled when using PRESSURE SUPPORT as soon as inspiratory flow rate decays to 25% of the PEAK FLOW setting. If a leak prevents flow from decreasing to 25%, the breath will be time cycled after 3 seconds or two breath periods, whichever comes first. There is a TERMINATION SENSITIVITY control (used in conjunction with the Bird Partner volume monitor) that may be used in TIME CYCLED modes. This allows pressure-limited mandatory breaths to be flow cycled based on a percentage of peak flow. The range of settings for flow termination is 5% to 25% of peak flow in 5% increments. If flow fails to drop to the percent set, as might occur with lower settings and the presence of a leak around the artificial airway, the breath will be time cycled based on the INSPIRATORY TIME control setting. Inspiration is time cycled according to the INSPIRATORY TIME control setting in TIME CYCLED modes.

Baseline pressure may be adjusted from 0 to 24 cm H_2O using the PEEP/CPAP knob.

Control Subsystems

CONTROL CIRCUIT. The Bird V.I.P. uses only electronic control components, although there is a pneumatically driven safety valve that allows the patient to inspire room air in the event of an electrical power failure or a ventilator inoperative state (Fig. 14-22). A microprocessor accepts input signals relating to airway pressure and control variable settings and outputs control signals to the output control valves.

Pressure is measured both at the airway opening and inside the ventilator. Feedback from the proximal airway pressure transducer is used to provide triggering, cycling, display, and alarm signals and to control the airway pressure waveform during pressure-controlled breaths. Proximal airway pressure is also measured with a redundant aneroid pressure gauge. A machine pressure transducer monitors machine outlet pressure and compares it to the proximal airway pressure. If the two signals do not agree within a specified tolerance, a CIRCUIT FAULT alarm is activated.

Flow information is obtained by sensing the position of the stepper motor inside the flow control valve (see Output Control Valves). Signals from the flow control valve are used for adjusting volume and flow.

DRIVE MECHANISM. The Bird V.I.P. uses either external compressed gas (for air and oxygen) or an electric motor and compressor (for air) in conjunction with a pressure regulator. Compressed gas from the blender (an internally mounted Bird 3800 Micro Blender) passes into a 1.1-L rigid chamber accumulator. The purpose of the accumulator is to store pressurized gas for augmenting the blender flow during high inspiratory flow demands. The blender is capable of delivering approximately 75 L/min with inlet and outlet pressures of 50 and 35 psig, respectively, while the accumulator allows the ventilator to deliver up to 120 L/min. This extra flow capacity is provided from gas stored in the accumulator during the expiratory phase.

Gas from the accumulator flows through a regulator that sets the driving pressure of the flow control valve to 25 psig. Between the regulator and the flow control valve is another accumulator, referred to as a pulsation dampener, with a volume of about 200 mL. This device compensates for transient pressure fluctuations caused by the regulator's slow response time (relative to flow rate changes during a ventilatory cycle) and thus helps to maintain a constant driving pressure to the flow control valve. A constant pressure is necessary to maintain the accuracy of the delivered flow rates and tidal volumes.

OUTPUT CONTROL VALVES. Gas flow to the patient is regulated by two electromechanical valves. For the main flow control valve, rotary motion of a stepper motor is transformed to linear motion required for controlling flow through a variable poppet type orifice. One valve controls the instantaneous flow rate of gas during inspiration. This valve is designed and calibrated to obtain a known relationship between position and orifice opening. With the system pressure at 25 psig, flow through the variable orifice is unaffected by downstream patient circuit pressures up to 350 cm H_2O. The range of the valve is 0 to 120 L/min with an approximate resolution of 0.1 L/min. An optical sensor detects the zero flow position.

The second output control valve is used to occlude the expiratory path during inspiration and when PEEP/CPAP are used. The microprocessor coordinates the activity of both valves such that the exhalation valve closes as the flow control valves begin to deliver flow to the patient circuit.

A jet solenoid is used to drive the exhalation valve jet venturi. This valve is used only for TIME CYCLED

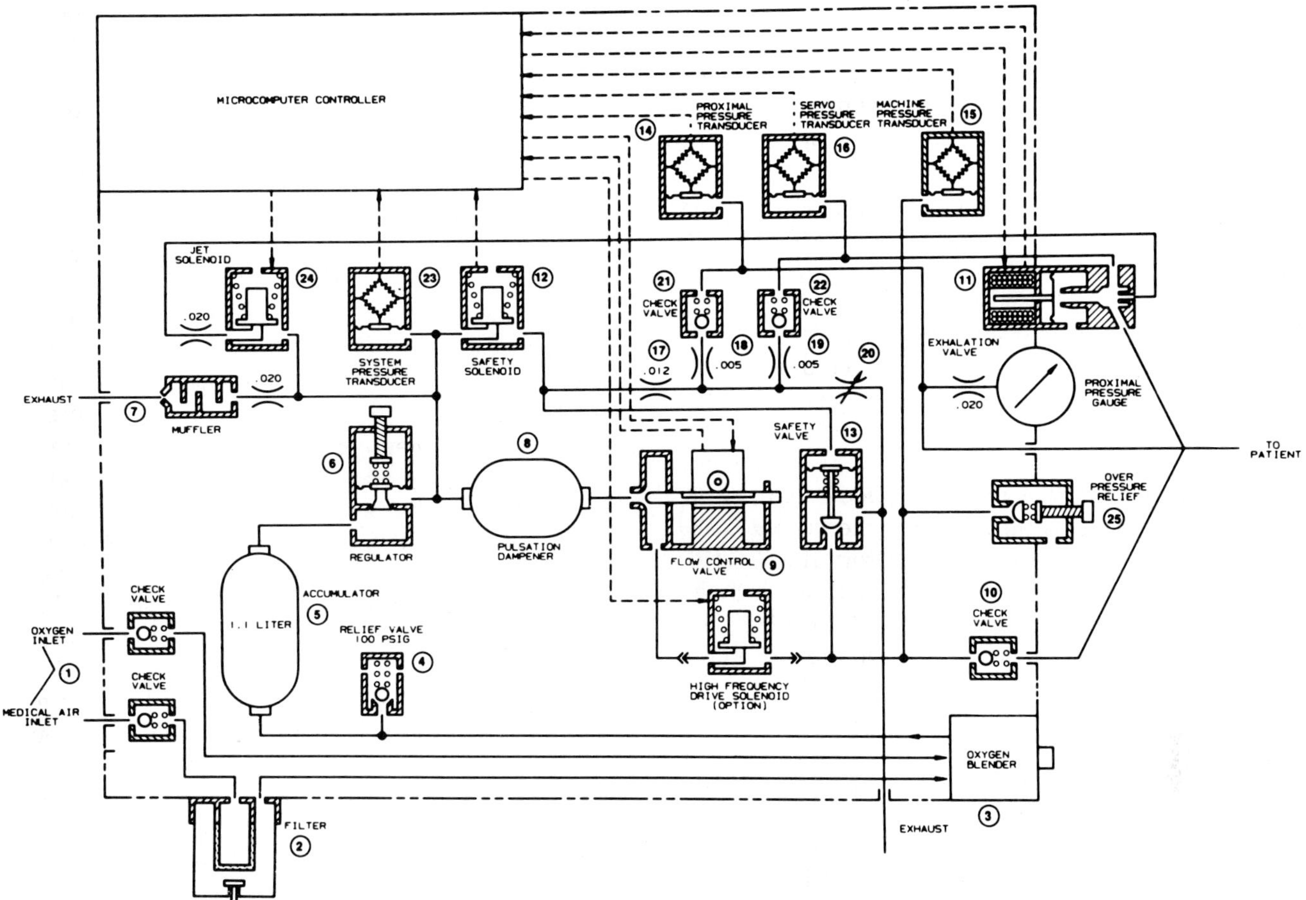

Figure 14-22. Internal components of the Bird V.I.P. ventilator control circuit. (Courtesy of Bird Products Corporation, Palm Springs, CA)

modes to overcome the inadvertent PEEP created by continuous flow through the exhalation leg of the patient circuit.

Output Displays

In addition to the various control settings, the front panel digital displays include PIP, mean airway pressure, breath rate, inspiratory time, I:E ratio, patient effort (indicates patient inspiratory effort that exceeds the ASSIST SENSITIVITY setting), and demand (indicates that a patient inspiratory effort has exceeded the pre-set trigger sensitivity during TIME CYCLED IMV). Airway pressures are also displayed on an aneroid pressure gauge.

Modes of Operation

The mode selector switch is labeled with two groups of modes. The TIME CYCLED group includes (S)IMV/CPAP and ASSIST/CONTROL. The VOLUME CYCLED group includes ASSIST/CONTROL and SIMV/CPAP.

Volume-Cycled Modes

ASSIST/CONTROL. In this mode, inspiration is flow controlled, pressure triggered (according to the ASSIST SENSITIVITY setting) or time triggered (according to the BREATH RATE setting), flow limited (by PEAK FLOW setting), and volume cycled (by TIDAL VOLUME setting).

SIMV/CPAP. In SIMV, mandatory breaths are flow controlled, pressure triggered (depending on the presence of spontaneous breathing efforts and the ASSIST SENSITIVITY setting), or time triggered (according to the BREATH RATE setting), flow limited (by PEAK FLOW setting), and volume cycled (by TIDAL VOLUME setting).

Spontaneous inspirations between mandatory breaths are pressure controlled (ie, inspiratory flow varies to maintain the set PEEP value), pressure triggered, and normally pressure cycled. Inspiration is flow cycled when the PRESSURE SUPPORT setting is above zero.

A mandatory breath is pressure triggered the first time a spontaneous breathing effort is detected during each ventilatory period (the time equal to the reciprocal of the BREATH RATE setting). Subsequent breathing efforts during the same period will not trigger another mandatory breath. If a breathing effort is not detected during a given ventilatory period, a mandatory breath will be delivered at the beginning of the next period. The ventilator will then deliver another mandatory breath the first time a spontaneous inspiratory effort is detected at which time the sequence of events repeats itself.

If the breath rate is set at zero, the mode is CPAP by definition and all breaths are pressure triggered, pressure limited, and pressure cycled.

Time-Cycled Modes

(S)IMV/CPAP. In IMV, mandatory breaths are pressure controlled, time triggered (according to the BREATH RATE setting), pressure limited (HIGH PRESSURE LIMIT setting), and time cycled (INSPIRATORY TIME SETTING). Spontaneous breaths are supported by a continuous flow (determined by the FLOW RATE setting) and the demand flow system (if spontaneous inspiratory flow exceeds the set flow rate such that airway pressure drops 1 cm H_2O below baseline). Breaths activating demand flow are pressure triggered, pressure limited, and pressure cycled. In (S)IMV/CPAP (using the Bird Partner volume monitor option), mandatory breaths are pressure controlled, flow triggered (depending on the presence of spontaneous breathing efforts and the ASSIST SENSITIVITY setting), pressure limited, and time cycled. If the TERMINATION SENSITIVITY is set to a value other than off, one spontaneous breath will be pressure supported per ventilatory cycle. That is, the first spontaneous breath in each period (period length is determined by BREATH RATE setting) will be flow triggered, pressure limited, and flow cycled. All other spontaneous breaths during the period will be supported by the continuous flow or the demand system.

ASSIST/CONTROL. (optional) In this mode, inspiration is pressure controlled, flow triggered (depending on the presence of spontaneous breathing efforts and the ASSIST SENSITIVITY setting) or time triggered (according to the BREATH RATE setting), pressure limited, and flow cycled (according to the TERMINATION SENSITIVITY setting).

Alarms

INPUT POWER ALARMS. Alarms are activated if the AC power supply fails or if the compressed gas supply drops below 22.5 psig or rises above 27.5 psig. An audible blender input gas alarm is activated whenever the pressure differential between the input air pressure and input oxygen pressure exceeds 20 psig. During this alarm, the higher of the two pressures is "bypassed" through to the ventilator (ie, either 21% or 100% oxygen).

CONTROL VARIABLE ALARMS. There are several alarms associated with ventilating pressures. One is a LOW PEEP/CPAP alarm that is adjustable from −9 to 24 cm H_2O. It is activated if the proximal airway pressure drops below the alarm setting for longer than 0.5 second at any time during the ventilatory cycle. A high inspiratory pressure alarm is adjustable from 3 to 120 cm H_2O. The HIGH PRESSURE LIMIT setting acts as the alarm in the VOLUME CYCLED modes (actually a high pressure alarm and cycling mechanism, not a pressure limit). The same dial behaves as a true pressure limit setting in the TIME CYCLED modes. A HIGH PRESSURE alarm is activated (and inspiration is cycled off) if the proximal airway pressure exceeds the HIGH PEAK PRESSURE LIMIT setting by 10 cm H_2O in the TIME CYCLED modes. This same alarm will activate (but no action is taken) in all modes if the proximal airway pressure exceeds PEEP + 6 cm H_2O continuously for 250 ms commencing 500 ms after the start of the expiratory phase. A low inspiratory pressure alarm is triggered if the airway pressure fails to exceed the alarm setting during inspiration (adjustable from 3 to 120 cm H_2O and may be turned off). This alarm is active for mandatory breaths only (eg, is not active for pressure supported breaths).

An APNEA alarm is triggered if the interval between any mechanical or spontaneous breath exceeds an internally set interval of 20, 40, or 60 seconds. This is active in the VOLUME CYCLED modes only.

CONTROL CIRCUIT ALARMS. A VENTILATOR INOPERATIVE alarm is activated if any of the following conditions occur:

- Electrical power supply voltages out of range
- System gas pressure, less than 20 psig or greater than 30 psig for longer than 1 second
- Software detection of an out of tolerance condition

When activated, this alarm causes the ventilator to cease operation and vent the patient circuit to room air. When the first and second conditions in the previous list no longer exist, the ventilator will run a self-test and resume normal operation. The third condition requires that the power switch be turned off and back on to reset the ventilator.

A CIRCUIT FAULT alarm is activated if proximal airway–machine outlet pressure difference or proximal airway–exhalation valve pressure difference is out of tolerance. Once activated, the ventilator is cycled off. If the condition continues for greater than 8 seconds, the patient circuit will be vented to room air. This alarm is active during all modes of ventilation except during the inspiratory phase of a pressure supported breath.

EMERSON 3MV

The Emerson 3MV ventilator (J. H. Emerson, Cambridge, MA) (Fig. 14-23) is a pressure or volume controller that is time or manually triggered, may be pressure limited, and is volume or time cycled. It requires an external air–oxygen blender.

Input Variables

The Emerson 3MV uses 115 volts AC at 60 Hz to power the control circuitry and drive mechanism. An external air–oxygen blender is required to provide a continuous flow of gas for IMV operation and for control of FIO_2.

The front panel of the Emerson 3MV is illustrated in Figure 14-24. The operator may select the tidal volume, inspiratory time, and total cycle time.

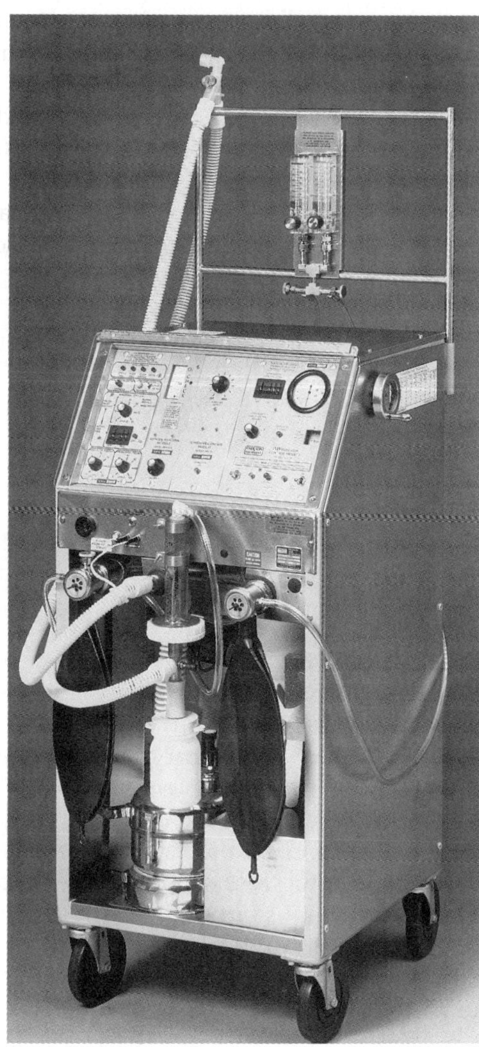

Figure 14-23. The Emerson 3MV ventilator. (Courtesy of J. H. Emerson, Cambridge, MA)

Control Variables

The Emerson 3MV controls either inspiratory pressure or volume. It controls inspiratory pressure if the pressure pop-off valve (located on top of the humidifier) is set to vent inspiratory pressure at a level below that which would normally be achieved as a result of the set tidal volume and inspiratory flow rate (the latter is indirectly determined by the set tidal volume and inspiratory time). If the pop-off valve is not used, ventilation is volume controlled.

INSPIRATORY WAVEFORMS. Under some conditions, it is possible to achieve an approximately rectangular pressure waveform. More commonly, the ventilator is operated to achieve a sinusoidal inspiratory volume waveform (and hence, a sinusoidal inspiratory flow waveform).

PHASE VARIABLES. Inspiration is time triggered as a function of the set total cycle time. Total cycle time may be adjusted from 2.3 seconds to 5 minutes (1.3 seconds to 5 minutes with the pediatric module). The Emerson 3MV may also be manually triggered.

Inspiration may be pressure limited if the inspiratory pressure is vented to atmosphere by the pressure relief valve (uncalibrated but controllable over a range of 20 to 140 cm H_2O). Flow is limited indirectly as a function of inspiratory time and tidal volume. Volume is not limited as there is no provision for an inspiratory pause.

Although the inspiratory time is adjustable from 1 to 5 seconds (0.5 to 2.5 seconds with the pediatric module), the Emerson 3MV is normally volume cycled (see Chapter 13). Inspiration is terminated when the ventilator's piston reaches the end of its stroke. Tidal volume may be set from 0 to 2000 mL (0 to 1000 mL with pediatric module). Inspiration may be considered to be time cycled if the pressure relief valve is used to limit inspiratory pressure. In this situation, the volume delivered to the patient will be a function of the airway pressures and lung mechanics and inspiration will be held constant at the set inspiratory time regardless of the load imposed by the patient's respiratory system. The combination of adjustable inspiratory time and total cycle time allows a maximum ventilatory frequency of 26 cycles/ min (45 cycles/min with pediatric module).

Baseline pressure may be adjusted from 0 to 25 cm H_2O using an external water-column PEEP/CPAP valve.

Control Subsystems

CONTROL CIRCUIT. The Emerson 3MV uses pneumatic and electronic control components (Fig. 14-25).

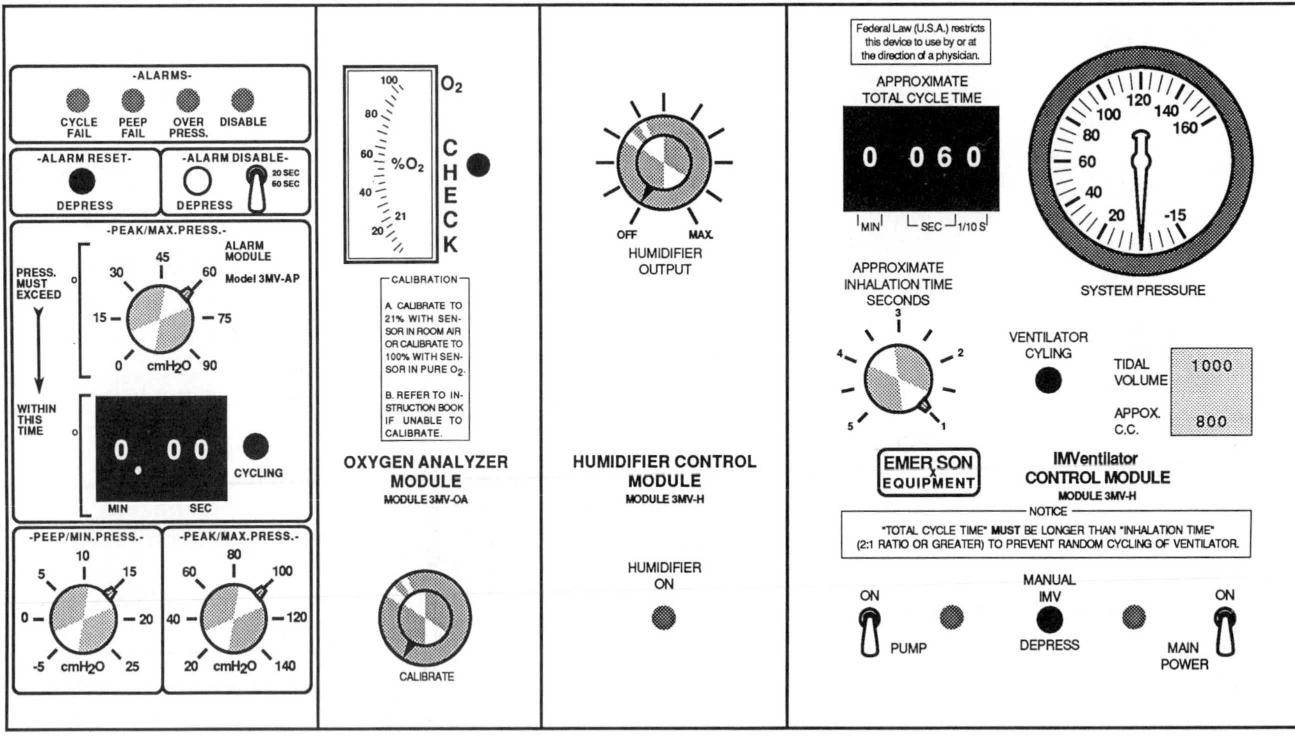

Figure 14-24. Control panel of the Emerson 3MV ventilator.

The electronic control circuitry determines the speed of the forward and backward motion of the ventilator's piston. The forward speed (ie, inspiratory time) is determined by the set inspiratory time. The backward speed (ie, expiratory time) is adjustable to control the ventilatory frequency. A pneumatic signal is taken from the inlet of the humidifier and used to force the PEEP/CPAP valve closed during inspiration.

DRIVE MECHANISM. The Emerson 3MV uses a piston inside a cylinder driven by an AC brushless motor to force gas through the patient circuit.

OUTPUT CONTROL VALVES. The only output control valve is the PEEP/CPAP valve, which also functions as the exhalation manifold. A column of water resting on a rubber manifold determines the backpressure (ie, PEEP) during exhalation. The PEEP level (indicated by the height of the water column) is adjusted by adding or draining off water.

Output Displays

In addition to the tidal volume, total cycle time, and inspiratory time control settings, the Emerson 3MV displays airway pressure on an aneroid pressure gauge (−15 to 160 cm H_2O). The humidifier temperature is adjustable from the front panel (with an uncalibrated dial) and accessory modules allow display of FIO_2 and airway pressure–based alarm conditions.

Modes of Operation

The Emerson 3MV operates exclusively in the continuous-flow IMV mode in which mandatory inspiration is time triggered and volume cycled. As mentioned earlier, a pressure pop-off valve allows inspiration to be time triggered, pressure limited, and time cycled. Spontaneous breaths are drawn from a reservoir bag fed by the external blender.

Alarms

INPUT POWER ALARMS. Audible alarms are activated if the electrical or pneumatic power supplies drop below pre-set levels (110 volts AC and 35 psig, respectively).

CONTROL VARIABLE ALARMS. There are visual and audible alarms associated with high and low ventilating pressures available with an accessory module. The low-pressure threshold is adjustable from −5 to 25 cm H_2O and the high-pressure threshold is adjustable from 0 to 120 cm H_2O. A visual and audible alarm is available that is activated if the measured FIO_2 goes 5% above or 5% below the set threshold (adjustable from 0% to 99 %). The accuracy of the alarm's oxygen analyzer is rated at ±2 % of full scale

CONTROL CIRCUIT ALARMS. A normal cycle alarm is activated if airway pressure fails to exceed a set pressure threshold (adjustable from 0 to 90 cm H_2O) within a specified time window (adjustable from 1 second to 5 minutes).

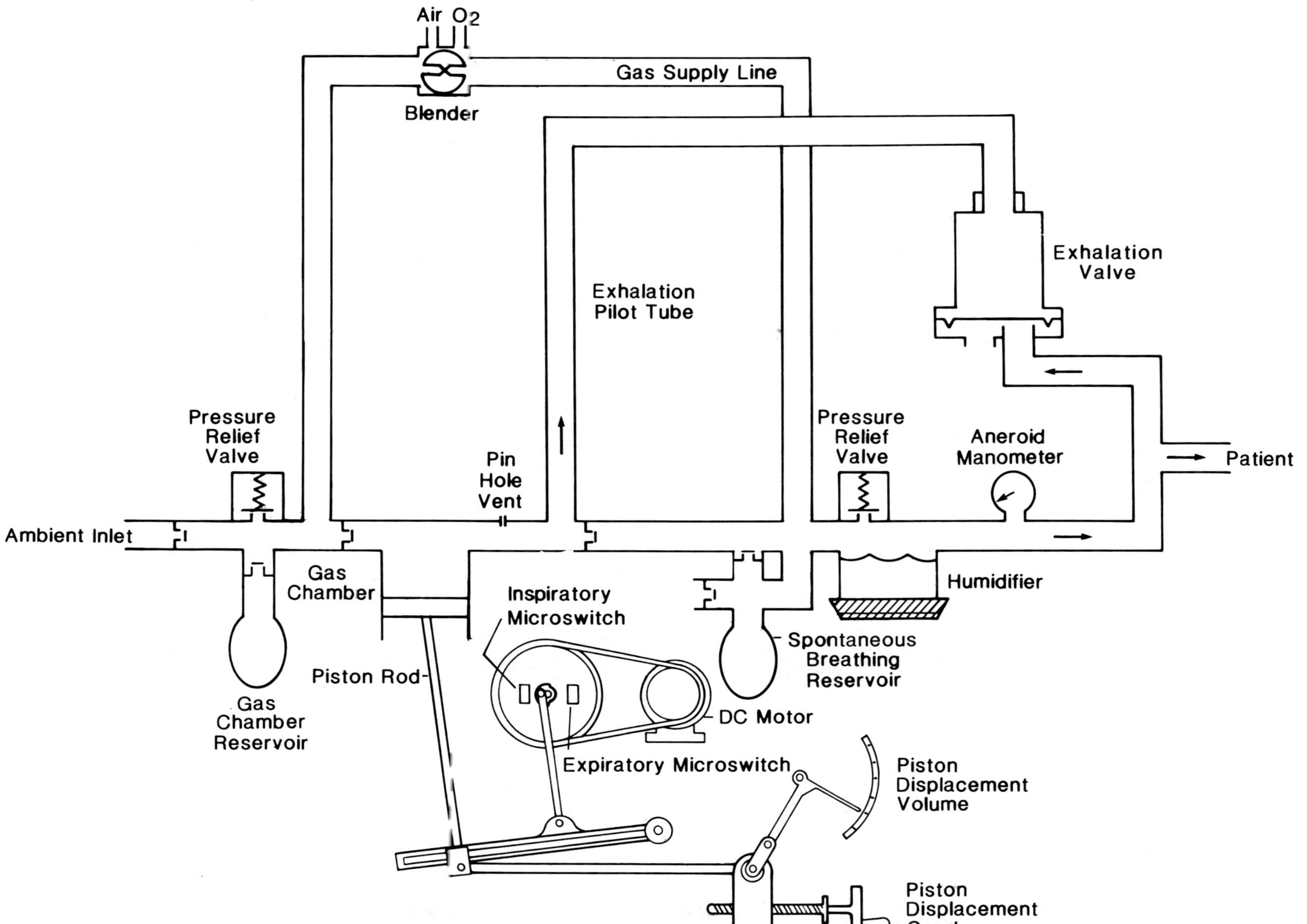

Figure 14-25. Internal components of the Emerson 3MV control circuit.

HAMILTON VEOLAR

The Hamilton Veolar ventilator (Hamilton Medical Corporation, Reno, NV) (Fig. 14-26) is a pressure or flow controller that may be pressure, time, or manually triggered; pressure, volume, or flow limited; and pressure, flow, or time cycled. It has an integral air–oxygen blender and a gas outlet port that will power a nebulizer during inspiration.

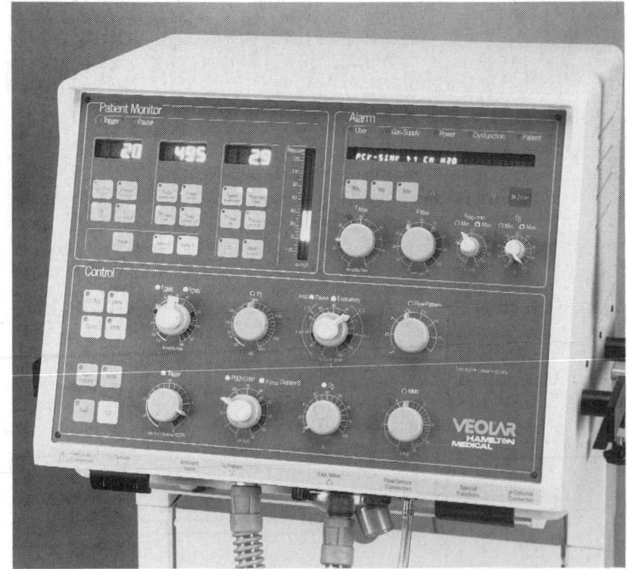

Figure 14-26. The Hamilton Veolar ventilator. (Courtesy of Hamilton Medical Corporation, Reno, NV)

Input Variables

The Veolar uses 115 volts AC at 60 Hz to power the control circuitry. The pneumatic circuit, which includes an integral air–oxygen blender, operates on external compressed gas sources (ie, air and oxygen) at 29 to 116 psig.

The front panel of the Veolar is illustrated in Figure 14-27. The operator may select the mode of ventilation; pressure-triggering, pressure-limiting, and pressure-cycling thresholds; PEEP/CPAP; tidal volume; I:E ratio; flow waveform; ventilatory frequency; inspiratory pause time; and F_{IO_2}. Ventilatory modes are selected using membrane switches (ie, touch key pushbuttons), and control settings are adjusted with calibrated dials.

Control Variables

The Veolar controls either inspiratory pressure or flow. It controls inspiratory pressure in the spontaneous and MMV modes. It controls flow in the CMV mode and switches between pressure control (for spontaneous breaths) and flow control (for mandatory breaths) in the SIMV mode.

INSPIRATORY WAVEFORMS. The Veolar offers one inspiratory pressure and four inspiratory flow waveforms. A rectangular pressure waveform can be achieved in the MMV mode or when pressure support is activated in the SIMV or spontaneous modes. Flow waveforms include ascending ramp, rectangular, descending ramp, and sine. Gas delivery with the rectangular waveform is relatively constant, and peak inspiratory flow rate is equivalent to the mean inspiratory flow rate, which is estimated from the tidal volume, frequency, and inspiratory time settings:

$$\begin{array}{c}\text{Mean inspiratory}\\ \text{flow rate (L/min)}\end{array} = \frac{\text{Tidal volume (L)} \times \text{frequency}}{\text{\% Cycle time/100}}$$

Note that inspiratory pause % (if used) is not included in the % cycle time. When the ascending ramp waveform is selected, flow starts out at its peak value (twice the mean inspiratory flow rate) and decreases linearly to zero. With the descending ramp waveform, inspiratory flow begins at zero and increases linearly to peak flow (twice the mean inspiratory flow rate). When the sine waveform is selected, inspiratory flow goes from zero to peak flow (1.57 times the mean inspiratory flow rate) and back to zero in a sinusoidal fashion.

PHASE VARIABLES. Inspiration is pressure triggered when a spontaneous ventilatory effort removes enough gas from the patient circuit to drop the pressure below the trigger setting. The threshold for triggering a mandatory breath is adjustable from 1.0 to 15.0 cm H_2O below the baseline pressure and may be turned off. Inspiration is time triggered as a function of the ventilator frequency, which is adjustable from 5 to 60 cycles/min in the CMV mode or 0.5 to 30 cycles/min in the SIMV mode. The Veolar may also be manually triggered.

Inspiration is pressure limited during spontaneous breaths in the SIMV, MMV, and the spontaneous modes. A demand flow system controls inspiratory pressure by attempting to maintain the set PEEP/CPAP level, which is adjustable from 0 to 50 cm H_2O, if pressure support is not used. If pressure support is used, the pressure limit may be set from 0 to 50 cm H_2O above the PEEP/CPAP level. Inspiration is volume limited whenever the inspiratory pause time is greater than zero. Inspiration is flow limited for mandatory breaths. Peak inspiratory flow rate is indirectly controlled by the tidal volume, frequency, % cycle time, and waveform settings (see Inspiratory Waveforms earlier). A peak flow of up to 180 L/min is available.

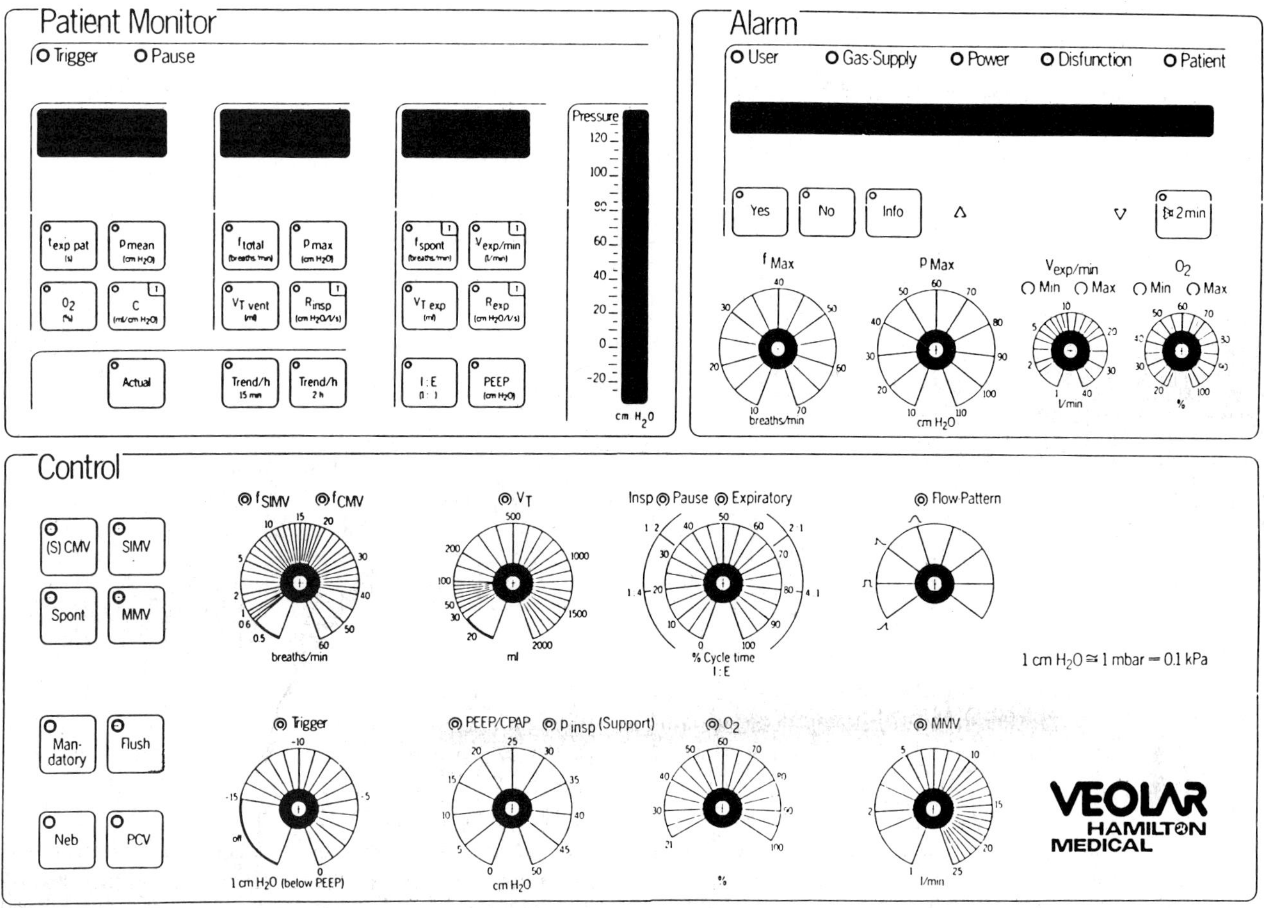

Figure 14-27. Control panel of the Hamilton Veolar ventilator. (Courtesy of Hamilton Medical Corporation, Reno, NV)

Inspiration is terminated when one of three variables reaches a pre-set threshold. Inspiration may be pressure cycled when the maximum inspiratory pressure threshold is violated. It may be set over a range of 10 to 110 cm H_2O. Active inspiratory flow is also pressure cycled for spontaneous breaths when pressure support is not used (when expiration causes airway pressure to rise above the PEEP setting). Inspiration cannot be volume cycled because the Veolar measures instantaneous flow rather than volume. However, when inspiration is flow controlled, tidal volume may be set from 20 to 2000 mL. Inspiration is flow cycled when using pressure support (ie, when Pinsp is set above zero) as soon as inspiratory flow rate decays to 25% of the peak flow rate for the breath. Inspiration is time cycled for flow-controlled breaths whenever the inspiratory time reaches the value determined by frequency and % cycle time settings (% inspiration is adjustable from 20% to 80%, equivalent to I:E ratios of 1:4 to 4:1). Inspiratory time is extended when the inspiratory pause time is set above zero. Inspiratory pause time is set as a percentage of the total ventilatory cycle using the % cycle time dual knob control (eg, with the insp dial set at 30 % and the expiratory dial set at 50 %, a 20 % inspiratory time will result).

Baseline pressure may be adjusted from 0 to 50 cm H_2O using the PEEP/CPAP function.

Control Subsystems

CONTROL CIRCUIT. The Veolar uses only electronic control components (Fig. 14-28). A pair of Intel 8031 microprocessors operating in parallel accept input signals relating to airway pressure and inspiratory flow as well as control variable settings and outputs control signals to the output control valves. The pressure transducer measures airway pressure from inside the ventilator. An optional transducer is available to measure pressure at any location outside the ventilator such as the airway opening. Feedback signals from the airway pressure transducer are used to provide triggering, cycling, and alarm signals and to control the airway pressure waveform during pressure-controlled breaths.

Flow information is obtained by measuring the pressure across the servo-controlled flow valve along with feedback from a high-precision linear potentiometer that senses the position of the valve's piston (see Output Control Valve). Signals from the servo-

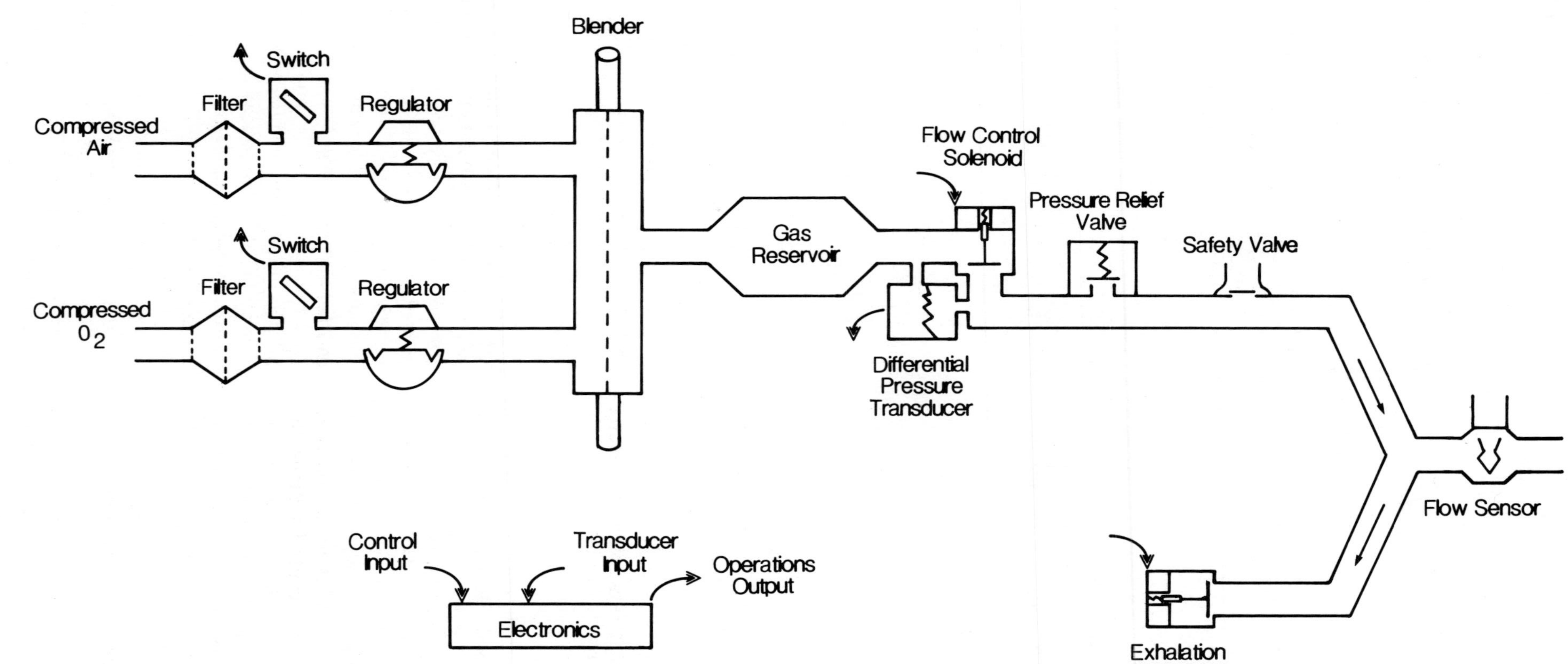

Figure 14-28. Internal components of the Hamilton Veolar control circuit. (Courtesy of Hamilton Medical Corporation, Reno, NV)

controlled flow valve are used for shaping the inspiratory flow waveform and maintaining the desired tidal volume.

The inspired oxygen concentration is also controlled by the microprocessor by adjusting the ratio of air flow to oxygen flow from compressed sources. The oxygen control system is accurate to within ± 5% of the set FIO_2.

DRIVE MECHANISM. The Veolar uses either external compressed gas (for air and oxygen) or an electric motor and compressor (for air) in conjunction with a pressure regulator. Gas pressure is regulated internally to about 22 psig for use by the gas mixer. Gas from the mixer is sent to a pressurized reservoir tank which holds a volume of about 8 L at a pressure of 350 cm H_2O. The flow control system is driven by the pressure from the accumulator. During a flow demand, the volume stored in the accumulator is exhausted quickly, reducing the instantaneous flow demand required of the blending system and upstream pressure regulating system. This action allows a wide range of peak flows, reduces the flow required of the compressed gas supply, and improves response time. The accumulator also acts as a mixing chamber, which helps to stabilize the delivered oxygen concentration within a given breath. A flush control button is provided on the front panel display. When activated, the expiratory valve opens full and the inspiratory valve produces 60 L/min of continuous flow to purge the gas reservoir tank, shortening the response time for large changes in FIO_2.

OUTPUT CONTROL VALVES. Gas flow to the patient is regulated by two electromechanical valves consisting of an electrodynamic motor (similar to a music speaker) connected to a piston. One valve controls the instantaneous flow rate of gas during inspiration. Connected to this valve's piston is a plunger that has a triangular orifice. The triangular shape was chosen because there is a specific relationship between the height of the triangular opening, the pressure on either side of the plunger, and the resulting flow. A high-precision linear potentiometer provides feedback to the microprocessor indicating the height of the opening, and a differential pressure transducer provides feedback for the pressure across the plunger. Based on the control settings, the microprocessor determines the correct current to send to the motor to raise the plunger. The resulting height and pressure drop across the plunger are used to calculate the flow rate. The flow control system is capable of delivering peak flows up to 180 L/min. Peak inspiratory flow is set indirectly as a function of the tidal volume, frequency, % cycle time, and waveform settings (see Inspiratory Waveforms).

The second electrodynamic motor and piston are used in conjunction with a large surface silicone membrane to occlude the expiratory path during inspiration and when PEEP/CPAP is used. The microprocessor coordinates the activity of both valves such that the exhalation valve closes as the flow control valves begin to deliver flow to the patient circuit.

Output Displays

In addition to the various control settings, the front panel displays include total (spontaneous and mandatory) and spontaneous ventilatory frequencies; delivered and exhaled tidal volumes; exhaled minute volume; peak, mean, and baseline airway pressures; a bar graph display of dynamic ventilatory pressure; and a wide variety of alarm and special operational help messages. The Veolar is unique in that it measures actual exhaled volumes at the airway opening with a small, disposable pneumotachometer (flow sensor). Several of the control variable and control circuit alarms are based on measurements made by the flow sensor.

The Veolar also calculates and displays respiratory system compliance and resistance. Static mechanics are calculated from tidal volume and inspiratory flow rate along with peak inspiratory, plateau, and baseline pressures by initiating an inspiratory pause during a volume-controlled breath. Because these variables can be measured at the airway opening, the values for compliance and resistance reflect only respiratory system (and endotracheal tube) mechanics uncontaminated by patient delivery circuit effects.

Several measured variables can be stored and later recalled for trend analysis. These include compliance, resistance, spontaneous breathing frequency, and expiratory minute volume. Both 15-minute and 2-hour trends are available.

Analog pressure, volume, and flow signals along with an inspiratory/expiratory time signal and an alarm relay (for remote alarms) may be obtained from the back of the ventilator using a standard DB-9 female connector. Most of the data available on the front of the ventilator can also be output to a serial printer through an RS 232C connector.

Modes of Operation

The following modes are those named on the control panel of the Veolar:

CMV. During continuous mechanical ventilation, inspiration is flow controlled, is pressure triggered (depending on the presence of spontaneous breathing efforts and the trigger setting) or time triggered (according to the CMV frequency setting), is flow limited, and time cycled. Tidal volume remains relatively constant from breath to breath, as determined by the tidal volume setting.

SIMV. In SIMV, mandatory breaths are flow controlled, pressure triggered (depending on the presence of spontaneous breathing efforts and the trigger setting) or time triggered (according to the SIMV frequency setting), flow limited, and time cycled.

Spontaneous inspirations between mandatory breaths are pressure controlled (ie, inspiratory flow varies to maintain the set PEEP value), pressure triggered, and normally pressure cycled. Inspiration is flow cycled when the Pinsp (ie, pressure support) setting is above zero.

A mandatory breath is pressure triggered the first time a spontaneous breathing effort is detected during each CMV ventilatory period (the time equal to the reciprocal of the CMV frequency). Subsequent breathing efforts during the same period will not trigger another mandatory breath. If a breathing effort is not detected during a given SIMV ventilatory period (the time equal to the reciprocal of the SIMV frequency), a mandatory breath will be delivered at the beginning of the next period. The ventilator will continue to deliver mandatory breaths according to the SIMV frequency setting until a spontaneous breath is detected, and the sequence of events repeats itself.

SPONTANEOUS. All inspirations are pressure controlled (ie, inspiratory flow varies to maintain either the set CPAP value or the pressure support value if this option is used), pressure triggered, and normally pressure cycled. Inspiration is flow cycled when using pressure support.

MMV. Minimum minute ventilation is a spontaneous breathing mode with pressure support. The difference between the spontaneous mode and MMV is in the control of the pressure support level. In the spontaneous mode, the operator manually selects the level of pressure support. In MMV, the ventilator determines the level of pressure support based on the exhaled minute volume. Once MMV is selected, the Veolar provides pressure support at the level set by the pressure support control for the first eight breaths. From the tidal volume of these eight breaths, the ventilator calculates an expected minute volume and compares that with the desired level as set on the MMV control. If the patient's expected minute volume is less than desired, the ventilator will begin to add pressure support. If the patient's minute volume is larger than the desired amount, the pressure support will drop. The amount of pressure support change is dependent on the difference between the desired minute volume and the expected minute volume. Any changes in pressure support are gradual, usually 1 to 2 cm H_2O at a time. The maximum increase in pressure support allowed is 30 cm H_2O above CPAP or 50 cm H_2O above atmospheric pressure. In the event of an alarm, the pressure support will remain frozen until all alarms have cleared.

Emergency Mode of Ventilation

The following emergency mode of ventilation is automatically triggered if the operator initially selects this option immediately after startup.

APNEA BACKUP VENTILATION. Apnea ventilation is triggered during the SIMV, spontaneous, or MMV modes if apnea is detected or if the measured expired minute volume drops below 1.0 L/min. The mode used during backup depends on which mode the patient was in before the apnea occurred. If the patient was in SIMV, the ventilator will switch to CMV. If the patient was in the spontaneous or MMV mode, the ventilator will switch to SIMV. In all cases, the patient will be ventilated at the current operator-selected values for frequency, tidal volume, inspiratory time, and flow waveform.

Alarms

All alarms are visual and audible.

INPUT POWER ALARMS. Alarms are activated if the AC power supply fails, if the compressed gas supply drops below 29 psig, or if the pressure in the internal reservoir tank drops below 200 cm H_2O. Separate alarms are provided for the air and oxygen sources.

Note: Several of the control variable and control circuit alarms are based on measurements made by the disposable flow sensor attached to the patient's airway opening.

CONTROL VARIABLE ALARMS. There are two alarms associated with ventilating pressures. One is a low PEEP/CPAP alarm that is nonadjustable and automatically triggered if pressure has fallen 3 cm H_2O below the set PEEP level. The other is a high inspiratory pressure alarm adjustable from 10 to 120 cm H_2O.

There are two alarms associated with exhaled volumes. Low or high exhaled minute volume alarms are activated if the minute volume measured at the airway opening passes through the set threshold (both adjustable from 1 to 40 L/min).

There are alarms for high ventilatory frequency (adjustable from 0 to 70 cycles/min) and apnea. The apnea alarm is triggered if the patient has not exhaled through the flow sensor during the last 15 seconds (nonadjustable). The apnea is detected, and the backup ventilation mode is automatically triggered (if this option has been activated by the operator). A nonadjustable fail to cycle alarm is triggered if there has been no inspiratory flow through the servo flow valve during the last 20 seconds. The usual cause is a failure of the patient to trigger the ventilator due to prolonged exhalation and then apnea.

Low- or high-oxygen alarms are triggered if the measured inspired oxygen concentration passes through the set threshold (both adjustable from 18% to 103%).

CONTROL CIRCUIT ALARMS. A nonadjustable alarm is triggered if the desired peak inspiratory flow rate is beyond the 180 L/min capability of the ventilator. This usually occurs if the set % inspiratory time is too short for the set CMV frequency and tidal volume.

A set trigger alarm is activated if the trigger is set to the off position and the operator tries to activate the SIMV, spontaneous, or MMV modes. Under these conditions, the ventilator will switch to the selected mode then automatically trigger at −5 cm H_2O and alarm until the trigger level is set by the operator.

Two nonadjustable disconnection alarms are provided. A disconnect ventilator side alarm is triggered if the volume measured by the flow sensor during inspiration is less than one half the volume leaving the ventilator servo flow valve, minus 9 mL, for two breaths in a row. A disconnection patient side alarm is triggered if the volume measured by the flow sensor during expiration is less than one-eighth of the volume leaving the servo flow valve, minus 3 mL, for two breaths in a row.

Two nonadjustable tidal volume mismatch alarms are provided. A VT insp mismatch alarm is triggered if the volume measured by the flow sensor during inspiration is more than twice the volume leaving the servo flow valve for three breaths in a row. The usual cause is an incorrect flow sensor measurement (ie, damaged sensor) or disconnection of the flow sensor pressure tubing. A VT exp mismatch alarm is triggered if the volume measured by the flow sensor during expiration is more than one-half the volume leaving the servo flow valve plus 25 mL, for two breaths in a row. The usual cause is that the flow sensor is placed backward at the airway opening.

A technical fault alarm is activated in the event of an internal electronic system failure.

INFRASONICS INFANT STAR

The Infant Star (Infrasonics, San Diego, CA) (Fig. 14-29) is a pressure controller or flow controller that is time triggered and time cycled. It operates in continuous-flow IMV, continuous-flow CPAP, demand-flow IMV, and demand-flow CPAP modes. Because it can control flow, the Infant Star is capable of volume-controlled ventilatory modes (ie, directly controlling flow indirectly controls volume) if operated in such a fashion that it does not limit airway pressure. Additionally, the Infant Star is capable of varying flow in response to negative pressure generated at the patient airway. It has an integral air–oxygen blender and a gas outlet that can power a separate flowmeter that can be mounted on the side of the ventilator.

Input Variables

The Infant Star requires 105 to 123 volts AC at 50 to 60 Hz to power the control circuitry. The main power switch is a recessed, rocker-type located on the back of the electronic module (upper portion). The pneumatic module (lower portion) contains the pneumatic circuit, which includes an integral air–oxygen blender and operates on external compressed gas sources (ie, air and oxygen) at 45 to 90 psig. The Infant Star has no internal compressor.

The front panel of the Infant Star is illustrated in Figure 14.30. The operator may select mode of ventilation, desired peak airway pressure (PIP), desired baseline pressure (PEEP), ventilatory frequency, inspiratory time, and flow rate.

Actual airway pressures are displayed by both an analog pressure gauge and digital displays for PIP, PEEP, and Paw. There are also digital displays for the control variables (desired) PIP, PEEP, inspiratory time, expiratory time, ventilator frequency, and flow rate. In addition, there are digital displays for duration of positive pressure and low inspiratory pressure alarm

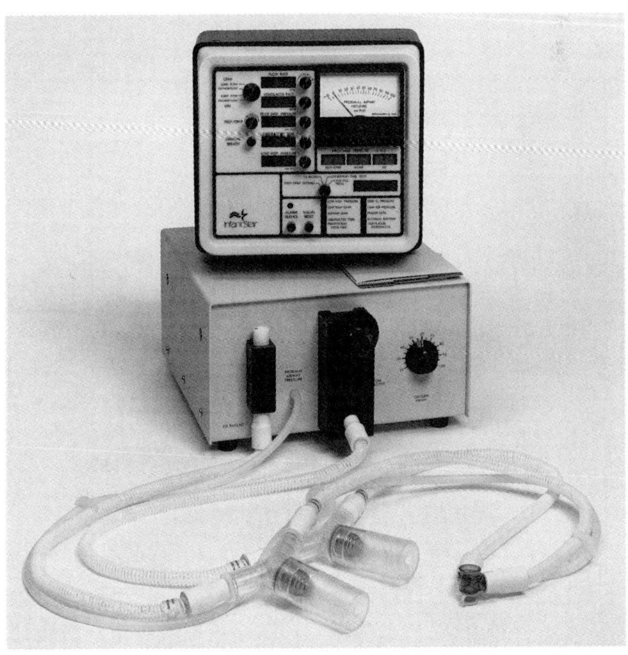

Figure 14-29. The Infrasonics Infant Star ventilator. (Courtesy of Infrasonics, San Diego, CA)

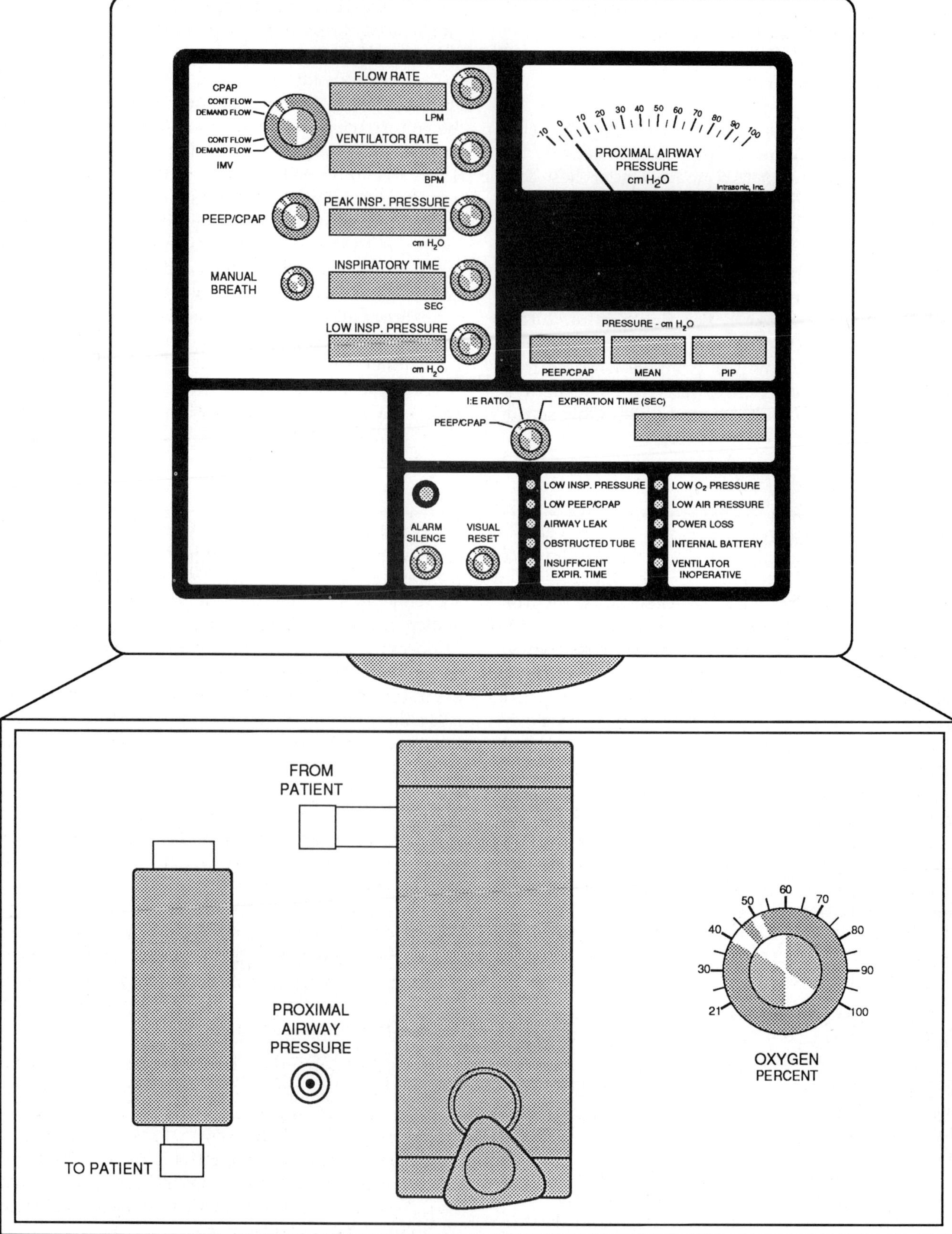

Figure 14-30. Control panel of the Infrasonics Infant Star ventilator.

limit. There are 10 LEDs indicating ventilator status and operating and alarm conditions.

Control Variables

The Infant Star is normally set to control inspiratory pressure. However, as with most infant ventilators, the Infant Star is designed more to limit rather than truly to control inspiratory pressure. This is because the peak inspiratory flow rate is always limited to the value set on the flowmeter. For a given inspiratory time, this flow rate may not be sufficient to achieve the set inspiratory pressure limit in the allotted inspiratory time (depending also on the compliance and resistance of the patient's respiratory system). Thus, in this situation, the Infant Star becomes a flow controller by default.

Flow rate is continuous at an operator set level in continuous flow IMV and continuous flow CPAP modes, unless the patient's spontaneous inspiratory flow rate exceeds that delivered by the ventilator, in which case the negative airway pressure generated by the patient will cause the ventilator to increase the flow rate incrementally until airway pressure returns to baseline values (PEEP level). In addition, the Infant Star can vary flow rate during inspiration and expiration in demand flow IMV and demand flow CPAP. When operating in either one of these modes the Infant Star keeps flow constant at 4 L/min between mechanical breaths, but during the time-triggered, time-cycled IMV breaths, flow delivered by the ventilator is increased to the operator selected level. At the end of inspiration, flow again decreases to 4 L/min. Between mechanical breaths, if the patient's spontaneous inspiratory flow rate exceeds the amount delivered by the ventilator, the negative airway pressure generated by the patient will cause the ventilator to increase flow rate incrementally until airway pressure returns to baseline values (PEEP level).

All control knobs on the Infant Star are designed so that they cannot be accidentally rotated. To set the controls, knobs must be depressed before turning.

INSPIRATORY WAVEFORMS. The Infant Star is most often operated with a rectangular pressure waveform.

If the PIP control is set high enough that the PIP is not limited, then the Infant Star can be operated in a flow-controlled fashion with an approximately rectangular flow waveform.

PHASE VARIABLES. Inspiration is time triggered and is a function of the set ventilator frequency, which is variable from 1 to 150 breaths per minute. From frequencies of 1 to 60, one-breath increments are available, while two-breath increments are available from rates of 61 to 130, and five-breath increments from 131 to 150. The Infant Star may also be manually triggered.

Inspiration may be pressure limited from 5 to 90 cm H_2O. If inspiration is not pressure limited, it is flow limited. The continuous flow rate may be adjusted from 4 to 40 L/min.

Inspiration is time cycled as a function of the set inspiratory time (adjustable from 0.1 to 3.0 seconds). Incremental changes of inspiratory time available are 0.01 second for settings from 0.10 to 0.60 second, 0.02 second for settings from 0.61 to 1.0 second, and 0.1 second for settings from 1.1 to 3.0 seconds. Inspiration is normally pressure cycled if measured peak airway pressure exceeds the control setting for PIP by more than 5 cm H_2O. When this happens the ventilator terminates all flow, activates a visual and audible alarm, and then resumes normal operation. However, this function can be overridden by a mechanical pressure-limiting pop-off valve.

Baseline pressure may be adjusted over the range of 0 to 24 cm H_2O using the PEEP/CPAP control knob.

Control Subsystems

CONTROL CIRCUIT. The Infant Star is electronically controlled by dual Intel type 8085 microprocessors. One microprocessor controls ventilator operations while the other provides display information. A schematic of the Infant Star's internal components is shown in Figure 14-31. Pressure is measured at the airway opening (the point of connection to the patient) and inside the ventilator by two pressure transducers. The airway pressures displayed on the control panel are those measured at the airway opening and are used by the pressure alarm systems.

Feedback signals from the transducer measuring pressure at the airway opening are used to adjust flow rates to achieve and maintain desired PIP and to control a venturi jet in the exhalation block to compensate automatically for inadvertent PEEP.

In addition, peak air pressure may be manually controlled by adjusting a spring-loaded pressure relief valve located at the output of the ventilator. Using the manual pressure relief valve in this fashion incapacitates many of the Infant Star's alarms that are activated in over-pressure situations.

DRIVE MECHANISM. The Infant Star requires an external pneumatic power source (compressed air and oxygen at 45 to 90 psig) to power a blender capable of delivering 21% to 100% oxygen. This blender employs a storage system and an electronic snap-acting regulator that turns the blender on and off, thus reducing waste of gas. The flow of this blended gas is controlled by a series of flow solenoids.

OUTPUT CONTROL VALVES. The Infant Star has six solenoid valves controlling flow. Three valves are preset to deliver 16 L/min: one is set at 8 L/min, one at 4

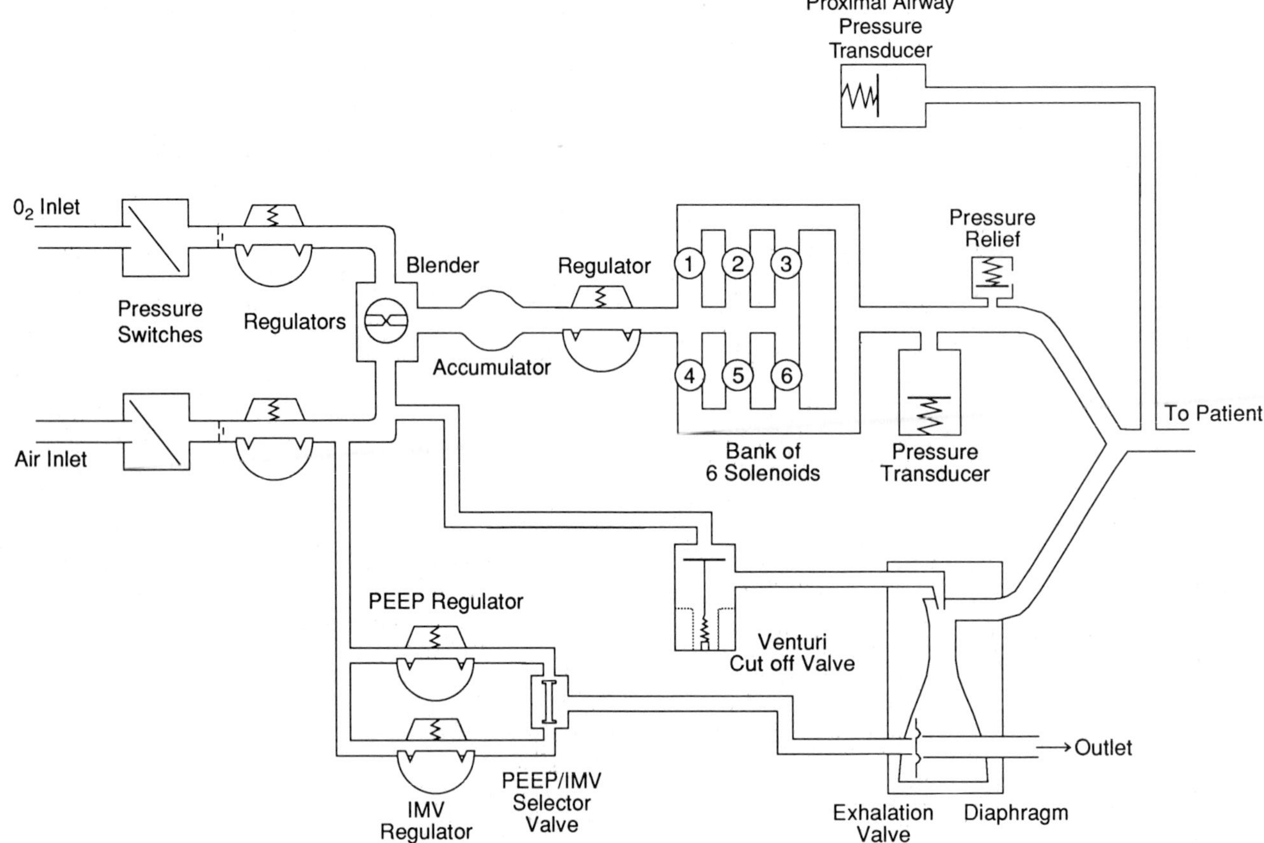

Figure 14-31. Internal components of the Infrasonics Infant Star control circuit.

L/min, and one at 2 L/min. By opening these solenoids in various combinations, flow rates from 4 to 40 L/min are available in 2-L/min increments. During a mandatory breath, another solenoid valve directs a pneumatic signal to one side of a diaphragm valve in the exhalation manifold. This occludes the expiratory limb of the patient circuit, diverting gas into the patient's airway. The pressure in the patient circuit increases until it matches the level determined by the inspiratory pressure limit control. As the measured airway pressure approaches about 75% of the set pressure limit, the flow valves begin to close and slow the inspiratory flow rate to avoid overshooting the desired airway pressure. When the measured airway pressure matches the set pressure, all flow is terminated. The flow valves can turn on again if needed during the pressure plateau portion of the inspiratory time (ie, if a drop in airway pressure is detected) to keep airway pressure constant.

During the expiratory phase, the flow valves switch on again and the exhalation manifold permits gas from the valves and the patient to exit to the atmosphere. However, a bias pressure remains on one side of the diaphragm to create PEEP/CPAP.

Output Displays

Digital displays on the Infant Star are color coded, with ventilator control settings in red and patient monitoring parameters in amber. Ventilators manufactured before December 1, 1986, may have red displays for monitored pressures instead of amber. Digital output displays include PIP, PEEP, mean airway pressure, inspiratory time, expiratory time, and I:E ratio.

Modes of Operation

The mode selector switch on the Infant Star is divided into two sections labeled CPAP and IMV, each of which has a continuous-flow and a demand-flow capability.

CONTINUOUS-FLOW IMV. Inspiration is pressure controlled, time triggered (based on the set ventilator rate), and time cycled (based on the set inspiratory time). There is a continuous flow of gas from the ventilator between mandatory breaths at the rate set on the flow rate control knob. If inspiration is not pressure limited (due to insufficient flow or inspiratory time), it is flow limited, time triggered, and time cycled.

If, during spontaneous breaths, the patient's inspiratory flow rate exceeds that delivered by the ventilator such that airway pressure drops more than 1 cm H_2O below the baseline pressure, the Infant Star will incrementally increase flow from 4 to 40 L/m to keep baseline pressure (PEEP) constant. It does this in all available modes.

DEMAND-FLOW IMV. Inspiration is pressure controlled, time triggered (based on the set ventilator rate), and time cycled (based on the set inspiratory time). Between mandatory breaths there is a continuous flow of gas at 4 L/min, but this increases to the value set on the flow rate control knob during the inspiratory portion of the mandatory breath. At end-inspiration, flow rate again drops to a factory pre-set value of 4 L/min. If inspiration is not pressure limited, it is flow limited, time triggered, and time cycled.

CONTINUOUS-FLOW CPAP. Spontaneous inspirations are pressure controlled (ie, flow rate can be varied to maintain the baseline pressure). If the patient's spontaneous inspiratory flow rate exceeds that supplied by the ventilator such that airway pressure drops more than 1 cm H_2O below the baseline pressure, the ventilator will vary inspiratory flow rate to keep baseline pressure constant. Otherwise the flow rate will remain constant at the level set on the flow rate control knob.

DEMAND-FLOW CPAP. This is the same as for continuous-flow CPAP except that flow rate delivered by the ventilator between spontaneous breaths is always at the pre-set level of 4 L/min, unless the patient generates an inspiratory flow rate large enough that airway pressure drops more than 1 cm H_2O below the baseline pressure, in which case the ventilator will vary flow rate to keep baseline pressure constant.

Alarms

INPUT POWER ALARMS. When external electrical power supply to the Infant Star is interrupted, the internal battery light goes on and the ventilator automatically switches to an internal battery and will operate for up to 30 minutes. Additionally, the ventilator beeps an audible alarm and alternately illuminates the power loss and internal battery lights when there are only 5 to 10 minutes remaining until full battery discharge. When the battery fully discharges, the ventilator inoperative and power loss light activates and there is an audible alarm.

A drop of oxygen inlet pressure to <45 psig results in an audible alarm and an activation of the low O_2 light. The ventilator will continue to operate, delivering an FIO_2 of 0.21. If the set FIO_2 is more than 0.80, ventilator performance may be compromised.

A drop of air inlet pressure to less than 45 psig results in an audible alarm and an activation of the low air light. Additionally, the ventilator stops cycling, gas flow stops, and the internal vent valve and the exhalation valve open, allowing the patient to breathe spontaneously from room air.

CONTROL VARIABLE ALARMS. There is an audible alarm and the "low insp" pressure light is activated if airway pressure does not meet an operator-established minimum level during the mandatory breath.

The low PEEP/CPAP light is activated and an audible alarm sounds when the measured PEEP falls below the alarm threshold for a 25-second period. The threshold for this alarm is automatically set by the microprocessor, based on the PEEP/CPAP setting. If the PEEP/CPAP setting is from 0 to 5 cm H_2O, the measured PEEP must be more than 2 cm H_2O below the set level to activate the alarm. If the PEEP/CPAP setting is from 6 to 8 cm H_2O, then the measured PEEP must be more than 3 cm H_2O below the set level. If the PEEP/CPAP setting is from 9 to 12 cm H_2O, then the measured PEEP must be more than 4 cm H_2O below the set level. If the PEEP/CPAP setting is from 13 to 24 cm H_2O, then the measured PEEP must be more than 5 cm H_2O below the set level. This feature is designed to allow for normal variations in PEEP associated with spontaneous breathing to occur without activating the alarm.

The airway leak light is activated and an audible alarm sounds if the demand flow rate exceeds the continuous flow rate by at least 8 L/min for more than 4 seconds. This is most likely to occur in demand flow IMV or demand flow CPAP and is designed to identify gross airway leaks.

The obstructed tube alarm is designed to activate under five different conditions. When any of these conditions occur, the obstructed tube light is activated, a variety of audible alarms sound (depending on the type of condition), and a message appears in the select display window identifying the problem. If airway pressure rises to more than 5 cm H_2O above the set PIP level during a mandatory breath, there is a single audible beep, the message "HI-PP-AO1" appears, flow is terminated, and both the inspiratory and expiratory side of the circuit are vented to room air to allow pressure to return to zero. PEEP is very quickly restored (usually within 200 ms), and the ventilator continues to cycle. This reaction of the ventilator will result in a loss of tidal volume.

If airway pressure during the mandatory breath rises to more than 10 cm H_2O above the set PIP level, there are multiple audible beeps, the message "HI-PP-AO2" appears, and the ventilator responds as described for the HI-PP-AO1.

The "HI-PP-AO3" message appears (and an audible alarm sounds) if there is an obstruction to exhalation in the patient's airway or the ventilator circuit.

The ventilator monitors how quickly pressure returns to baseline after a mandatory breath. Peak airway pressure must drop more than 50% of the difference between peak airway pressure and baseline pressure in less than 200 ms after the end of inspiration or the alarm will be activated.

When baseline pressure rises 6 cm H_2O above the set PEEP level for more than 5 seconds, the "HI-CP-AO4" message appears and an audible alarm sounds.

As stated earlier, the Infant Star measures pressures both at the airway opening (proximal airway) and inside the ventilator on the inspiratory side. If the machine pressure exceeds the proximal airway pressure by more than 15 cm H_2O, the "HI-PP-AO5" message appears, an audible alarm sounds, flow is terminated, and both the inspiratory and expiratory side of the circuit are vented to room air to allow pressure to return to zero, following which PEEP is restored and the ventilator continues to cycle.

The insufficient expiratory time alarm will activate if the inspiratory time and ventilator rate settings are incompatible, resulting in an unacceptably short expiratory time. For rates from 0 to 100 the minimum allowable expiratory time is 0.3 second, while for rates from 100 to 150 it is 0.2 second. If these threshold values are violated, the ventilator will automatically decrease the ventilator rate until the minimum allowable expiratory time is achieved. The alarm light will be activated, an audible alarm will sound, and the ventilator rate display will flash, indicating the set rate is not being delivered.

All of the Infant Star's audible alarms can be temporarily silenced (for 60 seconds) except the ventilator inoperative alarm. After 24 hours of continuous operation, activation of the alarm silence initiates a re-zero of the pressure transducers.

In the event of an accidental occlusion of the expiratory limb of the ventilator circuit, the Infant Star will sound an alarm, interrupt flow, and vent both sides of the circuit to the atmosphere, allowing the patient to breathe spontaneously from ambient.

CONTROL CIRCUIT ALARMS. When the computer detects an error in the electronic function or exhalation valve function, the ventilator inoperative light is activated, a continuous audible alarm sounds, the machine stops cycling, gas flow is interrupted, and both inspiratory and expiratory sides of the circuit are vented to the atmosphere, allowing the patient to breathe spontaneously from ambient.

INFRASONICS ADULT STAR

The Infrasonics Adult Star ventilator (Fig. 14-32) is a pressure or flow controller that may be pressure, time, or manually triggered; pressure, volume, or flow limited; and pressure, flow, or time cycled. It has an optional compressor, an integral air–oxygen blending system, and a gas outlet port that will power a nebulizer during inspiration. The nebulizer port is designed such that its output does not alter the set delivered volume.

Input Variables

The Adult Star uses 107 to 132 volts AC at 60 Hz to power the control circuitry. The pneumatic circuit operates on external compressed gas sources (ie, air and oxygen) at 30 to 90 psig and 160 L/min.

The front panel of the Adult Star is illustrated in Figure 14-33. The operator communicates with the ventilator by means of a control panel and three screen formats displayed on a CRT. The operator may select the mode of ventilation; pressure-triggering, pressure-limiting, and pressure-cycling thresholds; PEEP/CPAP; tidal volume; sigh volume; peak inspiratory flow rate; flow waveform; ventilatory frequency; inspiratory pause time; and F_{IO_2}.

Settings are selected using a control panel in conjunction with a CRT display. The control panel has pushbuttons and an optical encoder in the form of a large rotary knob (ie, the "select" knob, which is similar in function to the "mouse" used with some personal computers). As the select knob is rotated, ventilator parameters are highlighted by a cursor (yellow bar) on the CRT. When the select knob has aligned the cursor with the desired variable, the enter button is depressed. This action allows adjustment of the value of the variable by again rotating the select knob and depressing the enter button again. For example, the select knob may be rotated until peak flow is highlighted by the cursor. The enter button is depressed to select this variable, and the cursor then highlights the current numerical value of the variable. Now the select knob is rotated to adjust flow to the desired value and the enter button is depressed a second time to activate the current setting. The alarms are set in a similar fashion.

Control Variables

The Adult Star controls either inspiratory pressure or flow. It controls inspiratory pressure in the POSITIVE

PRESSURE SUPPORT and CPAP modes and flow in the ASSIST/CONTROL, and AUGMENTED MINUTE VOLUME modes. It switches between pressure control (for spontaneous breaths) and flow control (for mandatory breaths) in the SIMV mode.

INSPIRATORY WAVEFORMS. The Adult Star offers one inspiratory pressure and four inspiratory flow waveforms. A rectangular pressure waveform can be achieved in the pressure support mode. Flow waveforms include square (rectangular), accelerating (ascending ramp), decelerating (descending ramp), and sine. Gas delivery with the rectangular waveform is relatively constant at the peak flow setting. With the ascending ramp waveform, inspiratory flow begins at 30% of the peak flow setting and increases linearly to peak flow. Conversely, with the descending ramp waveform, it begins at the peak flow value and decreases linearly to 30% of peak flow by end-inspiration. When the sine waveform is selected, inspiratory flow goes from 30% of the peak flow setting to peak flow and back to 30% of peak flow in a sinusoidal fashion.

PHASE VARIABLES. Inspiration is pressure triggered when a spontaneous ventilatory effort removes enough gas from the patient circuit to drop the pressure below the sensitivity threshold. The threshold for triggering a mandatory or spontaneous breath is adjustable from 0.5 to 20.0 cm H_2O below the baseline pressure. Inspiration is time triggered as a function of the ventilator frequency or machine rate, which is adjustable from 0.5 to 80 cycles/min. Time triggering is also in effect when using the sigh rate and multiple

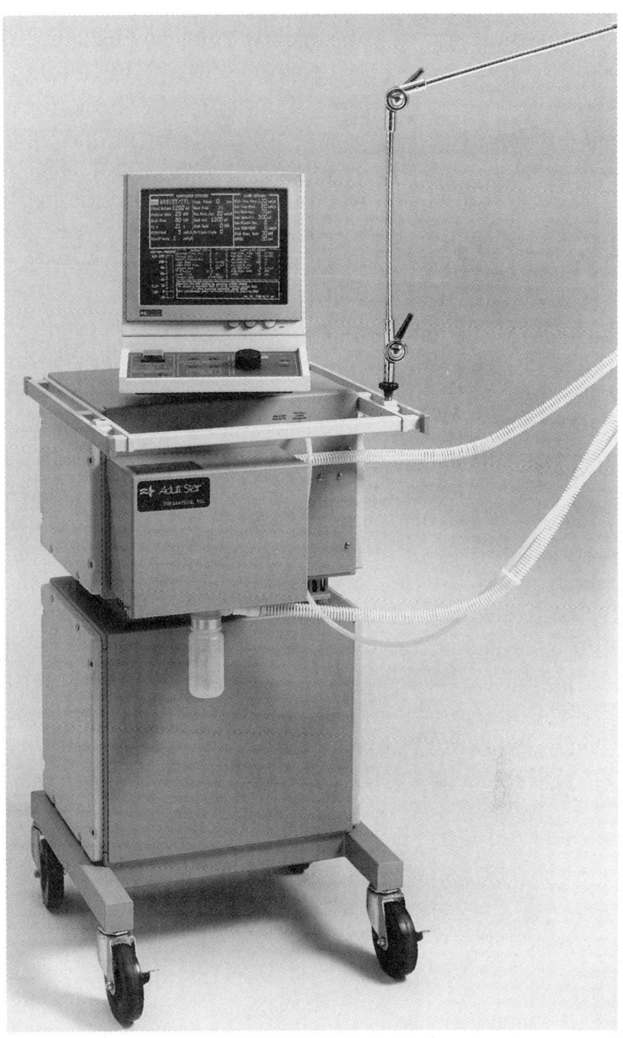

Figure 14-32. The Infrasonics Adult Star ventilator. (Courtesy of Infrasonics, San Diego, CA)

Control Panel

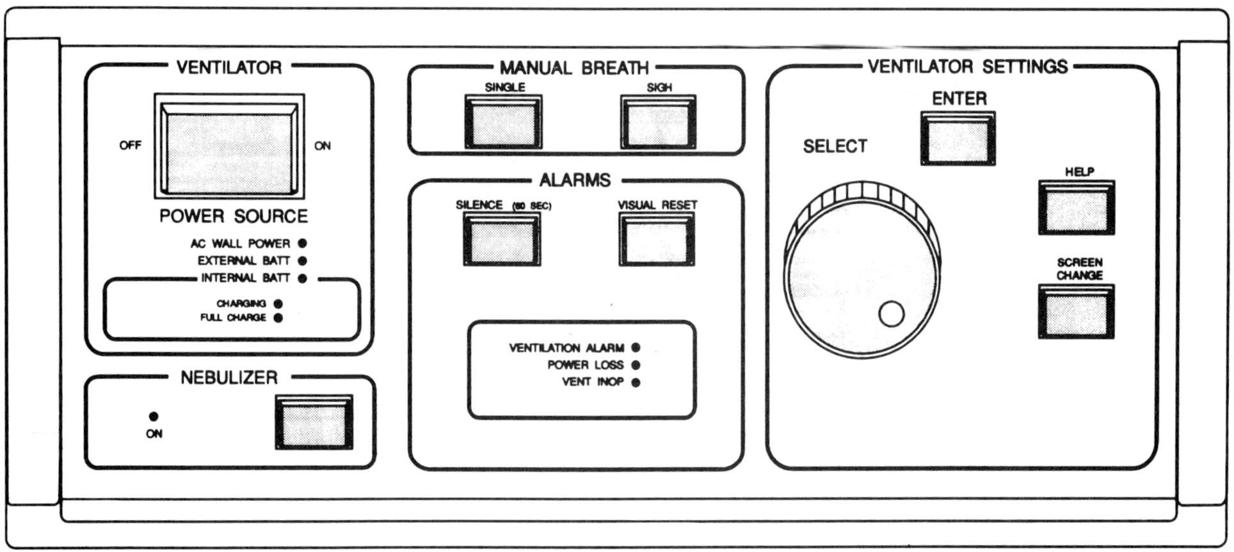

Figure 14-33. Control panel of the Infrasonics Adult Star ventilator. (Courtesy of Infrasonics, San Diego, CA)

sighs functions. The sigh rate works in all modes and is adjustable from 0 to 20 sighs per hour. The multiple sigh function allows two or three sighs to be delivered in a row, with each set delivered at the frequency set by the sigh rate. The Adult Star may also be manually triggered.

Inspiration is pressure limited during spontaneous breaths in the PRESSURE SUPPORT and the PEEP/CPAP modes. A demand valve controls inspiratory pressure by attempting to maintain the set PEEP/CPAP level, which is adjustable from 0 to 30 cm H_2O, if pressure support is not used. If pressure support is used, the pressure limit may be set from 0 to 70 cm H_2O above the PEEP/CPAP level. Inspiration is volume limited whenever the inspiratory pause time is greater than zero. Inspiration is flow limited for mandatory breaths. Peak inspiratory flow rate can be pre-set over a range of 10 to 120 L/min, though peak flow for a spontaneous breath can be as high as 150 L/min.

Inspiration is terminated when one of three variables reaches a pre-set threshold. Inspiration will be pressure cycled when the high inspiratory pressure threshold is violated (adjustable from 10 to 120 cm H_2O). Active inspiratory flow is also pressure cycled for spontaneous breaths when pressure support is not used (when expiration causes airway pressure to rise above the PEEP/CPAP setting). Inspiration is not volume cycled because the Adult Star does not measure instantaneous volume. However, when inspiration is flow controlled, tidal and sigh volumes may be set from 100 to 2500 mL. Inspiration is flow cycled in the PRESSURE SUPPORT mode when inspiratory flow rate decays to a flow rate of 4 L/min. Inspiration is time cycled for flow-controlled breaths whenever the inspiratory time reaches the value determined by the volume and flow rate settings. Inspiratory time is extended when the inspiratory pause time is set above zero. Inspiratory pause time is adjustable from 0 to 2.0 seconds.

Baseline pressure may be adjusted from 0 to 30 cm H_2O using the PEEP/CPAP function.

Control Subsystems

CONTROL CIRCUIT. The Adult Star uses pneumatic and electronic control components (Fig. 14-34). Five microprocessors (Main Processor, Graphics Processor, A/D Processor, and two Stepper Motor Processors) provide control and display functions. The Main Processor controls the pneumatics by direct I/O interface to the valve driver board and by a serial interface to the two stepper motor driver processors. The main processor accepts input from several pressure transducers (one differential pressure transducer across

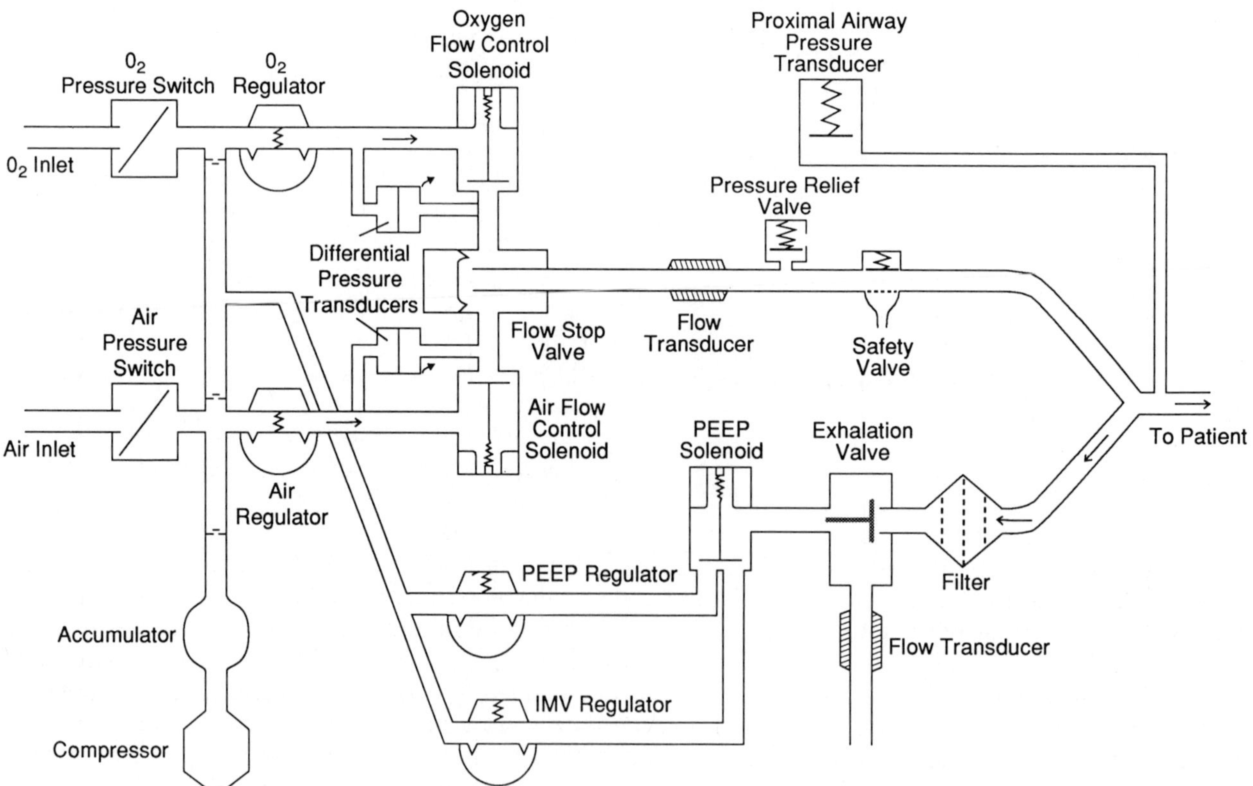

Figure 14-34. Internal components of the Infrasonics Adult Star control circuit.

both air and oxygen proportional valves, one internal system pressure transducer, and one proximal airway pressure transducer), two internal flow transducers (pneumotachometers), and the control variable settings and outputs control signals to the output control valves. Feedback from the airway pressure transducer is used to provide triggering, cycling, and alarm signals and to control the airway pressure waveform during pressure-controlled breaths. A pneumatic signal is directed to the exhalation manifold to control inspiratory pressure and PEEP.

Information from the inspiratory flow transducer provides the feedback for shaping the inspiratory flow waveform and for calculating delivered volume. A second flow transducer is used to measure exhaled volumes for display and for alarm functions.

The inspired oxygen concentration is controlled by microprocessor adjustment of the relative flows from the air and oxygen proportional valves according to the set FIO_2.

Drive Mechanism

The Adult Star uses either external compressed gas (for air and oxygen) or an electric motor and rotary vane-type compressor (for air) in conjunction with a pressure regulator. Gas pressure is initially regulated to 6.5 to 7.5 psig before reaching the air and oxygen proportional valves.

OUTPUT CONTROL VALVES. Gas flow to the patient is regulated by the air and oxygen proportional valves, which are driven by stepper motors. A pneumatic interface valve is connected to the pilot pressure control valve that supplies a pneumatic signal to the exhalation valve (a pneumatic diaphragm-type valve). The microprocessor coordinates the activity of all valves such that the exhalation valve closes as the proportional valves begin to deliver flow to the patient circuit.

The flow control system is capable of delivering calibrated peak flow up to 120 L/min and demand flow (in response to spontaneous inspiratory efforts) up to 150 L/min.

Output Displays

The CRT displays three different screens of information. Screen #1 (Ventilator Settings) shows the mode of ventilation, pressure, volume, flow, ventilatory frequency, FIO_2, and sensitivity settings. In addition, it shows apnea, pressure, volume, and frequency alarm settings. Screen #2 (Patient Monitoring) shows the patient's status in terms of measured exhaled tidal and minute volumes, spontaneous minute volume, and the source of the breath trigger (ie, spontaneous or controlled). Measured values for peak, mean, plateau, and PEEP/CPAP pressure are displayed digitally along with values for ventilatory frequency, I:E ratio, and inspiratory time. A dynamic representation of airway pressure is displayed by an analog bar graph, which also shows the high inspiratory pressure, low inspiratory pressure, and low PEEP/CPAP alarm settings. This screen also provides a summary of the other alarm limit settings and ventilator settings. Screen #3 (Graphics Monitoring) displays real-time pressure, volume, and flow waveforms. Like screen #2, this screen also provides a summary of the other alarm limit settings and ventilator settings.

The Adult Star's display screens are unique in that by pressing the help button on the control panel, the definition of a selected ventilatory variable or alarm is given along with available setting ranges. For alarm variables, possible causes of alarm activation are suggested. In effect, the important parts of the user manual are programmed into the ventilator for quick and easy access.

Modes of Operation

The following modes are those named on the output display of the Adult Star:

ASSIST/CONTROL. During continuous mechanical ventilation, inspiration is flow controlled, pressure triggered (depending on the presence of spontaneous breathing efforts and the sensitivity setting), or time triggered (according to the the machine rate setting); may be volume limited (when using an inspiratory pause); is flow limited, and time cycled. Tidal volume remains relatively constant from breath to breath as determined by the tidal volume and sigh volume settings.

SIMV. In SIMV, mandatory breaths are flow controlled, pressure triggered (depending on the presence of spontaneous breathing efforts and the sensitivity setting), or time triggered (according to the sigh rate and multiple sigh settings) and (time cycled).

Spontaneous inspirations between mandatory breaths are pressure controlled (ie, inspiratory flow varies to maintain the set PEEP/CPAP value), pressure triggered, and either pressure or flow cycled depending on whether the pressure support function is used.

A mandatory breath is pressure triggered the first time a spontaneous breathing effort is detected during each ventilatory period (the time equal to the reciprocal of the machine rate). Subsequent breathing efforts during the same period will not trigger another mandatory breath. If a breathing effort is not detected during a given ventilatory period, a mandatory breath will be delivered at the beginning of the next period. The ventilator will continue to deliver mandatory breaths according to the machine rate setting until a spontaneous breath is detected, and the sequence of events repeats itself.

CPAP. Spontaneous inspirations are pressure controlled (ie, inspiratory flow varies to maintain either the set CPAP or pressure support value), pressure triggered, and pressure or flow cycled depending on whether pressure support is activated.

POSITIVE-PRESSURE SUPPORT. Unlike some other ventilators, the Adult Star does not treat pressure support as a separate mode of ventilation. Rather, it is used to assist spontaneous breaths in the SIMV and CPAP modes. If a spontaneous effort drops the airway opening pressure below the sensitivity threshold, then inspiration is pressure limited to the pressure support setting, and flow cycled when the inspiratory flow rate decays to a flow rate of less than 6 L/min.

Alarms

INPUT POWER ALARMS. Visual and audible alarms are activated if the electrical or pneumatic power supplies drop below pre-set levels (102 volts and 30 psig, respectively). Separate visual and audible alarms are provided for the air and oxygen sources. A low-battery alarm activates when the internal battery is low and the available power to run the ventilator is expected to last less than 5 minutes. The self-contained battery and charger ensures uninterrupted operation for at least 20 minutes after external electrical power failure.

CONTROL VARIABLE ALARMS. There are four visual and audible alarms associated with ventilating pressures. These include low PEEP/CPAP (adjustable from 0 to 25 cm H_2O), high PEEP/CPAP (automatically triggered if baseline pressure exceeds set PEEP/CPAP by 10 cm H_2O for 2 seconds or if the baseline has fluctuated between 5 and 10 cm H_2O above the set PEEP/CPAP for more than 5 seconds), low inspiratory pressure (adjustable from 3 to 60 cm H_2O), and high inspiratory pressure (adjustable from 10 to 120 cm H_2O).

There are three visual and audible alarms associated with exhaled volumes. There are low mechanical volume and low spontaneous volume alarms, both adjustable from 0 to 2500 mL. There is also a low minute volume alarm, adjustable from 0 to 60 L/min.

There is a visual and audible alarm for low respiratory rate, adjustable from 0 to 90 cycles/min.

CONTROL CIRCUIT ALARMS. Visual and audible alarms indicate insufficient inspiratory and expiratory times.

Inverse I:E ratios are indicated by inverse video on the CRT.

A visual and audible apnea alarm is activated if an inspiration is not triggered within the operator-selected apnea period (adjustable from 5 to 60 seconds).

A visual and audible exhalation valve leak alarm indicates that the exhalation valve diaphragm is not sealing. The alarm is triggered if the exhaled flow transducer measures a flow greater than 10% of the inspired flow and that flow is greater than 4 L/min for 60 ms during the time that the exhalation valve is closed.

An obstructed tube alarm indicates that a condition exists that may be obstructing flow to the patient or that the airway pressure line is obstructed. This alarm is triggered during inspiration if

- The internal pressure transducer reads a pressure greater than the set high inspiratory pressure limit
- The internal pressure transducer reads a pressure greater than the pressure support setting and CPAP
- During a spontaneous breath the airway pressure is greater than 10 cm H_2O above the set PEEP/CPAP level for longer than 3 seconds

NEWPORT BREEZE

The Newport Breeze (Newport Medical Instruments, Newport Beach, CA) (Fig. 14-35) is a pressure or flow controller that is time or manually triggered and time cycled. It has an integral air–oxygen blender and a nebulizer output port.

Input Variables

The Breeze requires 100 to 120 volts AC at 60 Hz to power the control circuitry. The ventilator also requires pneumatic power and operates on external compressed air and oxygen sources at 35 to 70 psig. The Breeze has no internal compressor.

The front panel of the Breeze is illustrated in Figure 14-36 The operator may select mode of ventilation, desired pressure limit (PIP), desired baseline pressure (PEEP), trigger threshold, inspiratory time, ventilatory frequency, FIO_2, two separate flow rates (one for mechanical breaths, one for spontaneous breaths), and airway pressure alarm settings.

Control Variables

The Breeze is unique among infant ventilators in that it is designed to facilitate flow-controlled ventilation with pre-set tidal volumes as well as to perform pressure-controlled ventilation in both the SIMV and ASSIST/CONTROL modes.

In the pressure-limited ventilatory mode, the Breeze is designed more to limit rather than to control inspiratory pressure. In the first place, the inspiratory pressure limit knob is uncalibrated. But more to the point, the peak inspiratory flow rate is always limited to the value set on the flowmeter. For a given inspiratory time, this flow rate may not be sufficient to achieve the set inspiratory pressure limit in the allotted inspiratory time (depending also on the compliance and resistance of the patient's respiratory system). Thus, in this situation, the Breeze becomes a flow controller by default.

As a flow controller, the Breeze is similar to adult ventilators in that it displays the tidal volume that re-

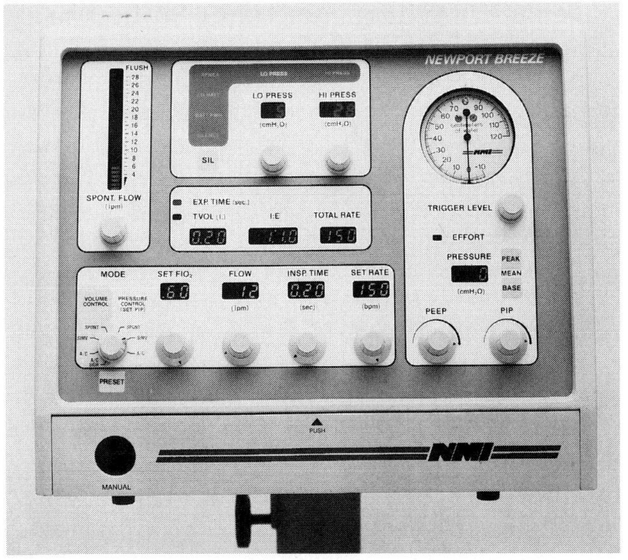

Figure 14-35. The Newport Breeze ventilator. (Courtesy of Newport Medical Instruments, Newport Beach, CA)

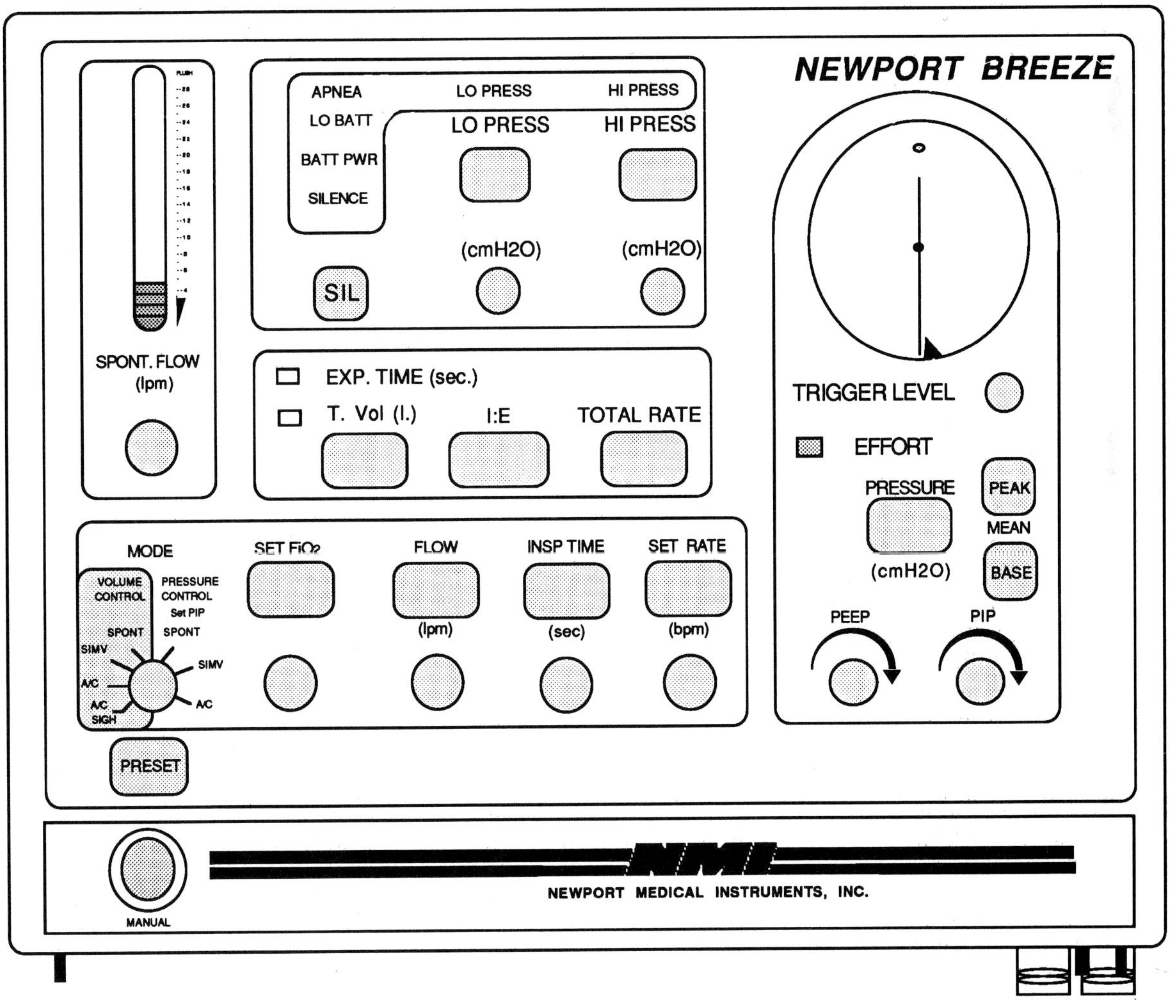

Figure 14-36. Control panel of the Newport Breeze ventilator. (Courtesy of Newport Medical Instruments, Newport Beach, CA)

sults from the set inspiratory time and inspiratory flow rate. One problem with other infant ventilators when used as flow controllers is that the flow rate required for a mechanical breath may be less than that demanded by the patient during spontaneous breaths. But because there is only one source of flow, the patient's demands are not met. On the other hand, the inspiratory flow rate required for a mechanical breath may be much larger than is needed for spontaneous breaths. The extra flow during spontaneous breathing periods may contribute to turbulence in the expiratory limb of the patient circuit, leading to inadvertent PEEP or increased work of breathing (for active exhalations).

The Breeze addresses these problems by splitting the flow control into mechanical and spontaneous breathing periods with its "Duoflow" system. Thus, for example, the flow into the lungs during the inspiratory time may be set at 12 L/min with the FLOW control knob, while the continuous flow through the patient circuit during the expiratory time may be set at 6 L/min using the SPONTANEOUS FLOW control knob.

INSPIRATORY WAVEFORMS. The Breeze is capable of producing a rectangular pressure waveform in PRESSURE CONTROL modes. It produces a rectangular flow waveform in the VOLUME CONTROL modes.

PHASE VARIABLES. Inspiration is normally time triggered and is a function of the set ventilatory frequency (labeled the "SET RATE," adjustable from 1 to 150 cycles/min). Inspiration may also be pressure triggered if the airway pressure falls below the set trigger level (adjustable from −10 to +60 cm H_2O). Inspiration may also be manually triggered.

Inspiration may be pressure limited from 0 to 60 cm H_2O. If inspiration is not pressure limited, it is flow limited. Inspiratory flow rate may be adjusted from 1 to 120 L/min. The continuous flow through the patient circuit, available for spontaneous breaths during the expiratory time, may be adjusted from 0 to 50 L/min (calibrated flow range is 0 to 28 L/min).

Inspiration is time cycled as a result of the set inspiratory time (adjustable from 0.1 to 3.0 seconds). Manual inspirations will be time cycled at 2 seconds. Inspiration is also pressure cycled if the airway pressure exceeds the set high pressure alarm threshold (adjustable from 10 to 120 cm H_2O).

Baseline pressure may be adjusted over the range of 0 to 60 cm H_2O using the (uncalibrated) PEEP knob.

Control Subsystems

CONTROL CIRCUIT. The control circuit of the Breeze uses electronic and pneumatic components (Fig. 14-37).

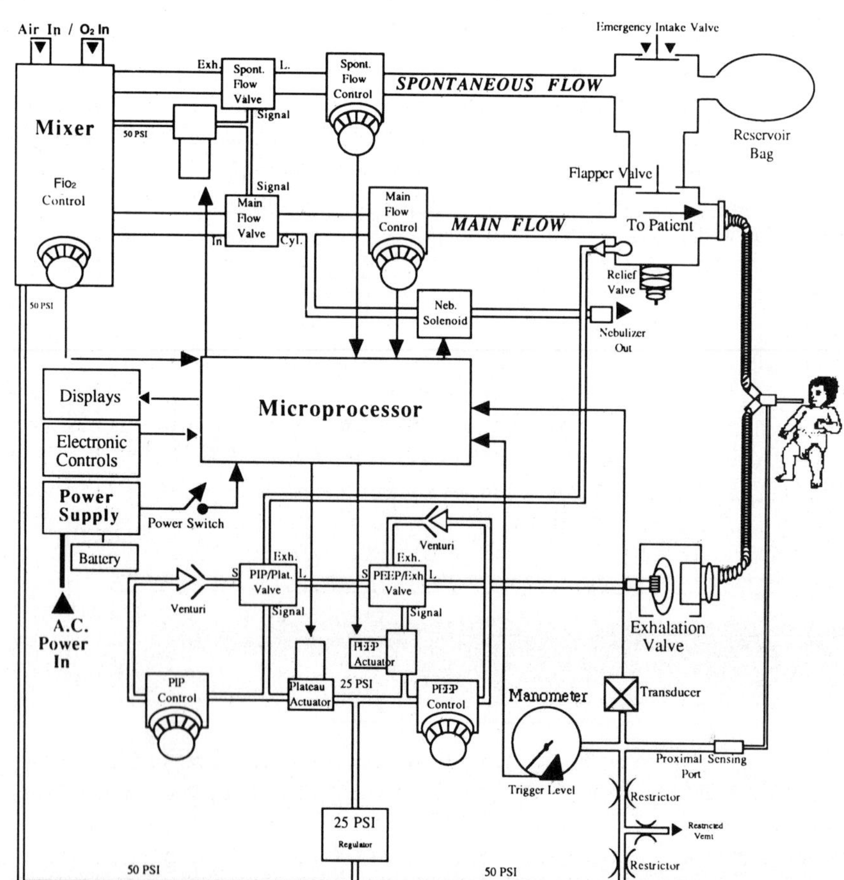

Figure 14-37. Internal components of the Newport Breeze ventilator control circuit. (Courtesy of Newport Medical Instruments, Newport Beach, CA)

A microprocessor sends timing signals to a variety of solenoid valves that use pneumatic signals to activate flow and pressure control valves and the exhalation manifold. An internal pressure transducer monitors airway pressure and generates signals for the high and low airway pressure alarms.

DRIVE MECHANISM. The Breeze requires an external pneumatic source to power an air–oxygen blender. This blender delivers pressurized gas to a flowmeter, which then routes a continuous flow of gas to the patient circuit.

OUTPUT CONTROL VALVES. The output control valves include both the spontaneous and main (ie, mechanical breath) flow-switching valves and flow-regulating needle valves, inspiratory and expiratory pressure-switching valves and pressure-regulating needle valves, and a diaphragm exhalation valve.

During a flow-controlled inspiration, the flow pilot solenoid is turned on by the microprocessor. This sends a pneumatic signal to open the master flow valve, directing gas from the blender through the inspiratory flow control needle valve. At the same time, a pneumatic signal from the inspiratory limb (inside the ventilator) is directed through the PIP and PEEP valves to the exhalation valve. Since this pressure is always greater than the pressure at the airway opening (because of the pressure drop due to flow resistance along the inspiratory portion of the patient circuit), the exhalation valve stays closed until the end of the inspiratory time. When inspiration is cycled off, the main flow valve is turned off and the spontaneous flow valve is turned on. At the same time, the PEEP solenoid switches on the PEEP valve, which cuts off the high-pressure pneumatic signal and directs a PEEP signal (from the PEEP control needle valve/venturi mechanism) to the exhalation manifold.

During a pressure-controlled inspiration, the main flow valve switches on as before but the plateau solenoid causes the PIP valve to direct a pneumatic signal from the PIP control needle valve/venturi mechanism through the PEEP valve to the exhalation valve. Thus, when airway pressure rises to the same pressure as that generated in the exhalation valve (ie, essentially the set PIP limit), excess flow from the main flow valve is vented to the atmosphere. When inspiration cycles off, the PIP valve is deactivated and the PEEP valve directs a pneumatic signal from the PEEP mechanism to the exhalation valve.

Output Displays

Airway pressure is displayed by an aneroid pressure gauge over the range of -10 to 120 cm H_2O. There are also digital displays for peak, mean, and baseline pressure; FIO_2; peak inspiratory flow rate; inspiratory time; expiratory time (when any of the PRESSURE CONTROL modes are selected); ventilatory frequency; calculated tidal volume (inspiratory flow × inspiratory time; displayed when any of the VOLUME CONTROL modes are selected); I:E ratio; total ventilatory frequency (spontaneous plus machine breaths); and for high and low airway pressure alarm thresholds. Continuous flow for spontaneous breaths is indicated on an LED bar graph display.

Modes of Operation

The mode selector switch on the Breeze is divided into two sections: VOLUME CONTROL (meaning flow controlled) and PRESSURE CONTROL. The following modes are those named under these sections:

Volume Control

A/C. Inspiration is normally flow controlled, time triggered (based on the ventilatory rate), or pressure triggered (depending on the patient's inspiratory effort and the set trigger level), flow limited (at the set FLOW rate), and time cycled (based on the inspiratory time).

A/C SIGH. Same as A/C with the addition of a mechanical sigh breath equal to 150% of the pre-set tidal volume (actually 150% of the inspiratory time) delivered once every 100 breaths.

SIMV. Mandatory inspiration is normally flow controlled, time triggered (based on the ventilatory rate) or pressure triggered (depending on the patient's inspiratory effort and the set trigger level), flow limited (at the set FLOW rate), and time cycled (based on the inspiratory time).

The number and timing of the mandatory breaths is determined by the set ventilatory frequency. During the first 75% of the ventilatory period (ventilatory period = 60/set frequency), inspiration cannot be triggered. During the last 25%, inspiration will be pressure triggered if the patient's ventilatory effort drops the airway pressure below the set TRIGGER LEVEL. If the patient is apneic for the duration of the ventilatory period, the Breeze will deliver the mandatory breath at the end of each ventilatory period.

If, during spontaneous breaths, the patient's inspiratory flow rate exceeds the set SPONTANEOUS FLOW rate, additional flow is available from a reservoir bag placed in the inspiratory limb of the patient circuit.

SPONT. Inspiration is not controlled in the SPONT mode. The patient breathes from the continuous flow set by the SPONT FLOW control and from the reservoir bag in the inspiratory limb of the patient circuit. The pressure at the airway opening during inspiration fluctuates as a function of the fixed resistance through the exhalation manifold (determined mainly by the PEEP setting) and the surplus inspiratory flow. Surplus inspiratory flow is the difference between the flow rate available from the patient circuit and the patient's instantaneous inspiratory flow rate.

If the MANUAL BREATH button is depressed in the SPONT mode, the ventilator will deliver a breath whose characteristics depend on the ventilator settings as displayed by pressing the PRESET switch. In the VOLUME LIMITED SPONT mode, the ventilator will deliver a flow-controlled breath with a tidal volume determined by the FLOW setting and the set inspiratory time. In the PRESSURE LIMITED SPONT mode, it will deliver a pressure-controlled breath with the PIP determined by the PIP setting (assuming that the FLOW and inspiratory time settings are large enough to reach the set PIP).

Pressure Control

A/C. Inspiration is normally pressure controlled, time triggered (based on the ventilatory rate), or pressure triggered (depending on the patient's inspiratory effort and the set trigger level), and time cycled (based on the inspiratory time). If inspiration is not pressure limited (owing to insufficient flow or inspiratory time), it is flow limited, time or pressure triggered, and time cycled.

SIMV Inspiration is normally pressure controlled, time triggered (based on the ventilatory rate), and time cycled (based on the inspiratory time). The timing of mandatory breaths is the same as for the VOLUME CONTROL SIMV mode. If inspiration is not pressure limited (owing to insufficient flow or inspiratory time), it is flow limited, time triggered, and time cycled.

There is a continuous flow of gas from the ventilator at the rate set on the SPONT FLOW control knob to allow for spontaneous breathing between mandatory breaths.

If, during spontaneous breaths, the patient's inspiratory flow rate exceeds the set SPONTANEOUS FLOW rate, additional flow is available from a reservoir bag placed in the inspiratory limb of the patient circuit.

Alarms

INPUT POWER ALARMS. When external electrical power supply to the Breeze is interrupted, there is an audible alarm. A drop of air or oxygen inlet pressure to less than 35 psig results in an audible alarm.

CONTROL VARIABLE ALARMS. The Breeze provides visual and audible alarms for high inspiratory pressure (HI PRESS, adjustable from 10 to 120 cm H_2O) and low inspiratory pressure (LO PRESS, adjustable from 3 to 99 cm H_2O).

CONTROL CIRCUIT ALARMS. An APNEA/LOW CPAP alarm monitors patient breaths in all modes. If the interval between breaths detected by ventilator exceeds the set delay period (adjustable from 5 to 60 seconds), audible and visual alarms are activated. Activation of the APNEA alarm depends on setting the TRIGGER LEVEL correctly so that the EFFORT LED lights with each breath. When the alarm is set to LOW CPAP in the SPONT mode, an audible alarm is triggered if the baseline pressure drops below the LO PRESS setting for more than 4 seconds.

NEWPORT E100i

The Newport E100i ventilator (Newport Medical Instruments, Newport Beach, CA) (Fig. 14-38) is a pressure or flow controller that may be pressure, time, or manually triggered; pressure or flow limited; and pressure or time cycled. It has an optional compressor, an external air–oxygen blender, and a gas outlet port that will power a nebulizer during inspiration.

Input Variables

The E100i uses 115 volts AC at 60 Hz to power the control circuitry (European voltages optional). There is an optional battery backup unit (lead-acid batteries and charger) that will power the E100i for about 4 hours. The pneumatic circuit, which includes an external air–oxygen blender, operates on external compressed gas sources (ie, air and oxygen) at 35 to 100 psig.

The front panel of the E100i is illustrated in Figure 14-39. The operator may select the mode of ventilation; pressure-triggering, pressure-limiting, and pressure-cycling thresholds; PEEP/CPAP; peak inspiratory flow rate; inspiratory time; ventilatory frequency; and F_{IO_2}.

Control Variables

The E100i controls either inspiratory pressure or flow. It controls inspiratory pressure in the spontaneous mode and whenever the peak pressure is limited by the relief valve setting in the ASSIST/CONTROL and SIMV modes. It normally controls flow in the ASSIST/CONTROL and SIMV modes.

INSPIRATORY WAVEFORMS. The E100i offers one inspiratory pressure and one inspiratory flow waveform. A rectangular pressure waveform can be achieved in the ASSIST/CONTROL and SIMV modes by using the pressure relief valve. Otherwise, a rectangular flow waveform will be delivered.

PHASE VARIABLES. Inspiration is pressure triggered when a spontaneous ventilatory effort removes enough gas from the patient circuit to drop the pressure below the trigger level. The threshold for triggering a mandatory breath is adjustable from 0 to −10 cm H_2O below the baseline pressure. Spontaneous breaths during SIMV are drawn from a continuous flow circuit containing a reservoir bag. Continuous flow may be selected by activating the constant flow switch (which re-

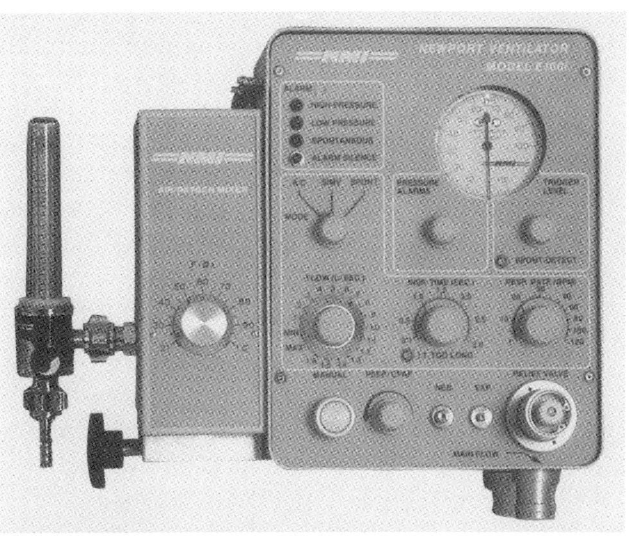

Figure 14-38. The Newport E100i ventilator. (Courtesy of Newport Medical Instruments, Newport Beach, CA)

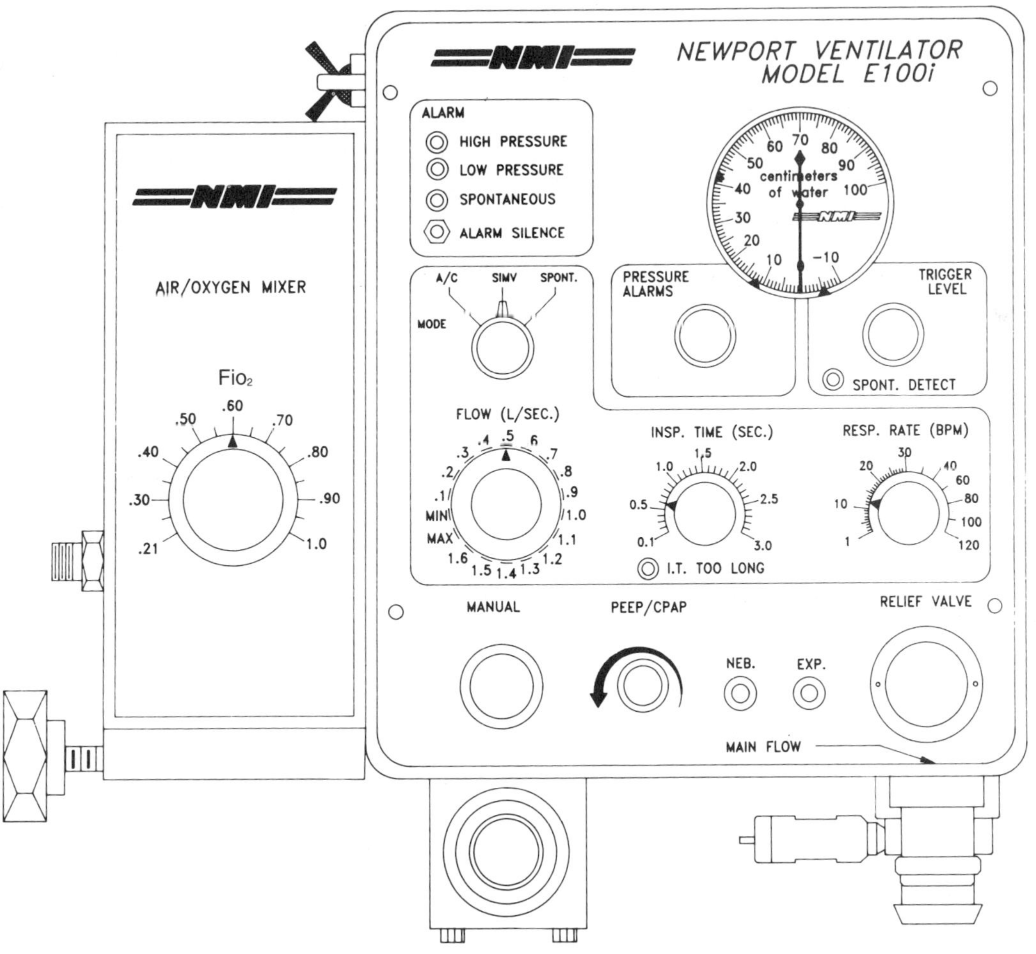

Figure 14-39. Control panel of the Newport E100i ventilator. (Courtesy of Newport Medical Instruments, Newport Beach, CA)

sults in a flow of 9 to 12 L/min). Alternatively, an external auxiliary flowmeter can be used to control the continuous flow rate through the patient circuit. Inspiration is time triggered as a function of the ventilator frequency or respiratory rate, which is adjustable from 1 to 120 cycles/min. The E100i may also be manually triggered. One advantage of the E100i's design is that the manual trigger system is pneumatically operated. This means that the operator can use the ventilator during an emergency when electrical power is not available (eg, when the ventilator's transport batteries have run low and there is no AC power). A manually triggered breath is flow limited but will last as long as the button is held down (ie, inspiration is manually cycled). Under these conditions, the pressure relief valve should be set to limit inspiratory pressure.

Inspiration is pressure limited during ASSIST/CONTROL and SIMV modes whenever the PIP determined by the pressure relief valve setting (uncalibrated but controllable over a range of 0–100 cm H_2O) is lower than that which would result from the inspiratory flow rate and inspiratory time settings. Otherwise, inspiration is flow limited. Inspiratory flow rate may be set from 0.1 to 1.6 L/s (3–100 L/min). The E100i cannot be volume limited because it does not allow for an inspiratory pause setting.

Inspiration is terminated when one of three variables reaches a pre-set threshold. Inspiration may be pressure cycled when the high inspiratory pressure alarm threshold is violated. It may be set over a range of 0 to 100 cm H_2O. Inspiration cannot be volume cycled because the E100i does not measure instantaneous volume. In practice, tidal volume is estimated by calculating the product of the set inspiratory flow rate and the set inspiratory time (see Fig. 14-36) and subtracting the compressed gas volume. The E100i is capable of delivering tidal volumes of 10 to 2000 mL. Inspiration is normally time cycled according to the inspiratory time setting (adjustable from 0.1 to 3.0 seconds).

Baseline pressure may be adjusted from 0 to 25 cm H_2O using the PEEP/CPAP dial.

Control Subsystems

CONTROL CIRCUIT. The E100i uses pneumatic and electronic control components (Fig. 14-40). The electronic control circuitry accepts input triggering and cycling signals from the inspiratory time and ventilatory frequency settings as well as from the pressure manometer alarm system. Output control signals go to a solenoid valve that drives the master control valve (a pneumatic interface valve) that directs gas through a

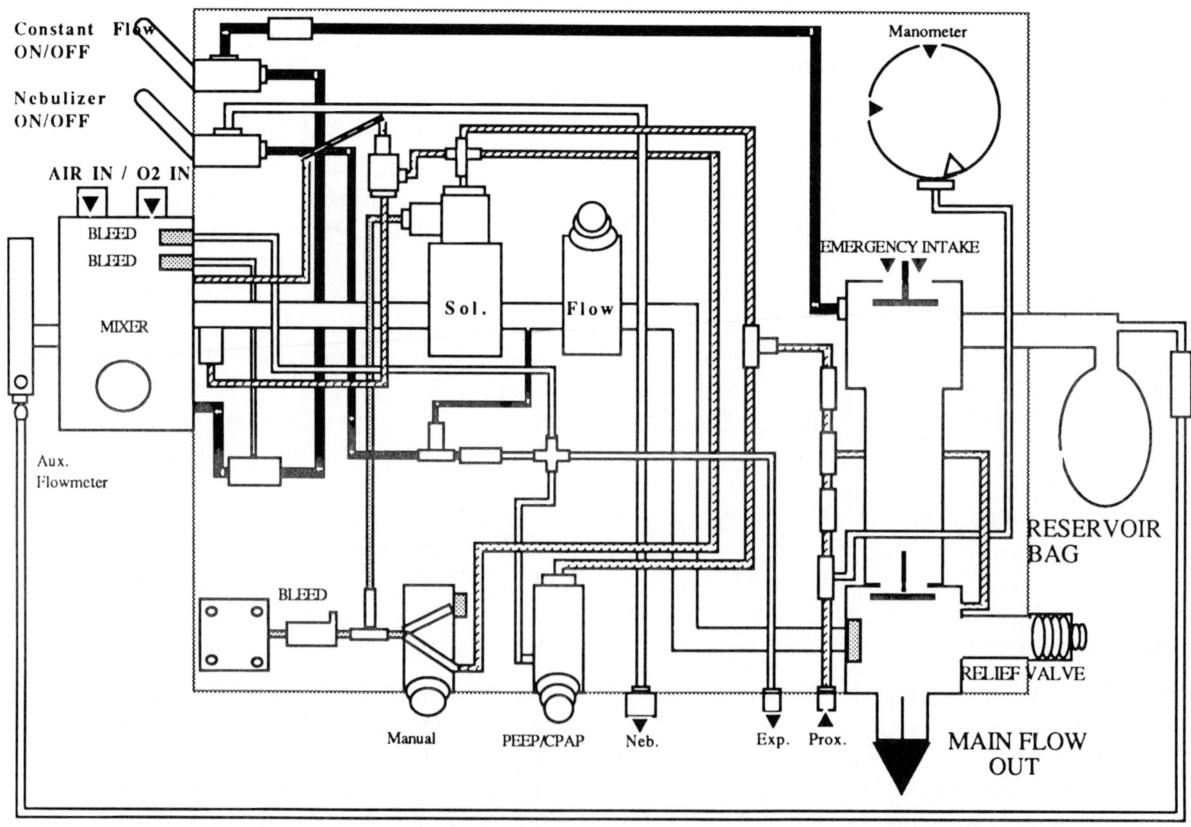

Figure 14-40. Internal components of the Newport E100i control circuit. (Courtesy of Newport Medical Instruments, Newport Beach, CA)

needle valve flowmeter. The manual inspiration button generates a pneumatic trigger signal. The exhalation manifold is controlled pneumatically.

DRIVE MECHANISM. The E100i uses either external compressed gas (for air and oxygen) or an electric motor and rotary vane-type compressor (for air) in conjunction with a pressure regulator. Gas pressure is regulated to about 29 psig by the air–oxygen blender. Mixed gas leaves the blender and enters the master control valves.

OUTPUT CONTROL VALVES. All gas flow to the patient is regulated by the master flow control valve, which is a pneumatic valve activated by a pilot valve. The pilot valve generates a pneumatic signal in response to electronic trigger signals from the control circuit or pneumatic trigger signals from the manual breath pushbutton.

Inspiratory flow rate is adjusted by directing the gas from the master control valve through a needle valve-type flowmeter.

When inspiration is triggered on, a pneumatic signal is sent to the exhalation manifold that closes to direct gas to the patient. During exhalation, the signal level drops to the value set by the PEEP/CPAP control to maintain end-expiratory pressure.

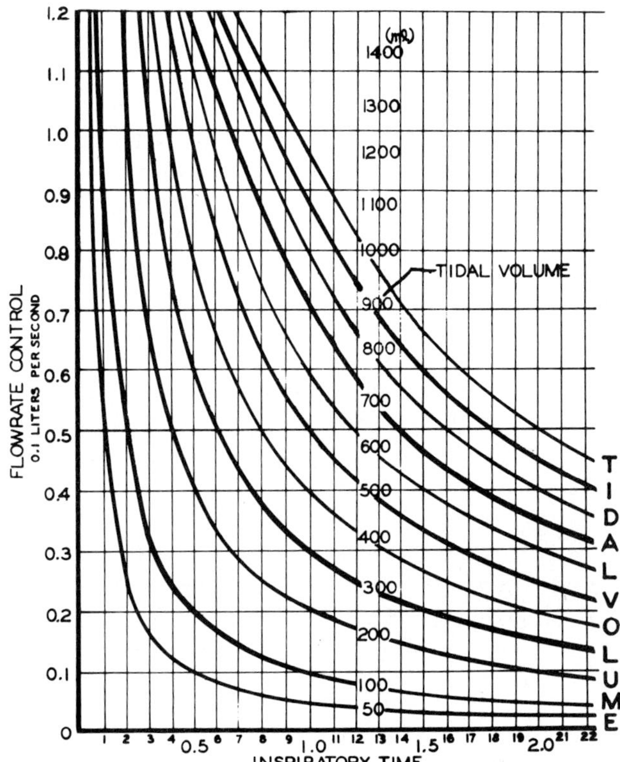

Figure 14-41. Chart to calculate tidal volume based on inspiratory time and inspiratory flow setting. (Courtesy of Newport Medical Instruments, Newport Beach, CA)

Output Displays

In addition to the various control settings, the E100i displays include visual alarm indicators (LEDs) and a visual (LED) indicator for spontaneously triggered breaths. An aneroid pressure gauge provides airway pressure measurement over the range of −10 to 100 cm H_2O.

Modes of Operation

The following modes are those named on the control panel of the E100i:

ASSIST/CONTROL. During continuous mechanical ventilation, inspiration is flow controlled, pressure triggered (depending on the presence of spontaneous breathing efforts and the sensitivity setting) or time triggered (according to the the respiratory rate setting), flow limited, and time cycled. Tidal volume remains relatively constant from breath to breath as determined by the inspiratory flow rate and inspiratory time settings (Fig. 14-41)

SIMV. In SIMV, mandatory breaths are flow controlled, pressure triggered (depending on the presence of spontaneous breathing efforts and the sensitivity setting) or time triggered (according to the frequency setting), flow limited, and time cycled.

A mandatory breath is pressure triggered the first time a spontaneous breathing effort is detected within the last 25% of each ventilatory period (the ventilatory period is equal to the reciprocal of the respiratory rate). Subsequent breathing efforts during the same period will not trigger another mandatory breath. If a breathing effort is not detected during a given ventilatory period, a mandatory breath will be delivered at the beginning of the next period. The ventilator will continue to deliver mandatory breaths according to the respiratory rate setting until a spontaneous breath is detected, and the sequence of events repeats itself. For SIMV rates above 20 cycles/min, some mandatory breaths may not be synchronous. It is recommended that for rates above 20 cycles/min, the trigger level should be set at −10 cm H_2O, thus changing SIMV to IMV.

Spontaneous inspirations between mandatory breaths are controlled for baseline pressure (ie, PEEP/CPAP) only. Spontaneous breaths are drawn from the continuous flow through the circuit and reservoir bag.

SPONTANEOUS. Inspiration is not controlled in the spontaneous mode. The patient breaths the continuous flow of gas from the flowmeter. The pressure at the airway opening during inspiration fluctuates as function of the fixed resistance through the exhalation manifold (determined mainly by the PEEP/CPAP setting) and the surplus inspiratory flow. Surplus inspiratory flow is the difference between the flow rate set on the flowmeter and the patient's instantaneous inspiratory flow rate. The continuous flow controlled by the constant flow switch (9–12 L/min) may be supplemented by an auxiliary flowmeter attached to the blender to keep the reservoir inflated and thus meet the patient's peak inspiratory flow demands.

Alarms

INPUT POWER ALARMS. Audible alarms are activated if the electrical or pneumatic power supplies drop below pre-set levels (100 volts AC and 35 psig, respectively).

CONTROL VARIABLE ALARMS. There are visual and audible alarms associated with high and low ventilating pressures. These are adjustable from 0 to 100 cm H_2O.

CONTROL CIRCUIT ALARMS. A visual inspiratory pressure too long alarm is activated if the inspiratory time and ventilatory rate settings result in an I:E ratio greater than 1:1. When activated, the ventilator will override the inspiratory time setting to limit the I:E ratio at 1:1.

A visual and audible alarm is activated if the time between breaths exceeds the selected delay time (15 or 30 seconds, adjustable on the rear panel) in the spontaneous mode.

NEWPORT WAVE

The Wave ventilator (Newport Medical Instruments, Newport Beach, CA) (Fig. 14-42) is a pressure or flow controller that may be pressure, time, or manually triggered; pressure, or flow limited; and pressure or time cycled. It has an optional compressor, an internal air–oxygen blender, and a gas outlet port that will power a nebulizer during inspiration.

Input Variables

The Wave uses 100 to 110 volts AC at 60 Hz to power the control circuitry (European voltages optional). The pneumatic circuit operates on external compressed gas sources (ie, air and oxygen) at 40 to 70 psig.

The front panel of the Wave is illustrated in Figure 14-43 The operator may select the mode of ventilation; pressure-triggering, pressure-limiting, and pressure-cycling thresholds; PEEP/CPAP; peak inspiratory flow rate; inspiratory time; ventilatory frequency; bias flow; and F_{IO_2}.

Control Variables

The Wave controls either inspiratory pressure or flow. It controls inspiratory pressure in the SPONTANEOUS mode and whenever the peak pressure is limited using the PRESSURE CONTROL knob. Otherwise it controls flow.

INSPIRATORY WAVEFORMS. The Wave delivers a rectangular flow waveform when set for volume control, that is, if the natural PIP is below the setting of the PRESSURE CONTROL knob or if this knob is set to "off." If PIP is limited using the PRESSURE CONTROL knob, a variety of pressure waveforms can be achieved, ranging from rectangular to triangular depending on the respiratory system mechanics and the inspiratory flow rate.

PHASE VARIABLES. Inspiration is pressure triggered when a spontaneous ventilatory effort removes enough gas from the patient circuit to drop the pressure below the SENSITIVITY setting. The threshold for triggering a mandatory breath is adjustable from 0.1 to 5 cm H_2O below the baseline pressure. The Wave may also be manually triggered.

Inspiration is pressure limited during ASSIST/CONTROL and SIMV modes whenever the PRES-

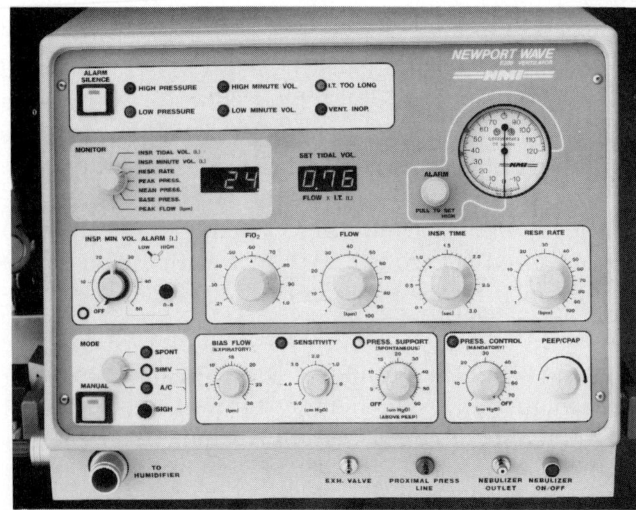

Figure 14-42. The Newport Wave ventilator. (Courtesy of Newport Medical Instruments, Newport Beach, CA)

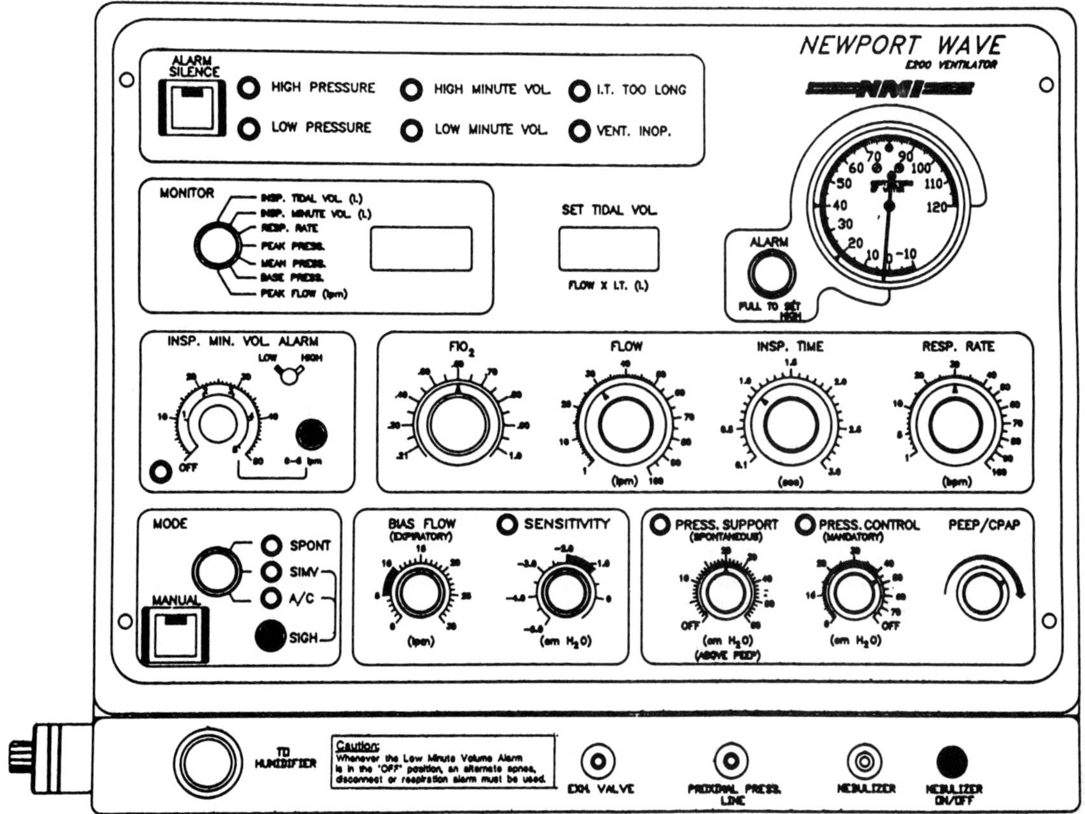

Figure 14-43. Control panel of the Newport Wave ventilator. (Courtesy of Newport Medical Instruments, Newport Beach, CA)

SURE CONTROL setting (0–80 cm H_2O) is lower than the natural PIP that would result from the FLOW and INSPIRATORY TIME settings. Inspiratory pressure may also be limited by a mechanical pressure relief valve, adjustable from 0 to 120 H_2O. Otherwise, inspiration is flow limited. Inspiratory flow rate may be set from 1 to 100 L/min. The Wave cannot be volume limited because it does not allow for an inspiratory pause setting.

Inspiration is terminated when one of three variables reaches a pre-set threshold. Inspiration may be pressure cycled when the high inspiratory pressure alarm threshold is violated. It may be set over a range of 5 to 120 cm H_2O. Inspiration cannot be volume cycled because the Wave does not measure instantaneous volume. In practice, tidal volume is estimated by calculating the product of the set inspiratory flow rate and the set inspiratory time and subtracting the compressed gas volume. The Wave is capable of delivering tidal volumes of 30 to 2000 mL. Spontaneous breaths are flow cycled when using pressure support. Inspiration is normally time cycled according to the INSPIRATORY TIME setting (adjustable from 0.1 to 3.0 seconds).

Baseline pressure may be adjusted from 0 to 25 cm H_2O using the PEEP/CPAP dial. Bias flow may be set from 0 to 30 L/min.

Control Subsystems

CONTROL CIRCUIT. The Wave uses pneumatic and electronic control components (Fig. 14-44). The electronic control circuitry accepts input triggering and cycling signals from the inspiratory time and ventilatory frequency settings as well as signals from the airway pressure transducer. Output control signals from two pressure transducers (one monitors airway pressure and one monitors pressure in the exhalation valve) and two redundant flow transducers (monitoring the output of the master flow control valve) are used to control flow. The exhalation manifold is controlled pneumatically.

DRIVE MECHANISM. The Wave uses either external compressed gas (for air and oxygen) or an electric motor and compressor (for air) in conjunction with a pressure regulator. Gas from supply lines is fed to an internal air–oxygen blender. Mixed gas leaves the blender at 28 psig and enters a rigid-walled vessel (the "accumulator"). The flow control system is driven by the pressure from the accumulator. During a flow demand, the volume stored in the accumulator is exhausted quickly, reducing the instantaneous flow demand required of the blending system. This action allows a wide range of peak flow settings, reduces the

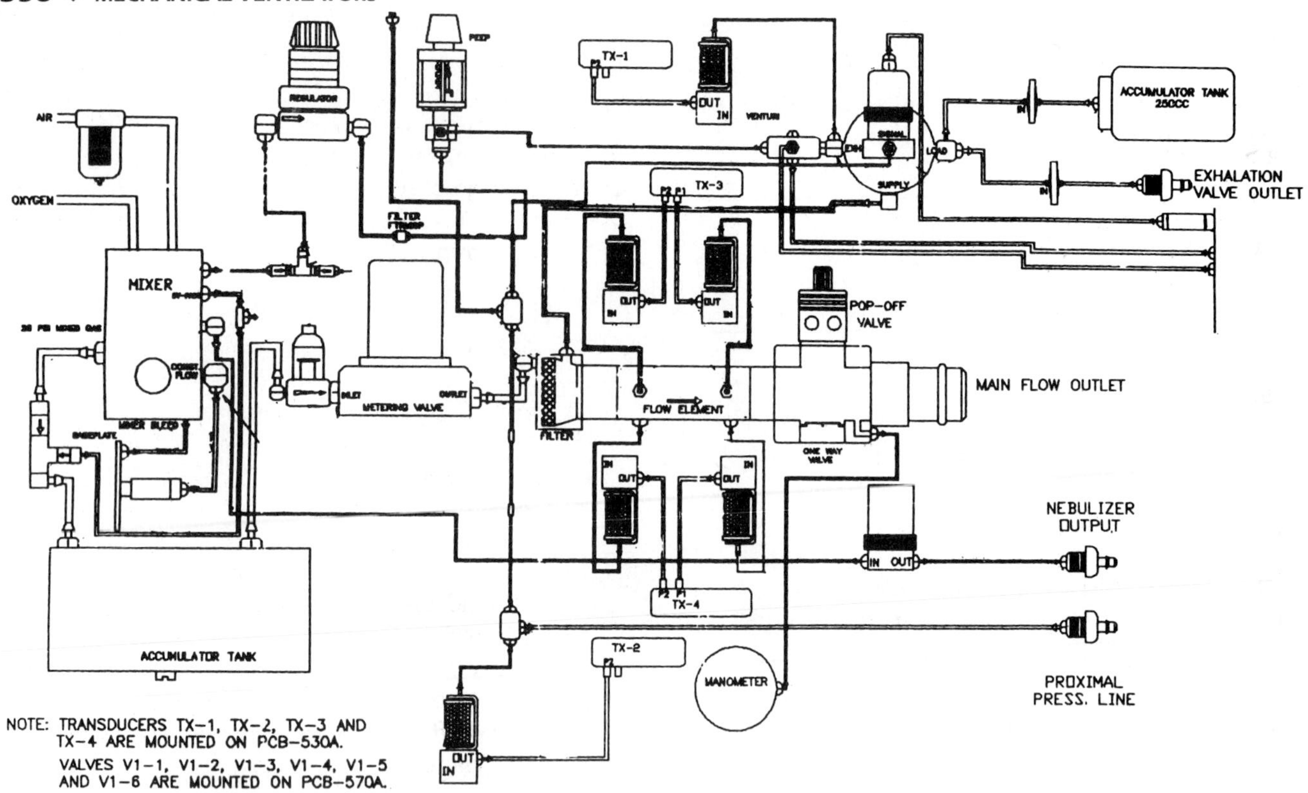

Figure 14-44. Internal components of the Newport Wave control circuit. (Courtesy of Newport Medical Instruments, Newport Beach, CA)

flow required of the compressed gas supply, and improves response time. The accumulator also acts as a mixing chamber, which helps to stabilize the delivered oxygen concentration within a given breath.

OUTPUT CONTROL VALVES. All gas flow to the patient is regulated by the main flow control valve, which is a proportional solenoid valve. An electromagnetic poppet valve switches between two sources of a pneumatic signal to the exhalation valve. One source comes from the output of the master flow control valve and keeps a diaphragm-type exhalation manifold closed during assisted breaths. The other source is a pressure regulator that generates an adjustable pressure signal to control baseline pressure (ie, PEEP/CPAP). The microprocessor coordinates the activity of both valves such that the exhalation valve closes as the flow control valve begins to deliver flow to the patient circuit.

Output Displays

In addition to the various control settings, the Wave displays include visual alarm indicators (LEDs) and digital display of tidal volume (calculated based on flow and inspiratory time settings); minute volume; ventilatory rate; peak, mean, and baseline airway pressures; and peak flow. An aneroid pressure gauge provides airway pressure measurement over the range of 0 to 120 cm H_2O.

Modes of Operation

The following modes are those named on the control panel of the Wave:

ASSIST/CONTROL. During continuous mechanical ventilation, inspiration is pressure triggered (depending on the presence of spontaneous breathing efforts and the sensitivity setting) or time triggered (according to the the RESPIRATORY RATE setting), may be pressure or flow limited, and is time cycled.

SIMV. In SIMV, mandatory breaths are pressure triggered (depending on the presence of spontaneous breathing efforts and the sensitivity setting) or time triggered (according to the frequency setting), may be pressure or flow limited, and is time cycled.

A mandatory breath is pressure triggered the first time a spontaneous breathing effort is detected within the last 25% of each ventilatory period (the ventilatory period is equal to the reciprocal of the RESPIRATORY RATE). Subsequent breathing efforts during the same period will not trigger another mandatory breath. If a breathing effort is not detected during a given ventilatory period, a mandatory breath will be delivered at the beginning of the next period. The ventilator will continue to deliver mandatory breaths according to the RESPIRATORY RATE setting until a spontaneous breath is detected, and the sequence of events repeats itself. For SIMV rates above 20 cycles/min, some mandatory breaths may not be synchronous. It is recommended that for rates above 20 cycles/min, the trigger level should be set at −10 cm H_2O, thus changing SIMV to IMV.

Spontaneous inspirations between mandatory breaths are controlled for baseline pressure (ie, PEEP/CPAP) and may be assisted if the PRESSURE SUPPORT setting is above zero. Spontaneous breaths are drawn from a continuous flow through the circuit when the BIAS FLOW setting is above zero.

SPONTANEOUS. Inspiration is pressure controlled in the SPONTANEOUS mode at the set PEEP/CPAP level. A PRESSURE SUPPORT level may also be set.

Alarms

INPUT POWER ALARMS. An audible alarm is activated if the electrical power is interrupted or if the air or oxygen supply falls below 32 psig.

CONTROL VARIABLE ALARMS. There are visual and audible alarms associated with high and low ventilating pressures. The low-pressure alarm is adjustable from 0 to 110 cm H_2O, and the high-pressure alarm is adjustable from 5 to 120 cm H_2O. High and low minute volume alarms are adjustable from 1 to 50 and 0 to 49 L/min, respectively. Resolution is 0.1 L/min over the range of minute volumes from 0 to 5 L/min. Resolution is 1.0 L/min over the minute volume range of 5 to 50 L/min.

CONTROL CIRCUIT ALARMS. A visual INSPIRATORY TIME TOO LONG alarm is activated if the inspiratory time and ventilatory rate settings result in an I:E ratio greater than the pre-set maximum. There are two selectable maximum ratios: 1:1 and 3:1. When the inspiratory time is set such that the pre-set maximum I:E ratio is violated, the ventilator will override the inspiratory time setting to restrict the I:E to the pre-set value.

Audible and visual VENTILATOR INOPERATIVE alarms are activated when malfunction of the integrated circuit or ventilator occurs.

There are two pressure and two flow sensors in the Wave. If the drift between the pressure or flow sensors is large, the visual display flashes automatically.

PURITAN-BENNETT MA-1

The Puritan-Bennett MA-1 ventilator (Puritan-Bennett Corporation, Carlsbad, CA) (Fig. 14-45) is a volume controller that may be pressure, time, or manually triggered; volume, or flow limited; and pressure, volume, or time cycled. It has an integral compressor, an air–oxygen blender, and a gas outlet port that will power a nebulizer during inspiration.

Input Variables

The MA-1 uses 115 volts AC at 60 Hz to power the control circuitry. The main electrical power switch is located on the front panel. The pneumatic circuit, which includes an integral air–oxygen blender, operates on external oxygen source at 35 to 100 psig. It has an internal compressor that will supply air to the bellows chamber at 7 psig.

The front panel of the MA-1 is illustrated in Figure 14-46. The operator may select the pressure-triggering and pressure-cycling thresholds, tidal volume, sigh volume, peak inspiratory flow rate, ventilatory frequency, and F_{IO_2}. Expiratory resistance and a short inspiratory hold may also be selected. A separate attachment that fits on the side of the ventilator allows adjustment of PEEP.

Control Variables

The MA-1 controls inspiratory volume rather than pressure or flow. The gas that is delivered to the patient comes from a bellows that empties in response to the force generated by the drive mechanism. The inspiratory volume is controlled by controlling the volume change of the bellows. The volume change of the bellows is sensed by a cable and pulley mechanism connecting the bellows to a potentiometer. As the volume of the bellows changes, the resistance of the potentiometer changes, which generates a changing electrical signal. The volume knobs are connected to similar potentiometers that establish an electrical reference value or threshold. The signal from the bellows is compared with the reference value(s) and when the threshold is met, inspiration is terminated.

INSPIRATORY WAVEFORMS. The MA-1 generates (approximately) an ascending ramp volume waveform. As a result, the inspiratory flow waveform is approximately rectangular but might be more accurately described as a descending ramp waveform under certain conditions. Peak flow usually decays during inspiration due to the design of the drive mechanism. Flow decay may be substantial under high ventilatory loads.

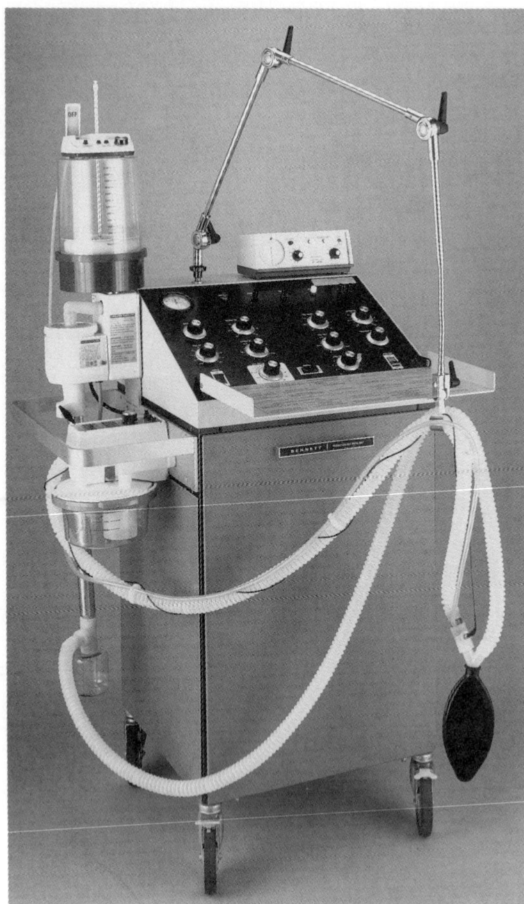

Figure 14-45. The Puritan-Bennett MA-1 ventilator. (Courtesy of Puritan-Bennett Corporation, Carlsbad, CA)

PHASE VARIABLES. Inspiration is pressure triggered when a spontaneous ventilatory effort removes enough gas from the patient circuit to drop the pressure below a threshold set by the sensitivity dial. The dial is uncalibrated, and sensitivity is only relatively increased or decreased. At the least sensitive setting the patient is not able to trigger inspiration. Time triggering is a function of the ventilator frequency, which is set with the rate knob from 6 to 60 breaths per minute. Time triggering is also in effect when using the sighs per hour and multi-sigh functions. Sigh frequencies of 4 to 15 sighs per hour may be selected. The multi-sigh switch allows two or three sighs to be delivered in a row, with each set delivered at the frequency set by the sighs per hour knob. The MA-1 may be manually triggered using either the normal or the sigh pushbutton.

Inspiration is volume limited any time the expiratory resistance knob is at the maximum resistance setting. In this case, the opening of the exhalation manifold is delayed briefly to create a short inspiratory hold. Peak inspiratory flow rate can be set over a calibrated range of 20 to 100 L/min, although it can be set slightly below 20 L/min.

Inspiration is terminated when one of three variables reaches a pre-set threshold. Inspiration may be pressure cycled using either the normal pressure limit or the sigh pressure limit knobs. Both may be set over a range of 20 to 80 H_2O. Inspiration may be volume cycled using either the normal volume or the sigh volume knobs. The tidal and sigh volume dials are calibrated from 0 to 2000 mL, with an actual minimum volume of approximately 100 mL. Inspiration is time cycled when the expiratory resistance knob is set to deliver an inspiratory hold.

Baseline pressure may be adjusted over an approximate range of 0 to 15 cm H_2O with a separate attachment that has an uncalibrated dial. The rate at which PIP decays to the baseline pressure may be adjusted using the expiratory resistance knob. Negative baseline pressures of approximately −9 to 0 cm H_2O may be achieved with a separate attachment.

Control Subsystems

CONTROL CIRCUIT. The MA-1 uses pneumatic, mechanical, and electronic control components (Fig. 14-47). The electronic control circuit accepts input triggering signals from the sensitivity mechanism and the ventilatory frequency control. Cycling signals are input from the volume control settings (both tidal and sigh volumes) and the normal pressure limit setting. Trigger and cycling signals control the main pneumatic solenoid that switches pressure to the bellows (see Drive Mechanism later).

Volume control is achieved by measuring the motion of the bellows. A pulley system attached to the bellows drives a potentiometer that creates an electrical signal proportional to the bellows excursion. The signal caused by the bellows motion is calibrated to function as a volume signal. When the delivered volume signal reaches the threshold set by the tidal volume or sigh volume controls, inspiration is cycled off.

DRIVE MECHANISM. The MA-1 uses an electric motor and rotary vane-type compressor to provide power for inspiration. Gas from the compressor is directed to a jet injector. The injector supplies the peak flow valve (a variable pneumatic resistor) with a driving pressure of about 1.8 psig (127 cm H_2O). This driving pressure in conjunction with the resistance set on the peak flow valve establishes the maximum (no load) inspiratory flow rate. However, the gas (air) from the injector does not go directly to the patient, since this would not allow for control of inspired oxygen concentration. Rather, it is used to drive a bellows that fills from a separate system including the air–oxygen blender.

The effect of loading on this type of drive mechanism can be illustrated using a simple model. First, we

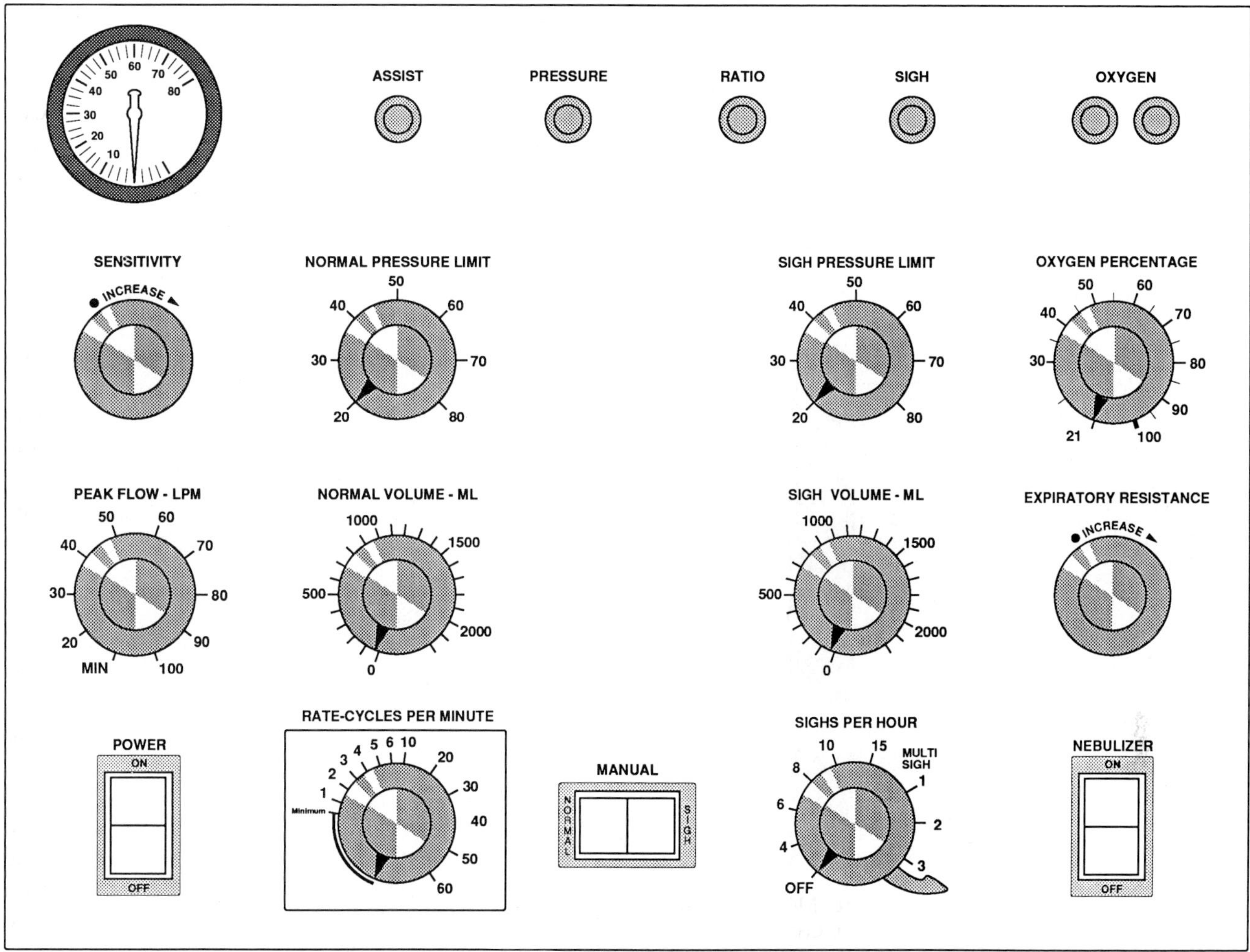

Figure 14-46. Control panel of the Puritan-Bennett MA-1 ventilator.

will assume that the driving pressure from the jet remains constant and that the ventilatory load can be represented as a single resistance connected in series with a single compliance. Inspiratory flow rate as a function of time can then be modeled by the equation:

$$\text{Inspiratory flow rate} = \left(\frac{\text{Driving pressure} - \text{baseline pressure}}{\text{R}}\right) e^{-t/RC}$$

where R is the combined total resistance of the peak flow valve, patient circuit, and respiratory system; C is the combined total compliance of the patient circuit and respiratory system; t is time from the start of inspiration; and e is the base of the natural logarithm ($\approx$ 2.72). For simplicity, we will neglect the effects of the patient circuit, assume zero baseline pressure, and assume that the peak flow dial is calibrated under zero load (ie, the ventilator's flow output port "sees" essentially zero resistance and infinite compliance). Using standard (American National Standards Institute) values for adult resistance, compliance, and tidal volume yields the data shown in Table 14-2.

Some general conclusions can be inferred from the equation and Table 14-2.

- Inspiratory flow rate remains relatively constant (less than 10% change) under small loads, with small tidal volumes, and at low peak flow settings.
- Actual flow rate may differ considerably from the set flow rate and may decay significantly during inspiration with large loads, large tidal volumes, and high peak flow settings.

From the previous equation, we would also expect that high PEEP settings would further corrupt ventilator performance. Because inspiratory flow rate at any moment during inspiration is directly proportional to the difference between driving pressure and airway pressure, and inversely proportional to the total system resistance, inspiratory flow rate may be expressed as a function of ventilating pressure.

OUTPUT CONTROL VALVES. There are three main control valves that work together to shape the inspira-

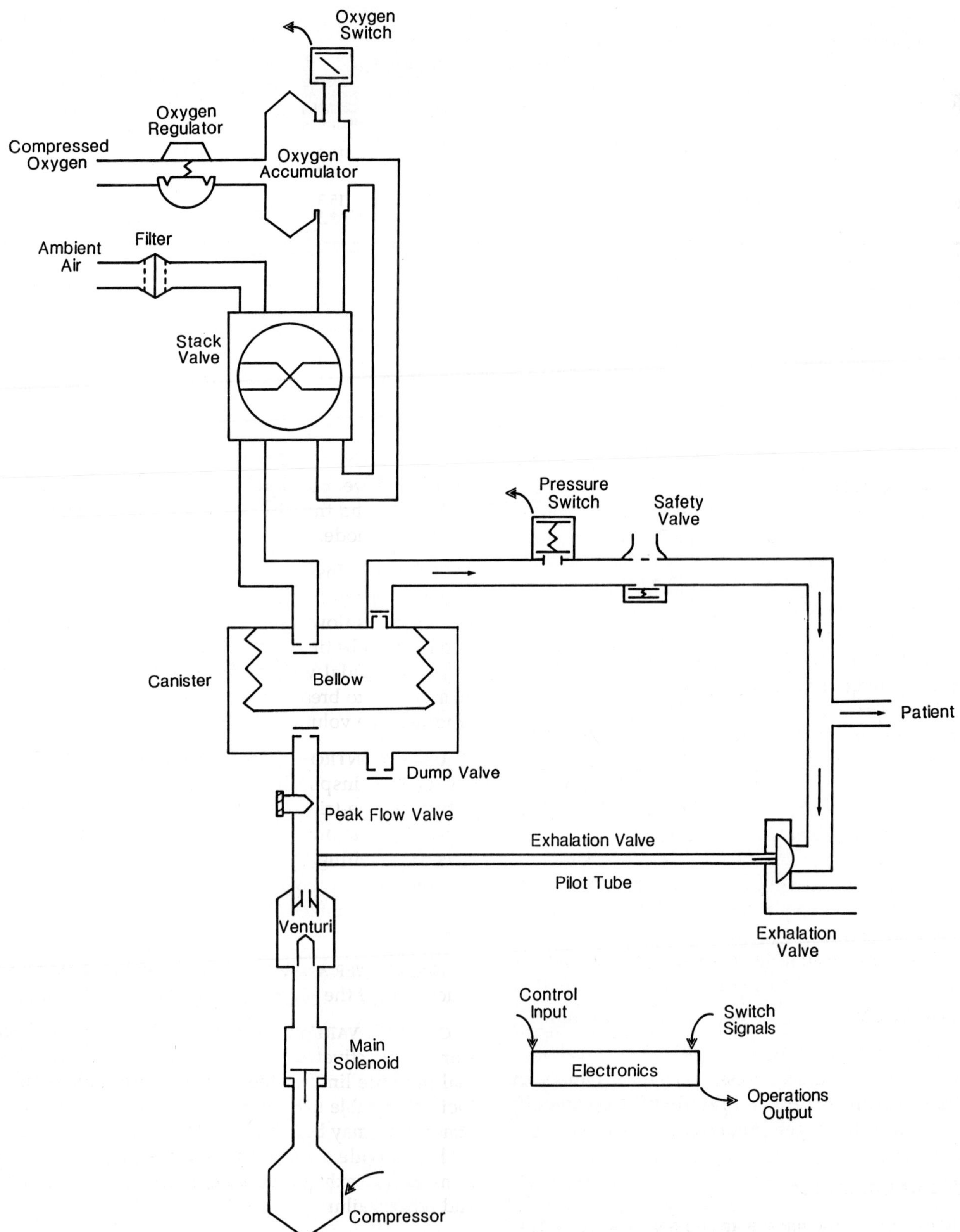

Figure 14-47. Internal components of the Puritan-Bennett MA-1 control circuit.

Table 14-2. Effects of Loading on the Performance of the MA-1 Ventilator.

Load	R*	C†	VT‡	Set Flow§	Actual Flow Initial	Actual Flow Final	Δ (%)‖	TI¶	PIP#
Small	5	0.05	0.5	20	19.8	18.2	6	1.58	12
				100	94.1	86.7	8	0.33	17
Large	20	0.02	0.5	20	19.1	15.3	20	1.75	30
				100	79.4	58.7	26	0.58	53

*R = resistance (cm H_2O/L/s).
†C = compliance (L/H_2O).
‡Vt = tidal volume (L).
§Flow is in L/min.
‖Δ (%) is the drop in flow rate during inspiration expressed as a percentage of initial flow.
¶Ti - inspiratory time (s).
#PIP = peak inspiratory pressure (H_2O).

tory flow waveform. A main solenoid valve controls flow to the peak flow valve. At the same time that the main solenoid valve turns flow on, a pneumatic signal is sent to a mushroom-valve type exhalation manifold (outside the ventilator) that blocks gas from leaving the exhalation side of the patient circuit, thus forcing gas into the patient's lungs. Inspiratory flow rate is adjusted mechanically by a variable-orifice restrictor valve connected to the peak flow knob.

During expiration, the main solenoid valve is off and the pressure in the mushroom valve bleeds off through an accumulator (a pneumatic capacitance) and the expiratory resistance valve (a variable-orifice restrictor valve). The combination of accumulator and resistor acts to slow the deflation of the mushroom valve, and hence provides resistance to exhalation. At the maximum resistance setting, there is a short delay after the tidal volume has been delivered before the mushroom valve expiratory flow. This causes an inspiratory hold along with the subsequent expiratory resistance.

Output Displays

An analog meter displays ventilating pressures. Miniature lamps indicate pressure-triggered and sigh breaths, overpressure and inverse I:E ratio conditions, and loss of oxygen pressure.

Modes of Operation

The MA-1 does not have a mode selector switch. It provides either CONTROL or ASSIST/CONTROL modes depending on the sensitivity setting. In the least sensitive position, the patient cannot trigger inspiration and thus, by definition, the ventilator is in the control mode.

CONTROL. Inspiration is volume controlled, is time triggered (according to the frequency set on the normal rate knob), is flow limited, and is usually volume cycled but may be time cycled (ie, when using an inspiratory hold). Tidal volume remains relatively constant from breath to breath, as determined by the tidal volume and sigh volume settings.

ASSIST/CONTROL. This is the same as CONTROL except that inspiration may be pressure triggered between time-triggered breaths, depending on the presence of spontaneous breathing efforts and the sensitivity setting.

Alarms

INPUT POWER ALARMS. A visual and audible alarm is activated if the source of compressed oxygen fails.

CONTROL VARIABLE ALARMS. Visual and audible alarms are activated if the PIP exceeds either the normal pressure limit or the sigh pressure limit settings (both adjustable from 20 to 80 cm H_2O). A spirometer attachment may be connected to the exhalation manifold to provide a visual and audible alarm for conditions of low exhaled volume, patient disconnection, and power failure.

CONTROL CIRCUIT ALARMS. A light is illuminated if the I:E ratio is greater than 1:1.

PURITAN-BENNETT 7200

The basic Puritan-Bennett 7200 ventilator (Puritan-Bennett Corporation, Carlsbad, CA) (Fig. 14-48) is a pressure or flow controller that may be pressure, time, or manually triggered; pressure, volume, or flow limited; and pressure or time cycled. It has an optional compressor, an integral air–oxygen blender, and a gas outlet port that will power a nebulizer during inspiration. The basic ventilator may be upgraded to allow flow triggering and flow cycling along with PRESSURE SUPPORT and continuous-flow IMV modes. The following description assumes that these options are installed.

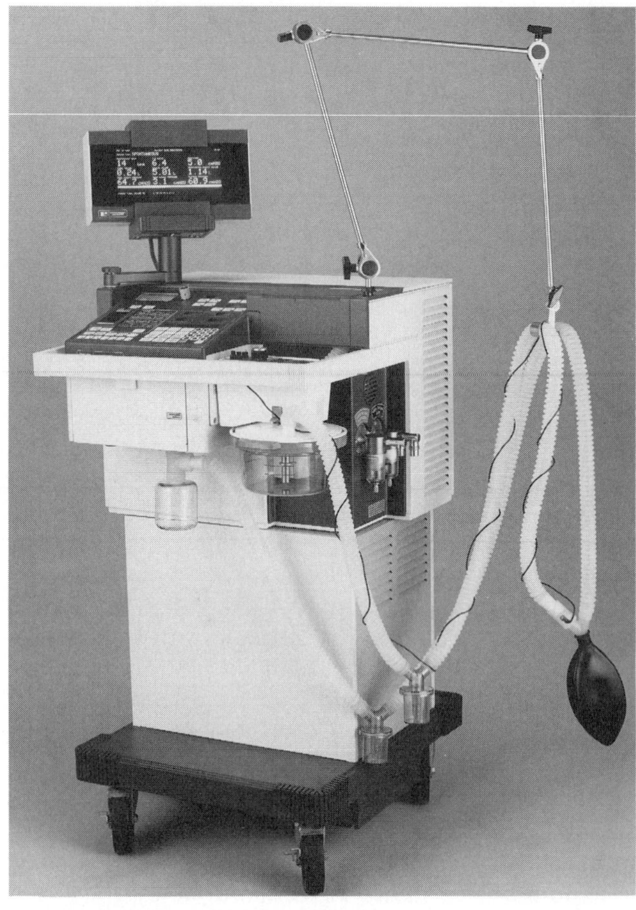

Figure 14-48. The Puritan-Bennett 7200 ventilator. (Courtesy of Puritan-Bennett Corporation, Carlsbad, CA)

Input Variables

The 7200 uses 115 volts AC at 60 Hz to power the control circuitry. The pneumatic circuit, which includes an integral air–oxygen blender, operates on external compressed gas sources (ie, air and oxygen) at 35 to 100 psig.

The front panel of the 7200 is illustrated in Figure 14-49. The operator may select the mode of ventilation; pressure-triggering, pressure-limiting, and pressure-cycling thresholds; PEEP/CPAP; tidal volume; sigh volume; flow-triggering threshold; peak inspiratory flow rate; flow waveform; ventilatory frequency; inspiratory pause time; and FIO_2. Settings are selected using a keypad in conjunction with alphanumeric LED displays or an optional electroluminescent flat-panel display module.

Control Variables

The 7200 controls either inspiratory pressure or flow. It controls inspiratory pressure in the PRESSURE SUPPORT and CPAP modes. It controls flow in the CONTROL and ASSIST/CONTROL modes and switches between pressure control (for spontaneous breaths) and flow control (for mandatory breaths) in the SIMV mode.

INSPIRATORY WAVEFORMS. The 7200 offers one inspiratory pressure and three inspiratory flow waveforms. A rectangular pressure waveform can be achieved in the PRESSURE SUPPORT mode. Flow waveforms include square (rectangular), descending ramp, and sine. Gas delivery with the rectangular waveform is relatively constant at the PEAK FLOW setting. With the descending ramp waveform, inspiratory flow begins at 5 L/min and increases linearly to peak flow. When the sine waveform is selected, inspiratory flow goes from 5 L/min to peak flow and back to 5 L/min in a sinusoidal fashion.

PHASE VARIABLES. Inspiration is pressure triggered when a spontaneous ventilatory effort removes enough gas from the patient circuit to drop the pressure below the SENSITIVITY threshold. The threshold for triggering a mandatory breath is adjustable from 0.5 to 20.0 cm H_2O below the baseline pressure. Inspiration is flow triggered when the FLOW-BY mode is activated. Inspiration is time triggered as a function of the ventilator frequency or RESPIRATORY RATE, which is adjustable from 0.5 to 70 cycles/min. Time triggering is also in effect when using the SIGH RATE and MULTIPLE SIGH functions. The SIGH RATE is adjustable from 1 to 15 sighs per minute. The MULTIPLE SIGH function allows two or three sighs to be delivered in a row, with each set delivered at the frequency set by the SIGH RATE. The Puritan-Bennett 7200 may also be manually triggered.

Inspiration is pressure limited during spontaneous breaths in the PRESSURE SUPPORT and the CPAP

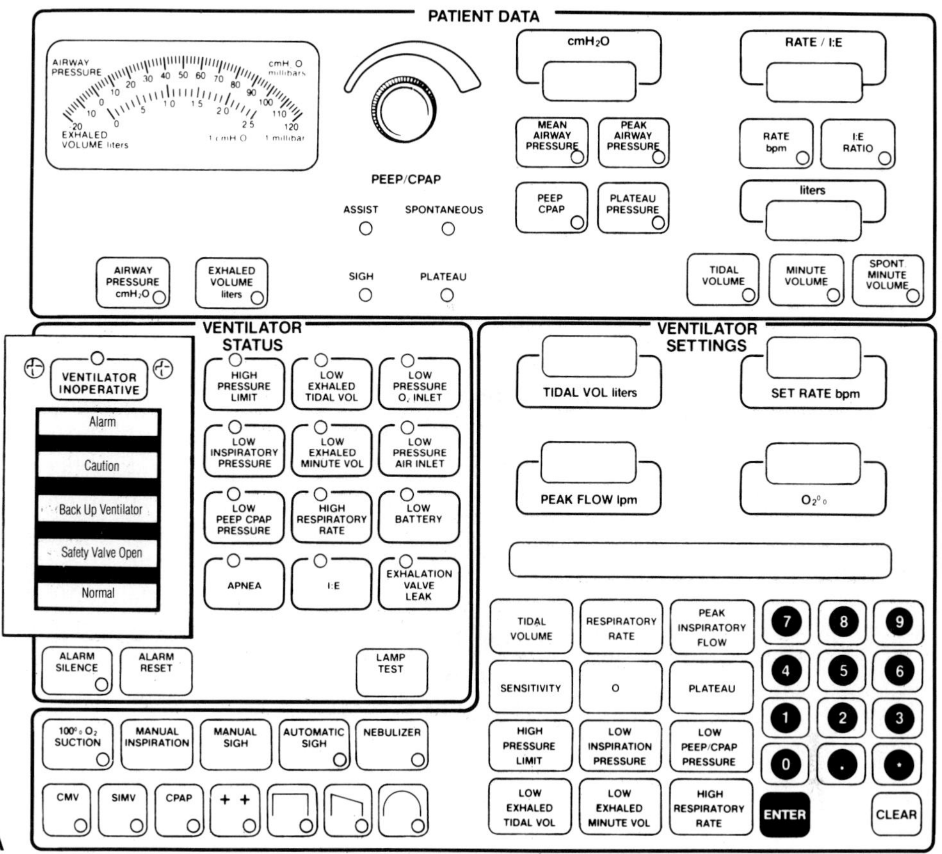

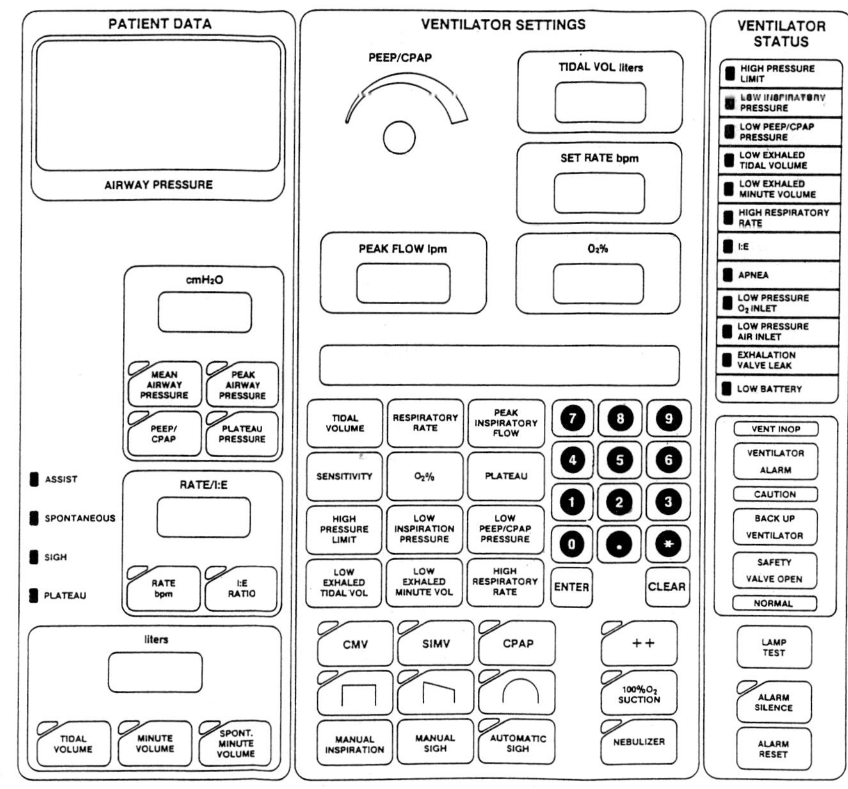

Figure 14-49. A and B. Two versions of the control panel of the Puritan-Bennett 7200 ventilator. (Courtesy of Puritan-Bennett Corporation, Carlsbad, CA)

modes. A demand flow system controls inspiratory pressure by attempting to maintain the set PEEP/CPAP level, which is adjustable from 0 to 45 cm H_2O, if PRESSURE SUPPORT is not used. If PRESSURE SUPPORT is used, the pressure limit may be set from 0 to 70 cm H_2O above the PEEP/CPAP level. Inspiration is pressure limited in the PRESSURE CONTROL mode (adjustable from 5 to 100 cm H_2O above PEEP/CPAP). Inspiration is volume limited whenever the inspiratory pause time is greater than zero. Inspiration is flow limited for mandatory flow-controlled breaths. Peak inspiratory flow rate can be pre-set over a range of 10 to 120 L/min, though peak flow for a spontaneous breath can be as high as 180 L/min. Using the FLOW-BY option, the continuous flow rate can be adjusted from 5 to 20 L/min, although flow of up to 180 L/min is available if the patient tries to inspire at a flow rate higher than the pre-set value.

Inspiration is terminated when one of three variables reaches a pre-set threshold. Inspiration may be pressure cycled when the HIGH PRESSURE LIMIT is violated. It may be set over a range of 10 to 120 cm H_2O. Active inspiratory flow is also pressure cycled for spontaneous breaths when PRESSURE SUPPORT is not used (when expiration causes airway pressure to rise above the PEEP setting). Inspiration cannot be volume cycled because the 7200 does not measure instantaneous volume. However, when inspiration is flow controlled, tidal volume and sigh volume may be set from 100 to 2500 mL. Inspiration is flow cycled in the PRESSURE SUPPORT mode when inspiratory flow rate decays to 5 L/min. Inspiration is time cycled for flow-controlled breaths whenever the inspiratory time reaches the value determined by the volume and flow rate settings. Inspiratory time is extended when the inspiratory pause time is set above zero. Inspiratory pause time is adjustable from 0 to 2.0 seconds.

Baseline pressure may be adjusted from 0 to 45 cm H_2O using the PEEP/CPAP function.

Control Subsystems

CONTROL CIRCUIT. The 7200 uses pneumatic and electronic control components (Fig. 14-50). A microprocessor accepts input signals from a pressure transducer (which measures pressure at the airway opening), two internal (hot film anemometer) flow transducers (one for air, one for oxygen), and the control variable settings and outputs control signals to the output control valves. Feedback from the airway pressure transducer is used to provide triggering, cycling, and alarm signals and to control the airway pressure waveform during pressure controlled breaths.

Information from the flow transducers provide the feedback for shaping the inspiratory flow waveform and for adjusting volume. A temperature sensor (thermistor) is paired with each of the flow transducers. They generate signals used by the microprocessor to correct the flow transducers for the effects of gas temperature.

The ventilator will automatically adjust the delivered volume to correct for BTPS (body temperature and pressure, saturated). This correction assumes that the gas delivered to the patient through the humidifier is 100% saturated at 37°C.

The 7200 will also compensate for the volume normally compressed in the patient circuit. Under these conditions, the inspiratory time (determined by the TIDAL VOLUME and PEAK FLOW settings) is held constant and the ventilator adds volume by increasing the inspiratory flow rate by an amount determined by the patient circuit compliance (ie, volume added = [compliance factor × end inspiratory pressure of previous breath]/inspiratory time). In this way, both the pre-set tidal volume and peak flow rate are delivered to the airway opening, assuming that the compliance factor is accurate.

An additional flow transducer (hot film anemometer) is used to measure exhaled volumes for display and alarm functions. Measured exhaled volumes displayed on the analog meter are not corrected for BTPS or for the additional volume compressed in the patient circuit. Therefore, inspired and exhaled volume readings may differ. Digital displays of exhaled volumes are corrected for BTPS and compressed volume.

The inspired oxygen concentration is also controlled by the microprocessor by adjusting the ratio of air flow to oxygen flow from compressed sources during each breath.

DRIVE MECHANISM. The 7200 uses either external compressed gas (for air and oxygen) or an electric motor and rotary vane-type compressor (for air) in conjunction with a pressure regulator. Gas pressure is regulated internally to about 10 psig, which drives the proportional valves (see Output Control Valves). Gas from the proportional valves is delivered directly to the patient circuit.

OUTPUT CONTROL VALVES. Gas flow to the patient is regulated by two proportional (ie, mass flow control) valves. One valve controls the instantaneous flow rate of air and the other the flow rate of oxygen. Both valves operate together during a breath, blending the source gases to achieve the F_{IO_2} setting. An additional solenoid valve directs a pneumatic signal to the exhalation valve. The microprocessor coordinates the activity of both valves such that the exhalation valve closes as the flow control valve begins to deliver flow to the patient circuit.

The flow control system is capable of delivering calibrated peak flow up to 120 L/min and demand flow (in response to spontaneous inspiratory efforts) up to 180 L/min.

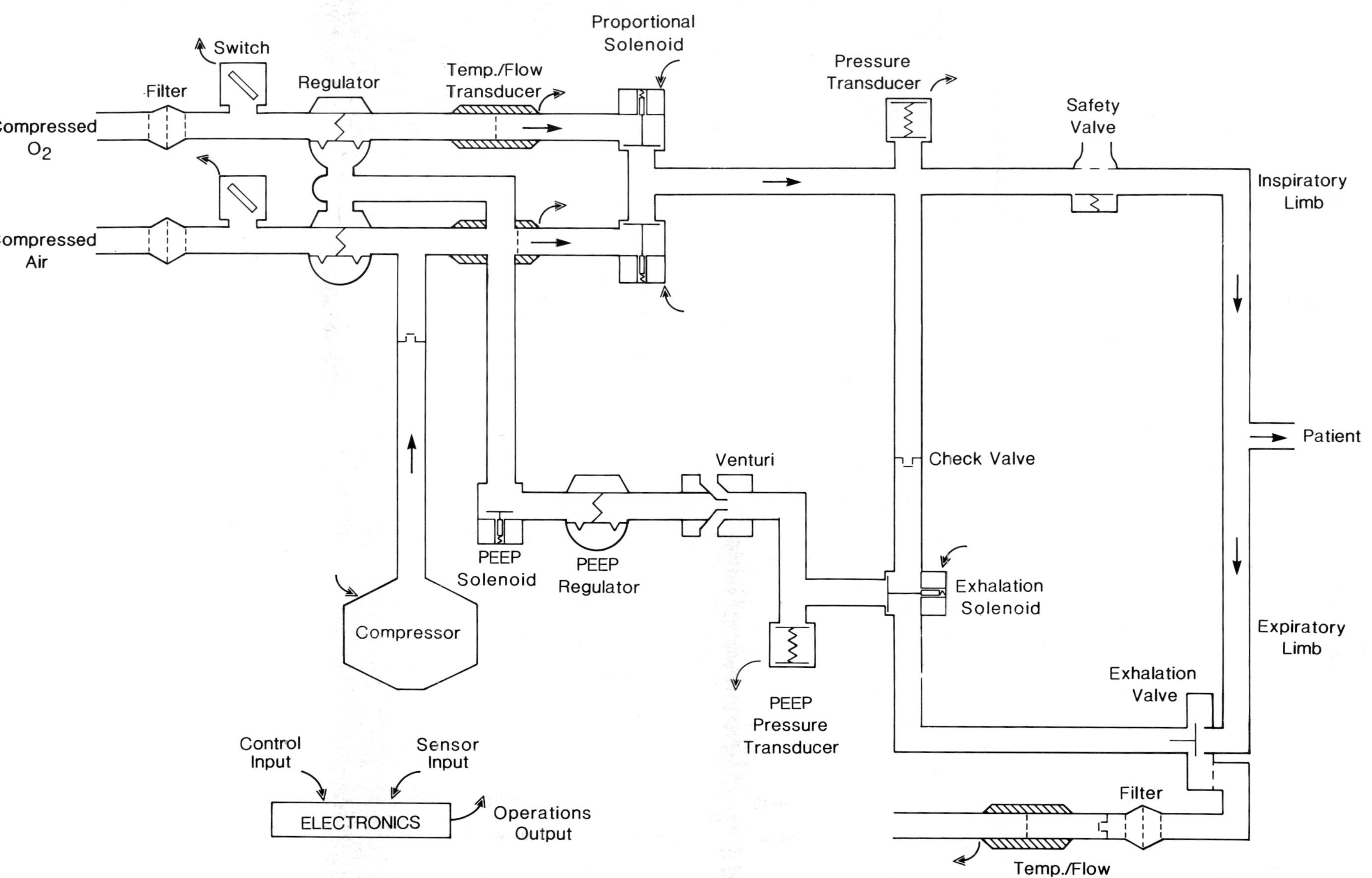

Figure 14-50. Internal components of the Puritan-Bennett 7200 ventilator control circuit.

Output Displays

In addition to the various control settings, the front panel displays include inspiratory source indicators (ie, whether a breath was assisted, spontaneous, sigh, etc.); ventilatory frequency; mandatory and spontaneous tidal volumes and minute volumes; peak, mean, plateau, and baseline airway pressures; and a wide variety of alarm and special operational help messages. An analog meter provides redundant airway pressure and exhaled volume measurements over the range of −20 to 120 cm H_2O and 0 to 2.5 L, respectively.

Digital exhaled volume displays are converted to BTPS and corrected for the volume of gas compressed in the patient circuit during inspiration (ie, to provide an accurate estimate of true exhaled volume).

The 7200 also calculates and displays respiratory system mechanics using two different algorithms. Static mechanics are calculated from tidal volume and inspiratory flow rate along with peak inspiratory, plateau, and baseline pressures by initiating an inspiratory pause during a volume-controlled breath. Dynamic mechanics are evaluated by sampling pressure, volume, and flow repeatedly during inspiration and then fitting the equation of motion to the resulting data set using a least squares statistical analysis. The equation of motion is a mathematical model of the form:

$$P_{TR} = \frac{V}{C} + R\dot{V}$$

where PTR is the change in transrespiratory system pressure (ie, airway pressure) relative to baseline pressure, V is inspired volume relative to FRC (ie, tidal volume), C is respiratory system compliance, R is respiratory system resistance (including the endotracheal tube), and $\dot{V}$ is inspiratory flow rate.

Analog pressure and flow signals may be obtained from a nine-pin connector on the back of the ventilator.

Modes of Operation

The following modes are those named on the control panel of the 7200:

CONTINUOUS MECHANICAL VENTILATION (CMV). During continuous mechanical ventilation, inspiration is flow controlled; is pressure triggered (depending on the presence of spontaneous breathing efforts and the sensitivity setting), flow triggered (if the FLOW-BY option is used), or time triggered (according to the normal or sigh frequency settings); may be volume limited (when using an inspiratory pause); is flow limited; and time cycled. Tidal volume remains relatively constant from breath to breath as determined by the TIDAL VOLUME and SIGH TIDAL VOLUME settings.

PRESSURE CONTROL. Same as CMV except that inspiration is pressure controlled, pressure limited, and time cycled.

SIMV. In SIMV, mandatory breaths are flow controlled; pressure triggered (depending on the presence of spontaneous breathing efforts and the sensitivity setting), flow triggered (if the FLOW-BY option is used), or time triggered (according to the frequency setting); and time cycled.

Spontaneous inspirations between mandatory breaths are pressure controlled (ie, inspiratory flow varies to maintain the set PEEP value), pressure triggered or flow triggered (if the FLOW-BY option is used), and normally pressure cycled. Inspiration is flow cycled when using the FLOW-BY or PRESSURE SUPPORT functions.

A mandatory breath is pressure triggered the first time a spontaneous breathing effort is detected during each ventilatory period (the time equal to the reciprocal of the RESPIRATORY RATE). Subsequent breathing efforts during the same period will not trigger another mandatory breath. If a breathing effort is not detected during a given ventilatory period, a mandatory breath will be delivered at the beginning of the next period. The ventilator will continue to deliver mandatory breaths according to the RESPIRATORY RATE setting until a spontaneous breath is detected, and the sequence of events repeats itself.

CPAP. Spontaneous inspirations are pressure controlled (ie, inspiratory flow varies to maintain either the set CPAP or PRESSURE SUPPORT value), pressure triggered or flow triggered (if the FLOW-BY option is used), and normally pressure cycled. Inspiration is flow cycled when using the FLOW-BY or PRESSURE SUPPORT functions.

PRESSURE SUPPORT. Unlike some other ventilators, the 7200 does not treat PRESSURE SUPPORT as a separate mode of ventilation. Rather, it is used to assist spontaneous breaths in the SIMV and CPAP modes. If a spontaneous effort drops the airway opening pressure below the SENSITIVITY threshold, then inspiration is pressure limited to the PRESSURE SUPPORT setting and flow cycled when the inspiratory flow rate decays to 5 L/min.

FLOW-BY. Like PRESSURE SUPPORT, FLOW-BY is not a separate mode of ventilation but rather a set of conditions designed to decrease the patient effort required to obtain gas for either spontaneous or mandatory breaths. When activated, FLOW-BY provides a continuous background flow past the airway opening and through the expiratory flow sensor and exhalation valve. This continuous flow may be adjusted from 5 to 20 L/min. The unique feature of this option is that inspiration is flow triggered. The sensitivity may be set from 1 to 10 L/min below baseline (eg, a spontaneous inspiratory flow rate of 2 L/min would drop the set continuous flow of 10 L/min to 8 L/min through the expiratory flow sensor and thus trigger a mandatory breath). Spontaneous inspirations are flow cycled when the ventilator detects a net flow through the expiratory flow sensor of greater than 2 L/min above the continuous-flow rate setting. When this happens, the background flow is reduced to 5 L/min to reduce expiratory resistance. The set background flow is re-established when the flow through the expiratory sensor decays to less than 2 L/min.

Emergency Modes of Ventilation

The following modes of ventilation support the patient when the ventilator detects certain problem conditions:

APNEA VENTILATION. Apnea ventilation is automatically activated whenever apnea is detected by the ventilator (based on the operator-selected apnea interval) and no LOW INSPIRATORY PRESSURE alarm exists. During this mode, the ventilator operates with the factory pre-set values equal to those for the BACKUP VENTILATION mode. The patient can cause the ventilator to deactivate this mode by initiating two consecutive inspirations, each of which returns 50% of the delivered volume of gas through the exhalation flow sensor.

DISCONNECT VENTILATION. This mode is automatically activated whenever the microprocessor detects inconsistencies among airway pressure, PEEP, and the gas delivery pressure in the pneumatic system. These may be caused by disconnected or plugged tubing. The ventilator will ignore spontaneous breathing efforts during this mode.

BACKUP VENTILATION. This mode is automatically activated if the ventilator's self-test program detects three system errors within 24 hours or whenever AC voltage falls below 90% of the rated input voltage. In this mode, the ventilator is time triggered, flow limited (at 45 L/min), and time cycled (at 0.5 L tidal volume) or pressure cycled (at 30 cm H_2O above the set PEEP level).

Alarms

INPUT POWER ALARMS. Visual and audible alarms are activated if the AC power supply fails or if the compressed gas supply drops below 35 psig. Separate visual and audible alarms are provided for the air and oxygen sources. A visual indicator is activated if the voltage of the internal batteries is too low to sustain 1 hour of audible alarm and battery-backed operation.

CONTROL VARIABLE ALARMS. There are several visual and audible alarms associated with ventilating pressures. These include LOW PEEP/CPAP (adjustable from 0 to 45 cm H_2O; also activated if $\geq$ 5 L has been delivered during a spontaneous breath), LOW INSPIRATORY PRESSURE (3 to 99 cm H_2O), and HIGH PRESSURE LIMIT (10 to 120 H_2O).

There are two visual and audible alarms associated with exhaled volumes. The LOW EXHALED TIDAL VOLUME alarm indicates that the four-breath running average for tidal volume is less than the set threshold (adjustable from 0 to 2500 mL). The LOW EXHALED MINUTE VOLUME alarm is adjustable over the range of 0 to 60 L.

There are visual and audible alarms for HIGH RESPIRATORY RATE (adjustable from 0 to 70 cycles/min) and APNEA. The APNEA alarm is triggered if the ventilator does not detect initiation of an exhalation during the operator-selected apnea interval (from 10 to 60 seconds).

CONTROL CIRCUIT ALARMS. A visual indicator is activated if the duration of inspiration is 50% or more of the ventilatory period (ie, the I:E ratio $\geq$ 1:1). Visual and audible EXHALATION VALVE LEAK alarms are triggered if more than 10% of the tidal volume (or 50 mL, whichever is greater) passes through the exhalation flow sensor during inspiration.

PPG IRISA

The PPG IRISA (Intelligent Respiratory Integrated System Advantage) ventilator (PPG Biomedical Systems, Lenexa, KS) (Fig. 14-51) is a pressure and flow controller that may be pressure, time, or manually triggered; pressure, volume, or flow limited; and pressure, flow, or time cycled. It has an integral air–oxygen blender and a gas outlet port that will power a nebulizer during inspiration.

Input Variables

The IRISA uses 120 volts AC at 60 Hz (or optional European voltages) to power the control circuitry. The pneumatic circuit operates on external compressed gas sources (ie, air and oxygen) at 40 to 87 psig.

The front panel of the IRISA is illustrated in Figure 14-52. The operator may select the mode of ventila-

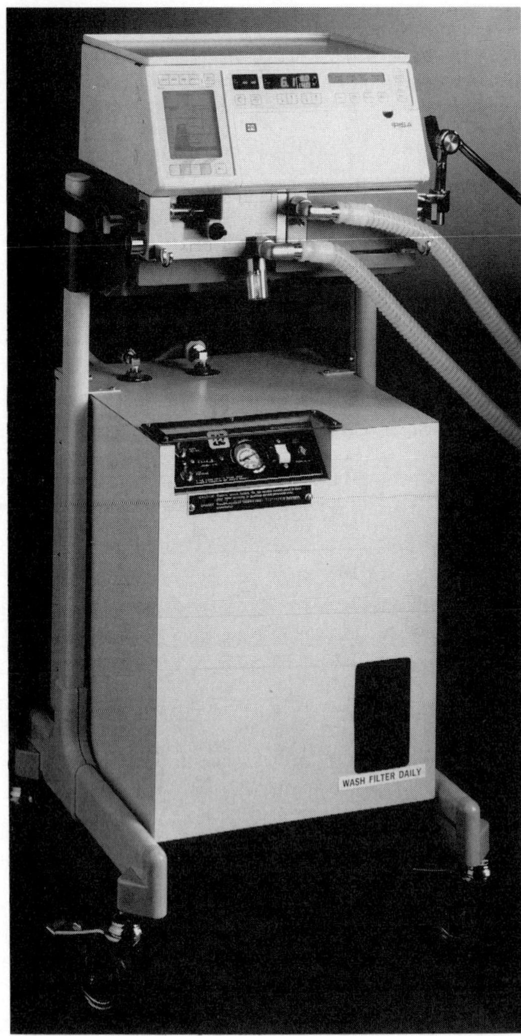

Figure 14-51. The PPG IRISA ventilator. (Courtesy of PPG Biomedical Systems, Lenexa, KS)

tion; pressure-triggering, pressure-limiting, and pressure-cycling thresholds; PEEP/CPAP; tidal volume; peak inspiratory flow rate; pressure support flow rate; flow waveform; ventilatory frequency; and I:E ratio. Settings are selected using calibrated dials.

Control Variables

The IRISA controls either inspiratory pressure or flow. It controls inspiratory pressure in the spontaneous mode. It also controls inspiratory pressure in the other modes any time the pressure control level is set to a value below the PIP that would occur during a flow-controlled breath. It controls flow in the CMV mode and switches between pressure control (for spontaneous breaths) and flow control (for mandatory breaths) in the SIMV and MMV modes.

INSPIRATORY WAVEFORMS. The IRISA offers a continuously adjustable inspiratory pressure waveform and one inspiratory flow waveform. A rectangular pressure waveform can be achieved when the pressure control option is activated. It can also be achieved in the SIMV or spontaneous modes when pressure support is activated. However, there is a pressure support flow control that modifies the flow waveform for a pressure-supported breath by setting the time it takes to reach the set level of pressure support. When inspiration is flow controlled, the waveform is rectangular only. Gas delivery with the rectangular waveform is relatively constant, and peak inspiratory flow rate is operator selectable.

PHASE VARIABLES. Inspiration is pressure triggered when a spontaneous ventilatory effort removes enough gas from the patient circuit to drop the pressure below the sensitivity setting. The threshold for triggering a mandatory breath is adjustable from 0.5 to 5.0 cm H_2O below the baseline pressure and may be turned off. Sensitivity is automatically set at 0.7 cm H_2O below baseline during SIMV. Inspiration is time triggered as a function of the ventilator frequency, which is adjustable from 5 to 60 cycles/min in the CMV mode and from 0.5 to 20 cycles/min in the SIMV mode. The IRISA may also be manually triggered.

Inspiration is pressure limited during spontaneous breaths in the spontaneous and SIMV modes. A demand flow system controls inspiratory pressure by attempting to maintain the set PEEP/CPAP level, which is adjustable from 0 to 35 cm H_2O if pressure support is not used. If pressure support is used, the pressure limit may be set from 0 to 80 cm H_2O above the PEEP/CPAP level. Pressure support begins when the demand flow generator has delivered a volume of at least 25 mL and reached a minimum flow of 1.5 L/min. Pressure limiting also occurs in the other modes whenever the pressure control setting is adjusted to a value below the PIP of a flow-controlled breath. If the pressure control setting is below the PIP but above the plateau pressure (ie, the static pressure during an inspiratory hold after a complete tidal volume is delivered), the ventilator is designed to automatically adjust flow to maintain the set tidal volume and I:E ratio, a unique feature among ventilator control schemes. If, however, the pressure control setting is adjusted to a value below the plateau pressure, it will be impossible for the ventilator to deliver the set tidal volume. The pressure control level can be adjusted from 10 to 100 cm H_2O. Inspiration is volume limited any time an inspiratory hold is set. Unlike ventilators that allow direct setting of an inspiratory hold interval, an inspiratory hold on the IRISA is an indirect result of the tidal volume, inspiratory flow rate, frequency, and I:E ratio settings. That is, whenever the inspiratory time determined by the frequency and I:E settings:

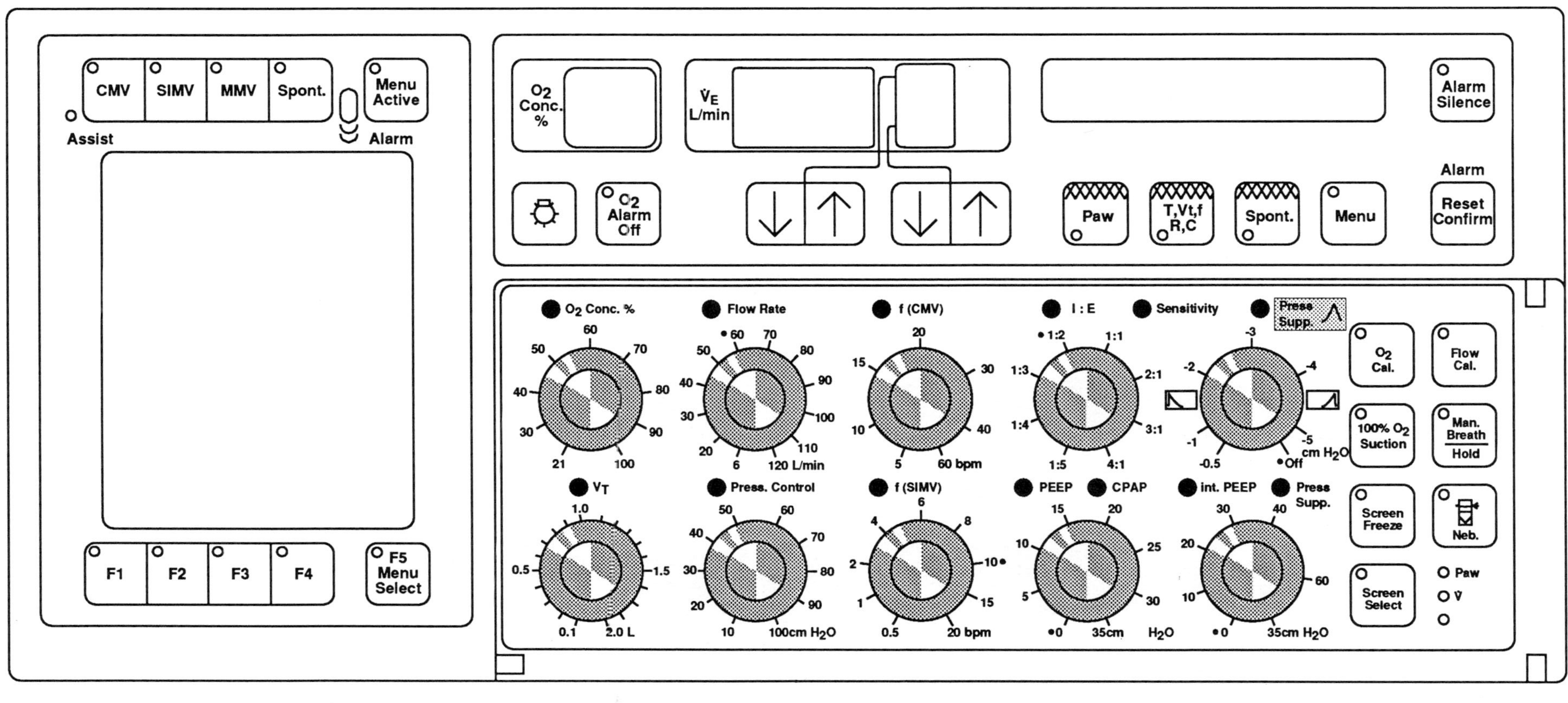

Figure 14-52. Control panel of the PPG IRISA ventilator.

$$\text{Inspiratory time(s)} = \frac{60}{\text{Frequency (cycles/min)}} \times \frac{I}{I + E}$$

is longer than the inspiratory time determined by the tidal volume and flow rate settings:

$$\text{Inspiratory time(s)} = \frac{60 \times \text{tidal volume (L)}}{\text{Peak flow (L/min)}}$$

An inspiratory hold occurs that lasts for an interval equal to the difference between the two inspiratory times. Inspiration is flow limited for all flow-controlled breaths. Peak inspiratory flow rate (in this case the same as mean inspiratory flow rate) is adjustable from 6 to 120 L/min.

Inspiration is terminated when one of three variables reaches a pre-set threshold. Inspiration may be pressure cycled when the maximum inspiratory pressure threshold is violated. This threshold is automatically set at 10 cm H_2O above the pressure control setting (adjustable from 10 to 100 cm H_2O). Active inspiratory flow is also pressure cycled for spontaneous breaths when pressure support is not used (when expiration causes airway pressure to rise above the PEEP setting). Inspiration cannot be volume cycled because the IRISA does not measure instantaneous volume. However, when inspiration is flow controlled, tidal volume may be set from 100 to 2000 mL. Inspiration is flow cycled when using pressure support as soon as inspiratory flow rate decays to 25% of the peak flow for the breath. Inspiration is time cycled for flow-controlled breaths whenever the inspiratory time reaches the value determined by the volume and flow rate settings. Inspiratory time is extended when an inspiratory hold is created. Inspiration will also be time cycled if the set flow rate is not large enough to deliver the set tidal volume in the inspiratory time determined by the I:E ratio and frequency settings. The I:E ratio may be adjusted from 1:5 to 4:1. Finally, inspiration may be time cycled by depressing and holding down the manual breath/hold button, which will cause an inspiratory hold for up to 15 seconds.

Baseline pressure may be adjusted from 0 to 35 cm H_2O using the PEEP/CPAP function. However, there is a unique intermittent PEEP control. This feature is activated when the control is set greater than zero. Two breaths every 3 minutes are delivered with a baseline pressure equal to the intermittent PEEP setting rather than the PEEP setting. Intermittent PEEP may be adjusted from 0 to 35 cm H_2O.

Control Subsystems

CONTROL CIRCUIT. The IRISA control circuit is a hybrid of electric, electronic, and pneumatic components (Fig. 14-53). Both solenoid valves (controlled by a microprocessor) and pneumatic interface valves are

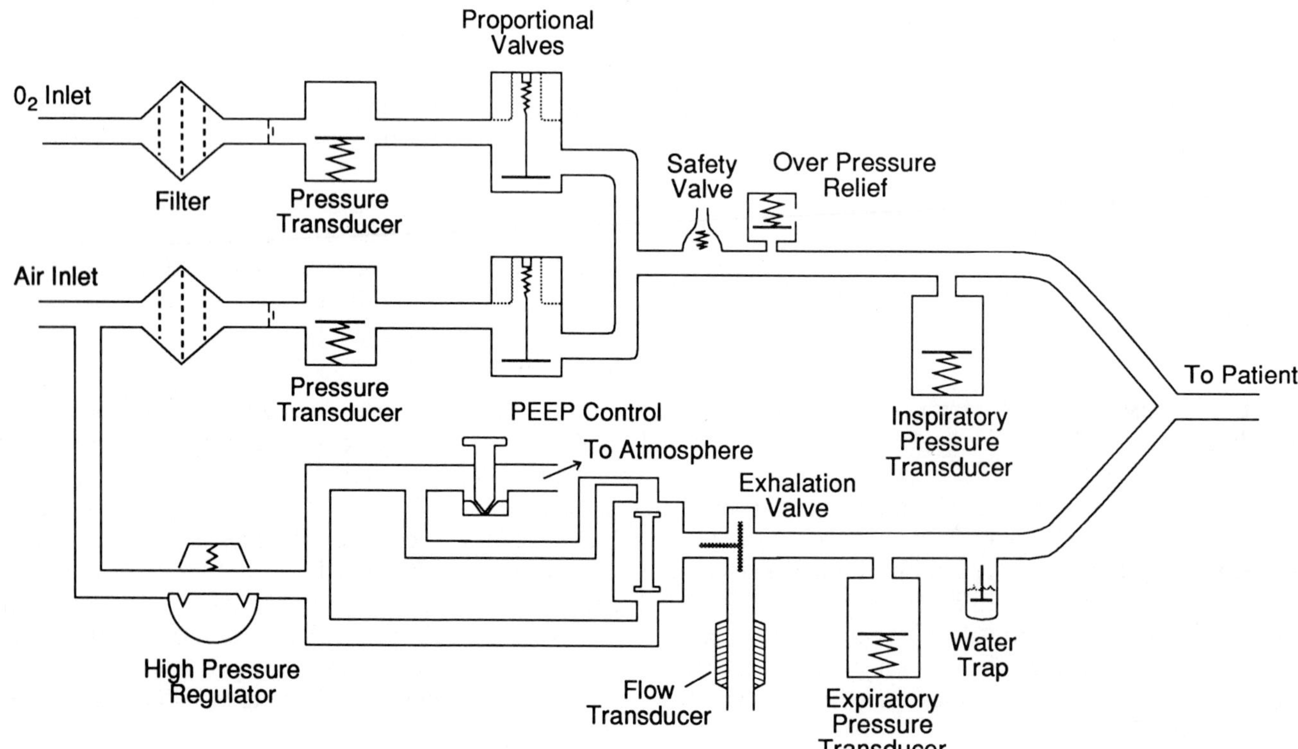

Figure 14-53. Internal components of the PPG IRISA control circuit.

used to actuate various parts of the control circuit. The microprocessor accepts input signals relating to airway pressure and flow as well as controls variable settings and outputs control signals to the output control valves.

The IRISA uses two pressure transducers inside the ventilator in a unique way to estimate airway opening pressure. One transducer, located near the port conducting gas from the patient circuit to the exhalation manifold, measures pressure during inspiration. Because the gas between this point and the patient's airway opening is stagnant during inspiration, this pressure approximates inspiratory pressure at the airway opening. This avoids the added pressure (due to airflow resistance of the delivery circuit) that would be seen if pressure was measured inside the ventilator on the inspiratory side of the delivery circuit (as some other ventilators do). Another transducer measures pressure near the port conducting gas from the ventilator to the delivery circuit. Because the gas between this point and the patient's airway opening is stagnant during expiration, pressures measured here approximate airway opening pressure during expiration and hence reflect any added pressure due to the flow resistance of the expiratory side of the delivery circuit and the exhalation manifold. Feedback from the airway pressure transducers are used to provide cycling and alarm signals and to control the airway pressure waveform during pressure-controlled breaths. A third pressure transducer, located inside the ventilator on the expiratory side of the delivery circuit, senses the patient's ventilatory efforts (ie, establishes sensitivity control) and detects leaks.

Flow information is obtained from the flow control valves and is used for shaping the inspiratory flow waveforms and for adjusting volume.

DRIVE MECHANISM. The IRISA uses either external compressed gas (for air and oxygen) or an electric motor and compressor (for air). Compressed gas from the external sources is delivered directly to the proportional valves, which control the inspiratory pressure or flow waveforms.

OUTPUT CONTROL VALVES. Gas flow to the patient is regulated by two proportional valves, a solenoid valve, and a pneumatically controlled exhalation valve. The two proportional valves are driven by the external gas sources (ie, air and oxygen). Each valve has a pressure transducer that relays information about the driving pressure of the source gas to the microprocessor. Based on the instantaneous driving pressures, the microprocessor adjusts the orifice openings inside the proportional valves to generate the desired instantaneous flow rate and FIO_2.

The solenoid valve controls the exhalation valve by switching that valve's driving pressure between a 150 cm H_2O source (during inspiration) and a variable PEEP/CPAP pressure source (for exhalation).

The exhalation valve is used to occlude the expiratory path during inspiration and when PEEP/CPAP is used. The microprocessor coordinates the activity of all valves such that the exhalation valve closes as the flow control valves begin to deliver flow to the patient circuit.

Output Displays

In addition to the various control settings, the front panel displays include peak, plateau, mean, and end-expiratory pressures; inspired gas temperature and measured oxygen concentration; set tidal volume; set frequency; compliance; resistance; spontaneous expired minute volume and frequency; and alarm indicators. In addition, there is a screen for menu-driven displays of pressure or flow waveforms and alphanumeric messages regarding settings and alarm conditions.

An optional analog output of all ventilator parameters is available. An RS 232C digital output is standard.

Modes of Operation

The following modes are those named on the control panel of the IRISA:

CMV. In the CMV mode the ventilator delivers either IMV or assist/control depending on whether the sensitivity is turned on or off. When the sensitivity is turned on, all breaths are mandatory and flow controlled, time triggered (according to the CMV frequency setting) or pressure triggered (depending on the presence of spontaneous breathing efforts and the sensitivity setting), flow limited, and time cycled. When the sensitivity is turned off, spontaneous breaths are permitted between mandatory breaths. Spontaneous breaths are pressure controlled (ie, inspiratory flow varies to maintain the set PEEP value), pressure triggered (sensitivity is automatically defaulted to 0.7 cm H_2O), and pressure cycled.

SIMV. In SIMV, mandatory breaths are flow controlled, pressure triggered (depending on the presence of spontaneous breathing efforts, sensitivity is automatically set a 0.7 cm H_2O) or time triggered (according to the SIMV frequency setting), and time cycled.

Spontaneous inspirations between mandatory breaths are pressure controlled (ie, inspiratory flow varies to maintain the set PEEP value), pressure triggered, and normally pressure cycled. Inspiration is flow cycled when the PRESSURE SUPPORT setting is above zero.

If a spontaneous inspiratory effort is observed during the trigger window phase, a synchronized mandatory breath is delivered. The duration of the trigger window is influenced by the CMV frequency, I:E, and SIMV frequency settings and may last up to 2.5 seconds.

SPONTANEOUS. All inspirations are pressure controlled (ie, inspiratory flow varies to maintain either the set CPAP value or the pressure support value if this option is used), pressure triggered, and normally pressure cycled. Inspiration is flow cycled when using pressure support.

MMV. MMV is the same as spontaneous except that time-triggered (determined by the SIMV frequency setting), time-cycled breaths are delivered whenever the patient's minute volume falls below the desired minimum minute volume (determined as tidal volume times SIMV frequency). The patient is credited only with spontaneous volumes up to 1.5 times the desired minute volume. This removes the risk of undetected apnea.

Alarms

All alarms are visual and audible.

INPUT POWER ALARMS. Alarms are activated if the AC power supply fails or if the compressed gas supply drops below 40 psig.

CONTROL VARIABLE ALARMS. There are two alarms associated with ventilating pressures. A high inspiratory pressure alarm is automatically set at 10 cm H_2O above the pressure control setting. A low inspiratory pressure alarm is triggered if the airway pressure fails to exceed the set PEEP + 5 cm H_2O for two cycles.

There are low and high minute volume alarms, both adjustable from 0 to 41 L/min.

There is a high ventilatory frequency alarm adjustable from 5 to 80 cycles/min.

There are low and high oxygen concentration alarms automatically set at 4% below and above the oxygen concentration setting.

There is a high inspired gas temperature alarm set at 40°C.

CONTROL CIRCUIT ALARMS. Alarm messages are displayed in the event of the following system failures:

- Fail to cycle
- Mixer inoperative
- O_2 measurement inoperative
- Expiration valve inoperative
- Pressure measurement inoperative
- Fan defective
- Device failure
- Apnea (if interval between breaths exceeds 15 seconds)

SECHRIST IV-100B

The Sechrist IV-100B (Sechrist Industries, Anaheim, CA) (Fig. 14-54) is a pressure or flow controller that is time or manually triggered and time cycled. It uses an external air–oxygen blender/flowmeter module.

Input Variables

The Sechrist IV-100B requires 117 volts AC at 60 Hz to power the control circuitry. The ventilator also requires pneumatic power and operates on external compressed air and oxygen sources at 11 to 100 psig. The Sechrist IV-100B has no internal compressor.

The front panel of the Sechrist IV-100B is illustrated in Figure 14-55. The operator may select mode of ventilation, desired pressure limit (PIP), desired baseline pressure (PEEP), inspiratory time, expiratory time, and flow rate.

Control Variables

The Sechrist IV-100B is normally set to control inspiratory pressure. However, as with most infant ventilators, the Sechrist IV-100B is designed more to limit rather than truly control inspiratory pressure. In the first place, the pressure limit control knob is uncalibrated. But more to the point, the peak inspiratory flow rate is always limited to the value set on the flowmeter. For a given inspiratory time, this flow rate may not be sufficient to achieve the set inspiratory pressure limit in the allotted inspiratory time (depending also on the compliance and resistance of the patient's respiratory system). Thus, in this situation, the Sechrist IV-100B becomes a flow controller by default.

INSPIRATORY WAVEFORMS. The Sechrist IV-100B is capable of producing either a rectangular pressure or a flow waveform. It is most often operated with a rectangular pressure waveform in a pressure-controlled (ie, pressure-limited) mode. However, there is a waveform control valve that can be used to create quasi-sinusoidal pressure and flow waveforms. A rectangular flow waveform may be obtained by setting the PIP limit high enough to achieve flow control.

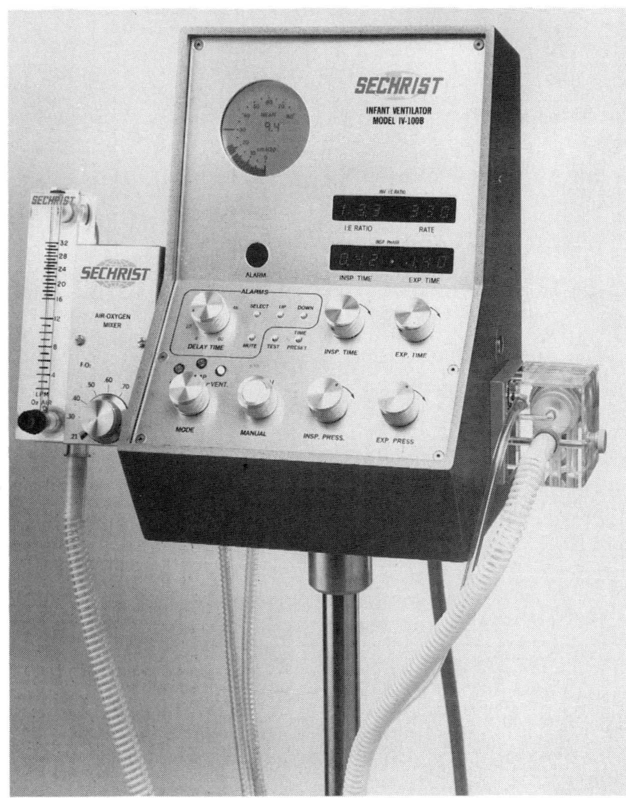

Figure 14-54. The Sechrist IV-100B ventilator. (Courtesy of Sechrist Industries, Anaheim, CA)

PHASE VARIABLES. Inspiration is normally time triggered and is a function of the set inspiratory time (adjustable from 0.1 to 2.9 seconds) and expiratory time (adjustable from 0.3 to 60.0 seconds). These ranges yield a ventilatory frequency range of 1 to 150 cycles/min. Inspiration may also be manually triggered.

Inspiration may be pressure limited from 7 to 70 cm H_2O. If inspiration is not pressure limited, it is flow limited. Inspiratory flow rate may be adjusted from 0 to 20 L/min.

Inspiration is time cycled as a result of the set inspiratory time.

Baseline pressure may be adjusted over the range of −2 to 15 cm H_2O using the (uncalibrated) expiratory pressure knob.

Control Subsystems

CONTROL CIRCUIT. The control circuit of the Sechrist IV-100B uses electronic, pneumatic, and fluidic components (Fig. 14-56). A microprocessor sends timing signals to a solenoid valve, which drives two fluidic components, a back-pressure switch, and an or/nor gate. A pneumatic signal from the fluidic components drives a diaphragm-type valve in the exhalation manifold.

DRIVE MECHANISM. The Sechrist IV-100B requires an external pneumatic source to power an air–oxygen blender. This blender delivers pressurized gas to a flowmeter, which then routes a continuous flow of gas to the patient circuit.

OUTPUT CONTROL VALVES. The output control valves include the flow control needle valve, inspiratory and expiratory pressure control needle valves, a plunger-type solenoid valve, a waveform adjust needle valve, and a diaphragm exhalation valve. During inspiration, a timing signal from a microprocessor (or from the manual breath pushbutton) drives a solenoid that directs a pneumatic signal to a fluidic back-pressure switch. The back-pressure switch sends a pneumatic signal to a fluidic or/nor gate. The output pneumatic signal from the or/nor gate is directed through the inspiratory pressure needle valve, which adjusts the pressure applied to the exhalation valve diaphragm, and hence the peak inspiratory airway pressure limit.

During expiration, the solenoid valve removes the pneumatic signal from the back-pressure switch. The back-pressure switch changes its output, causing the or/nor gate to remove its pneumatic signal from the inspiratory pressure valve and apply it through the expiratory pressure needle valve. This valve sets the baseline pressure applied to the exhalation valve, which determines the PEEP/CPAP level.

The waveform adjustment needle valve adjusts the time constant of the pressure build-up and decay (ie, during inspiratory and expiratory times) in the exhalation valve. If the time constant is short, the pressure builds up rapidly during the inspiratory phase and decays rapidly after inspiration cycles off so that the inspiratory pressure waveform tends to be rectangular. If the time constant is long, the opposite occurs and the inspiratory pressure waveform appears more rounded or sinusoidal.

Both the PIP and the PEEP/CPAP level are set by observing an aneroid pressure gauge while adjusting the uncalibrated control knobs.

Output Displays

Airway pressure is displayed by an aneroid pressure gauge over the range of −10 to 80 cm H_2O. There are also digital displays for inspiratory time, expiratory time, I:E ratio, and ventilatory frequency, as well as indicators for inspiratory phase and inverse I:E ratio. Flow is indicated on a Thorpe-tube flowmeter.

Modes of Operation

The following modes are those named on the control panel of the Sechrist IV-100B:

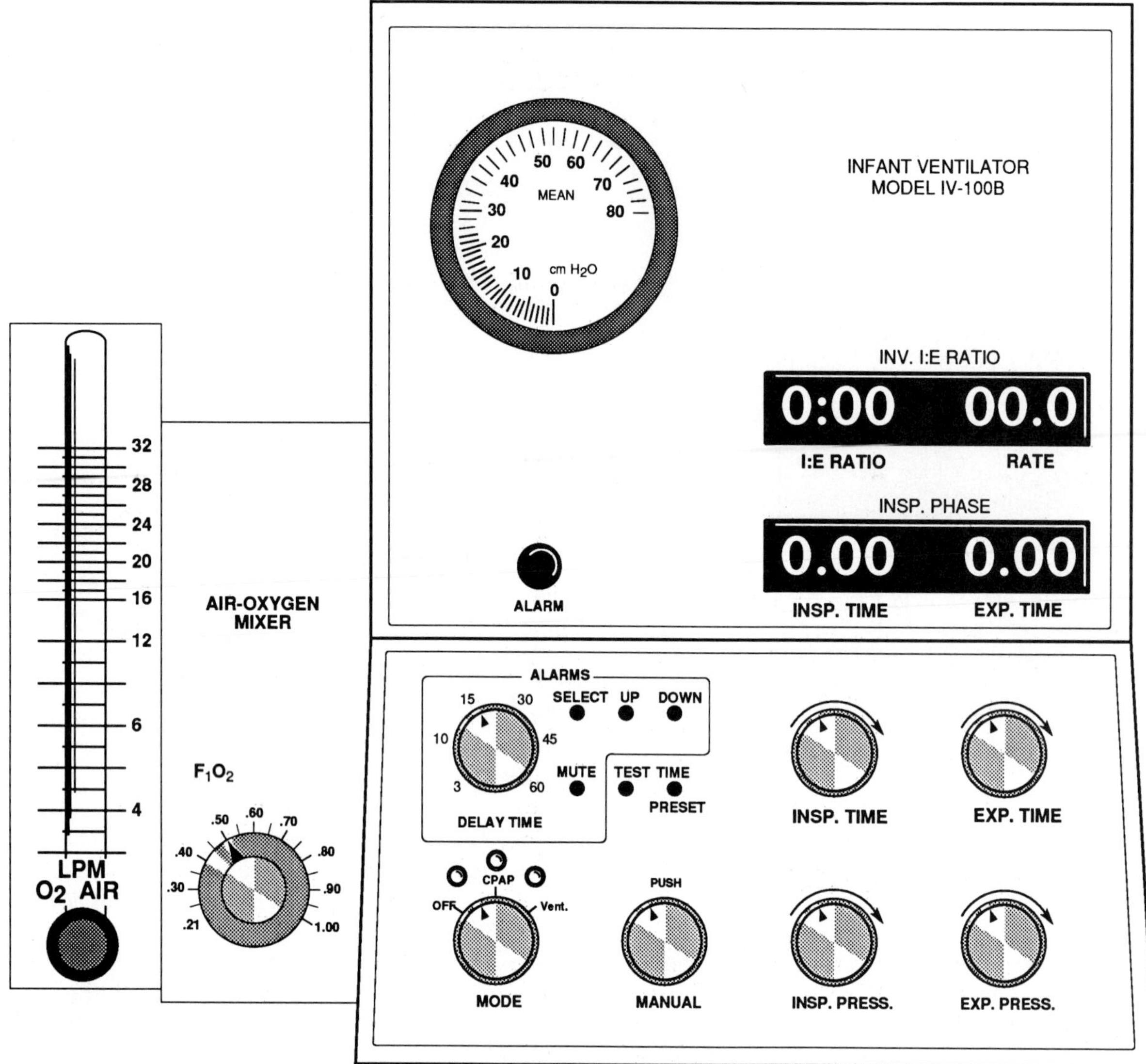

Figure 14-55. Control panel of the Sechrist IV-100B ventilator.

VENTILATION. Inspiration is normally pressure controlled, time triggered (based on the ventilatory rate), and time cycled (based on the inspiratory time). There is a continuous flow of gas from the ventilator at the rate set on the flow control knob to allow for spontaneous breathing between mandatory breaths. If inspiration is not pressure limited (owing to insufficient flow or inspiratory time), it is flow limited, time triggered, and time cycled.

If, during spontaneous breaths, the patient's inspiratory flow rate exceeds that delivered by the ventilator such that negative airway pressure is generated below the baseline pressure, the Sechrist IV-100B is incapable of varying flow rate to meet the patients demand. It is therefore important that the operator have the continuous flow rate set sufficiently high to meet all the patient's demand.

CPAP. Inspiration is not controlled in the CPAP mode. The patient breathes the continuous flow of gas from the flowmeter. The pressure at the airway opening during inspiration fluctuates as a function of the fixed resistance through the exhalation manifold (determined mainly by the PEEP/CPAP setting) and the surplus inspiratory flow. Surplus inspiratory flow is the difference between the flow rate set on the flowmeter and the patient's instantaneous inspiratory flow rate.

Alarms

INPUT POWER ALARMS. When external electrical power supply to the Sechrist IV-100B is interrupted there is an audible and visual alarm. A drop of air or oxygen inlet pressure to less than 15 psig results in an audible alarm.

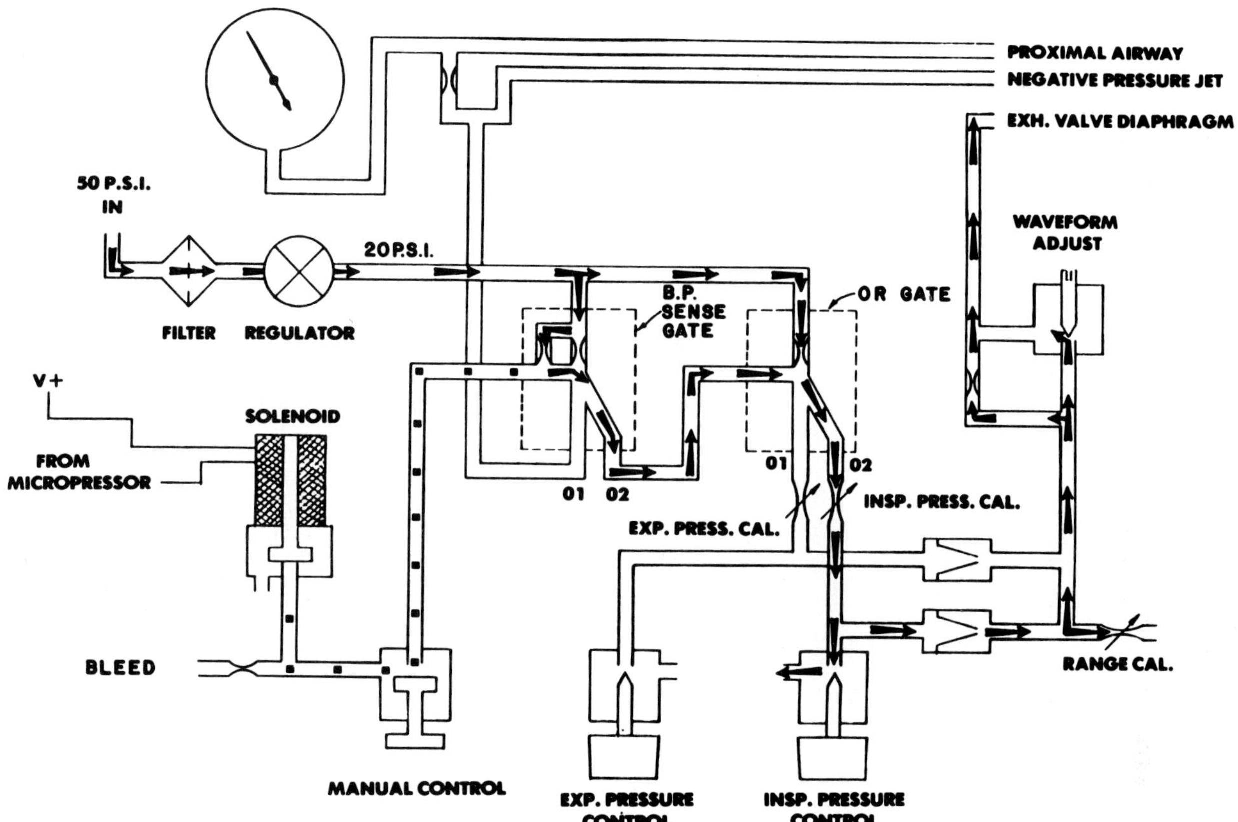

Figure 14-56. Internal components of the Sechrist IV-100B control circuit. (Courtesy of Sechrist Industries, Anaheim, CA)

CONTROL VARIABLE ALARMS. The Sechrist IV-100B provides a visual and audible alarm based on the presence or absence of an inspiratory pressure signal. To sense the airway pressure signal, a movable sensor is located on the periphery of the airway pressure manometer. The sensor consists of an infrared emitter and a photo transistor detector. If the sensor is located so that the manometer needle passes through the infrared light beam during each inspiration, a signal is sent to the alarm circuit. If the signal is not sensed, visual and audible alarms are triggered, indicating such conditions as a leak in the patient circuit, source gas failure, microprocessor failure, prolonged inspiration, or patient circuit disconnection.

CONTROL CIRCUIT ALARMS. The Sechrist IV-100B has no control circuit alarms.

SECHRIST 2200B

The Sechrist 2200B ventilator (Sechrist Industries, Anaheim, CA) (Fig. 14-57) is a pressure or volume controller that may be pressure, time, or manually triggered; pressure, volume, or flow limited; and pressure, volume, flow, or time cycled. The Sechrist 2200B has an optional compressor, an integral air–oxygen blender, and a gas outlet port that will power a nebulizer during inspiration.

Input Variables

The Sechrist 2200B uses 115 volts AC at 60 Hz to power the control circuitry. The pneumatic circuit, which includes an integral air–oxygen blender, operates on external compressed gas sources (ie, air and oxygen) at 40 to 60 psig.

The front panel of the Sechrist 2200B is illustrated in Figure 14-58. Control variables are adjusted by individ-

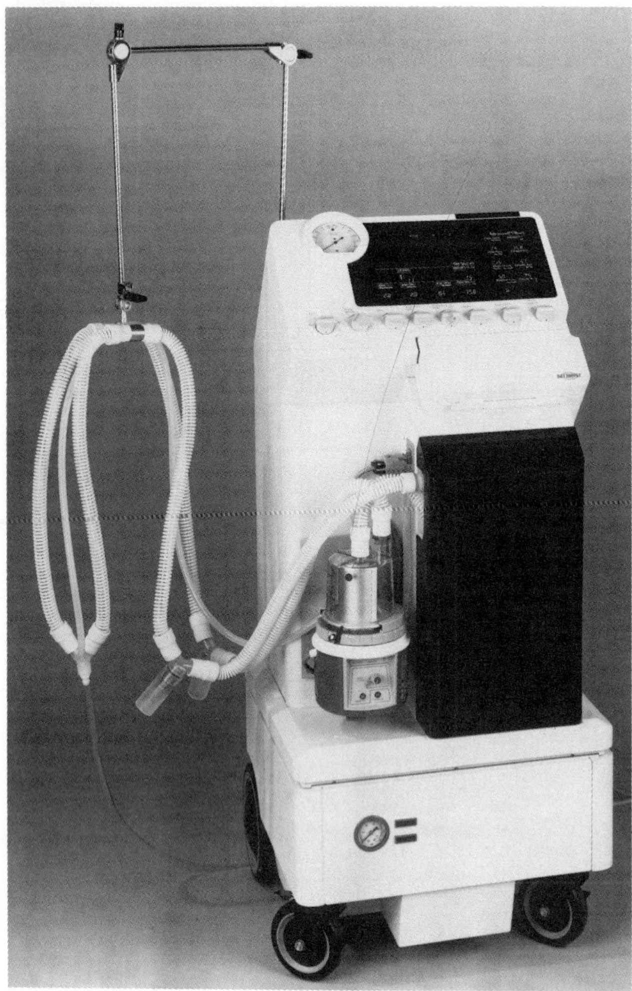

Figure 14-57. The Sechrist 2200B ventilator. (Courtesy of Sechrist Industries, Anaheim, CA)

ual knobs with the set values shown in a separate digital display area. There is also a keypad used to set alarms, parameters for sighs and MMV, set patient circuit compliance correction, select flow waveforms, and set various auxiliary/diagnostic functions. The keypad offers a unique help routine that calculates a nominal patient minute volume based on the Radford nomogram.

The operator may select the mode of ventilation, pressure triggering and pressure limiting thresholds, PEEP/CPAP, tidal volume, compliance compensation factor (adds to set tidal volume to compensate for patient circuit compliance), inspiratory flow waveform, MMV, ventilatory frequency, inspiratory time, inspiratory pause time, and F_{IO_2}.

Control Variables

The Sechrist 2200B controls either inspiratory pressure or volume. It controls inspiratory pressure in the CPAP and PRESSURE CONTROL modes and volume in the ASSIST/CONTROL, SIMV, and MMV modes. It switches between pressure control (for spontaneous breaths) and flow control (for mandatory breaths) in the SIMV and MMV modes.

INSPIRATORY WAVEFORMS. The Sechrist 2200B offers one inspiratory pressure and four inspiratory flow waveforms. A rectangular pressure waveform can be achieved in the PRESSURE CONTROL mode and when pressure support is used to assist spontaneous breaths. Flow waveforms include square (rectangular), accelerating (ascending ramp), decelerating (descending ramp), and sine.

PHASE VARIABLES. Inspiration is pressure triggered when a spontaneous ventilatory effort removes enough gas from the patient circuit to drop the pressure below the TRIGGER SENSITIVITY threshold. The threshold for triggering all assisted breaths is adjustable from 0.5 to over 5.0 cm H_2O below the baseline pressure (may be turned off). Unassisted breaths can access demand flow with a pressure drop of less than 1.0 cm H_2O. Inspiration is time triggered as a function of the ventilator frequency, or rate, which is adjustable from 0.5 to 60 cycles/min. Time triggering is also in effect when using sighs. Single sighs may be set from 1 to 10 sighs per hour. Multiple sighs (two or three) may also be selected. The Sechrist 2200B may also be manually triggered for both regular and sigh breaths.

Inspiration is pressure limited for mandatory breaths in the PRESSURE CONTROL mode and for all spontaneous breaths. A demand valve controls inspiratory pressure by attempting to maintain the set PEEP/CPAP level, which is adjustable from 0 to 30 cm H_2O. If PRESSURE LEVEL is set above zero (range 0–50 H_2O above baseline), spontaneous breaths will be pressure supported. (Note that there is no explicit mode selection for pressure support.) Inspiration is volume limited whenever the INSPIRATORY HOLD is greater than zero. Inspiration is flow limited for volume-controlled breaths. Inspiratory flow rate cannot be directly pre-set; it is a function of the VOLUME and INSPIRATORY TIME settings for volume-controlled breaths. The ventilator can deliver flows from 2 to 120 L/min.

Inspiration is terminated when one of three variables reaches a pre-set threshold. Inspiration may be pressure cycled when either the high inspiratory pressure alarm threshold is violated. Inspiration is also pressure cycled for spontaneous breaths when pressure support is not used (when expiration causes airway pressure to rise above the PEEP setting). Inspiration is volume cycled in the ASSIST/CONTROL and SIMV modes. Tidal volume may be set from 100 to 2200 mL. Inspiration is flow cycled for pressure-supported spontaneous breaths when inspiratory flow rate decays to 25% of the peak inspiratory flow rate.

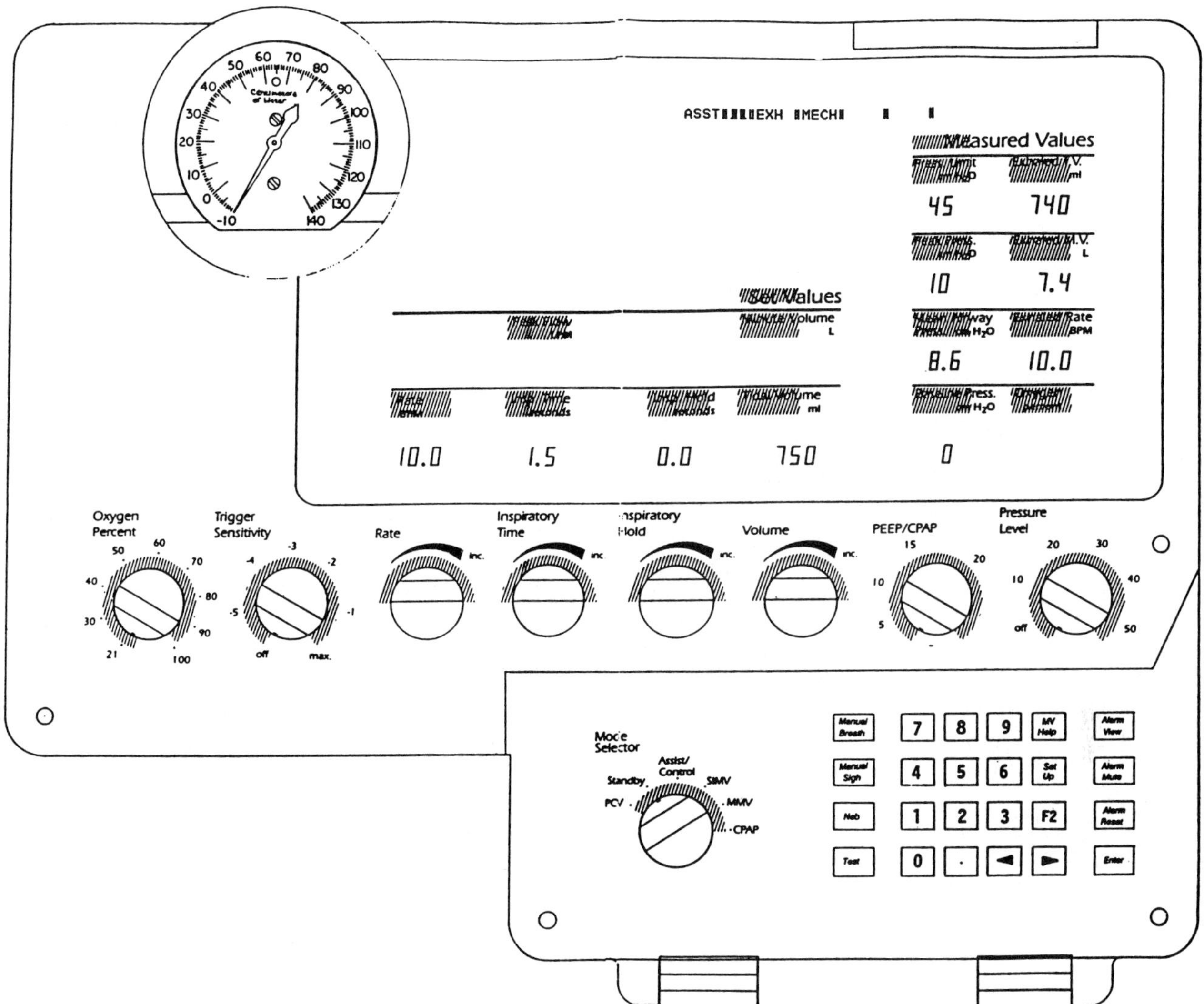

Figure 14-58. Control panel of the Sechrist 2200B ventilator. (Courtesy of Sechrist Industries, Anaheim, CA)

Inspiration is time cycled for mandatory breaths in the PRESSURE CONTROL mode. The INSPIRATORY TIME may be set from 0.2 to 3.0 seconds. Inspiration is also time cycled when INSPIRATORY HOLD is set above zero (adjustable from 0 to 2.0 seconds).

Baseline pressure may be adjusted from 0 to 30 cm H_2O using the PEEP/CPAP knob.

Control Subsystems

CONTROL CIRCUIT. The Sechrist 2200B uses pneumatic and electronic control signals (Fig. 14-59). The microprocessor accepts input from three pressure transducers (proximal airway measured at the exhalation manifold, machine pressure, and proximal/PEEP differential pressure). Input signals also come from an external flow sensor to measure exhaled flow. Output control signals go to the flow control valve, nebulizer solenoid valve, exhalation solenoid valve, and others. The exhalation solenoid valve outputs pneumatic signals to the exhalation valve that allows control of peak inspiratory and baseline pressures.

DRIVE MECHANISM. The Sechrist 2200B uses either external compressed gas (for air and oxygen) or an electric motor and compressor (for air). Gas pressure is balanced before reaching the air–oxygen blender mechanism. Mixed gas leaves the blender and enters a rigid-walled vessel (the "accumulator") with an internal volume of about 0.46 L. The flow control system is driven by the pressure from the accumulator. Volume stored in the accumulator reduces the instantaneous flow demand required of the blending system and upstream pressure-regulating system. This action allows a wide range of peak flows, reduces the flow required of the compressed gas supply, and improves response time. The accumulator also acts as a mixing chamber, which helps to stabilize the delivered oxygen concentration within a given breath.

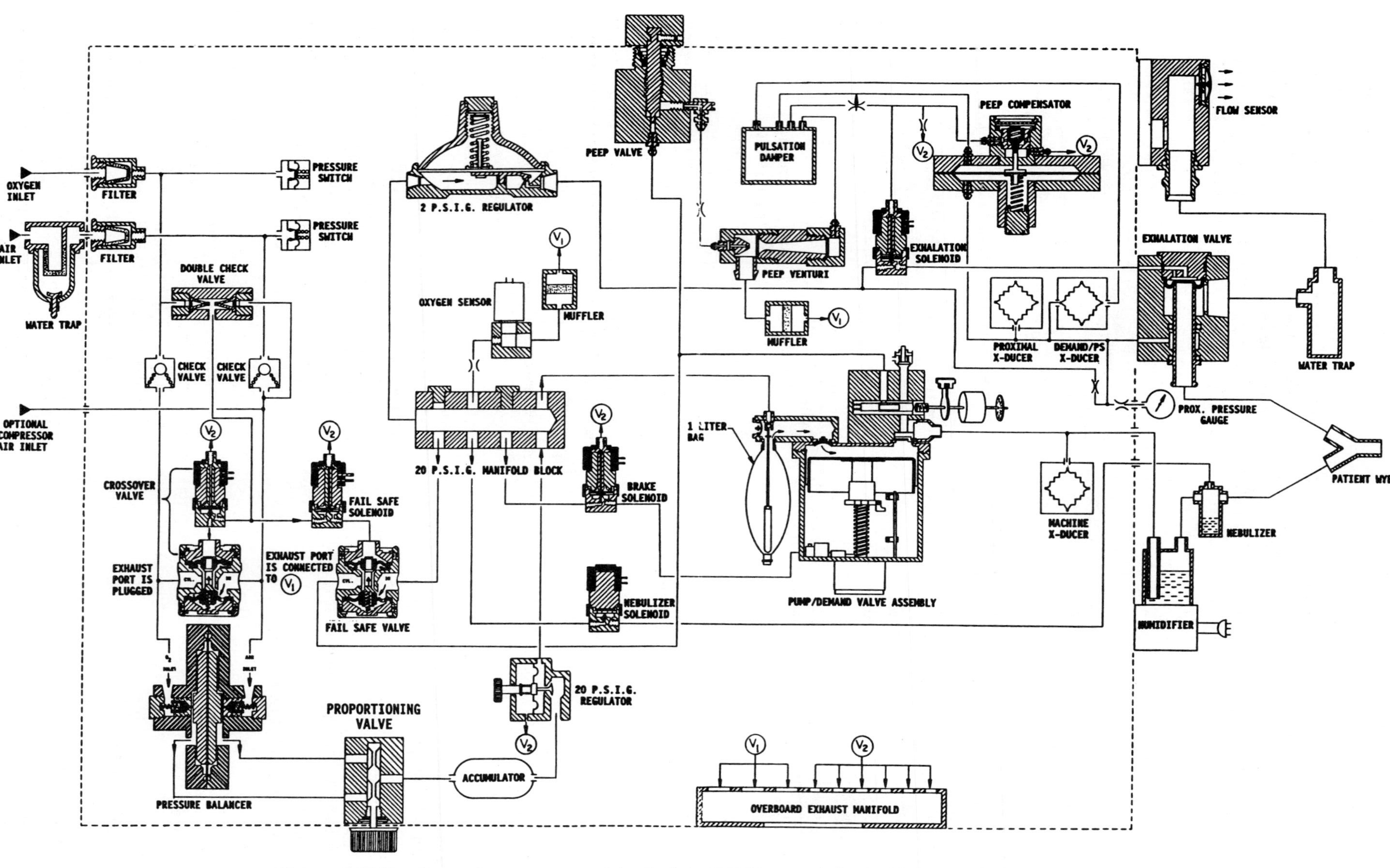

Figure 14-59. Internal components of the Sechrist 2200B control circuit. (Courtesy of Sechrist Industries, Anaheim, CA)

OUTPUT CONTROL VALVES. Gas flow to the patient is regulated by a main flow control valve (for control of mandatory breaths) and a demand valve (for control of spontaneous breaths). The main flow control valve is a piston pump connected to a stepper motor. A 1.0 L reservoir bag is connected to the inlet of the flow control valve. The demand valve is a proportional solenoid valve (driven by a stepper motor) connected to a 20-psig source of blended gas. An electromagnetic poppet valve switches between two sources of a pneumatic signal to the exhalation valve. One source is a 2-psig pressure regulator that keeps a diaphragm-type exhalation manifold closed during assisted breaths. The other source is a jet venturi that generates an adjustable pressure signal to control baseline pressure (ie, PEEP/CPAP). The microprocessor coordinates the activity of both valves such that the exhalation valve closes as the flow control valve begins to deliver flow to the patient circuit.

OUTPUT DISPLAYS The main output displays for the Sechrist 2200B include a "Status Line" and a digital display of measured variables. There is also an aneroid pressure gauge. The Status Line is divided into seven "cells," or sections.

- Cell 1 displays the mode of ventilation.
- Cell 2 displays a graphic representation of the selected flow waveform.
- Cell 3 indicates the current phase of each breath (ie, inspiration and expiration).
- Cell 4 indicates the current type of breath using a rather arbitrary nomenclature: MECH = mandatory breaths in the ASSIST/CONTROL, SIMV, MMV, or PRESSURE CONTROL modes; PSV = pressure supported breaths; and SPON = an unassisted spontaneous breath.
- Cell 5 indicates when the nebulizer is on.
- Cell 6 shows when a sigh is delivered.
- Cell 7 displays the current I:E ratio.

The Status Line is also used to display alarm messages.

Measured values displayed include the following:

- Pressure limit
- Peak, mean, and baseline pressures
- Exhaled tidal volume
- Exhaled minute volume
- Total breath rate (mandatory and spontaneous)
- Oxygen concentration

Modes of Operation

The following modes are those named on the control panel of the Sechrist 2200B:

STANDBY. In this mode the clinician can perform pre-operational checkout procedures before placing the patient on the ventilator. Ventilation parameters and alarms can be set or changed without actually generating flow. When the ventilator is in standby, it will not ventilate the patient. However, the MANUAL BREATH button can be used to deliver a single breath according to the pre-set INSPIRATORY TIME, INSPIRATORY HOLD (if any), VOLUME, and WAVEFORM.

ASSIST/CONTROL. Inspiration is volume controlled, is pressure triggered (depending on the presence of spontaneous breathing efforts and the TRIGGER SENSITIVITY setting) or time triggered (according to the RATE setting), may be volume limited (when INSPIRATORY HOLD is set above zero), is flow limited, and volume cycled (according to the TIDAL VOLUME setting) or time cycled (when INSPIRATORY HOLD is set above zero).

SIMV. In SIMV, mandatory breaths are volume controlled, are pressure triggered (depending on the presence of spontaneous breathing efforts and the TRIGGER SENSITIVITY setting) or time triggered (according to the RATE setting), may be volume limited (when INSPIRATORY HOLD is set above zero), are flow limited, and are volume cycled (according to the TIDAL VOLUME setting) or time cycled (when INSPIRATORY HOLD is set above zero).

A mandatory breath is pressure triggered the first time a spontaneous breathing effort is detected during each ventilatory period (the time equal to the reciprocal of the RATE). Subsequent breathing efforts during the same period will not trigger another mandatory breath. If a breathing effort is not detected during a given ventilatory period, a mandatory breath will be delivered at the beginning of the next period. The ventilator will continue to deliver mandatory breaths according to the RATE setting until a spontaneous breath is detected, and the sequence of events repeats itself.

Spontaneous inspirations between mandatory breaths are pressure limited (ie, inspiratory flow varies to maintain the set PEEP value), pressure triggered (depending on the presence of spontaneous breathing efforts and the TRIGGER SENSITIVITY setting), and pressure cycled. They are flow cycled and assisted by pressure support if PRESSURE LEVEL is set above zero.

MMV. MMV is identical to SIMV except that the average exhaled minute volume must exceed the threshold determined by the MMV LEVEL setting. If it does not, a new backup rate (greater than the RATE setting) is established according to the equation:

$$\begin{array}{c}\text{Backup rate}\\ \text{(cycles/min)}\end{array} = \frac{\text{MMV level (L/min)}}{\text{Tidal volume (L/cycle)}}$$

The ventilator will resume operation at the RATE setting when the average exhaled minute volume meets or exceeds the MMV LEVEL setting.

PRESSURE CONTROL. Mandatory breaths are pressure controlled, pressure triggered (depending on the presence of spontaneous breathing efforts and the TRIGGER SENSITIVITY setting) or time triggered (according to the RATE setting), pressure limited, and time cycled (according to the INSPIRATORY TIME setting).

CPAP. Spontaneous breaths are pressure limited (ie, inspiratory flow varies to maintain the set PEEP value), pressure triggered (depending on the presence of spontaneous breathing efforts and the TRIGGER SENSITIVITY setting), and pressure cycled. They are flow cycled and assisted by pressure support if PRESSURE LEVEL is set above zero.

SIGH. Sigh frequency can be set from 1 to 10 sighs per hour, in multiples of one to three, and at volumes from 100% to 150% of set tidal volume.

Alarms

INPUT POWER ALARMS. Visual and audible alarms are activated if there is an electrical power failure or if the pneumatic power supply falls outside of 25 ± 3 psig.

CONTROL VARIABLE ALARMS. Low (5–118 cm H_2O) and high (5–118 cm H_2O) alarm thresholds can be set for PIP. Activation of the high-pressure alarm terminates inspiration. The ventilator also compares airway pressure (measured at the exhalation valve) and machine pressure (measured at the outlet of the flow control valve) to detect possible patient circuit occlusions. The default value of the measured pressure difference is set to 10 cm H_2O but is user adjustable from 5 to 40 H_2O.

There is an alarm for "no detectable exhalation flow" acting as the primary disconnect or apnea alarm.

There are alarms for low (30–5000 mL) and high (30–5000 mL) tidal volume, low (1–75 L) and high (1–75 L) minute volume, low and high breath rates (both 5–99.9 breaths per minute), and low and high FIO_2 (both 16%–105%).

CONTROL CIRCUIT ALARMS. Visual and audible alarms are activated in the case of electronic or mechanical failures. There are nine different alarm conditions (seven of which terminate inspiration) and 17 alerts. Each condition is described by a brief message in the Status Line on the front panel display.

SIEMENS SERVO 900C

The Siemens Servo 900C (Siemens Life Support Systems, Iselin, NJ) (Fig. 14-60) is a pressure or flow controller that may be pressure, time, or manually triggered; pressure, volume, or flow limited; and pressure, flow, or time cycled. A separate blender is required to control FIO_2.

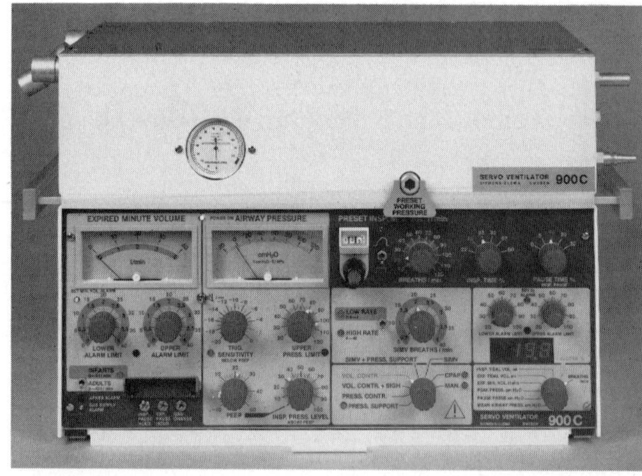

Figure 14-60. The Siemens Servo 900C ventilator. (Courtesy of Siemens Life Support Systems, Iselin, NJ)

Input Variables

The 900C uses 115 volts AC at 60 Hz to power the control circuitry. The main electrical power switch is located on the rear panel. The pneumatic circuit has two input ports, although only one is active at a time. A low-pressure port is available for input from a flowmeter or anesthesia circuit. A high-pressure port is for input from a compressed gas source, which is usually provided by a Bird-type blender.

The front control panel is divided into several sections of control/display knobs (Fig. 14-61). The operator may select manual, volume (ie, flow), or pressure control using a mode selector switch. There are also control knobs for minute volume, ventilatory frequency, inspiratory time (as a percentage of the ventilatory cycle), inspiratory pause time (as a percentage of the ventilatory cycle), trigger sensitivity, inspiratory pressure limit, inspiratory flow limit (and waveform), inspiratory pressure-cycling threshold, and end expiratory pressure level (ie, PEEP).

Control Variables

The 900C can control either inspiratory pressure or flow. The ventilator controls inspiratory pressure in the pressure control and pressure support modes. It

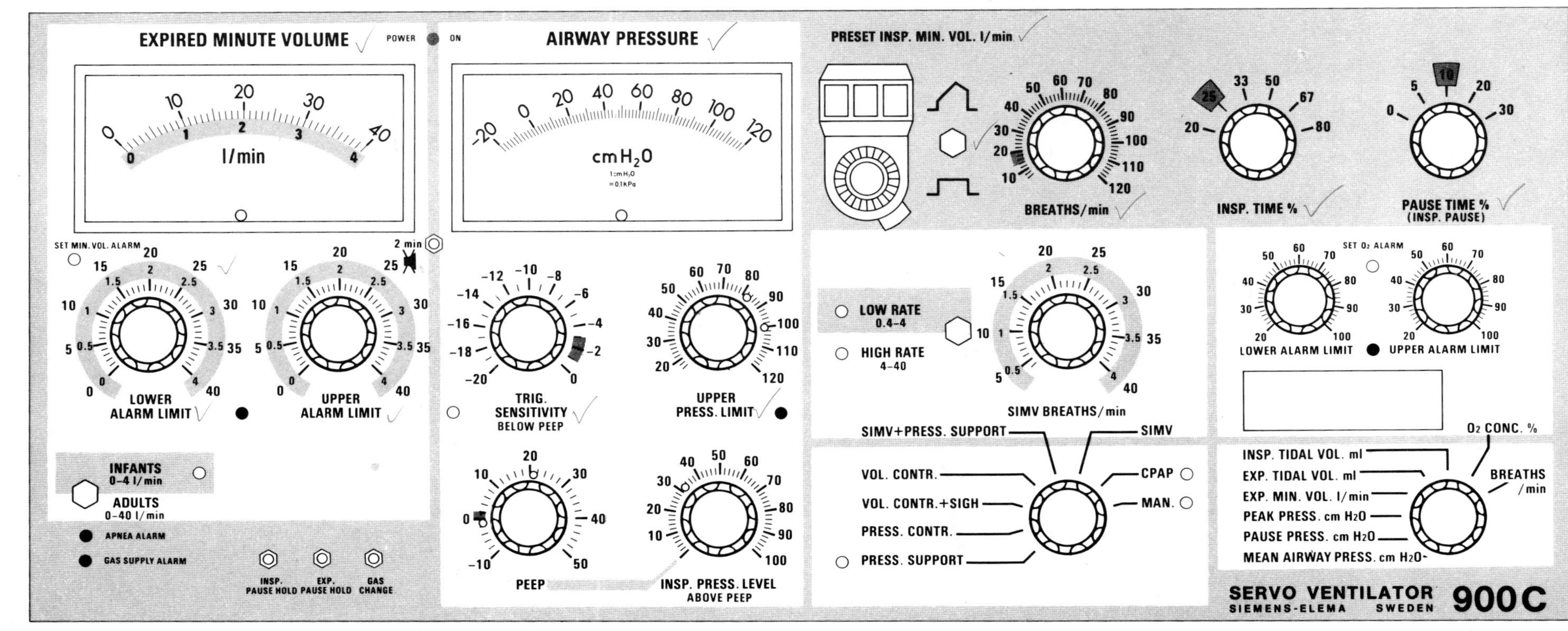

Figure 14-61. Control panel of the Siemens Servo 900C ventilator. (Courtesy of Siemens Life Support Systems, Iselin, NJ)

controls inspiratory flow in the volume control and volume control + sigh modes. It switches between pressure control (for spontaneous breaths) and flow control (for mandatory breaths) in the SIMV and SIMV + PRESS. SUPPORT modes.

INSPIRATORY WAVEFORMS. Pressure control is provided with a rectangular pressure waveform only. However, for flow, the operator may select either a rectangular or a simulated sine waveform (ie, an ascending-descending ramp). It is also possible to approximate a descending ramp flow waveform by first selecting a rectangular flow waveform and then adjusting the working pressure to a level equal to or slightly higher than the PIP associated with the desired tidal volume.

PHASE VARIABLES. Inspiration is pressure triggered when the patient inspires enough volume from the patient circuit to drop the baseline pressure to the triggering threshold. The triggering threshold can be set from 0 to 20 cm H_2O below the set PEEP level using the trigger sensitivity knob. Time triggering occurs as a function of the set ventilatory frequency. The frequency of mandatory breaths is set with either the breaths knob (over a range of 10 to 120 breaths per minute) or the SIMV breaths knob (ranging from 0.5 to 4 breaths per minute or 4 to 40 breaths per minute depending on which scale is used; a toggle switch selects the desired scale). When selected, a sigh breath is automatically triggered once every 100 mandatory breaths.

Inspiration is pressure limited in both the pressure control and the pressure support mode. A demand valve controls inspiratory pressure by attempting to maintain the set PEEP/CPAP level if pressure control or pressure support is not used. If pressure control or pressure support is used, the pressure limit may be set from 0 to 100 cm H_2O above the set PEEP level (ie, the PIP may be set as high as 120 cm H_2O) using the inspiratory pressure level knob. Inspiration is volume limited whenever the pause time knob is set above 0. The available range for pause time is 0% to 30%. Pause time increases the I:E ratio, which may be calculated as:

$$\text{I:E} = \text{Inspiratory time \%} + \text{pause time \%}: (100 - \text{inspiratory time \%} + \text{pause time \%})$$

For example, an inspiratory time of 20% plus a pause time of 5% yields:

$$\begin{aligned}\text{I:E} &= (20\% + 5\%) : [100\% - (20\% + 5\%)] \\ &= 25\% : 75\% \\ &= 1{:}3\end{aligned}$$

Inspiration is flow limited in volume control modes waveform, the peak value is the same as the mean value during the inspiratory phase. The mean inspiratory flow rate is indirectly controlled by the pre-set inspiratory minute volume and inspiratory time settings according to the equation:

$$\frac{\text{Mean inspiratory}}{\text{flow rate (L/min)}} = \frac{\text{Minute volume (L/min)}}{\text{Inspiratory time (as decimal)}}$$

For example, if the pre-set inspiratory minute volume is set at 12 L/min and the inspiratory time at 20%, then the peak inspiratory flow rate is 60 L/min. The above equation holds for the pseudo sine wave setting also. However, when using this setting, the peak value is different from the mean value. Because the mean value of the inspiratory portion of a sine waveform is 1.57 times the peak value, the peak inspiratory flow rate in this setting can be estimated as:

$$\frac{\text{Peak inspiratory}}{\text{flow rate (L/min)}} = \frac{1.57 \times \text{minute volume (L/min)}}{\text{Inspiratory time (as decimal)}}$$

The pre-set inspiratory minute volume may be set from 0.5 to 40 L/min, and inspiratory time may be set to 20%, 25%, 33%, 50%, 67%, or 80%.

Inspiration is terminated when one of three variables reaches a pre-set threshold value. Inspiration may be pressure cycled using the upper pressure limit knob, which adjusts the pressure cycling threshold over the range of 16 to 120 cm H_2O above ambient. Active inspiratory flow is also pressure cycled for spontaneous breaths when pressure support is not used (when expiration causes airway pressure to rise above the PEEP setting). Inspiration is flow cycled in the pressure support mode when inspiratory flow rate decays to 25% of the set peak flow rate. Inspiration is time cycled, in the pressure control, volume control, and SIMV modes. When selected, a tidal volume of approximately twice the normal tidal volume is delivered by doubling the inspiratory time.

Baseline pressure, either negative or positive end-expiratory pressure (NEEP or PEEP), may be adjusted over the range of 210 to 50 cm H_2O using the PEEP control knob. A vacuum source must be connected to the expiratory side of the patient circuit to provide NEEP.

Control Subsystems

CONTROL CIRCUIT. The Siemens Servo 900C is electronically controlled but does not use a microprocessor (Fig. 14-62). Pressure and flow are measured by two (inspiratory and expiratory line) pressure transducers and two (inspiratory and expiratory line) flow transducers. The "airway" pressures that are measured and displayed are not airway opening pressures because they are measured inside the ventilator rather than at the point of connection to the patient. Feedback signals from the flow transducers are electronically integrated to measure volume. The volume signals are used to display inspired tidal volume and expired tidal volume. The inspiratory pressure signal generates the

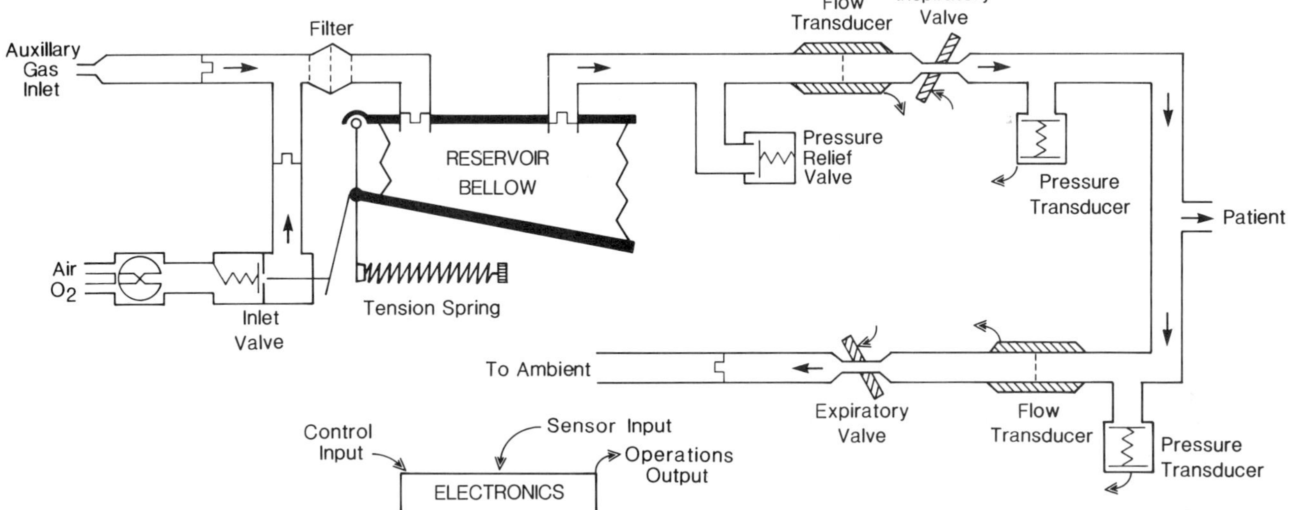

Figure 14-62. Internal components of the Siemens Servo 900C control circuit.

reading on the airway pressure display and is used by the pressure alarm systems.

Feedback signals from the pressure and flow transducers on the inspiratory side are used to control the scissors valve to shape the output pressure and flow waveforms during inspiration.

The feedback signals from the pressure transducer on the expiratory side closes the expiratory scissors valve when the pressure at that point drops to the value set on the PEEP dial.

DRIVE MECHANISM. The Siemens Servo 900C has an internal compressor composed of a plastic bellows that is placed under tension by an adjustable spring. The force exerted by the spring sets the ventilator's working pressure, which may be varied over a range of 0 to 120 cm H_2O. Thus, the spring assembly acts as the motor that causes movement of gas out of the bellows into the patient circuit. The ventilator requires an external pneumatic power source (ie, compressed gas from a flowmeter or blender) to fill the bellows against the force of the spring.

OUTPUT CONTROL VALVES. There are two scissors valves located in the inspiratory and expiratory sections of the delivery circuit inside the ventilator. During inspiration, the valve on the expiratory side is closed and the valve on the inspiratory side shapes either the pressure or the flow waveform. During expiration, the valve on the inspiratory side is closed and the valve on the expiratory side controls the baseline pressure.

Output Displays

Digital displays include inspired and expired tidal volume, expired minute volume, PIP, pause pressure, mean airway pressure, and inspired oxygen concentration. Three analog meters display expired minute volume, ventilating pressure, and working pressure.

Modes of Operation

The following modes are those named on the mode selector switch of the Siemens Servo 900C:

VOLUME CONTROL. Inspiration is flow controlled, time triggered (according to the frequency set on the breaths knob) or pressure triggered (depending on the presence of spontaneous breathing efforts and the trigger sensitivity setting), flow limited, and time cycled. The tidal volume, which remains constant from breath to breath, is calculated as

$$\text{Tidal volume (L)} = \frac{\text{Minute volume (L/min)}}{\text{Frequency (breaths per minute)}}$$

VOLUME CONTROL + SIGH. This is the same as VOLUME CONTROL except that a sigh is automatically delivered every 100 breaths. The sigh volume is automatically set at twice the tidal volume.

SIMV. Mandatory breaths are flow controlled, time triggered (according to the frequency set on the SIMV BREATHS knob) or pressure triggered (depending on the presence of spontaneous breathing efforts and the trigger sensitivity setting), flow limited, and time cycled. The mandatory tidal volume and inspiratory flow rate are determined by the pre-set inspiratory minute volume, breaths, and inspiratory time settings. Spontaneous inspirations between mandatory breaths are pressure controlled (ie, inspiratory flow rate varies to maintain the set PEEP level), pressure triggered, and flow cycled. Flow delivery during a spontaneous inspiration is terminated the same as for pressure support.

Each SIMV total cycle time (ie, the reciprocal of the SIMV BREATHS setting) is divided into two parts, the first (temporally) is the "SIMV period," and the second is the "spontaneous period." The SIMV period is equal to the ventilatory period set by the BREATHS knob (not the SIMV BREATHS knob). The spontaneous period is equal to the difference between the SIMV period and the spontaneous period. If a sufficiently large spontaneous effort (ie, one large enough to pass the threshold set by the TRIGGER SENSITIVITY knob) is detected during the SIMV period, then a mandatory breath will be pressure triggered. If not, a mandatory breath is time triggered at the end of the SIMV period. The patient may breathe freely without triggering a mandatory breath during the spontaneous period.

For example, suppose that the SIMV BREATHS knob were set at 6, the BREATHS knob were set at 15, and the INSPIRATORY TIME knob were set at 25% (with no pause time). The maximum time between mandatory breaths would be 12 seconds, the inspiratory time would be 1 second, and the SIMV period available for pressure-triggering the next mandatory breath would be 4 seconds. After a mandatory breath, the patient has 10 − 4 = 6 seconds (the spontaneous period) in which to pressure-trigger spontaneous breaths at his or her own frequency before pressure-triggering another mandatory breath. Suppose the patient does not pressure-trigger the next mandatory breath at the end of the SIMV total cycle time (ie, 12 seconds after the first). Then a new SIMV total cycle time begins and the ventilator will wait 4 seconds (the SIMV period) for a spontaneous effort before time-triggering a mandatory breath and the cycle repeats itself.

SIMV + PRESSURE SUPPORT. This is the same as SIMV except that spontaneous breaths are pressure controlled (in the PRESSURE SUPPORT mode) to maintain the value set on the INSPIRATORY PRESSURE level knob rather than to the set PEEP level.

PRESSURE CONTROL. This indicates a form of assist/control in which breaths are pressure controlled (to maintain the value set on the INSPIRATORY PRESSURE LEVEL knob), time triggered (according to the frequency set on the breaths knob) or pressure triggered (depending on the presence of spontaneous breathing efforts and the sensitivity setting), and time cycled.

The pre-set inspiratory minute volume setting is inactivated in the PRESSURE CONTROL mode. Tidal volume and inspiratory flow rate are dependent primarily on the magnitude of the change in airway pressure (ie, inspiratory pressure level minus PEEP), the inspiratory time (determined by the settings of the BREATHS, INSPIRATORY TIME, and PAUSE TIME dials), and the compliance and resistance of the patient circuit and respiratory system.

PRESSURE SUPPORT. Inspiration is pressure controlled, pressure triggered (depending on the presence of spontaneous breathing efforts and the trigger sensitivity setting), pressure limited, and flow cycled. Inspiratory flow rate varies to maintain airway pressure at the value set by the INSPIRATORY PRESSURE LEVEL knob. Inspiration is terminated when the inspiratory flow rate drops to 25% of the peak inspiratory flow rate generated on that breath. If inspiratory flow does not drop to 25% of the peak value (eg, due to a leak in the system), then inspiration is terminated when airway pressure reaches 3 cm H_2O above the set inspiratory pressure level or when inspiration lasts more than 80% of the set ventilatory period. The ventilatory period is the reciprocal of the ventilatory frequency set by the BREATHS knob:

$$\text{Ventilatory period(s)} = \frac{60}{\text{Frequency (breaths per minute)}}$$

The pre-set inspiratory minute volume setting is inactivated in the PRESSURE SUPPORT mode, and tidal volume during mandatory breaths is dependent on many factors. These include the magnitude of the change in airway pressure (ie, inspiratory pressure level minus PEEP), the contribution to transrespiratory pressure change made by the ventilatory muscles, the inspiratory time, and the compliance and resistance of the patient circuit and respiratory system.

MANUAL. This mode is designed for anesthesia and requires an accessory circuit. The circuit consists of a reservoir bag and a manual ventilation valve. This assembly is connected to the inspiratory outlet port. Flow into the bag is regulated by the pre-set inspiratory minute volume control. Ventilation is achieved by manually compressing the bag. The patient may breathe spontaneously from the bag provided he or she can generate the 2 cm H_2O pressure drop required to open the valve. The trigger sensitivity is disabled in this mode.

CPAP. Spontaneous inspirations are pressure controlled (ie, inspiratory flow rate varies to maintain the set PEEP level), pressure triggered (depending on the presence of spontaneous breathing efforts and the trigger sensitivity setting), and flow cycled. Flow delivery is terminated the same as for pressure support.

Alarms

INPUT POWER ALARMS. The green power on-light goes out and an audible alarm is activated when the electrical power supply to the ventilator is interrupted. A flashing red gas supply alarm light and an audible alarm are activated if the gas supply does not meet the demands imposed by the ventilator settings.

CONTROL VARIABLE ALARMS. A red flashing light and an audible alarm are activated if airway pressure exceeds the threshold set on the upper pressure limit knob.

Red flashing lights and audible alarms are activated if the expired minute volume crosses either the lower alarm limit or the upper alarm limit. The lower limit is adjustable from 0 to 37 L/min (for adults) or 0 to 3.7 L/min (for infants). The upper limit can be set over the range of 3 to 43 L/min (for adults) or 0 to 4.3 L/min (for infants). Both knobs have dual scales that are selected by a toggle switch.

Red flashing lights and audible alarms are activated if the inspired oxygen concentration crosses either the lower alarm limit or the upper alarm limit. The lower limit is adjustable from 18% to 90% and the upper limit is adjustable from 30% to 100%.

A red flashing apnea light and an audible alarm are activated if no attempt (ie, negative airway pressure deflection) to inspire is detected for 15 seconds. This alarm is disabled in the manual ventilation mode.

CONTROL CIRCUIT ALARMS. This device has no control circuit alarms.

SIEMENS SERVO 300

The Siemens Servo 300 (Siemens Life Support Systems, Iselin, NJ) (Fig. 14-63) is a pressure or flow controller that may be pressure, time, or manually triggered; pressure, volume, or flow limited; and pressure, flow, or time cycled. Unlike previous Servo models, the 300 has an integral air–oxygen blender.

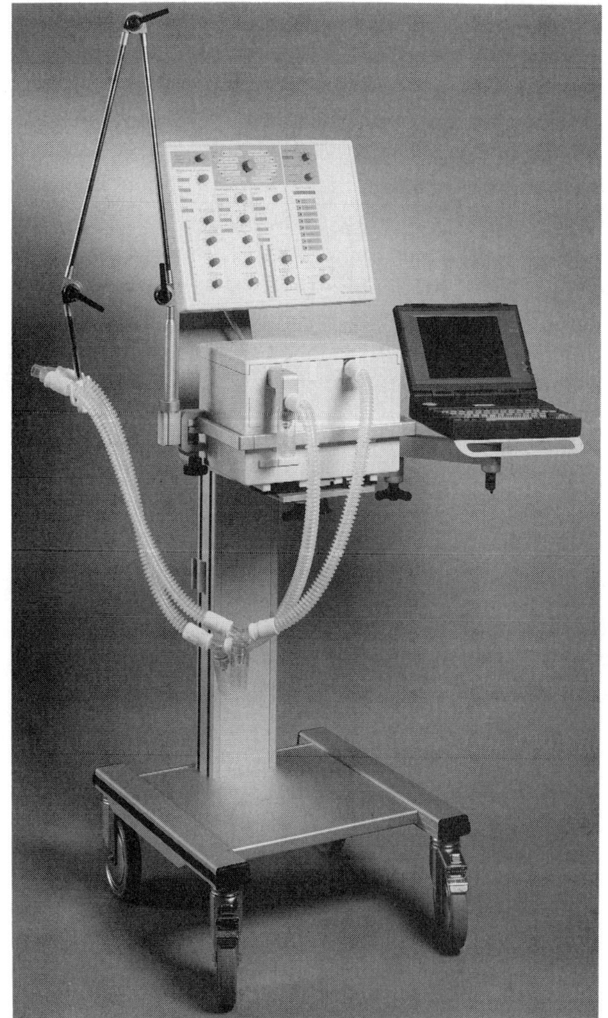

Figure 14-63. The Siemens Servo 300 ventilator. (Courtesy of Siemens Life Support Systems, Iselin, NJ)

Input Variables

The Siemens Servo 300 uses 115 volts AC at 60 Hz to power the control circuitry. The pneumatic circuit operates on external compressed gas sources (ie, air and oxygen) at 29 to 100 psig.

On the control panel (Fig. 14-64) the operator may select the patient type (ie, adult, pediatric, neonate), mode of ventilation, pressure or flow triggering, pressure limit and baseline pressure, minute volume (MMV), ventilatory frequency, inspiratory time (%), inspiratory pause time (%), rise time of inspiratory pressure or flow (% of ventilatory cycle), and FIO_2. The operator may also select to deliver a pre-set group of "oxygen breaths" with 100% oxygen. A momentary inspiratory and expiratory pause function is available to measure static transrespiratory pressures.

Control Variables

The Siemens Servo 300 can control either inspiratory pressure or flow. The ventilator controls inspiratory pressure in the following modes

- PRESSURE CONTROL
- PRESSURE SUPPORT
- SIMV (PRESSURE CONTROL) + PRESSURE SUPPORT
- PRESSURE REGULATED VOLUME CONTROL

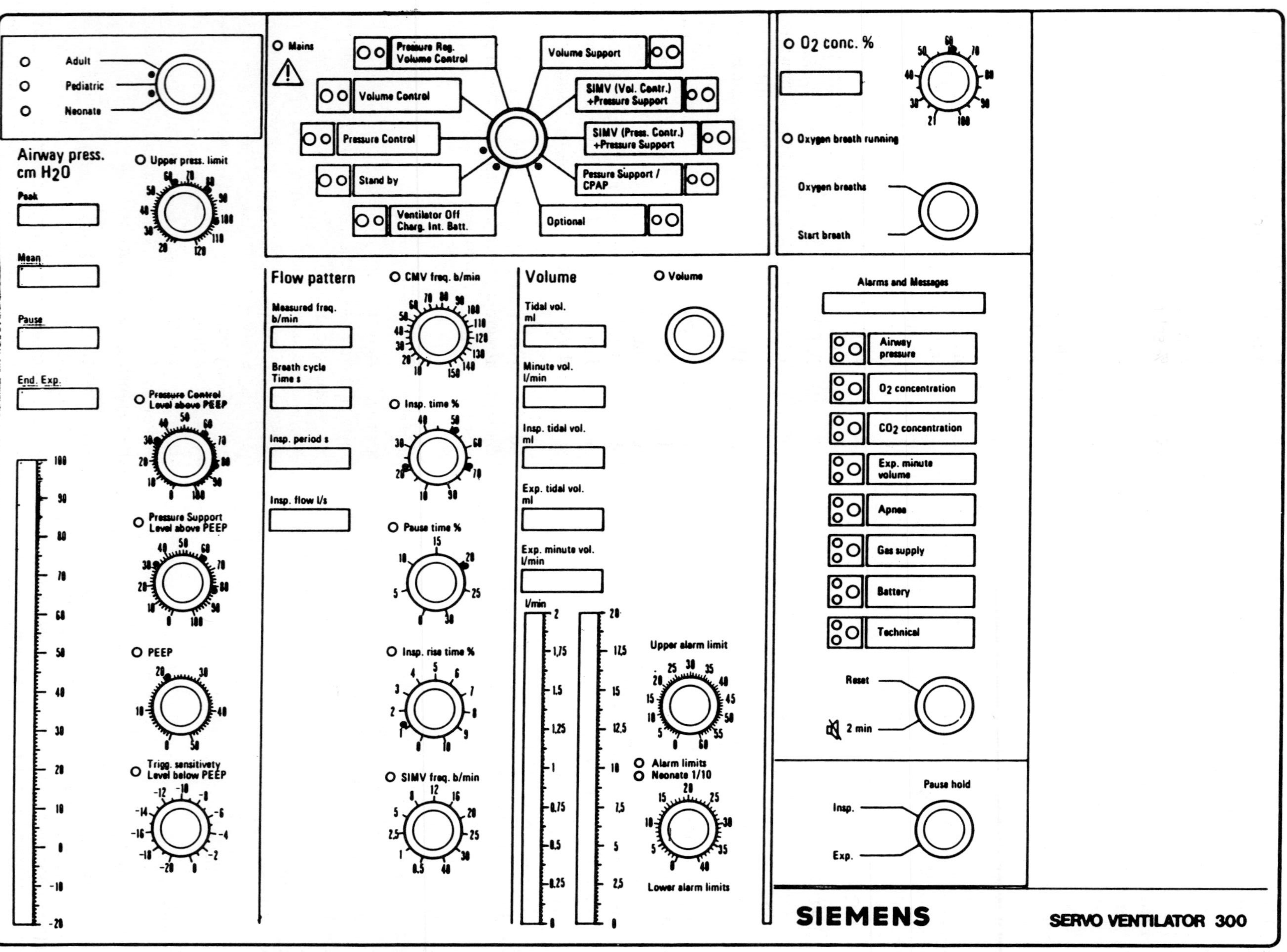

Figure 14-64. Control panel of the Siemens Servo 300 ventilator. (Courtesy of Siemens Life Support Systems, Iselin, NJ)

- VOLUME SUPPORT
- CPAP

The Siemens Servo 300 controls inspiratory flow in the remaining modes

- VOLUME CONTROL
- SIMV (VOLUME CONTROL) + PRESSURE SUPPORT when not using pressure support

The ventilator switches between inspiratory pressure control (for spontaneous breaths) and inspiratory flow control (for mandatory breaths) in the SIMV (VOLUME CONTROL) + PRESSURE SUPPORT mode. The ventilator will switch from flow control to pressure control within a breath if the patient demands more flow than is set, thus dropping airway pressure below the set PEEP. In this case, the ventilator will increase flow to maintain the PEEP level. The set tidal volume acts as a feedback control variable to automatically adjust the pressure limit between breaths in the VOLUME SUPPORT and PRESSURE REGULATED VOLUME CONTROL modes (see Modes).

INSPIRATORY WAVEFORMS. The default setting for pressure and flow waveforms is rectangular. However, the INSPIRATORY RISE TIME (%) sets the time period during which pressure or flow (depending on the mode) increases to the pre-set limit in the beginning of inspiration. The range is from 0% to 10% of the ventilatory period. Thus, the rise time control allows shaping of the leading edge of pressure and flow waveforms to promote patient comfort and avoid premature cycling of inspiration.

PHASE VARIABLES. Inspiration is pressure triggered when the patient inspires enough volume from the patient circuit to drop the baseline pressure to the TRIGGER SENSITIVITY LEVEL, adjustable from 0 to 20 cm H_2O below PEEP. The ventilator can also be set to flow trigger, with default sensitivity settings depending on the patient type selected (adult: 0.6–2.0 L/min; pediatric: 0.3–1.0 L/min; neonate: 0.15–0.5 L/min). Time triggering occurs as a function of the set ventilatory frequency. The frequency of mandatory breaths is set with either the CMV FREQUENCY knob (over a range of 5 to 150 breaths per minute) or the SIMV FREQUENCY knob (ranging from 0.5 to 40 breaths per minute). A manual trigger can be initiated using the START BREATH switch. Normal triggering can be manually overridden with an inspiratory PAUSE HOLD switch to obtain static expiratory pressure.

Inspiration is pressure limited in all modes except VOLUME CONTROL and SIMV (VOLUME CONTROL). The pressure limit may be set from 0 to 100 cm H_2O above the set PEEP level using the PRESSURE CONTROL LEVEL ABOVE PEEP or PRESSURE SUPPORT LEVEL ABOVE PEEP control knobs. The shape of the pressure waveform can be adjusted using the INSP. RISE TIME % control knob. Inspiration is volume limited whenever the PAUSE TIME knob is set above 0 for a flow-controlled breath. The available range for PAUSE TIME is 0% to 30%.

Inspiration is flow limited in the VOLUME CONTROL and SIMV (VOLUME CONTROL) modes. The mean inspiratory flow rate in this mode is indirectly controlled by the CMV FREQUENCY and INSPIRATORY TIME % settings according to the equation:

$$\frac{\text{Mean inspiratory}}{\text{flow rate (L/min)}} = \frac{\text{Minute volume (L/min)}}{\text{Inspiratory time \% (as decimal)}}$$

For example, if the PRESET INSPIRATORY MINUTE VOLUME is set at 12 L/min and the inspiratory time at 20%, then the peak inspiratory flow rate is 60 L/min.

The minute volume ranges from 0.2 to 60 L/min, and inspiratory times are adjustable from 10% to 80% of the ventilatory period. The resultant tidal volumes range from 2 to 4000 mL.

Inspiration will be pressure cycled when the upper pressure alarm threshold is violated. Inspiratory flow is also pressure cycled for spontaneous breaths when PRESSURE SUPPORT is not used (when expiration causes airway pressure to rise above the PEEP setting). Inspiration is flow cycled in the PRESSURE SUPPORT and VOLUME SUPPORT modes when inspiratory flow rate decays to 5% of the set peak flow rate. Inspiration is time cycled in the PRESSURE CONTROL, VOLUME CONTROL, and SIMV modes. Inspiratory time is determined by the INSP. TIME %, PAUSE TIME %, and CMV FREQUENCY settings. Inspiration is time cycled in the PRESSURE SUPPORT mode after 80% of the set ventilatory period. Normal cycling can be manually overridden with an expiratory "Pause Hold" switch to obtain static inspiratory pressure.

Baseline pressure may be adjusted over the range of 0 to 50 cm H_2O using the PEEP control knob.

Control Subsystems

CONTROL CIRCUIT. The Siemens Servo 300 is electronically controlled using a microprocessor. Pressure is measured inside the ventilator in two locations (Fig. 14-65). Inspiratory pressure is measured just after gas leaves the mixing chamber on the inspiratory side. Expiratory pressure is measured just before gas enters the expiratory valve. Flow is measured on the expiratory side just before the expiratory valve. These signals are used to control the pressure and flow waveforms. Oxygen concentration is also measured before entering the patient circuit.

DRIVE MECHANISM. The Siemens Servo 300 uses either external compressed gas (for air and oxygen) or an electric motor and compressor (for air) in conjunction with a pressure regulator. It accepts compressed gas at 28 to 91 psig into two flow control modules.

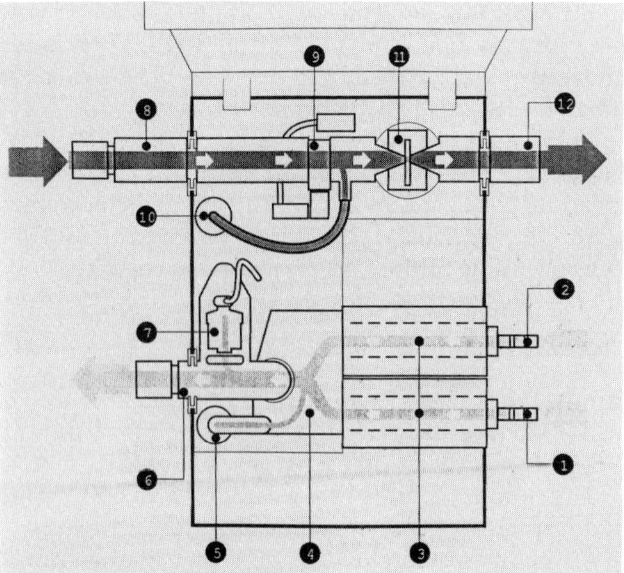

Figure 14-65. Internal components of the Siemens Servo 300 ventilator:

1. Gas inlet for air. The connected air must have a pressure between 2 and 6.5 bar.
2. Gas inlet for O_2. The connected O_2 must have a pressure between 2 and 6.5 bar.
3. The flow of the gas delivered is regulated by the gas modules.
4. The gases are mixed in the inspiratory mixing port.
5. The pressure of the mixed gas delivered to the patient is measured by a pressure transducer. The transducer is protected by a bacteria filter.
6. The inspiratory pipe leads the mixed gas from the inspiratory mixing port to the patient system. The inspiratory pipe also contains the safety valve, a holder for the O_2 cell and the inspiratory outlet.
7. The oxygen concentration is measured by an O_2 cell. The O_2 cell is protected by a bacteria filter.
8. The patient systems' expiratory gas tube is connected at the expiratory inlet. The expiratory inlet also contains a moisture tap.
9. The gas flow through the expiratory channel is measured by the expiratory flow transducer. Patient trigger efforts are sensed as a decrease in the continuous expiratory flow or a decrease in pressure.
10. The expiratory pressure is measured by the expiratory pressure transducer. The transducer is protected by a bacteria filter. Patient trigger efforts are sensed by this expiratory pressure transducer.
11. The pressure of the gas (PEEP pressure) in the patient system is regulated by the expiratory valve.
12. The gas from the patient system leaves the ventilator through the expiratory outlet. The outlet contains a nonreturn valve.

(Courtesy of Siemens Life Support Systems, Iselin, NJ)

These modules control both the oxygen concentration and flow waveform of inspired gas.

OUTPUT CONTROL VALVES. Gas flow to the patient is regulated by two flow control valves. The exhalation valve is a scissors type, similar to previous versions of the Siemens Servo ventilator. The microprocessor coordinates the activity of the valves such that the exhalation valve closes as the flow control valves begin to deliver flow to the patient circuit.

Output Display

The front panel of the Siemens Servo 300 is divided into eight sections: (1) patient range selection, (2) airway pressures, (3) mode selection, (4) respiratory pattern, (5) volumes, (6) oxygen concentration/manual breath, (7) alarms and messages, and (8) inspiratory and expiratory hold. Peak, mean, pause, and baseline pressures are shown in digital displays. In addition, an analog bar graph display shows instantaneous airway pressure along with alarm and trigger sensitivity settings using colored lights. The "Respiratory Pattern" section has digital displays for measured and set frequencies, inspiratory time, inspiratory flow rate, ventilatory period, and I:E ratio. The "Volumes" section has digital displays for set tidal volume and minute ventilation along with measured values for inspired and expired volumes and minute ventilation. There is also an analog bar graph showing the set and measured values for minute ventilation along with the set minute ventilation alarm thresholds. The set oxygen concentration is digitally displayed in section 6.

Modes of Operation

The following modes are those named on the mode selector switch of the Siemens Servo 300:

PRESSURE CONTROL. Inspiration is pressure controlled, time triggered (according to the frequency set on the CMV FREQUENCY knob) or patient triggered (depending on the presence of spontaneous breathing efforts and the sensitivity setting), pressure limited (at the PRESSURE CONTROL LEVEL ABOVE PEEP), and time cycled (determined by the INSP. TIME % and CMV FREQUENCY settings; PAUSE TIME % is not active).

VOLUME CONTROL. Inspiration is flow controlled, is time triggered (according to the set frequency) or patient triggered (depending on the presence of spontaneous breathing efforts and the sensitivity setting), may be volume limited, is flow limited, and is time cycled (determined by the INSP. TIME %, PAUSE TIME %, and CMV FREQUENCY settings). Inspiratory time may be no longer than 80% of set ventilatory period. The tidal volume, which remains constant from breath to breath, is calculated as:

$$\text{Tidal volume (L)} = \frac{\text{Minute volume (L/min)}}{\text{CMV frequency (breaths per minute)}}$$

If the patient needs higher flow than pre-set, and by inspiratory efforts creates a pressure below the set PEEP level during inspiration, the ventilator will switch to pressure control, providing enough flow to maintain the set PEEP level. In this case, inspiration will be terminated when the delivered tidal volume exceeds 125% of the set tidal volume.

PRESSURE-REGULATED VOLUME CONTROL. Inspiration is pressure controlled, time triggered (according to CMV FREQUENCY setting), pressure limited (automatically controlled by ventilator), and time cycled (determined by the INSP. TIME % and CMV FREQUENCY settings). The first breath will be delivered at an inspiratory pressure of 5 cm H_2O. The delivered volume at this pressure is measured, and compliance is calculated by the ventilator. The following three breaths will be delivered at a pressure of 75% of the calculated pressure needed to deliver the pre-set tidal volume (determined by CMV FREQUENCY and VOLUME settings). For each of the following breaths, the inspiratory pressure will be regulated to a value based on the compliance calculation for the previous breath compared with the pre-set tidal volume. The pressure will then never change more than 3 cm H_2O from one breath to the next. Inspiratory pressure is automatically regulated between 0 cm H_2O above PEEP and 5 cm H_2O below the set UPPER PRESS LIMIT.

VOLUME SUPPORT. Inspiration is pressure controlled, pressure or flow triggered (depending on the presence of spontaneous breathing efforts and the sensitivity setting), pressure limited (automatically controlled by ventilator), and flow cycled (when flow has decreased to 5% of peak flow), time cycled (after 80% of the set ventilatory period), or volume cycled (if delivered tidal volume exceeds 175% of set tidal volume). The pressure limit is automatically set as in the PRESSURE REGULATED VOLUME CONTROL mode. If the apnea alarm is triggered, the ventilator will automatically switch to the PRESSURE REGULATED VOLUME CONTROL mode.

SIMV (VOLUME CONTROL) + PRESSURE SUPPORT. Mandatory breaths are flow controlled, are time triggered (according to the SIMV FREQ setting) or pressure or flow triggered (depending on the presence of spontaneous breathing efforts and the sensitivity setting), may be volume limited, are flow limited, and are time cycled (determined by the INSP TIME %, PAUSE TIME %, and CMV FREQUENCY settings) or volume cycled (if delivered tidal volume exceeds 125% of set tidal volume). Spontaneous breaths are pressure controlled, pressure or flow triggered (depending on the presence of spontaneous breathing efforts and the sensitivity setting), pressure limited (to either the PEEP or PRESSURE SUPPORT LEVEL ABOVE PEEP setting), and pressure cycled (if pressure exceeds pre-set level by 20 cm H_2O), flow cycled (at 5% of the peak flow), or time cycled (at 80% of the set SIMV period).

Each SIMV cycle time (ie, the reciprocal of the SIMV FREQ setting) is divided into two parts, the first is the "SIMV period," and the second is the "spontaneous period". The SIMV period is equal to the ventilatory period set by the CMV FREQ knob. The spontaneous period is equal to the difference between the SIMV period and the spontaneous period. If a sufficiently large spontaneous effort is detected during the SIMV period, then a mandatory breath will be patient triggered. If not, a mandatory breath is time triggered at the end of the SIMV period. The patient may breathe freely without triggering a mandatory breath during the spontaneous period.

SIMV (PRESSURE CONTROL) + PRESSURE SUPPORT. This is the same as SIMV (VOLUME CONTROL) + PRESSURE SUPPORT except that mandatory breaths are pressure controlled (see PRESSURE CONTROL mode).

PRESSURE SUPPORT/CPAP. Inspiration is pressure controlled, pressure or flow triggered (depending on the presence of spontaneous breathing efforts and the sensitivity setting), pressure limited (to either the PEEP or PRESSURE SUPPORT LEVEL ABOVE PEEP setting), and pressure cycled (if pressure exceeds preset level by 20 cm H_2O), flow cycled (at 5 % of the peak flow), or time cycled (at 80% of the set SIMV period).

CPAP. Spontaneous breaths are pressure controlled, pressure or flow triggered (depending on the presence of spontaneous breathing efforts and the sensitivity setting), pressure limited (to the PEEP setting), and pressure cycled (if pressure exceeds pre-set level by 20 cm H_2O), flow cycled (at 5% of the peak flow), or time cycled (at 80% of the set SIMV period).

Alarms

The alarm display on the Siemens Servo 300 is composed of an alphanumeric ALARMS AND MESSAGES display and eight labeled touchpad/light displays. A red flashing light in an alarm section touchpad (accompanied by an audio alarm) indicates a high priority alarm and is associated with a text message in the ALARMS AND MESSAGES display. A flashing yellow light indicates that certain alarms have been deliberately overridden by means of a manual reset action or that a previous high-priority alarm condition has been corrected.

INPUT POWER ALARMS. A BATTERY alarm indicates that the main electrical power has failed and the ventilator has switched to battery backup power. Alarm messages will also alert the operator of low-battery power. A GAS SUPPLY alarm is activated if the inlet gas pressure is outside the range of 29 to 94 psig.

CONTROL VARIABLE ALARMS. The AIRWAY PRESSURE alarm is activated if the set UPPER PRESSURE LIMIT is exceeded or if the airway pressure is higher than the set PEEP level plus 15 cm H_2O continuously for more than 15 seconds. An O_2 CONCENTRATION alarm is activated if the FIO_2 falls above or below 6% of the set alarm value or if the oxygen fuel cell is not connected. The EXP MINUTE VOLUME alarm is activated if the exhaled minute volume exceeds the set value or if it falls below the default values of 0.3 L/min for adults and children and 0.06 L/min for neonates. An APNEA alarm is activated if the time between two patient-triggered breaths exceeds the default values of 10 seconds for adults; 15 seconds for children, and 20 seconds for neonates.

CONTROL CIRCUIT ALARMS. A TECHNICAL alarm is activated for a wide variety of technical problems. Most are not described in the operator's manual and indicate the need for repair service.

AARC Clinical Practice Guideline

Patient-Ventilator System Checks: Indications, Contraindications, Hazards and Complications

A patient-ventilator system check is a documented evaluation of a mechanical ventilator and of the patient's response to ventilatory support.

- Indications: Patient-ventilator system checks must be performed on a scheduled basis and should also be performed:
  - prior to obtaining samples for analysis of blood gases and pH
  - prior to obtaining hemodynamic or bedside pulmonary function data
  - following any change in ventilator settings
  - as soon as possible following an acute deterioration in a patient's condition
  - any time that ventilator performance is questionable
- Contraindications: There are no absolute contraindications to the performance of a patient-ventilator system check. However, portions of the check requiring patient disconnection from the ventilator may be contraindicated in unstable patients.
- Hazards/Complications:
  - Disconnecting the patient from the ventilator may result in hypoventilation, hypoxemia, bradycardia, and hypotension.
  - Prior to disconnection, preoxygenation and hyperventilation may minimize these complications.
  - When disconnected from the patient, some ventilators generate a high flow through the patient circuit that may aerosolize contaminated condensate, putting both the patient and clinician at risk for nosocomial infection.

(Adapted from AARC Clinical Practice Guideline, published in August, 1992, issue of Respiratory Care; see original publication for complete text)

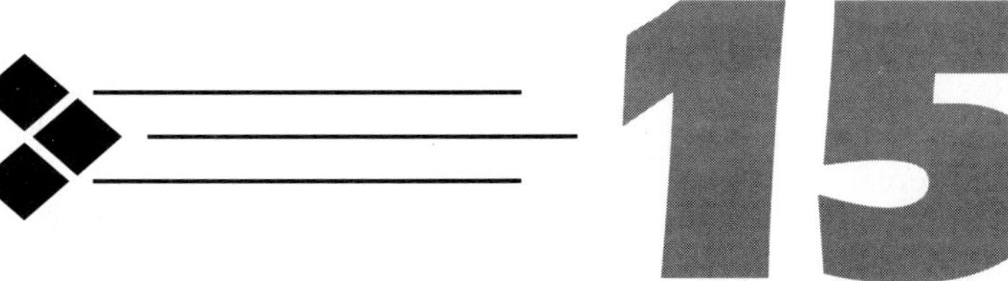

15 Transport Ventilators

Richard D. Branson

OBJECTIVES

1. Describe the operation of transport ventilators according to the classification system in Chapter 13.
2. Explain the advantages and disadvantages of using a transport ventilator compared with manual ventilation with a self-inflating bag.
3. Describe the desirable characteristics of a transport ventilator used in pre-hospital care.
4. Describe the desirable characteristics of a transport ventilator used for in-hospital transport.

Introduction

Ventilatory support of patients during transport can present unique technical challenges. A transport ventilator must be rugged and compact, yet it must also be capable of mimicking ventilatory support provided by larger, more expensive intensive care unit ventilators. Of course, tradeoffs must be made with respect to complexity to meet size and weight requirements.

Transport ventilators are frequently used in pre-hospital care by paramedics, in fixed- and rotor-wing aircraft for inter-hospital transport, and in the hospital for transport of critically ill patients from intensive care units to diagnostic testing facilities. The requirements in each situation are different. The available transport ventilators are reviewed in this chapter with recommendations given for their suitability in these situations.

Pre-Hospital Ventilators

Ventilators for pre-hospital use are subjected to extremes of environmental conditions and will be used in situations not typically encountered in the hospital. The typical ventilator used in this situation should be compact, simple to operate, safe, and extremely durable. Desirable characteristics of ventilators used in pre-hospital care include the following.

Portability

Size and weight are two of the chief concerns in pre-hospital care. Ideally, the ventilator should weigh less than 4 kg and provide some mounting or carrying bracket. Orientation of the control panel such that all adjustments can be made from the same plane is also desirable.

Power Source

Pneumatically powered ventilators have been preferred to their electronic counterparts for some time. A pneumatically powered ventilator only requires compressed gas for operation. An electronically powered ventilator requires both compressed gas and a power source (battery); thus two perishable power sources are required. However, pneumatically powered ventilators generally consume gas to operate and are sensitive to changes in source gas pressure. That is, a pneumatically powered ventilator calibrated to work at 50 psi may not deliver the selected rate and tidal volume when operated at 40 psi or 60 psi. Electronic ventilators offer more precise control of variables and do not consume gas to operate. Either type of ventilator is adequate as long as the shortcomings are understood.

Operational Characteristics

Ventilators used for pre-hospital care should be simple and time or flow cycled. Pressure-cycled devices should be avoided. Delivered tidal volume should be relatively unaffected by changes in lung–thorax compliance ($< 10\%$ change). Gas consumption to power the ventilator's system components should ideally be zero. Low-level gas consumption (< 5 L/min) is acceptable but will decrease the life of the gas source.

Ease of Operation

A minimum number of easily identifiable controls should be used, and each should be labeled as to function and effects. If possible, a diagram of the ventilator circuit and its proper connection should be printed on the ventilator. Pre-hospital ventilators do not require a variable FIO_2, CPAP/PEEP, or a variety of ventilatory modes. Demand valves for spontaneous breathing add size, weight, and complexity to the ventilator. Although a few select patients may benefit from the presence of a demand valve, my experience suggests that the overwhelming majority of patients ventilated in the pre-hospital setting ($> 95\%$) never regain spontaneous breathing during transport.[1]

Although simplicity is desirable, my experience suggests that a minimum of a tidal volume (flow) and rate control be available.[2] A manual breath button is also desirable. This allows the operator to control ventilation independently of ventilator settings and is useful during auscultation of breath sounds to confirm proper endotracheal tube placement.

Assembly and Disassembly

The breathing circuit should be simple, and incorrect assembly should be impossible. Many transport ventilators use a "patient-valve," which may be a simple non-rebreathing valve or may contain an exhalation valve, antiasphyxia valve, and pressure relief valve. If a patient valve is used, it should be easily cleaned of vomitus, blood, and secretions.

Durability

Extremes of temperature and humidity should not adversely effect the function of pre-hospital ventilators. Pre-hospital ventilators should be operable at a moment's notice, even after prolonged storage, and should withstand physical abuse without affecting proper function. Ventilators used in hazardous environments should have protective cases that withstand erosion by chemicals.

Maintenance

A preventative maintenance schedule should be set up by the manufacturer and owner to ensure safe operation. Routine maintenance should be minimal.

In-Hospital Transport Ventilators

Many of the desirable characteristics of in-hospital transport ventilators have been mentioned earlier. These ventilators should be compact, lightweight, time or flow cycled, durable, pneumatically and/or electronically powered, and easy to operate and require little maintenance. The biggest difference should be in operational characteristics.

Operational Characteristics

An in-hospital transport ventilator should be capable of providing ventilatory support equal to that provided in the intensive care unit. As such, transport ventilators should be capable of operating in the AMV or IMV mode, allow spontaneous breathing through a demand valve, allow for the application of PEEP with PEEP-compensation of the demand system, and allow separate adjustments for respiratory rate and tidal volume. A minimum number of alarms should be available, including low- and high-pressure, apnea, and disconnect alarms. In adults, use of 100% oxygen for transport is desirable and poses no threat to the patient. In neonates, an external blender should be provided to allow adjustments of F_{IO_2} and prevention of hyperoxia.

Inter-Hospital Transport

Ventilators used in aeromedical ambulances or ground ambulances for inter-hospital transport should be chosen based on the patient population. For scene runs, a simple, rugged ventilator should be used. If transport of a critically ill, mechanically ventilated patient is required, then a more sophisticated in-hospital ventilator should be used. The effects of altitude on pneumatic ventilators can be of concern but are usually insignificant at altitudes flown in rotor-wing aircraft. At higher altitudes the effects on ventilators are related to the changing density of gas. Pneumatically powered ventilators, when effected by altitude, will typically deliver a slower rate and longer inspiratory time than the control settings. This problem can be overcome by close monitoring by a skilled respiratory care practitioner.

Why Use a Ventilator During Transport?

Several studies have shown that manual ventilation with a self-inflating bag during transport can lead to unintentional hyperventilation and subsequent respiratory alkalosis.[3–5] The result can be hypotension and cardiac dysrhythmias. Table 15-1 depicts the results from the study by Hurst and colleagues[3] demonstrating the untoward effects of manual ventilation.

TABLE 15-1. Effects of Manual Versus Conventional Ventilation

	Conventional Ventilation	After Manual Ventilation	Conventional Ventilation	After Transport Ventilation
pH	7.39 ± 0.03	7.51 ± 0.02*	7.41 ± 0.02	7.40 ± 0.03
Pa_{CO_2} (mm Hg)	39 ± 4	30 ± 3*	38 ± 2	39 ± 3
Pa_{O_2} (mm Hg)	116 ± 17	109 ± 24	120 ± 12	117 ± 20
Heart rate (beats per minute)	106 ± 23	115 ± 19	104 ± 26	109 ± 25
Systolic blood pressure (mm Hg)	130 ± 36	112 ± 12	128 ± 24	136 ± 31
Diastolic blood pressure (mm Hg)	86 ± 12	73 ± 10	80 ± 16	81 ± 20

Average transport time = 9 ± 3 minutes during manual ventilation and 8 ± 3 minutes during transport ventilation.

*$P < .05$ compared with conventional ventilation.

Transport Ventilators

BIO-MED IC-2A

The Bio-Med IC-2A (Bio-Med Devices, Stamford, CT) (Fig. 15-1) is a flow controller that can be pressure, time, or manually triggered, pressure or flow limited, and time cycled. It requires a compressed gas source for delivery to the patient as well as for the fluidic logic circuit. The IC-2A delivers 100% source gas to the patient. It does not have an integral air–oxygen blender.

Input Variables

The IC-2A is pneumatically powered, operating on external compressed gases at 45 to 55 psig. On the front panel, the operator may select the mode of ventilation, inspiratory time, expiratory time, inspiratory flow rate, sensitivity, and PEEP/CPAP level. A single control on the rear panel adjusts the pressure limit. Mode of ventilation is selected by two toggle switches and inspiratory flow, inspiratory time, and expiratory time are adjusted with calibrated dials. Controls for sensitivity, PEEP/CPAP, and pressure limit are set with uncalibrated controls.

Control Variables

The IC-2A controls flow during mandatory as well as spontaneous breaths.

INSPIRATORY WAVEFORMS. The IC-2A can produce a rectangular pressure waveform when the set pressure limit is exceeded and inspiratory flow rate is sufficient. When peak pressure is below the set pressure limit, the IC-2A delivers a rectangular flow waveform.

PHASE VARIABLES. Inspiration is time triggered in the CMV mode and is a function of the set inspiratory and expiratory time. Inspiratory time is adjustable from 0.4 to 2.0 seconds and expiratory time is adjustable from 0.5 to 4.0 seconds in the CMV mode and up to 45 seconds in the SIMV mode. Respiratory frequency is adjustable from 1 to 66 breaths per minute. Inspiration may be pressure triggered in the SIMV and CPAP modes when the patient creates a negative inspiratory effort equal to or greater than the sensitivity setting. The sensitivity control is uncalibrated and must be reset when changes in end-expiratory pressures are made. Inspiration may also be manually triggered by depressing the manual cycle button. Inspiration can be pressure limited when the peak inspiratory pressure exceeds the set pressure limit, but it is normally flow limited. Inspiratory flow rate is adjustable from 20 to 75 L/min. Tidal volume is set by setting inspiratory time and inspiratory flow and calculated as

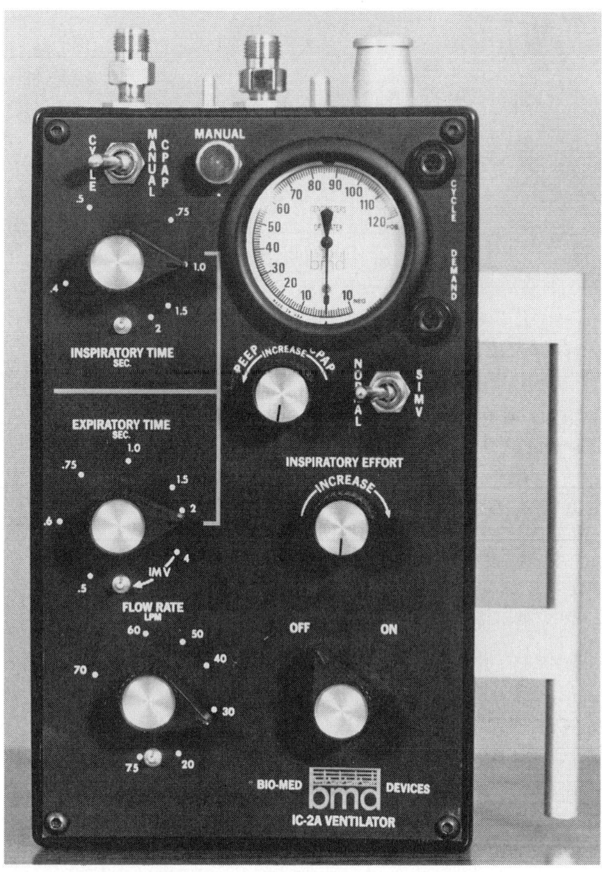

Figure 15-1. The Bio-Med IC-2A. (Courtesy of Bio-Med Devices, Stamford, CT)

$$\text{Tidal volume (mL)} = \text{Inspiratory time(s)} \times \text{inspiratory flow rate (mL/s)}$$

Tidal volume is adjustable up to 3000 mL. Activation of the manual cycle delivers gas to the patient at the set flow rate for the length of time the button is depressed.

Inspiration is time cycled as a result of set inspiratory time for both mandatory and spontaneous breaths. Baseline pressure is controlled by the uncalibrated PEEP/CPAP control from 0 to 25 cm H_2O.

Control Subsystems

CONTROL CIRCUIT. The IC-2A is pneumatically powered and fluidically controlled (Fig. 15-2). The fluidic logic controls the flow of gas to the patient and to the exhalation valve.

DRIVE MECHANISM. The IC-2A requires a 45 to 55 psig source of pressurized gas to power the fluidic logic circuit and provide gas to the patient. Gas powering the fluidic logic circuit travels through the

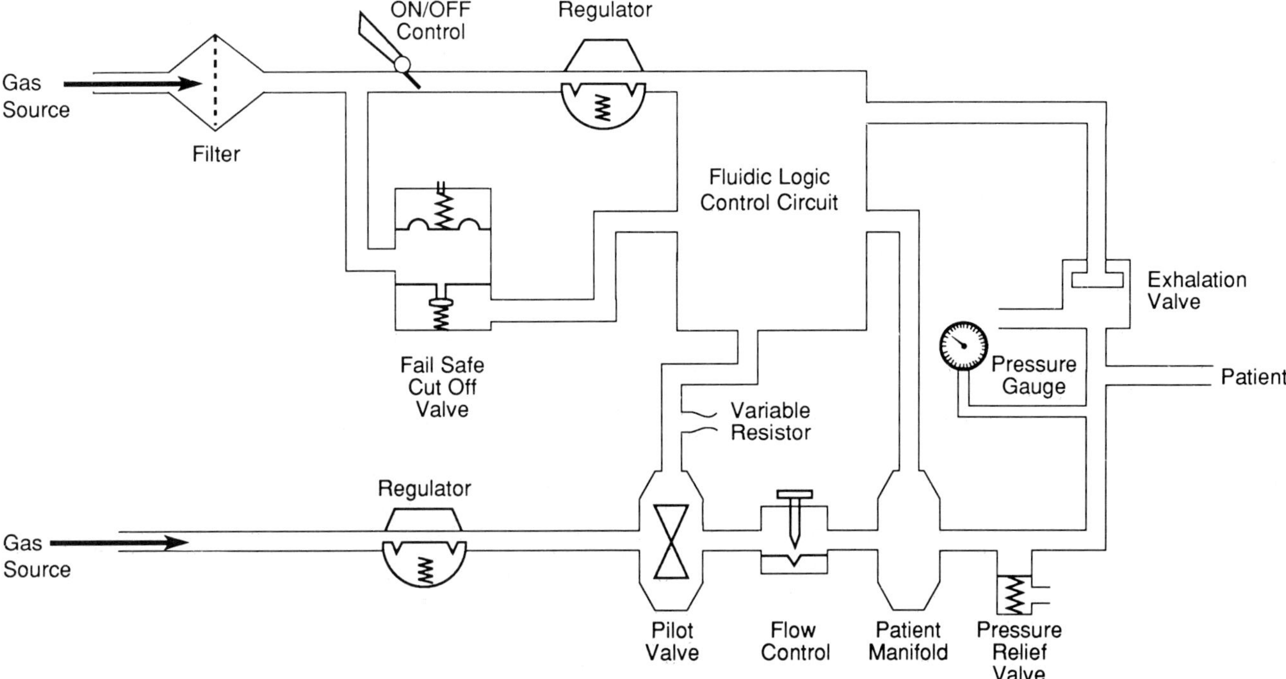

Figure 15-2. Pneumatic components of the Bio-Med IC-2A.

on/off switch and is then reduced to 30 psig, while gas to be delivered to the patient remains at 50 psig. If gas powering the fluidic logic falls below 30 psig, a fail-safe valve prevents flow to the exhalation valve, preventing it from being activated. This mechanism protects the patient from prolonged delivery of peak pressure. The fluidic logic circuit is calibrated using 100% oxygen at 20°C and 1 atm.

Powering the fluidic logic with less than 100% oxygen will alter calibration slightly. Likewise, use of the IC-2A at altitude will cause an increase in set inspiratory and expiratory times by approximately 2.5% per 1000 feet. Gas consumption of the fluidic logic circuit is approximately 12 L/min.

OUTPUT CONTROL VALVES. Output control valves of the IC-2A include a pilot valve (solenoid), flow control needle valve, and peak inspiratory and end-expiratory pressure needle valves. During inspiration a timing signal from the fluidic logic (or from the manual cycle control) opens the pilot valve, which allows gas to flow through the inspiratory flow control valve to the patient, while simultaneously charging the exhalation valve line and pressurizing the exhalation valve.

During exhalation, the fluidic logic closes the pilot valve, preventing gas flow to the patient. End-expiratory pressure is set by adjusting the PEEP/CPAP needle valve, which allows gas to partially pressurize the exhalation valve. The peak inspiratory pressure limit is also set by an uncalibrated needle valve, which limits the amount of flow to the exhalation valve. Both PEEP/CPAP and pressure limit levels should be set by observing the integral aneroid pressure gauge.

In the event of failure of the pressure-limiting valve a nonadjustable pressure relief valve in the patient manifold will limit pressure to 120 cm H_2O. Additionally, if the patient's spontaneous effort is greater than −4 cm H_2O, an antiasphyxia valve will open to allow spontaneous breathing from ambient.

Output Displays

Airway pressure is displayed by an aneroid pressure gauge over the range of −10 to 120 cm H_2O. Pressure-activated indicators alert the operator as to the type of breath delivered: mandatory (cycle indicator) or spontaneous (demand indicator).

Modes of Operation

The following modes are those named on the IC-2A. Each requires the correct combination of toggle switch settings.

CYCLE/NORMAL (CMV). Inspiration is normally flow controlled, time triggered (based on inspiratory and expiratory time settings), and time cycled (based on inspiratory time settings). If inspiration is not pressure limited, it is flow limited.

CYCLE/SIMV. Inspiration is time (mandatory breaths) or pressure triggered (spontaneous breaths), flow or pressure limited, and time cycled. The system for delivering gas during spontaneous breaths is not truly a demand valve and is unique to the IC-2A. Between mandatory breaths, if the patient's inspiratory effort exceeds the sensitivity setting, the IC-2A will deliver gas at the set inspiratory flow and inspiratory time on the ventilator. In fact, the only difference between a mandatory and spontaneous breath is that the latter is pressure triggered and the fluidic logic prevents pressurization of the exhalation valve.

CYCLE/CPAP. Inspiration is pressure triggered, flow limited, and time cycled. The cycle/CPAP mode operates identically to the cycle/SIMV mode except that no mandatory breaths are delivered. In the case of apnea, the IC-2A has no provision for switching to a backup rate.

MANUAL. When the Cycle/Manual CPAP toggle switch is switched to the manual position, the manual pushbutton becomes active. During a manual breath, inspiration is manually triggered, may be pressure or flow limited, and cycles off when the pushbutton is released.

ALARMS. The IC-2A has no audible or visual alarms.

Critical Comment

The IC-2A is a sophisticated transport ventilator intended for inter- and intra-hospital use. It is too sophisticated for pre-hospital care. The flexibility of the IC-2A makes it a useful in-hospital ventilator. Its excessive gas consumption should be considered before embarking on a transport where gas supplies are limited. The "demand" system may be a problem in patients with a large spontaneous minute ventilation requiring PEEP.

BIO-MED MVP-10

The Bio-Med MVP-10 (Bio-Med Devices, Stamford, CT) (Fig. 15-3) is a pressure or flow controller that is time triggered and time cycled. Integral air and oxygen flowmeters are used to control inspired oxygen concentration.

Input Variables

The MVP-10 is pneumatically powered by external sources of air and oxygen (45–55 psig) and fluidically controlled. The MVP-10 has no blender or internal compressor. The operator may select mode of ventilation, inspiratory time, expiratory time, pressure limit (PIP), PEEP/CPAP level, and oxygen and air flow rates.

Control Variables

The MVP-10 is normally set to control inspiratory pressure. However, like other neonatal/pediatric ventilators, if inspiratory flow and inspiratory time settings are insufficient to allow the peak pressure setting to be reached, it becomes a flow controller.

INSPIRATORY WAVEFORMS. The MVP-10 is capable of producing either a rectangular pressure or a flow waveform. When used to control pressure (pressure limited) the MVP-10 produces a rectangular pressure waveform. A rectangular flow waveform results when flow is insufficient to achieve the desired PIP.

PHASE VARIABLES. Inspiration is time triggered and is a function of the set inspiratory time (adjustable from 0.2 to 2.0 seconds) and expiratory time (adjustable from 0.25 to 30 seconds). Respiratory frequency is also a function of inspiratory and expiratory

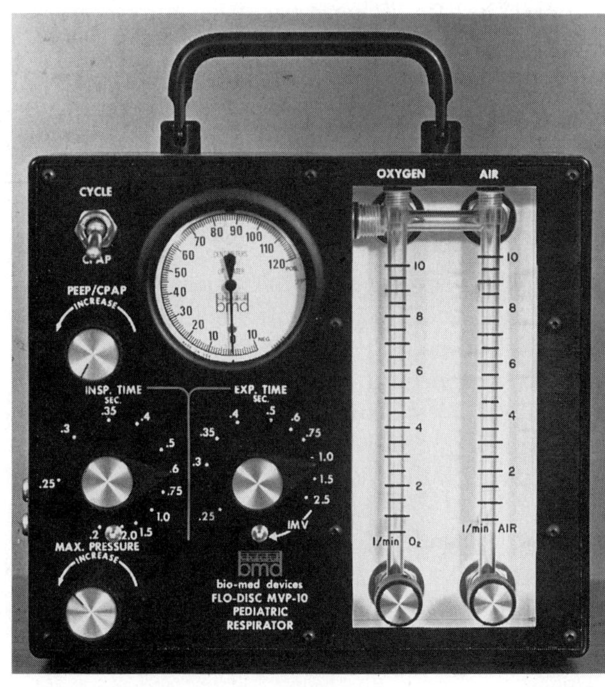

Figure 15-3. The Bio-Med MVP-10. (Courtesy of Bio-Med Devices, Stamford, CT)

times and is adjustable from 0 to 120 breaths per minute. The MVP-10 cannot be manually triggered.

Inspiration can be pressure limited from 0 to 80 cm H_2O. When the pressure limit is not reached, flow-limiting occurs. Inspiratory flow is adjustable through flowmeters for air and oxygen adjustable from 1.2 to 12 L/min.

Inspiration is always time cycled as a result of the set inspiratory time.

Baseline pressure is controlled by the uncalibrated PEEP/CPAP control and is adjustable from 0 to 18 cm H_2O.

Control Subsystems

CONTROL CIRCUIT. The control circuit of the MVP-10 (Fig. 15-4) is pneumatically powered and fluidically controlled.

DRIVE MECHANISM. The MVP-10 requires air and oxygen gas sources at 45 to 55 psig be delivered to dual flowmeters. The air and oxygen flowmeters are set to deliver the appropriate continuous gas flow and oxygen concentration.

OUTPUT CONTROL VALVES. The output control valves include the two flow control needle valves (flowmeters), a series of pneumatic cartridges,[3] needle valves to control PIP and PEEP/CPAP, and a diaphragm-type exhalation valve.

Air and oxygen enter the MVP-10 where regulators reduce the inlet pressure to 50 psig. Gas then passes through the respective flowmeters to the patient and/or out through the exhalation valve. The pneumatic cartridges act to control closure (inspiration) and opening (exhalation) of the exhalation valve. Each cartridge consists of a variable resistor and poppet valve. Adjustment of the inspiratory and expiratory time controls serves to change how quickly gas pressurizes within the cartridges, which causes the poppets to change position. The more open the inspiratory time control (reduced resistance), the more quickly pressure builds and terminates inspiration. As the expiratory time control is increased, the pressure in the expiratory cartridge is removed more slowly, increasing expiratory time. When the inspiratory timer is open, gas flows through the pressure limit control and on to close the exhalation valve. Gas in the logic circuit that closes the exhalation valve is completely separate

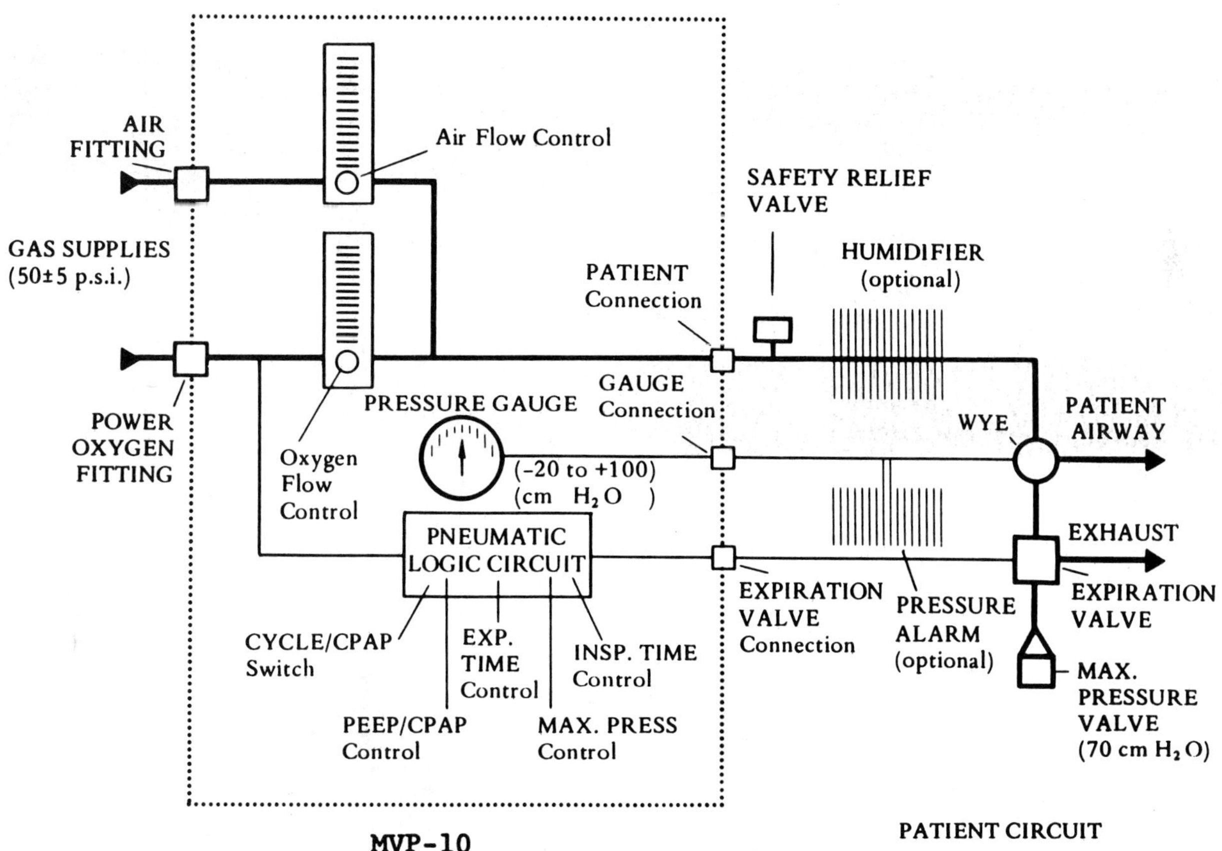

Figure 15-4. Pneumatic components of the Bio-Med MVP-10. (Courtesy of Bio-Med Devices, Stamford, CT)

from gas breathed by the patient. Likewise, gas from the patient does not enter the logic circuit. Gas consumption of the fluidic logic circuit is dependent on respiratory rate, PIP, and PEEP/CPAP level. At 50 breaths per minute, gas consumption of the fluidic logic is approximately 4 L/min.

Output Displays

Airway pressure is displayed by an aneroid gauge over the range of −10 to 120 cm H_2O. Air and oxygen flow rate are displayed on Thorpe-tube flowmeters.

Modes of Operation

The following modes are those named on the control panel of the MVP-10:

CYCLE (IMV). Inspiration is pressure controlled, time triggered (based on ventilation rate), pressure limited and time cycled (based on inspiratory time setting). A continuous flow, controlled by the air and oxygen flowmeters, allows for spontaneous breathing between mandatory breaths. If flow-limiting occurs, mandatory breaths remain time triggered and time cycled.

CPAP. Inspiration is not controlled in the CPAP mode. Spontaneous breathing occurs from the continuous gas flow. Airway pressure is set by adjusting the uncalibrated PEEP/CPAP valve until the desired end-expiratory pressure is displayed on the aneroid gauge.

ALARMS. The MVP-10 has no alarms.

Critical Comment

The MVP-10 is intended for inter- and intra-hospital transport of neonatal and pediatric patients. Its simple operation and reliability are desirable qualities in this type of ventilator. Like the IC-2A, gas consumption of the fluidic logic should be considered before this ventilator is used. The lack of alarms is undesirable, but external pressure monitoring/alarm systems are available.

BIRD SPACE TECHNOLOGIES MINI-TXP

The Mini-TXP (Percussionaire, Sandpoint, ID) (Fig. 15-5) is a flow controller that is time triggered, flow limited, and time cycled. It does not use an external air–oxygen blender or compressor. However, the patient valve consists of a sliding venturi that entrains room air during normal operation.

Input Variables

The Mini-TXP operates pneumatically from external compressed gas sources of 20 to 100 psig. The control panel consists of a respiratory rate control and "breath size" (flow) control. It also has a pushbutton for delivery of a mandatory breath.

Control Variables

The Mini-TXP only controls inspiratory flow.

INSPIRATORY WAVEFORMS. During inspiration the Mini-TXP provides gas to the patient through a venturi. As pressure builds up in the patient's respiratory system (distal to the venturi) entrainment of room air by the venturi is reduced until flow reaches a point of equilibrium. As such, the Mini-TXP normally delivers a descending ramp waveform that can be altered by changes in driving pressure of the venturi and/or patient respiratory system mechanics.

PHASE VARIABLES. Inspiration is always time triggered and is a function of set respiratory rate, which is adjustable from 6 to 150 breaths per minute. The inspiratory:expiratory (I:E) ratio is controlled by the rate control and ranges from 1:1 to 1:5.

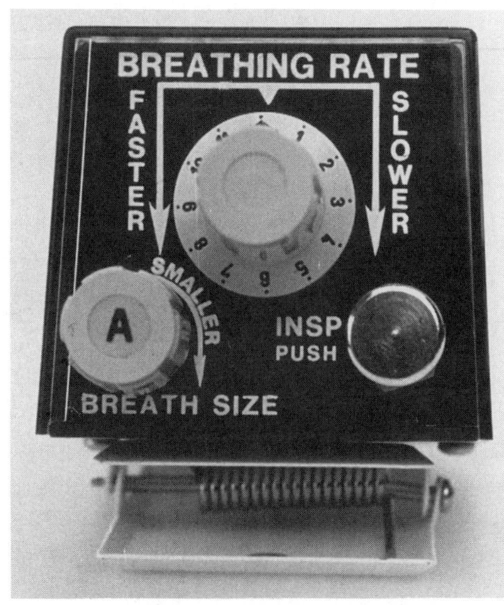

Figure 15-5. Control module of the Mini-TXP transport ventilator. (Courtesy of Percussionaire, Sandpoint, ID)

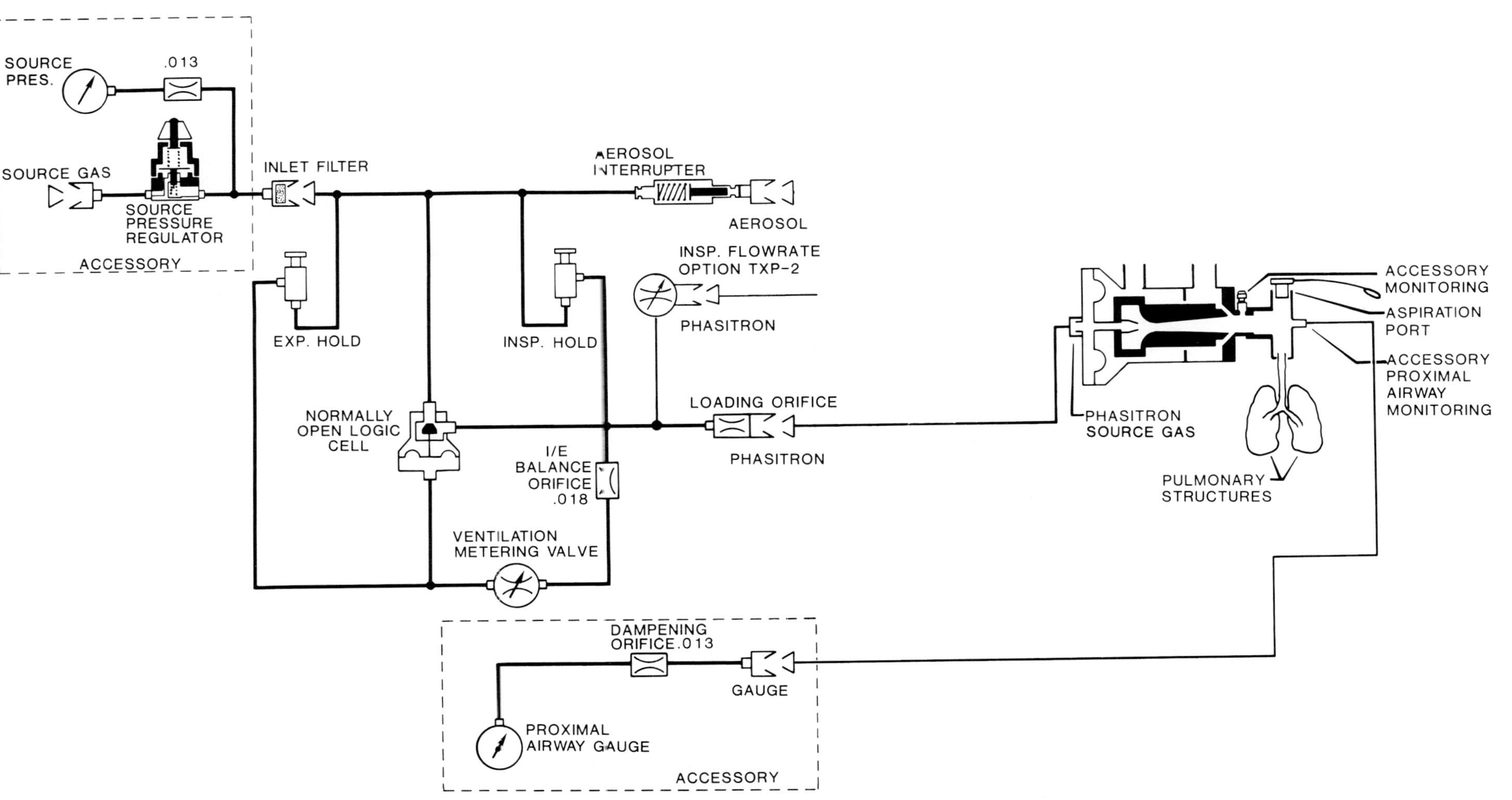

Figure 15-6. Pneumatic components of the Mini-TXP. (Courtesy of Percussionaire, Sandpoint, ID)

Inspiration is flow limited, and peak inspiratory flow is adjustable from 10 to 120 L/min.

Inspiration is time cycled as a result of the ventilatory rate setting.

No control for baseline pressure is available; however, end-expiratory pressure may be applied by a suitable PEEP/CPAP valve.

Control Subsystems

CONTROL CIRCUIT. The control circuit of the Mini-TXP is pneumatically powered and pneumatically controlled (Fig. 15-6). A "pneumatic cam" consisting of a poppet, spring, and several diaphragms controls gas movement.

DRIVE MECHANISM. An external pneumatic power source serves to power the Mini-TXP.

OUTPUT CONTROL VALVES. The output control valves include the rate control (a needle valve), the flow control needle valve, and the sliding venturi valve (Fig. 15-7). Gas from the compressed gas source enters the pneumatic cam, which during inspiration allows gas to travel through the flow control needle valve to the sliding venturi. The rate control is a needle valve that controls how quickly pressure builds up on the opposite side of the main diaphragm in the pneumatic cam. As the pressure rises the diaphragm shifts, seating the poppet and cycling inspiration off. Gas delivered to the venturi during a mandatory inspiration entrains room air at a ratio of 1:5 down to 1:1, depending on back-pressure. As such, the FIO_2 (assuming the Mini-TXP is operated from 100% oxygen) changes with back-pressure within a range of 0.45 to 0.80. An optional nebulizer can be added that provides a continuous flow of 100% source gas (20 L/min) to the sliding venturi for entrainment. This allows an FIO_2 of nearly 100% to be delivered.

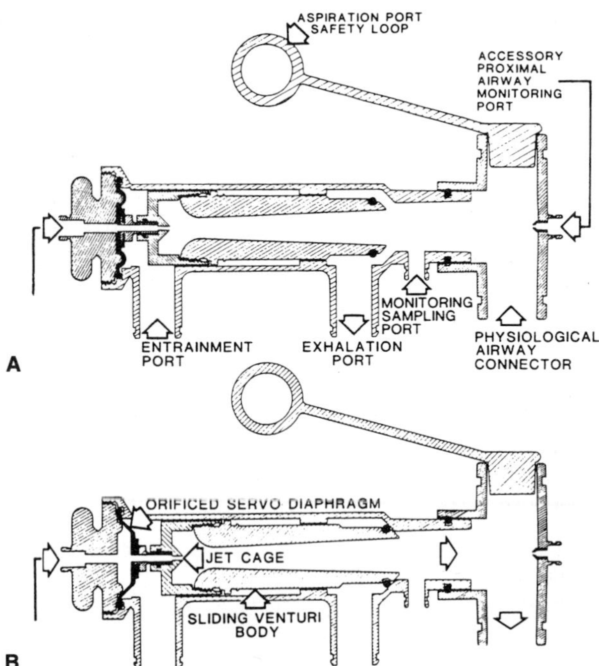

Figure 15-7. The sliding Venturi (in cross section) used to entrain ambient air and control inspiratory and expiratory gas flows. The top (A) demonstrates the expiratory phase, where the patient exhales through the exhalation port. In (B), gas from the control module enters the top of the sliding Venturi, inflating the diaphragm and seating the venturi. Gas is entrained through the entrainment port and delivered to the patient.

Output Displays

An optional aneroid gauge can be added to the Mini-TXP to display airway pressure from −10 to 120 cm H_2O.

Modes of Operation

The Mini-TXP only operates in the CMV mode, and there is no mode selection control.

CMV. Inspiration is time triggered, flow limited, and time cycled. Between mandatory breaths the patient may inspire ambient air through the exhalation port of the venturi. This mechanism also allows spontaneous breathing in the event of a gas source failure. A manual breath may be delivered by depressing the manual inspiration button. A manual breath is manually triggered, flow limited, and manually cycled (inspiration continues at the set flow rate until the pushbutton is released).

ALARMS. The Mini-TXP has no alarm system.

Critical Comment

The Mini-TXP is easy to operate and capable of ventilating a wide range of patients. Because the controls are uncalibrated, a portable respirometer should be used to set tidal volume. When PEEP is added, spontaneous breathing from ambient is equivalent to an EPAP system, which may increase the patient work of breathing. The Mini-TXP has been shown to be an effective ventilator in the hospital and in pre-hospital care.[1,3]

HAMILTON MAX

The Hamilton MAX (Hamilton Medical Corporation, Reno, NV) (Fig. 15-8) is a pressure or flow controller that is time, pressure, or manually triggered and time or pressure cycled. It operates on 100% source gas.

Input Variables

The MAX operates on electric as well as pneumatic power. Electric power is supplied by four 1.5-V AA alkaline batteries, and pneumatic power is supplied by external compressed gas at 50 to 90 psig. The MAX has no internal compressor or air–oxygen blender.

The front panel of the MAX allows the operator to select respiratory rate and tidal volume and also allows a manual breath to be triggered.

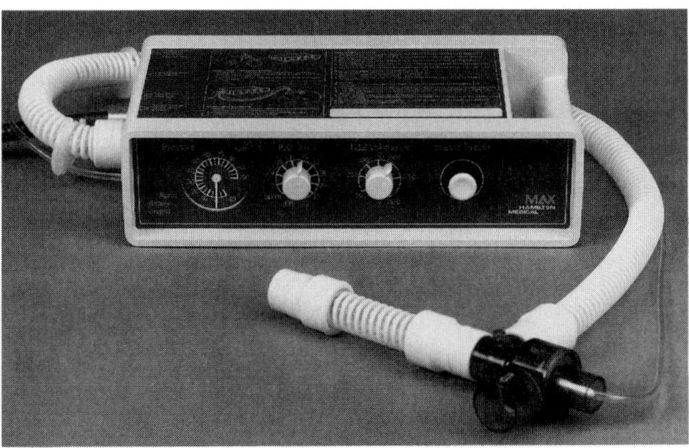

Figure 15-8. The Hamilton MAX transport ventilator. (Courtesy of Hamilton Medical Corporation, Reno, NV)

Control Variables

The MAX is a flow controller during mandatory breaths and a pressure controller during spontaneous breaths.

INSPIRATORY WAVEFORMS. The MAX offers a rectangular flow waveform during normal operation. A rectangular pressure waveform can occur if tidal volume and patient respiratory mechanics cause pressure to exceed the pre-set pressure limit. The pressure waveform, however, is not truly controlled by the ventilator.

PHASE VARIABLES. Mandatory breaths are time triggered according to the set ventilator rate (adjustable from 2 to 30 cycles/min). Inspiration may also be manually triggered. During spontaneous breathing, inspiration is pressure triggered when a negative pressure (< -2 cm H_2O) is created by the patient across the pneumatic demand valve.

Inspiration is normally flow limited (30 to 90 L/min) during mandatory breaths but may be pressure limited (10 to 100 cm H_2O) by an internally adjustable pressure relief or through a factory pre-set pressure relief (120 cm H_2O). Mandatory breaths are flow limited but may also become pressure limited if the peak pressure limit is violated. Spontaneous breaths are pressure limited.

Inspiration is time cycled during mandatory breaths according to a fixed inspiratory time of 1 second. Manually triggered breaths are delivered as long as the manual breath button is depressed. Spontaneous breaths are pressure cycled when the end-expiratory pressure rises 2 cm H_2O above ambient. There is no control for baseline pressure, but an external PEEP/ CPAP valve can be used to deliver end-expiratory pressure.

Control Subsystems

CONTROL CIRCUIT. The MAX uses both electronic and pneumatic components (Fig. 15-9) to direct gas flow to the patient. Mandatory breaths are pneumatically powered and electronically controlled, while spontaneous and manual breaths are pneumatically powered and pneumatically controlled.

DRIVE MECHANISM. The MAX requires an external gas source to power the pneumatic components. Gas delivered to the MAX is reduced by an internal regulator to 50 psig.

OUTPUT CONTROL VALVES. The output control valves include an electronic solenoid, a needle valve flow control, and a pneumatic demand valve. External gas is delivered to the MAX where an internal pressure regulator reduces pressure to 50 psig. During a mandatory breath, the solenoid opens for a fixed time of 1 second and gas travels through the flow control to the patient. Prior to the flow control, some gas is diverted to an adjustable pressure regulator, which sets the peak pressure limit by controlling pressurization of the exhalation diaphragm. Manual inspirations are solely a pneumatic function. When the manual breath switch is depressed, gas bypasses the solenoid and travels through the flow control and on to the patient. In this manner, manual ventilation can be accomplished without the need for electric power.

Spontaneous breaths are controlled by the pneumatic demand valve. Gas powering the demand valve is at source gas pressure (50 psig), which allows a peak

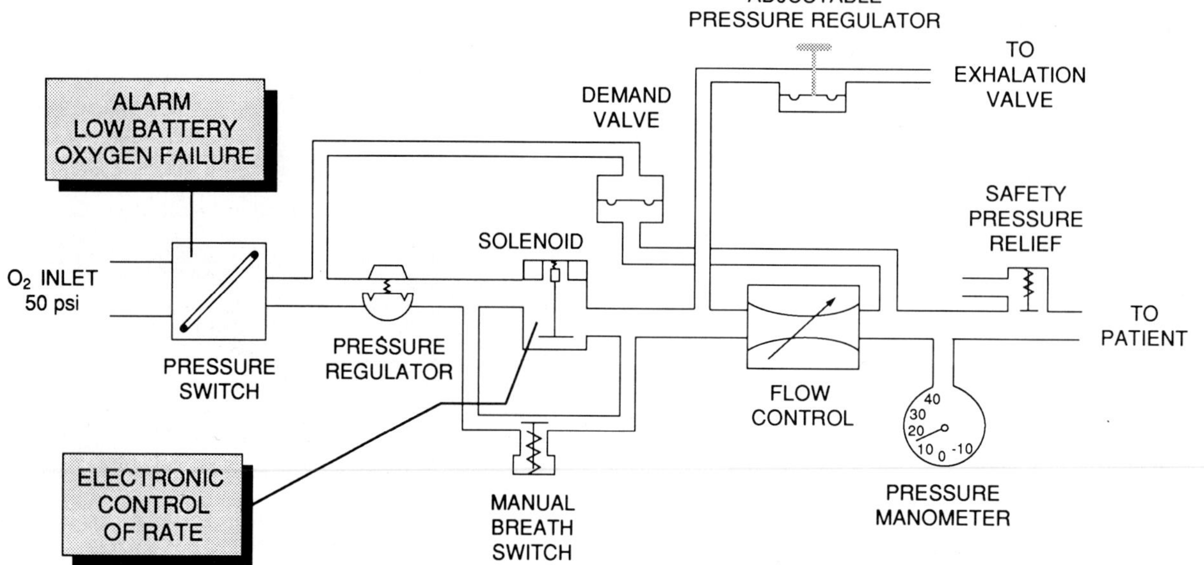

Figure 15-9. Internal schematic of the Hamilton MAX transport ventilator.

inspiratory flow up to 145 L/min. The demand valve is triggered on by a −2 cm H_2O deflation in airway pressure and is referenced to ambient pressure. Demand flow is cycled off when airway pressure rises 2 cm H_2O above ambient pressure. There is no control for baseline pressure, but PEEP/CPAP can be provided with an external PEEP/CPAP valve. When PEEP/CPAP is used, triggering of the demand valve remains at −2 cm H_2O from ambient (not PEEP compensated).

Output Displays

Airway pressure is displayed by an aneroid gauge over the range of −10 to 100 cm H_2O.

Modes of Operation

The MAX operates strictly in the IMV mode. There is no mode selector switch.

IMV. Mandatory breaths are time triggered (based on ventilatory rate), pressure or flow limited, and time cycled (based on the fixed 1 second inspiratory time). Spontaneous breaths from the demand valve are pressure triggered, pressure limited, and pressure cycled.

Alarms

INPUT POWER ALARMS. When less than 30 minutes of battery power remain, the low-battery alarm will illuminate. If battery power becomes disconnected, no alarm will be activated. A pressure switch located prior to the pressure regulator will cause the oxygen alarm to illuminate when gas pressure is disconnected or falls below 27 psig.

CONTROL CIRCUIT ALARMS. The MAX has no control circuit alarms.

Critical Comment

The MAX is intended for both in-hospital and pre-hospital transport. It has been shown to be a reliable ventilator for in-hospital transport. It has no gas consumption due to electronic control and allows spontaneous breathing through a demand valve. Johannigman and associates[6] list the shortcomings of the MAX as (1) no low-pressure alarm; (2) the demand system is not PEEP compensated; and (3) the adjustable pressure limit control is only accessible by removing the ventilator's cover.

IMPACT UNI-VENT 706

The Impact Uni-Vent 706 (Impact Medical Corporation, West Caldwell, NJ) (Fig. 15-10) is a flow or pressure controller that is time or manually triggered and time cycled. It operates from 100% source gas. It has no air–oxygen blender, air-entrainment mechanism, or compressor.

Input Variables

The Uni-Vent 706 uses 115 volts AC at 60 Hz, 230 volts AC at 50 Hz, or internal lead acid batteries (12 volts DC) to power the control circuitry. External compressed gas at 50 to 100 psig is used as the pneumatic power source.

The front panel allows control of inspiratory flow and a series of respiratory rate, inspiratory time, and I:E ratio settings named in Table 15-2. The patient valve contains two pressure relief valves that limit peak inspiratory pressure.

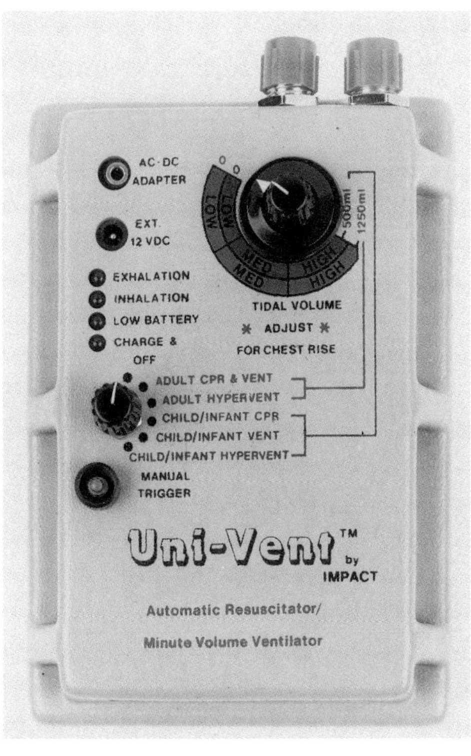

Figure 15-10. The Uni-Vent 706 ventilator. (Courtesy of Impact Medical Corporation, West Caldwell, NJ)

Control Variables

The Uni-Vent 706 is normally a flow controller, but if peak inspiratory pressure relief settings are violated, it controls pressure.

INSPIRATORY WAVEFORMS. The Uni-Vent 706 produces a rectangular flow waveform during normal operation. In instances when tidal volume settings and patient respiratory system mechanics cause the pressure relief valve to be activated, the Uni-Vent 706 will produce a rectangular pressure waveform.

PHASE VARIABLES. Inspiration is time triggered depending on the respiratory rate, inspiratory time, and I:E ratio setting chosen.

Inspiration is flow limited from 0 to 90 L/min during normal operation. Pressure limiting can be achieved by selecting either the 60 or 80 cm H_2O pressure relief setting on the patient valve.

Inspiration is always time cycled. Baseline pressure is not controlled, but an external PEEP/CPAP valve can be used to create elevated end-expiratory pressure.

Control Subsystems

CONTROL CIRCUIT. The control circuit of the Uni-Vent 706 is electronically controlled and consists of both electronic and pneumatic components (Fig. 15-11).

DRIVE MECHANISM. The Uni-Vent 706 is pneumatically powered from an external compressed gas source at 50 to 100 psig.

TABLE 15-2. Respiratory Frequency, Inspiratory Time and I:E Settings Used by the Impact 706

	Ventilation Rate (breaths per minute)	Inspiration Time(s)	I:E
Adult cardiopulmonary resuscitation	12	1.5	1:2.3
Adult hyperventilation	18	1.5	1:1.2
Child/infant cardiopulmonary resuscitation	14	1.5	1:1.8
Child/infant ventilation	20	1.0	1:2.0
Child/infant hyperventilation	30	0.75	1:1.6

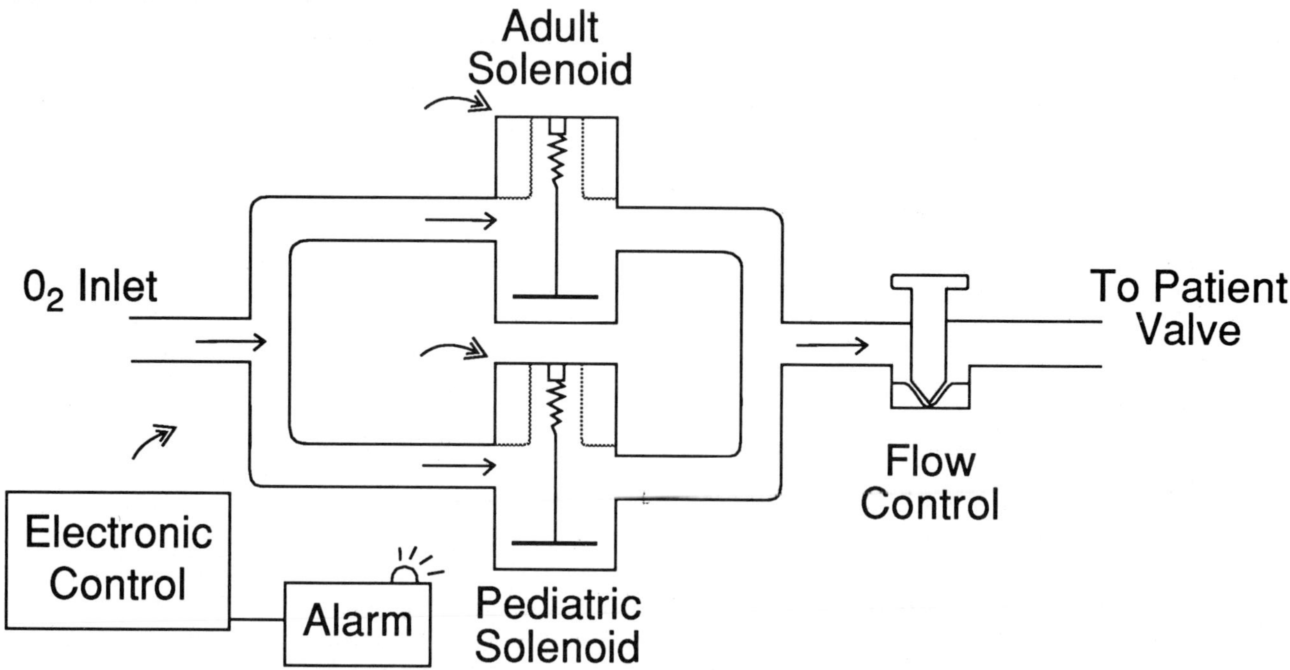

Figure 15-11. The internal components of the Uni-Vent 706 ventilator.

OUTPUT CONTROL VALVES. The output control valves include two solenoids, a flow control needle valve and the patient valve, which contains a mushroom-type exhalation valve, spring-loaded pressure limiting valves, and an antiasphyxia valve (one-way valve). During inspiration, a timing signal from the electronic control circuit board opens the appropriate solenoid for the settings selected. Gas travels from the solenoid through the needle valve flow control and to the patient valve. At the patient valve, gas pressurizes the exhalation valve and inspiration occurs. If peak inspiratory pressure exceeds the set pressure relief (60 or 80 cm H_2O), gas exits to ambient through the pressure relief valve, creating a low-pitch audible signal that pressure limiting has occurred.

Inspiration is cycled off according to the selected inspiratory time and the solenoid is closed, preventing gas flow to the patient. When gas flow to the patient valve is interrupted, the exhalation valve deflates and allows passive exhalation.

Output Displays

Indicator lamps (inhalation, exhalation) illuminate during the respective parts of the ventilatory cycle.

Modes of Operation

The Uni-Vent 706 operates only in the CONTROL mode. There is no mode selection control.

CMV. Inspiration is normally flow controlled, time triggered, flow limited, and time cycled. Between mandatory breaths the patient may respire ambient gases through the antiasphyxia valve in the patient valve. As described earlier, inspiration can also be pressure limited under some circumstances.

A manual breath may also be delivered. Manual breaths are manually triggered, flow limited, and manually cycled. That is, gas passes through the flow control and to the patient as long as the manual trigger button is activated.

Alarms

INPUT POWER ALARMS. When less than 5 hours of operation remain in the internal batteries, the low-battery light will illuminate.

CONTROL VARIABLE ALARM. If during normal ventilation the peak inspiratory pressure relief setting is exceeded, an audible, mechanical alarm will sound as pressure is released through the relief valve. Pressure relief settings are controlled at the patient valve at either 60 or 80 cm H_2O.

Critical Comment

The Uni-Vent 706 is intended for use in pre-hospital care. Its simplicity and separate volume and rate controls meet the demands of pre-hospital providers. Johannigman and colleagues[2] have demonstrated the effective use of the Uni-Vent 706 by paramedics. Addition of a low-gas inlet pressure alarm to warn of gas pressure failure or disconnect would be useful in the Uni-Vent 706.

IMPACT UNI-VENT 750

The Impact Uni-Vent 750 (Impact Medical Corporation, West Caldwell, NJ) (Fig. 15-12) is a flow or pressure controller that is pressure, time, or manually triggered and time or pressure cycled. It does not have an integral blender or compressor.

Input Variables

The Uni-Vent 750's electronic control circuitry will accept 12 volts DC from internal rechargeable batteries or 12 volts DC through an optional 115/230 volts AC, 11 to 30 volts AC/DC converter at 50 to 400 Hz. Pneumatic power is supplied by external compressed gas at 50 to 100 psig.

The front panel of the Uni-Vent 750 is shown in Figure 15-13. The operator may select mode of ventilation, ventilator rate, inspiratory time, inspiratory flow, pressure triggering (sensitivity), and peak inspiratory pressure limit. Calibrated dials and membrane switches are used as the operator interface.

Control Variables

The Uni-Vent 750 controls inspiratory pressure or inspiratory flow. Mandatory breaths are flow controlled while spontaneous breaths are pressure controlled.

INSPIRATORY FLOW WAVEFORM. The Uni-Vent 750 offers a rectangular flow waveform during normal operation. A rectangular pressure waveform can be accomplished when pressure limiting occurs.

PHASE VARIABLES. In the CONTROL mode (CMV), inspiration is time triggered according to the set ventilatory rate, adjustable from 1 to 150 breaths per minute. Inspiration can be time or pressure triggered in the ASSIST (AMV) and SIMV modes. The threshold for triggering a breath in AMV and SIMV is adjustable from −2 to −8 cm H_2O in 2-cm H_2O increments. Pressure triggering is PEEP compensated. Manual triggering is also available.

Inspiration is flow limited for mandatory breaths and pressure limited for spontaneous breaths in the SIMV mode. Pressure limiting can occur during delivery of a mandatory breath if the high-pressure limit setting is violated. Flow is controlled by a calibrated dial and is adjustable from 0 to 100 L/min.

All mandatory breaths are time cycled as a result of the set inspiratory time, adjustable from 0.1 to 3.0 seconds. Spontaneous breaths are pressure cycled when airway pressure exceeds the baseline pressure setting by 2 cm H_2O.

Baseline pressure is not controlled by the Uni-Vent 750. Application of PEEP/CPAP requires an external PEEP/CPAP valve.

Control Subsystems

CONTROL CIRCUIT. The Uni-Vent 750 uses both pneumatic and electronic control components (Fig. 15-14). A microprocessor controls the ventilatory rate and inspiratory time by sending signals to the appropriate

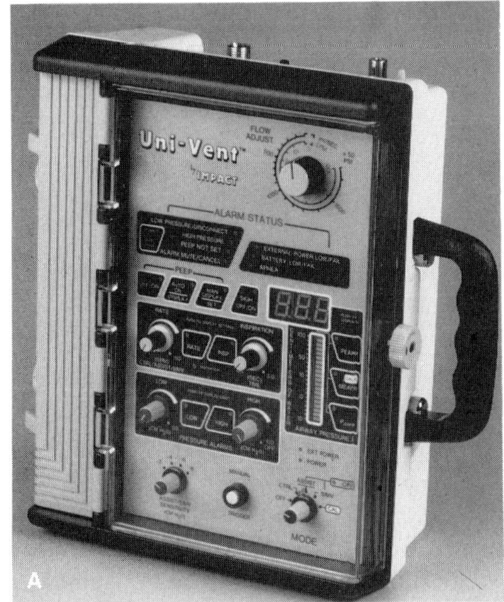

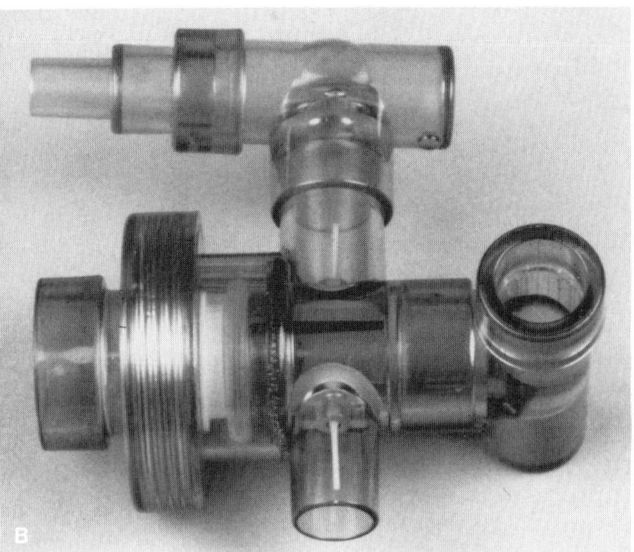

Figure 15-12. (A.) Control module of the Uni-Vent 750. (Courtesy of Impact Medical Corporation, West Caldwell, NJ) (B.) Patient valve assembly of the Uni-Vent 750. (Courtesy of Impact Medical Corporation, West Caldwell, NJ)

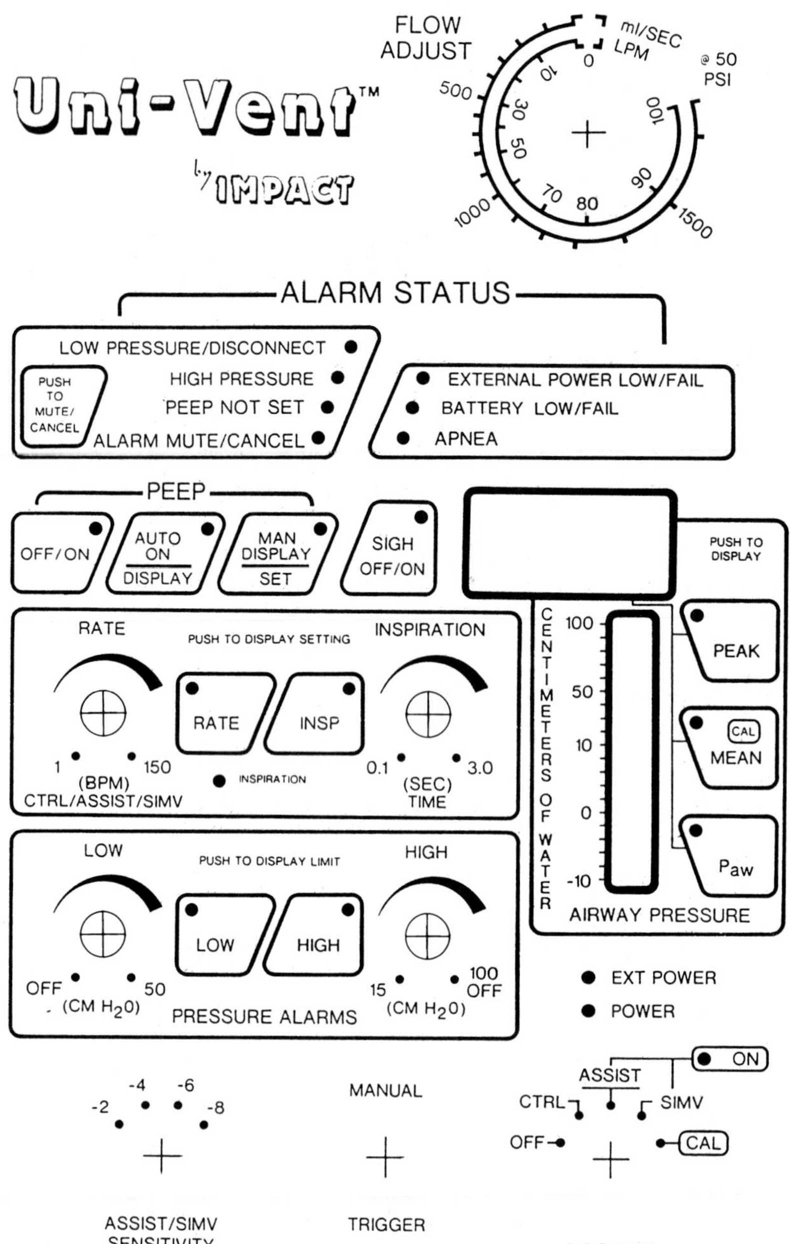

Figure 15-13. Control panel of the Uni-Vent 750. (Courtesy of Impact Medical Corporation, West Caldwell, NJ)

solenoids and accepts signals from a pressure transducer for triggering assisted breaths, monitoring, and controlling alarm functions.

DRIVE MECHANISM. The Uni-Vent 750 uses external compressed gas at 50 psig to deliver gas to the patient. It has no external compressor, air–oxygen blender, or air-entrainment system.

OUTPUT CONTROL VALVES. The output control valves include the solenoid valves, flow control needle valve, and exhalation diaphragm. Gas entering the Uni-Vent 750 passes through a regulator set at 50 psig and is delivered to the inspiratory solenoids and demand flow solenoid. During a mandatory breath, the inspiratory solenoids open at the selected inspiratory time and direct gas to the flow control needle valve. Gas exiting the ventilator travels through the main circuit to the patient valve where it pressurizes the mushroom-type exhalation valve and ventilates the patient. During exhalation, pressure from the mushroom valve is released and expiratory gas traverses a one-way valve to ambient.

During IMV, an internal pressure transducer monitors airway pressure. When a spontaneous breath reduces circuit pressure below the pressure triggering threshold (adjustable from −2 to 8 cm H_2O) the demand flow solenoid is opened to provide flow up to 150 L/min. Gas from the demand flow solenoid is delivered through a separate circuit to the patient valve, which prevents pressurization of the exhalation valve.

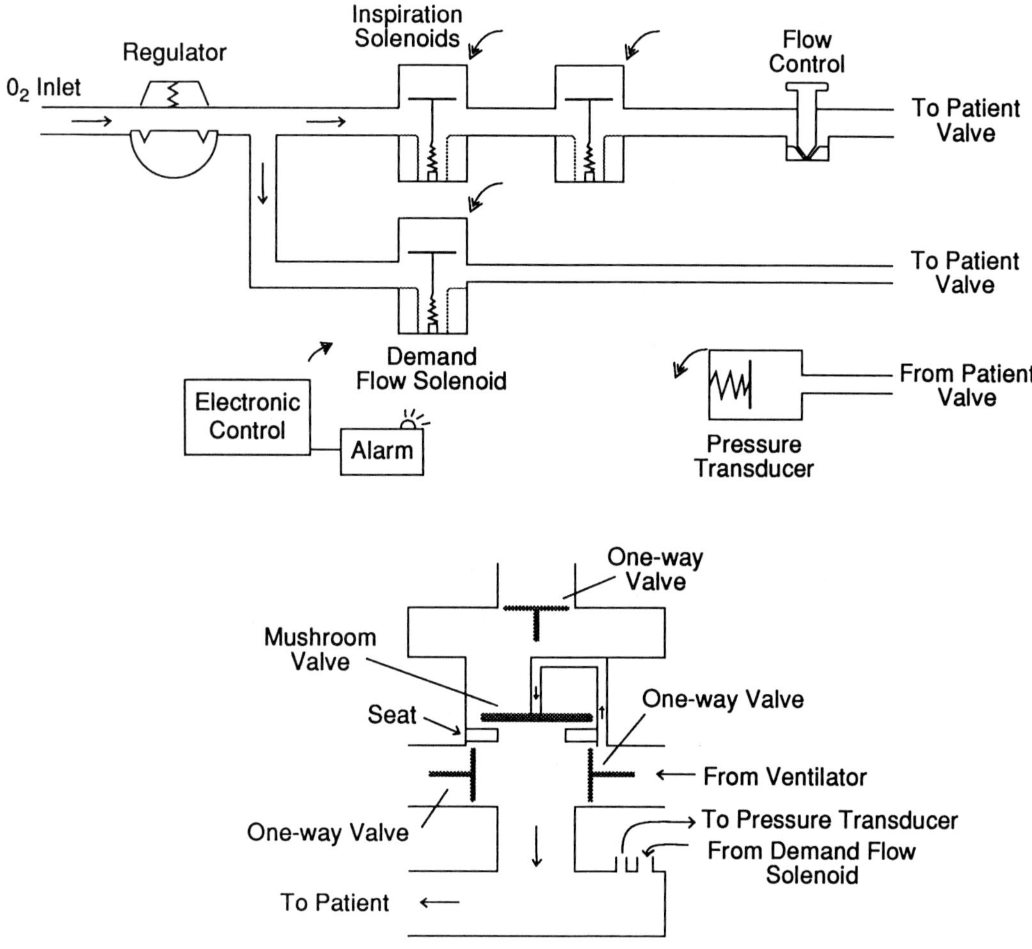

Figure 15-14. Schematic of the internal components (top) and patient valve (bottom) of the Uni-Vent 750.

Output Displays

The Uni-Vent 750 uses a display window to display ventilator and alarm settings as well as airway pressures. Whenever a control is adjusted or its corresponding membrane pad is depressed, its setting will be shown in the display window. Variables that are displayed include ventilator rate, inspiratory time, sensitivity, high-pressure alarm settings, low-pressure alarm setting, peak inspiratory pressure, mean airway pressure, and baseline pressure. A bar graph display of dynamic airway pressure from -10 to 100 cm H_2O is also included. Additionally, indicator lights illuminate next to the selected functions (sigh on/off, PEEP on/off, power, external power), and during a mandatory breath the inspiration indicator light illuminates during the inspiratory time.

Modes of Operation

The following modes are those named on the control panel of the Uni-Vent 750:

CONTROL (CMV). During CMV, inspiration is time triggered (according to set ventilation rate), flow or pressure limited, and time cycled (according to set inspiratory time). Spontaneous breathing in the CMV mode can occur through the antiasphyxia valve in the patient valve.

ASSIST (AMV). During AMV, inspiration is either time triggered or pressure triggered (depending on sensitivity setting), flow or pressure limited, and time cycled.

SIMV. In SIMV, mandatory breaths are flow controlled, time or pressure triggered, flow or pressure limited, and time cycled. Spontaneous breaths are pressure controlled, pressure triggered, pressure limited, and pressure cycled. If PEEP or CPAP is used, the Uni-Vent 750 allows PEEP compensation of triggered breaths through two methods. The first occurs by depressing the AUTO-ON-PEEP membrane pad. In this case the pressure transducer monitors baseline pressure and pressure triggering will occur at the sensitivity setting minus baseline pressure. The second is by depressing the MAN-DISPLAY PEEP membrane pad, which allows the clinician to enter the appropriate baseline pressure value. With this method pressure triggering occurs at the sensitivity setting below the manually entered baseline pressure.

SIGH. A sigh may be added in all three modes of ventilation. When activated by depressing the SIGH membrane pad, a sigh breath is delivered every 7 minutes or every 100 ventilator breaths at an inspiratory time 50% greater than set inspiratory time (limit 3 seconds). Sigh breaths are then time triggered, flow or pressure limited, and time cycled.

Emergency Modes of Ventilation

If apnea is detected in the AMV or SIMV mode (defined as no spontaneous or mandatory breaths for 19 seconds) the apnea alarm will sound and the Uni-Vent 750 will default to a ventilation rate of 12 breaths per minute at the current inspiratory time and inspiratory flow settings.

Alarms

All alarms are visual and audible.

INPUT POWER ALARM. Alarms are activated if the external power source fails or is disconnected and when the internal battery voltage falls below 11 volts DC or is defective. If the Uni-Vent 750 is operating from external power and is disconnected, it will immediately switch to internal battery power.

CONTROL VARIABLE ALARMS. All control variable alarms are activated by the microprocessor based on signals received from the pressure transducer. The low-pressure/disconnect alarm sounds when airway pressure falls below the low-pressure alarm setting (adjustable from 0 to 50 cm H_2O) or when airway pressure fails to exceed 1 cm H_2O within a window surrounding the next scheduled mandatory breath. If the latter occurs, the ventilator will deliver a mandatory breath at 50% greater than the set inspiratory time. If pressure is detected, the apnea alarm is activated. If pressure is not detected, the disconnect alarm is activated. The high-pressure alarm is activated when airway pressure exceeds the set high-pressure limit (adjustable from 15 to 100 cm H_2O) for 2 seconds during a single breath or for 50 ms during four consecutive breaths. The apnea alarm is functional only in the Assist and SIMV modes and is activated when no mandatory or spontaneous breaths are detected for 19 seconds.

When inspiratory time is set longer than expiratory time the display window will flash I:E to alert the operator of a reverse I:E ratio. During activation of the I:E alarm the Uni-Vent 750 will not deliver a mandatory breath.

The PEEP not set alarm will sound when baseline pressure is $\pm$ 2 cm H_2O from the set baseline pressure for three consecutive breaths.

All alarms can be muted by depressing the alarm mute membrane keypad, but indicator lights next to the violated alarms remain on.

CONTROL CIRCUIT ALARMS. If during a self-check the microprocessor detects a RAM or ROM failure, a nonmutable alarm will sound and the display window will read FAL (for Fail). During this time the ventilator will not deliver a mandatory breath. Two other control circuit alarms concern the pressure transducer. If the pressure transducer calibration is prematurely stopped or transducer calibration fails, the display window will flash "–" and an audible alarm will sound. Proper calibration of the transducer will deactivate the alarm.

Critical Comment

The Uni-Vent 750 is intended for inter- and intra-hospital transport. It is too sophisticated for pre-hospital use. The ability of the Uni-Vent 750 to provide three modes of ventilation, allow PEEP compensation of the demand valve, and provide an essential alarm package is unique among transport ventilators. Campbell and colleagues[7] have demonstrated the effectiveness of the Uni-Vent 750 during the in-hospital transport. They also recommend that sensitivity remain set at −2 cm H_2O, since they noticed that as sensitivity was decreased (−6 or −8 cm H_2O) inspiratory effort was not detected by the transducer because gas was inspired through the antiasphyxia valve.

LIFE SUPPORT PRODUCTS AUTOVENT 2000 AND AUTOVENT 3000

The AutoVent 2000 and AutoVent 3000 transport ventilators (Life Support Products, Irvine, CA) (Figs. 15-15 and 15-16) are flow or pressure controllers that are time or pressure triggered, flow or pressure limited, and time cycled. They do not have an external blender, compressor, or air-mixing system.

Input Variables

The AutoVent ventilators are pneumatically powered and pneumatically operated. They will accept external compressed gas at 40 to 90 psig.

The control panel of the AutoVent 2000 allows the operator to select ventilator rate and tidal volume, while the AutoVent 3000 allows ventilator rate, inspiratory time, and tidal volume to be set.

Control Variables

The AutoVent ventilators are normally set to control inspiratory flow. However, the patient valve has a preset, nonadjustable pressure limit set at 55 cm H_2O. When ventilator settings and patient respiratory mechanics cause peak pressure to exceed this pressure limit, mandatory breaths are pressure controlled. Spontaneous breaths are pressure controlled.

INSPIRATORY WAVEFORMS. The AutoVent ventilators normally produce a rectangular flow waveform. When the pressure limit is violated, a rectangular pressure waveform may be observed.

PHASE VARIABLES. Mandatory breaths are time triggered as a function of ventilator rate, and spontaneous breaths from the pneumatic demand valve are

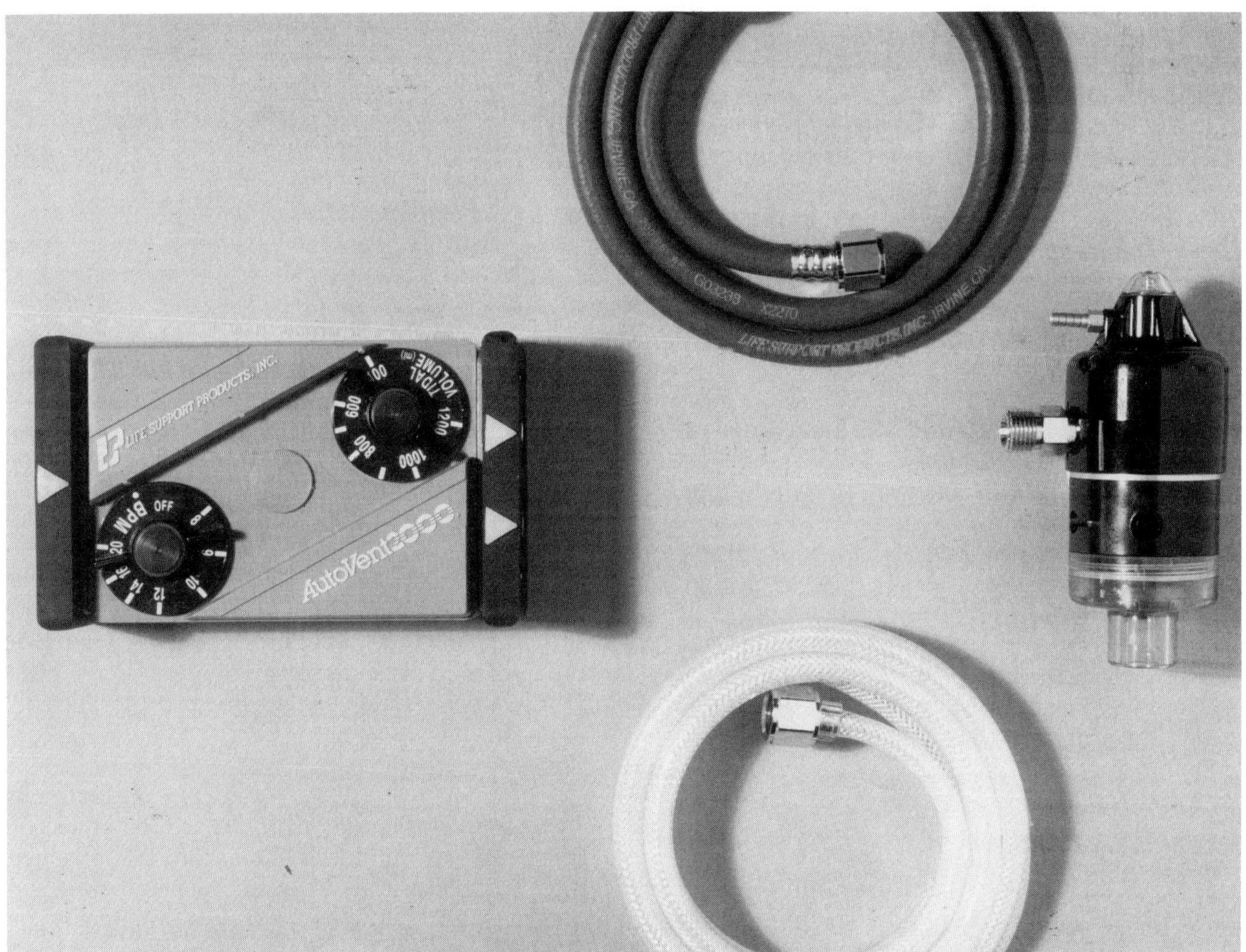

Figure 15-15. The AutoVent 2000 transport ventilator, connecting hoses, and demand valve. (Courtesy of Life Support Products, Irvine, CA)

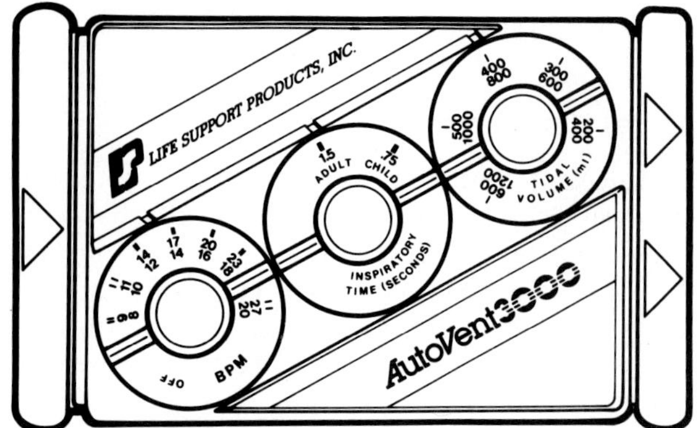

Figure 15-16. Control module of the AutoVent 3000 ventilator. (Courtesy of Life Support Products, Irvine, CA)

pressure triggered. The AutoVent 2000 has seven ventilator rate settings (8, 9, 10, 12, 14, 16, and 20 breaths per minute), and the AutoVent 3000 has 14 ventilator rate settings (Adult 8, 10, 12, 14, 16, 18, and 20 breaths per minute; Child 9, 11, 14, 17, 20, 23, and 27 breaths per minute). Spontaneous breaths are pressure triggered.

Inspiration is normally flow limited (16 to 48 L/min) but may be pressure limited (50 ± 5 cm H_2O). Tidal volume can be set at 400, 600, 800, 1000, and 1200 mL with the AutoVent 2000 and at 200, 300, 400, 500, 600 (child setting) and 400, 600, 800, 1000, and 1200 mL (adult setting) with the AutoVent 3000.

Inspiration is time cycled according to set inspiratory time (AutoVent 2000, 1.5 second; AutoVent 3000, 0.75 and 1.5 seconds) during mandatory breaths. Spontaneous breaths are pressure cycled.

There is no control for baseline pressure and PEEP/CPAP cannot be added to the exhalation port of the patient valve.

Control Subsystems

CONTROL CIRCUIT. The control circuit of the AutoVent ventilators uses only pneumatic components (Fig. 15-17). Gas flow and inspiratory and expiratory time are controlled by movement of a spool valve.

DRIVE MECHANISM. The AutoVent ventilators require a pneumatic source to power the pneumatic circuit.

OUTPUT CONTROL VALVES. The output control valves include needle valves for control of inspiratory time, ventilator rate and tidal volume, the spool valve, and the pneumatic demand valve (Fig. 15-18). Compressed gas from an external source passes through a filter to a pressure regulator, which reduces pressure to 30 psig. Gas then travels bidirectionally to the patient through the tidal volume control (actually controls flow) and to the spool valve and inspiratory time control. The AutoVent 2000 has a fixed inspiratory time (1.5 seconds), while the AutoVent 3000 has a variable inspiratory time (0.75 and 1.5 seconds). Gas passing through the timer fills a volume chamber and begins to increase pressure on the spool valve. Adjustment of the inspiratory time setting simply controls how quickly the pressure increases. As pressure builds in the patient circuit, the spool valve slides into the expiratory position. During the expiratory phase the spool valve directs gas to the rate control, which truly controls expiratory time by changing the speed at which pressure fills the expiratory volume chamber and slides the spool valve back to the inspiratory position. The pneumatic demand valve controls pressure during spontaneous breaths. A patient inspiratory effort greater than −2 cm H_2O below ambient causes the demand valve to open and deliver a flow rate of 48 L/min. As pressure rises above ambient, the demand valve closes, pressure cycling the breath. The patient valve also allows ambient air to be drawn into the patient valve if patient spontaneous inspiratory flow demand is greater than 48 L/min. A pressure relief (limit) valve is also located in the patient valve, which limits peak pressure to 50 ± 5 cm H_2O.

Output Displays

The AutoVent ventilators have a pneumatic indicator on top of the patient valve that flashes green during the inspiratory phase.

Modes of Operation

The AutoVent ventilators operate solely in the IMV mode. There is no mode selector switch.

IMV. Mandatory breaths are time triggered, flow or pressure limited, and time cycled. Spontaneous breaths from the pneumatic demand valve are pressure triggered, pressure limited, and pressure cycled.

Alarms

CONTROL VARIABLE ALARMS. When the pre-set 50 ± 5 cm H_2O pressure limit is reached, gas is vented through a mechanical pressure relief valve. As gas passes through the pressure relief valve it creates an audible alarm.

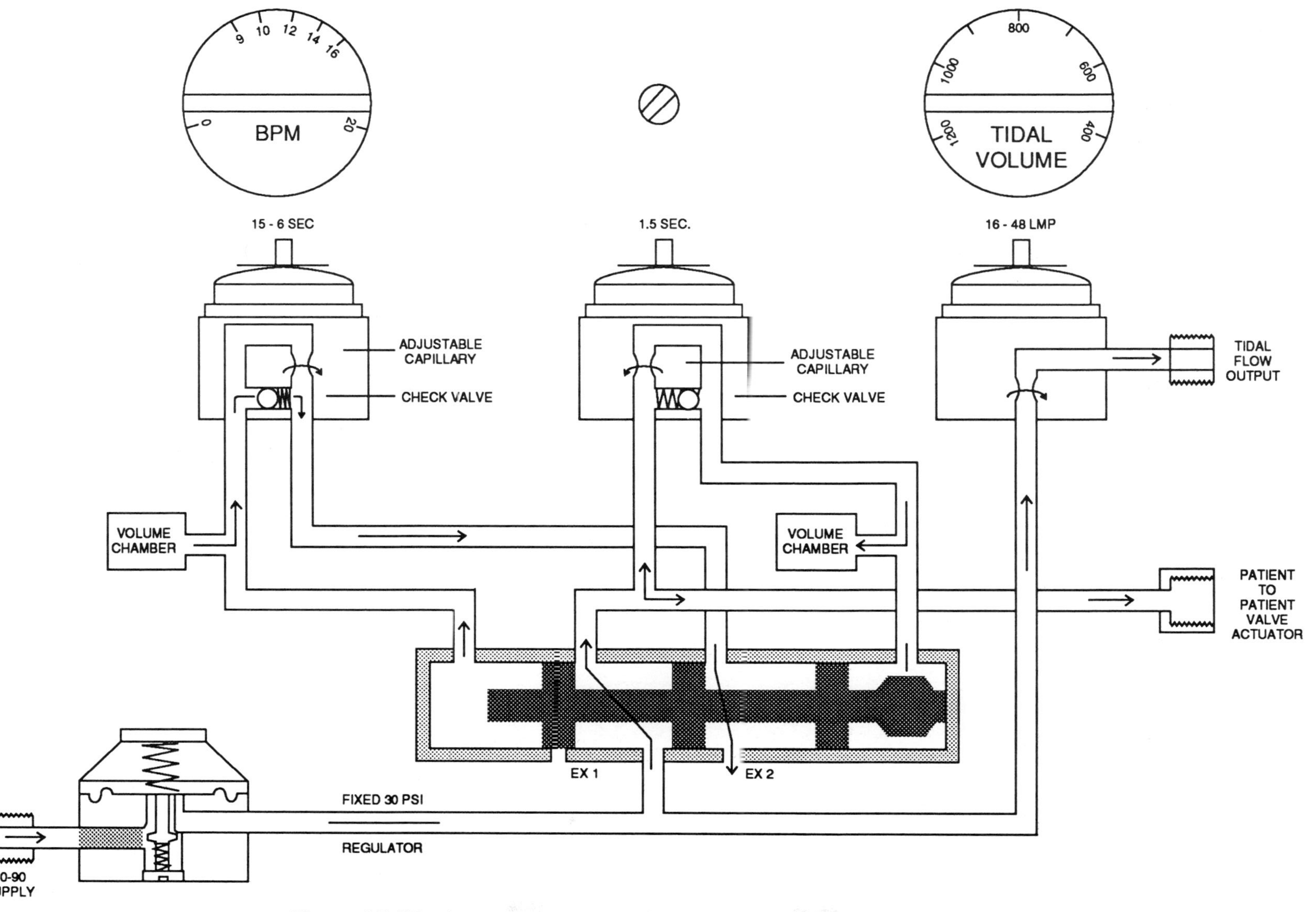

Figure 15-17. Internal components of the AutoVent 2000 transport ventilator.

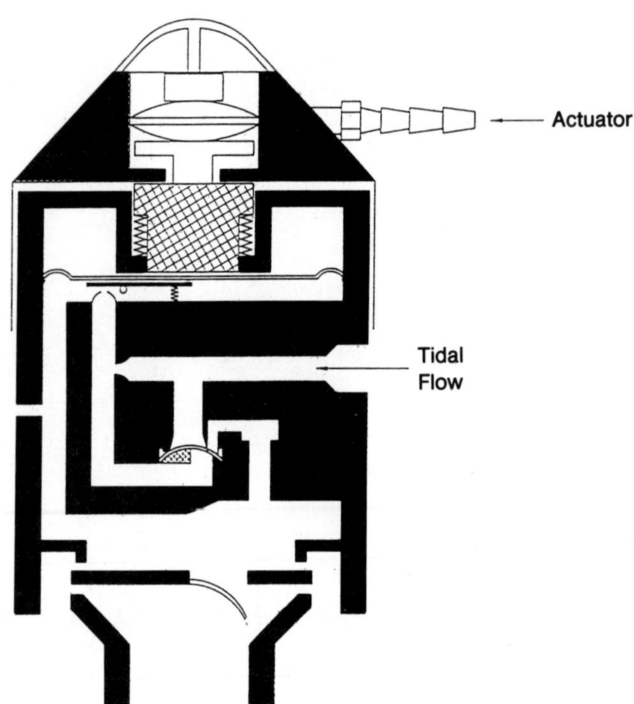

Figure 15-18. Cross-section of the LSP demand valve used with the AutoVent 2000 and 3000. (Courtesy of Life Support Products, Irvine, CA)

Critical Comment

The AutoVent 2000 and 3000 ventilators are intended for pre-hospital care and lack the flexibility and sophistication to be used with critically ill patients. Both meet most of the demands of pre-hospital care. Weight of the patient valve on the endotracheal tube may be of concern. Additionally, the demand flow is fixed (48 L/min), which means if the patient breathes spontaneously at a flow greater than 48 L/min, gas will have to be entrained from ambient through the patient valve. This increases the work of breathing and may prove intolerable by an alert patient.

OHMEDA LOGIC 07

The Ohmeda Logic 07 (Ohmeda, Madison, WI) (Fig. 15-19) is a pressure or flow controller that is time triggered, flow or pressure limited, and time cycled. It has no internal blender or compressor but may deliver 100% or 50% oxygen through a venturi mechanism.

Input Variables

The Logic 07 requires pneumatic power and operates from an external compressed gas source at 44 to 88 psig.

The operator may select ventilator frequency, ventilator minute volume, peak pressure limit, and F_{IO_2} (100% or 50%). Ventilator frequency and minute volume are controlled by calibrated dials, F_{IO_2} by a toggle switch, and pressure limit by an uncalibrated dial.

Control Variables

The Logic 07 normally controls inspiratory flow but can control inspiratory pressure.

INSPIRATORY WAVEFORMS. During flow control, the Logic 07 produces a rectangular flow waveform. When pressure controlled, a rectangular pressure waveform may be produced.

PHASE VARIABLES. Inspiration is time triggered according to set ventilator rate (adjustable from 10 to 40 breaths per minute) and is either flow (12 to 65 L/min) or pressure limited (20 to 90 cm H_2O). Inspiration is time cycled based on the ventilator rate setting. I:E is constant at 1:2 regardless of ventilator frequency.

Baseline pressure is not controlled but can be added with a PEEP/CPAP valve.

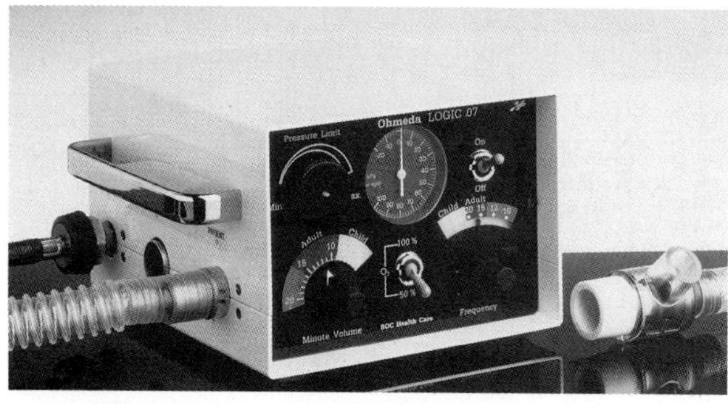

Figure 15-19. The Ohmeda Logic 07 transport ventilator. (Courtesy of Ohmeda, Madison, WI)

Control Subsystems

CONTROL CIRCUIT. The control circuit of the Logic 07 is pneumatically powered and fluidically controlled (Fig. 15-20). The timing circuit is a flip-flop valve, and all other components are pneumatic.

DRIVE MECHANISM. External compressed gas serves as the driving mechanism for the Logic 07. Gas delivered to the patient may be at 100% source gas or 50%, through use of a venturi and air entrainment.

OUTPUT CONTROL VALVES. The output control valves include the ventilator frequency needle valve, the FIO_2 toggle switch, the pressure limiting valve, and minute volume control. Gas entering the ventilator is reduced to 44 psig by a pressure regulator. From this regulator, gas flows bidirectionally: one source is further reduced to 22 psig by a second regulator and is used to power the pneumatic circuit, and the other travels to a flow regulator. The timing circuit is a flip-flop valve (Fig. 15-21) that uses timing reservoirs and pre-set restrictions to control signals to the flow regulator. During inspiration, the flow regulator is activated and the internal expiratory valve closed by the flip-flop signal. When pressure in the timing reservoir causes the ball valve to move, inspiration is terminated. Gas then passes through the expiratory timing reservoir and restrictor where pressure will eventually rise to move the expiratory ball valve. This causes the input gas to travel to the flow regulator, closing it (expiration), or to the expiratory valve, closing it (inspiration). Gas from the flow regulator travels to the venturi system. The FIO_2 toggle switch controls operation of the venturi (100% no venturi flow, 50% gas flow through the venturi). When FIO_2 is changed from 100% to 50%, an increase in minute volume of approximately 15% will occur. Gas then travels to the flow control, which operates like a needle valve. The PRESSURE LIMIT control is set by adjusting the control until pressure is vented to atmosphere of the desired pressure (monitored on the aneroid gauge). The PRESSURE LIMIT control operates by increasing spring tension on a diaphragm.

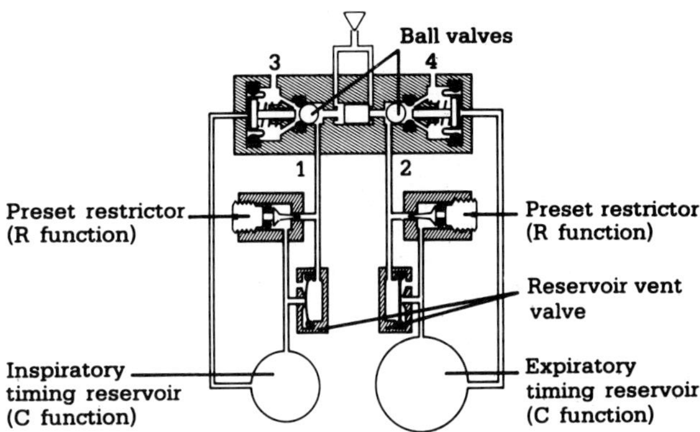

Figure 15-21. Timing circuit of the Logic 07 ventilator. (Courtesy of Ohmeda, Madison, WI)

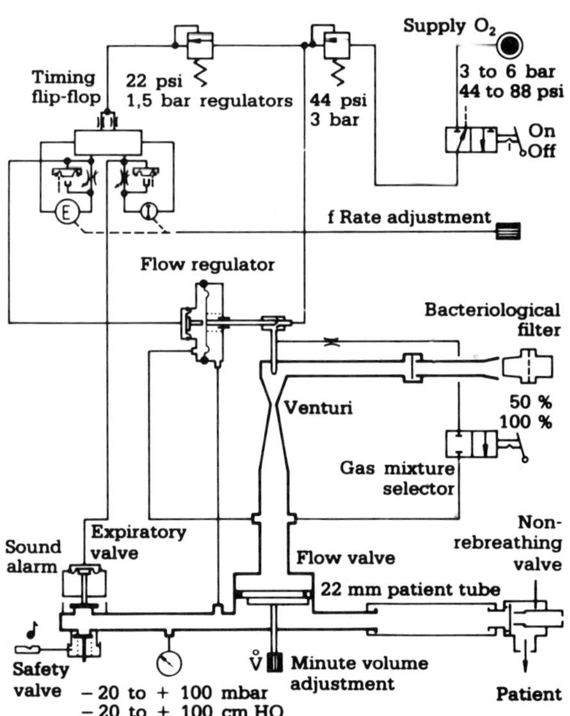

Figure 15-20. Pneumatic circuit of the Logic 07. (Courtesy of Ohmeda, Madison, WI)

Output Displays

Airway pressure is displayed on an aneroid pressure gauge over the range of −20 to 100 cm H_2O.

Modes of Operation

The Logic 07 operates solely in the control mode.

CMV. Inspiration is time triggered, flow or pressure limited, and time cycled. Between mandatory breaths, spontaneous breathing through the expiratory port of the non-rebreathing valve is possible.

Alarms

CONTROL VARIABLE ALARMS. When the pressure limit is exceeded, the escape of gas from the spring-loaded, diaphragm mechanism creates an audible alarm.

Critical Comment

The Logic 07 is intended for inter- and intra-hospital transport. Its ability to change FIO_2 is a unique feature that helps to prolong gas source life. The adjustment of tidal volume by manipulating rate and minute volume is disturbing to some operators. Morash and colleagues[8] found the Logic 07 to be simple to operate but also found that there was up to a 30% variance in actual volume and rate versus set volume and rate as patient compliance fell. They believed this variance was "clinically unacceptable." Spontaneous breathing occurs from ambient (through the non-rebreathing valve) unless PEEP is used. With a PEEP valve attached, spontaneous breathing occurs through the length of the patient circuit through the entrainment part of the venturi mechanism. Patients on PEEP who are spontaneously breathing may find this increase in the work of breathing intolerable.

OHMEDA HARV (PNEUPAC 2-R)

The Ohmeda HARV (Hope Anesthesia Resuscitator/Ventilator) (Ohmeda Emergency Care, Orchard Park, NY) is a flow or pressure controller that is time triggered, flow or pressure limited, and time cycled (Fig. 15-22).

Input Variables

The HARV has an optional compressor but is normally operated from external sources of compressed gas at 40–90 psig.

A single control knob serves to control both ventilator rate and tidal volume (Fig. 15-23). Pressure can be limited through a nonadjustable mechanical pressure relief in the patient valve.

Control Variables

The HARV is normally set to control inspiratory flow. When inspiratory pressure exceeds the pressure relief (limiting) valve, inspiration is pressure controlled.

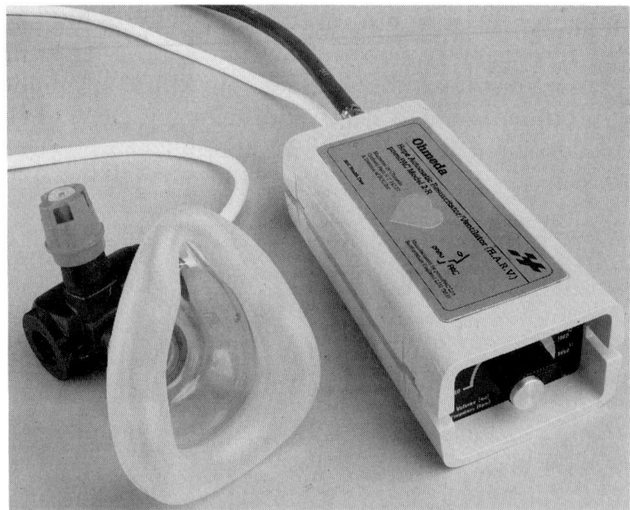

Figure 15-22. The Ohmeda HARV (PneuPac 2-R) transport ventilator and patient valve. (Courtesy of Ohmeda Emergency Care, Orchard Park, NY)

INSPIRATORY WAVEFORMS. During normal operation the HARV produces a rectangular flow waveform. When the pressure limit is breached, a rectangular pressure waveform may be produced.

PHASE VARIABLES. Inspiration is time triggered, as a function of respiratory frequency, adjustable to 11, 12, 13, 14, 16, 19 and 21 breaths per minute.

Inspiration is normally flow limited (40 L/min) but may be pressure limited (60 cm H_2O).

Inspiration is time cycled, and inspiratory time varies according to set ventilator rate from 0.5 to 2.2 seconds.

There is no control for baseline pressure, but a PEEP/CPAP valve available from the manufacturer can create end-expiratory pressure up to 10 cm H_2O.

Control Subsystems

CONTROL CIRCUIT. The HARV is pneumatically powered and pneumatically controlled (Fig. 15-24). The control circuit is similar to the AutoVent ventilators.

DRIVE MECHANISM. The HARV operates from an external pneumatic source that powers the pneumatic circuit.

OUTPUT CONTROL VALVES. The output control valves include the rate/volume control needle valve and the pressure relief valve. During inspiration, gas traverses a filter and is delivered to a pressure regulator where pressure is reduced to 30 psig. Gas then travels through the spool valve to a nonadjustable flow control (40 L/min) and to the patient valve. Gas also flows to the inspiratory and expiratory timers, each of which consists of a gas reservoir, one-way check valve, and piston. Like the AutoVent Ventilators, timing depends on how quickly the reservoir fills, which increases pressure and moves the piston. The expiratory timer is not adjustable, and when the reservoir is filled pressure causes the piston to slide upward. This allows gas to travel to the spool valve, sliding it into the expiratory position. The inspiratory

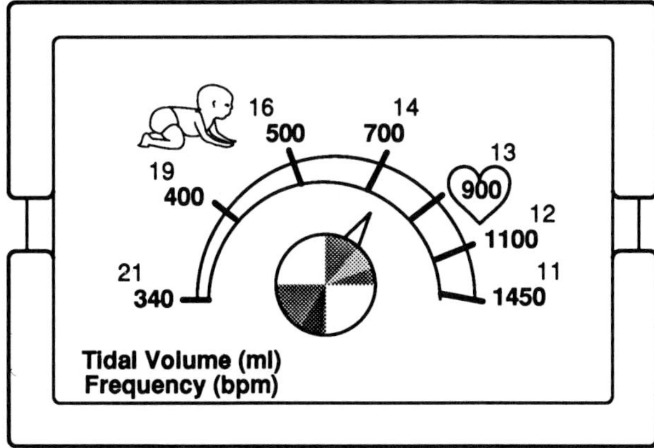

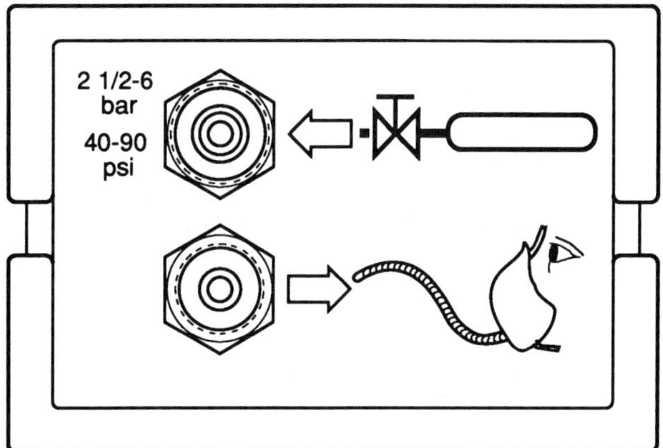

Figure 15-23. Front (left) and rear (right) panels of the HARV. The front panel has a single control that sets one of seven rate/tidal volume combinations. The rear panel has threaded outlets for connection of compressed gas (top) and connection of the hose to the patient valve (bottom).

timer can be adjusted by the rate/volume control needle, which changes the speed at which pressure rises in the reservoir, lifts the piston, and causes the spool valve to slide into the inspiratory position. Gas then travels to the patient valve (Fig. 15-25). The patient valve consists of a piston and spring within a durable housing. During inspiration, gas pressure moves the piston forward, closing the expiratory port and allowing gas flow to the patient. When inspiration is terminated, the piston returns to its resting position (due to spring tension) and the patient can exhale through the expiratory port. During the expiratory time, spontaneous breathing from ambient may occur through the exhaust port.

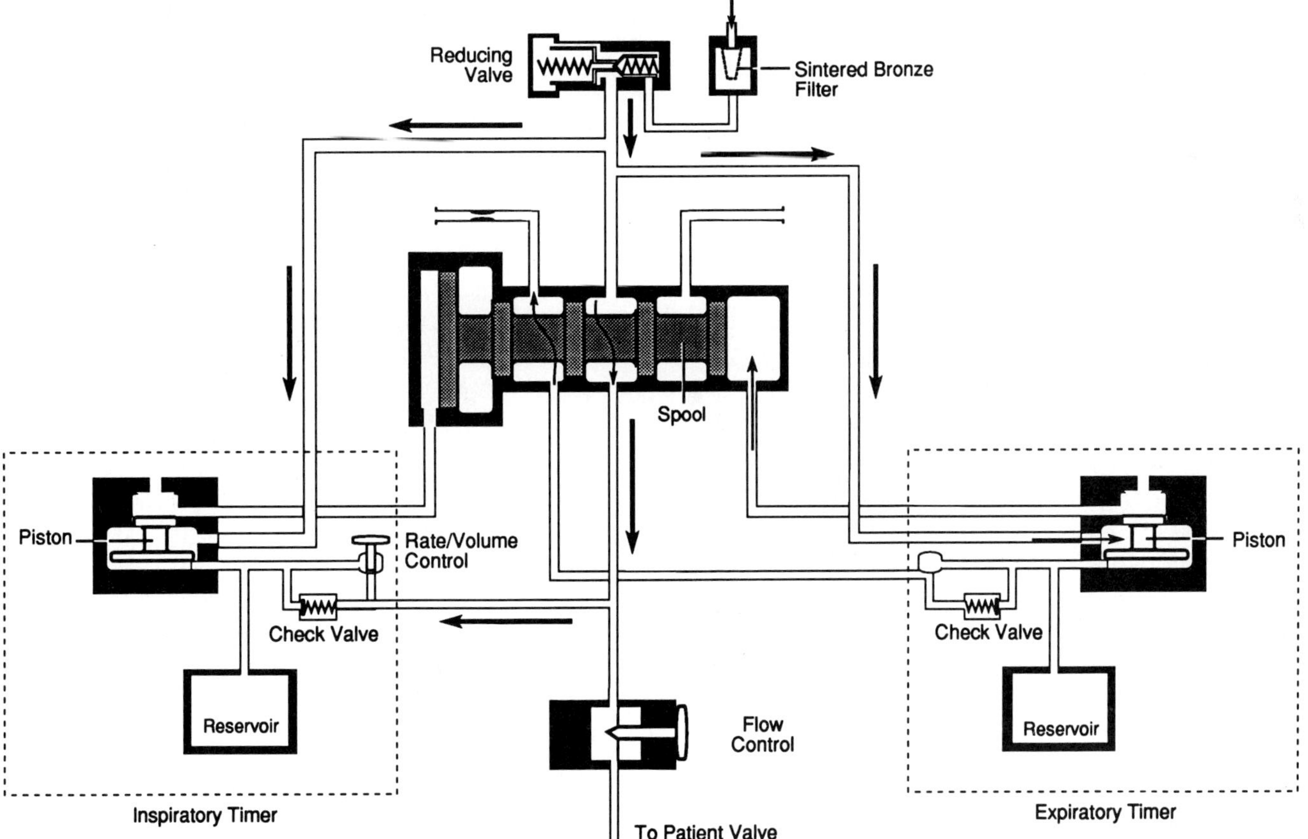

Figure 15-24. The internal components of the HARV.

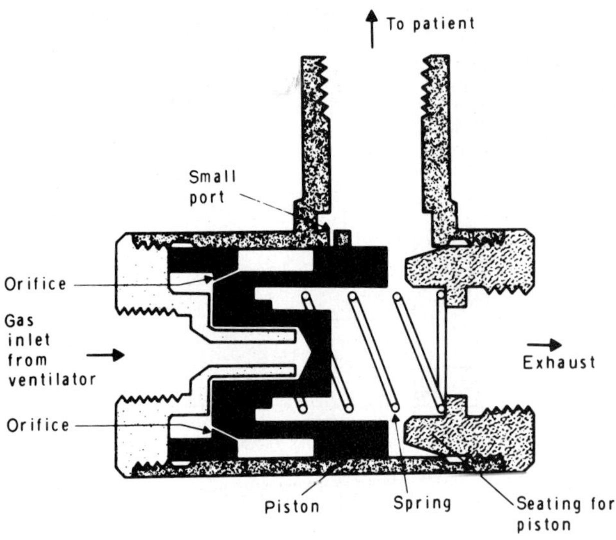

Figure 15-25. The patient valve assembly of the HARV.

Output Displays

There are normally no output displays on the HARV. An external aneroid pressure gauge can be mounted on the ventilator, but this is optional.

Modes of Operation

The HARV only allows controlled ventilation.

CMV. Inspiration is time triggered, flow or pressure limited, and time cycled. Spontaneous breathing between mandatory breaths can occur from ambient through the exhalation port of the patient valve (this is not possible if PEEP/CPAP is applied).

Alarms

CONTROL VARIABLE ALARMS. When the pressure relief (limiting) valve is activated a mechanical audible alarm sounds as gas passes through the spring-loaded valve.

Critical Comment

The HARV is intended for pre-hospital use, although its successful use in inter-hospital and intra-hospital transport has been reported in intubated subjects.[9–11] However, because tidal volume and ventilator rate are not independently adjustable, Johannigman and associates[2] found that the tidal volume delivered through the PneuPAC to an unintubated model was less than 500 mL. The simplicity of the PneuPac is both its greatest asset and hindrance.

PENLON 350

The Penlon 350 (Bear Medical Corporation, Riverside, CA) is a flow or pressure controller that is time triggered, flow or pressure limited, and time cycled. It does not have an integral air–oxygen blender or compressor. It can be operated in two configurations: child/adult or neonatal/pediatric (Fig. 15-26).

Input Variables

The Penlon 350 requires a pneumatic power source and operates from external compressed gas at 36 to 100 psig.

The front panel allows control of inspiratory time, expiratory time, and inspiratory flow rate (child/adult) or pressure (neonatal/pediatric). In the child/adult configuration a mechanical pressure-limiting valve within the patient valve allows control of peak pressure.

Control Variables

In the child/adult mode the Penlon 350 controls either flow or pressure, while in the neonatal/pediatric configuration only pressure is controlled. In the latter a continuous flow of gas from an external flowmeter is required.

INSPIRATORY WAVEFORMS. A rectangular flow waveform is produced during normal operation in the child/adult configuration. In the neonatal/pediatric configuration a rectangular pressure waveform is produced.

PHASE VARIABLES. Inspiration is time triggered as a function of inspiratory time (adjustable from 0.2 to 2.0 seconds) and expiratory time (adjustable from 0.5 to 4.0 seconds). This allows for cycling frequencies of 10 to 85 breaths per minute.

Inspiration is pressure limited in the neonatal/pediatric configuration (0 to 40 cm H_2O) and pressure (60 cm H_2O) or flow limited (15 to 60 L/min) in the child/adult configuration.

Inspiration is always time cycled according to set inspiratory time.

Baseline pressure may be added with an external PEEP/CPAP valve.

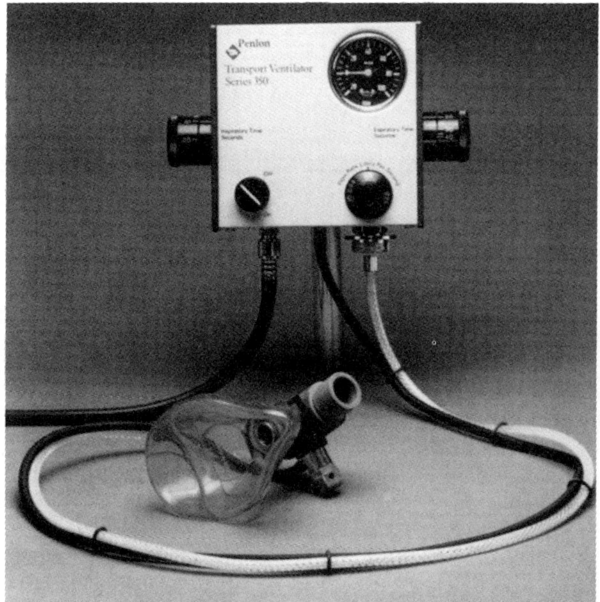

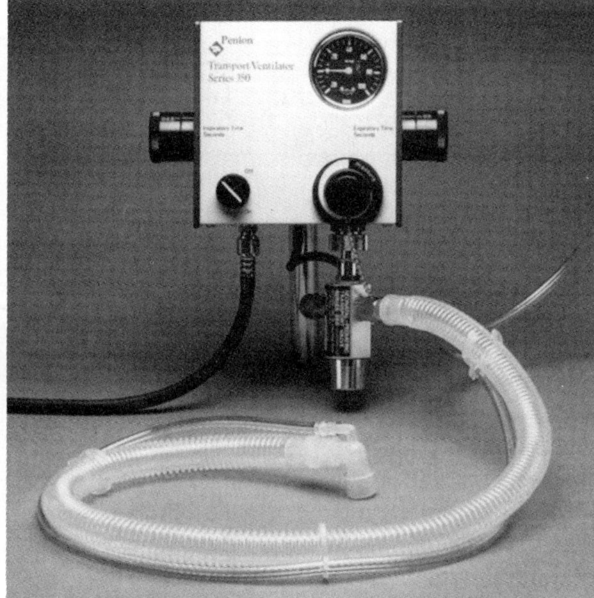

Figure 15-26. The Penlon 350 ventilator child/adult (left) and neonatal/pediatric (right) configurations. (Courtesy of Bear Medical Corporation, Riverside, CA)

Control Subsystems

CONTROL CIRCUIT The Penlon 350 is pneumatically powered and pneumatically controlled (Fig. 15-27).

DRIVE MECHANISM. The Penlon 350 requires an external pneumatic power source to power the components.

OUTPUT CONTROL VALVES. The output control valves include the inspiratory and expiratory time controls and the flow rate control. All three are needle valves.

The Penlon 350 operates identically to the HARV, except that the variable resistances that control the speed at which the timing reservoirs fill are adjustable needle valves (inspiratory and expiratory time). Gas entering the ventilator is reduced to 30 psig and delivered through the spool valve to the adjustable inspiratory flow control valve and to the patient. When pressure builds in the inspiratory timer (as controlled by the inspiratory time needle valve and reservoir), the piston on the inspiratory side is lifted, pressurizing the spool valve and initiating inspiration by connecting gas from the reducing valve to the flow control. This also diverts flow to the expiratory timer, which according to the needle valve setting will lift the expiratory piston and return the spool to its original resting position.

When the neonatal/pediatric configuration is used a continuous flow of gas from an external flowmeter is provided to the patient. The timing circuit operates as described previously. However, a mechanical valve is added to the outlet of the ventilator that serves as an exhalation valve and the flow control is changed to a pressure control. Increasing the pressure control causes a greater flow to the exhalation valve, which allows peak inspiratory pressure to be increased.

Output Displays

Airway pressure is displayed by an aneroid gauge over the range of −20 to 100 cm H_2O.

Modes of Operation

The Penlon 350 operates in the control mode.

CMV (CHILD/ADULT). Inspiration is time triggered, pressure or flow limited, and time cycled. Spontaneous breathing can occur through the expiratory part of the patient valve.

CMV (NEONATAL/PEDIATRIC). Inspiration is time triggered, pressure limited, and time cycled. Spontaneous breathing from the continuous flow of gas is possible, but the ventilator does not control flow to meet the patient's demand.

Alarms

CONTROL/VARIABLE ALARMS. In the CHILD/ADULT mode, the mechanical pressure relief valve emits an audible tone when violated.

Critical Comment

The Penlon 350 transport ventilator is intended to ventilate neonates and adults during inter- or intra-hospi-

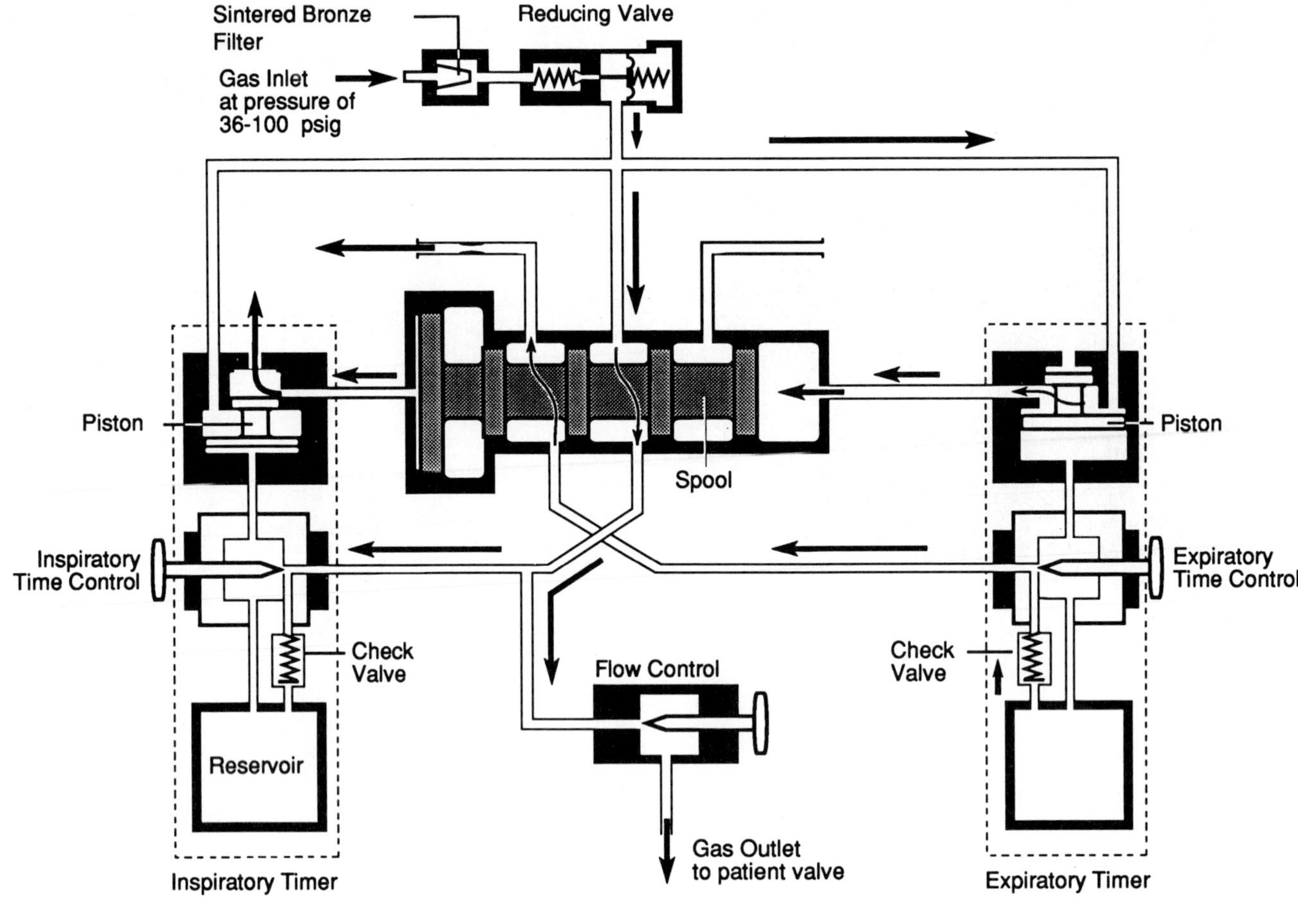

Figure 15-27. Internal schematic of the Penlon 350 transport ventilator.

tal transport. In the adult configuration there is no demand valve, and when PEEP is attached to the outlet of the patient valve, spontaneous breathing is prevented.

The neonatal configuration allows greater flexibility and control but does require an external blender and flowmeter. The lack of alarms must also be considered.

STEIN GATES OMNI-VENT D/MRI

The Stein Gates Omni-Vent (Stein Gates, Atchinson, KS) (Fig. 15-28) is a flow controller that is time triggered, flow limited, and time cycled. It does not have an integral blender or compressor.

Input Variables

The Omni-Vent requires pneumatic power from external sources of compressed gas at 40 to 140 psig.

The operator can set inspiratory time, expiratory time, and inspiratory flow rate with uncalibrated dials on the control panel.

Control Variables

The Omni-Vent controls flow during normal operation. An external pressure relief valve can be fitted to the gas outlet that allows pressure to be controlled.

INSPIRATORY WAVEFORMS. A rectangular flow waveform is produced during normal operation. When the external pressure relief is added, a rectangular pressure waveform may be produced.

PHASE VARIABLES. Inspiration is time triggered according to the inspiratory time (0.2 to 3.0 seconds) and expiratory time (0.2 to 6.0 seconds). Ventilator rate can be adjusted from 1 to 150 breaths per minute.

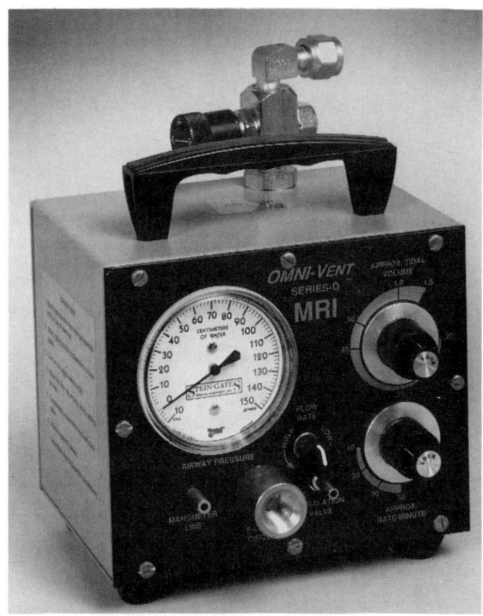

Figure 15-28. The Stein Gates Omni-Vent series D-MRI. This ventilator is made specifically for use in MRI. It has a minimum of metal components. (Courtesy of Stein Gates, Atchinson, KS)

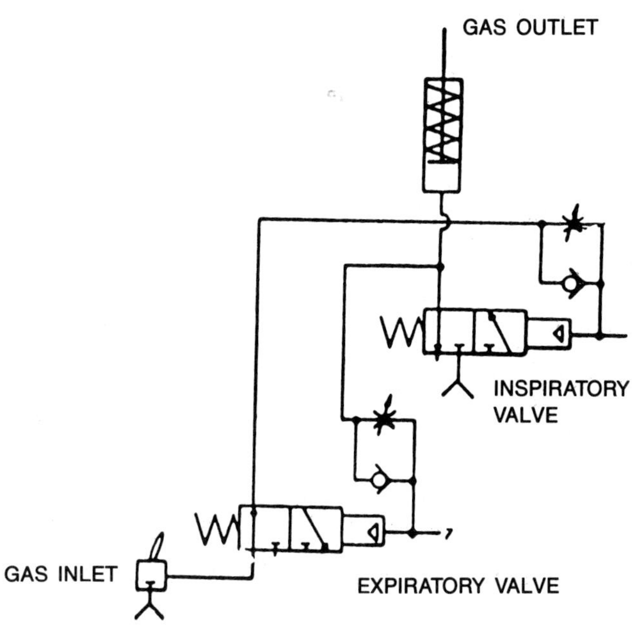

Figure 15-29. Control circuit of the Omni-Vent transport ventilator. (Courtesy of Stein Gates, Atchinson, KS)

Inspiration is flow limited (0 to 98 L/min) during normal operation but may be pressure limited (20 to 120 cm H_2O) by addition of the external pressure relief valve.

Inspiration is time cycled according to the set inspiratory time. Baseline pressure is not controlled but may be added by an external PEEP/CPAP valve.

Control Subsystems

CONTROL CIRCUIT. The control circuit of the Omni-Vent uses pneumatic components (Fig. 15-29).

DRIVE MECHANISM. The Omni-Vent is powered by external compressed gas.

OUTPUT CONTROL VALVES. The output control valves include the flow control needle valve, the inspiratory and expiratory time control needle valves, and the external spring-loaded pressure relief valve. Gas travels through the on/off switch to the inspiratory and expiratory time valves. These are pneumatic valves that control timing by the build-up and release of pressure inside the valve. During inspiration the inspiratory timer allows flow to travel to the patient through the flow control valve while simultaneously pressurizing the disposable, mushroom-type exhalation valve in the ventilator circuit. Expiration occurs when control is switched from the inspiratory timer and flow to the flow control valve is interrupted.

Output Displays

Airway pressure is displayed on an aneroid pressure gauge from −10 to 150 cm H_2O.

Modes of Operation

The Omni-Vent operates in the control mode.

CMV. Inspiration is time triggered, flow or pressure limited, and time cycled. During normal operation spontaneous breathing cannot occur. The addition of an external continuous flow of gas to a reservoir bag is recommended by the manufacturer if spontaneous breathing is allowed.

Alarms

The Omni-Vent has no alarms.

Critical Comment

The Omni-Vent is a flexible ventilator that, owing to uncalibrated controls, is sometimes difficult to set up. Its ability to be used in a magnetic resonance scanner is unique. The Omni-Vent should always be used with the external pressure-limiting valve. Spontaneous breathing cannot occur unless an optional continuous flow of gas is provided.

Comparisons of the physical and operational characteristics of the transport ventilators discussed in this chapter are shown in Tables 15-3 and 15-4.

(Text continues on page 424)

TABLE 15-3. Physical Characteristics of Transport Ventilators

Type of Ventilator	Ventilator Dimensions (cm)	Ventilator Weight (kg)	Supply Pressure (psig)	Operating Temperature	Gas Consumption (L/min)	Battery	Battery Dimensional (cm)	Battery Weight (kg)	Duration
Bio-Med IC-2A	8.6×15.6×26	4.1	45–55	NS	12	No	—	—	—
Bio-Med MVP-10	20×23×7.4	2.3	45–55	NS	4*	No	—	—	—
Bird Space Technologies Mini-TXP	7×6×8.5	1.2	20–100	−40°C–60°C	0	No	—	—	—
Hamilton MAX	30×8×16.5	5.0	50–90	−18°C–50°C	0	Yes Internal	4 1.5AA	0.1	Rechargeable 8-h alkaline 30 h
Impact 706	20×13×5.5	1.45	50–100	−60°C–60°C	0	Yes Internal	6×12×5	0.75	10 h
Impact 750	23.9×11.5×4.5	4.4	45–55	−60°C–60°C	0	Yes Internal	22.9×4.5×4.5	2.6	12 h
Life Support Products Autovent 2000	15×9×4.5	0.68	40–90	−34°C–46°C	0.5	No	—	—	—
Life Support Products Autovent 3000	15×9×4.5	0.68	40–90	−34°C–46°C	0.5	No	—	—	—
Ohmeda Logic 07	18×13×21	5	44–88	NS	0.4–2.0	No	—	—	—
Ohmeda HARV	18×9×6	1.3	40–60	−18°C–65°C	2.0	No	—	—	—
Penlon 350	17×24×10	3.5	36–100	NS	0.1/cycle	No	—	—	—
Stein Gates Omnivent	10×13×15	2.5	40–140	NS	NS	No	—	—	—

NS, Not specified.

*Changes with breaths per minute.

TABLE 15-4. Operational Characteristics of Transport Ventilators

Type of Ventilator	Cycling Variables	Modes	Rate (breaths per minute)	Tidal Volume (mL)	Maximum Minute Volume (L/min)*	Inspiratory Time(s)	Peak Inspiratory Flow (L/min)	FIO_2 %	PEEP† (cm H_2O)	PEEP Compensation	Alarms	Monitoring	Demand Flow Valve	Manual Breath
Bio-Med IC-2A	Time—C Pressure—S	SIMV, CMV/CPAP	1–66	130–2500	37.5	0.4–2.0	75	1.0	Yes	Yes	None	Airway pressure	Yes	Yes
Bio-Med MVP-10	Time—C	IMV, CMV	0–120	–	–	0.2–2.0	12	1.0	18	No demand valve	None	Airway pressure	No continuous flow	No
Bird Space Technologies Mini-TXP	Time—C	CMV	2–60	50–2500	30.0	0.3–4.0	120	0.45–0.8	No	No	None	Optional Airway pressure	No	Yes
Hamilton MAX	Time—C Pressure—S	IMV, CMV	2–30	50–1500	45.0	1.0	90	1.0	No	No	Low gas Inlet pressure Low battery	Airway pressure	Yes	Yes
Impact 706	Time—C	CMV	14, 20, 30 (child) 12, 18 (adult)	10–1250	22.5	0.75–2.7 (child) 1.5–3.5 (adult)	90	1.0	No	No	Low battery	None	No	Yes
Impact 750	Time—C Pressure—S	CMV, SIMV, AMV	1–150	10–3000	45.0	0.1–3.0	100	1.0	No	Yes	‡	Airway pressure	Yes	Yes
Life Support Products Autovent 2000	Time—C Pressure—S	CMV IMV	8–20	400–1200	24.0	1.5	48	1.0	No	No	High pressure	None	Yes	No
Life Support Products Autovent 3000	Time—C Pressure—S	CMV IMV	9–27 (child) 8–20 (adult)	200–600 (child) 400–1200 (adult)	16.0 (child) 24.0 (adult)	0.75 (child) 1.5 (adult)	48	1.0	No	No	High pressure	None	Yes	No
Ohmeda Logic 07	Time—C	CMV	10–40	100–2000	20.0	0.5–2.0	65	0.5 or 1.0	No	No	High pressure	Airway pressure	No	No
Ohmeda HARV	Time—C	CMV	11–21	340–1450	16.0	0.5–2.5	40	0.45 or 1.0	No	No	High pressure	None	No	No
Penlon 350	Time—C	CMV	10–85	10–300 (child) 50–2000 (adult)	9.0 (child) 30.0 (adult)	0.2–2.0	60	1.0	No	No	High pressure	Airway pressure	No	No
Stein Gates OmniVent	Time—C	CMV	1–150	30–3000	30.0	0.2–3.0	45	1.0	No	No	None	Airway pressure	No	No

C = Control Breaths, S = Spontaneous

* I:E = 1:1

† PEEP is available with all ventilators with an external PEEP valve.

‡ Low battery, external power failure, low-pressure disconnect, high pressure, apnea PEEP not set, inverse I:E

AARC Clinical Practice Guideline

Transport of the Mechanically Ventilated Patient: Indications, Contraindications, Hazards and Complications

Transportation of mechanically ventilated patients for diagnosis or therapeutic procedures is always associated with a degree or risk. Every attempt should be made to assure that monitoring, ventilation, oxygenation, and patient care remain constant during movement. Patient transport includes preparation, movement to and from, and time spent at destination.

- Indications:
  - Transportation of mechanically ventilated patients should only be undertaken following a careful evaluation of the risk-benefit ratio.
  - Transportation should be undertaken on the attending physician's order.
- Contraindications:
  - Inability to provide adequate oxygenation and ventilation during transport either by manual ventilation or portable ventilator
  - Inability to maintain acceptable hemodynamic performance during transport
  - Inability to monitor patient's cardiopulmonary status during transport
  - Inability to maintain airway control during transport
  - Transport should not be undertaken unless all the necessary members of the transport team are present.
- Hazards/Complications:
  - Hyperventilation during manual ventilation may cause respiratory alkalosis, cardiac dysrhythmias, and hypotension.
  - Loss of PEEP/CPAP may result in hypoxemia.
  - Position changes may result in hypotension, hypercarbia, and hypoxemia.
  - Tachycardia and other dysrhythmias have been associated with transport.
  - Equipment failure can result in inaccurate data or loss of monitoring capabilities.
  - Inadvertent disconnection of intravenous pharmacologic agents may result in hemodynamic instability.
  - Movement may cause disconnection from ventilatory support and respiratory compromise.
  - Movement may result in accidental extubation.
  - Movement may result in accidental removal of vascular access.
  - Loss of oxygen supply may lead to hypoxemia.

(Adapted from AARC Clinical Practice Guideline, published in December, 1993, issue of Respiratory Care; see original publication for complete text)

References

1. Hurst JM, Davis K, Branson RD, et al. Ventilatory support in the field: A prospective study. Crit Care Med 1989;17:527.
2. Johannigman JA, Branson RD, Davis K, et al. Techniques of emergency ventilation: A model to evaluate tidal volume, airway pressure, and gastric insufflation. J Trauma 1991;31:93–98.
3. Hurst JM, Davis K, Branson RD, et al. Comparison of blood gases during transport using two methods of ventilatory support. J Trauma 1989;29:1637–1640.
4. Gervais HW, Eberle B, Konietzke D, et al. Comparison of blood gases of ventilated patients during transport. Crit Care Med 1987;15:761–764.
5. Braman SS, Dunn SM, Amico C, et al. Complications of interhospital transport in critically ill patients. Ann Intern Med 1987;107:469–473.
6. Johannigman JA, Branson RD, Campbell RS, et al. Laboratory and clinical evaluation of the MAX transport ventilator. Respir Care 1990;35:952–959.
7. Campbell RS, Davis K, Johnson DJ, et al. Laboratory and clinical evaluation of the Uni-Vent 750 portable ventilator. Respir Care 1992;37:29–36.
8. Morash C, Potash RJ, Kacmarek RM. Performance evaluation of the Ohmeda Logic 07 transport ventilator. Respir Care 1986; 31:937.
9. Adams AP, Henville JD. A new generation of anaesthetic ventilators: The PneuPAC and Penlon A.P. Anaesthesia 1977;32:34–40.
10. Park GR, Manara AR, Bodenham AR, Moss CJ. The PneuPAC ventilator with new patient valve and air compressors. Anaesthesia 1989;44:419–424.
11. Melker RJ. A clinical evaluation of the PneuPAC ventilator. Presented before the 4th World Congress on Intensive Care Medicine, 1985.

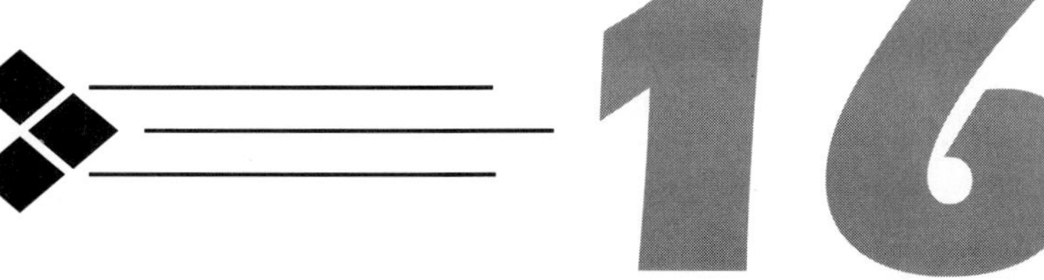

Home Mechanical Ventilation Equipment

Robert M. Kacmarek

OBJECTIVES

1. Describe the operation of a pneumobelt and a rocking bed.
2. Compare the following negative-pressure chambers: full-body chambers, chest cuirass, raincoat wrap, and pneumosuit.
3. Compare the following negative-pressure generators: Emerson Iron Lung, Emerson Negative-Pressure Generators, Lifecare 170C, Lifecare NEV-100, and Puritan-Bennett Thompson Maxivent.
4. Describe the ideal home positive-pressure ventilator.
5. Compare the following positive pressure ventilators: Puritan-Bennett Companion 2800, Puritan-Bennett Companion 2801, Puritan-Bennett 2500, Aequitron Medical LP-6, Aequitron Medical LP-10, Aequitron Medical LP-6 Plus, Lifecare PLV-100, Lifecare PLV-102, and Intermed Bear 33.
6. Compare the following nasal ventilation devices: Respironics BiPAP ST, Respironics BiPAP ST-D, and Puritan-Bennett Companion 320 I/E.

(continued)

OBJECTIVES, (continued)

7. Discuss the following common features of all portable positive-pressure ventilators: delivery of increased FIO_2, SIMV/IMV and work of breathing, humidification, application of PEEP, and pediatric ventilation.

8. Compare the following facial appliances for noninvasive ventilation: full-face masks, nasal masks, nasal pillows, and mouthpieces.

KEY TERMS

cuirass
full-face mask
iron lung
mouthpiece
nasal mask
nasal pillows
nasal ventilation device
negative-pressure chamber
negative-pressure generator
pneumobelt
pneumosuit
oxygen accumulator
raincoat wrap
rocking bed

Introduction

There has been increased interest in ventilation of patients in the home in recent years. All of the available approaches to ventilatory support have been used successfully for long-term maintenance of patients with respiratory failure from both neuromuscular disease and primary pulmonary disease.[1–7] These include negative-pressure techniques and, more commonly, invasive and noninvasive positive pressure. Long-term mechanical ventilation has been used in two ways: (1) it is mandatory for use during true life support, and (2) it is elective for managing chronic ventilatory failure.[8,9] Although some patients requiring mandatory ventilation can be maintained with noninvasive methods,[10–12] invasive approaches are most commonly used. Patients with slowly progressive chronic ventilatory failure and the ability to sustain spontaneous breathing for some period during the day can be managed noninvasively.[5] In this chapter the discussion focuses on the technical aspects of equipment used to provide ventilatory support in the home.

Pneumobelt and Rocking Bed

Pneumobelt

The pneumobelt (Fig. 16-1) is an adjustable corset containing an inflatable bladder. It functions by exerting a positive pressure on the abdomen, forcing the diaphragm cephalad, and assisting exhalation[13,14] (Fig. 16-2). Inspiration proceeds under the patient's own efforts. With proper application of the pneumobelt, functional residual capacity (FRC) is reduced and the elastic recoil of reexpansion to FRC increases tidal volume. For proper function, the appropriate-size pneumobelt should be selected and fitted tightly over the abdomen from the xiphoid process to just about the pelvic arch. Fit is important to prevent paradoxical movement of the rib cage during exhalation. Depending on the patient, 30 to 50 cm H_2O must be applied to the bladder, and the patient should ideally be seated at a 75-degree angle.[12] As the angle from supine decreases, the effectiveness of the belt also decreases. The pneumobelt may be powered by any positive-pressure generator.

Rocking Bed

The rocking bed (Fig. 16-3) bases its operation on the effect gravity has on the abdominal contents.[14] As the bed rocks, the abdominal contents assist the movement of the diaphragm. When the bed tilts head down, exhalation is assisted and when the head tilts up, inspiration is assisted. The rocking bed can move through a total arc of up to 60 degrees (30 degrees head down and 30 degrees head up). A 15-degree head-down and 30-degree head-up tilt is sufficient for most patients.[14] Rate can be

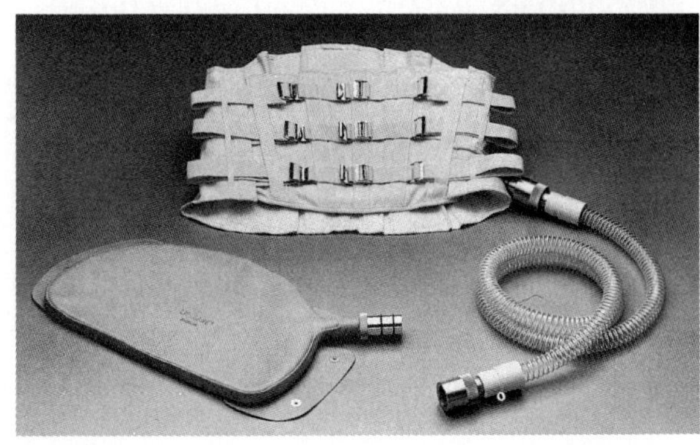

Figure 16-1. Pneumobelt with its internal inflatable bladder. (Courtesy of Lifecare, Boulder, CO)

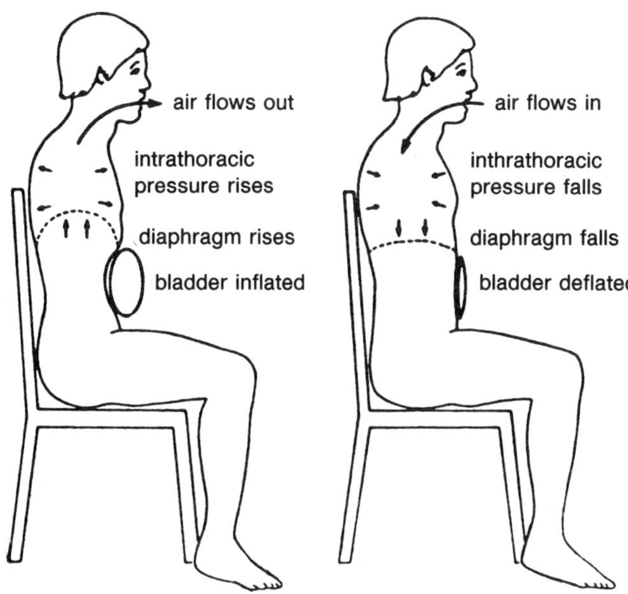

Figure 16-2. The pneumobelt functions by exerting pressure on the abdominal contents by inflation of a rubber bladder, forcing the diaphragm upward and assisting exhalation (left). When the bladder deflates, gravity pulls the diaphragm back down, assisting inhalation (right). (From Hill NS. Clinical application of body ventilators. Chest 1986;90: 897–905)

adjusted from 8 to 34/min. A break at the knee can be used to prevent sliding. Some patients develop motion sickness with the rocking bed and require appropriate medication. However, most patients can tolerate the motion and comfortably sleep in the rocking bed.

Analysis of Pneumobelt and Rocking Bed

Both of these noninvasive approaches to ventilatory support have limited application, but they may be beneficial in some patients. Neither functions well in patients with chronic lung disease. However, patients with primary neuromuscular or neurologic disorders may benefit. The pneumobelt and rocking bed are used primarily for daytime ventilatory assistance in patients requiring other forms of ventilatory support at the night. Because the pneumobelt requires a sitting position, it is rarely used at night. Because both of these units function as controllers, patients who are anxious and frequently change their ventilatory rate rarely tolerate either.

Negative-Pressure Chambers

Full-Body Chambers

The Porta-Lung (Fig. 16-4) is a full-body chamber without a negative-pressure generator. It is manufactured by the Massachusetts Rehabilitation Services, is lightweight and easy to use, and can be driven by any negative-pressure generator. It is available in child and adolescent sizes. Its major limitation is the requirement of an assistant to operate it.

Chest Cuirass

The chest cuirass (Fig. 16-5) is designed to be placed over the patient's thorax and abdomen and is secured with wide straps. A negative-pressure generator is attached at the opening on the top of the shell. Each shell is designed with a cushion of 2 to 3 inches of air between the patient's maximum chest rise and shell to ensure that the chest wall of the patient does not come directly into contact with the top of the shell, which would prevent further thoracic expansion. Most patients find the shell reasonably comfortable. The major problem with commercial shells is fit. In many cases

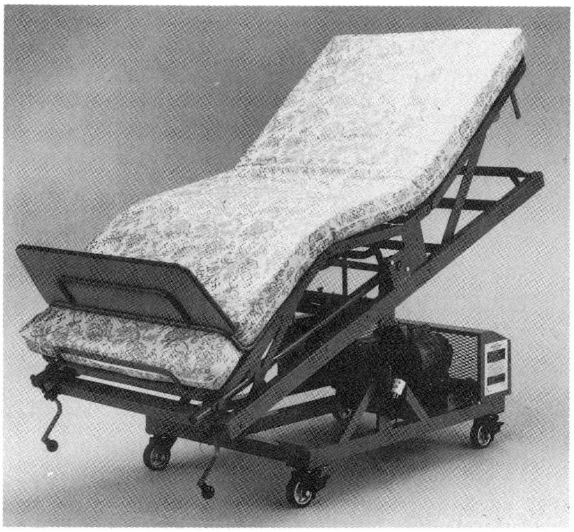

Figure 16-3. The Emerson Rocking Bed. (Courtesy of J. H. Emerson, Cambridge, MA)

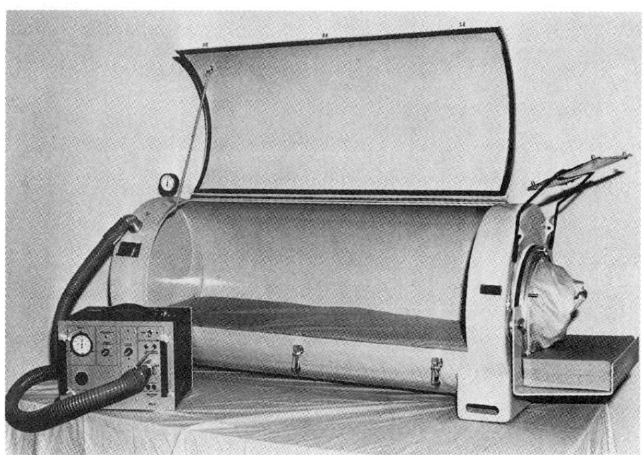

Figure 16-4. The Porta-Lung with an Emerson 33-CRE Negative Pressure Ventilator. (From Kacmarek RM, Spearman CB. Equipment used for ventilatory support in the home. Respir Care 1986;31:311–328).

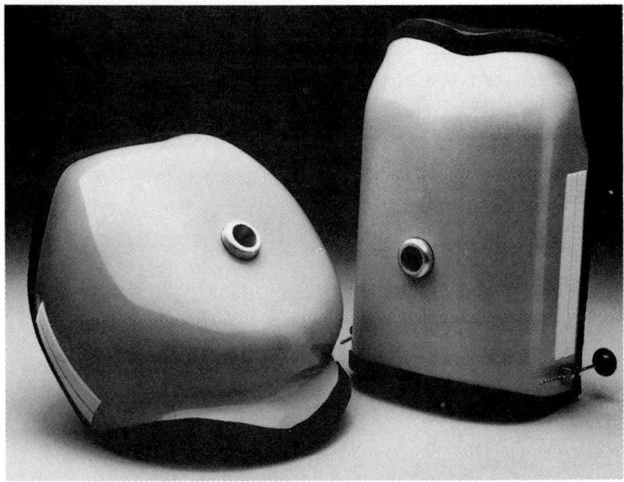

Figure 16-5. Commercially available chest cuirass. (Courtesy of Lifecare, Boulder, CO)

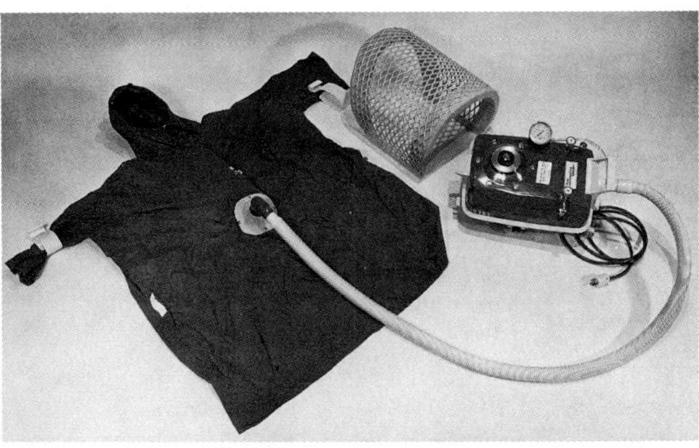

Figure 16-7. The "raincoat" or wrap, with shell-like grid and Emerson 33-CRE Negative Pressure Ventilator. (From Kacmarek RM, Spearman CB. Equipment used for ventilatory support in the home. Respir Care 1986;31:311–328)

towels must be stuffed between the shell and the patient to ensure a seal, or foam rubber is added. Leaks most often occur at the neck and pelvis. It is best to have a shell customized to the patient. Figure 16-6 is a cast of a patient's chest and abdomen from which a customized shell is designed. Customized shells are particularly important in patients with thoracic deformities.

To fit well, the shell should extend from the clavicle to the pelvic arch and along the sides of the chest wall. Ideally, the shell should not rest on the bed but should extend about halfway down the chest wall. Of all the negative-pressure chambers available, the chest cuirass is the easiest for the patient to use independently.

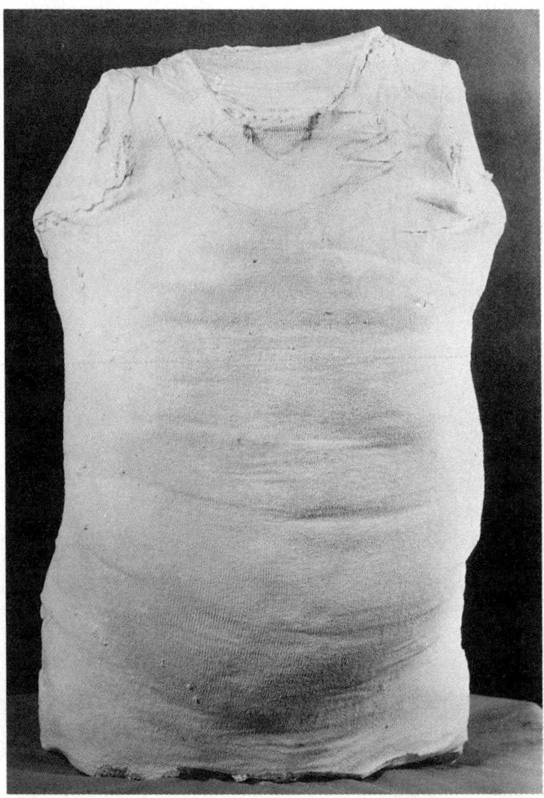

Figure 16-6. Cast of the thorax used to make a customized chest cuirass. (From Kacmarek RM, Spearman CB. Equipment used for ventilatory support in the home. Respir Care 1986;31:311–328)

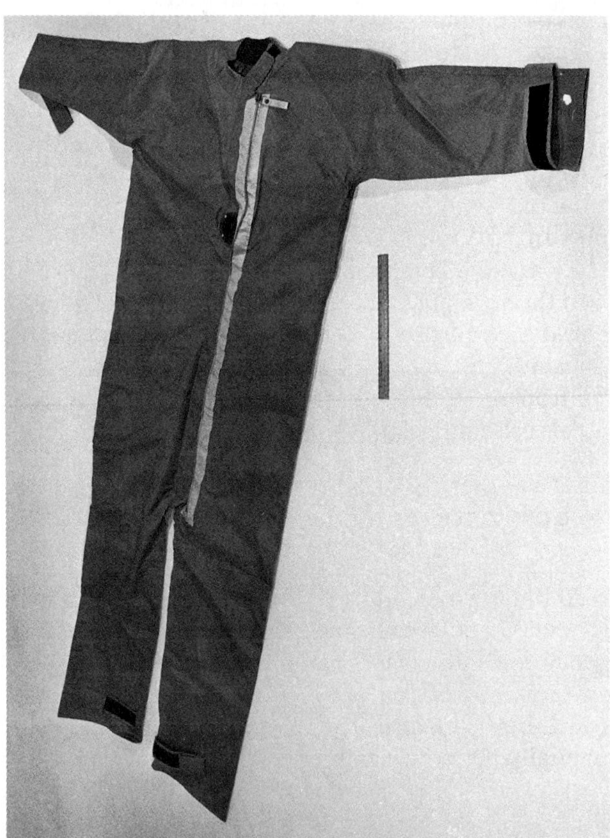

Figure 16-8. The pneumosuit used for negative pressure ventilation. (From Kacmarek RM, Spearman CB. Equipment used for ventilatory support in the home. Respir Care 1986;31:311–328)

Raincoat

The raincoat, with its shell-like grid, and an Emerson negative-pressure generator are shown in Figure 16-7. The raincoat is actually a modified poncho that is worn over the grid. The grid is necessary to prevent the negative-pressure attachment from directly being applied to the thorax. It maintains a 2- to 3-inch cushion of air that can be decompressed during inspiration. When applied, the raincoat is secured at the neck with a tie string and at the arms and hips with Velcro straps. The primary problem with this chamber is leakage. Many patients complain of being cold when using the raincoat, because room air is drawn into it when negative pressure is generated. Leaks are most common at the hips and neck.

Pneumosuit

The pneumosuit is shown in Figure 16-8. This chamber is similar to the raincoat. It also requires the use of the shell-like grid but has fewer problems with leaks because of its design. Major leaks occur only at the neck. Seals at the arms and legs are accomplished with Velcro wraps. Many patients experience difficulty getting into and out of the suit, particularly during the night.

Analysis of Negative-Pressure Chambers

Acceptance and acclimation to a negative-pressure chamber is primarily dependent on patient preference. The chest cuirass is usually best tolerated, particularly if the patient is claustrophobic. A customized cuirass is preferable in most situations. The full-body chamber seems to work best with children and adolescents. However, many adult polio victims and kyphoscoliosis patients still use iron lungs or Porta-Lungs. The raincoat and the pneumosuit are cumbersome for patients to use, and many patients become claustrophobic in them. However, all approaches should be considered and tried clinically before deciding on one method for a given patient.

Negative-Pressure Generators

EMERSON IRON LUNG

The Emerson Iron Lung (J.H. Emerson, Cambridge, MA) (Figs. 16-9 and 16-10), first manufactured in 1931, is the oldest commercially available mechanical ventilator in the United States. It consists of a large, relatively airtight chamber in which the patient is placed, with the patient's head exposed to the atmosphere.[15–17] A seal around the patient's neck is achieved with an adjustable plastic ring. Locking ports on each side of the Iron Lung allow access to the patient, and glass panels are configured across the top of the unit.

Input Variables

With the adult Iron Lung the operator can set rate at 10 to 30 breaths per minute, and greater rates are available with adolescent and pediatric units. The inspiratory:expiratory (I:E) ratio is fixed at 1:1. Negative pressures as great as −60 cm H_2O can be obtained. The Iron Lung is electrically powered and can be cycled manually if a power failure occurs.

Control and Phase Variables

The Iron Lung is a negative-pressure controller. Inspiration is time triggered, time cycled, and pressure limited. All breaths are mandatory.

Control Systems

At the foot end of the Iron Lung, a flexible diaphragm is attached to an electrical motor. The motor drives a variable-size wheel (actual diameter varies from one end to the other) by means of a fan belt. A transfer case

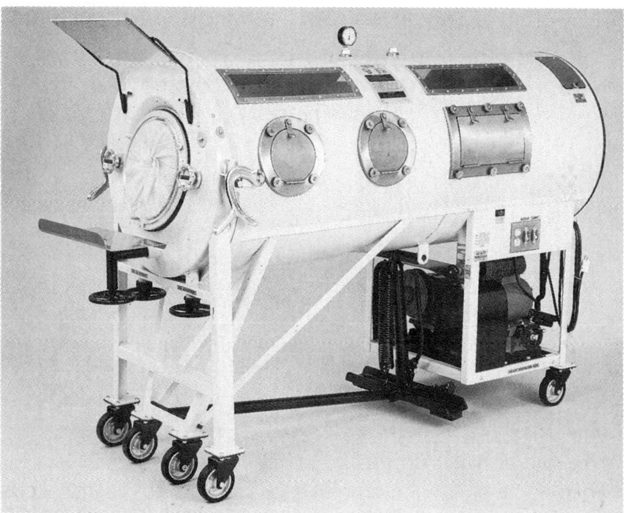

Figure 16-9. Emerson iron lung. (Courtesy of J. H. Emerson, Cambridge, MA)

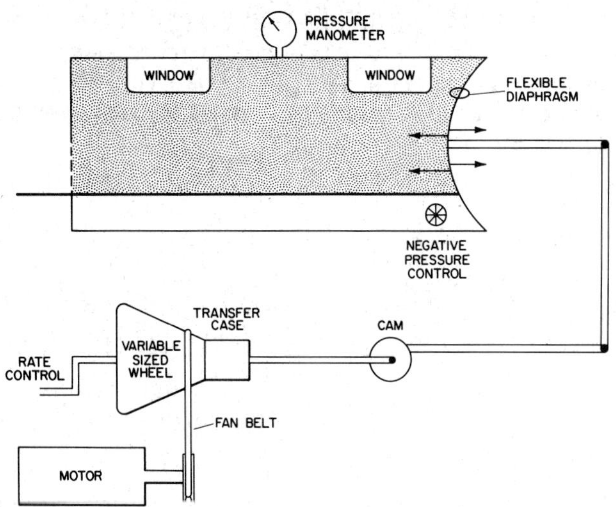

Figure 16-10. Operation of iron lung.

translates the motion of the wheel to the cam. The cam is connected by a series of linkages and arms to the movable leather/rubber diaphragm at the rear of the lung. The movement of the diaphragm is constant, and the level of negative pressure is controlled by the size of an adjustable leak. Rate is adjusted by varying the position of the variable-size wheel.

Output Displays

A pressure manometer on the top of the Iron Lung allows the amount of negative pressure to be monitored.

Alarms

The Iron Lung incorporates no alarms.

EMERSON NEGATIVE-PRESSURE GENERATORS

The 33 CRE (J. H. Emerson, Cambridge, MA) (Fig. 16-11) is the standard Emerson negative-pressure generator.[18] The 33 CRE (Fig. 16-12) is the newest of the Emerson negative-pressure generators and is capable of providing controlled ventilation, assisted ventilation, or assist/control ventilation.[17,19]

Input Variables

The 33 CRE is capable of achieving rates of 30 to 40 breaths per minute at pressures as great as −50 cm H_2O, and is capable of a range of I:E ratios (1:3 to inverse ratios). With the 33 CRE, a maximum of −90 cm H_2O can be applied at a rate of 0 to 49 breaths per minute with an inspiratory time up to 5 seconds. These units are electrically powered and have no battery capabilities.

Control and Phase Variables

These are negative-pressure controllers. The 33 CRE is time triggered, time cycled, and pressure limited. The 33 CR is also a negative-pressure, pressure-limited device. It is time cycled or pressure cycled. Because inspiration can be time or pressure triggered, it is capable of control, assist/control, or assisted ventilation.

During CONTROL mode in the 33 CRE, the operator sets the rate, negative pressure, minimum inspiratory time, and fixed or variable inspiratory time. If the fixed time is selected, inspiratory time is equal to that

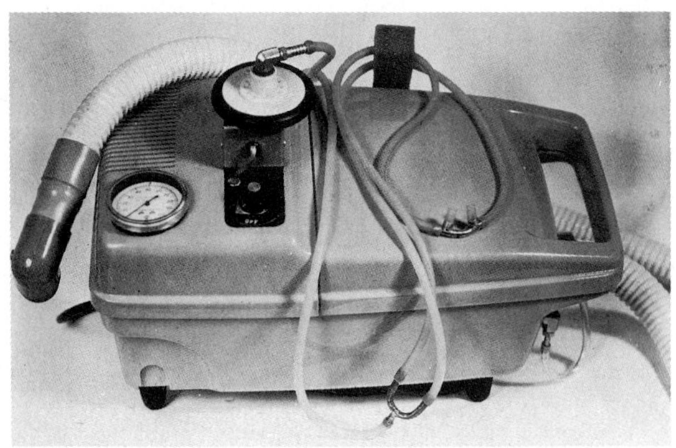

Figure 16-11. Emerson 33 CRE Negative Pressure Ventilator. (Courtesy of J. H. Emerson, Cambridge, MA)

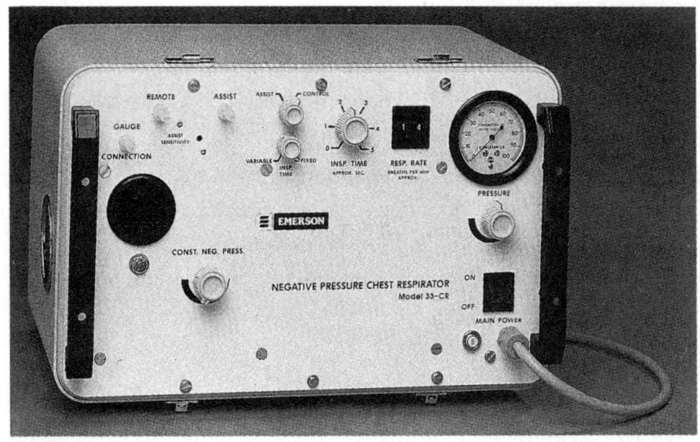

Figure 16-12. Emerson 33 CR Negative Pressure Ventilator. (Courtesy of J. H. Emerson, Cambridge, MA)

selected on every breath. If the variable time position is set, the remote pressure sensing cannula is used. This requires a standard nasal cannula attached to the front of the machine and the patient's face, which allows inspiratory time to exceed that set if the ventilator continues to sense negative pressure. Inspiration ends when no negative pressure is sensed. Although this may allow better coordination of inspiration with patient demand, it also results in highly variable I:E ratio with the potential of an inverse I:E ratio. For patient-triggered inspiration, the nasal cannula must be in place and the sensitivity set on the ventilator. During assist/control ventilation, inspiratory time may be set at the fixed or variable time setting. Total assisted ventilation, at a fixed or variable inspiratory time, can also be set. Constant negative pressure can also be applied to the airway by setting the rate control to zero and sensitivity to its most insensitive setting.

Control Systems

With these units, a turbine is used to create negative pressure. The amount of negative pressure developed is controlled by the speed of the turbine, and rate is controlled by alternately opening and closing a master control valve.

Output Displays

System pressure is monitored at the patient and displayed on a pressure manometer.

Alarms

No alarms are included.

LIFECARE 170C

This is a compact, lightweight, portable negative- and positive-pressure generator (Lifecare, Boulder, CO) (Fig. 16-13).[20]

Input Variables

Rate can vary between 10 and 40 breaths per minute, I:E ratio is fixed at 1:1.5, and as much as −60 cm H_2O positive or negative pressure can be applied. The unit only has three basic controls: rate, positive pressure, and negative pressure. It can be powered with standard household current or a 12-volt battery.

Control and Phase Variables

This unit is a negative- and positive-pressure controller and is time triggered, time cycled, and pressure limited. It only functions as a controller, either providing negative pressure to the thorax during inhalation, negative pressure during inhalation with positive pressure during exhalation, or positive pressure to the airway during inspiration. It may also be used to power a pneumobelt.

Control Systems

The unit operates as a continuous-flow turbine creating positive or negative pressure, depending on the position of its main valve. Adjustment of the variable speed control results in either atmospheric pressure or positive pressure being produced. The negative-pressure level depends on the turbine speed, and the respiratory rate is controlled by the variable main valve speed control.

Output Display

System pressure is displayed on a manometer.

Alarms

This unit has alarms for power loss.

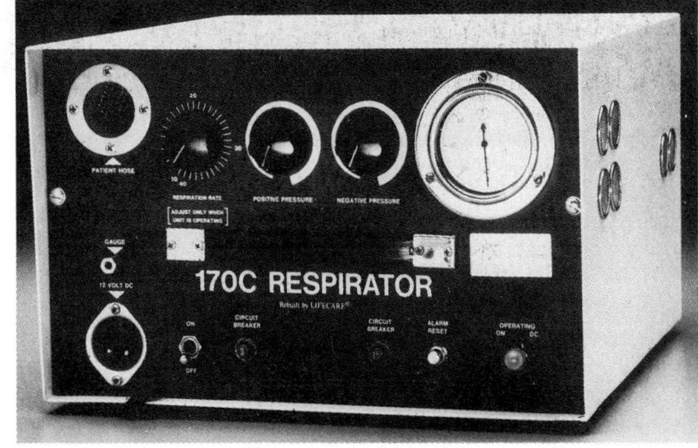

Figure 16-13. Lifecare 170C Negative Pressure Ventilator. (Courtesy of Lifecare, Boulder, CO)

LIFECARE NEV-100

This is the most sophisticated of the negative-pressure ventilators currently available (Lifecare, Boulder, CO).[21]

Input Variables

The front panel has three buttons (manual sigh, 30-second alarm silence, and panel lock/unlock), a computer screen menu display, and a single rotary parameter controller. All setting adjustments are made with the rotary controller, which must be unlocked before use (it automatically locks 30 seconds after use). Three different menus are available on the computer screen. One menu displays and sets mode, negative inspiratory pressure (−5 to −100 cm H_2O), base pressure (−30 to +30 cm H_2O), rate (4 to 60 breaths per minute), inspiratory time (0.5 to 5.0 seconds), I:E ratio (1:0.5 to 1:29.1), sigh pressure (−5 to −100 cm H_2O), sigh multiple breaths (1, 2, or 3), sigh frequency (1 to 20 sighs per hour), and low-pressure alarm setting. The second menu indicates frequency of output to printer, units of pressure displayed (cm H_2O, kPa, mbar) alarm history, screen brightness, date and time, alarm volume, assist sensitivity (levels 1 to 10 without units), alarm pitch, and remote alarm status. The final menu is for the setting of continuous negative extrathoracic pressure (CNEP) and low-pressure alarm. In the four ventilation modes the clinician must set the rate, negative inspiratory pressure, base pressure, inspiratory time, and I:E ratio. Sigh pressure, multiples and frequency, and sensitivity are set if indicated by the mode. Although I:E ratio can be set, it is dependent on rate and inspiratory time and will default to that ratio indicated by the combination of these variables. It operates from household current and is incapable of being operated with a battery.

Control and Phase Variables

This unit is a negative-pressure controller, is time or pressure triggered, and is pressure limited. Five modes are available: CONTROL, CONTROL WITH SIGH, ASSIST/CONTROL, ASSIST/CONTROL WITH SIGH, and CNEP. In all but the CNEP mode, a negative or positive base pressure (expiratory pressure) can also be set.

Control Systems

This unit is microprocessor controlled and turbine driven.

Output Displays

A variety of parameters can be displayed on the computer screen, as described earlier. The unit is capable of being attached to a recorder for the display of alarms and ventilation variables, as well as diagnostic information.

Alarms

This unit has 13 alarms. Only one, the low-pressure alarm, is set by the clinician from −1 cm H_2O below to +1 cm above the base pressure setting. If system pressure is below the set level for a 20-second period, audio and visual alarms are activated. Both audio and visual alarms are activated if excessive negative pressure or base pressure develops or if the inspiratory CNEP or base pressure is out of range. Internal system failure, constant pressure failure, missing parameter, and high or low internal temperature alarms are also present. A continuous audio alarm sounds if a power failure occurs, and an information message is displayed if an inverse ratio is set. This unit has a remote alarm.

PURITAN-BENNETT THOMPSON MAXIVENT

This unit (Puritan-Bennett Corporation, Lenexa, KS) is shown in Figure 16-14.[22]

Input Variables

The only three controls on the unit are positive pressure, negative pressure, and rate. The unit is electrically powered by household current and cannot be battery powered.

Control and Phase Variables

This unit is a positive- or negative-pressure controller and is time triggered, time cycled, and pressure limited. It operates only in the CONTROL mode with a fixed I:E ratio of 1:2. Rate can be adjusted from 8 to 24 breaths per minute. Negative pressure as great as −70 cm H_2O and positive pressure 0 to 80 cm H_2O can be produced. Positive pressure may also be applied to the

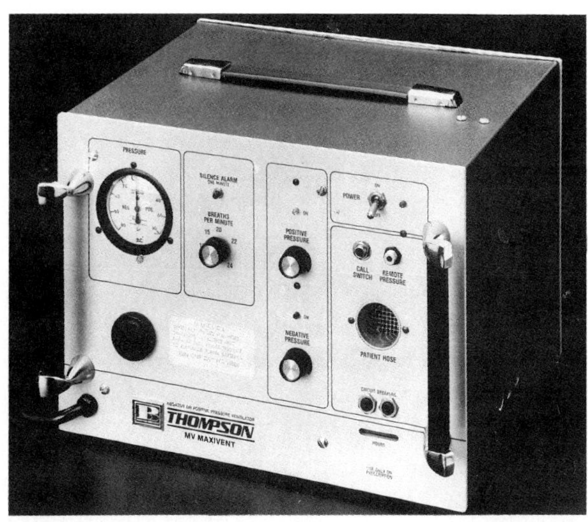

Figure 16-14. Puritan-Bennett Thompson Maxivent Negative Pressure Ventilator. (Courtesy of Puritan-Bennett Corporation, Lenexa, KS)

thorax during expiration. The manufacturer recommends that the total pressure applied (positive plus absolute negative value) should not exceed 70 cm H_2O.

Control Systems

This unit operates by means of a turbine to control positive pressure, negative pressure, and rate.

Output Displays

System pressure is displayed.

Alarms

A low-pressure/fail-to-cycle alarm is activated if the machine does not cycle for a 12-second period, which is detected if a positive pressure does not exceed 10 cm H_2O or a negative pressure is not less than -10 cm H_2O for a 12-second period. A power failure alarm is also included.

Analysis of Negative-Pressure Generators

The Iron Lung is still the standard for negative-pressure ventilation and is the most reliable and effective method of providing negative-pressure ventilation. However, its size, weight, and lack of access to the patient has forced the development of other units. The other major weaknesses of the Iron Lung are its lack of alarms and its fixed I:E ratio of 1:1.[17] Negative-pressure ventilation is now being used with a wider variety of patients,[2,3,23–27] and therefore ability to vary I:E ratio and provide assisted ventilation has become important to ensure patient acceptance of the apparatus.

Functionally, all of the portable negative-pressure units are similar. The only differences are in the areas of alarms, variability in I:E ratio, and capability of assisted ventilation. For the patient with neuromuscular or neurologic disease in whom a 1:1.5 or 1:2 fixed ratio is acceptable and in whom negative-pressure ventilation for a fixed number of hours per day is imperative, the Lifecare 170C or Puritan-Bennett Thompson Maxivent may be most appropriate because of their alarm packages. For the patient with chronic pulmonary disease where negative-pressure ventilation is used to periodically rest the diaphragm,[23–25] the Emerson 33 CRE and the Lifecare NEV-100 may be more appropriate because of their variability in I:E ratio and assist capabilities. The positive expiratory pressure available on some of these units is designed to assist the patient with exhalation by compressing the thorax. In most cases, its application is unnecessary and patients frequently find the alternating of negative and positive pressure distressing.

The Ideal Home Positive-Pressure Ventilator

Whether there is an ideal home mechanical ventilator is questionable. This description is based on the assumption that adult patients on home mechanical ventilation have stable conditions and are not weanable. The two key words that describe such a unit are simplicity and reliability.[17] Since the operation of this unit is primarily by non–health care workers, its design must be straightforward and its operation user-friendly. It should only incorporate a single mode (ASSIST/CONTROL) and should have a reasonable range of operation: rate, 6 to 40 breaths per minute; tidal volume, 200 to 2000 mL; peak flow, 30 to 100 L/min; or inspiratory time, 0.5 to 2.0 seconds. It should also have an appropriate sensitivity control.[17] It should be alarmed with only the following: high pressure, low pressure/apnea, ventilator failure, and power switch over.[17] In addition, a simple method of increasing the F_{IO_2} to 0.40 should be included. SIMV, sigh, additional alarms, and the ability to apply PEEP only complicates the unit's operation, increasing the difficulty home care givers and patients have in learning to operate the unit and increasing cost.[17] Furthermore, these additional features are generally unnecessary in the majority of patients dependent on home ventilators.

Positive-Pressure Ventilators

A number of positive-pressure ventilators have been designed specifically for use in the home. The features of these are described here. Settings ranges and alarms for these are summarized in Tables 16-1 and 16-2.

(Text continues on page 436)

TABLE 16-1. Setting Ranges for Volume-Targeted Home Care Positive-Pressure Ventilations

	Puritan-Bennett 2800	Puritan-Bennett 2801	Puritan-Bennett 2500	Aequitron LP-6	Aequitron LP-10	Aequitron LP-6 Plus	Lifecare PLV-100	Lifecare PLV-102	Intermed Bear 33
Modes	Control, assist/control, pressure limited plateau	Control, assist/control, pressure limited plateau	Control, assist/control	Control, assist/control, pressure limited (no plateau)	Control, assist/control, pressure limited (with or without plateau)	Control, assist/control, pressure limited (no plateau)	Control, assist/control, SIMV	Control, assist/control, SIMV	Control, assist/control, SIMV
Tidal volume	50–2800 mL	50–2800 mL	300–2500 mL	100–2200 mL	100–2200 mL	100–2200 mL	50–3000 mL	50–1800 mL	100–2200 mL
Rate	1–69/min	1–69/min	<4->20/min	1–38/min	1–38/min	1–38/min	2–40/min	2–40/min	2–40/min
Peak flow	40–125 L/min	20–120 L/min	—	—	—	—	10–120 L/min	10–120 L/min	20–120 L/min
Inspiratory time (seconds)	—	—	0.8–1.5 minimum to 5 maximum	0.5–5.5	0.5–5.5	0.5–5.5	—	—	0.25–4.99
Sensitivity	–5 to 10 cm H_2O	–10 to +10 cm H_2O	–1 cm H_2O pre-set	–10 to +10 cm H_2O	–10 to +10 cm H_2O	–10 to +10 cm H_2O	–6 to +3 cm H_2O	–6 to +18 cm H_2O	–9 to +9 cm H_2O
Sigh volume	125–2800 mL	125–2800 mL	—	—	—	—	—	1.5 times set tidal volume	1.5 times set tidal volume
Sigh rate	3/10 min	3/10 min	—	—	—	—	—	—	6/h

TABLE 16-2. Alarm Systems of Volume-Targeted Home Care Positive-Pressure Ventilators

Function	Puritan-Bennett 2800	Puritan-Bennett 2801	Puritan-Bennett 2500	Aequitron LP-6	Aequitron LP-10	Aequitron LP-6 Plus	Lifecare PLV-100	Lifecare PLV-102	Intermed Bear 33
High inspiratory pressure alarm	20–60 cm H_2O	25–100 cm H_2O	60–70 cm H_2O	25–100 cm H_2O	25–100 cm H_2O	25–100 cm H_2O	5–95 cm H_2O	5–95 cm H_2O	10–80 cm H_2O
High inspiratory pressure limit	10–70 cm H_2O	10–100 cm H_2O	No	25–100 cm H_2O	25–100 cm H_2O	25–100 cm H_2O	5–95 cm H_2O	5–95 cm H_2O	10–80 cm H_2O
Low inspiratory pressure	3–20 cm H_2O	2–32 cm H_2O	11–14 cm H_2O	2–50 cm H_2O	2–50 cm H_2O	2–50 cm H_2O	2–50 cm H_2O	2–50 cm H_2O	3–70 cm H_2O
Apnea	Yes	Yes	No	Yes	Yes	Yes	Yes	Yes	Yes
Low battery	Yes	Yes	Yes	Yes	Yes	Yes	Yes	Yes	Yes
Inverse I:E ratio	Yes	Yes	No	Yes	Yes	Yes	Yes	Yes	No
Ventilator malfunction	Yes	Yes	No	No	Yes	Yes	Yes	Yes	Yes
Low inspiratory flow	No	No	No	No	Yes	Yes	Yes	Yes	No
Reverse external battery connections	No	No	No	No	No	No	Yes	Yes	No
Microprocessor failure	No	No	No	No	Yes	Yes	Yes	Yes	No
Switch to battery	No	Yes	No	No	Yes	Yes	Yes	Yes	Yes
Power failure	No	No	No	No	Yes	Yes	Yes	Yes	No
Oxygen	No	No	No	No	No	No	No	Yes	No
Minimum minute ventilation	No	No	No	No	No	No	No	No	No

PURITAN-BENNETT COMPANION 2800

The Companion 2800 (Puritan-Bennett Corporation, Lenexa, KS) (Fig. 16-15) is a lightweight (31 lbs), compact (11⅜″ × 10″ × 12″), microprocessor-based, positive-pressure ventilator.[28]

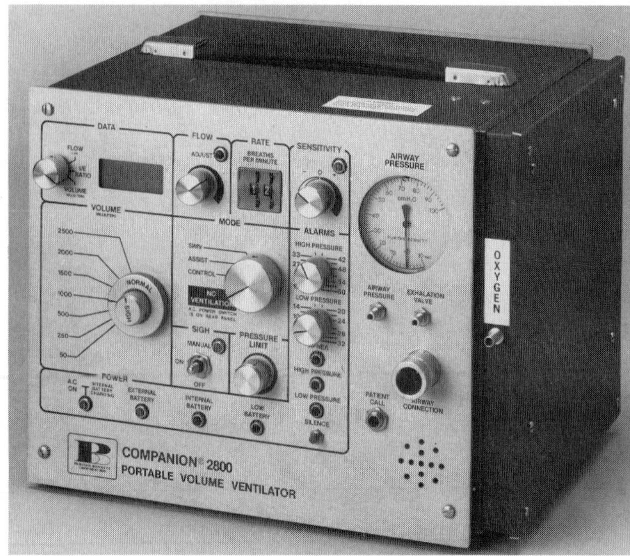

Figure 16-15. The Puritan-Bennett Companion 2800. (Courtesy of Puritan-Bennett, Lenexa, KS)

Input Variables

The pneumatic control of this ventilator is rotary piston driven. The 2800 can be operated by household AC, external DC, and internal DC current. If plugged into an AC outlet, the unit is always powered by AC current. If a power failure should occur, the unit will automatically switch to external DC power, if attached, then to internal DC power. To recharge the internal battery, the unit must be plugged in and the mode switch turned to "INTERNAL BATTERY CHARGING."

During use, the internal battery is also recharged. Recharging time is about ten times actual battery use time. If totally discharged, recharging time is approximately 10 hours. The internal battery can operate the unit for 20 to 60 minutes, depending on ventilator setup (a more rapid rate and larger tidal volume results in shorter battery life). If the ventilator automatically switches from a high priority power source to a lower priority power source (AC to external DC to internal DC) a repetitive short audible alarm is activated.

Control Variables, Phase Variables, and Modes

The Companion 2800 is an electrically powered, rotary piston-driven, microprocessor controlled, positive-pressure ventilator, incorporating a single gas delivery circuit. It is a volume controller and produces a sine wave flow and sigmoidal pressure patterns. It is either time or pressure triggered and volume cycled. Inspiration can also be pressure limited. No expiratory maneuvers (eg, PEEP) are available. An inspiratory sigh can be used.

The Companion 2800 incorporates three primary volume-targeted or pressure-limited ventilatory modes: CONTROL, ASSIST/CONTROL, and SIMV. In the CONTROL mode, the operator sets the tidal volume, inspiratory flow, and the positive-pressure breath rate. In this mode the sensitivity is locked out and no assisted breaths can be delivered. However, the patient can inspire spontaneously through the piston chamber and the exhalation valve between control breaths, simulating the intermittent mandatory ventilation mode. This ventilator does not contain a demand valve, nor is it configured with a continuous gas flow system.

In the ASSIST mode (actually ASSIST/CONTROL) the operator sets tidal volume, inspiratory flow, back-up rate, and sensitivity. Patient-triggered positive-pressure breaths are delivered unless the patient's rate falls below the back-up rate. If no patient inspiratory effort is sensed for two back-up control rate breathing cycles, the ventilator reverts to the control mode at the set rate. The patient may, however, resume spontaneous triggering of ventilation at any time.

With SIMV, a periodic assist/control, volume-targeted or pressure limited breath is delivered at an operator-selected rate. If the machine does not sense patient effort by the end of a ventilatory cycle (length in seconds determined by the SIMV rate setting) the unit delivers a positive-pressure breath. If no patient effort occurs for 45 seconds, the ventilator automatically switches to apnea ventilation at a rate of 12 breaths per minute, or higher if the SIMV rate is set greater than 12 breaths per minute. Between SIMV mandatory breaths, the patient may breathe spontaneously by means of the unit's piston chamber or exhalation valve. Because the Companion 2800 does not incorporate a demand system, during spontaneous ventilation gas can enter the circuit only through the piston chamber or through the exhalation valve.

Sigh breaths may be delivered in all modes: CONTROL, ASSIST/CONTROL, and SIMV. A separate sigh volume control determines delivered volume. When the sigh switch is placed in the "on" position, three consecutive sigh breaths are delivered every 10 minutes. In addition, by repositioning, a single sigh breath or multiple sigh breaths may be delivered manually.

Pressure-controlled ventilation can also be achieved in all three primary modes by adjustment of the high-pressure limit and tidal volume. This is achieved by adjusting the high-pressure limit to the desired peak airway pressure, and while connected to the patient, adjusting the tidal volume to achieve the desired plateau time. A change in the patient's compliance/resistance or obstruction of the system results in an altered tidal volume, of which the home care provider may not be aware (eg, no alarms). The high airway pressure alarm would be set differently from that during standard operation, that is, at a pressure higher than the pressure limit. Therefore, this alarm would only sound if the high-pressure limit failed. In spite of this approach being commonly used in pediatric home ventilation, it cannot be recommended without additional alarms guaranteeing gas delivery.

Control Systems

Gas flow through the Companion 2800 is illustrated in Figure 16-16. Gas enters the piston chamber from the right side of the ventilator (when facing unit) through an intake filter designed to remove particulate matter.[17] An optional oxygen accumulator can be attached over the total right side of the unit. Oxygen can be titrated into the accumulator for the delivery of increased FIO_2. One-way valves directing gas flow are located at the intake filter (A) and distal to the unit's piston chamber (B). From the intake filter, gas enters the piston chamber during its back stroke. During the piston's forward stroke, gas exits the piston chamber through a one-way valve (B). This valve prevents gas from being drawn into the piston chamber from the patient's breathing circuit during the piston's back stroke. In addition, a pop-off valve is located in the piston chamber to prevent excessive chamber pressurization should an obstruction at the piston outlet develop. Once gas exits the piston chamber, it passes the inspiratory adjustable pressure limit valve and proceeds through the inspiratory circuit to the patient. Before the circuit exiting the unit, a tee is positioned for charging the exhalation valve. A proximal airway pressure line is interfaced within the ventilator circuit near the patient's airway and leads to the unit's microprocessor and pressure manometer. In turn, signals programmed by the unit's control panel are received by the microprocessor and directed to the piston motor. Pressure sensed through the proximal pressure line is used to trigger assisted positive-pressure breaths. The one-way gas inlet valve located at C is not included in the Companion 2800 circuitry.

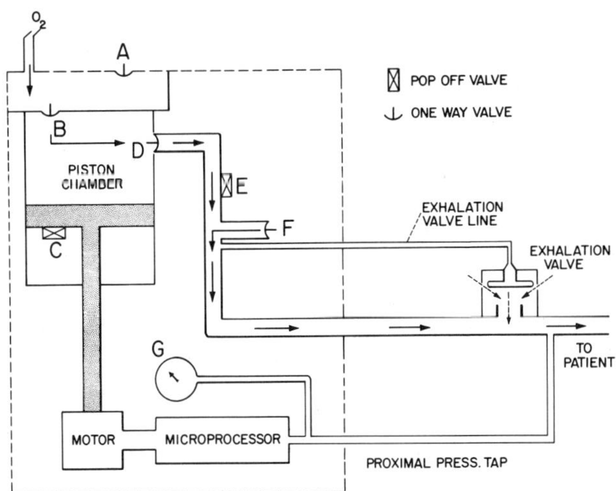

Figure 16-16. Generalized gas flow routes through typical home care ventilators. A one-way check valve (A) allows gas entry into the piston chamber during the piston backstroke. One-way check valve (B) prevents subatmospheric pressure from developing in the ventilator circuit during the backstroke of the piston. One-way check valve (antisuffocation valve) (C) allows patient to inspire spontaneously during closure of B when piston backstroke is in progress. Some gas may enter system at the exhalation valve during spontaneous breathing. Arrows depict gas flow possible during spontaneous inspiration. (From Kacmarek RM, Stanek KS, McMahon KM, Wilson RS. Imposed work of breathing during synchronized intermittent mandatory ventilation: Provided by Five Home Care Ventilators. Respir Care 1990;35:405–414)

Output Display

Airway pressure is displayed on a calibrated analog meter. Average flow, volume, or I:E ratio can be displayed. Colored lights on the front panel indicate pressure triggering and sigh breaths, source power, low battery, high and low airway pressure, I:E ratio less than 1:0.8, and apnea.

Alarms

Six alarms are incorporated in the Companion 2800: high inspiratory pressure, low inspiratory pressure, apnea, low battery, inverse I:E ratio, and ventilator malfunction. A 60-second alarm silence is also included. The high-pressure alarm is variable from 20 to 60 cm H_2O and produces an intermittent audio and visual alarm when activated but does not end the inspiratory phase. A separately set high-pressure limit prevents system pressure from exceeding a preselected level from 10 to 70 cm H_2O. When the set level is reached, inspiration continues until the selected tidal volume is delivered, while continually releasing excess pressure and venting delivered volume. During normal operation the high inspiratory pressure alarm should be set at a pressure lower than the high-pressure limit. This ensures the activation of the high-pressure alarm before the delivered tidal volume is dumped from the system. The only time these settings should be reversed is during pressure-limited plateau ventilation.

The low-pressure alarm is both audio and visual and can be set between 3 and 20 cm H_2O. It is activated when the set pressure is not exceeded within 15 seconds or two breath periods, whichever is sooner, when the CONTROL or ASSIST/CONTROL mode is used. In the SIMV mode it occurs if pressure is not reached within two breath periods, regardless of duration.

The apnea alarm is also an audio and visual alarm, functioning primarily in the SIMV mode. If the unit does not sense patient inspiratory effort within 15 seconds, the alarm is activated and mandatory breaths are delivered at the set rate after two breath periods. If the SIMV mode fails and the patient does not activate the unit within a 45-second period, a back-up rate of 12 breaths per minute (or at the operator set rate if higher than 12 breaths per minute) is provided. Tidal volume delivery is that pre-set by the operator. To return to the SIMV mode, the patient must trigger two breaths within a 10-second period or the mode selector control must be manually switched out of and back into the SIMV mode. In addition, the apnea alarm sounds in all modes if the airway pressure is greater than the low-pressure control set point for 15 seconds.

The low-battery audio and visual alarm sounds if either the internal DC battery or external DC battery charge is below acceptable limits. Inverse I:E ratio, or low flow alarm, is activated if the ratio falls below 1:0.85. This alarm is both audio and visual. The ventilator malfunction alarm, a constant audio alarm, is activated if the circuit breakers are open, the microprocessor malfunctions, the piston is out of range, or a problem in the software is detected. A remote alarm jack is available as an option for attachment to a secondary alarm system. An auxiliary remote alarm and patient call are available as options. The unit also incorporates a 60-second alarm silence, an alarm volume control, and an hour meter.

Analysis

In general, this is a well-designed, easy-to-operate ventilator with a wide range of capabilities. However, a few specific features require comment. The sensitivity, flow, pressure limit, and airway pressure alarms are not calibrated, which make it difficult for the user to determine actual settings.[17] These controls, and the flow control, are very easy to turn and readjust. The likelihood of inadvertent change in these settings is high. There is no face cover for the control panel. All controls are easily accessible, and the potential for change by children is high. An inverse ratio may be inadvertently set; if the ratio is inverted, the flow adjust lamp flashes, alarm sounds, and the set rate may decrease depending on actual ratio. The exhalation port tubing attachment and proximal pressure port are the same size; as a result, it is easy to inadvertently confuse their attachment. As a result of a separate control for pressure limit and high-pressure alarm, the high-pressure limiting may occur without practitioner notification if the high-pressure alarm is set above the high-pressure limit.[17]

PURITAN-BENNETT COMPANION 2801

The Companion 2801 (Puritan-Bennett Corporation, Lenexa, KS) (Fig. 16-17) is an upgrade of the Companion 2800.[29] It is 12¾ × 10⅝ × 13¼ inches and weighs 35.5 lbs. The control panels of the Companion 2800 and Companion 2801 are arranged differently, although essentially all of the same controls are on the front panel. They differ in that the power "off" switch of the Companion 2801 has been moved to the back of the ventilator, a battery charge indicator is incorporated with the pressure manometer, a battery test is included with the alarm silence button, the connectors for the airway pressure tap and exhalation valves are of different sizes, the high and low airway pressure alarm controls are calibrated (flow, sensitivity, and pressure limit controls are still uncalibrated), the patient call attachment has been eliminated, the panel face has been indented approximately 1 inch, and a removable plastic panel cover is available. The control and phase variables, modes, and gas delivery system are the same as for the Companion 2800. Larger ranges for the following parameters are available for the Companion 2801: peak flow, peak inspiratory pressure limit, peak inspiratory pressure alarm, low inspiratory pressure limit, and sensitivity. Some of the problems with the Companion 2800 have been corrected in the Companion 2801. However, a number still exist: the sensitivity, flow, and pressure limit controls are not calibrated; an inverse ratio may be inadvertently set; and the high-pressure alarm may still be set above the high-pressure limit in volume-targeted ventilation.

The alarms are the same as the 2800, with the exception of redesign of the apnea alarm. A visual alarm warns that the ventilator has failed to sense patient effort for 15 seconds when in the SIMV mode. If the SIMV rate is also less than 8 breaths per minute, then an audio alarm will sound and in another 30 seconds the ventilator automatically switches to a backup rate of 12 breaths per minute. To return to SIMV the patient must trigger the ventilator twice in 10 seconds or the mode switch must be switched out of, then into, SIMV. If the ventilator rate is 8 breaths per minute or greater, the visual alarm is activated without an audio alarm or backup rate. One additional alarm has been added—a power switch over; a pulsing audio alarm sounds when the ventilator automatically switches from AC to external or internal DC or from external DC to internal DC.

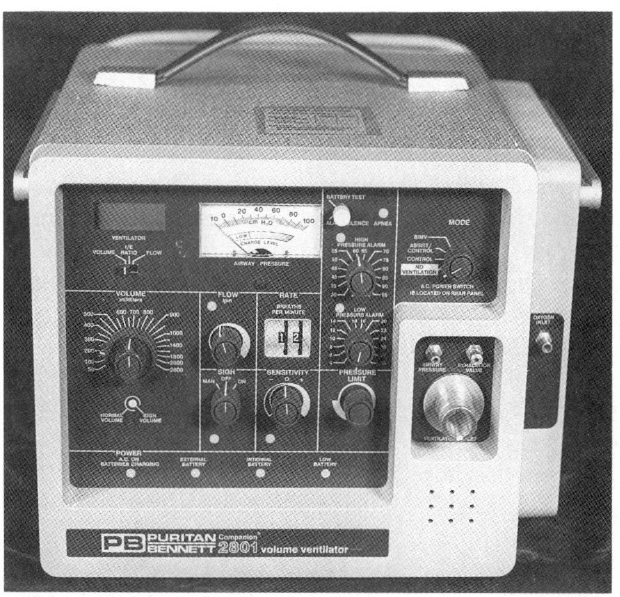

Figure 16-17. The Puritan-Bennett Companion 2801. (Courtesy of Puritan-Bennett Corporation, Lenexa, KS)

PURITAN-BENNETT COMPANION 2500

This ventilator is the oldest of the Puritan-Bennett group.[30] It is 16 × 8 × 9 inches and weighs 27 lbs. It is not microprocessor controlled.

Input Variables

The ventilator is piston-driven by a brushed motor. The unit can be operated by either AC current, external DC current, or internal DC battery. When operating, the internal battery is recharging. If an AC power failure occurs, the unit switches to external battery, then to internal battery. The internal battery lasts about 1 hour, depending on actual ventilator set-up.

Control Variables, Phase Variables, and Modes

The Companion 2500 is an electrically powered, rotary piston-driven, positive-pressure ventilator, incorporating a single gas delivery system and delivering a sine wave flow pattern with a sigmoidal pressure curve. It is a volume controller and is time or pressure triggered and volume cycled. Volume-targeted control or assist/control ventilation is available, but no expiratory maneuvers are present.

During CONTROL mode, the operator sets a tidal volume, inspiratory time and positive-pressure breathing rate. As with the 2800 or 2801, spontaneous breathing does not trigger an additional breath, but nonpressurized gas can be drawn from valve C (Figure 16-16) or the piston chamber in between control breaths. In the ASSIST/ CONTROL mode, the factory-set sensitivity of −1 cm H_2O is activated. This unit also incorporates a PRESSURE LIMIT control, allowing pressure plateau ventilation by setting a large tidal volume in conjunction with the pressure limit. When the pressure limit is reached, inspiratory time continues to completion, dumping excess volume to atmosphere. Pressure-limited ventilation may be set in either the CONTROL or the ASSIST/CONTROL mode.

Control System

Figure 16-16 illustrates the gas delivery pattern of the Companion 2500. Gas enters the piston chamber at A and proceeds from the chamber past a one-way valve (B) into the inspiratory circuit. Pressure taps for the exhalation valve and the monitoring of system pressure come off the inspiratory limb internal to the ventilator.

Output Display

Airway pressure is displayed on an aneroid manometer.

Alarms

Three alarms are included: low pressure, high pressure, and low battery. The low-pressure alarm is factory pre-set at 11 to 14 cm H_2O. An audio alarm is activated if circuit pressure does not reach this pressure within 15 to 20 seconds. The high-pressure alarm is also factory pre-set at 60 to 70 cm H_2O. As pressures exceed this level, an audio alarm is sounded. Both high- and low-pressure alarms must be reset after activation, and both may be adjusted to different levels by the dealer. The low-battery alarm is activated if either an external or the internal battery falls below 11.0 to 10.5 volts DC. In addition, if an inverse ratio is established by the set parameters and insufficient time is available for exhalation to maintain at least a 1:1 I:E ratio, a red visual alarm is activated.

Analysis

This unit is a redesign of one of the earliest home care ventilators and, consequently, does not present the range of operational capabilities of the newer units. Its tidal volume and rate range limits its use to adults, while its limited alarm capability and pre-set high- and low-pressure alarms require more intense monitoring of patients who are truly ventilator dependent.[17] Generally, this unit is not recommended for use in patients who require continuous (24 hours a day) invasive positive-pressure ventilation. However, it is useful for the operation of a pneumobelt or for the provision of periodic mouth ventilation to wheelchair-dependent patients who are maintained by negative pressure at night.

AEQUITRON MEDICAL LP-6

The LP-6 (Aequitron Medical, Minneapolis, MN) (Fig. 16-18) is a lightweight (32 lbs), compact (9¼″ × 13½″ × 12½″), microprocessor-based, positive-pressure mechanical ventilator.[31] The internal gas flow pathway in this unit is similar to that of the Puritan-Bennett Companion 2800 (see Fig. 16-16).

Input Variables

The LP-6 is a microprocessor-controlled, electrically powered, and rotary piston-driven via a brushless motor positive-pressure home care ventilator. The LP-6 can be operated by household AC, external DC, and internal DC current. The unit always selects the highest power source available: AC, then external DC, then internal DC. When connected to an electrical outlet, the internal DC battery is automatically charged, unless the unit is turned off. It takes 2 to 3 hours to recharge a discharged internal battery. The internal battery can operate the LP-6 for up to 1 hour, depending on the actual ventilator set-up. The unit automatically converts from AC to DC sources, if required. The power switch-over alarm is activated when switchover occurs.

Control Systems

Gas enters the unit from atmosphere or through a reservoir bag assembly attached to the gas inlet port on the back panel of the machine. From here, through a one-way valve (see Fig. 16-16*A*), gas enters the piston chamber; gas exits the piston chamber at a second one-way valve (B) from which it proceeds into the inspiratory circuit. Within the internal inspiratory circuit, a gas tap supplying flow to the exhalation valve is configured. Additionally, a manufacturer-set nonadjustable pressure pop-off valve is located internally on the inspiratory limb (this is different from the high pressure limit as noted in the Companion 2800). A proximal pressure tap leads from the patient's airways to the ventilator front panel and on to the microprocessor. The system's pressure gauge attaches to this line. The high-pressure limit is identified by the micro-

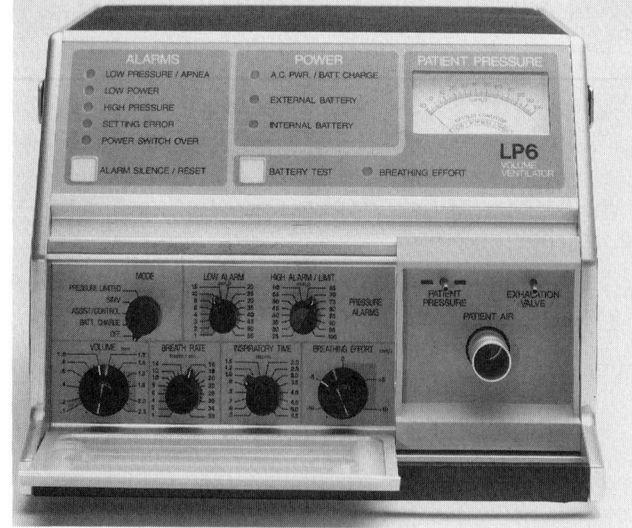

Figure 16-18. The Aequitron Medical LP-6. (Courtesy of Aequitron Medical, Minneapolis, MN)

processor and, when reached, an alarm is activated and the inspiratory phase is terminated.

Parameters set on the control panel are relayed to the piston motor by means of the microprocessor. Patient effort during assisted ventilation is sensed through the proximal pressure tap. The one-way gas inlet valve located at C (see Fig. 16-16) is not included in the LP-6 gas flow path. The oxygen accumulating apparatus used on the LP-6 is more elaborate than that used on the other units presented here. The suggested configuration is depicted in Figure 16-19. To the gas inlet port on the back of the machine, a 30×22-mm adapter is used to attach a large bore connecting tube that affixes to a specifically designed T-piece attached to the unit's accessory side rail on the right side panel of the unit. This T-piece is configured with an O_2 tap and a reservoir bag. A detailed discussion of oxygen delivery is provided later in the chapter.

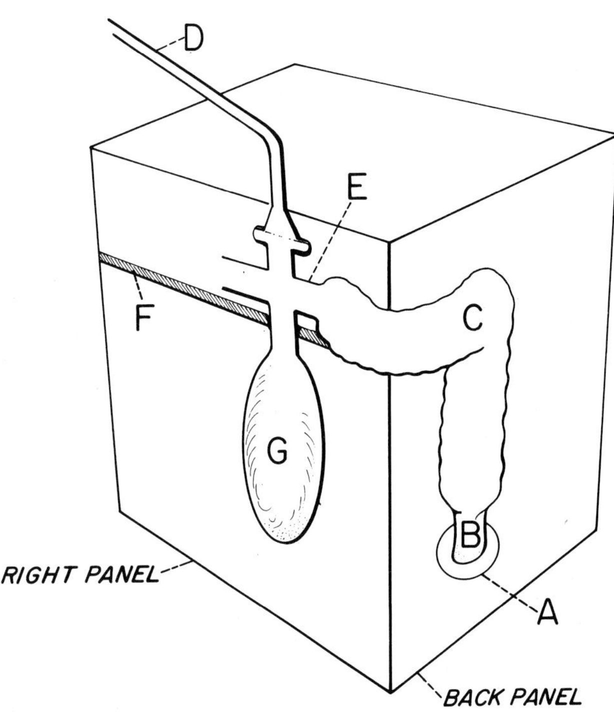

Figure 16-19. The oxygen accumulator used on the LP series ventilators. See text for discussion. (From Aequitron LP-6 Compact Volume Ventilator: User's Guide and Instruction Manual. Minneapolis, MN: Aequitron Medical Inc., 1985)

Control Variables, Phase Variables, and Modes

The LP-6 ventilator is a volume controller. Inspiration is either time triggered or pressure triggered and can be either volume cycled or pressure cycled. As the result of the piston-driving mechanism, the unit is a non–constant-flow generator, producing a sigmoidal pressure pattern. Apnea ventilation is available, but no inspiratory sigh or expiratory maneuvers are included.

ASSIST/CONTROL, SIMV, and PRESSURE LIMIT are the primary modes available with the LP-6. In the ASSIST/CONTROL mode, the operator sets breath rate, tidal volume, inspiratory time, and breathing effort (patient-triggered sensitivity). During SIMV, the operator must also set breath rate, tidal volume, inspiratory time, and breathing effort. Between SIMV positive-pressure breaths, the patient may breathe spontaneously, drawing gas from the piston chamber or through the exhalation valve. As with all ventilators in this group, the LP-6 does not have a demand system, nor is it configured with a continuous flow system. If the patient fails to create sufficient inspiratory force to be sensed by the ventilator for a 20-second period, the unit goes into back-up ventilation at a rate of 10 breaths per minute and the pre-set tidal volume. If the SIMV breath rate is set at 6 breaths per minute or greater, the apnea alarm will sound but the machine will not revert to back-up ventilation.

The PRESSURE LIMIT mode functions exactly the same as the ASSIST/CONTROL mode, except that inspiration is terminated when the set high pressure limit is reached. This mode does *not* result in a pressure plateau. As in all pressure-cycled approaches to ventilation, actual tidal volume delivered depends on ventilator settings and patient's airways resistance and compliance. When this mode is used, the high-pressure alarm is inactivated. Thus, any acute change in system compliance or airways resistance may go unnoticed because no method of monitoring tidal volume or minute ventilation is available.

Output Displays

Airway pressure is displayed. LEDs indicate pressure triggering and power source (AC, external battery, internal battery). Flashing red LEDs indicate low pressure or apnea, high pressure, low power, setting error, and power switch over.

Alarms

Five alarms are incorporated into the LP-6: low pressure, apnea, low power, high pressure, and setting error. The low-pressure alarm sounds if the peak airway pressure fails to reach the pre-set level, and automatically corrects itself if the low-pressure setting is exceeded on subsequent breaths. The high-pressure alarm terminates the inspiratory phase when activated. If the condition activating this alarm is spontaneously corrected, the alarm is deactivated. Setting error is activated if the ventilator controls are set outside the capabilities of the ventilator. Once corrected, this alarm is silenced. The LP-6 will not allow an inverse I:E ratio to be delivered. The low-power alarm is activated when the internal DC battery is the primary power source and its voltage is low, almost inadequate to ensure proper machine function.

The apnea alarm functions in all modes. If the set rate is less than 6 breaths per minute and the patient is apneic for 10 seconds, the apnea alarm will sound. If apnea persists for 20 seconds, the unit provides backup ventilation at a rate of 10 breaths per minute, delivering the set tidal volume or pressure limit. If the unit is set at a rate greater than 6 breaths per minute, apnea of 10 seconds or longer results only in an alarm.

A remote alarm and accessory printer capable of tracking alarm conditions and monitoring ventilator performance is available. A 60-second alarm silence is included, however no reset is provided; alarms are reset once alarm conditions are resolved.

Analysis

This unit may not be appropriate for pediatric use.[17] Its minimal VT is 100 mL and VT can only be changed in 100-mL increments. It has many features that make it attractive for use with adults. Inadvertent parameter change is decreased by design of the control panel, which is recessed and covered by a door. The design of the control panel is very simple and straightforward, improving user-friendliness. Of major concern is the similarity in size of the ports at the ventilator for attachment of the exhalation valve line and the proximal pressure line.

AEQUITRON MEDICAL LP-10

The LP-10 (Aequitron Medical, Minneapolis, MN) (Fig. 16-20) is an enhanced LP-6.[32] The LP-10 looks like the LP-6; its control panel is designed the same as the LP-6, but it is slightly larger (9¾″ × 14½″ × 13¼″) and weighs 34 lbs. The two obvious changes are variations in size of the connections for airway pressure and the exhalation valve lines (airway pressure larger diameter) and the addition of a PRESSURE LIMIT control. Its classification is the same as the LP-6. All modes available on the LP-6 are also available on the LP-10 plus the PRESSURE LIMIT control. During either SIMV or ASSIST/CONTROL, a large tidal volume can be set in association with a specific pressure limit. During inspiration, the ventilator delivers the complete tidal volume. However, pressure will not be allowed to exceed the pressure limit. Volume delivered after the limit has been reached is dumped to atmosphere. In addition, the high-pressure alarm limit is not affected by the PRESSURE LIMIT control. If the high-pressure alarm limit is reached, the ventilator alarms and dumps additional volume to atmosphere without altering inspiratory time.

Alarms

This is the area of greatest difference between the LP-6 and LP-10. The actual number of specific alarm conditions identifiable with the LP-10 is 23. These conditions are categorized under five major alarm conditions: high pressure, low pressure/apnea, low power, power switch over, and setting error. Audio and visual indicators are available for these five major categories. No other information except these five indicators is available to the practitioner unless the optional printer is set up and active during ventilation. When the printer is in use, a specific description of the alarm, along with an indication of why the alarm occurred is provided.

There are six individual alarm specifications in the category low pressure/apnea: low pressure (system pressure below limit for two consecutive breaths), valley alarm (system pressure does not drop below

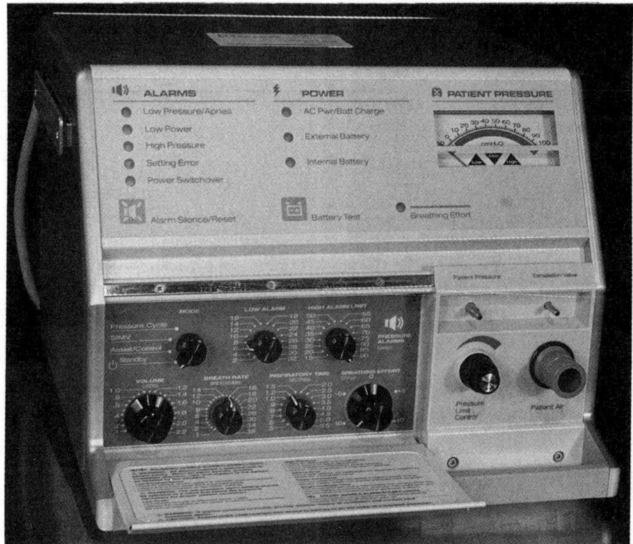

Figure 16-20. The Aequitron LP-10 ventilator. (Courtesy of Aequitron Medical, Minneapolis, MN)

the low pressure setting for two consecutive breaths), exhale fail (system pressure is above the low pressure alarm setting at the beginning of a breath), apnea (same as LP-6), stall (failure to complete a breathing cycle in 14 seconds) and failure of system leak self-test.

The power failure alarm results from two distinct conditions: internal battery voltage below 11.6 volts and failure of the battery charger. The power switchover alarm is the same as the LP-6. Under the high-pressure alarm, three situations are identified: (1) system pressure is above set level, (2) system pressure exceeds set level by 10 cm H_2O and (3) failure of over-pressure relief valve during self-test. With the setting error alarm, 11 different user or machine operational errors are identified.

The unit has a remote alarm access port and a communication port for an optional printer. If the communications port is used, access to detailed monitoring data is available based on alarm activation. That is, each alarm condition is categorized, a description of the alarm condition is provided, and an indication of why the condition occurred is detailed.

Analysis

As with the LP-6, minimal VT is 100 mL and VT changes are in 100-mL increments, which limits the unit's use in pediatrics. The addition of the PRESSURE LIMIT control offsets this concern in some settings. However, because volume monitoring is not provided, extreme care must be exercised when the PRESSURE LIMIT control is used. This includes proper setting of the high- and low-pressure alarms. An additional concern with the PRESSURE LIMIT control is the fact that it is not calibrated. Inadvertent parameter change is decreased (except for the PRESSURE LIMIT control) by the design of the unit (the recession of the control panel and its door). The design of the control panel is simple and straightforward, improving user-friendliness. The communication port enhances the monitoring of, and appropriate response to, alarm conditions.

AEQUITRON LP-6 PLUS

This unit is exactly the same as the LP-10, except that the pressure limit control is not included.

LIFECARE PLV-100

The Lifecare PLV-100 (Lifecare, Boulder, CO) weighs 28.2 lbs and measures 9″ × 12.5″ × 12.25″ (Fig. 16-21).[33] It is thus a compact and highly portable microprocessor-based home care ventilator.

Input Variables

The PLV-100 is electrically powered, rotary piston-driven by means of an electric motor, and under the control of a microprocessor. It is operational with three distinct power sources: AC, external DC, and internal DC. This unit always selects AC power if the powering mechanism is available. If the unit must switch to either DC source, a 3-second alarm is activated. When functioning on a DC source, the voltage level of the source can be rapidly evaluated by the "READ BAT-

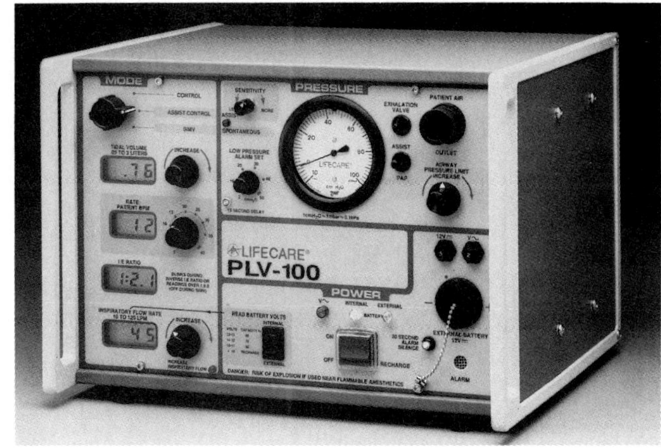

Figure 16-21. The Lifecare PLV-100 ventilator. (Courtesy of Lifecare, Boulder, CO)

TERY VOLTS" indicator on the front panel. The internal battery is capable of providing up to 60 minutes of power, depending on the actual ventilator settings. The higher the demand, the shorter the time period. The internal battery is charging whenever the unit is plugged into an AC outlet, regardless of activation.

During machine power up, a complete unit diagnostic check of all systems occurs. This lasts about 5 seconds, during which time LEDs are active and alarms sound.

Control Variables, Phase Variables, and Modes

The PLV-100 is a volume controller, and its rotary piston design produces a sine wave gas flow pattern with a sigmoidal pressure curve. Inspiration is either time or pressure triggered, volume cycled, and pressure limited. System pressure is limited by the high airway pressure alarm, which, when reached, dumps the remaining gas in the piston chamber to atmosphere without altering inspiratory time.

CONTROL, ASSIST/CONTROL, and SIMV modes are available on the PLV-100. In the CONTROL mode, rate, tidal volume, and inspiratory flow are set. The unit determines inspiratory time based on these settings and displays an I:E ratio. In the CONTROL mode the patient is unable to activate a positive-pressure breath but can breathe spontaneously through the piston chamber or the exhalation valve. In the ASSIST/CONTROL mode all settings are identical to the CONTROL mode, with the addition of the sensitivity setting. The inspiratory time remains constant with each positive-pressure breath but the I:E ratio display indicates a varied ratio dependent on the rate the patient is assisting. In the SIMV mode the machine set-up is identical to the ASSIST/CONTROL mode. However, because of the patient's spontaneous breathing efforts, the I:E ratio display is inactivated. A 6-second window of time is available for patient triggering of the SIMV mandatory breath; as a result of this large window, delivered positive-pressure rate may vary. The PLV-100 does not contain a demand system. Thus, unless the unit is configured with a continuous-flow system, the patient must draw air during spontaneous ventilation either from the piston chamber or from the exhalation valve.

Control System

The basic gas flow pattern for the PLV-100 is illustrated in Figure 16-16. This figure appropriately represents gas flow, with two major exceptions. First, no oxygen accumulator is available for attachment to the unit's gas entry port A; and, second, the one-way valve at C, allowing gas inflow during spontaneous breathing when the piston in its backstroke, is not present. Essentially, gas enters the piston chamber at A and is moved from the chamber into the internal gas delivery system at B. A pressure pop-off valve is also located inside the piston chamber. From B, gas proceeds past an inspiratory pressure limit valve, out of the ventilator, through the inspiratory circuitry and on to the patient. The exhalation valve line originates from the internal ventilator circuitry. A proximal airway pressure line provides input to the microprocessor (the system manometer is tapped off this line). Oxygen may be administered through an adapter interfaced with the unit between the external circuitry and the unit itself (an increase in delivered tidal volume, as well as F_{IO_2} results) or through an accumulator placed at the gas intake port.

Output Displays

Airway pressure is displayed on an aneroid gauge. Digital readouts of tidal volume, rate, I:E ratio, and inspiratory flow rate are provided. A number of alarm conditions are also displayed, as described below.

Alarms

The PLV-100 incorporates 11 system alarms: low pressure/apnea, high pressure, inverse I:E ratio, increase inspiratory flow, low internal battery, low external battery, reverse external battery connection, switch to battery, power failure, microprocessor failure, and ventilator malfunction. The low-pressure audio alarm is activated if the set low airway pressure is not exceeded within a 15-second period. A front panel LED flashes with each breath as pressure passes the set level. In SIMV, the low-pressure alarm also acts as an apnea alarm. The patient's spontaneous inspiratory efforts are sensed by the low pressure mechanism and the 15-second delay is reset. Thus, if either the machine does not sense a spontaneous breath, or the positive-pressure level does not exceed the set mark within a 15-second period, the alarm is activated.

The high airway pressure alarm (audio only) is activated each time the patient's peak airway pressure exceeds the alarm setting. When this occurs, tidal volume remaining in the piston chamber is dumped to atmosphere as the piston continues its forward motion. As a result, inspiratory time remains unaltered. The alarm automatically resets each breath.

The inverse I:E ratio alarm is a visual flashing alarm that is activated whenever the inspiratory time exceeds the expiratory time. No action on the part of the practitioner is indicated if an inverse I:E ratio is desired.

The increase inspiratory flow alarm is a visual alarm activated if inspiratory flow is insufficient to meet other set parameters. When activated, the inspiratory flow display will flash "Increase Inspiratory

Flow" while the inspiratory flow is automatically increased. However, inspiratory flow will not increase to a level to prevent an inverse I:E ratio.

The low internal battery alarm is both an audio and visual alarm, activated if the internal battery falls below 9.5 volts. The external battery alarm functions in precisely the same manner. If an attempt is made to reverse the external battery connection, an alarm sounds until the connection is corrected. Whenever the power source switches from AC to either external DC or internal DC, a 3-second audible alarm sounds. Additionally, if the power switch is in the "on" position and no power is applied to the unit, an audible alarm is activated.

If the microprocessor fails to pass its diagnostic self-test, an audio alarm is activated and the piston motor is locked, preventing uncontrolled function. In addition, if the unit's pressure transducer fails or the piston system fails to properly cycle a "fast beep," audible alarm is continuously activated if attempts are made to use the unit.

Analysis

The overall physical layout of the control panel is very busy, making the machine appear intimidating and increasing the difficulty in initially teaching its operation.[17] The sensitivity and high airway pressure limit control knobs are not calibrated, making them difficult to set. To determine the high airway pressure limit setting, the patient must be removed from the ventilator. It is possible to provide inverse ratio ventilation, an approach that is not indicated in the home. The attachment for the exhalation valve line and the proximal airway pressure line is of a different size to avoid inadvertent misconnection.

LIFECARE PLV-102

The Lifecare PLV-102 (Lifecare, Boulder, CO) (Fig. 16-22) is an update of the PLV-100.[34] The internal gas flow path is the same as with the PLV-100, with the addition of an oxygen proportioning valve and a 50-psig oxygen attachment. A standard DISS oxygen connector exists on the back of the ventilator, and from here oxygen enters a proportional valve from which it proceeds to a flow sensor, then into the internal inspiratory circuit, bypassing the piston chamber and allowing a delivered F_{IO_2} up to 0.90. In ASSIST/CONTROL and CONTROL mode ventilation, the oxygen percent is simply set on the front panel. An appropriate amount of oxygen enters the system to maintain F_{IO_2}. However, the accuracy of oxygen delivery decreases at tidal volume setting less than 300 mL and F_{IO_2} greater than 0.40. During SIMV, the manufacturer recommends using the unit's oxygen sensor. The sensor cable originates from the front of the machine and is interfaced between the humidifier and the ventilator at least 18 inches proximal to any H-valve set-up or the unit itself. The sensor is necessary to ensure consistent F_{IO_2} during spontaneous ventilation. If the sensor is not present during SIMV, room air is inspired during spontaneous ventilation.

In addition to the CONTROL, ASSIST/CONTROL, and SIMV modes, the PLV-102 incorporates CONTROL + SIGH and ASSIST/CONTROL + SIGH modes. During both of these modes the ventilator automatically delivers a sigh breath at 150% of the set tidal volume once every 100 breaths.

The PLV-102 incorporates the 11 alarms included on the PLV-100, with the addition of an oxygen alarm that is activated if (1) O_2 source pressure is less than 45 psig; (2) O_2 source pressure is greater than 55 psig; (3) the ventilator oxygen valve is stuck open; (4) the oxygen sensor is defective; and (5) the ventilatory demand exceeds oxygen valve capability (>90 L/min). In addition, the PLV-102 displays alarm codes in the peak flow digital readout window. A decal with code definitions is attached to the machine. A 30-second alarm silence has also been included.

The PLV-102 has two options not available on the PLV-100: a remote alarm and printer hook-up. In addition, a manual sigh button allows for sighs upon user's discretion.

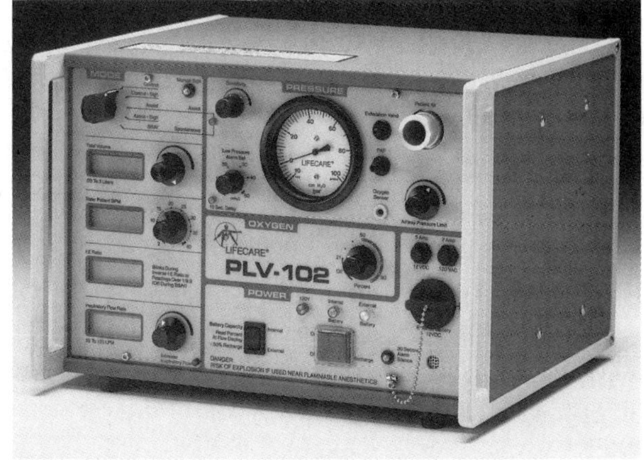

Figure 16-22. The Lifecare PLV-102 ventilator. (Courtesy of Lifecare, Boulder, CO)

Analysis

The PLV-102 is even more complex than the PLV-100 and less user-friendly. In addition, the 50-psig oxygen attachment and FIO_2 delivery system makes it even less practical for home use. However, this add-on makes the unit a very attractive ventilator for use in long-term care facilities or hospitals. The sensitivity and high-pressure limit control knobs are not calibrated, and inverse I:E ratio ventilation is also feasible, as in the PLV-100.

INTERMED BEAR 33

The Bear 33 (Bear Medical Corporation, Riverside, CA) (Fig. 16-23) functions similarly to all other home care ventilators but appears distinctly different.[35] It is the only unit of this class that has a computer touch pad keyboard for its control panel. A double-entry procedure is required to change panel settings. On the lower left-hand corner of the machine is a panel unlock button that must be pressed before making any change. Once the panel is unlocked, simultaneous depression of one of two arrows (↑ or ↓) and the parameter to be altered must be performed. The sequence required for parameter change virtually eliminates the likelihood of inadvertent parameter changes. However, it also increases the difficulty in teaching patients and caregivers the basics of operating this unit. As with all of the units discussed, the Bear 33 is a lightweight (32 lbs) and compact (7.5″ × 14″ × 12.8″) microprocessor-based home care ventilator.

Input Variables

The Bear 33 is an electrically powered, microprocessor-controlled, rotary piston-driven (brushless motor) home care positive-pressure ventilator. Three power sources are available with the Bear 33: AC, DC external battery, and DC internal battery. The unit always uses the highest power source available: AC before external DC and before internal DC. When a power changeover occurs, an audiovisual alarm is activated and must be manually silenced. The internal battery can function for up to 60 minutes, depending on actual ventilator settings. The internal battery is recharged when the unit is plugged into an electrical outlet. The machine does not have to be turned on for charging to occur. Battery charge indicators for the internal and external batteries are located on the front lower left-hand portion of the machine.

Control Variables, Phase Variables, and Modes

As a result of the rotary piston-driving mechanism, this ventilator is a volume controller, and sine wave flow and sigmoidal pressure patterns are produced. Inspiration is time or pressure triggered,and volume-cycled or pressure cycled. Sighs can be programmed, but no expiratory maneuvers are included.

Three modes are incorporated into the Bear 33: CONTROL, ASSIST/CONTROL, and SIMV. In addition, sigh breaths can be programmed. In the CONTROL mode, the operator sets the tidal volume, rate, and peak flow. The sensitivity control is not functional in this mode; however, its last setting is always displayed. The tidal volume can be changed in increments of 10 mL; the rate by 0.5 breath per minute, from 2 to 10 breaths per minute, and by one breath from 10 to 40 breaths per minute; and the peak flow by 10 L/min. Once parameters have been set, the inspiratory time is calculated and displayed in the inspiratory time digital readout. This unit is designed to prevent an inverse I:E ratio from being programmed. If selected parameters result in an inverse I:E ratio, the LED displaying the parameters will stop changing and begin to flash, indicating the limit preventing inverting the I:E ratio. The maximum inspiratory time during positive-pressure breaths is 4.99 seconds, with a minimum of 0.25 second. Minimum expiratory time during CONTROL and ASSIST/CONTROL ventilation is 0.75 second. When the unit is set for control ventilation, IMV is available if the patient is breathing spontaneously. Gas may be drawn from the internal gas flow system and exhalation valve in exactly the same manner as in SIMV.

During ASSIST/CONTROL the unit is set as in control, with the addition of setting the sensitivity. Assisted breaths may be delivered up to a rate of 40 breaths per minute. If the patient were to become apneic, the set rate would provide back-up ventilation.

In the SIMV mode, the unit periodically delivers a mandatory breath between which the ventilator becomes insensitive to patient inspiratory efforts and forces the patient to draw gas from the exhalation valve or the ventilator internal circuitry. As outlined earlier, a piston bypass one-way valve is located on the internal inspiratory circuit. Patient spontaneous tidal volume is normally achieved by the patient

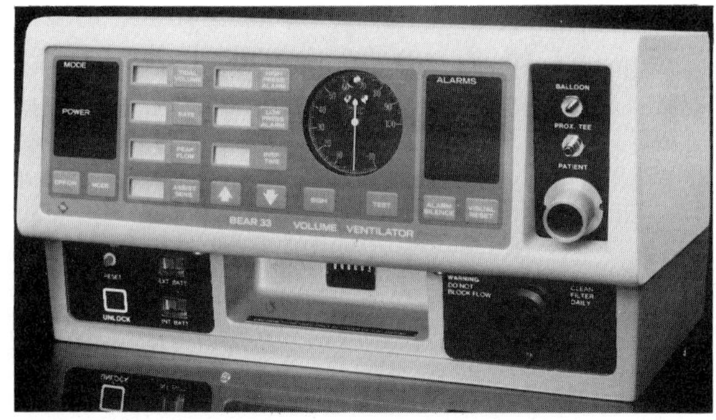

A

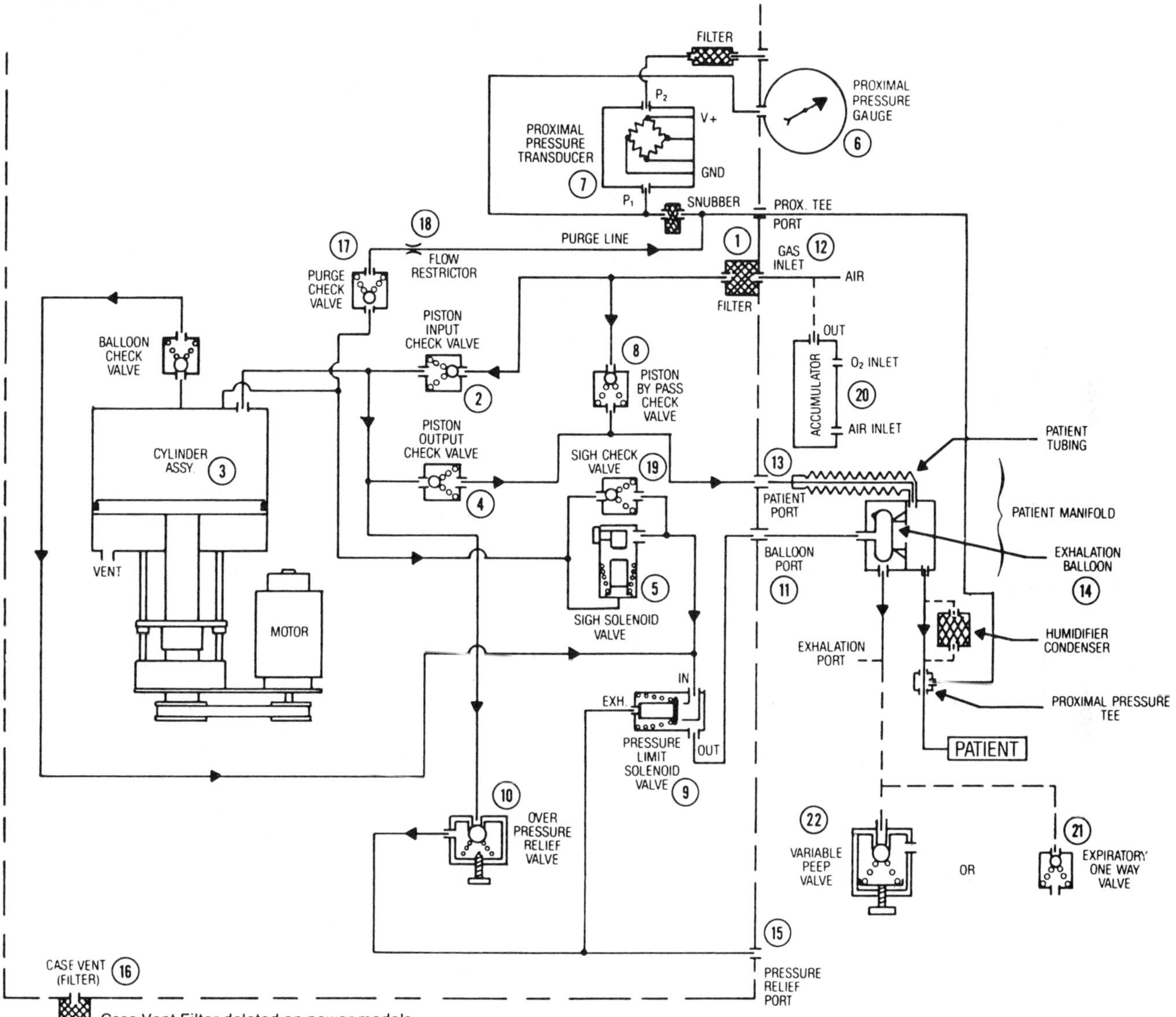

FILTER
PROXIMAL PRESSURE GAUGE (6)
P_2
V+
PROXIMAL PRESSURE TRANSDUCER (7)
GND
P_1
SNUBBER
PROX. TEE PORT
(18)
PURGE LINE
(17)
FLOW RESTRICTOR
PURGE CHECK VALVE
(1)
GAS INLET (12)
AIR
FILTER
BALLOON CHECK VALVE
PISTON INPUT CHECK VALVE (2)
(8)
PISTON BY PASS CHECK VALVE
OUT
ACCUMULATOR
O_2 INLET
(20)
AIR INLET
CYLINDER ASSY. (3)
PISTON OUTPUT CHECK VALVE (4)
SIGH CHECK VALVE (19)
(13)
PATIENT PORT
PATIENT TUBING
PATIENT MANIFOLD
BALLOON PORT (11)
EXHALATION BALLOON (14)
VENT
(5)
MOTOR
SIGH SOLENOID VALVE
EXHALATION PORT
HUMIDIFIER CONDENSER
IN
EXH.
PRESSURE LIMIT SOLENOID VALVE (9)
OUT
PROXIMAL PRESSURE TEE
PATIENT
(10)
OVER PRESSURE RELIEF VALVE
(22)
VARIABLE PEEP VALVE
OR
(21)
EXPIRATORY ONE WAY VALVE
(15)
CASE VENT (FILTER) (16)
PRESSURE RELIEF PORT
Case Vent Filter deleted on newer models.

B

Figure 16-23. A. The Intermed Bear 33 ventilator. B. Schematic diagram of Intermed Bear 33 ventilator. (A and B, courtesy of Bear Medical Corporation, Riverside, CA)

drawing gas through the piston bypass one-way valve and the piston chamber. None of the volume-limited home care ventilators incorporate a demand system.

When the sigh control is activated, a volume equal to one and one-half times the set tidal volume is delivered at a rate of 6 sighs per hour. During sigh breaths the high-pressure alarm setting and expiratory time are increased one and one-half times. A manual sigh can be administered by first unlocking the panel, then activating the sigh control. For multiple sighs the sigh control must be repeatedly activated and deactivated.

Control System

Figure 16-23*B* illustrates the internal gas flow system of the Bear 33. Gas enters the unit at A, the one-way gas entry port of the piston chamber or the optional oxygen accumulator. The accumulator is attached under the basic unit. Gas exits from the piston chamber through the one-way valve at B. If excessive pressure is generated in the piston chamber it is released by a pop-off valve or vent. From B, gas flows into the inspiratory limb to the patient. On the internal aspect of the inspiratory limb a manufacturer's set pressure relief valve is included to dump pressure if it should exceed 85 cm H_2O. In addition, a tee for gas to inflate the exhalation valve and a piston bypass one-way valve (C) are located in the internal ventilation circuit. The bypass valve allows the patient to inspire spontaneously from the circuit when the piston is in its backstroke, closing valve A. This gas entry route is used during SIMV ventilation. At the patient airway is a pressure tap for attachment of the proximal airway pressure line. This line leads to a pressure transducer and provides information to the microprocessor to determine patient triggering effort and pressure alarm activation. Activation of the high-pressure alarm/limit results in termination of the inspiratory phase and release of excessive system pressure. All control panel settings are evaluated by the unit's microprocessor, which, in turn, provides output for overall operation of the ventilator.

The Bear 33 contains an hour meter activated when the unit is turned on. It also has a remote alarm, PEEP valve, and one-way valve for attachment to the exhalation port available as accessories. The one-way exhalation valve is recommended by the manufacturer during ASSIST/CONTROL to decrease gas entry through the exhalation valve.

Output Display

Digital displays of set tidal volume, rate, peak flow, assist sensitivity, high-pressure and low-pressure alarm settings, and inspiratory time are included on the Bear 33.

Alarms

Six alarms are included in the Bear 33: high pressure alarm/limit, low pressure, ventilator inoperative, apnea, low internal battery, and power source change. The high-pressure alarm/limit, when activated, cycles the unit to expiration. It can be set from 10 to 80 cm H_2O. On the first breath that the limit is exceeded, inspiration is terminated and a flashing visual alarm is activated. If during the subsequent breath pressure remains below the limit, the alarm resets itself. If, however, the pressure limit is again exceeded, the audio portion of the alarm is activated. If on subsequent breaths the condition is corrected, the audio portion is reset; however, the visual alarm must be manually reset. If, after activation of the alarm system, pressure does not reduce to below the low-pressure limit within 3 seconds, the machine ceases delivering positive-pressure breaths. If the condition is not resolved in 20 seconds, the apnea alarm is activated; and after 61 seconds the ventilator inoperative alarm is activated.

The low-pressure alarm is adjustable from 3 to 70 cm H_2O. Its function is similar to the high-pressure alarm. If violated for one breath a visual alarm is activated and reset on subsequent breaths. If violated for two consecutive breaths, the audio portion is activated. After audio activation, elimination of the condition results in resetting of the audio portion but the visual portion of the alarm requires manual reset.

The ventilator inoperative alarm is activated if the unit fails to cycle, the inspiratory time limits during positive-pressure ventilation are exceeded, the microprocessor's timing clock fails, the internal power supply fails, or the internal battery power is insufficient to drive the ventilator.

The apnea alarm (audio and visual) is activated if patient inspiratory effort is not sensed for a 20-second period. Detection of patient effort by the ventilator is dependent on the setting of the sensitivity control.

The low internal battery alarm is activated if the internal battery operating capacity is below 25%. This alarm is both visual and audio. If all power were to fail, the machine's internal capacitor would activate the audio alarm for a period of 60 seconds, with the loudness of the alarm diminishing as time proceeded.

The power source change alarm is both an audio and visual alarm that is activated whenever the power source is changed. This alarm must be reset manually.

The Bear 33 also incorporates a 60-second alarm silence that silences audio alarms for all conditions except "Ventilator Inoperative."

Analysis

The unit is designed in a straightforward manner, making it easy to teach patients and caregivers how to operate it. On the other hand, the panel unlock and simultaneous depression of directional arrows and parameters to be changed increases difficulty during patient teaching.[17] These features, however, virtually eliminate inadvertent parameter change. Different-sized ports for attachment of the exhalation port line and the proximal airway pressure are incorporated. The ventilator does not allow the delivery of inverse I:E ratios, which is an advantage for home care use. Finally, this unit may not be appropriate for infant use because tidal volume limit is 100 mL; however, since its tidal volume can be changed in 10-mL increments, it can be used with older pediatric cases.

Nasal Ventilation Devices

RESPIRONICS BIPAP ST

The Respironics BiPAP ST (Respironics, Murrysville, PA) was designed specifically for noninvasive use (Fig. 16-24) by means of a nasal mask.[36] The Respironics ventilator is 7.75″ × 9″ × 12.2″ and weighs 9.5 lbs.

Input Variables

This unit only operates off AC current. It does not have an internal battery; however, it may be attached to an external DC battery.

Control Variables, Phase Variables, and Modes

The Respironics ventilator is an electrically powered, compressor-blower–driven, microprocessor-controlled ventilator that incorporates a single gas flow delivery system producing a decelerating gas flow pattern and a square wave pressure pattern. It is a flow controller. Inspiration is either time (control) or flow (assist/control or assist) triggered and either flow (assist/control, assist) or time (control) cycled.

This unit includes five separate controls: mode selector, inspiratory positive airway pressure (IPAP) level, expiratory positive airway pressure (EPAP) or continuous positive airway pressure (CPAP), rate, and inspiratory time percent. As a result of system design, CPAP is provided, regardless of mode. Even when the EPAP control is set at minimum, a low level of CPAP/PEEP (2 cm H_2O) is maintained in the airway. The mode selector control can be set in seven different positions. The "zero" and "cal" positions are for adjustment and verification of unit function. In either the IPAP or the EPAP position, CPAP is applied to the patient. The level of CPAP is controlled by the corresponding pressure selector. The three other settings are SPONTANEOUS (ASSIST), SPONTANEOUS/TIMED (ASSIST/CONTROL), and TIMED (CONTROL).

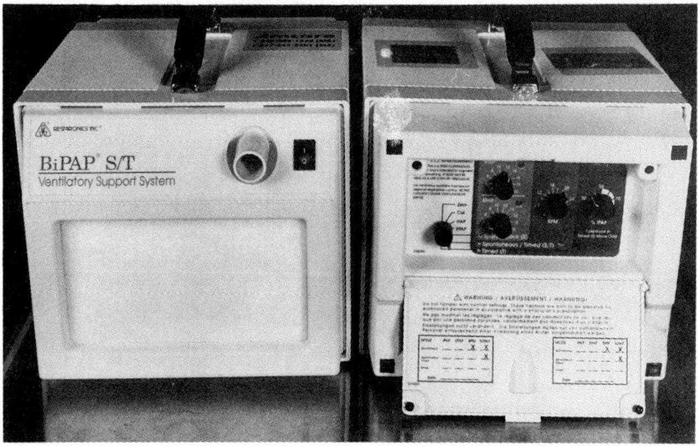

Figure 16-24. The Respironics BiPAP S/T-D ventilator. (Courtesy of Respironics, Murrysville, PA)

In the ASSIST mode the unit essentially functions like pressure support with CPAP, the only other operational controls being the EPAP and IPAP level selectors. When the SPONTANEOUS/TIMED mode is selected, the ventilator operates as if it were applying pressure support with a modified pressure control backup rate. In this mode the EPAP, IPAP, and rate selector, are operational. Here expiration is always flow cycled, with inspiration being flow-triggered if the patient is assisting and time cycled if the backup rate is used.

During TIMED mode ventilation, all controls (IPAP, EPAP, rate, and percent inspiratory time) are operational. In this mode the machine provides pressure control, time-triggered, pressure-limited, time cycled ventilation.

Control System

Instead of being operated by a piston, this ventilator is operated by a compressor-blower and is designed to provide a continuous flow of gas. Delivery gas is drawn into the unit from the filtered back panel by a compressor-blower and then passes through an electromagnetically operated solenoid valve (Fig. 16-25) that controls flow, pressure level, and inspiratory and expiratory time by means of a microprocessor. Before gas leaves the unit it traverses a flow transducer that provides feedback through the microprocessor to the

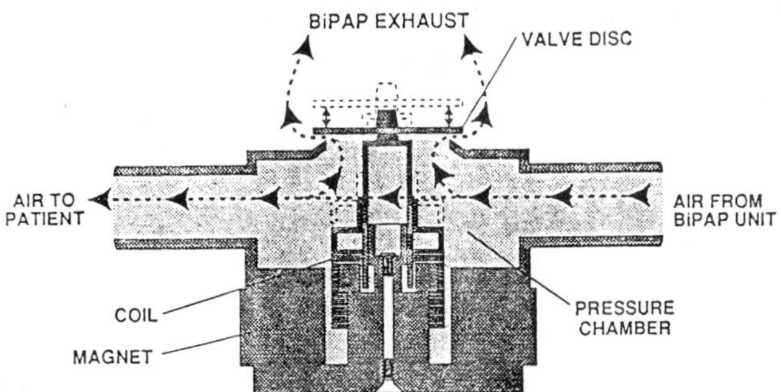

Figure 16-25. The BiPAP pressure/flow control mechanism. The electrical coil and magnet cyclically apply a force to the valve disk that is equal to the IPAP and EPAP settings. Excess pressure is vented to the room, allowing for maintenance of stable pressures despite changes in flow rate. (From BiPAP Ventilatory Support System, Clinical Manual for Models S/T and S/T-D. Form Number 336051, 10/20/89. Respironics, Murrysville, PA)

control solenoid valve. Increased F_{IO_2} can be delivered by continuously bleeding oxygen into the circuit at the ventilator or at the nasal mask.

Alarms

The BiPAP ST ventilator does not incorporate any alarms.

Analysis

This unit is designed only for use in patients who can sustain spontaneous ventilation independent of the unit for prolonged periods of time.[17] It was originally designed for elective nocturnal use to augment nasal CPAP in patients with obstructive sleep apnea.[37] However, it has also been used in acute settings.[38,39] The major factor limiting its use is the fact that no alarms are included in the basic design of the ventilator. Although the unit is designed to be used without a humidifier, the addition of a humidifier does not alter its operation.[40] For reliable function, the whisper swivel (Fig. 16-26) valve which allows a continuous leak, must be included.

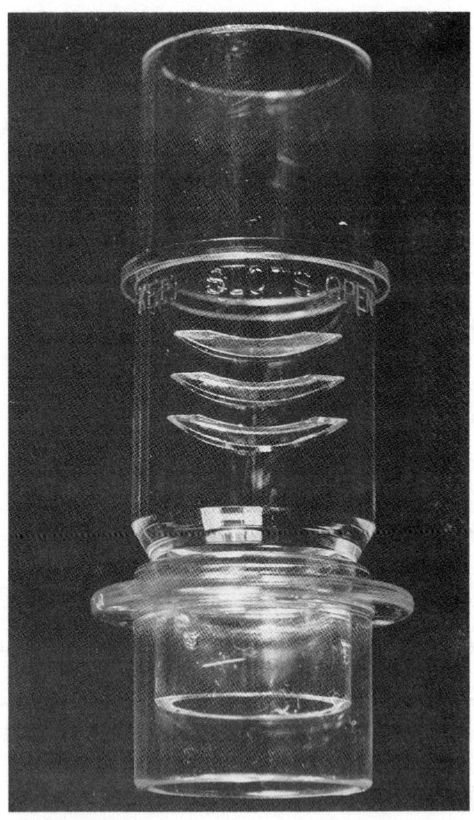

Figure 16-26. Respironics whisper swivel valve provides a fixed leak during use. (From Kacmarek RM, Hess D. Equipment required for home mechanical ventilation. In: Tobin MJ, ed. Principles and Practice of Mechanical Ventilation. New York: McGraw-Hill, 1994)

RESPIRONICS BIPAP ST-D

This unit is exactly the same as the ST model, except that it provides output signals that can be interfaced with a recorder or oscilloscope and has an optional alarm/monitor that monitors high and low airway pressure with up to a 60-second alarm delay. In addition, an optional detachable control panel, which provides calculated estimates of tidal volume and leak, is available for use during set-up or in the sleep laboratory. This unit also displays calculated IPAP and EPAP levels on a breath-by-breath basis.

PURITAN-BENNETT COMPANION 320 I/E

The Puritan-Bennett Companion 320 I/E (Puritan-Bennett Corporation, Lenexa, KS) is a unit designed for nasal ventilation of patients who can sustain spontaneous breathing.[41] This unit is very small ($7 \times 9 \times 7.5$ inches) and is lightweight (8.5 lbs).

Input Variables

The Companion 320 I/E is operated only by AC current.

Control Variables, Phase Variables, and Modes

This is an electrically powered, compressor-blower–driven, microprocessor-controlled ventilator that incorporates a single gas delivery system, producing a decelerating gas flow pattern with a square wave pressure pattern. It is a flow controller. Inspiration is flow triggered and flow cycled.

Only assisted ventilation and CPAP are available with this unit. During assisted ventilation, the clinician has the option of not only setting IPAP and EPAP levels but also of inspiratory and expiratory sensitivity, as well as the use of the delay/ramp option. This option allows the clinician to set the speed of pressure increase to set CPAP level over time, after the completion of a delay period of up to 30 minutes. During the delay period, system pressure is maintained at 3.5 cm H_2O. Once ramping of pressure begins, the rate of rise can be set at 1, 2, or 3 cm H_2O/min. Controls for pressure settings and delay/ramp are located under a panel on the bottom of the machine (adjustable dip switches), while sensitivity controls are located at the back of the machine and accessible to the patient. In addition, a "DELAY ADJUST" control is located next to the sensitivity controls, which allows the patient to vary the delay time from zero minutes to the level set by the clinician. If CPAP is used, IPAP and EPAP are set at the same level.

Control Systems

Room air enters this unit from the back panel directly into a compressor-blower assembly. From there it passes a pressure regulator and flow sensor on its way out of the unit to the patient. Feedback between the unit's microprocessor, pressure regulator, and flow sensor allows the unit to compensate for leaks during gas delivery. A single gas delivery tube leads to the patient. No exhalation valve is included in the circuit. The normal leak at the patient's airway allows exhaled gas to leave the circuit.

Alarms

This unit has no built-in or optional alarms.

Analysis

The Companion 320 I/E is designed only for use in patients capable of breathing spontaneously for prolonged periods of time. The incorporation of both inspiratory and expiratory sensitivity controls, as well as the delay/ramp features during CPAP should greatly assist some patients in acclimating to the machine, both initially and on a daily basis.[17] Since the unit provides only assisted ventilation, complete unloading of ventilatory work and the provision of controlled ventilation is impossible to achieve.

Common Features of All Positive-Pressure Home Care Ventilators

Delivery of Increased F_{IO_2}

The typical home mechanical ventilator is not designed to provide a precise F_{IO_2} above 0.21. The reason for this is that few patients receiving home ventilation require a precise or high F_{IO_2}. Typically, an F_{IO_2} of 0.25 to 0.35 is needed, and a 0.05 variation in F_{IO_2} is clinically acceptable in these patients.

Only the Lifecare PLV-102, by the use of a proportioning solenoid valve, is capable of setting and maintaining a precise F_{IO_2}. The other ventilators increase F_{IO_2} by the attachment of an O_2 accumulator to the gas entry port or the titration of O_2 into the inspiratory limb between the ventilator and the humidifier (or internally). The one exception occurs if nasal mask ventilation is performed. In this case, oxygen may be delivered directly into masks that include pressure monitoring and O_2 delivery ports. If this option is used, it is difficult to approximate, and impossible to measure, F_{IO_2}.

An O_2 accumulator is a large, rectangular box attached to the gas entry port within which oxygen and room air mix to establish a desired F_{IO_2}. Oxygen is bled into the accumulator while room air is drawn into the accumulator during the backstroke of the piston. In spite of the fact that all manufacturers provide elaborate formulas to calculate F_{IO_2} delivered in this way, these formulas are only correct if the patient is ventilated in the CONTROL mode. Variation in the ventilator rate, tidal volume, oxygen flow, and level of spontaneous breathing all affect the breath-by-breath F_{IO_2} delivered. Oxygen accumulators are available on the Companion 2800, Companion 2801, PLV-100, Bear

33, LP-6, LP-6 Plus, and LP-10. Figure 16-19 depicts the accumulator used on the LP-6.

F_{IO_2} may be increased in all units (including pressure-limited units) by the use of an O_2 delivery elbow (Fig. 16-27) between the ventilator and the humidifier. As with the O_2 accumulator, the F_{IO_2} delivered is affected by all ventilatory variables. In general, a more stable F_{IO_2} is possible with the accumulator than with the O_2 delivery elbow. In addition, a bias flow added at the outflow port of the ventilator increases the effort required to trigger the ventilator to inspiration during ASSIST/CONTROL ventilation.

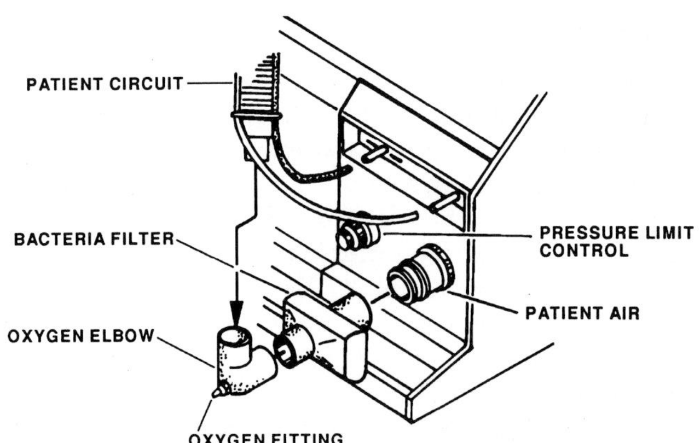

Figure 16-27. Oxygen delivery elbow used on the LP series ventilators; however, this type of adaptor may be used on any of the home care ventilators. Oxygen is titrated directly into the inspiratory limb, bypassing the piston chamber. (From Aequitron LP-6 Compact Volume Ventilator: User's Guide and Instruction Manual. Minneapolis, MN: Aequitron Medical Inc, 1985)

SIMV/IMV and Work of Breathing

None of the volume-controlled home care ventilators incorporates a demand system. Thus, during the spontaneous breathing phase of SIMV, the patient must draw gas from either the piston chamber, a piston chamber bypass valve, or through the exhalation valve. As a result, even with the use of an optimal humidifying system (passover humidifier) a large amount of work is imposed by the ventilator system.[42,43] This work increases as patient peak spontaneous inspiratory flow rate increases and by the use of a bubble-through humidifier. The use of a cascade humidifier can more than double the work imposed by the ventilator during the spontaneous breathing phase of SIMV.[42]

Whenever the SIMV mode is used, it is recommended that a passover humidifier is used as well as the incorporation of a one-way H-valve between the ventilator and the humidifier. This set-up reduces the inspiratory work imposed during the spontaneous breathing phase of SIMV.[42] If an increased F_{IO_2} is required, a reservoir bag system should be added to the H-valve setup. (See Chapter 18.)

The addition of a one-way H-valve, particularly if an increased F_{IO_2} is desired, complicates the ventilator set-up, limits portability, and wastes oxygen. Because of the difficulty in oxygen delivery and the increased workload, the use of the SIMV mode on home care ventilators should be avoided. Until these units incorporate demand systems that reduce the imposed work of breathing, it seems best to maintain patients at home in the ASSIST/CONTROL mode.

Humidification

Three basic humidification systems may be used with home care ventilators: bubble, passover, and artificial noses. Bubble humidifiers should never be used during SIMV. During control (patient not breathing around control breath) and assist/control ventilation, bubble humidifiers function well. Artificial noses, while not recommended on a continuous basis, are very useful during transport and periods of time away from home. The use of these devices greatly simplifies the ventilator set-up on a wheelchair or in a car. When the patient returns home, changing to a bubble or passover humidifier is recommended. The ventilatory load of artificial noses increases with time and varies from one unit to another.[43,44] There are no published data to support the use of artificial noses as the sole source of humidity for mechanically ventilated patients in the home.

Application of PEEP

A PEEP device can be added to the ventilator circuit of any home care ventilator. Unless control ventilation is used, the increased work of breathing is great, since none of these units automatically compensates for PEEP.[17] In the ASSIST/CONTROL mode, the sensitivity must be adjusted to decrease the pressure gradient necessary to trigger the unit. That is, if 5 cm H_2O PEEP is applied, the sensitivity must be set to about +4 cm H_2O (1 cm H_2O below baseline required to trigger inspiration). However, many patients at home do not maintain a tight seal at the tracheostomy cuff, which increases the likelihood of auto-triggering when PEEP is used.

PEEP should not be used in the SIMV mode. Appropriate setting of the sensitivity may allow for triggering during positive-pressure breaths. However, the work of breathing during spontaneous breaths is markedly increased. The pressure gradient required to inspire is increased by the amount of PEEP applied. If indications for the use of PEEP arise, use of the ASSIST/CONTROL mode with appropriate sensitivity setting is recommended.

Pediatric Ventilation

The ventilation of pediatric patients is a challenge with the present generation of home care ventilators. Systems almost always require modifications to ensure proper gas delivery. Pressure-limited ventilation is commonly used.[45] Pop-off or pressure limiting valves attached in the circuit between the ventilator and the humidifier accomplish the same result. With many small infants the addition of a continuous-flow system is essential to allow the child to interface with the ventilator.[46] None of the home care ventilators is designed for the pediatric patient, and extreme care and diligent monitoring is required for successful ventilation of this population.

Facial Appliances for Noninvasive Positive-Pressure Ventilation

The most difficult aspect of establishing noninvasive positive-pressure ventilation (NIPPV) is finding a properly fitting appliance. Four different approaches are in use: full-face mask, nasal mask, nasal pillows, and mouthpieces. Each of these approaches should be considered with every patient, although there are different problems with each appliance.

Full-Face Masks

Full-face masks have been the appliance of choice for the delivery of NIPPV in acutely ill patients[46–48] and patients[47–49] requiring long-term ventilatory support (Fig. 16-28).[50–53] There are many face masks available, and most work well, provided that a proper fit is achieved. The ideal face mask for long-term ventilation is made of clear plastic to allow visual assessment of secretions, has a soft inflatable cuff that conforms to the anatomy of the patient's face, is easily deformed from its factory shape as needed to fit the patient, and has memory so it maintains its deformed shape when the mask is removed.[17] Ideally, a number of different masks of varying sizes should be available when attempting to fit a mask to a particular patient.

Once an appropriate mask is chosen, proper fit of the mask is essential. Leaks at the bridge of the nose, causing air to blow into the patient's eyes, will result in NIPPV failure owing to patient intolerance. The mask should fit comfortably from just below the lower lip to near the top of the bridge of the nose. The exact fit depends on the patient. Patient comfort is essential, and the patient is always the final judge of proper fit.

The most common error in securing the mask to the patient's face is exerting excessive pressure.[17] With NIPPV, low peak airway pressures (generally 15 to 20 cm H_2O) are usually used. Because some leak is expected, masks do not need to be secured so tightly that pressure sores develop. Firm, evenly distributed pressure over the entire mask is usually sufficient to make a seal. If a patient cannot tolerate the facial pressure, the whole process may fail.

Nasal Masks

The most popular approach to the application of NIPPV is the use of nasal masks. Ideally, these masks are customized for the patient (Fig. 16-29), and they can be created from a mold of the patient's face. However, numerous commercial nasal masks are available that work well on most patients. One such

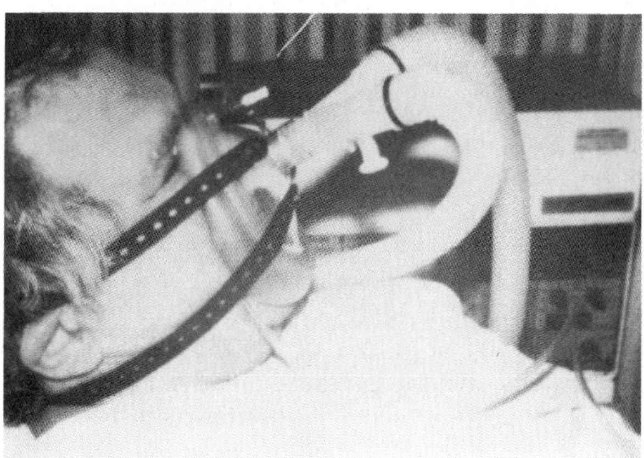

Figure 16-28. Application of NIPPV by means of full face mask. (From Meduri GU, Conoscenti CC, Menashe PH, Nair S. Noninvasive face mask ventilation in patients with acute respiratory failure. Chest 1989;95:865–870)

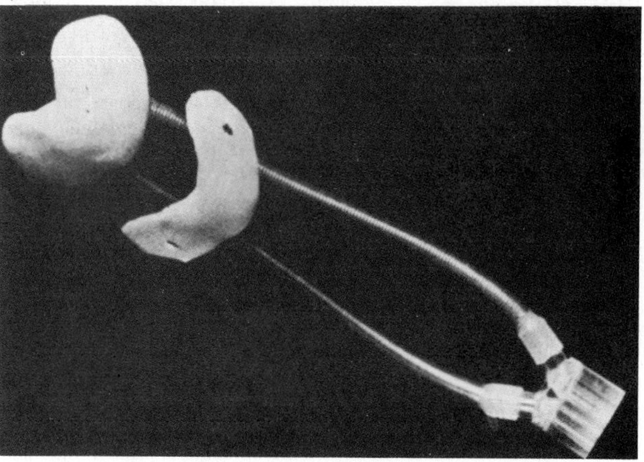

Figure 16-29. Customized nasal positive-pressure mask. (From Leger P, Jennequin J, Gerard M, Robert D. Home positive-pressure ventilation via nasal mask for patients with neuromuscular weakness or restrictive lung or chest wall disease. Respir Care 1989;34:73–79)

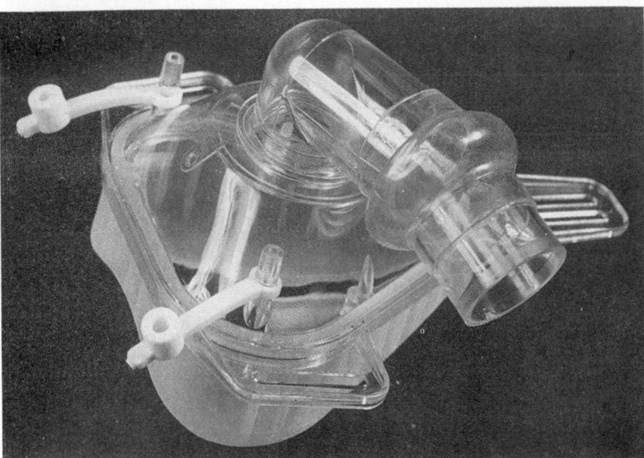

Figure 16-30. Respironics nasal positive-pressure mask. (From Kacmarek RM, Hess D. Equipment required for home mechanical ventilation. In: Tobin MJ, ed. Principles and Practice of Mechanical Ventilation. New York: McGraw-Hill, 1994)

mask is the Respironics nasal mask (Fig. 16-30). It is made of clear plastic and instead of using an inflatable cuff, it has an inner lip of ¼ to ½ inch that forms an open space between the inner and outer wall of the mask. When positive pressure is applied, force is exerted between the inner and outer folds, creating a better seal during the application of the inspiratory pressure. Because of this, only low to moderate pressure is needed to secure the mask. As with the full-face mask, pressure must be applied equally at the three points of connection to the head gear; at the bridge of the nose and at each side of the mask. If a proper fitting mask is chosen, and moderate but equal pressure is applied at each connection, a very comfortable fit is achieved.

Choosing the proper size mask is critical. As a general rule, the smaller the mask the better the fit.[17] There are about six sizes of masks available from Respironics. However, nearly all patients are fitted with the three smallest masks. Respironics provides a template (Fig. 16-31) that greatly helps in proper sizing of masks. The ideal mask fits closely to the lateral contour of the nose, extending from just under the external nares to near the top of the bridge of the nose.

Chin straps are also available to reduce mouth leak. Although they are frequently tried, they infrequently reduce mouth leak. If patients are actively opposing nasal NIPPV, nothing eliminates mouth leak. In many patients, the extent of the mouth leak decreases as they acclimate to ventilation. Many patients who have a large leak while awake demonstrate little or no leak while sleeping, or vice versa. Since peak pressures are

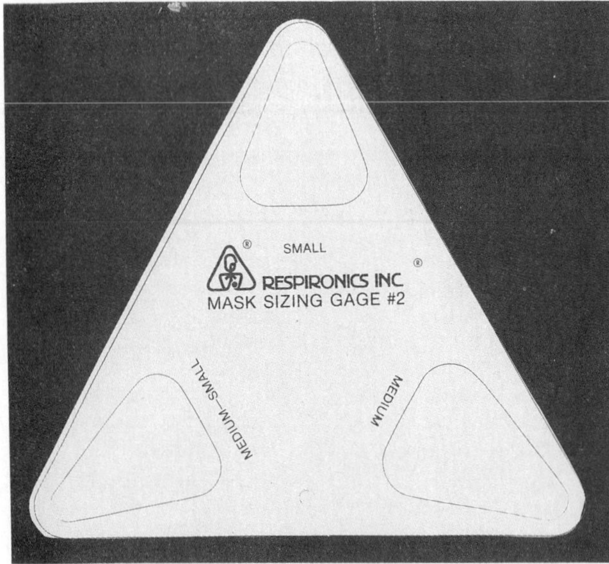

Figure 16-31. Respironics nasal positive-pressure mask sizing template. (From Kacmarek RM, Hess D. Equipment required for home mechanical ventilation. In: Tobin MJ, ed. Principles and Practice of Mechanical Ventilation. New York: McGraw-Hill, 1994)

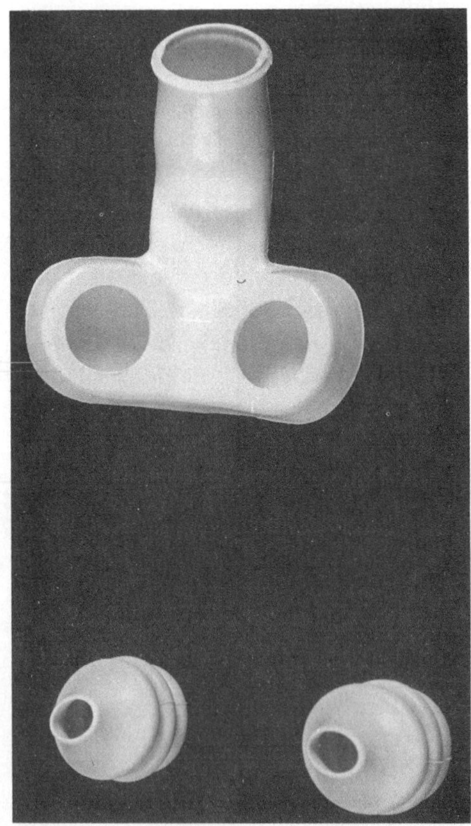

Figure 16-32. Individual Puritan-Bennett nasal pillows with manifold for attachment to large bore tubing. (From Kacmarek RM, Hess D. Equipment required for home mechanical ventilation. In: Tobin MJ, ed. Principles and Practice of Mechanical Ventilation. New York: McGraw-Hill, 1994)

usually 15 to 20 cm H_2O, during sleep the soft palate and the base of the tongue are elevated sufficiently to prevent excessive leak.

Nasal Pillows

A variation on the application of nasal ventilation, nasal pillows (Fig. 16-32), are available from several manufacturers. The individual pillows fit into a manifold that is attached over the top of the patient's head (Fig. 16-33). Some patients actually prefer this approach over the nasal mask, while others who are sensitive to face pressure actually use both nasal masks and nasal pillows, switching back and forth as irritation develops. Because of difference in design, the points of pressure differ greatly between the two approaches. There are three sizes of pillows, corresponding to the size of an individual's external nares.

Mouthpieces

Many patients who use negative-pressure ventilation at night use periodic positive-pressure ventilation during the day. In others, mouthpiece positive-pressure ventilation has been applied 24 hours per day.[54] This requires more than the use of a standard mouthpiece. Some commercially available mouthpieces with inner flanges are available (Fig. 16-34). However, patients do best when an acrylic customized mouthpiece is made from an impression of the patient's mouth (Fig. 16-35). With a customized mouthpiece, many patients are capable of comfortably maintaining ventilation for indefinite periods. Most do not experience significant nasal

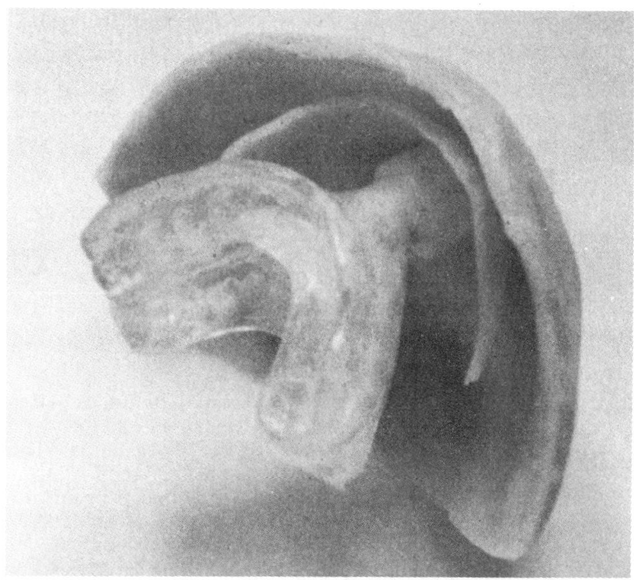

Figure 16-34. Commercially available flanged mouthpiece. (From Back JR, Alba A, Saporito LR. Intermittent positive-pressure ventilation via the mouth as an alternative to tracheostomy for 257 ventilator users. Chest 1993;103: 174–182)

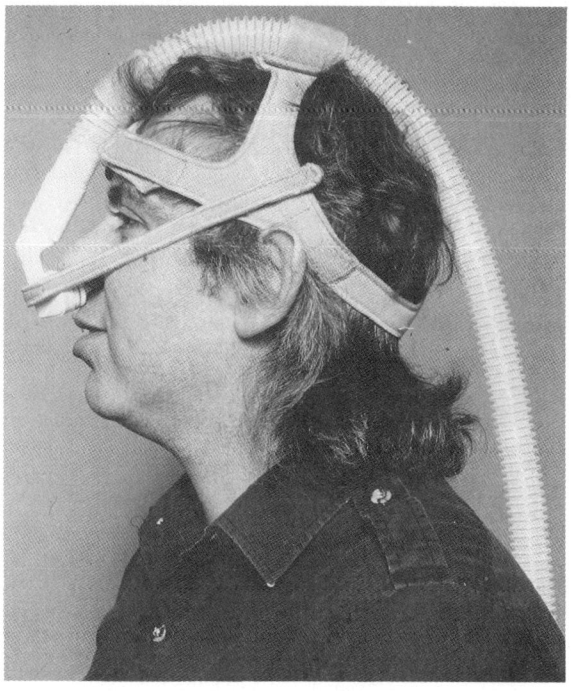

Figure 16-33. Method of attaching nasal pillows and manifold to a patient. (Courtesy of Puritan-Bennett Corporation, Lenexa, KS)

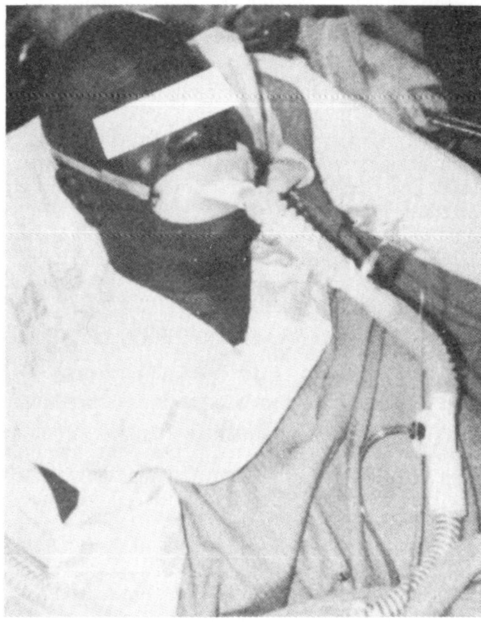

Figure 16-35. Customized mouthpiece for continuous positive-pressure ventilation. (From Back JR, Alba A, Saporito LR. Intermittent positive-pressure ventilation via the mouth as an alternative to tracheostomy for 257 ventilator users. Chest 1993;103:174–182)

leaks during sleep, while others also require nasal plugs or nose clips. With this approach, monitoring for sores on the gum line is necessary.

References

1. Leger P, Bedicarn JM, Cornette A, et al. Nasal intermittent positive-pressure ventilation: Long-term follow-up in patients with severe respiratory insufficiency. Chest 1994;105:100–105.
2. Gigliotti F, Spinelli A, Duranti R, Gorini M, Goti G, Scano G. Four-week negative-pressure ventilation improves respiratory function in severe hypercapnic COPD patients. Chest 1994;105: 87–94.
3. Corrado A, DePaola E, Messori A, Bruscoli G, Nutino S. The effect of intermittent negative-pressure ventilation and long-term oxygen therapy for patients with COPD: A 4-year study. Chest 1994;105:95–99.
4. Yang GW, Alba A, Lee M. Pneumobelt for sleep in the ventilator user: Clinical experience. Arch Phys Med Rehabil 1989;20: 707–711.
5. Leger P, Jennequin J, Gerard M, Robert D. Home positive-pressure ventilation via nasal mask for patients with neuromuscular weakness or restrictive lung or chest wall disease. Respir Care 1989;34:23–77.
6. Corrado A, Bruscoli G, DePaola E, Ciardi-Dupre GF, Baccini A, Taddei M. Respiratory muscle insufficiency in acute respiratory failure of subject with severe COPD: Treatment with intermittent negative-pressure ventilation. Eur Respir J 1990;3:644–648.
7. Cropp A, DiMarco AF. Affects of intermittent negative-pressure ventilation on respiratory muscle function in patient with severe chronic obstructive pulmonary disease. Am Rev Respir Dis 1987;135:1056–1061.
8. Kacmarek RM. The practical application of home mechanical ventilatory equipment. J Neurol Rehabil 1992;6:103–112.
9. Pierson DJ, Kacmarek RM. Home ventilator care. In: Casoburi R, Petty T, eds. Principles and Practice of Pulmonary Rehabilitation, 2nd ed. Philadelphia: WB Saunders, 1993:274–288.
10. Bach JR, Alba AS. Non-invasive options for ventilatory support of the traumatic high-level quadriplegic patient. Chest 1990; 98:613–619.
11. Back JA, Alba AS. Management of chronic alveolar hypoventilation by nasal ventilation. Chest 1990;97:52–57.
12. Hill NS. Clinical application of body ventilators. Chest 1986; 90:897–905.
13. Adamson JP, Lewis L, Stein JD. Application of abdominal pressure for artificial respiration. JAMA 1959;169:1613–1617.
14. Kacmarek RM, Spearman CB. Equipment used for ventilatory support in the home. Respir Care 1986;31:311–328.
15. Drinker PA, Shaw LA. An apparatus for the prolonged administration of artificial ventilation. J Clin Invest 1926;7:229–247.
16. Drinker PA, McKhann CF. The iron lung, first practical means of respiratory support. JAMA 1986;255:1476–1480.
17. Kacmarek RM, Hess D. Equipment required for home mechanical ventilation. In: Tobin MJ, ed. Principles and Practice of Mechanical Ventilation. New York: McGraw-Hill, 1994.
18. Emerson Negative-Pressure Ventilator (product literature 33-CRE). Cambridge, MA: J.H. Emerson Co.
19. Emerson Negative-Pressure Ventilator (product literature 33-CR Form No. 910-1098-0). Cambridge, MA: J.H. Emerson Co.
20. Lifecare 170C Respirator Operation and Maintenance Manual. Boulder, CO: Lifecare, 1980.
21. Lifecare NEV-100 Operating Manual (Form #12500A). Lafayette, CO: Lifecare International, 1992.
22. Puritan-Bennett Thompson Maxivent (product and operation literature). Lenexa, KS: Puritan-Bennett Corporation, 1979.
23. Guitierrez M, Berioza T, Contraras G, et al. Weekly cuirass ventilation improves blood gases and inspiratory muscle strength in patients with chronic airflow limitation and hypercarbia. Am Rev Respir Dis 1988;138:617–623.
24. Cropp A, Dimarro AF. Effects of intermittent negative-pressure ventilation on respiratory muscle function in patients with severe chronic obstructive pulmonary disease. Am Rev Respir Dis 1987;135:1056–1061.
25. Scano G, Gigliotti F, Duranti R, Spinelli A. Gorini M, Schlavina M. Changes in ventilatory muscle function with negative ventilation in patients with severe COPD. Chest 1990;97:322–327.
26. Shapiro SH, Ernst P, Gray-Donald K, et al. Effect of negative pressure ventilation in severe pulmonary disease. Lancet 1992; 340:1425–1429.
27. Hill NS, Redine S, Carskadon M, Curran FJ, Millman RP. Sleep-disordered breathing in patients with Duchenne muscular dystrophy using negative pressure ventilators. Chest 1992;102: 1656–1662.
28. Puritan-Bennett Companion 2800 Clinician Guide. Lenexa, KS: Puritan-Bennett Corporation, 1985.
29. Puritan-Bennett Companion 2801 Volume Ventilator, Operating Instruction Manual, Form No. T12963 Issue B. Lenexa, KS: Puritan-Bennett Corporation, 1990.
30. Puritan-Bennett Companion 2500 Portable Volume Ventilator, Form T No. T12650. Lenexa, KS: Puritan-Bennett Corporation, 1988.
31. Aequitron LP-6 Compact Volume Ventilator: User's Guide and Instruction Manual. Minneapolis, MN: Aequitron Medical, 1985.
32. Aequitron LP-10 Volume Ventilator with Pressure Limit Clinician's Manual. Minneapolis, MN: Aequitron Medical, 1991.
33. Lifecare PLV-100 Operating Manual. Lafayette, CO: Lifecare, 1986.
34. Lifecare PLV-102 Operating Manual. Form #37-500E. Lafayette, CO: Lifecare, 1991.
35. Intermed Bear 33 Clinical Instruction Manual. Riverside, CA: Bear Medical Corporation, 1987.
36. BiPAP Ventilatory Support System, Clinical Manual for Models S/T and S/T-D. Form Number 336051, 10/20/89. Murrysville, PA: Respironics.
37. Strumpf DA, Carlisle CC, Millman RP, Smith KW, Hill NS. An evaluation of the Respironics BiPAP Bilevel CPAP device for delivery of assisted ventilation. Respir Care 1990;35:415–422.
38. Marino W. Intermittent volume-cycled mechanical ventilation via nasal mask in patients with respiratory failure due to COPD. Chest 1991;99:681–684.
39. Sanders MH, Kern N. Obstructive sleep apnea treated by independently adjusted inspiratory and expiratory positive airway pressures via nasal mask: Physiologic and clinical implications. Chest 1990;98:317–324.
40. Hirsch C, Robart P, Barker S, Kacmarek RM. Inspiratory work of breathing imposed (WOBI) by the Respironics BiPAP ventilator (abstract). Respir Care 1992;37:1315.
41. Puritan-Bennett Companion 320 I/E ventilator Form No. 799855 Rev. A. Lenexa, KS: Puritan-Bennett Corporation, 1993.
42. Kacmarek RM, Stanek KS, McMahon KM, Wilson RS. Imposed work of breathing during synchronized intermittent mandatory ventilation: Provided by five home care ventilators. Respir Care 1990;35:405–414.
43. Robart P, Hirsch C, Barker S, Kacmarek RM. Work of breathing imposed during spontaneous breathing in the SIMV mode of the newest home care ventilators (abstract). Respir Care 1192; 37:1358.
44. Ploysongsang Y, Branson RD, Rashkin MC, Hurst JM. Effect of flow rate and duration of use on the pressure drop across six artificial noses. Respir Care 1989;34:902–907.
45. Kacmarek RM, Thompson JE. Respiratory care of the ventilator-assisted infant in the home. Respir Care 1986;31:605–614.
46. O'Donohue WJ, Giovannoni RM, Goldberg AL, et al. Long-term mechanical ventilation: Guidelines for management in the home and at alternate community sites (consensus report). Chest 1986;Supplement 1S-37S.
47. Brochard L, Isabey D, Piquet J, et al. Reversal of acute exacerbations of chronic obstructive lung disease by inspiratory assistance with a face mask. N Engl J Med 1990;323:1523–1529.
48. Meduri GU, Abou-Shala N, Fox RC, Jones CB, Leeper KV, Wunderink RG. Noninvasive face mask mechanical ventilation in patients with acute respiratory failure. Chest 1991;100:445–454.
49. Meduri GU, Conoscenti CC, Menashe PH, Nair S. Noninvasive

face mask ventilation in patients with acute respiratory failure. Chest 1989;95:865–870.
50. Back JR, O'Brien J, Krotenberg R, Alba A. Management of end stage respiratory failure in Duchenne muscular dystrophy. Muscle Nerve 1987;10:177–182.
51. Alexander MA, Johnson EW, Petty J, Stauch D. Mechanical ventilation of patients with late-stage Duchenne muscular dystrophy: Management in the home. Arch Phys Med Rehabil 1979; 60:289–292.
52. Goldstein RS, Avendano MA. Long-term mechanical ventilation as elective therapy: Clinical status and future prospects. Respir Care 1991;36:297–304.
53. Branthwaite MA. Noninvasive and domiciliary ventilation: Positive-pressure techniques. Thorax 1991;46:208–212.
54. Back JR, Alba A, Saporito LR. Intermittent positive-pressure ventilation via the mouth as an alternative to tracheostomy for 257 ventilator users. Chest 1993;103:174–182

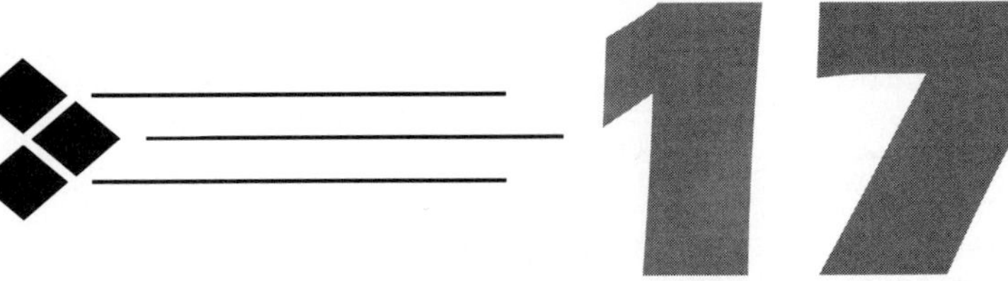

17 High-Frequency Ventilators

Richard D. Branson

OBJECTIVES

1. Compare and contrast high-frequency ventilation with conventional ventilation.
2. Describe the differences in high-frequency ventilation techniques.
3. List the potential advantages and disadvantages of high-frequency ventilation.
4. List the complications associated with high-frequency ventilation.
5. Describe the theories of gas movement during high-frequency ventilation.

KEY TERMS

bias flow
hertz (Hz)
high-frequency flow interrupter
high-frequency jet ventilation
high-frequency oscillation
high-frequency percussive ventilation
high-frequency positive-pressure ventilation
high-frequency ventilation
low pass filter

Introduction

The future of high-frequency ventilation (HFV) in clinical practice is unclear. Advocates believe HFV is firmly entrenched in the critical care armamentarium, whereas skeptics are anxious to see HFV condemned to the museum of medical history. All, however, agree that concentrated research into every aspect of HFV has stimulated clinicians to reevaluate the ways in which we look at gas exchange, control of ventilation, and cardiopulmonary interactions.

During the period from 1970 to 1985, some 800 papers were published on varying aspects of HFV. Comparisons of results have been extremely difficult since investigators have used different HFV techniques, varied the equipment, and have studied everything from fowl (geese, ducks, chickens) through the evolutionary chain to rabbits, cats, dogs, horses, monkeys, and, finally, humans. This proliferation of research prompted Froese to suggest that "this flurry of activity appears to have generated more noise than light."[1]

The aim of this chapter is to acquaint the reader with the different techniques of HFV and the principles of operation and to describe briefly the potential clinical uses and complications of HFV.

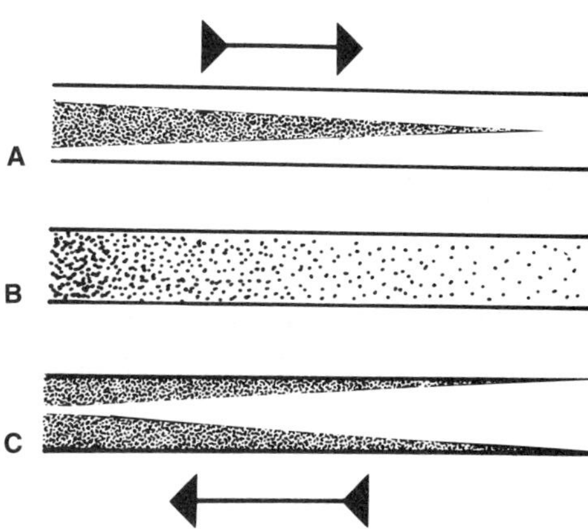

Figure 17-1. The parabolic spike as described by Henderson. When smoke is forcefully blown into one end, it does not immediately fill the tube. Instead, a spike of smoke travels radially toward the other end. The volume of the smoke is less than the tube, yet it crosses the entire length. When the end of the tube is blocked, smoke fills the entire tube. A rapid withdrawal of gas creates a spike of fresh air traveling back through the tube. The faster the injection, the smaller the spike that is produced.

Historical Aspects

The relevant history of HFV really starts in the early 1970s. Before this, however, there are two contributions that deserve mention. In 1915, Henderson and colleagues found that ventilation could be maintained with tidal volumes less than anatomical deadspace.[2] This work was performed on "panting" dogs and led the investigators to believe there must be alternative mechanisms of gas transport in major airways. To test their hypothesis, Henderson and associates[2] constructed a series of glass tubes (stimulating the tracheobronchial tree) and injected smoke into the mouth of the tube. They observed a "parabolic spike" of smoke during rapid injections. The "parabolic spike" is the foundation of the axial diffusion theory of gas transport (Fig. 17-1).[3]

In 1959, Emerson patented a device to "vibrate" gas in the airway during conventional ventilation, hoping to improve intrapulmonary gas mixing. To quote from Emerson, "vibrating the column of gas undoubtedly causes the gas to diffuse more rapidly within the airway and, therefore, aids in the breathing function by circulating the gas more thoroughly."[4] This device is still used today and represents the first true high-frequency ventilator devised.

Types of High-Frequency Ventilation

Among the most confounding aspects of HFV is the lack of uniform classification and standardized nomenclature. Authors have suggested there are as few as three varieties of HFV and as many as nine. Generically, the term refers to any of these techniques whose major characteristic is a respiratory frequency of four times normal.[5]

Early attempts at classifying HFV were based on cycling frequency: (1) high-frequency positive-pressure ventilation: 60–110 cpm, (2) high-frequency jet ventilation: 110–400 cpm, and (3) high-frequency oscillation: 400–2400 cpm.[6] This system fell apart quickly as investigators used high-frequency jet ventilators in the high-frequency oscillation range and vice versa. Froese and Bryan[5] have suggested that techniques be placed into two main categories on the basis of the expiratory phase: (1) active (A), or (2) passive (P). This system is helpful but does not cover the techniques in sufficient detail.

In an effort to clarify the types of HFV (and not to further confuse), five varieties of HFV are listed: (1) high-frequency positive pressure ventilation (HFPPV), (2) high-frequency jet ventilation (HFJV), (3) high-frequency flow interruption (HFFI), (4) high-frequency oscillation (HFO), and (5) high-frequency percussive ventilation (HFPV).

High-Frequency Positive-Pressure Ventilation

HFPPV was developed by Sjöstrand in Sweden around 1967.[7] While studying the carotid sinus reflex, Sjostrand was faced with the problem of eliminating respiration-related alternation in blood pressure. He devised a low deadspace system (50 mL) and used a circuit with minimal compressible volume. It was hypothesized that if tidal volume was reduced and the ventilator rate increased, CO_2 elimination would be adequate for at least the 30 minutes required for the investigation. In fact, this new mode of ventilation was capable of maintaining normal gas exchange in healthy animals indefinitely.[7]

The hardware used for HFPPV consists of a specially designed, time-triggered, time-cycled, volume-limited ventilator with minimal compressible volume (< 0.06 mL/cm H_2O), capable of delivering gas at high flow rates (175–250 L/min). The ventilator/airway interface consists of a fluidic valve, based on the Coanda or wall attachment effect (Fig. 17-2). This system permits delivery of gas from the ventilator through a side-arm and exhalation through a larger main channel. An exhalation valve, attached to the main channel of the fluidic valve, allows for the application of end-expiratory pressure and control of mean airway pressure. Gas entrainment does not occur during HFPPV. This permits accurate control of tidal volume. Optimum operating frequency is between 60 and 110 cpm with a tidal volume of 2.5 to 3.5 mL/kg. Inspiratory time is 15% to 35% of the respiratory cycle; expiration is passive; and the I:E ratio is generally 1:3 or greater. A schematic of a HFPPV system is shown in Figure 17-3.

Commercially available devices in Europe allow for independent control of tidal volume, frequency, pressure limit, and I:E ratio. These devices are not marketed in the United States. Humidification is accomplished with a standard humidifier in the main gas flow. The use of modified conventional ventilators to deliver HFPPV has been described in the literature.[8] Many of these ventilators do not possess the flow capabilities necessary to deliver HFPPV effectively. An inadequate flow rate coupled with excessive resistance from commercially available exhalation valves could result in the development of auto-PEEP and pulmonary barotrauma. Most HFV options of pediatric and neonatal ventilators are a form of HFPPV.

Clinical Uses

The major advantages of HFPPV have been seen in the operating theater. HFPPV has been used extensively during laryngoscopy, bronchoscopy, and upper airway surgery.[9] In this setting, the unique fluidic value allows ventilation through a small catheter, allowing the surgeon an improved operative view. The use of HFPPV in acute respiratory failure has been described, but no concrete advantages have been proven.[10,11]

High-Frequency Jet Ventilation

High-frequency jet ventilation was developed in the United States by Klain and Smith in 1977.[12] The simple design of jet ventilators combined with commercial availability has made HFJV the most popular of HFV techniques.

HFJV provides intermittent delivery of gas from a high-pressure source (20–50 psig) through a cannula situated in the airway or endotracheal tube. The ventilator consists of an air–oxygen blender, a system for regulating inlet pressure (psig), and a cycling mechanism (usually an electronically controlled solenoid valve or a fluidic valve). High-pressure gas at the desired F_{IO_2} and driving pressure is delivered to the cycling mechanism. In the case of a solenoid valve, control is limited to frequency (the number of times the solenoid valve opens and closes) and percent inspiratory time (% T_I) (the amount of time the solenoid stays open relative to the entire cycle). An example would be if f = 100 cpm and % T_I was 30%, then one cycle would be 0.6 second and T_I = 0.18 second.

After exiting the solenoid, gas travels into the low compressible volume circuit to the airway or "jet" catheter. Inside the endotracheal tube, high-pressure gas exits the catheter into the larger opening. The resulting rapid reduction in pressure causes ambient air to be entrained into the airway (Fig. 17-4). This is not a venturi system but rather works by the principle of

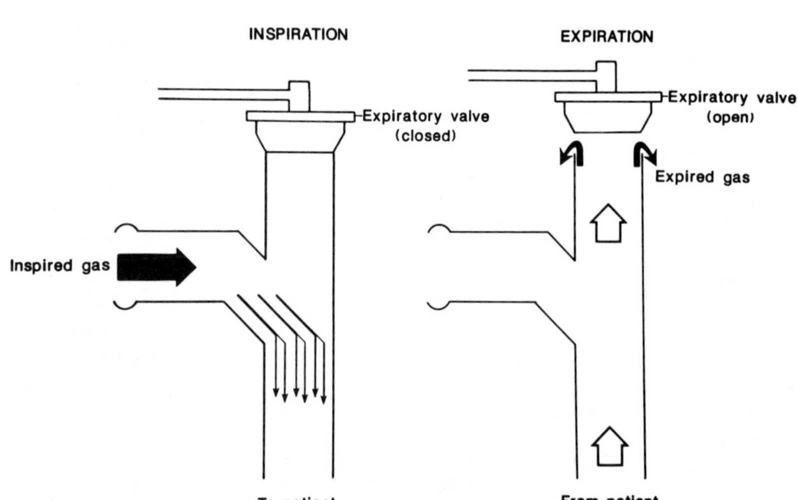

Figure 17-2. Fluidic valve used during HFPPV. See text for description.

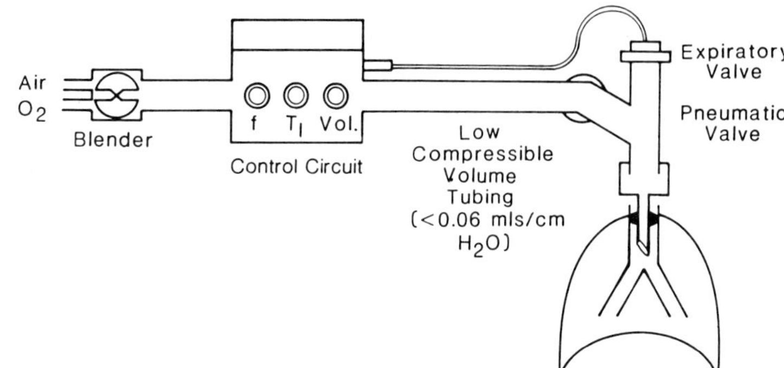

Figure 17-3. The essential parts of an HFPPV system. See text for description.

"jet mixing." Jet mixing occurs when high-flowing gas contacts stagnant gas in the airway. Viscous shearing between the two "layers" causes the stagnant gas to be "dragged" into the airway.[13] The result is an increase in the total volume delivered to the patient. This can be measured by placing volume-measuring devices at the site of entrainment and at the expiratory valve. Total expired volume minus the entrained volume equals the volume delivered by the jet ventilator. Delivered volume is a somewhat precarious relationship between driving pressure, % Tɪ, catheter size, and the patient's pulmonary mechanics (resistance and compliance).[14,15] Since entrainment is a feature, when back pressure increases, entrainment will decrease. As such, sudden changes in compliance and resistance will result in delivery of inconsistent tidal volumes. Mean airway pressure and, hence, oxygenation are controlled by driving pressure, I:E ratio, and PEEP.

The optimum position of the catheter in the airway has been a subject of some debate. Authors have advocated positions as low as 1 to 2 cm above the carina, mid-airway, and proximal airway positions. Entrainment appears to be best with a proximal jet position. Low jet positions were thought to be beneficial since the tracheal deadspace volume was bypassed. Generally, low jet positions have been abandoned since distal migration of the catheter drastically reduces entrainment. There was also a concern by some investigators that trauma to the tracheal epithelium from high-velocity gases was occurring.[16,17]

Optimum HFJV frequency appears to be between 100 and 200 cpm in adults, with higher frequencies being used in infants and neonates. % Tɪ is usually maintained between 0.20 and 0.50 second, providing an I:E ratio of no less than 1:1. At Tɪ of 0.50 or greater, unacceptable levels of inadvertent PEEP may develop resulting in hemodynamic compromise, CO_2, and potentially barotrauma.[18]

There are several HFJV devices marketed in the United States. Indications for HFJV include (1) during laryngoscopy, (2) during bronchoscopy, and (3) in patients with "pulmonary air leaks" (pneumothorax, bronchopleural fistulae, pulmonary interstitial emphysema).

One of the confounding problems during HFJV has been achieving adequate humidification. Early in its use, only entrained gas was humidified. This was adequate in subjects with normal lungs, but as patients who were more seriously ill were studied, and lung compliance fell, entrainment was reduced. The result was inadequate humidification, drying of secretions, damage to the airway epithelium, and resultant plugging of endotracheal tubes.[15,19] At present, humidification of the entrained gases is coupled with pumping fluid (usually at 15 to 25 mL/h) into the jet stream of gas. This fluid may be warmed before being placed into the gas stream to improve water-carrying capacity.

Another problem associated with HFJV has been airway pressure measurement. Initially, measurements

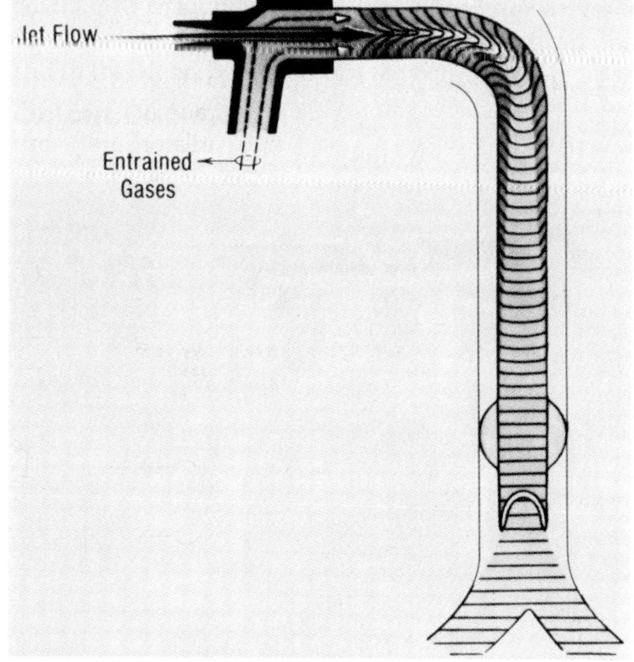

Figure 17-4. When gas exits the jet catheter in the airway, a rapid reduction in pressure causes humidified gas to be entrained into the system, modifying the tidal volume.

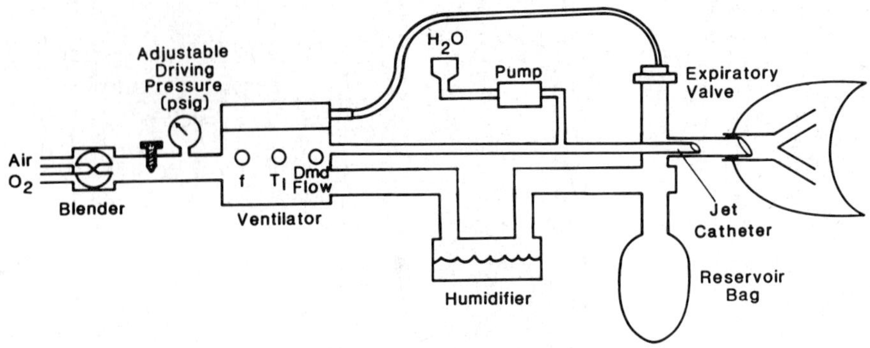

Figure 17-5. The essential parts of an HFJV system. See text for description.

were made next to the "jet" catheter. Since pressure becomes negative when gas exits the jet (producing entrainment), airway pressures measured at this position are less than actual pressure. Heard and Banner found that a position 9 to 10 cm distal to the jet was optimal for measurement of true airway pressure. A schematic of an HFJV system is shown in Figure 17-5. A commercially available jet ventilator is shown in Figure 17-6.

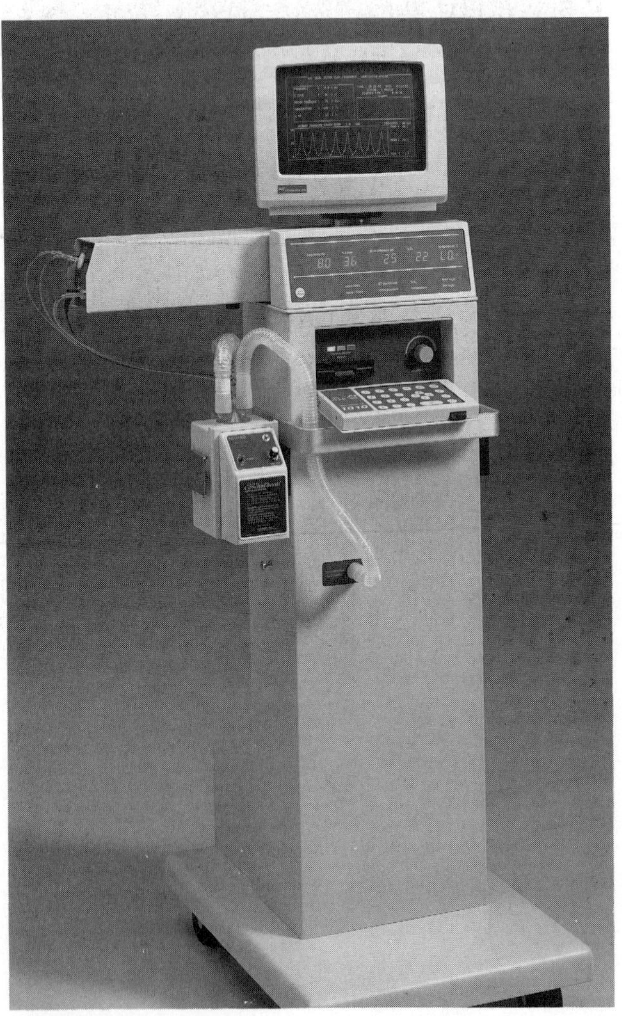

Figure 17-6. Infrasonics Adult Star 1010 high-frequency jet ventilator. (Courtesy of Infrasonics, San Diego, CA)

Clinical Uses

The plethora of reports and studies comparing HFJV to conventional ventilation prevents a listing of all potential and proposed benefits from being included here. Clinical use of HFJV may be divided into five categories: (1) use during airway procedures, (2) use in established pulmonary barotrauma, (3) use in surgery, (4) use in head-injured patients, and (5) use in respiratory distress syndrome (adult or neonatal).

HFJV is ideally suited for use during laryngoscopy, bronchoscopy, and tracheal surgery. The small catheter allows the surgeon an improved view of the airway while providing adequate oxygenation and ventilation.[20] The use of HFJV in established barotrauma was one of its most promising features. Lower airway pressures generated during HFJV reduced flow through bronchopleural fistulae and was lifesaving in many situations.[21,22] Initial experience was carried out many times in patients with normal lungs after surgery. When patients with adult respiratory distress syndrome (ARDS) and air leaks were studied, results were not nearly as dramatic.[23] At present, however, use of HFJV in the presence of bronchopulmonary fistulae, pulmonary interstitial emphysema, and undefined air leaks is approved by the FDA and may be more effective than conventional ventilation in many situations.

Aside from use during airway surgery, HFV has been shown to be useful during lithotripsy.[24] Diminished movement of the diaphragm provides a more stable abdomen and reduces respiration-related stone displacement. Although proven effective in this situation, critics suggest alternate methods using standard equipment are just as successful without the inherent dangers of becoming accustomed to new technology.

Several authors have found HFJV to be effective in reducing intracranial pressure in patients requiring hyperventilation for closed-head injuries.[25–27] Todd and associates[28] found that during HFJV there were reduced brain surface movements in cats compared with continuous mandatory ventilation (CMV). They postulated that HFJV may be useful during intracranial surgery, particularly microsurgery with a laser.

Findings by Hurst et al.[27] suggest that HFJV, by means of a reduction in peak and mean airway pressure, improves venous return from the head and lowers intracranial pressure while maintaining comparable oxygenation and ventilation. The use of HFJV to control intracranial pressure in all patients is unnecessary. HFJV should be reserved for those patients who are the most difficult to ventilate and who have failed to maintain intracranial pressures of less than 20 mm Hg despite optimum medical management.

Perhaps the most often explored application has been for the treatment of ARDS. Despite volumes of information compiled on this subject, there remains considerable disagreement. Conclusions have ranged from no significant difference to the vast superiority of HFJV. It is reasonable to assume that HFJV can provide comparable oxygenation and ventilation to CMV at lower peak airway pressures. When lower peak airway pressures may be advantageous (reduce barotrauma and hemodynamic compromise), a trial of HFJV may be warranted.[29,30]

High-Frequency Flow Interruption

High-frequency flow interruption is a close relative of HFJV (Fig. 17-7}. Both provide a high-pressure gas source intermittently applied to the airway by an electronically controlled valve. HFFI, however, may or may not use an airway catheter. The best known high-frequency interruptor is the Emerson rotating ball ventilator. The ball, with a single, fixed conduit through it, "chops" or "interrupts" the gas stream, creating periodic flow interruptions. In this device, the % Ti is fixed at 30%. Frequency (110–200 cpm) and driving pressure have separate, independent controls. The inspiratory:expiratory (I:E) ratio is a function of the fixed % Ti and frequency (cpm). HFFI uses a secondary of "bias" flow directed at the airway to "amplify" delivered tidal volume. This concept is described more completely in the section on high-frequency oscillation. As gas is delivered to the patient from the ventilator, bias flow is entrained into the stream, increasing the tidal volume. Mean airway pressure is controlled by driving pressure, frequency, and PEEP. Some HFFI systems use a standard exhalation valve, while others use a low pass filter (LPF). An LPF allows continuous low flows to exit the expiratory port relatively unimpeded. During high-flow situations the LPF creates an end-expiratory pressure effect by increasing resistance. Tidal volume is determined by driving pressure, bias flow, frequency, and impedance of the patient's respiratory system relative to the impedance caused by the LPF.

Humidification is accomplished by directing the bias flow through a conventional humidifier or adding water directly into the gas stream after the cycling mechanism, similar to HFJV.

Clinical Uses

The majority of work in this area has been done using the Emerson ventilator. Frantz and colleagues[31] have reported excellent results in treating neonates with established pulmonary barotrauma.[31] Gettinger and Glass[10] have described its use in adults for the treatment of ARDS and bronchopulmonary fistulae. Their results have been good, with 76% of patients (n = 50) showing an improvement in oxygenation. A detailed description of the system used by Gettinger and colleagues is shown in Figure 17-8. Presently, HFFI remains investigational and clinical studies are few compared with HFJV.

High-Frequency Oscillation

Like HFPPV, HFO was discovered serendipitously. During studies of cardiac function using transtracheal pressure oscillations to measure transmyocardial pressure transmission, Lukenheimer and colleagues[32] found that paralyzed canines remained normocarbic despite several minutes of apnea. These initial observations led Lukenheimer's group to pursue the mechanism of gas exchange in this situation.

Mechanically, the system used to provide HFO may be a loudspeaker, diaphragm, or reciprocating pump (usually a piston). The common characteristics of each

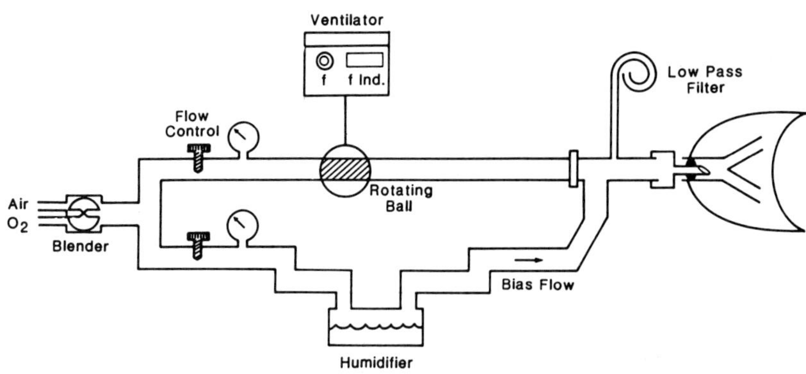

Figure 17-7. The HFFI system. See text for description

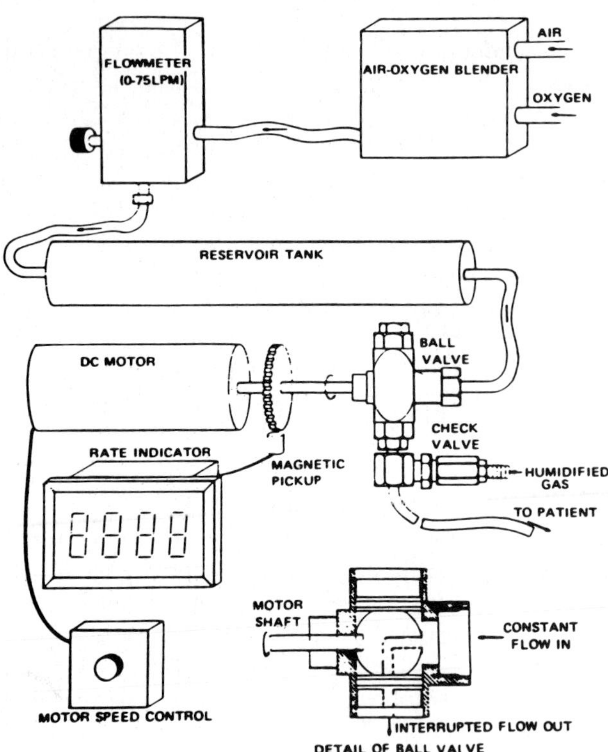

Figure 17-8. Detailed drawing of the HFFI system used by Gettinger and Glass. (From Gettinger A, Glass DD. High frequency positive pressure ventilation. In: Carlon GC, Howland WS, eds. High-Frequency Ventilation in Intensive Care and During Surgery. New York: Marcel Dekker, 1985)

are (1) an approximate sinusoidal gas flow with active inspiration and expiration and (2) an I:E ratio of 1:1. Initially, systems merely consisted of the oscillator situated at the airway. Although effective for short periods of time, during long-term ventilation, hypercarbia and acidosis developed. To prevent CO_2 retention, a steady supply of oxygen was supplied between the oscillating membrane and the patient. This was termed *bias flow* and served as a means of supplying humidified oxygen and removing excess CO_2. On the opposite end of the bias flow (where gas exits) an LPF is used to control mean airway pressure. The LPF is usually a long, narrow tube that provides a high impedance to gas flow at high frequencies and very little impedance to gas flows at low frequencies. With the LPF, Paw may be altered by either increasing the bias flow or changing the resistance characteristics of the LPF. A byproduct of the bias flow is amplification of tidal volume. As the bias flow enters the oscillating system, the forward stroke volume of the piston plus a quantity of bias flow gas enters the airway. During active expiration (backward displacement of the piston), part of the bias flow is drawn into the piston. The end result is a larger volume delivered during inspiration then is removed during inspiration. This also explains why alveolar pressures during HFO exceed proximal airway pressures.

Tidal volumes delivered during HFO are reported to be 0.8 to 2.0 mL/kg, with frequencies most commonly being used between 3 to 20 Hz (180–1200 cpm). Delivered tidal volumes are dependent on the piston stroke volume, compressible volume of the circuitry, bias flow, endotracheal tube size, impedance of the LPF, and respiratory system compliance and resistance. Humidification of the bias flow is adequate during HFO and easily accomplished. A representative HFO system is shown in Figure 17-9.

The SensorMedics high-frequency oscillator (Yorba Linda, CA) (Fig. 17-10) is the only commercially available HFO device. This HFO device uses an electromagnetic valve to control the piston assembly (Fig. 17-11). This device is unique in that it has the ability to vary I:E.

Clinical Uses

The efficiency of HFO is inversely proportional to the size of the subject; therefore, most clinical experience with HFO has been done in neonates. As with other HFV techniques, HFO has been described as equal to, vastly superior to, and inferior to standard conventional ventilation.[33,34]

Advocates insist that, despite increases in Paw during HFO, the reduction in peak inspiratory pressure allows equal or improved oxygenation without

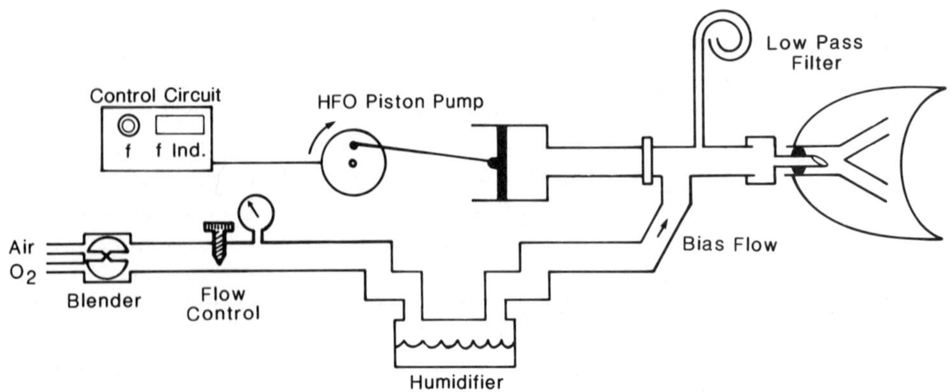

Figure 17-9. The essential parts of an HFO system. See text for description.

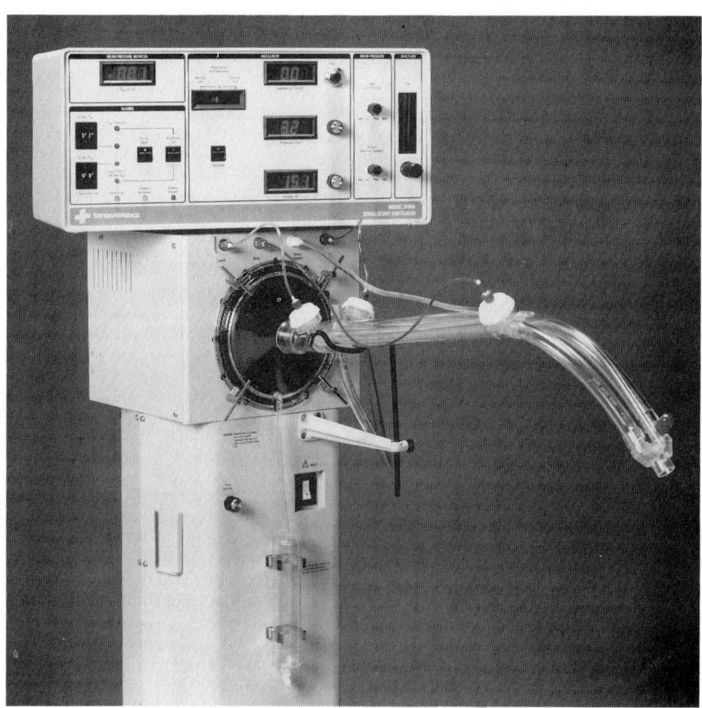

Figure 17-10. SensorMedics 3100 oscillatory ventilator. (Courtesy of SensorMedics Corporation, Yorba Linda, CA)

hemodynamic interference. Marchak and associates[35] demonstrated this in a group of infants with respiratory distress syndrome, in whom, despite an increase in Paw from 10 to 15 cm H_2O, FIO_2 was able to be reduced from 0.66 to 0.41 during HFO. A multi-institutional trial of HFO in neonatal respiratory distress syndrome has been completed. The results failed to demonstrate any superiority of HFO. On the contrary, the neonates treated with HFO had a higher incidence of intracranial hemorrhage than those treated conventionally. The mechanism by which this occurs appears to be related to the higher lung volumes and lack of intrathoracic pressure fluctuations.[36]

Unique to HFO is the variety of ways it has been applied. Investigators have used the system described earlier, as well as modifications using a CO_2 absorber or rotating valve. Interestingly, HFO has been used externally on the chest wall (high-frequency chest wall vibration) and on animals in a body box (whole-body high-frequency vibration). It is thought that high-frequency chest wall oscillation may facilitate removal of secretions much like percussion and postural drainage. HFO has also been combined with conventional ventilation. Figure 17-12 represents the six different techniques of HFO.

High-Frequency Percussive Ventilation

High-frequency percussive ventilation was devised by Forrest M. Bird. This mode is an attempt to combine the most desirable attributes of HFJV, HFO, and conventional ventilation into one ventilator. Others have described HFPV as HFFI, while Bunnell has referred to it as a "setback jet." Neither is completely accurate.

The control module of HFPV is a pneumatically controlled, time-triggered, time-cycled, pressure-limited ventilator referred to as a high-frequency pulse generator. The pneumatic system inside the HFPG allows programming of inspiratory time, expiratory time, peak airway pressure, CPAP or PEEP, and frequency. A sample of the pressure waveforms that can be created are shown in Figure 17-13.

Like HFPPV, HFPV uses a specially designed valve at the airway to deliver gases. In the case of HFPV, a sliding nongated venturi serves to separate inspired and expired gases and produce end-expiratory pressure. During inspiration, gas is delivered from the HFPG to the sliding venturi. The diaphragm on top of the venturi fills with gas, moving the venturi cage forward and closing off the expiratory port. A continuous flow of gas from a nebulizer, already warmed and humidified is the source of entrained gas. The degree of entrainment is reduced as back-pressure increases and delivered volume falls. This is similar to HFJV, except the venturi is more efficient at entraining gases than the jet mixing effect of jet ventilation. At the end of inspiration, the diaphragm above the venturi collapses and displaces the venturi cage backward, clearing the way for gases to exit the expiratory port passively (Fig. 17-14). End-expiratory pressure is accomplished by using the sliding venturi as an opposing flow apparatus. A demand valve allows the patient to breathe spontaneously during HFPV, in either the inspiratory or expiratory phase.

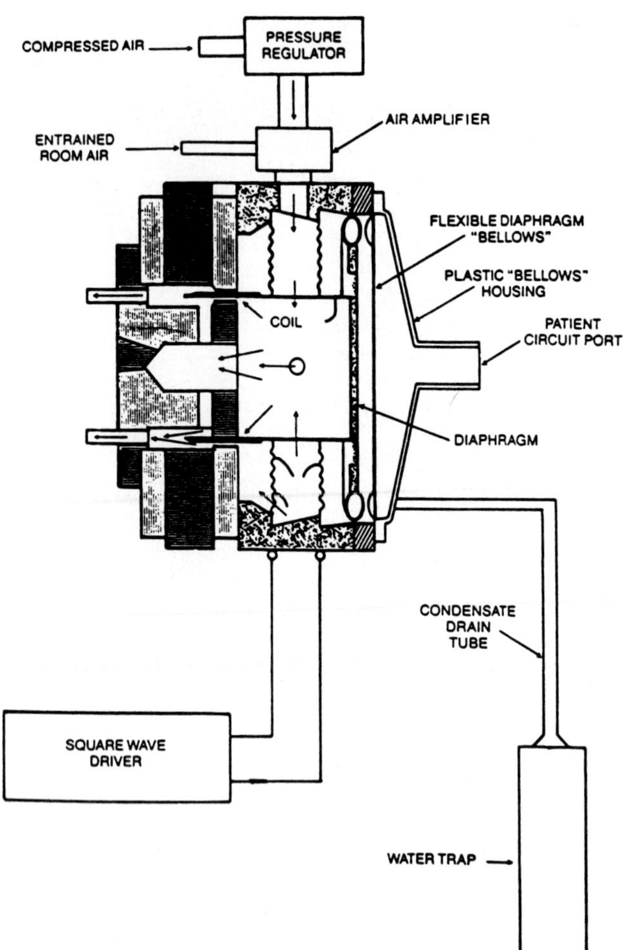

Figure 17-11. Oscillator components of the SensorMedics 3100 HFV device. The square wave driver controls timing of the motor that drives the piston. During positive displacement (inspiration) the motor moves the piston toward the patient circuit port. The compressed air is used to cool the electric coil. (Courtesy of SensorMedics, Yorba Linda, CA)

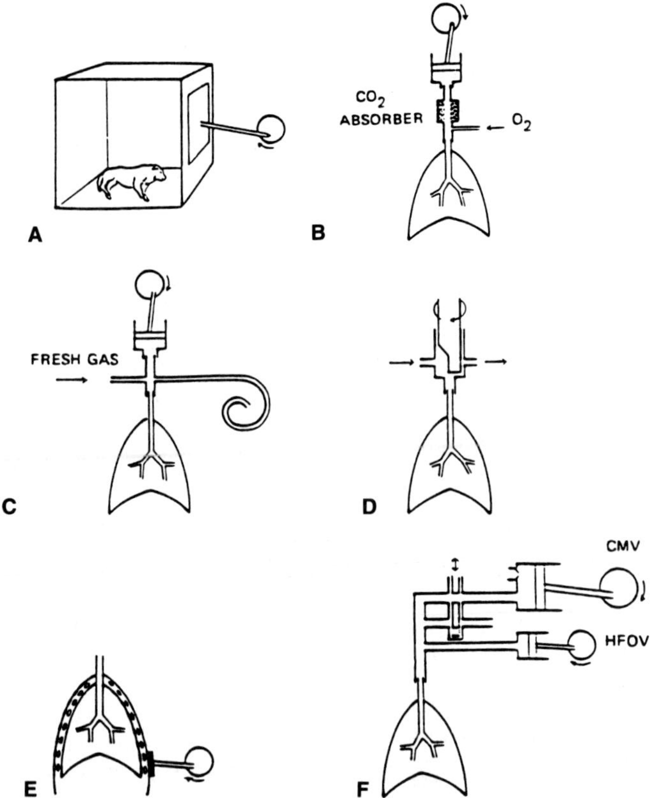

Figure 17-12. Six different types of HFOV. (A.) Whole-body oscillation administered either in a dynamic pressure chamber or by whole-body mechanical vibrations. (B.) A "closed" system in which CO_2 is absorbed and O_2 added to meet metabolic demand. (C.) Bias flow oscillator circuit. As with B, the pump may be a piston–cylinder combination, loudspeaker cone, or other vibrating membrane. The bias-flow circuit can utilize a long, low-impedance exhaust or high-impedance tube with positive source and negative sink pressures. It may be directed down the airway rather than across the airway opening. (D.) Rotating valve that interrupts a high-pressure gas source. (E.) Oscillations coupled to the thorax either by a vibrating disc or a pressure cuff. (F.) HFOV, combined with CMV, as shown, or spontaneous ventilation. (From McEvoy RD. High frequency oscillatory ventilation. In: Carlon GC, Howland WS, eds. High Frequency Ventilation in Intensive Care and During Surgery. New York: Marcel Dekker, 1985)

As with conventional, time-cycled, pressure-limited ventilation, CO_2 removal is controlled by respiratory frequency and peak airway pressure. Oxygenation is controlled by peak airway pressure, inspiratory time, I:E ratio, and end-expiratory pressure. Changing the frequency of the percussions can also effect gas exchange. At low rates, 180 to 240 cpm, CO_2 elimination is improved, whereas with higher frequencies, 300 to 600 cpm, oxygenation is augmented. HFPV is similar to HFJV in its entrainment principle and to conventional ventilation in the way which "breaths" are delivered. In fact, some have suggested that HFPV is HFJV superimposed on conventional ventilation. A schematic of the HFPV system is shown in Figure 17-15.

Clinical Uses

HFPV has been advocated in the treatment of neonates with respiratory distress syndrome, in adults with respiratory distress syndrome, and in both groups of patients with concomitant pulmonary air leaks. Most work in neonates has been done in Europe. Several investigators have shown improvement in gas exchange at lowered peak inspiratory pressure compared with conventional ventilation.[37,38]

Gallagher and colleagues[39] compared HFPV with intermittent mandatory ventilation in a group of adults with ARDS and showed an improvement in oxygenation. Hurst and associates[40] have demonstrated improved oxygenation and CO_2 elimination at lower peak airway pressures. No difference in cardiovascular parameters were identified.[40]

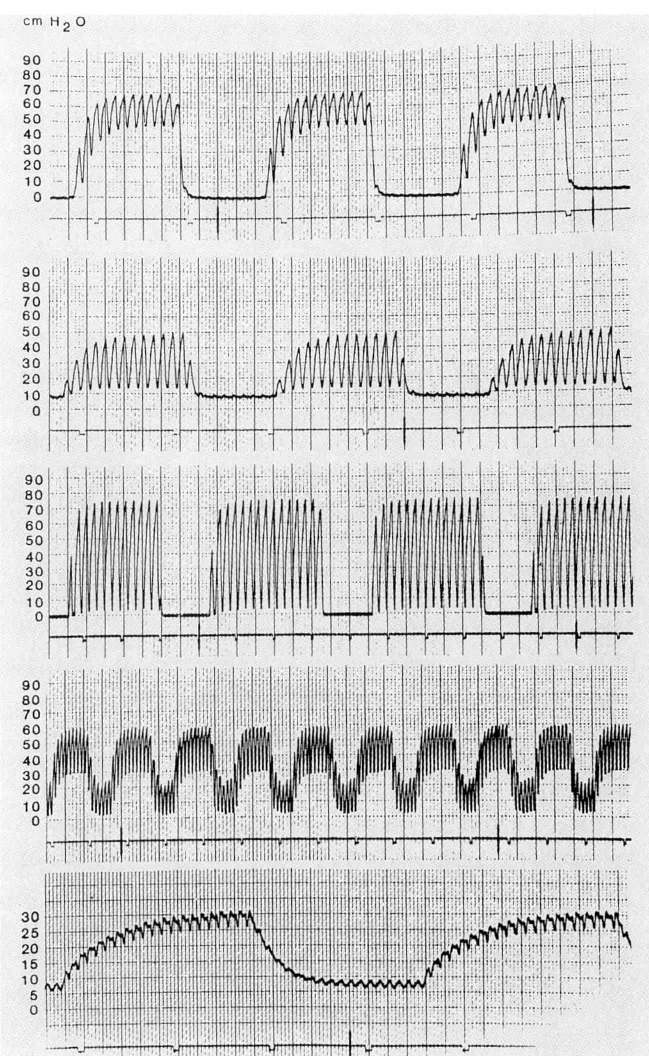

Figure 17-13. Pressure waveforms created by HFPV.

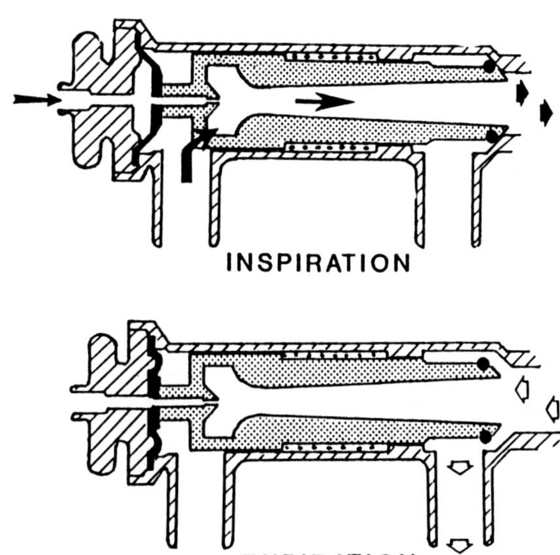

Figure 17-14. The sliding venturi used for delivery of HFPV.

Gas Transport During High-Frequency Ventilation

No discussion of HFV is complete without mentioning the numerous gas transport theories. Although detailed description is beyond the scope of this chapter, some of the basic proposed mechanisms are addressed.

In Figure 17-16, six of the most popular theories are presented. The first is direct alveolar ventilation or bulk gas flow.[1] This, of course, is the simplest and most common type of alveolar ventilation associated with spontaneous as well as conventional mechanical ventilation. Direct alveolar ventilation is thought to play the major role in gas transport during HFPPV, HFJV, and HFPV.

The second theory is a "buzz word" of HFV—facilitated diffusion.[2] This theory suggests that the high-frequency pulsations, or vibrations, in the airway increase the kinetic energy of gas molecules and enhance diffusion across the alveolar-capillary membrane. In actual fact, diffusion across the alveolar-capillary membrane only represents a small portion of total gas transport during HFV.

The third theory represents what is commonly referred to as the Taylor dispersion theories. Taylor described both turbulent and laminar dispersion occurring in a model of pulmonary airways. During turbulent flow, eddies are formed and mixing of gases

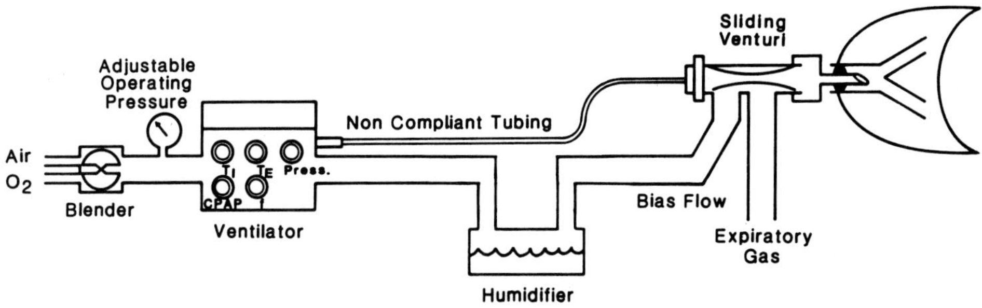

Figure 17-15. The essential parts of an HFPV system.

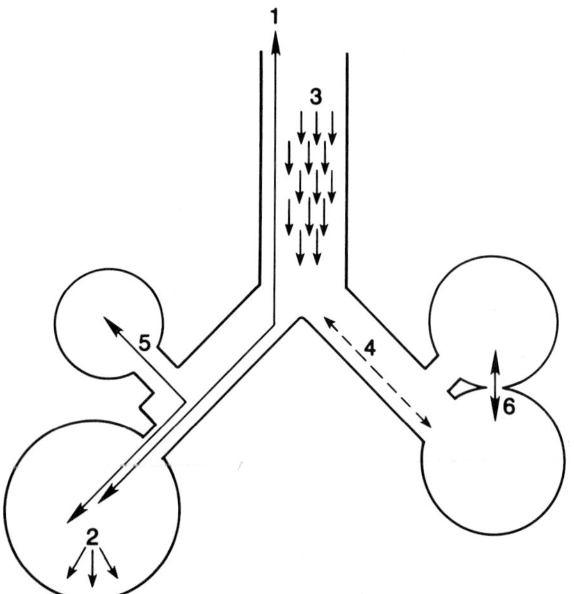

Figure 17-16. Representation of gas transport theories thought to be operable during HFV. See text for description.

between the central airway and periphery is enhanced.[3] It has also been suggested that some gas exchange may occur across the airway epithelium in these situations. During laminar flow dispersion, particularly during HFO, to and fro movement of the piston creates an acceleration/deceleration phenomena. Inertia of the molecules moving forward with a certain axial velocity will be resistant to changing direction during backward movement of the piston. As a result, molecules continue to travel forward (out of phase with the piston) and improve gas mixing with small tidal volumes.

The fourth theory represents asymmetric velocity profiles. In this situation, inspiratory gas travels down the center of the airway while expired gas travels proximally around the periphery of the airway.[4] In essence, inspired and expired gas travel in their respective directions simultaneously.

The fifth mechanism is clearly operative during HFO and represents sharing of gases between alveolar units with short time constants and those with longer time constants.[5] This pendelluft effect occurs when the lung region with the short time constant empties into the airway and is then transferred to a slow filling lung region. The result is improved gas exchange by creating a state of homogeneity in the lung.

The last proposed mechanism is improved collateral ventilation through the pores of Kohn and canals of Lambert.[6] The impact of interregional mixing through collateral channels during HFV, however, is unknown.[1] Comparison of high-frequency techniques is difficult for many reasons described earlier. Figure 17-17 demonstrates the effects of increasing frequency on mean airway pressure and on the variation between end-inspiratory and end-expiratory pressure. Conventional ventilation is represented at the far left and HFO to the far right.

HFV is a group of sophisticated ventilatory techniques destined to be around for many years to come. Only time will determine whether its final position is at the forefront of ventilatory support or encased in dust on the back shelf of the respiratory care department.

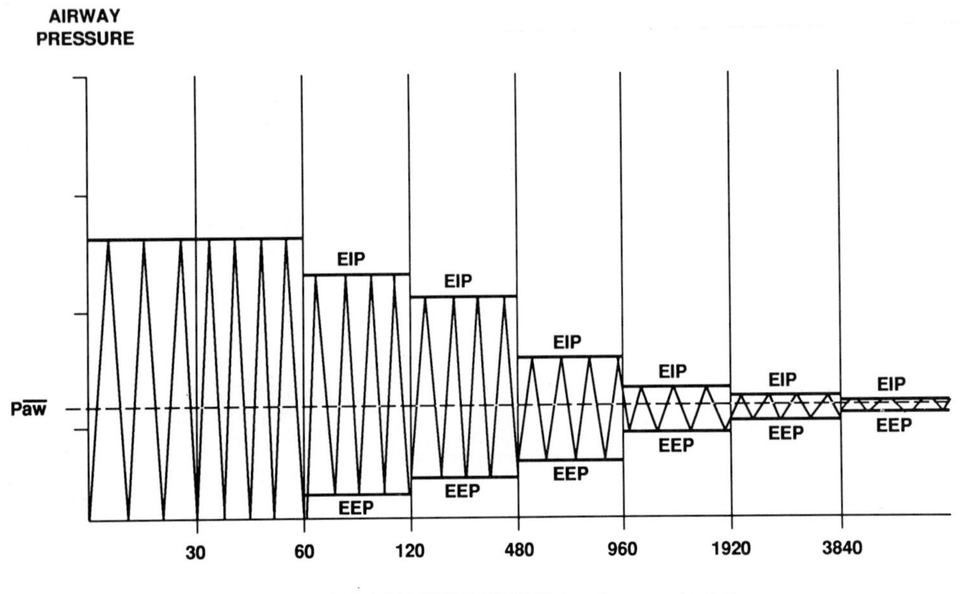

Figure 17-17. Changes in airway pressures as frequency increases from conventional ranges (far left) and HFO (far right).

References

1. Froese AB. High-frequency ventilation: A critical assessment. In: Shoemaker WC, ed. Critical Care: State of the Art, vol 5. Fullerton, CA: Society of Critical Care Medicine, 1984:A3–A51.
2. Henderson Y, Chillingworth FD, Whitney JL. The respiratory deadspace. Am J Physiol 1915;38:1.
3. Crawford MR. High frequency ventilation. Anaesth Intens Care 1986;14:281.
4. Emerson JH. Apparatus for vibrating portions of a patients airway. Patent No. 2918197. Washington, DC: US Patent Office, December 29, 1959.
5. Froese AB, Bryan AC. High-frequency ventilation. Am Rev Respir Dis 1987;135:1363–1374.
6. Smith RB. Ventilation at high respiratory frequencies. Anaesthesia 1982;37:1011–1018.
7. Sjostrand U. High-frequency positive-pressure ventilation (HFPPV): A review. Crit Care Med 1980;8:345–364.
8. Abu-Dbai J, Flatau E, Lev A, Kohn D, Monis-Hass I, Barzilay E. The use of conventional ventilators for high-frequency positive-pressure ventilation. Crit Care Med 1983;11:356–358.
9. Borg U, Erikson I, Sjostrand U. High-frequency positive-pressure ventilation (HFPPV): A review based upon its use during bronchoscopy and for laryngoscopy and microlaryngeal surgery under general anesthesia. Anesth Analg 1980;59:594–603.
10. Gettinger A, Glass DD. High-frequency positive-pressure ventilation. In: Lenfant C, ed. Lung Biology in Health and Disease. New York: Marcel Dekker, 1985;63–76.
11. Wattwil LM, Sjostrand UH, Borg UR. Comparative studies of IPPV and HFPPV with PEEP in critical care patients: I. A clinical evaluation. Crit Care Med 1983;11:30–37.
12. Klain M, Smith RB. High-frequency percutaneous transtracheal jet ventilation. Crit Care Med 1977;5:280–287.
13. Rubini A, Travan M. Gas dynamic principles. In Chiaranda M, Giron G, eds. High-Frequency Jet Ventilation. Padua, Italy: Piccin/Ishiyaku, 1985;18–33.
14. Baum ML, Benzer HR, Geyer AM, Muntz NJ. Theoretical evaluation of gas exchange mechanisms. In: Carlon GC, Howland WS, eds. High-Frequency Ventilation in Intensive Care and During Surgery. New York: Marcel Dekker, 1985;25–36.
15. Carlon GC, Miodownik S, Ray C Jr. High-frequency jet ventilation: Technical evaluation and device characterization. In: Carlon GC, Howland WS, eds. High-Frequency Ventilation in Intensive Care and During Surgery. New York: Marcel Dekker, 1985;77–110.
16. Calkins JM. High-frequency jet ventilation. Experimental evaluation. In: Carlon GC, Howlan WS, eds. High-frequency ventilation in intensive care and during surgery. New York: Marcel Dekker, 1985;111–135.
17. Banner MJ, Boysen PG. Comparison of two flow injector devices to deliver high-frequency jet ventilation. Crit Care Med 1986; 14:374.
18. Banner MJ, Gallagher TJ, Banner TC. Frequency and percent inspiratory time for high-frequency jet ventilation. Crit Care Med 1985;13:395–398.
19. Ophoven JP, Mammel MC, Gordon MJ, Boros SJ. Tracheobronchial histopathology associated with high-frequency jet ventilation. Crit Care Med 1984;12:829–832.
20. El-Baz N, Holinger L, El-Ganzouri A, Gottschalk W, Ivankovich AD. High-frequency positive pressure ventilation for tracheal reconstruction supported by tracheal T-tube. Anesth Analg 1982;61:796–800.
21. Carlon GC, Kahn RC, Howland WS, Ray C Jr, Turnbull AD. Clinical experience with high-frequency jet ventilation. Crit Care Med 1981;9:1–6.
22. Turnbull AD, Carlon G, Howland WS, Beattie EJ. High-frequency jet ventilation in major airway or pulmonary disruption. Ann Thorac Surg 1981;32:468–474.
23. Ritz R, Benson M, Bishop MJ, Measuring gas leakage from bronchopleural fistulas during high-frequency jet ventilation. Crit Care Med 1984;12:836–837.
24. Schulte EJ, Kochs E, Meyer WH. Use of high-frequency jet ventilation in extracorporeal shockwave lithotripsy. Anaesthesist 1985;34:294–298.
25. O'Donnell JM, Thompson DR, Layotn TR. The effect of high-frequency jet ventilation on intracranial pressure in patients with closed head injuries. J Trauma 1984;24:73–75.
26. Branson RD, Hurst JM, DeHaven CB. Use of high-frequency jet ventilation during mechanical hyperventilation for control of elevated intracranial pressure: A case report. Respir Care 1984;29: 1221–1225.
27. Hurst JM, Saul TG, DeHaven CB, Branson RD. Use of high-frequency jet ventilation during mechanical hyperventilation to reduce intracranial pressure in patients with multiple organ system injury. Neurosurgery 1984;15:530–534.
28. Todd MM, Toutant SM, Shapiro HM. The effects of HFPPV on ICP and brain surface movements in cats. Crit Care Med 1981; 54:496–500.
29. Carlon GC, Howland WS, Ray C, Miodownik S, Griffin JP, Groeger JS. High-frequency jet ventilation: A prospective randomized evaluation. Chest 1983;84:551–559.
30. Schuster DP, Klain M, Snyder JV. Comparison of high-frequency jet ventilation to conventional ventilation during severe acute respiratory failure in humans. Crit Care Med 1982; 10:625–630.
31. Frantz ID III, Werthammer J, Stark AR. High-frequency ventilation in premature infants with lung disease: Adequate gas exchange at low tracheal pressure. Pediatrics 1983;71:483–488.
32. Lukenheimer PP, Frank I, Ising H, Keller H, Dickhut HH. Intrapulmonaler Gaswechsel unter simulierter Apnoe durch transtrachealen, periodischen intrathorakalen Druckwechsel. Anaesthesist 1973;22:232–238.
33. Slutsky AS, Brown R, Lehr J, Rossing T, Drazen JM. High-frequency ventilation: A promising new approach to mechanical ventilation. Med Instrum 1981;15:229–233.
34. Kolton M. A review of high-frequency oscillation. Can Anaesth Soc J 1984;31:416–429.
35. Marchak BE, Thompson WK, Duffy P, et al. Treatment of RDS by high-frequency oscillatory ventilation: A preliminary report. J Pediatr 1981;99:287–291.
36. HFFI Study group. High-frequency oscillatory ventilation compared with conventional mechanical ventilation in the treatment of respiratory failure in preterm infants. N Engl J Med 1989; 320:88–93.
37. Biarent D, Steppe F, Muller G, et al. High-frequency jet percussive ventilation in newborns with damaged lungs. Acta Anaesth Belg 1985;3:122–128.
38. Pfenninger J, Gerber AC. HFV in hyaline membrane disease: A preliminary report. Intens Care Med 1987;13:71–75.
39. Gallagher TJ, Boysen PG, Davidson DD, et al. HFPV compared with CMV. Crit Care Med 1985;13:312.
40. Hurst JM, Branson RD, DeHaven CB. The role of HFV in posttraumatic respiratory insufficiency. J Trauma 1987;27:236–242.

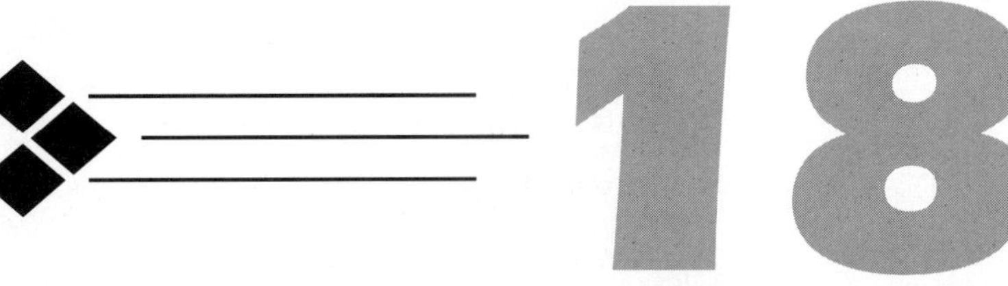

Spontaneous Breathing Systems: IMV and CPAP

Richard D. Branson

OBJECTIVES

1. Demonstrate the methods of providing a continuous flow of gas to a mechanical ventilator allowing intermittent mandatory ventilation to be accomplished.
2. Compare open-circuit and closed-circuit intermittent mandatory ventilation systems.
3. Describe the effects of open- and closed-circuit intermittent mandatory ventilation systems on the work of breathing.
4. Explain the function of a demand valve.
5. Compare pressure triggering and flow triggering.
6. Describe the systems used to provide spontaneous positive end-expiratory pressure (sPEEP) and continuous positive airway pressure (CPAP).

KEY TERMS

closed-circuit IMV system
continuous positive airway pressure (CPAP)
demand valve
intermittent mandatory ventilation (IMV)
open circuit IMV system
spontaneous PEEP system
trigger
- flow trigger
- pressure trigger

Introduction

Intermittent mandatory ventilation (IMV) was introduced in 1971 as a means of ventilatory support for infants with hyaline membrane disease[1] and subsequently employed as a method of weaning adult patients from mechanical ventilation.[2] Initially, IMV was described as a combination of spontaneous and controlled ventilation (Fig. 18-1). However, many ventilators provide a mechanism for patient-triggered IMV or synchronized IMV (SIMV). In SIMV mode, the mandatory tidal volume (VT) delivery can be initiated by spontaneous inspiratory effort and thus represents a form of "assisted" ventilation.

Most ventilators incorporate IMV/SIMV as an integral feature. However, older models (ie, Bennett MA-1, Emerson 3PV) and some home care ventilators must be modified to provide this mode. Because many nursing homes and extended care facilities rely on these older ventilators, the appropriate application of these modifications is described in this chapter along with a review of demand flow systems.

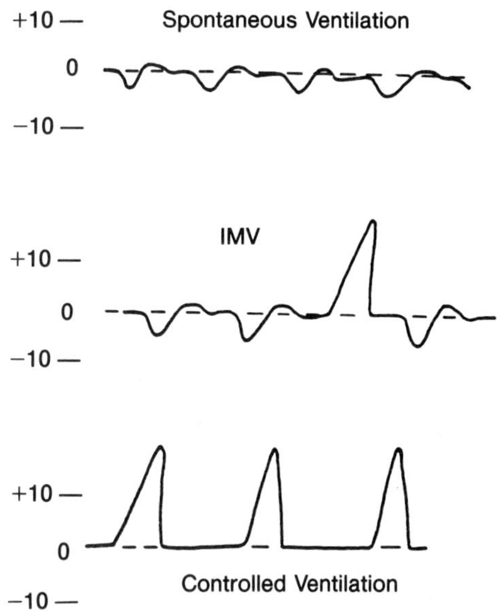

Figure 18-1. Airway pressure patterns during IMV illustrating the combination of spontaneous and controlled ventilation.

Intermittent Mandatory Ventilation Systems

Three mechanisms are employed to allow IMV: (1) parallel flow or open-circuit, (2) continuous-flow or closed-circuit, and (3) demand-valve systems.

Open-Circuit Systems

An open-circuit system (Fig. 18-2) is the simplest and least expensive IMV modification. A one-way valve assembly is attached to the inspiratory limb of the patient circuit. The valve-circuit interface should be near the proximal airway to minimize inspiratory resistance as a result of the circuitry. Humidified gas at the same FIO_2 provided by the mechanical ventilator is usually supplied by a wall-mounted aerosol generator. An air–oxygen blender or air–oxygen flowmeters may also be used. During spontaneous ventilation, the patient inspires from this parallel gas flow through the one-way valve.

The inspiratory effort required to open most one-way valves is from 0.5 to 2.0 cm H_2O. However, when the patient is receiving PEEP, the inspiratory effort necessary to open the valve is increased by the level of expiratory pressure employed. This increased inspiratory load occurs because the patient side of the valve is pressurized to the level of PEEP while the fresh gas side of the valve is at atmospheric pressure. To access parallel gas flow during spontaneous inspiration, the circuit pressure must be reduced below atmospheric pressure by an amount equal to the inherent opening pressure of the valve. For example, if a patient is receiving 10 cm H_2O PEEP and the opening pressure of the one-way valve is 2 cm H_2O, a total inspiratory

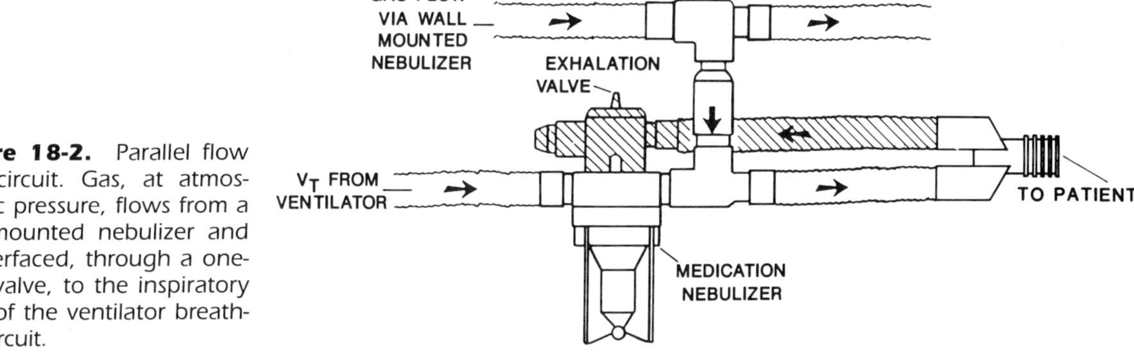

Figure 18-2. Parallel flow IMV circuit. Gas, at atmospheric pressure, flows from a wall-mounted nebulizer and is interfaced, through a one-way valve, to the inspiratory limb of the ventilator breathing circuit.

force of −12 cm H_2O is necessary. The patient must first overcome the difference in pressure between the ventilator circuit and the IMV flow circuit and then open the valve. In a parallel flow IMV system, work of breathing incurred by the patient is directly proportional to the opening pressure of the one-way valve and the PEEP level.[3]

Closed-Circuit Systems

A continuous-flow system can be adapted to any mechanical ventilator (Fig. 18-3). This modification requires a compressed air and oxygen blending system. Mixing of air and oxygen can be accomplished with an air–oxygen blender or by adjusting independent flows of air and oxygen to produce the desired F_{IO_2}. Continuous-flow IMV valve assemblies should always be attached proximal to the humidifier so that the patient does not breathe dry gas.

In a continuous-flow system, flow should be set to minimize pressure deflections seen on a proximal airway pressure manometer in an effort to reduce the work of breathing. It has been suggested that the optimum flow is three to four times the patient's minute ventilation. Subjective assessment of patient comfort may be the best method for determining the appropriate flow. Occasionally, enough flow can be delivered to the reservoir bag to maintain pressure above that in the circuit. Thus, spontaneous inspiratory effort can be minimized at any level of expiratory pressure by adjusting gas flow until the desired deflection on the airway pressure manometer is achieved. During IMV, as pressure develops in the circuit, the one-way valve closes to prevent retrograde flow of mechanical V_T into the reservoir bag. The continuous flow causes the reservoir bag to expand during mechanical inspiration. If the reservoir bag compliance is low, it is possible for pressure to develop that exceeds circuit pressure. Thus, the one-way valve would open and flow from the reservoir bag will add to the delivered mechanical V_T.[4] This potential complication can be avoided by placement of a pressure relief valve between the reservoir bag and humidifier. The relief valve can then be adjusted to vent continuous gas flow to the room when pressure in the bag approaches circuit pressure. An antiasphyxia valve should also be present. If there is a gas source failure or disconnection, the patient can breathe ambient air through the antiasphyxia valve.

When a continuous-flow IMV system is used and circuit pressure is monitored proximal to a cascade type humidifier, the recorded pressure is artificially elevated because of back-pressure developed by resistance to flow through the humidifier and circuit. This specifically refers to ventilators that measure airway pressure within the inspiratory limb of the ventilator. Correct circuit pressure can only be measured distal to the humidifier, preferably at the proximal airway. To prevent problems with measuring circuit pressure, some practitioners advocate cutting the tail off the reservoir bag. This allows excess pressure and flow to vent to atmosphere. This should never be done. Venting the flow reduces the amount of gas available to the patient and drastically increases the work of breathing.

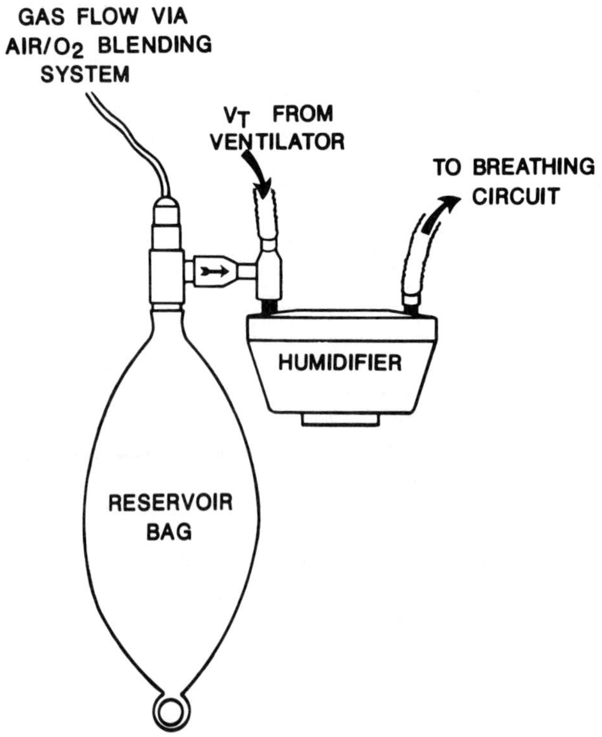

Figure 18-3. Continuous-flow IMV circuit. Blended compressed air and oxygen is metered into a reservoir bag and passes through a unidirectional valve and humidifier into the breathing circuit.

The resistance to flow through the humidifier poses another important problem. If patient demand for flow during inspiration exceeds that supplied, the patient must generate additional work to draw sufficient gas from the reservoir through the humidifier. In this instance, the inspiratory workload would increase proportionally to flow resistance through the circuit. The pressure gradient across most commonly employed humidifiers is 3 to 6 cm H_2O at a flow rate of 1 L/s (60 L/min). This resistance in and of itself may not impose significant work; however, in conjunction with the resistance provided by the one-way valve, it could cause an intolerable inspiratory workload for some patients.

Demand Valve Systems

Demand flow valves can be incorporated to provide gas for spontaneous inspiratory effort (Fig. 18-4). Current demand valves can be pressure or flow triggered.

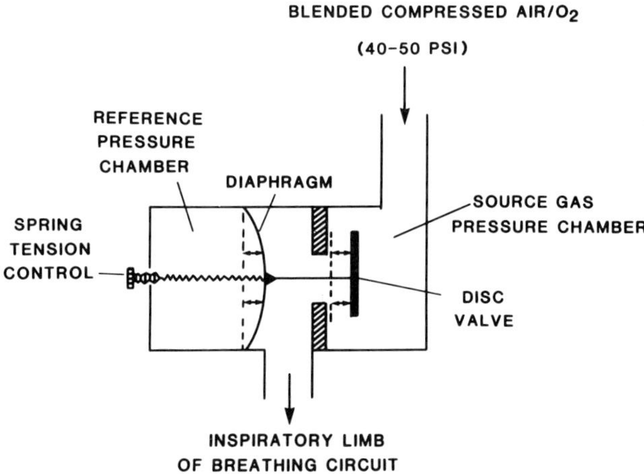

Figure 18-4. Cutaway of an Emerson demand valve. Spring tension is normally adjusted to exert sufficient force on diaphragm, necessitating only minimal inspiratory effort to overcome pressure in source gas chamber. As the diaphragm responds to spontaneous inspiratory effort, it migrates from a nominal (—) to displaced (--) position while unseating disk valve facilitating gas flow delivery to breathing circuit. When inspiration ceases, source gas pressure exceeds spring tension and the diaphragm returns to resting position and disk valve seats terminating demand flow.

Pressure Triggered

During pressure triggering, the opening or "trigger" pressure (usually set by the sensitivity control) is referenced to that in the patient's circuit. This is sometimes referred to as "PEEP compensation." This means that for a given sensitivity setting (-2 cm H_2O) the ventilator will trigger at that pressure change regardless of the set PEEP. For example, at a PEEP of 10 cm H_2O the ventilator would trigger when pressure fell below 8 cm H_2O. If the PEEP were changed to 6 cm H_2O, the ventilator would trigger a spontaneous breath when pressure fell below 4 cm H_2O. During patient exhalation, the circuit pressure increases slightly, thereby terminating gas flow.

Microprocessor-operated ventilators use a rapid response flow control valve as part of an inspiratory servo system (Fig. 18-5). When the airway pressure (Paw) transducer detects an inspiratory effort, a signal is "bused" to the microprocessor. The microprocessor modulates the control valve to provide sufficient gas to meet inspiratory flow demand.

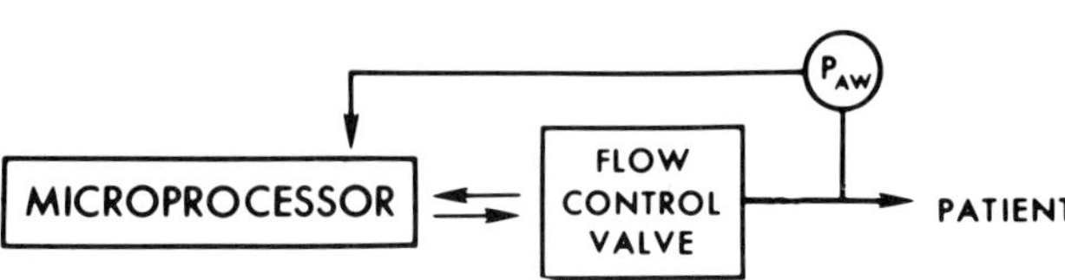

Figure 18-5. Servo-controlled demand flow valve. An airway pressure (Paw) transducer detects spontaneous inspiration and signals the microprocessor. The microprocessor activates the electronic flow control valve that supplies gas to satisfy inspiratory demand.

Flow Triggered

Another mechanism for initiating demand flow is by means of inspiratory flow rather than pressure triggering. This is known as flow triggering. Flow triggering is accomplished by creating a baseline flow of gas traveling through a flow measurement device (usually a pneumotachometer). This flow is set by the operator. A flow sensitivity setting is then set at a level less than the baseline flow. For example, if a baseline flow of 10 L/min is set, the ventilator will provide 10 L/min of flow through the ventilator circuit. This flow is measured by the proximal airway flow transducer (eg, Hamilton Veolar) or the expiratory flow transducer (eg, Bird 8400ST, Puritan Bennett 7200ae, Siemens Servo 300). When the patient's inspiratory effort causes flow through the flow transducer to change greater than the flow sensitivity setting, a spontaneous breath is triggered. With a baseline flow of 10 L/min and a flow sensitivity of 4 L/min, a spontaneous breath will be triggered when flow through the transducer falls to less than 6 L/min. The ventilator senses the end of inspiration when the flow exceeds the baseline flow, suggesting the patient is exhaling.

Problems With IMV Modifications

Many failures occurring with IMV-modified ventilators are caused by disconnections within the circuitry.[5] When a continuous-flow IMV system is employed with a Bennett MA-1, the only inherent ventilator circuit disconnect alarm, the exhaled volume spirometer is rendered inoperable in its normal configuration. The continuous flow fills the spirometer constantly, preventing it from operating the alarm system. Therefore, a low-pressure alarm should be placed in the circuit near the proximal airway to detect disconnections. Page and Downs[6] reported a complication associated with a continuous-flow IMV system. Excessive gas flow delivery to the spontaneous gas reservoir bag of an Emerson 3-PV ventilator resulted in inadvertent pressurization of the exhalation valve. Under this situation, the patient was unable to exhale either spontaneous or mechanical breaths. An adjustable pressure relief valve was placed between the reservoir bag and internal ventilator circuit, permitting excess gas to vent to atmosphere.

IMV may be administered with confidence, even when modified older ventilators are used. However, clinicians must ascertain that the modifications employed are safe and reliable and that appropriate alarms are incorporated.

Continuous Positive Airway Pressure (CPAP) Systems

Continuous positive airway pressure (CPAP) was employed as early as 1878 to treat pulmonary diseases characterized by reduced lung volume. Oertel[7] recognized that "the increase in the exchange of gases is of therapeutic importance, especially in cases in which the respiratory surface is diminished and shrunken." He also observed "that during expiration into compressed air even with slight pressure (averaging 10.6 cm H_2O), the respiratory air is increased."

In 1936, Poulton and Oxon[8] reported the use of CPAP therapy for congestive heart failure with pulmonary edema. In 1937, Bullowa[9] used up to 10 cm H_2O of CPAP to treat patients with pneumonia. During that same year, Barach and associates[10] described the use of CPAP for the treatment of pulmonary edema and to reduce airway resistance in obstructive pulmonary disease.

CPAP was applied by face mask in these initial reports but did not experience widespread use until Gregory and colleagues[11] reintroduced it in 1971 for the treatment of intubated infants with hyaline membrane disease. CPAP therapy improved the survival rate for 1000- to 1500-g infants with hyaline membrane disease from 11% to 83%. Since then, various forms of expiratory pressure therapy have been applied to spontaneously breathing adults with acute pulmonary dysfunction.

Spontaneous Positive End-Expiratory Pressure Systems (sPEEP)

Spontaneous PEEP (sPEEP) is the simplest and least expensive method for applying expiratory pressure therapy. Civetta and coworkers[12] introduced a sPEEP circuit (Fig. 18-6) for the management of acute respiratory insufficiency following near drowning. Humidified oxygen enriched gas is provided by a gas-powered aerosol generator. Gas flows freely to ambient through a reservoir tube. The length of the reservoir tube should be sufficient to prevent entrainment of room air during inspiration. Reservoir tube length must be substantially increased at FIO_2 less than 0.6 owing to reduced air dilution (entrainment flow) of oxygen source gas.

The patient inspires fresh gas through the one-way valve and exhales to ambient through an end-expiratory pressure valve. As the patient begins to exhale, the one-way valve in the inspiratory limb closes, preventing retrograde flow of expired gases. When expiratory recoil pressure equals that exerted by the water column PEEP valve, the valve closes, creating the desired end-expiratory pressure.

The inspiratory effort required to open most one-way valves is from 0.5 to 2.0 cm H_2O. However, when the patient receives end-expiratory pressure, the inspiratory force required to open the valve is increased by the level of PEEP employed. This increased effort is required because the patient side of the valve is pressurized to the level of PEEP while the fresh gas side of the valve is at atmospheric pressure. For the valve to open during spontaneous inspiration, the circuit pressure must be reduced below atmospheric pressure (Fig. 18-7). Thus the patient must generate an inspiratory force sufficient to create a "negative" pressure equal and opposite to the sum of PEEP and the opening pressure of the unidirectional valve. The work of breathing on an sPEEP system can be high, resulting in patient fatigue.

Spontaneous PEEP provides pressure only during exhalation, whereas a CPAP circuit is pressurized during the entire respiratory cycle (Fig. 18-8). The mechanical difference between sPEEP and CPAP is in how the fresh gas is supplied. CPAP requires a high

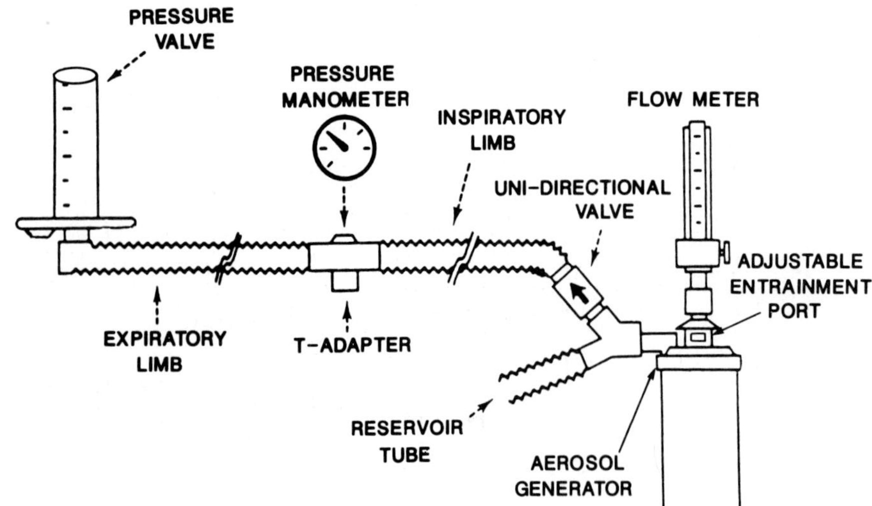

Figure 18-6. Schematic representation of a spontaneous PEEP circuit. See text for detailed description.

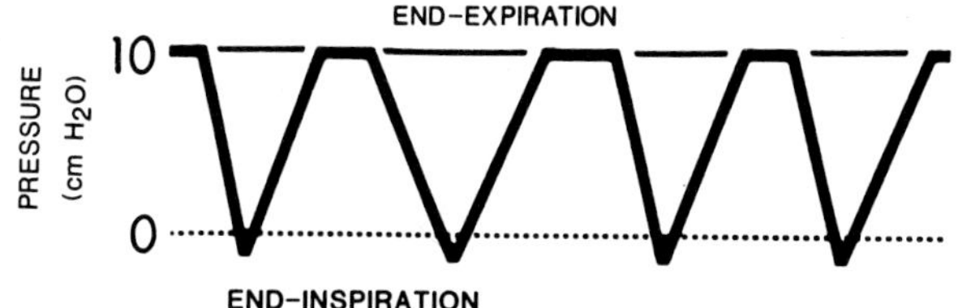

Figure 18-7. Airway pressure pattern associated with spontaneous PEEP therapy.

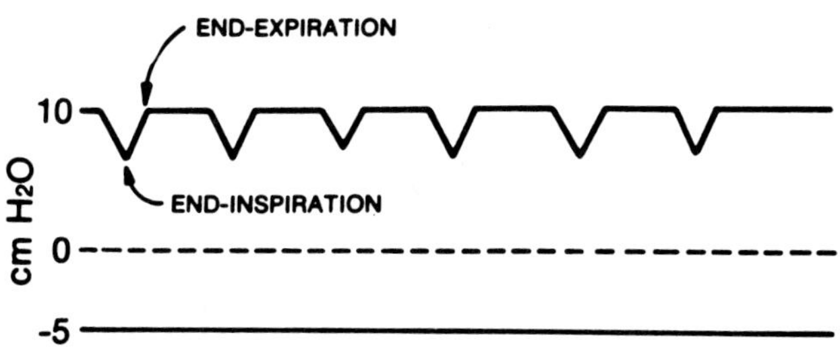

Figure 18-8. Continuous-flow CPAP circuit. See text for detailed explanation.

flow of gas, usually from a blender. Mixing of air and oxygen can be accomplished without a blender by regulating independent flows of air and oxygen to produce the desired FIO_2.

A commonly used CPAP circuit is shown in Figure 18-9. This homemade CPAP system has been used effectively by a number of investigators to deliver CPAP to patients with hypoxemia.

Commercially Available Devices

There are several commercially available CPAP systems. These can be divided into two groups: pneumatic and electronic devices.

PNEUMATIC DEVICES. The pneumatic devices operate from a 50-psi oxygen source and entrain room air through a venturi to produce the desired FIO_2. The Vital Signs Downs (Vital Signs Inc., Totowa, NJ) flow generator (Fig. 18-10) and AMBU CPAP system (Fig. 18-11) are commonly used pneumatic CPAP systems. The Vital Signs device is simply an adjustable-flow venturi. As the FIO_2 control is opened (to increase FIO_2) gas is diverted from the venturi to a side channel. This reduces entrainment of ambient air and FIO_2 rises. This also results in a slight reduction in total outflow, but the oxygen traveling through the side channel makes up for most of the decrease in entrainment. If the FIO_2 control is completely closed, all the source gas enters the venturi, FIO_2 falls, and total flow increases. The Vital Signs flow generator can deliver an FIO_2 from 0.30 to 1.0 at 95 to 105 L/min.

The AMBU CPAP system consists of an inlet venturi, a noncompliant 4-L reservoir bag, and a PEEP valve. Gas from the venturi enters the reservoir at an FIO_2 of 0.33. The reservoir fills, and the system is pressurized to the level set by the PEEP valve. During inspiration, the continuous flow from the venturi and the volume of gas in the reservoir meet the patient's inspiratory demands. The reservoir acts as a buffer, expanding and contracting with the respiratory cycle in an attempt to minimize end-inspiratory to end-expiratory pressure variations and hence the work of breathing. The maximum flow from the venturi is 25 L/min. If a higher flow is necessary, a blender and high-flow flowmeter (0 to 75 L/min) can be substituted for the venturi.

ELECTRONIC DEVICES. Electronic CPAP devices (Fig. 18-12) are most commonly used in the nighttime treatment of obstructive sleep apnea. They are simple devices that generally consist of a compressor, pressure gauge, and PEEP valve. The compressor draws air from the room through a filter and delivers it, at an accelerated flow, through corrugated tubing to the patient. Between the patient and the compressor a wye piece connects to a PEEP valve that creates the required end-expiratory pressure. Since ambient air is

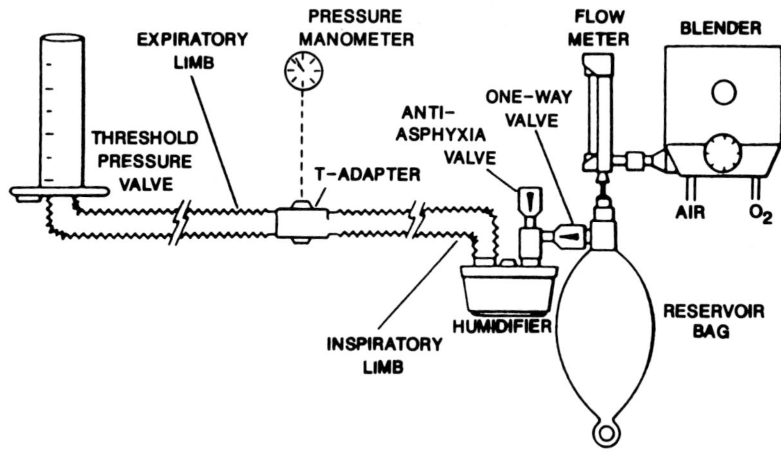

Figure 18-9. Airway pressure pattern encountered during CPAP therapy.

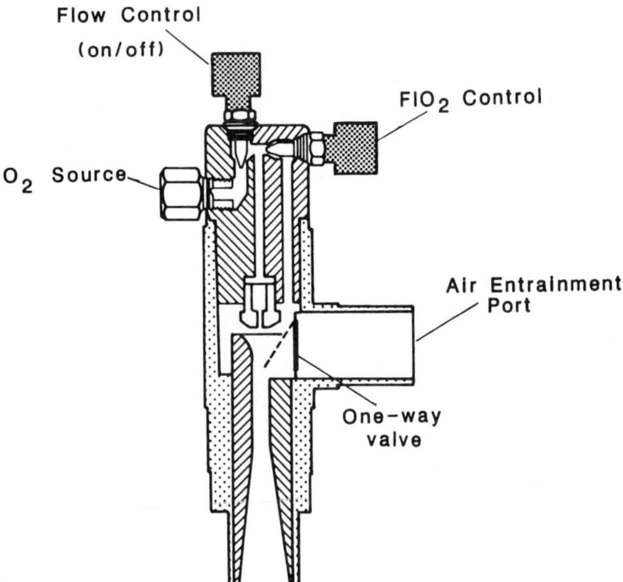

Figure 18-10. Schematic of the Vital Signs Flow Generator.

used to create the flow, a humidifier is generally not necessary. These devices are used at home throughout the night and therefore should operate quietly so sleep is not further interrupted by noise.

Problems With CPAP Systems

With a continuous-flow system, sufficient gas must be delivered to the reservoir bag to maintain pressure above that in the circuit. Thus, spontaneous inspiratory effort can be minimized at any level of expiratory pressure. Gas flow is adjusted until the desired inspiratory deflection of the airway pressure manometer is achieved (Fig. 18-13).

Demand systems similar to the spring-tension valve previously described may be substituted for the flowmeter and reservoir bag assembly in the CPAP circuitry. In this circumstance, the spring-tension can be adjusted to exceed source pressure so that the valve remains partially open, providing continuous circuit flow. The continuous flow satisfies initial inspiratory gas requirement, and inspiratory load may prove less with this configuration versus when the valve is employed as a strict demand flow system.

At least two physiologic differences exist between sPEEP and CPAP: (1) work of breathing and (2) venous return and cardiac output. Both effects are related to the transpulmonary pressure (PTP) during inspiration and the resultant mean pleural pressure (Ppl). Since the sPEEP system necessitates the generation of subambient airway pressure (Paw) to inspire fresh gas, inspiratory PTP is significantly greater than that required with CPAP (see Fig. 18-14).[13] Thus, the

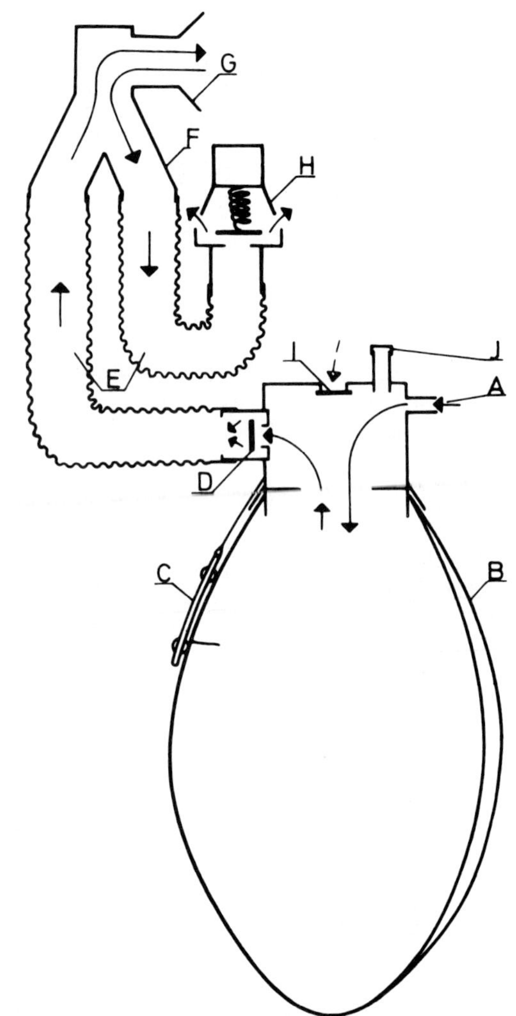

Figure 18-11. Schematic of the AMBU CPAP system. Gas enters the system from the Venturi at (A), filling the reservoir bag (B). A pressure indicator (C) displays approximate circuit pressure by changing position as the reservoir bag expands and contracts. A one-way valve (D) prevents rebreathing of gas from the patient circuit (E). The inspired and expired sides of the patient circuit are separated by a "Y" (F), which connects to the patient airway (G). The AMBU PEEP valve is a spring-loaded valve (H). An optional inlet (J) can be used to monitor pressure or to bleed in low flows of oxygen. An anti-asphyxia valve (I) allows the patient to breathe ambient air in case of gas source failure or accidental disconnection.

work of breathing is greater with sPEEP than CPAP at the same expiratory pressure. However, the larger PTP fluctuation (thoracic pump) with sPEEP augments venous return to the right side of the heart, and an increased stroke volume and cardiac output may result.

Continuous-flow rate or the demand valve sensitivity in the CPAP circuit can theoretically be regulated so that inspiratory effort and work of breathing are minimal. Since the patient's inspiratory PTP is small at an elevated mean Ppl, venous return may be impeded.

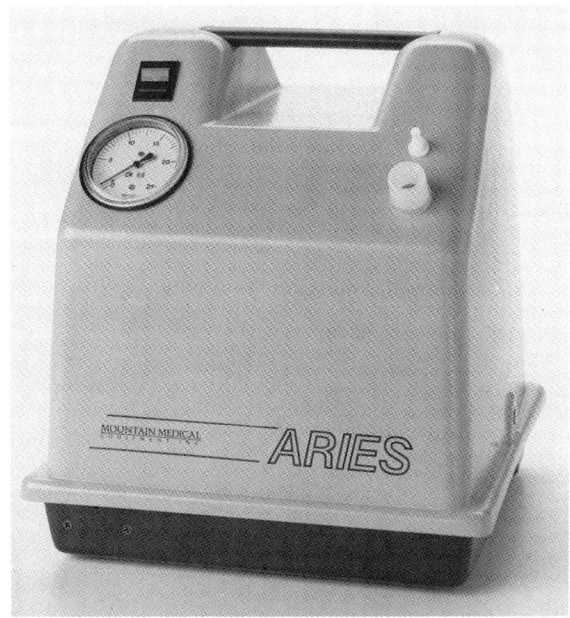

Figure 18-12. Aries nasal CPAP system. (Courtesy of Mountain Medical Equipment, Denver, CO)

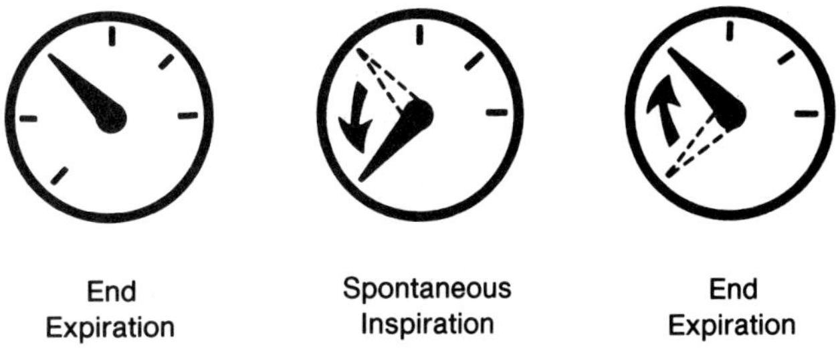

End Expiration | Spontaneous Inspiration | End Expiration

Figure 18-13. Aneroid pressure manometer can be employed to quantitate phasic alterations in circuit pressure during spontaneous positive-pressure therapy.

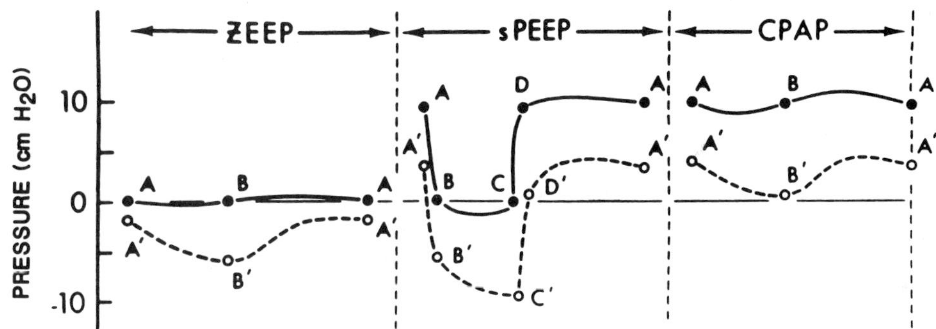

Figure 18-14. During normal spontaneous inspiration at zero end-expiratory pressure (ZEEP), airway pressure (Paw) (solid line) decreases slightly (A, B) and pleural pressure (PPL) (dotted line) is reduced by approximately 6 cm H_2O (A′, B′). However, during spontaneous PEEP (sPEEP), Paw must be reduced by an amount equal to PEEP (A, B) plus that required to open the unidirectional valve (B, C) with a parallel change in PPL (A′, B′, C′). Spontaneous ventilation with a minimal effort CPAP system should impose Paw and PPL changes similar in magnitude as ZEEP.

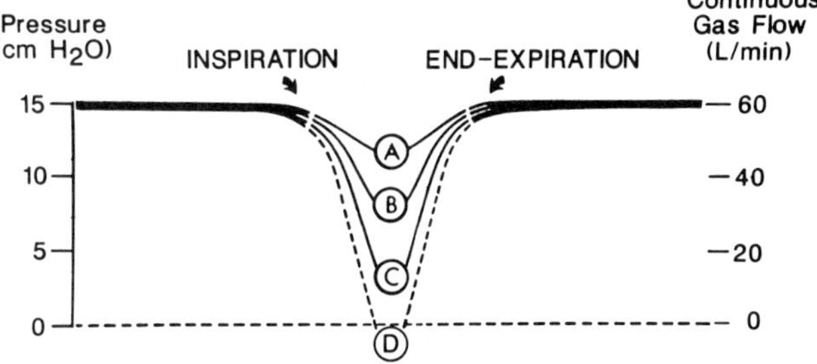

Figure 18-15. Curves A, B, and C are inspiratory pressure contours associated with various continuous flow rates in a CPAP system. When spontaneous inspiratory demand exceeds continuous flow rate, an airway pressure pattern approximating spontaneous PEEP (curve D) may occur. Although the end-expiratory pressure coincides for each pattern, the inspiratory effort is different.

Reports in healthy volunteers[14,15] and lung models[16,17] have shown significant variability in the functional performance of demand valves. Some studies have observed that a continuous-flow reservoir CPAP system at 60 L/min with an Emerson water column PEEP valve facilitates a lower inspiratory effort and lower expiratory resistance when compared with demand valve systems.[14-20] Some demand valves can impose a significant increase in the inspiratory work of breathing that may not be tolerated by some patients. Flow triggering appears to be more sensitive than pressure triggering and reduces the patient's work of breathing.[21-25] Often the "failure" of CPAP therapy is related to the mechanics rather than the technique. When "air hunger" is greater while a patient is attached to an sPEEP/CPAP circuit than when not, the mechanics or the appropriateness of the circuitry should be suspect. Some patients may tolerate and respond well to 10 to 15 cm H_2O sPEEP, whereas others may only be able to generate little inspiratory effort and require CPAP. Thus the circuitry/system should be tailored to the individual and clinical circumstances.

These patients also emphasize the importance of scrutinizing the end-expiratory pressure (EEP) to end-inspiratory (EIP) gradient, particularly when evaluating hemodynamic data during spontaneous positive-pressure breathing. In Figure 18-15, four examples of inspiratory pressure patterns with the same EEP are shown. Curves A, B and C represent CPAP, but the EIP is different. It is important to recognize that the wider the EEP-EIP gradient the greater is the inspiratory PTP. Curve D represents sPEEP (ie, the EIP is subambient).

References

1. Kirby RR, Robinson EJ, Schulz J, et al. A new pediatric volume ventilator. Anesth Analg 1971;50:533–537.
2. Downs JB, Klein EF, Desautels D, et al. Intermittent mandatory ventilation: A new approach to weaning patients from mechanical ventilators. Chest 1973;56:638–641.
3. Sturgeon CL, Douglas ME, Downs JB, et al. PEEP and CPAP: Cardiopulmonary effects during spontaneous ventilation. Anesth Analg 1978;56:638–641.
4. Parel A, Pachys F, Olshwang D, et al. Mechanical inspiratory peak flow as a determinant of tidal volume during IMV and PEEP. Anesthesiology 1978;48:290–292.
5. Banner MJ, Boysen PG. Demand valve improperly set resulting in barotrauma. Anesthesiology 1984;61:86–87.
6. Page BA, Downs JB. IMV and continuous gas flow: A complication. Anesthesiology 1977;46:72–73.
7. Oertel MJ. In: Van Ziemssen Handbook of Therapeutics (1878), vol 3. (Yeo JB, trans.) 1885:448–451.
8. Poulton EP, Oxon DM. Left-sided heart failure with pulmonary edema: Its treatment with the "pulmonary plus pressure machine." Lancet 1936;231:981–983.
9. Bullowa JGH. The Management of the Pneumonias. New York: Oxford University Press, 1937:88–90
10. Barach AL, Martin J, Eckman M. Positive pressure respiration and its application to the treatment of acute pulmonary edema. Ann Intern Med 1938;12:754–795.
11. Gregory G, Kitterman J, Phibbs RH, et al. Treatment of idiopathic respiratory-distress syndrome with continuous positive airway pressure. N Engl J Med 1971;284:1333–1340.
12. Civetta JM, Brons R, Gabel JC. A simple and effective method of employing spontaneous positive pressure ventilation. J Thorac Cardiovasc Surg 1972;63:312–313.
13. Douglas ME, Downs JB. Cardiopulmonary effects of PEEP and CPAP (letter to editor). Anesth Analg 1978;57:347–350.
14. Gibney RTN, Wilson RS, Pontoppidan H. Comparison of work of breathing on high gas flow and demand valve continuous positive airway pressure systems. Chest 1982;82:692–695.
15. Cox D, Niblett DJ. Studies on continuous positive airway pressure breathing systems. Br J Anaesth 1984;56:905–911.
16. Christopher KL, Neff TA, Eberle DJ, et al. Demand and continuous flow intermittent mandatory ventilation systems. Chest 1985;87:625–630.
17. Katz JA, Kraemer RW, Gjerde GE. Inspiratory work and airway pressure with continuous positive airway pressure delivery systems. Chest 1985;88:519–526.
18. Hirsch C, Kacmarek RM, Stanek K. Work of breathing during CPAP and PSV imposed by the new generation mechanical ventilators: A lung model study. Respir Care 1991;36:815–828.
19. Samodelov LF, Falke KJ. Total inspiratory work with modern demand valve devices compared to continuous flow CPAP. Intens Care Med 1988;14:632–639.
20. Moran JL, Homan S, O'Fathartaigh M, Jackson M, Leppard P. Inspiratory work imposed by continuous positive airway pressure (CPAP) machines: The effect of CPAP level and endotracheal tube size. Intens Care Med 1992;18:148–154.
21. Sassoon CSH. Mechanical ventilator design and function: The trigger variable. Respir Care 1992;37:1056–1069.
22. Sassoon CSH, Giran AE, Ely E, Light RW. Inspiratory work of breathing on flow-by and demand-flow continuous positive airway pressure. Crit Care 1989;17:1108–1114.
23. Sassoon CSH, Light RW, Lodia R, Sieck GC, Mahutte CK. Pressure-time product during continuous positive airway pressure, pressure support ventilation, and T-piece during weaning from mechanical ventilation. Am Rev Respir Dis 1991;143: 469–475.
24. Branson RD, Davis K Jr, Johnson DJ, Campbell RS. A comparison of flow and pressure triggering systems during CPAP. Respir Care 1993;38:1244.
25. Branson RD. Flow-triggering systems. Respir Care 1994;39:-138–144.

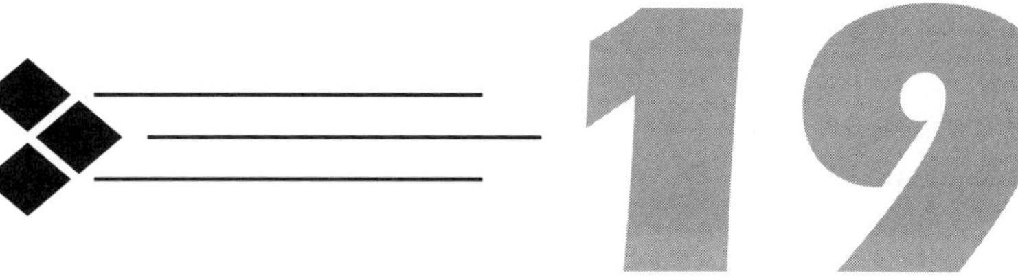

Expiratory Pressure Valves

Michael J. Banner
Samsun Lampotang

OBJECTIVES

1. Compare the characteristic features of threshold resistors and flow resistors.
2. Explain the difference between threshold resistors and flow resistors.
3. Describe the structure and function of water column, weighted ball, electromagnetic valve, and flexed spring threshold devices.
4. Describe the structure and function of adjustable orifice and scissors valve flow resistors.
5. Explain the effects of end-expiratory pressure valves on the work of breathing.

KEY TERMS

expiratory pressure valve
flow resistor
imposed work of breathing
scissors valve
threshold resistor
water column expiratory pressure valve

Introduction

Expiratory pressure valves regulate the level of airway pressure during spontaneous ventilation with continuous positive airway pressure (CPAP), as well as during mechanical ventilation with positive end-expiratory pressure (PEEP). These valves are characterized as threshold and flow resistors.[1,2]

Threshold Resistors

In theory, threshold resistors generate expiratory pressure (P) without associated flow resistance (Equation Box 19-1). Exhaled gas passes freely through the completely open threshold resistor orifice until the balance of forces on opposite sides of the valve mechanism is disrupted.[2] At this point, the valve closes abruptly, preventing further gas loss from the airways and lungs.

Various mechanisms have been employed in the design of threshold resistors (Table 19-1). The following are examples of some commercially available types.

Equation Box 19-1: Pressure Created in a Threshold Resistor

Pressure (P) in a threshold resistor results from a force (F), expressed in newtons (N), applied over a discrete surface area (SA), expressed in square meters (m^2):

$$P = \frac{F}{SA}$$

For example, a loading F of 10 N applied to SA of 0.01 m^2 generates a pressure of 1000 N/m^2 = 10 cm H_2O.

Water Column

The Emerson water column valve is a gravity-dependent device and uses the weight of a column of water to exert force over the surface area of a diaphragm. Expiratory pressure (level of CPAP) may be titrated by varying the amount of water (force) held in a column (Fig. 19-1).

Weighted Ball

The Boehringer weighted-ball valve is another example of a gravity-dependent threshold resistor. Pressure is generated by the weight of the ball applied over the surface area of the exhalation orifice. These valves are available in pre-set pressure levels of 2.5, 5, 10, and 15 cm H_2O.

TABLE 19-1. Expiratory Positive-Pressure Valves

Valve	Description
Threshold Resistors	
Non–gravity–dependent	
Vital Signs	Flexion of multiple springs against a disk
Ambu	Compression of a single spring against a disk
Hamilton Veolar and Amadeus	Electromagnetically activated piston over a diaphragm
Instrumentation Industries	Magnetic attraction of a metal disk valve
Bourns BP 200, Bear Cub, Ohmeda CPU-1, Puritan-Bennett 7200a	Venturi (jet pump) back-pressure against a diaphragm
IMV Bird	Pressure-loaded diaphragm–disk mechanism
Gravity-dependent	
Emerson	Water column hydrostatic force over a diaphragm
Boehringer	Weighted-ball valve over an orifice
Underwater valve	Hydrostatic force over the orifice of the exhalation tube
Flow Resistor	
Screw-clamp	Variable orifice
Flow resistor–like devices	Hinged clamp–"scissor valve"
Siemens 900B and 900C*	
Hybrid Valves†	
Balloon valves	
eg, Puritan-Bennett MA-1, MA-2, and Bear 1, 2 and 5	Inflatable balloon (mushroom) valve
Babybird outflow valve	Variable orifice

*Although the Siemens expiratory pressure valve is servo controlled, it responds as a flow resistor (ie, pressure drop across the valve increases as flow rate increases).[3-5]

†This design has characteristics of both threshold and flow resistors, although in theory it is a threshold resistor; flow resistance occurs primarily because of the limited opening area for exhalation.[2]

THRESHOLD RESISTOR $(P \propto F/SA)$

A. BEGINNING EXHALATION B. END–EXHALATION

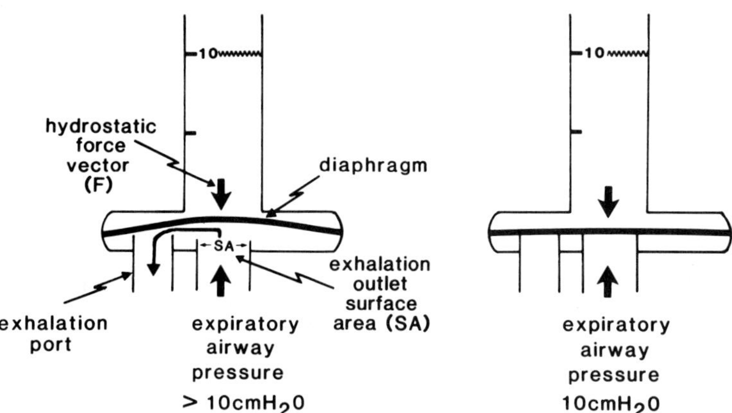

Figure 19-1. A and B. A threshold resistor expiratory pressure valve (Emerson) generates expiratory positive pressure (P) by exerting force (F) over a surface area (SA). (From Banner MJ, Lampotang S, Boysen PG, Hurd TE, Desautels DA. Flow resistance of expiratory positive pressure valve systems. Chest 1986; 90:212–217)

Electromagnetic Valve

The Hamilton threshold resistor (Hamilton Medical Veolar ventilator, Hamilton Medical Corporation, Reno, NV) produces pressure by relying on electromagnetic force, generated by a solenoid, applied over the surface area of a diaphragm. With this device, force and therefore expiratory pressure are proportional to the electric current supplied to the solenoid. By regulating the amount of current with a rheostat (control knob on ventilator panel), the level of CPAP is selected (Figs. 19-2 and 19-3).

Flexed Springs

The Vital Signs (Vital Signs Inc., Totowa, NJ) valve produces pressure by employing flexed, coiled springs that exert force against a plastic disk. A *flexing* rather than compressing action of the springs appears to maintain constant force irrespective of the degree of displacement (opening) of the plastic disk from the exhalation orifice, and thus nearly constant pressure is maintained (Fig. 19-4). In contrast, spring-loaded

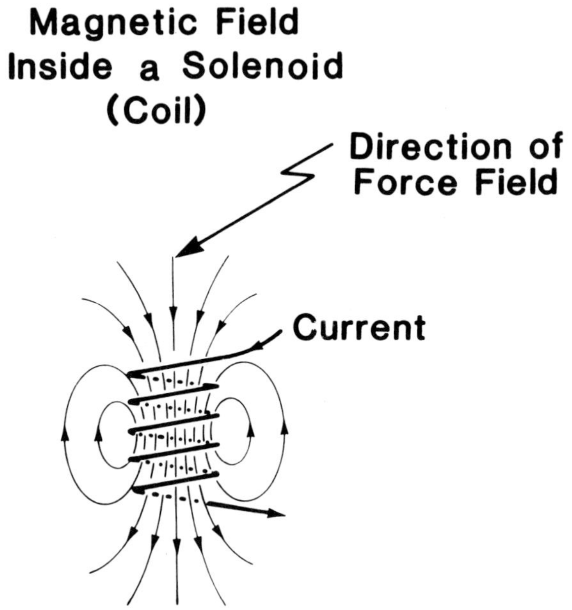

Magnetic Field Inside a Solenoid (Coil)
Direction of Force Field
Current

Figure 19-2. A solenoid is a coil of wire that produces a magnetic field when electric current flows through it. Force vectors are in the direction of the magnetic field pattern.

THRESHOLD RESISTOR:(Hamilton Veolar®)

EXPIRATORY PRESSURE ∝ ELECTRIC CURRENT

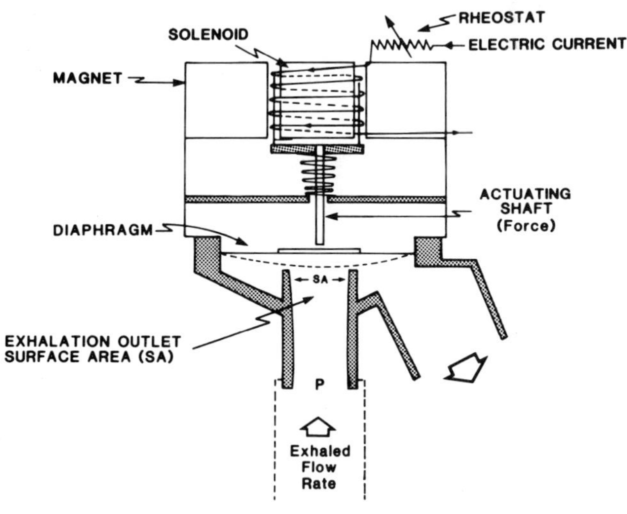

Figure 19-3. Threshold resistor expiratory pressure valve in the Hamilton Veolar ventilator (Hamilton Medical Corporation, Reno, NV). A rheostat regulates electric current to a solenoid. The force (F) transmitted downward, through an actuating shaft, to a diaphragm surface area (SA), is proportional to the amount of current supplied to the solenoid (see Figure 19-2).

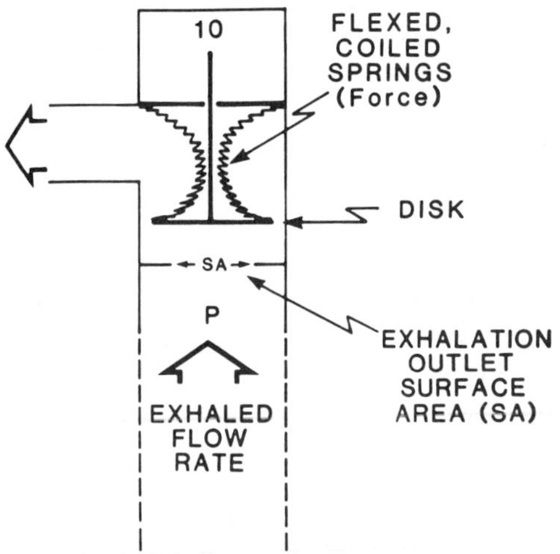

Figure 19-4. Threshold resistor expiratory pressure valve (Vital Signs Inc., Totowa, NJ). Expiratory positive pressure (P) is generated through force (F) exerted by the flexion of multiple coiled springs against a plastic disk (ie, exhalation out surface area [SA]) (P α F/SA). The orifice size of the valve is such that flow resistance is minimal.

valves that rely on *compression* of a spring result in an increase in force as the spring is compressed when the valve opens during exhalation. When exhaled flow rate is high, the valve opens wider and spring compression increases; thus force increases over surface area and therefore pressure increases. The Vital Signs valves are available in pre-set pressure levels of 2.5, 5, 7.5, 10, 12.5, 15, and 20 cm H_2O.

Jet Pump (Venturi) Diaphragm

Another type of threshold resistor found on the BP 200 and Bear Cub infant ventilators uses gas flow from a Venturi (jet pump) directed against a diaphragm. By regulating gas flow rate into the venturi, the back-pressure of the venturi is controlled. The back-pressure of the venturi applied to the surface area of the diaphragm is equivalent to force. Titrating gas flow rate to the jet regulates the level of CPAP (Fig. 19-5).

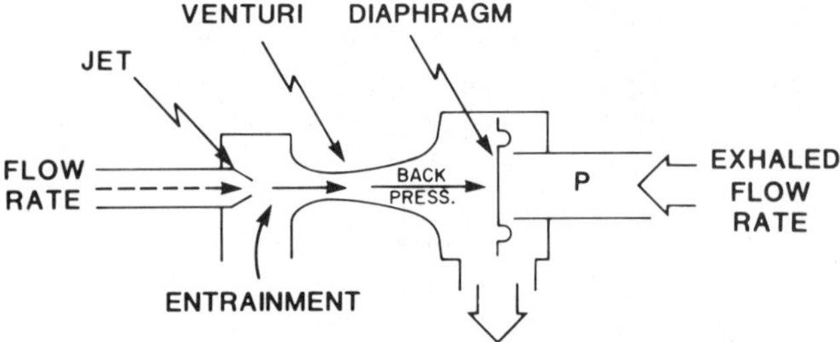

Figure 19-5. Venturi (ejector)–diaphragm threshold resistor expiratory positive-pressure valve, similar to that found on the BP 200 and BEAR Cub infant ventilators (Bear Medical Corporation, Riverside, CA). Expiratory positive pressure (P) is controlled by titrating the flow rate to the jet, which directly affects the back-pressure generated by the Venturi.

Equation Box 19-2: Pressure Created in a Flow Resistor

$$P = R\dot{V}$$

This relationship is congruent only under laminar flow conditions and a given range of flow rates (Fig. 19-6). For example, if R is 10 cm H_2O/L/s and exhaled $\dot{V}$ is 1 L/s, then P = 10 cm H_2O.

Flow Resistors

Flow resistor expiratory pressure valves generate pressure by imposing an adjustable orifice resistance (R) to exhaled flow rate ($\dot{V}$). Pressure (P) varies inversely with the orifice size, assuming exhaled flow rate is constant. Thus, the magnitude of the pressure generated is directly related to orifice resistance (Equation Box 19-2). If the adjustable exhalation ori-

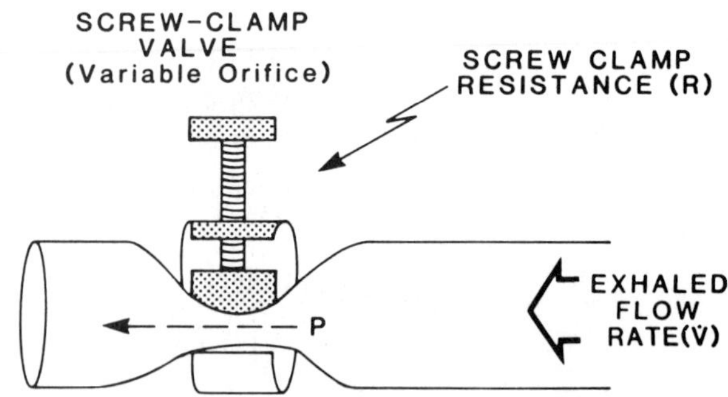

Figure 19-6. A flow resistor (screw–clamp variable orifice) determines expiratory positive pressure (P) by the product of resistance (R) and flow rate ($\dot{V}$) directed through the valve. The resistance is regulated by varying the orifice size with the screw-clamp and varies inversely with orifice size. The smaller the exhalation orifice, the greater the resistance and, thus, the greater the pressure. (From Banner MJ, Lampotang S, Boysen PG, Hurd TE, Desautels DA. Flow resistance of expiratory positive pressure valve systems. Chest 1986;90:212–217)

fice is narrowed, greater resistance to exhaled flow rate results. Hence greater pressure (ie, CPAP level) is generated in the breathing circuit.

The Siemens servo-controlled "scissor valve" found on the Siemens 900B and 900C ventilators (Siemens Life Support Systems, Iselin, NJ) appears to respond as a flow resistor–like valve.[3,4] With this device, the exhalation orifice is situated between a hinged clamp mechanism (Fig. 19-7).

Hybrid Valves

The Babybird variable orifice outflow valve is a component of the Babybird ventilator (Bird Products Corporation, Palm Springs, CA). With this device, expiratory pressure is regulated by directing gas flow through an orifice against a diaphragm. The exhalation orifice can be positioned closer to or farther away from the diaphragm, which, in turn, acts to increase or decrease resistance to flow, respectively. Force is also exerted by the elastic recoil properties of the diaphragm over the exhalation orifice and directly affects the expiratory pressure generated. It is increased as the diaphragm is displaced upward when the exhalation orifice is positioned closer to the diaphragm in a fashion analogous to compression of a coiled spring. At flow rates greater than approximately 30 L/min, expiratory pressure progressively increases, while at flow rates less than this, expiratory pressure is relatively stable. Therefore, the valve functions as a hybrid; that is, it has characteristics of both flow and threshold resistors. The valve was designed to be used at low flow rates (2–15 L/min) and for neonates. Because of its flow resistor characteristics at higher flow rates, it is not recommended for adult patients.

Another type of expiratory pressure valve uses a pressurized, inflatable balloon to obstruct the exhalation outlet. The balloon valve is pressurized through a charging line attached to a mechanical ventilator where a Venturi mechanism may be used to apply pressure to the balloon. By regulating the flow rate of gas supplied to the Venturi, the loading pressure to the balloon and hence the CPAP level is controlled. Balloon valves appear to function as a hybrid design; that is, they have characteristics of both threshold and flow resistors. Although in theory this type of valve was conceived as a threshold resistor, flow resistance occurs primarily because of the limited opening area of the balloon valve for exhalation.[2] An eccentric, partial deflation of the balloon during exhalation may occur, forming an orifice-like resistance to exhaled flow. As a result, nearly linear relationships between pressure and flow rate have been reported for these valves,[5] much like a flow resistor. Inflatable balloon valves generate pressure as the result of the loading pressure applied to the balloon and the resistance characteristics of the valve (Fig. 19-8). See Equation Box 19-3.

Ventilators incorporating inflatable balloon expiratory pressure valves are the Puritan-Bennett MA-1 and MA-2 and the Bear 1, 2, and 5 models.

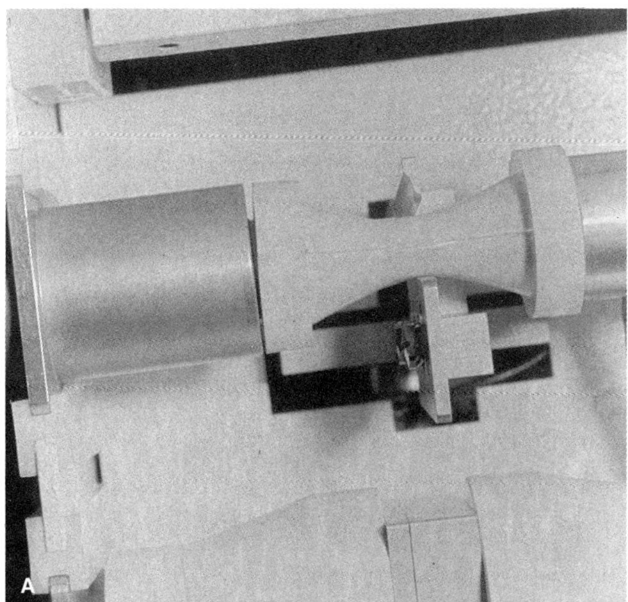

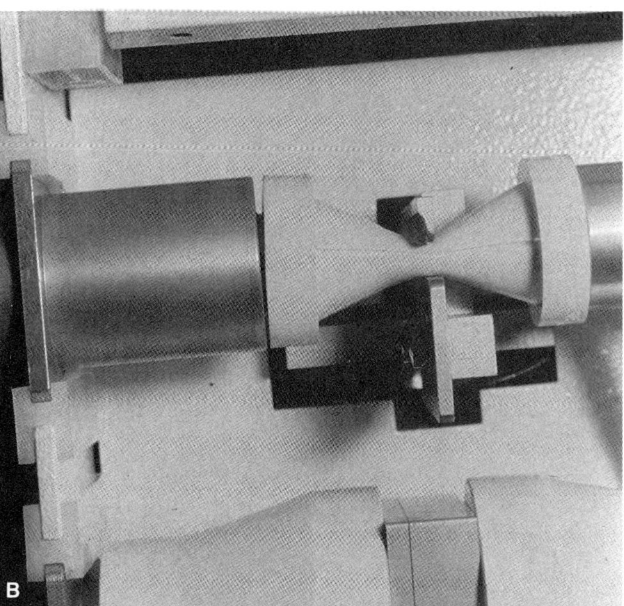

Figure 19-7. Siemens 900C expiratory pressure valve is servo-controlled; it responds as a flow resistor (ie, pressure drop across the valve increases as flow rate increases).[3,4] Under conditions of zero expiratory pressure, the valve is fully open (A). Under conditions of positive expiratory pressure, the exhalation orifice is narrowed by the "scissor-like" device (B).

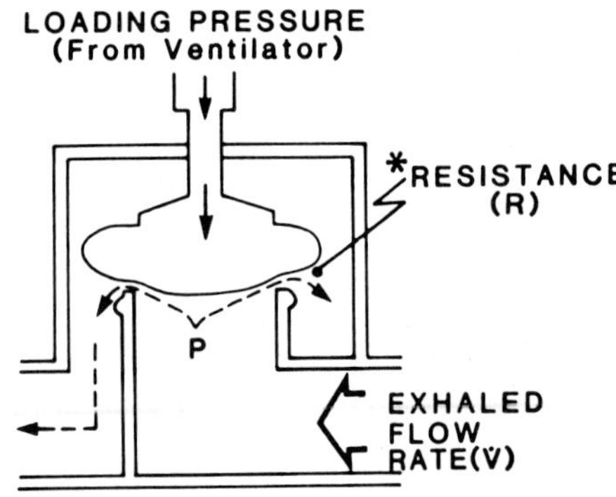

Figure 19-8. Inflatable balloon expiratory pressure valve. An inflatable balloon is pressurized by a loading pressure from the ventilator that is set by the operator. The exhalation orifice is thus obstructed and exhaled flow rate (V̇) is opposed by the balloon-loading pressure. Exhaled flow rate is directed through narrow openings between the bottom of the balloon and the valve seat, which give rise to resistance (R) to flow rate.

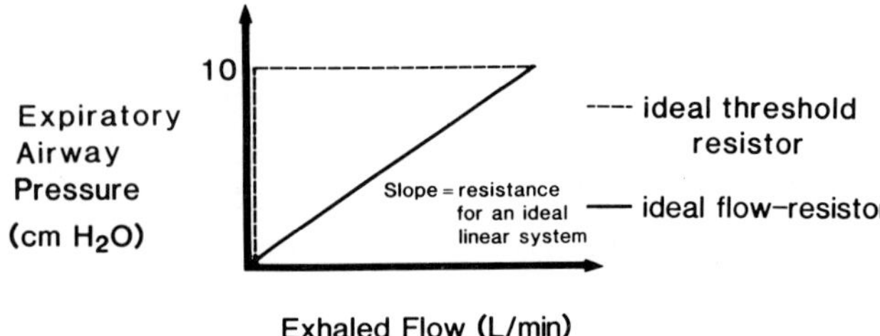

Figure 19-9. An ideal threshold resistor maintains a constant expiratory airway pressure under conditions of varying exhaled flow rate. In contrast, with an ideal flow resistor, expiratory airway pressure varies in a linear fashion with exhaled flow rate. (From Banner MJ. Expiratory positive pressure valves and work of breathing. Respir Care 1987; 32:431–436)

Resistance Characteristics

Theoretically, a threshold resistor should maintain a constant pressure regardless of variations in exhaled flow rate, as contrasted to a flow resistor, in which airway pressure deviations occur when the flow rate of gas through the CPAP system is changed (Fig. 19-9).[6]

Actually, resistance to exhaled flow occurs with both types of valves.[3–5,7,8] As a result, pressure increases above the desired level when the exhaled flow rate and/or the continuous flow rate through the CPAP system increases (Figs. 19-10 and 19-11). When exhaled flow rate is high (as during coughing), very high airway pressures may result (Fig. 19-12)and may increase the likelihood of barotrauma. When high-resistance valves are used, exhalation is no longer passive and expiratory work of breathing and oxygen consumption may increase. When high-resistance expiratory-pressure valves are combined with poorly designed demand-flow valves (ie, those with slow response time, substantial reduction in airway pressure required to initiate flow during spontaneous inhalation, and no provision for instantaneous, high flow rate on demand),[9] highly resistant humidifiers,[10] or low-flow rate air–oxygen blenders,[11] then intolerably high resistance to flow may result during spontaneous breathing.[12] Unless clinicians attempt to decrease resistance to flow throughout the breathing circuit, work of breathing may be intolerable. The presence of high resistance to flow may explain why CPAP and intermittent mandatory ventilation have failed in the hands of some clinicians.[13]

If an expiratory pressure valve with high flow resistance reduces the expiratory flow rate significantly, exhalation may not be complete before the next mechanical inflation begins. High flow resistance also increases peak and mean exhalation pressures[3] and may compromise thoracic venous blood inflow, preload, and cardiac output.

Equation Box 19-3: Pressure Created in an Inflatable Balloon PEEP Valve

$$P = \text{Loading pressure} + R\dot{V}$$

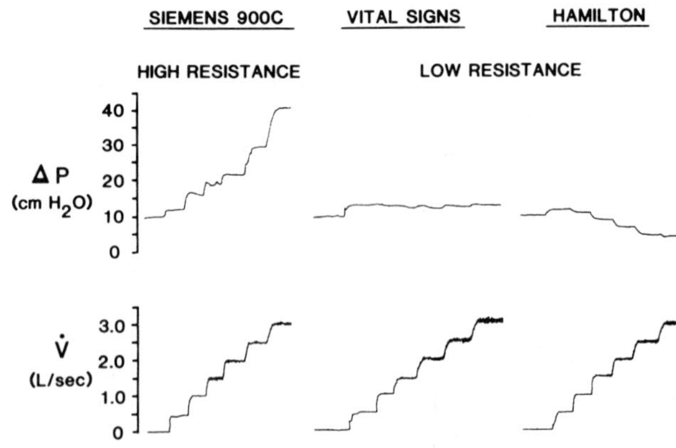

Figure 19-10. Comparison of the flow resistive characteristics of high- and low-resistance expiratory positive-pressure valves.

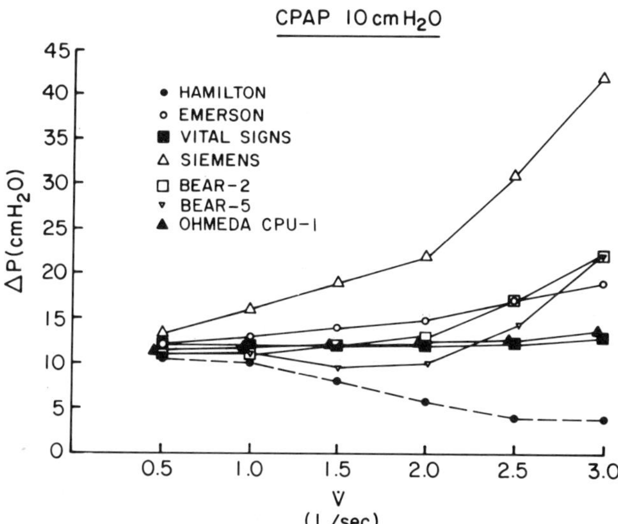

Figure 19-11. Comparison of the flow-resistance characteristics of various expiratory positive-pressure valves. The greater the slope, the greater the resistance and vice versa. (From Banner MJ. Expiratory positive pressure valves and work of breathing. Respir Care 1987;32:431–436)

The flow resistive characteristics of most threshold resistor expiratory pressure valves under sinusoidal flow rate conditions deviates from the ideal.[3,14] Resistance to exhaled flow varies widely, which further classifies them as high and low flow-resistant valves. The equation describing the operation of threshold resistors is thus revised as shown in Equation Box 19-4.

Low flow-resistant threshold resistors may decrease the incidence of barotrauma and other untoward airway pressure–related effects by avoiding acute increases in airway pressure. The Hamilton threshold resistor, which is an electromagnetically activated piston acting against a diaphragm, seems to open wider under conditions of high flow rate (*without* a concomitant increase in force applied to the diaphragm) and, thereby, vents the increased flow rate by increasing the effective exhalation area for gas efflux.[3,14] Since resistance is inversely proportional to exhalation area, as the exhalation area increases, resistance and, thus, pressure decrease. Rapid unloading of airway pressure during high flow rate conditions minimizes the potential danger of pulmonary barotrauma. The Vital Signs valve, which flexes multiple springs against a disk, appears to be another low flow-resistant threshold resistor.[3,14,15] The exhalation orifice size is such that flow resistance is minimal. This device has almost ideal threshold resistor characteristics because expiratory pressure increases only slightly above the set level, with constant flow rates up to 180 L/min (see Fig. 19-10) and peak sinusoidal flow rates up to 200 L/min[21] (see Fig. 19-12).

The Siemens 900C hinged-clamped "scissor" valve generates high expiratory pressures during intermittent high flow rate (eg, simulated coughing) and constant flow rate.[3] Increasing levels of flow resistance with increasing levels of end-expiratory pressure have also been demonstrated with this valve.[16,17]

Equation Box 19-4: Revised Equation Describing the Operation of a Threshold Resistor

$$P = F/SA + R(\dot{V}exh + \dot{V}sys)$$

where $\dot{V}exh$ is the patient's instantaneous exhaled flow rate and $\dot{V}sys$ is the constant rate of gas flow through the CPAP system. The $R\dot{V}$ component of this expression differentiates high-flow and low-flow resistant threshold resistors. For example, if two threshold resistor valves are set to exert a P of 10 cm H_2O and with valve No. 1, R is 10 cm H_2O/L/s and $\dot{V}exh$ and $\dot{V}sys$ are 0.5 L/s each, then total P = 20 cm H_2O (ie, P = 10 + 10 [0.5 + 0.5]). In contrast, with Valve No. 2, in which R is 1 cm H_2O/L/s and $\dot{V}exh$ and $\dot{V}sys$ are 0.5 L/s each, then P is only 11 cm H_2O (ie, P = 10 + 1 [0.5 + 0.5]). If Valve No. 1 were being used and the patient suddenly coughed and generated a peak $\dot{V}exh$ of 3 L/s (180 L/min), the expiratory pressure would peak at 45 cm H_2O, compared with only 13.5 cm H_2O peak expiratory pressure if Valve No. 2 were being used (assuming the resistances of Valve No. 1 and Valve No. 2 are linear).

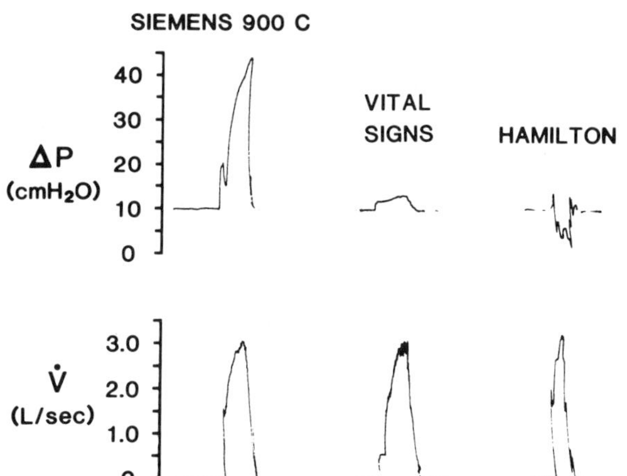

Figure 19-12. Effects of a simulated cough with high- and low-resistance expiratory pressure valves (see Fig. 19-11). All valves were set to a CPAP of 10 cm H_2O when the flow rate ($\dot{V}$) was zero.

"Passive" and "Active" Threshold Resistors

A threshold resistor that does not vary the obstructing force applied during the respiratory cycle may be defined as a "passive" threshold resistor. Such a valve acts as a rectilinear mechanical system with one degree of freedom. See Equation Box 19-5. Different designs of passive threshold resistors emphasize different terms of Equation Box 19-5. For example, the gravity-dependent valves (water column, submerged-outlet, and weighted-ball valve) develop force from the third term, mass × acceleration (ma: acceleration {a} is provided by gravity), with negligible contribution from the other two terms. In a spring-loaded valve, the spring constant (K) of the valve system times the displacement (1) of the valve face from its natural resting position is the dominant term.

An inflatable balloon valve that uses a pressurized balloon to obstruct the exhalation outlet may be considered an "active" threshold resistor–like device. The analysis of this design is more complex because the balloon acts as a miniature lung with its own dynamic characteristics, including flow resistance, compliance, and internal pressure. The obstructing force applied by the balloon can also be expressed mathematically. See Equation Box 19-6.

Rate of decrease of force exerted by the balloon during exhalation is affected mainly by the system resistance (Rsys), that is, the resistance to the displacement of the volume of air loading the balloon. When the balloon valve cannot recoil fast enough (excessive Rsys) at the beginning of exhalation, the exit area for gas efflux is small and resistance to flow is appreciable. This might be the case with ventilators employing an inflatable balloon pressurized by a Venturi that tends to apply constant pressure to the balloon (e.g., Bear 2, Puritan-Bennett MA-2). The force applied by the balloon *may* not decrease quickly enough at the onset of exhalation because the loading volume of gas cannot be quickly displaced from the balloon due to the constant pressure exerted by the Venturi and the flow resistance of the narrow throat in the Venturi (ie, high Rsys) mechanism. Thus, although in theory the inflatable balloon valves on these ventilators are sometimes referred to as "threshold resistors," they seem to function more as flow resistors.

Equation Box 19-5: Equation of Motion for a Rectilinear Mechanical System

The equation of motion for a rectilinear mechanical system provides a mathematical description of the mode of operation of a "passive" threshold resistor:

$$F = K\ell + cv + ma$$

where F is the force applied against the expiratory valve face (in newtons), K is the elastic modulus (spring constant) of the valve system (in newtons per centimeter), ℓ is the distance of compression or extension of the valve face from its natural resting position (in centimeters), c is the viscous resistance opposing valve face movement (in newtons per centimeter per second), v is the rate of valve face displacement (velocity, in centimeters per second), m is the inertia (mass, in kilograms) distributed among the moving parts of the valve system, and a is the system's acceleration (in meters per second squared). F represents the force exerted by physiologic airway pressure on the valve face that is obstructing the exhalation outlet. This force tends to set the system into motion (ie, opens the valve and allows exhalation). The terms on the right side of the equation oppose motion of the system (ie, keep the valve closed).

Equation Box 19-6: Equation for Force Generated by an Inflatable Balloon Valve

The obstructing force applied by an inflatable-balloon threshold resistor–like device can be expressed as

$$F = SA\left(\frac{V}{C} + Rsys\,\dot{V} + I\ddot{V}\right)k$$

where SA is that part of the internal surface area of the balloon that develops a force in a direction parallel to the exhalation outlet axis (in square centimeters), C is the compliance of the valve system (in liters per centimeter of water), V is the volume (proportional to the distance of movement of the valve face) for the opening and closing of the valve (in liters), Rsys is the system resistance of the balloon to "unloading" at the beginning of exhalation (in centimeters of water per liter per second), $\dot{V}$ is the rate of volume displacement (flow rate out of the balloon, in liters per second), I is the system inertia (in centimeters of water per liter per second squared) distributed among the wall of the valve and the fluid in motion contained within the balloon, and $\ddot{V}$ is the volume acceleration (in liters per second squared). The conversion constant, $k = 9.81 \times 10^{-3}$, is included so that F is in newtons.

Expiratory Pressure Valve Flow Resistance: Effects on Inspiratory Airway Pressure and Work of Breathing

Downs[12] has contended that the resistance of the expiratory pressure valve effects the inspiratory positive airway pressure level and inspiratory work of breathing during CPAP. A high flow-resistant expiratory pressure valve leads to a greater decrease in airway pressure than does a low flow-resistant one during spontaneous inhalation (if all other factors are constant.)[18–20]

In CPAP systems employing a continuous gas flow rate, part of the measured CPAP results from the resistance to flow rate as it passes through the expiratory pressure valve orifice ($P \propto R\dot{V}$). Valves that generate pressure in part by resistance times flow rate (e.g., balloon valve), or solely by resistance times flow rate (flow resistor), will lead to decreases in airway pressure during spontaneous inhalation on CPAP. The higher the contribution of resistance to airway pressure, the greater the decrease in airway pressure during spontaneous inhalation. When the patient inhales, part (or even all) of the continuous flow rate is diverted from the valve to the lungs. If flow rate through the valve is less, and assuming resistance is unchanged, then resistance times less flow rate yields less pressure. The greater the decrease in airway pressure, the greater the increase in imposed work of breathing, measured at the Y piece of the breathing circuit, since imposed work of the breathing circuit = ~ Paw × dV (where Paw is the pressure and dV is the volume change). Under these conditions, intrapleural pressure must decrease by a corresponding amount to generate appropriate changes in transpulmonary pressure (transpulmonary pressure = airway pressure − intrapleural pressure) during spontaneous inhalation.[20]

To evaluate imposed work during CPAP, a threshold resistor (Emerson) and a flow resistor (screw clamp) were examined during simulated spontaneous ventilation with a piston-driven mechanical model. Inspiratory and expiratory peak sinusoidal flow rates, inhalation-to-exhalation time ratio, breathing frequency, tidal volume, and end-expiratory pressure were held constant with both valves. A greater decrease in airway pressure and greater imposed work were noted with the flow resistor valve (Fig. 19-13). Thus, one can predict that high flow-resistant expiratory pressure valves will decrease airway pressure and increase imposed work more than will low flow-resistant valves for a given decrement of flow rate through the expiratory pressure valve.

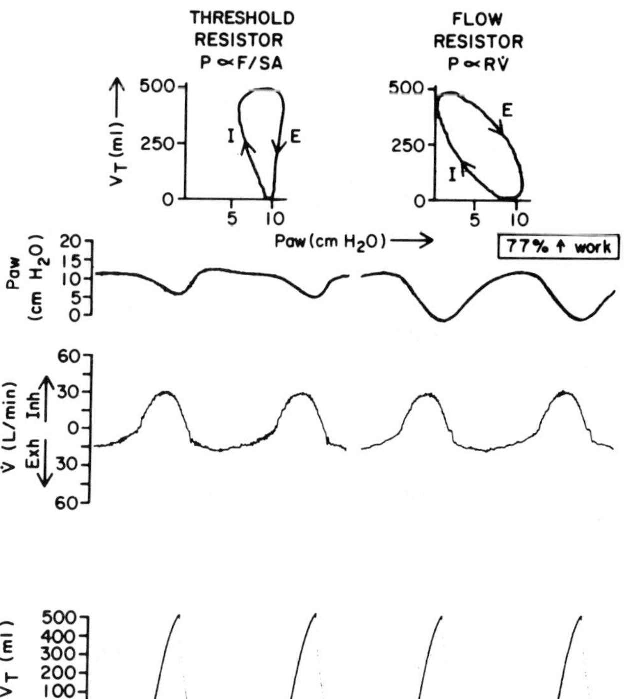

Figure 19-13. Comparison of the imposed work of breathing required to breathe through a CPAP system with a threshold resistor (Emerson) and a flow resistor (screw-clamp). (From Banner MJ. Expiratory positive pressure valves and work of breathing. Respir Care 1987;32:431–436)

Conclusion

Ideally, *only* low flow-resistant threshold resistors should be used in CPAP systems to maintain relatively constant airway pressure in the face of changing exhaled flow rate. The use of such valves may reduce the incidence of barotrauma and the work of breathing by minimizing acute increases in expiratory pressure and large decreases in inspiratory pressure, respectively.

Acknowledgments

The authors would like to thank Ms. Hope Olivo for her editorial assistance and Mr. Jake Fuller for graphics.

References

1. Kacmarek RM, Dimas S, Reynolds J, Shapiro BA. Technical aspects of positive end-expiratory pressure (PEEP): I. Physics of PEEP devices. Respir Care 1982;27:1478–1489.
2. Kirby RR: Positive airway pressure: System design and clinical application. In: Shoemaker WC, ed. Critical Care: State of the Art, vol 6. Fullerton, CA: Society of Critical Care Medicine, 1985:G1–G52.
3. Banner MJ. Expiratory positive pressure valves: Flow resistance and work of breathing. Respir Care 1987;32:431–436.
4. Banner MJ, Lampotang S, Boysen PB, et al. Resistance of expiratory positive pressure valves. Chest 1988;94:893–895.
5. Marini JJ, Culver BH, Kirk W. Flow resistance of exhalation valves and positive end-expiratory pressure devices used in mechanical ventilation. Am Rev Respir Dis 1985;131:850–854.

6. Mushin WW, Rendell-Baker L, Thompson PW. Automatic Ventilation of the Lungs, 3rd ed. Oxford: Blackwell Scientific Publications, 1969:105–127.
7. Hall JR, Rendleman DC, Downs JB. PEEP devices: Flow dependent increases in airway pressure (abstract). Crit Care Med 1978;6:100.
8. Nunn JF. Applied Respiratory Physiology, 2nd ed. London: Butterworths, 1977;100–103.
9. Viale JB, Annal G, Bertrand O, Ing D, Godard J, Motin J. Additional inspiratory work in intubated patients breathing with continuous positive airway pressure systems. Anesthesiology 1985;63:536–539.
10. Poulton TJ, Downs JB. Humidification of rapidly flowing gas. Crit Care Med 1981;9:59–63.
11. ECRI. Oxygen-air proportioners. Health Dev 1985;14:263–276.
12. Downs JB. Ventilatory patterns and modes of ventilation in acute respiratory failure. Respir Care 1983;28:586–591.
13. Downs JB. Inappropriate application of IMV (letter). Chest 1980;78:897.
14. Banner MJ, Lampotang S. Boysen PG, Kirby RR, Smith RA. Resistance characteristics of expiratory pressure valves (abstract). Anesthesiology 1986;65:A80.
15. Hillman DR, Finuane KE. Continuous positive airway pressure: A breathing system to minimize respiratory work. Crit Care Med 1985;13:8–43.
16. Cox D, Niblet DJ. Studies on continuous positive pressure breathing systems. Br J Anaesth 1984;56:905–911.
17. Link J. Increases in expiratory resistance of the PEEP valve of the servoventilator. Intens Care Med 1983;9:137–138.
18. Emergency Care Research Institute. PEEP valves. Health Dev 1985;14:387.
19. Banner MJ, Downs JB, Kirby RR, et al. Effects of expiratory flow resistance on inspiratory work of breathing. Chest 1988;93: 795–799.
20. Pinsky MR, Hrehocik D, Culpepper JA, et al. Flow resistance of expiratory positive pressure systems. Chest 1988;94:788.
21. Gal TJ. Effects of endotracheal tube intubation on normal cough performance. Anesthesiology 1980;52:324–329.

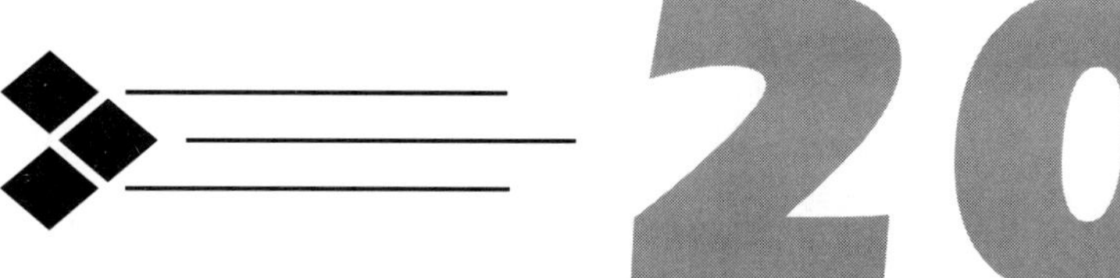

Decontamination of Respiratory Care Equipment: What Can Be Done, What Should Be Done

Robert L. Chatburn
Mark L. Simmons

OBJECTIVES

1. Classify the major microorganisms causing infection.
2. List the factors that affect microbial destruction.
3. Distinguish between cleaning, disinfection, and sterilization.
4. List the major techniques for each type of decontamination.

KEY TERMS

antiseptic
asepsis
bacteria filter
bactericidal
disinfectant
disinfection
HEPA
nosocomial
sporicidal
sporicide
sterile
sterilization
thermophilic
viricidal
viricide

Introduction

In the late 1960s and early 1970s, there was a great deal of concern about the role of what was then called "inhalation therapy" equipment in the spread of nosocomial infections. A number of studies[1–11] and literature reviews[12,13] called attention to contaminated aerosols, nebulizers, and resuscitation devices. In one study conducted by the Centers for Disease Control (CDC), 11% of all epidemics between 1970 and 1975 involved respiratory assistance devices.[14] As the scope and sophistication of respiratory care procedures evolved, so, too, has our understanding of infection control methodology. Consequently, infection related to respiratory care equipment has apparently decreased[15] to the point that, according to one study, these devices are infrequently the source of *endemic* nosocomial pneumonia.[16]

The purpose of this chapter is to describe the procedures used to decontaminate respiratory care equipment and to suggest guidelines for departmental infection control activities. First, however, it may be helpful to review the general principles of microbiology that apply to this topic.

Microbiology of Decontamination

Classification of Microorganisms

The microorganisms that cause infection can be grouped into four general categories: protozoa, fungi, viruses, and bacteria. Protozoa are single-celled eucaryotic (ie, they possess a distinct membrane-bounded nucleus) microbes ranging in size from 5 to 60 μm. Although protozoa do not commonly cause lung infections, they may manifest in immunosuppressed patients.

Fungi, generally molds or yeasts, are also eucaryotic microorganisms. Molds appear as branching multicellular filaments that form a mycelial mass. The mold, *Aspergillus fumigatus,* can be a systemic pathogen. Yeasts are unicellular, ranging in size from 2.5 to 6 μm. *Cryptococcus neoformans* and *Candida albicans* are fungi that are potentially pathogenic. Fungi are tenacious infective agents because their cellular functions are similar to those of human cells, which limits the pharmacologic attacks that can be used. Because of their eucaryotic nature they do not respond well to antibiotics that are effective against bacteria. Fungi can reproduce either sexually or asexually and spread by means of spores.

Viruses are submicroscopic, noncellular, parasitic particles composed of a protein shell and a nucleic acid core. Although they exhibit some characteristics of living organisms (such as the ability to reproduce with the help of living cells, and mutate), they lack other features, such as energy-generating mechanisms. They are resistant to common antimicrobial drugs and, because they have a shell rather than a membranous cell wall, can withstand many decontamination procedures.

Most cases of nosocomial infection are caused by bacteria. Bacteria are procaryotic (ie, they lack a membrane-bounded nucleus) cells, which exist in a wide range of shapes and sizes (0.5 to 6 μm). The three basic morphologies are spherical (coccus), rod shaped (bacillus), and spiral (spirochete)—each with several variations. Pneumonia-causing bacteria are often found in pairs of cells (diplococci). The cells of some spherical bacteria form chain-like aggregates (streptococci), while others form grape-like clusters (staphylococci). Bacteria are also classified according to their oxygen requirements (aerobic, anaerobic, or facultative) and how they react to staining. Bacteria that commonly cause nosocomial infections include species of *Staphylococcus, Klebsiella, and Enterobacter, Pseudomonas aeruginosa, Serratia marcescens,* and species of *Herellea, Mimi,* and *Flavobacterium.*[17] In general, aerobic gram-negative bacilli seem to be the most prevalent pneumonia-causing microbes.[18]

A unique characteristic of some bacteria is the ability to enter a dormant state when environmental conditions turn unfavorable and to enclose themselves in an almost indestructible coat. These *spores* can often withstand hours of boiling and can be frozen for decades or perhaps centuries without harm.[19]

Identification of Microorganisms

An initial microscopic observation of collected specimens provides information about the presence, type, and relative numbers of organisms. In addition, two useful techniques for identifying microorganisms are staining and culturing. Staining with various dyes allows differentiation of organisms that have different cell wall structures. For example, the commonly used Gram's stain separates organisms that retain crystal violet stain and appear blue (gram positive) from those that are decolorized by solvent and appear red from counter staining (gram negative). Another important stain is the acid-fast stain. The specimen is first stained red and then exposed to an acid-alcohol solvent; if the cell retains the red dye, it is called acid fast. This technique provides a fast screen for tubercle bacilli.

Staining helps in the initial identification of organisms involved in an infection. Definitive supporting evidence can only be obtained by culturing specimens in an environment that will grow the suspected species.[20] Most bacteria can be grown in liquid or on solid media made from broth, which is sometimes enriched with extra nutrients such as blood (viruses require living cell cultures). In the case of a solid medium (eg, broth solidified with agar) the specimen is spread over the surface and the plate incubated in a specific environment of temperature, oxygen, and carbon dioxide known to encourage the growth of the postulated organism. A distinct colony of organisms will form wherever at least a single microbe was deposited on the surface of the culture medium. Thus, it can be inferred that a given number of "colony-forming units" represents at least as many organisms that were present in the original sample placed on the culture plate. If the volume of the sample is known, a rough estimate of the density of the contaminating organisms can be calculated and expressed in units of colony-forming units per milliliter.

Killing Microorganisms

In general, microbes are killed by damaging their cell membrane, denaturing their protein, or disrupting cellular processes. Several factors affect microbial destruction[21]:

1. *Type of organism.* Organisms vary widely in their susceptibility to disinfection. Most bacteria, except acid-fast bacilli, can be rapidly killed by chemical disinfectants.[22] Some microbes are especially resistant and have even been found growing in disinfectants such as quaternary ammonium compounds[23–30] and hexachlorophene.[31] Spores are particularly resistant.
2. *Number of organisms.* As the number of organisms to be killed increases, the kill rate or the exposure time or both must increase.[20]
3. *Intensity of killing agent.* In general, the rate of kill of a bacterial population varies directly with the intensity or concentration of the germicidal agent. However, there are exceptions (eg, alcohol works most effectively when combined with water).[32]
4. *Temperature.* Microorganisms usually die faster at higher temperatures. One source states that the rate of killing doubles with every 10°C rise in temperature.[17]
5. *Environment.* The environment in which microbes exist can greatly affect the efficiency of the disinfection procedure. For example, porous surfaces are more difficult to decontaminate than smooth surfaces because deeply embedded organisms are shielded from killing agents. Air entrapment may prevent exposure to liquid agents. For the same reasons, dirt or organic matter on the surface of an object will decrease the effectiveness of disinfection procedures. Chemical contaminants in the environment may adversely affect disinfection by diluting or inactivating the killing agent. On the other hand, some substances may be intentionally added to potentiate the killing action of a particular agent.
6. *Time of exposure.* The time required for effective killing action varies from seconds to hours, depending on the other factors mentioned. For a given procedure, the kill rate is essentially fixed, so that the exposure time must increase as the number of contaminating organisms increases. It is important to understand the factors involved and to follow manufacturers' recommendations when using commercial preparations to ensure that the desired level of decontamination is achieved.

Disinfection

The various disinfection procedures can be placed in two categories: physical methods and chemical methods.

Physical Methods

Among the physical methods, *incineration* is the preferred method for materials contaminated with extremely virulent pathogens and for waste disposal. *Dry heat* is often used for glassware and substances such as powders and oils that cannot withstand moist heat. Dry heat kills by desiccation, alteration of osmotic pressure, coagulation of proteins, and the effects of oxidation. The standard procedure is a temperature of 160°C to 180°C applied for 1 to 2 hours.[32] *Moist heat,* in the form of hot water or steam, is generally more effective than dry heat because moisture conducts heat better than dry gas and because water has a higher specific heat (ie, heating capacity) than air. Moist heat can kill the same microbe in 4 minutes at 160°C that it takes dry heat 2 hours to kill at 160°C. Water at 100°C (ie, boiling at sea level) kills all vegetative forms of bacteria, some spores, and nearly all viruses after an exposure time of 30 minutes.[21] Because water boils at less than 100°C above sea level, the 30-minute exposure time should be extended by 5 minutes for each 1000 ft of altitude.[33] This method is probably of more interest to backpackers than to hospital cleaning personnel. The more practical techniques of pasteurization and steam autoclaving are discussed later.

Radiation, specifically gamma radiation (an electromagnetic wave produced during the decay of radioactive elements such as cobalt 60), is an effective agent for killing all microorganisms, including viruses and spores. Radiation ionizes water molecules, which, in turn, inactivate DNA molecules by increasing the rate of reaction of DNA with hydrogen and hydroxyl ions.[34] One advantage of gamma-radiation is that items can be prepackaged (the package does not interfere with the radiation) so that recontamination is avoided before use. Also, sterilization can take place at room temperature so that thermolabile materials will not be damaged. No aeration period is needed so treated items can be used immediately. Unfortunately, gamma-radiation is not practical for hospital use because it requires expensive equipment and is used primarily by manufacturers of disposable products. Gamma-radiation does cause changes in some plastics, like polyvinyl chloride (PVC). Gamma rays liberate chloride ions in PVC, which themselves cause no problems. However, if such an item is resterilized with ethylene oxide gas, ethylene chlorohydrin may be formed. This substance is extemely toxic to tissues and is not easily dissipated.[35]

Chemical Methods

Chemical disinfection methods include the use of ethylene oxide, aldehydes, alcohols, quaternary ammonium compounds, and acetic acid—all of which have been used with respiratory care equipment. Other chemicals, such as phenols and iodines, are commonly used but not for respiratory equipment. *Phenols* are a group of compounds derived from carbolic acid, the oldest of the germicides. The use of carbolic acid to prevent wound infection was first reported by Joseph Lister in *Lancet* in 1865. Phenols are good bactericides, and they are effective against the tubercle bacillus, but they do not kill spores. They are popular housekeeping agents and have a residual effect (with subsequent application of moisture) over prolonged periods. Phenols kill by penetrating the cell wall and precipitating cell protein or inactivating the cellular enzyme system.[32] *Iodine* is an effective germicide, especially when combined with alcohol (ie, tincture of iodine). Iodine can also be combined with a surface-active solvent (creating an iodophor) such as in the commercial product Betadine. Iodine is used as a skin preparation and is effective against vegetative bacteria, spores, fungi, and some viruses. Its presumed mechanism of action is to form salts with protein, thus killing the microbe.[32] *Oxidizing agents* such as hydrogen peroxide and potassium permanganate oxidize sulfhydryl groups, producing free chlorine, bromine, iodine, and fluoride, which are highly toxic to all bacteria. Oxidizing agents generally are not sporicidal when used alone.

Decontamination of Respiratory Care Equipment

So far in this discussion, the term *decontamination* has been used to mean simply the reduction of microbial contamination to some acceptable level. An acceptable level might imply anything from a modest reduction to complete eradication of microbes. Before describing specific decontamination policies and procedures used in respiratory care, it is necessary to introduce more specific terminology.

Cleaning is the process of removing foreign material such as blood, sputum, and dust from objects. Cleaning is an essential preliminary procedure intended to improve the physical access of germicides subsequently applied to any remaining contaminants. Sometimes the term *sanitization* is used to mean cleaning to reduce the health hazards of contaminated surfaces.

The suffix "cidal" means, to kill. An agent that is bactericidal can kill bacteria. An algacide kills algae. The suffix "static" means, to inhibit growth. An agent that is bacteriostatic prevents bacterial growth.

Disinfection means killing pathogenic organisms on inanimate objects. The CDC has adopted a classification system proposed by Spalding that distinguishes three levels of chemical disinfection: high, intermediate, and low (Table 20-1).[36] According to this scheme, high-level disinfectants are capable of sterilization if exposure times are long enough.

Sterilization is a process that completely destroys all microbial life, including viruses and spores. The use of the words "almost sterile" is inappropriate. An object is either sterile or it is not. Sterility is an ideal concept that is often sought as a goal but is seldom confirmed in practice.

TABLE 20-1. Levels of Disinfection

	Bacteria				Viruses	
Levels	Vegetative	Tubercle Bacillus	Spores	**Fungi***	Lipid and Medium Size	Nonlipid and Small
High	+†	+	+‡	+	+	+
Intermediate	+	+	±§	+	+	±‖
Low	+	−	−	±	+	−

*Includes asexual spores but not necessarily chlamydospores or sexual spores.

†Plus sign indicates that a killing effect can be expected when the normal-use concentrations of chemical disinfectants or pasteurization are properly employed; a negative sign indicates little or no killing effect.

‡Only with extended exposure times are high-level disinfectant chemicals capable of actual sterilization.

§Some intermediate-level disinfectants can be expected to exhibit some sporicidal action.

‖Some intermediate-level disinfectants may have limited virucidal activity.

Cleaning

Decontamination procedures should take place in a designated location that is divided into dirty and clean areas. All equipment used in patient care should be disassembled and examined for worn or defective parts. The main idea is to take apart each device as much as practical to expose the maximum surface area. Adhesive residue should be removed with a special solvent (eg, chlorothane). The parts should then be placed in a basin filled with hot water and soap or detergent. Hot water helps reduce surface tension.

Soaps are generally sodium salts of long-chain fatty acids whose principal actions are to lower surface tension and to form an emulsion with grease, thus helping to remove dirt. This action is accomplished by the dual nature of the soap molecule. One end is polarized and is water soluble (hydrophilic), while the other end is nonpolar and is not water soluble (hydrophobic). Molecules like this that have both polar and nonpolar ends and are big enough for each end to display its own solubility behavior are called *amphipathic*. Normally, water cannot dissolve fat and grease (hydrophobic substances) that make up and contain the dirt on soiled surfaces. When soap is present, the nonpolar ends of the molecules dissolve in the oil droplets (according to the rule "like dissolves like"), leaving the polar ends projecting into the surrounding water layer. Then, the repulsion between similar charges keeps the oil droplets from coalescing and a stable emulsion is formed.[37] Soap alone is not bactericidal, but disinfectants are often added to it during manufacture.

Detergents are salts of synthetic aliphatic compounds whose properties are similar to soaps. Although synthetic detergents vary greatly in chemical structure, their molecules are all amphipathic. Thus, detergents reduce the forces at the interface between water and oil, allowing the spread of germicidal compound over a greater surface area. The most widely used detergents are sodium salts of alkylbenzensulfonic acids (ie, a long-chain alkyl group attached to a benzene ring and an alkyl halide, an alkene, or an alcohol). Unlike soaps, detergents retain their efficiency in hard water. Also, detergents have some bactericidal effect, acting by dissolving the lipid in the plasma membrane and allowing cell contents to leak out. Detergents are most effective against gram-positive bacteria and are inactivated by contact with protein. They are not effective against tubercle bacilli and many viruses.[21] Commercial products (eg, blends of quaternary ammonium compounds with other additives) are available that provide the double action of cleaning and preliminary disinfection, thereby reducing health hazards during decontamination.

Dirty equipment should be allowed to soak long enough for the detergent solution to penetrate and loosen organic matter. Next, it should be scrubbed thoroughly inside and out to remove all debris. As an alternative to washing by hand, automatic washers, similar to kitchen dish washers, are commercially available. These devices go through several cycles to wash, rinse, and pasteurize or cold disinfect with glutaraldehyde. Either the hot water or chemical disinfectant is held in a side tank and is automatically pumped into the holding tub. After the disinfection cycle, the liquid is pumped back into the side tank for reuse.[38–40]

Small parts that have many crevices can be treated in an ultrasonic cleaner. This is a device similar to an ultrasonic nebulizer except that the vibrations are tuned to produce submicroscopic bubbles on the surface of the object to be cleaned. When these bubbles collapse, they generate tiny shock waves that knock dirt off surfaces that cannot be reached by hand.

After scrubbing, the equipment is rinsed and dried, unless it is to undergo heat sterilization. If rinse water is not completely removed, it may dilute the subsequent use of chemical disinfectant solutions. If the equipment is to be gas sterilized, water may combine with ethylene oxide gas to form ethylene glycol, which is toxic and difficult to remove. Drying is important even if no further disinfection procedures are used because a humid environment encourages the growth of gram-negative organisms.

Disinfection (Low/Intermediate)

Quaternary Ammonium Compounds

Quaternary ammonium compounds, or "quats," are a special class of synthetic detergents. They are the result of nucleophilic substitution reactions of alkyl halides with tertiary amines[37] that typically result in a product with 8 or 10 carbon molecules. Quats are thought to kill bacteria by dissolving the lipid in the plasma membrane and by attaching to anionic sites on active portions of enzymes. They are bactericidal, fungicidal, and viricidal at room temperature with-in 10 minutes but have not demonstrated sporicidal effects. Quats are only marginally effective against *Pseudomonas aeruginosa*,[41] and the use of low dilutions (1:1000) has often led to poor results, as mentioned previously. However, researchers have suggested that a new, third-generation, 12-carbon quaternary ammonium cationic surfactant (1:400 dilution) when mixed with a nonionic emulsifier, a nontoxic hydrocarbon compound, and readily available hydroxyl groups produces a synergistic effect far greater than any of the individual components. Such a mixture is said to have demonstrated effectiveness against a broad range of bacteria, fungi, and viruses (unpublished data furnished by Airshields, marketers of Vapaseptic and Kleenaseptic). Kleenaseptic, for example, consists of a third-generation quaternary ammonium compound potentiated with isopropanol and is available in spray can dispensers for cleaning countertops and devices that cannot be soaked, such as ventilators. Because quats are quick-acting, are relatively nontoxic, are noncaustic, and do not produce noxious fumes, they are useful for initial cleaning procedures. When kept free of foreign matter, aqueous quat solutions may retain their effectiveness for up to 14 days.

Acetic Acid

Acetic acid, in the form of white household vinegar, has been recommended as a disinfectant for both hospital and home care equipment.[42–44] Concentrations from 0.25% to 2% with an exposure time of 1 hour have been used with variable effects.[45,46] Acetic acid solutions, with a pH in the range of 2 to 3, presumably kill bacteria by lowering intracellular pH and inactivating enzymes. Also, in an acid environment, ionized compounds become nonionized and penetrate the cell more readily, thus disrupting cellular metabolism.[47] In a controlled study,[41] acetic acid was comparable to one commercial blend of quaternary ammonium compounds for disinfection of *Staphylococcus aureus* and *Pseudomonas cepacia* but was superior against *Pseudomonas aeruginosa.* In this study, the best concentration of acetic acid was 1.25% (ie, one part 5% household vinegar to three parts water). Acetic acid has long been used in food preparation to retard the formation of mold. However, there appear to be no data in the literature regarding sporicidal or viricidal effects. Based on the proposed mechanism of action, it is doubtful that any exist. Nevertheless, because of its universal availability, acetic acid is a practical emergency alternative to commercial disinfectants (eg, quaternary ammonium compounds or glutaraldehydes) for decontamination of home care equipment.

Alcohol

Both ethyl and isopropyl alcohol are good disinfectants when combined with water. Ethyl alcohol is best at a 70% concentration, while isopropyl alcohol is less dependent on water and the optimum concentration is 90%. Both solutions kill most bacteria within 1 to 5 minutes[48] by denaturing cellular proteins, particularly enzymes called dehydrogenases.[32] They do not destroy spores but are among the best agents for killing tubercle bacillus.[49] Their viricidal activity is variable, with ethyl alcohol being superior to isopropyl alcohol. The CDC recommends exposure to 70% ethanol for 15 minutes to inactivate the hepatitis virus, but shorter periods of time should be adequate for human immunodeficiency virus.[50] Alcohols are inactivated by protein and may cause swelling and hardening of rubber and certain plastics.

Pasteurization

Pasteurization of respiratory care equipment involves the application of heat (at least 62°C) for at least 30 minutes. These conditions will kill bacteria (including tubercle) and some viruses but are ineffective against spores.[20,51–53] The major disadvantage of this process is that equipment may become recontaminated during drying and repackaging. In addition, some materials may deform owing to the heat. CDC guidelines specifically refer to pasteurization as a high-level disinfection process,[54] although this is inconsistent with their classification system (see Table 20-1) because of the inability of the procedure to reliably kill spores and viruses. Ernst[55] states that very unrealistic times of exposure would be required for the destruction of spores even in boiling water; therefore, for all practical purposes, pasteurization should not be regarded as a sterilizing process.

Some respiratory care departments make use of commercially available machines that both wash and pasteurize. For example, one model (HR STERI•VERS, HR, Bellevue, WA) features full immersion and agitation during the wash cycle followed by two full-immersion rinses and an agitation drain cycle. It is claimed that agitation is so effective that manual prescrubbing is unnecessary. Next, the compartment is flooded with water and heated to 77°C for 30 minutes during the pasteurization cycle. As an alternative to pasteurization, the compartment can be flooded with a chemical disinfectant for 10 minutes, after which the solution is pumped back into a storage tank for reuse.

Glutaraldehydes

Glutaraldehydes are chemically related to formaldehyde, a fumigant that has been used for decades. Glutaraldehyde attacks the lipoproteins in bacterial cell membranes and cytoplasm. Glutaraldehydes are used extensively for disinfection of endoscopy equipment, respiratory therapy equipment, physical therapy equipment, and surgical instruments.[56] Alkaline glutaraldehyde was the first of this type of chemical available commercially. Typically, it is available as a mildly acidic, 2.0% solution that is activated with a 0.3% bicarbonate buffer, yielding a solution with a pH of 7.5 to 8.5. This solution is bactericidal, viricidal, and tuberculocidal at room temperature within 10 minutes and sporicidal in 3 to 10 hours.[57–65]

These solutions are reusable for 14 to 28 days, depending on the specific brand, and some are designed to be used with automatic machines (eg, the Cidematic, Surgikos, Arlington, TX). With short exposure times, alkaline glutaraldehyde is noncorrosive to metal, will not harm rubber or plastics, and can be used with rigid and flexible endoscopes. However, it has an irritating odor and rubber gloves should always be worn to avoid contact dermatitis.[66] Equipment should be thoroughly rinsed before use because residual glutaraldehyde is irritating to tissues. Pseudomembranous laryngitis has been associated with the usage of endotracheal tubes disinfected with this agent.[67]

Acid glutaraldehyde comes as a ready-to-use 2% solution with a pH of 2.7 to 3.7. Its action is the same as alkaline glutaraldehyde except that it requires 20 minutes to be tuberculocidal. It is not sporicidal at room temperature. At 60°C, it is bactericidal, viricidal, and fungicidal in 5 minutes, tuberculocidal in 20 minutes, and sporicidal in 60 minutes.[21] Acid glutaraldehyde is noncorrosive to most materials but is not recommended for plated metal instruments. It does not irritate the eyes or nose, and it is not necessary to wear gloves when using it.[21] Solutions can be effectively reused for up to 30 days.[68]

Neutral glutaraldehyde with a pH of 7.0 to 7.5 is used in a 2% solution. After liquid activation it has a useful life of 28 days. It kills bacteria (including tubercle bacilli), fungi, and some viruses within 10 minutes and spores in 10 hours.

Glutaraldehyde fumes have a pungent odor with a recognition threshold at 0.04 parts per million (ppm) by volume in air, and an irritation response level at 0.3 ppm.[56] Concentrations of 0.3 ppm or greater have demonstrated a significant risk of irritation to the eyes, nose, and throat. These effects include asthma, rhinitis, lung irritation, chest tightness, breathlessness, and reduced lung function.[56,69] Liquid glutaraldehyde is also a skin irritant and can cause contact dermatitis. For this reason, appropriate gloves should be worn when working with these solutions.

To help prevent the effects of the fumes, the Occupational Safety and Health Administration (OSHA)[69] has set 0.2 ppm as the maximum permissible exposure limit for inhaled fumes of glutaraldehyde, based on a time-weighted average concentration for a 15-minute period. To help keep environmental levels less than 0.2 ppm, the following are suggested: keep containers of glutaraldehyde covered when not in use and increase room ventilation or use an exhaust hood during processing. Glutaraldehyde solutions are also now available for hospital use that, when diluted, contain 0.13% glutaraldehyde. This reduced concentration would help reduce vapor content in the processing room.

Hydrogen Peroxide–Based Compounds

A product called ENDO-SPOR (Globe Medical, Clearwater FL) introduces an entirely new class of high-level disinfectants that have hydrogen peroxide–based formulas with added stabilizers and inhibitors. According to product literature, this product is bactericidal (including tubercle bacilli) and fungicidal in 10 minutes at 20°C and is also viricidal against influenza and herpes simplex viruses. It is sporicidal in 6 hours at 20°C or in 10 minutes at 50°C. Furthermore, it is reported to maintain effective germicidal activity after 6 weeks of continuous reuse in the presence of a heavy organic load. The advantage of this compound over glutaraldehydes is that it requires no mixing or activation and does not produce harsh fumes. It is said to be safe for use with rubber, plastic, and stainless steel.

All items subjected to high-level chemical disinfection should be rinsed in *sterile* water to remove toxic residues and then thoroughly dried. These objects should then be handled aseptically with sterile gloves and towels during the packaging process.[54]

Sterilization

Steam

At atmospheric pressure (at sea level), water and steam exist at 100°C. The efficiency of moist heat as a disinfecting agent can be increased by increasing its temperature. This can be accomplished by boiling water in a closed container so that as the pressure increases, the temperature of the steam also increases. The autoclave, allowing the application of Gay-Lussac's law, provides an environment for this to occur. Under these conditions, disinfection results due to the disruption of cell membranes and coagulation of proteins. Pressure per se contributes little or nothing to the sterilization process and is simply a variable used to control the temperature. Equipment to be sterilized is first cleaned and then packaged in muslin, linen, or paper. The steam easily penetrates these materials. After sterilization, the packaging materials help prevent recontamination during subsequent handling and storage.

Steam at 121°C and 15 psig sterilizes within 15 minutes.[70] If the temperature is increased to 126°C, the time is reduced to 10 minutes and is further reduced to only a few seconds at 150°C.[61] Because air is a poor conductor of heat, its presence within the autoclave or in the equipment bundle reduces the efficiency of the steam.[72] The same effect can result from overloading or improper packaging of the items to be sterilized. To help prevent this, most autoclaves are designed to evacuate the air before steam enters the chamber.[73,74]

Because several factors (ie, time, temperature and penetration) affect the thoroughness of sterilization by steam, both heat-sensitive and biologic monitors should be used to maintain quality control. Heat indicators help ensure that the necessary physical conditions have occurred, but biologic indicators help document actual sterilization. *Bacillus stearothermophilus* spores (in capsules containing 10^6 organisms) are often used because of their high resistance to moist heat. If culturing the capsule produces no growth, sterility can be assumed. The CDC recommends that steam sterilizers be checked with microbiologic indicators at least once a week,[54] or with each load when any implantable device is being sterilized.

The advantages of autoclaving include speed, economy, absence of toxic residues, and reliability. A major disadvantage is the fact that most respiratory care equipment is made from heat-sensitive material (including rubber and plastic) and can be damaged by the process. More than one fiberoptic bronchoscope has been ruined by steam autoclaving because the processor failed to realize the scope's vulnerability to high temperature.

Ethylene Oxide

Ethylene oxide is a poisonous gas, with an ether-like odor that is detectable at airborne concentrations of 700 ppm and greater. It is flammable and explosive in concentrations above 3% when mixed with room air. It is sometimes mixed with Freon or carbon dioxide to decrease the chance of fire or explosion. As a liquid, it is colorless, with a boiling point at approximately 10.8°C. The gas is presumed to kill microorganism by damaging genetic nucleic acids by a process known as alkylation. Alkylation is the result of hydrogen ions being replaced by hydroxyethyl radicals in protein molecules of the microbe. It is lethal to all known microbes when enough hydrogen ions are replaced.

Items to be sterilized must be disassembled and thoroughly cleaned to ensure adequate penetration of the gas. After cleaning, they should be dried to prevent ethylene oxide from combining with residual water to form ethylene glycol. The equipment should then be packaged in gas-permeable wrapping. Muslin and paper wrapping can be used, but heat-sealed polyethylene pouches are probably faster and easier to use. Packaging materials that should be avoided include aluminum foil, nylon film, Saran wrap, Mylar, cellophane, polyester, and polyvinylidene film because they may not be permeable to the gas.

Four major factors determine proper gas sterilization: gas concentration, temperature, humidity, and exposure time. Gas concentration is usually measured in milligrams of gas per liter of space. Concentrations of 450 mg/L or greater are required.[21] Some commercial sterilizers offer a selection of temperatures, such as 49°C to 60°C for a warm cycle and 29°C to 38°C for a cold cycle. Temperatures above 60°C should not be used because polymerization of the ethylene oxide takes place and its ability to act as a sterilant is removed.[32] Humidity is necessary to soften the walls of spores and to catalyze the reaction between ethylene oxide and bacterial proteins. Most sterilizers evacuate the chamber and then inject water vapor to attain a relative humidity of 30% to 60%. This conditioning may last for up to an hour before admitting the ethylene oxide (sometimes under pressure, ranging from 5 to 30 psig). Adequate exposure time will range from 1½ to 6 hours depending on the factors listed.

As with steam sterilization, it is necessary to monitor the effectiveness of gas sterilization with appropriate indicators. These include: physical, chemical, and biologic. Physical indicators include all sterilizer components that measure temperature, humidity, pressure, and exposure time. Chemical indicators, in the form of tapes, cards, or sheets, are designed to change color when the conditions necessary for sterilization have been met. These indicators change color in response to either a combination of gas concentration and moisture or heat and moisture. Chemical indicators should be used with each package that is sterilized and checked for the appropriate change in color before the equipment is used. Of course, physical and chemical devices do not indicate that sterilization has taken place, only that the appropriate conditions were present. Biologic indicators must be included with each load of equipment to be sterilized using ethylene oxide to ensure that complete decontamination has been achieved. For this purpose, cultures of *Bacillus subtilis* var. globigii or *niger* have been used.[32,34,54]

Ethylene oxide is absorbed into a variety of materials. For this reason, sterilized articles must be aerated to prevent residual gas from contacting skin and mucous membranes. Aeration may be accomplished passively in air, but there are advantages to the use of mechanical aerators. For example, devices that require 7 days of ambient aeration require only 8 to 12 hours in an aeration chamber at a temperature of 50°C to 60°C.[75,76] Although room air (shelf) aeration was commonly used in the past, it must now be used with caution. Shelf aeration may result in ethylene oxide concentrations exceeding the recommended levels in a room unless proper ventilation is present.

The factors that affect aeration include the composition of the sterilized article, its configuration and intended use, the gas diluent, the temperature of aeration, the air flow, the type of sterilizer used, and the time of aeration. Materials like glass and metal require little or no aeration, whereas plastic, rubber, cloth, and paper may absorb significant amounts of ethylene oxide. Thick items require more time to aerate than thin ones because they have a smaller ratio of surface area to volume that reduces the rate of gas diffusion. Aeration of devices intended for implantation or contact with mucous membranes is more critical than those that normally do not touch the body. Gas mixtures using a fluorocarbon diluent require a longer aeration time than those with carbon dioxide. Increasing the temperature decreases aeration time, with the usual range being 50°C to 60°C. Increasing the airflow around sterilized objects decreases aeration time. Sterilizers that use high temperatures and pressures may cause higher levels of gas to be present in sterilized objects.[77] Because so many factors affect aeration, it is difficult to establish one aeration time that is best for all materials. The minimum times recommended for materials that are difficult to aerate are 8 hours at 60°C or 12 hours at 50°C in a mechanical aeration chamber or 7 days at room temperatures.[78]

Inadequate aeration of gas-sterilized equipment, or the formation of ethylene glycol or ethylene chlorohydrin, can lead to skin reactions, anaphylaxis, and laryngotracheal inflammation.[79–82]. Ethylene oxide–treated materials may cause destruction of red blood cells.[83,84] Because of the potential for ethylene chlorhydrine formation, the American National Standards Institute at one time recommended that devices made of PVC and gamma-irradiated should never be resterilized with ethylene oxide.[76] However, several studies have failed to substantiate this fear.[84–87] Manufacturers' guidelines should be followed for resterilization procedures.

Perhaps a more common problem is the leaching of plasticizers from some materials after repeated exposure to heat and ethylene oxide gas.[88] This leads to structural weakness and cracking.

Ethylene oxide can be harmful if the vapors are inhaled, if contact is made with the skin or eyes, or if swallowed. Ethylene oxide in liquid form can cause eye irritation and injury to the cornea, frostbite, and severe irritation and blistering of the skin on prolonged or confined contact. Ingestion of ethylene oxide can cause gastric irritation and liver damage.

Inhalation of ethylene oxide gas can lead to acute toxic effects such as respiratory irritation, lung injury, nausea, vomiting, diarrhea, headache, dizziness, convulsions, shortness of breath and cyanosis.[89] Chronic exposure may lead to respiratory infection, anemia, neurotoxicity, and altered behavior.[90] Additional concerns include carcinogenic and possible mutagenic and teratogenic effects.[78,91] The current U.S. standard for a worker's exposure to ethylene oxide gas is 1 ppm for an 8 hour time-weighted average.[32] Further OSHA requirements limit the maximum short-time exposure to 5 ppm as averaged over a 15-minute period.[93] Dorsch and Dorsch have compiled a comprehensive list of recommendations to reduce exposure of hospital personnel to ethylene oxide gas.[21]

A summary of the capabilities of the various decontamination agents is shown in Table 20-2.

Recommendations

Rationales for decontaminating medical equipment are logically based on the perceived risk such equipment poses for patients. That is, devices that, in use, will bypass the normal body defenses need to be more thoroughly disinfected than those that are not expected to contact the body or will only touch the skin. Of course, exceptions should be kept in mind, such as the added precautions required for patients whose normal body defenses may be weakened or absent. To facilitate the classification of medical devices in terms of the risk of infection, the CDC has adopted three categories: *critical, semicritical,* and *noncritical*.[54]

Critical items are those that are introduced into the bloodstream or into other areas of the body by penetrating skin or mucous membranes. Examples include surgical devices, cardiac catheters, implants, and various components of heart-lung machines or hemodialyzers. These items must be sterile at the time of use.

Semicritical items are instruments that come in contact with intact mucous membranes, such as fiberoptic endoscopes, endotracheal tubes, and ventilator delivery circuits. Sterilization of these devices is not absolutely essential. However, Spector[94] states that endoscopes used on patients suspected of having hepatitis B or the acquired immunodeficiency syndrome *must* be gas sterilized. At minimum, a high-level disinfection process should be used with the goal of destroying vegetative microorganisms, most fungal spores, tubercle bacilli, and small nonlipid viruses. The reasoning is that "intact mucous membranes are generally resistant to infection by common bacterial spores but are not resistant to many other microorganisms,

TABLE 20-2. Capabilities of Disinfecting Agents Commonly Used in Respiratory Care

Disinfectant	Gram-Positive Bacteria	Gram-Negative Bacteria	Tubercle Bacillus	Spores	Viruses	Fungi
Soaps	0	0	0	0	0	0
Detergents	±	≠	0	0	0	0
Quaternary ammonium compounds	+	±	0	0	±	±
Acetic acid	?	+	?	?	?	+
Alcohols	+	+	+	0	±	±
Hot water (<100°C)	+	+	+	0	±	?
Glutaraldehydes	+	+	+	±	+	+
Steam (>100°C)	+	+	+	+	+	+
Ethylene oxide	+	+	+	+	+	+

+, good; ±, fair; ≠, poor; ?, unknown; 0, little or none.

such as viruses and tubercle bacilli; therefore, items that touch mucous membranes require a disinfection process that kills all but resistant bacterial spores."[54]

Noncritical items are those that are not expected to touch the patient or touch only intact skin. These include face masks, blood pressure cuffs, ventilators, and a variety of other medical equipment. They rarely, if ever, transmit disease so that washing with detergent may be sufficient depending on the particular item and its intended use.[54] The rationale is that "in general, intact skin acts as an effective barrier to most microorganisms; thus, items that touch only intact skin need only be clean."[54] Nevertheless, because of the availability of inexpensive and effective germicidals (eg, quats in spray dispensers), it is difficult to argue against the practice of routine low-intermediate level disinfection of noncritical items.

Respiratory care disinfection policies must take into consideration several factors: the intended use of the equipment to be decontaminated, the construction of the equipment (ie, material and configuration), the resources made available by the hospital (eg, autoclave or gas sterilizer in a central processing department), and cost (both labor and materials), roughly in that order. In practice, all equipment should undergo low- or intermediate-level disinfection during the initial cleaning process. There are essentially three choices for the further decontamination of semicritical respiratory care items; sterilization with ethylene oxide gas, high-level disinfection with glutaraldehydes, or pasteurization, in that order of preference (in terms of effectiveness of decontamination). The ideal situation is to be able to clean and package equipment in the respiratory care department and then send it to a central supply department for gas sterilization and aeration. From the respiratory manager's point of view, this provides the most efficient decontamination for the least expenditure of supplies, labor, and space. Unfortunately, such facilities are not universally available and are very expensive to set up. The next best approach may be to purchase a commercial washing/disinfection machine that provides a glutaraldehyde soak cycle. If operating costs are a major factor, glutaraldehyde disinfection can be replaced with a pasteurization cycle. Although pasteurization is recognized by the CDC as an appropriate procedure for respiratory care equipment, it does not provide as high a level of disinfection as does the glutaraldehyde procedure. However, there appears to be no data to support the belief that one procedure is superior for preventing nosocomial infection. In this era of cost containment, the issue of whether to disinfect and reuse disposable or single use items has become important. Disposable ventilator circuits are an example of typical high-volume and hence high-cost items. There appears to be little scientific data to support the practice of reuse, and the arguments for and against reuse have been summarized elsewhere.[95] CDC guidelines[54] state that "the recommendation against reprocessing and reusing single-use items has been removed." And furthermore, "Since there is a lack of evidence indicating increased risk of nosocomial infections associated with the reuse of all single-use items, a categorical recommendation against all types of reuse is not considered justifiable. Rather than recommending for or against reprocessing and reuse of all single-use items, it appears more prudent to recommend that hospitals consider the safety and efficacy of the reprocessing procedure of each item or device separately and the likelihood that the device will function as intended after reprocessing."[54] Thus, the burden of proof has been shifted to individual respiratory care departments and, in fact, to the profession as a whole. Clearly, more research in this area is indicated as manufacturers rarely provide reprocessing information.

The issue of microbiologic surveillance has not changed since 1982. At that time, the CDC recommended that the disinfection process for respiratory care equipment not be monitored by routine microbiologic sampling.[96] The reasoning seems to be based on the fact that rates of nosocomial infection have not been related to levels of general microbial contamination of environmental surfaces and that standards for permissible levels of contamination do not exist.[54] Such sampling is indicated during investigation of infection problems if environmental reservoirs are implicated. It is important that such culturing follow a written plan that specifies the objects to be sampled and the actions to be taken based on culture results.[54]

A noteworthy omission from a recent CDC guideline[54] specifically mentioned in the earlier version[96] is the recommended frequency for changing respiratory care equipment, specifically ventilator circuits and humidifiers. A wide variety of practices has been observed probably because of the scarcity of data.[97] Clearly, much work needs to be done to quantitatively describe the relationship among such variables as equipment design (eg, the presence or absence of heating wires), operating temperature, patient population, and the frequency of change and its effect on patient outcome.

References

1. Kresky B. Control of gram-negative bacilli in a hospital nursery. Am J Dis Child 1964;107:363–369.
2. Reinarz JA, Pierce AK, Mays BB, Sanford JP. The potential role of inhalation therapy equipment in nosocomial pulmonary infections. J Clin Invest 1965;44:831–839.
3. Bassett CDJ, Thompson SAS, Page B. Neonatal infections with *Pseudomonas aeruginosa* associated with contaminated resuscitation equipment. Lancet 1965;1:781–784.

4. Mertz JJ, Scharer L, McClement JH. A hospital outbreak of *Klebsiella pneumonia* from inhalation therapy with contaminated aerosol solution. Am Rev Respir Dis 1966;94:454–460.
5. Fierer J, Taylor PM, Gezon HM. *Pseudomonas aeruginosa* epidemic traced to delivery-room resuscitators. N Engl J Med 1967; 276:991–996.
6. McNamara MJ, Hill MC, Balows A, et al. A study of the bacteriologic patterns of hospital infections. Ann Intern Med 1967;66: 480–487.
7. Moffet HL, Allan D. Colonization of infants exposed to bacterially contaminated mists. Am J Dis Child 1967;114:21–25.
8. Ringrose RE, McKown B, Felton FG, et al. A hospital outbreak of *Serratia marcescens* associated with ultrasonic nebulizers. Ann Intern Med 1968;69:719–729.
9. Cabrera HA. An outbreak of *Serratia marcescens* and its control. Arch Intern Med 1969;123:650–655.
10. Grieble HG, Colton FR, Bird TJ, et al. Fine-particle humidifiers: Source of *Pseudomonas aeruginosa* infections in a respiratory-disease unit. N Engl J Med 1970;282:531–534.
11. Sanders CV Jr, Luby JP, Johanson WG Jr, et al. *Serratia marcescens* infections from inhalation therapy medications: Nosocomial outbreak. Ann Intern Med 1970;73:15–21.
12. Pierce AK, Sanford JP. Bacterial contamination of aerosols. Arch Intern Med 1973;13:156–159.
13. Pierce AK, Sanford JP. Aerobic gram-negative bacillary pneumonias. Am Rev Respir Dis 1974;110:647–658.
14. Stamm WE. Infections related to medical devices. Ann Intern Med 1978;89:764–769.
15. Masferrer R, DuPriest M. Six-year evaluation of decontamination of respiratory therapy equipment. Respir Care 1977;22:145–148.
16. Crosso AS, Roup B. Role of respiratory assistance devices in endemic nosocomial pneumonia. Am J Med 1981;70:681–685.
17. Eubanks DH, Bone RC. Comprehensive Respiratory Care. St. Louis: CV Mosby, 1985:237–255.
18. Simmons BP, Wong ES. Guide for prevention of nosocomial pneumonia. Infect Control 1982;3:327–333; reprinted in Respir Care 1983;28:221–232.
19. Keeton WT. Biological Science, 2nd ed. New York: WW Norton, 1972:713.
20. Elder HA, Sauer RL. Infectious disease aspects of respiratory therapy. In: Burton GG, Gee GN, Hodgkin JE, eds. Respiratory Care: A Guide to Clinical Practice. Philadelphia: JB Lippincott, 1977.
21. Dorsch JA, Dorsch SE. Understanding Anesthesia Equipment. 2nd ed. Baltimore: Williams & Wilkins, 1984:415–442.
22. Rice HM. Testing of air filters for hospital sterilizers. Lancet 1958;2:1275–1277.
23. Dixon RE, Kaslow RA, Maackel DC, Fulkerson CC, Mallison GF. Aqueous quaternary ammonium antiseptics and disinfectants. JAMA 1976;236:2415–2417.
24. Bacteria in antiseptic solutions. Br Med J 1958;2:436.
25. Lee JC, Fialkow PJ. Benzalkonium chloride: Source of hospital infection with gram-negative bacteria. JAMA 1961;177:708–710.
26. Malizia WF, Gangarosa EJ, Goley AF. Benzalkonium chloride as a source of infection. N Engl J Med 1960;263:800–802.
27. Plotkin SA, Austrian R. Bacteremia caused by *Pseudomonas* sp following the use of materials stored in solutions of a cationic surface-active agent. Am J Med Sci 1958;238:621–627.
28. Frank MJ, Schaffner W. Contaminated aqueous benzalkonium chloride: An unnecessary hospital infection hazard. JAMA 1976;236:2418–2419.
29. Failure of deterrents to disinfect. Lancet 1958;2:306.
30. Disinfectants and gram-negative bacteria. Lancet 1972;1:26–27.
31. Burdon DW, Whitby JL. Contamination of hospital disinfectants with *Pseudomonas* species. Br Med J 1967;1:153–155.
32. Edge RS. Infection control. In: Barnes TA, Lisbon A. Respiratory Care Practice. Chicago: Year Book Medical Publishers, 1988: 573–582.
33. Schnierson SS. Sterilization by heat. Int Anesthesiol Clin 1972; 10(2)67–83.
34. Kacmarek RM, Mack CW, Dimas S. The Essentials of Respiratory Therapy, 2nd ed. Chicago: Year Book Medical Publishers, 1985:584.
35. Artandi C. Sterilization by ionizing radiation. Int Anesthesiol Clin 1972;10(2):123–130.
36. Favero MS. Chemical disinfection of medical and surgical materials. In: Block SS, ed. Disinfection, Sterilization and Preservation, 3rd ed. Philadelphia: Lea & Febiger, 1983:469–492.
37. Morrison RT, Boyd RN. Organic Chemistry, 3rd ed. Boston: Allyn & Bacon, 1973:752:1059–1062.
38. Wilson RD, Traber DL, ALlen CR, Priano LL, Bass J. An evaluation of the Cidematic decontamination system for anesthesia equipment. Anesth Analg 1972;51:658–661.
39. Borick PM, Dondershine FH, Hollis RA. A new automated unit for cleaning and disinfecting anesthesia equipment and other medical instruments. Dev Ind Microbiol 1971;12:266–272.
40. Iddenden FR. New decontamination procedure cuts costs, reduces staff time. Can Hosp 1972;49:26–28.
41. Chatburn RL, Kallstrom TJ, Bajaksouzian MS. A comparison of acetic acid with a quaternary ammonium compound for disinfection of hand-held nebulizers. Respir Care 1988:33:179–187.
42. O'Ryan J, Burns D. Pulmonary Rehabilitation: From Hospital to Home. Chicago: Year Book Medical Publishers, 1984:227–229.
43. Blodgett D. Manual of Respiratory Care Procedures. Philadelphia: JB Lippincott, 1987:308–310.
44. Ziment I. Pharmacology of drugs used in respiratory therapy. In: Burton GG, Gee GN, Hodgkin JE, eds. Respiratory Care: A Guide to Clinical Practice. Philadelphia: JB Lippincott, 1977:493.
45. Edmondson E, Reinarz J, Pierce AK, Sanford J. Nebulization equipment: A potential source of infection in gram-negative pneumonia. Am J Dis Child 1966;3:357–360.
46. Rhoades E, Ringrose R, Mohr J, Brooks L, McKown B, Felton F. Contamination of ultrasonic nebulization equipment with gram-negative bacteria. Arch Intern Med 1971;127:228–232.
47. Brock TD. Biology of Microorganisms. Englewood Cliffs, NJ: Prentice Hall, 1970:213–214.
48. Spalding EH. Principles and application of chemical disinfection. Assoc Operating Room Nurses J 1963;1:36–46.
49. Spaulding EH. Chemical disinfection and antisepsis in the hospital. J Hosp Res 1972;9:7–31.
50. Ayliffe GAJ. Hospital disinfection and antibiotic policies. Chemotherapy 1987;6:228–233.
51. Roberts FJ, Cockcroft WH, Johnson HE. A hot water disinfection method for inhalation therapy equipment. Can Med Assoc J 1969;101:30–32.
52. Nelson EJ, Ryan KJ. A new use for pasteurization: Disinfection of inhalation therapy equipment. Respir Care 1971;16:97–103.
53. Harada S, Yoshiyama H, Yamamoto N. Effect of heat and fresh human serum on the infectivity of human T-cell lymphotropic virus type III evaluated with new bioassay systems. J Clin Microbiol 1985;22:908–911.
54. Garner JS, Favero MS. CDC guidelines for the prevention and control of nosocomial infections: Guideline for handwashing and hospital environmental control, 1985. Am J Infect Control 1986;14:110–129.
55. Ernst RR. Sterilization by heat. In: Block SS. Disinfection, Sterilization and Preservation. Philadelphia: Lea & Febiger, 1977:494.
56. Newman MA, Kachuba JB. Glutaraldehyde: A potential health risk to nurses. Soc Gastroenterol Nurses Associates 1983:19: 501–528.
57. Borik PM. Chemical sterilizers (chemosterilizers). Adv Appl Microbiol 1968;10:291–312.
58. Borik PM, Dondershine FH, Chandler VL. Alkalinized glutaraldehyde, a new antimicrobial agent. J Pharm Sci 1964;53: 1273–1275.
59. Borik PM. Antimicrobial agents as liquid chemosterilizers. Biotechnol Bioeng 1965;7:435–443.
60. Kelsey JC, Mackinnon IH, Maurer IM. Sporicidal activity of hospital disinfectants. J Clin Pathol 1974;27:632–638.
61. Haselhuhn DH, Brason FW, Borick PM. "In use" study of buffered glutaraldehyde for cold sterilization of anesthesia equipment. Anesth Analg 1967;46:468–474.
62. Pepper RE, Chandler VLI. Sporicidal activity of alkaline alcoholic saturated dialdehyde solutions. J Appl Microbiol 1968;11: 384–388.

63. Roberts RB. The anaesthetist, cross-infection and sterilization techniques: A review. Anaesth Intensive Care 1973;1:400–406.
64. Snyder RW, Cheatle EL. Alkaline glutaraldehyde as effective disinfectant. Am J Hosp Pharm 1965;22:321–327.
65. Stonehill AA, Krop S, Borick PM. Buffered glutaraldehyde, a new chemical sterilizing solution. Am J Hosp Pharm 1963;20: 458–465.
66. Fisher AA. Reactions to glutaraldehyde with particular reference to radiologists and x-ray technicians. Cutis 1981;28:113, 114, 119.
67. Belani KG, Priedkalns J. An epidemic of pseudomembranous laryngotracheitis. Anesthesiology 1977;47:530–531.
68. Boucher RMG. Cidex and Sonacide compared. Respir Care 1977;22:790–799.
69. Glutaraldehyde. Fed Register 1989;54(12):2464.
70. Medical Research Council. Sterilization by steam under increased pressure. Lancet 1959;1:425–435.
71. Rendell-Baker L, Roberts RB. Gas versus steam sterilization: When to use which. Med Surg Rev 1969;4th quarter:10–14.
72. Hoyt A, Chaney AL, Cavell K. Studies on steam sterilization and the effects of air in the autoclave. J Bacteriol 1938;36:639–652.
73. Fallon RJ. Factors concerned in the efficient steam sterilization of surgical dressings. J Clin Pathol 1961;14:505–511.
74. Kretz AP. High vacuum sterilization. Assoc Operating Room Nurses J 1964;2:35–40.
75. Rendell-Baker L. Ethylene oxide: II. Aeration. Int Anesthesiol Clin 1972;10:101–122.
76. American National Standards Institute Sectional Committee Z-79 and ASA Subcommittee on Standardization. Ethylene oxide sterilization of anesthesia apparatus. Anesthesiology 1970;33:120.
77. Anderson SR. Ethylene oxide residues in medical materials. Bull Parenter Drug Assoc 1973;27:49–57.
78. Association for the Advance of Medical Instrumentation. Good hospital practice: Ethylene oxide gas-ventilation recommendations and safe use. AAMI DO-VRSU 1981
79. Lipton B, Guitierrez R, Blaugrund S, Litwak RS, Rendall-Baker L. Irradiatied PVC plastic and gas sterilization in the production of tracheal stenosis following tracheostomy. Anesth Analg 1971;50:578–586.
80. Royce A, Moore WKS. Occupational dermatitis caused by ethylene oxide. Br J Ind Med 1955;12:169–171.
81. Poothullil J, Shimizu A, Dy Ro, Dolovish J. Anaphylaxis from the product(s) of ethylene oxide gas. Ann Intern Med 1975; 85:58–60.
82. Anderson SR. Ethylene oxide toxicity. J Lab Clin Med 1971;77: 346–355.
83. O'Leary RK, Guess WL. The toxiogenic potential of medical plastics sterilized with ethylene oxide vapors. J Biomed Mater Res 1968;2:297–311.
84. Hirose T, Goldstein R, Bailey CP. Hemolysis of blood due to exposure to different types of plastic tubing and the influence of ethylene oxide sterilization. J Thorac Cardiovasc Surg 1963;45: 245–251.
85. Roberts RB, Gamma rays + PVC + EO = OK. Respir Care 1976;21:223–224.
86. Stetson JB, Whitbourne JE, Eastman C. Ethylene oxide degassing of rubber and plastic materials. Anesthesiology 1976;44: 174–180.
87. Bogdansky S, Lehn PJ. Effects of gamma-irradiation on 2-chloro-ethanol formation in ethylene oxide–sterilized polyvinyl chloride. J Pharm Sci 1964;63:802–803.
88. Bryson TK, Saidman LJ, Nelson W. A potential hazard connected with the resterilization and reuse of disposable equipment. Anesthesiology 1979;50:370.
89. Gross JA, Haaas ML, Swift TR. Ethylene oxide neurotoxicity: Report of four cases and review of the literature. Neurology 1979;29:978–983.
90. Glaser ZR. Special occupation hazard review with control recommendations for the use of ethylene oxide as a sterilant in medical facilities. US Dept HEW DHEW (NIOSH), publication No. 77-200, August 1977.
91. US Department of Health and Human Services, DHSS (NIOSH). NIOSH current intelligence bulletin 35: Ethylene oxide. Publication No. 81-130, May 22, 1981.
92. CMP Publications Health Week: The Newspaper for America's Health Industry. Emoryville, CA: CMP Publications, 1987;1:6–7.
93. Occupational Safety and Health Administration, Department of Labor: Occupational exposure to ethylene oxide: Final standard (April 6, 1988) 29 CFR 1910.1047.
94. Spector GJ. Cleansing of endoscopic instruments to prevent spread of infectious disease (letter). Laryngoscope 1987;97:887.
95. Institute for Health Policy Analysis, Georgetown University Medical Center. Proceedings of International Conference on the Re-use of Disposable Medical Devices in the 1980s, March 29–30, 1984. Washington, DC: Institute for Health Policy Analysis, 1984.
96. Simmons BP, Wong ES. Guidelines for prevention of nosocomial pneumonia. Infect Control 1982;3:327–333.
97. Goularte TA, Craven DE. Results of a survey of infection control practices for respiratory therapy equipment. Infect Control 1986;7:327–330.
98. Emergency Care Research Institute. Personal protective equipment: I. Chemical protective clothing and respirators. HHMM 1989;3(1).
99. JAHCSM. EtO Sterilization and Aeration: Central Service Technical Manual 1986;9:79–101.
100. Perkins JJ. Sterilization of medical and surgical supplies with EtO: Principles and methods of sterilization in health sciences. 1983;19:501–528.

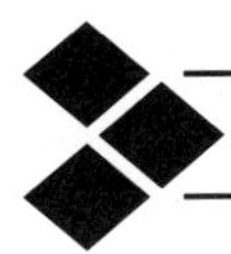

21

Computers and Respiratory Care Equipment

Christopher I. Maxwell
Dennis A. Silage

OBJECTIVES

1. Describe the basic components of a computer.
2. Compare random-access memory and read-only memory.
3. Compare a mainframe computer, personal computer, and portable computer.
4. Compare bits and bytes of computer information.
5. Explain the difference between hardware and software.
6. Describe the following types of software: word processing, spreadsheet, database, graphics, communications.
7. Explain the function of computer programming languages.
8. Describe the use of computers in the pulmonary function laboratory, in the blood gas laboratory, in the intensive care unit, with mechanical ventilators, with computerized control of mechanical ventilation, during monitoring, and with clinical information systems.
9. Describe stand-alone and management applications of computers.
10. Describe applications of hand-held computers.

KEY TERMS

bit
byte
central processing unit
clinical information systems
computer
- desktop computer
- hand-held computer
- laptop computer
- mainframe computer
- notebook computer

database
diskette
formatting
graphics
hard disk
hardware
keyboard
kilobyte
megabyte
modem
monitor
mouse
operating system
parallel transmission
printing device
programming languages
random-access memory
read-only memory
serial transmission
software
spreadsheet
word processing

Introduction

The current application of computers in respiratory care encompasses virtually all aspects of departmental operations, including utilization, clinical information management, patient monitoring, and charting. Computers are indispensable in the pulmonary function and blood gas laboratory. Current-generation mechanical ventilators, patient monitors, and portable instruments are microprocessor controlled. Moreover, the acquisitions of medical information systems that integrate mainframe, mini, micro, and hand-held computers are burgeoning.

In the midst of this computational and information management revolution, respiratory care practitioners are gaining experience through a variety of professional applications software, now available on many types of microprocessor-based computer systems. Many of these programs are of intense practical interest. Examples include those that calculate and interpret hemodynamic or other physiologic profiles and those that perform managerial tasks by manipulating spreadsheet templates. Educational software is also widely available for use on personal computers. Finally, the routine transfer of data from microprocessor-based computers to other computers, both large mainframe and small hand-held computers, implements an electronic network of medical information systems.

As a basis of understanding for this complex field, it is useful first to describe what computers can do (that, for example, a calculator cannot do) and to list what is reasonable to expect a computer to perform.

First, a computer has memory. This memory is composed of semiconductor circuits that are volatile (random-access memory) or nonvolatile (read-only memory) or a magnetic medium whose memory is transient (that is readable and/or writable, as in a disk drive or magnetic tape). Memory permits storage of both instructions (programs) and processed data (information).

A computer can process, organize, and present large amounts of information. This speed of execution permits the computation and presentation of complex data derived from the continuous (on-line) processing of electrocardiographic, electromyographic, electroencephalographic, or other bioelectric signals or the calculation of pulmonary mechanics from airflows, pressures, and gas concentrations.

The computer can interpret the information if a logical decision-making scheme is provided by a knowledgeable individual (the expert). Such a scheme, a set of clinical algorithms known as an expert computer system, provides the ranges and limits (the rules) assigned to each of the interpretive statements.

The introduction of the expert computer system into the respiratory care profession presents an opportunity for the advancement and refinement of interventions in respiratory care. Instead of simply decreasing the tedium of calculations, or merely making processed data available in numerical or graphical form, the expert computer system organizes and interprets information to give a useful and clinically rational description, which is the innovation.

How the Computer Works

Components of the Computer System

Computer systems can generally be classified as mainframe computers, personal computers, or portable computers. A mainframe computer is very large and essentially immobile. A personal computer is usually small enough to be placed on a desk or table. Portable computers can be notebook, laptop, or hand-held. One of the major revolutions that has occurred in computer science within the past 20 years is a decrease in the size and an increase in the power of computers. Thus, very powerful computer systems are available today in the personal computer and portable computer categories.

The principal components of a computer system are shown in Figure 21-1. At the heart of every computer system is the central processing unit (CPU). In the personal computer, the CPU (sometimes called the microprocessor) is a single semiconductor chip about an inch long. The CPU performs all of the commands of the computer, such as arithmetic and logical decisions.

The memory of the computer allows it to remember information. The integral memory capacity of the computer is in the form of ROM and RAM memory (see later). For memory storage, a diskette or hard disk (also called a hard drive) is used with most personal computer systems, and magnetic tape is used with mainframe systems. Information is usually entered into the computer by use of a keyboard or mouse. Information can also be entered into a computer using a modem (which is an acronym for modulator-demodulator). The output of a computer can be directed to either a monitor (video screen), printing device (printer or plotter), or another computer by use of a modem.

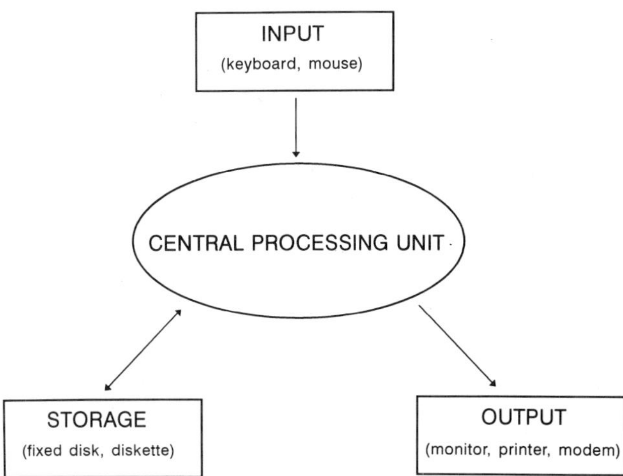

Figure 21-1. Components of a computer system.

Computer Memory

Computers think in binary digital terms of 1s and 0s. Everything that the computer does is based on these 1s and 0s, which actually represent two electrical states and are called bits. The computer generates characters by putting together eight or more bits for a byte. Generally, a byte represents a character (eg, a letter, digit, punctuation mark) and multiple bytes form a computer word. Different CPUs deal with words of differing length. Some, such as the original Apple II series, use 1 byte per word. Others, such as the IBM PC use 2 bytes per word. As a general rule, the larger the word size used by the computer, the more powerful will be the computer. Computers that process a large byte will be able to generate more characters and will be able to access more memory.

Computer memory is of two types. Random-access memory (RAM) is a nonpermanent type of memory that can be easily changed by the user. RAM is used when a program is loaded into a computer or when data or information is turned off unless that information is saved on a diskette or other storage device. Read-only memory (ROM), on the other hand, is permanent and cannot be changed by the user. A powerful computer system is one that provides the user with a lot of RAM and ROM. The amount of memory is stated as the number of bytes. A kilobyte (KB) is 1024 bytes, and a megabyte (MB) is 1,048,576 bytes. In other words, a computer that has a RAM capacity of 64 KB can store 65,536 characters of information, and a diskette that can store 1.2 MB can store 1,258,291 characters of information.

Information Storage

Most personal computers can store data on the magnetic material of a diskette. Diskettes are available in several sizes (3.5 inches and 5.25 inches), and are capable of holding anywhere from 360 KB to 2.88 MB of information. A diskette is a removable storage medium, meaning that diskettes can be removed from the disk drive and replaced with new information. The recording surfaces of a diskette are fragile and need to be handled with care. Damage to the recording surface of a diskette can result in the loss of important information. For this reason, the information is stored on more than one diskette. In that way, if the diskette is damaged, the information can be retrieved from the backup. Data are stored on the diskette in tracks and sectors. The diskette is divided into tracks and sectors in a process called formatting.

A hard drive (or fixed disk) is a magnetic storage device in the form of one or more circular platters that rotate within a sealed enclosure. Like the diskette, the hard drive must be formatted before it can be used by the computer. Unlike the diskette, the hard drive cannot be easily removed from the computer. Furthermore, the hard drive has a much higher storage capacity than the diskette, often in the range of 20 to 520 MB. The computer can also access information on a hard drive faster than it can access information from a diskette. As with the diskette, information stored on a hard drive should be backed up at regular intervals. Backups can be made to multiple diskettes or to a high-capacity tape.

Output Devices

Output from the computer is usually displayed on a video monitor. The monitor can display a single color (monochrome) or many colors. Computer monitors also often have a high resolution (sharpness) to facilitate the display of graphics.

A printing device is used to produce hard-copy output from the computer. A letter-quality printer uses a character-producing printwheel to produce output that is similar in appearance to that which comes from a typewriter. A dot-matrix printer produces characters as the result of a set of pins impacting on a ribbon. Although the quality of characters produced by original dot-matrix printers was poor, the quality of characters generated by many dot-matrix printers available today rivals that from letter quality printers. Unlike the letter quality printer, the dot-matrix printer can generate sophisticated characters and graphics and do so in multiple colors. The most sophisticated printing device is a laser printer. The laser printer produces high-quality text and graphics and does so with great speed.

Information can be sent from one computer to another using a modem. A modem allows computer-generated information to be sent from one computer to another using an ordinary telephone line. There are now many electronic bulletin boards and information services available that use a computer link via modem.

There are two commonly used methods of transmitting information from a computer: serial and parallel. Serial transmission sends data one bit at a time, whereas parallel transmission sends data in multibit clusters. A modem usually uses serial transmission. When serial transmission is used, a commonly accepted protocol for cable configuration is RS-232C. Using the RS-232C interface allows computers to interface with microprocessor-controlled devices such as ventilators, physiologic monitors, and pulmonary function equipment.

Hardware Versus Software

Hardware refers to that part of the computer system made of plastic and metal such as the disk drive, monitor, printer, and keyboard. Software refers to that part of the computer that consists of the useful programs. Software is usually stored on diskettes or hard drives. Some commonly used categories of software include the following

- Word processing: these programs allow manipulation of text.
- Spreadsheet: these programs produce columns of numbers that can be manipulated by the user; although originally developed for use in accounting, this software has application wherever groups of data need to be manipulated.
- Database: these programs allow filing and storage of data and information.
- Graphics: these programs are used to produce graphs.
- Communications: these programs allow computers to interact through a modem.

It is often possible to move information from one software package to another. This allows the user to make best use of the strengths of each program. For example, a database is useful to file data, a spreadsheet is useful to manipulate the data, and graphics software is useful to display graphs.

Operating System

The computer needs a system of instructions related to the interactions of the various components. In other words, the computer must know how to accept instructions from the keyboard, how to display information on the monitor, and how to send and receive information from the disk drive and hard drive. The operating instructions are included in special software called the operating system, or disk operating system (DOS). In addition to the operating system, a user interface can be used. A common user interface is the Windows Graphical User Interface.

Computer Programming Languages

Computer programming involves the writing of specific instructions that the computer can use to perform desired functions. It is this code that provides the "brains" of the computer. In other words, the computer can be no smarter than the person who writes the code (ie, the computer programmer). A common programming language is a BASIC (Beginner's All-purpose Symbolic Instruction Code). BASIC is a relatively easy programming language to learn and generally uses everyday English words to write the code. Other programming languages include FORTRAN (FORmula TRANslation), COBOL, LOGO, Pascal, C, and MUMPS.

The programming languages listed above are sometimes referred to as an interpreter, which is a program that translates source code into a format that the computer can use and then executes the code. A compiler, on the other hand, translates the code at the time of compilation. A language that uses an interpreter is usually easier to write and edit, whereas a language that uses a compiler executes much faster.

Computers in Clinical Respiratory Care

Computers in the Pulmonary Function Laboratory

In the pulmonary function laboratory, on-line interconnections between a spirometer or manual pulmonary function analyzers initially were made to a microcomputer through existing analog recorder outputs. This significantly increased the speed of testing while reducing tedium and error. The microcomputer was capable, even at its inception, of producing video display and hard copy graphics similar in resolution and presentation to the traditional pen-on-paper graphics, as well as an interpretation of the results. An early but relatively expensive pulmonary function computer system was based on the Tektronix 4051, which was in use at the Hospital of the University of Pennsylvania in 1975 (Fig. 21-2). However, with its hard copy unit, spirometric interface and applications software, the cost exceeded $20,000. By 1980, the Apple IIe microcomputer and the inexpensive dot matrix graphical printer lowered the cost to less than $4,000.

Although at first only performing calculations, analysis programs were soon employing the expert system concept to provide technical feedback as to the performance of the apparatus and the patient. Thus the quality of the laboratory testing improved and various laboratories were assured of uniform results.

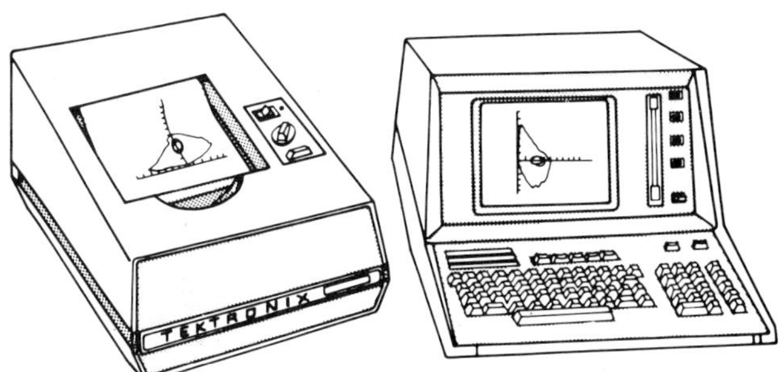

Figure 21-2. Early computerized pulmonary function system based on the Tektronix 4051, developed at the Hospital of the University of Pennsylvania (1975).

Furthermore, the expert system is ideally suited to instrument process control and made possible the automation of sophisticated lung volume analyzers. The ChesTech Prodigy (1983) lung volume analyzer was the first to feature no manual adjustments and complete control of the instrument by the microcomputer (Apple IIe and IBM PC) (Fig. 21-3).

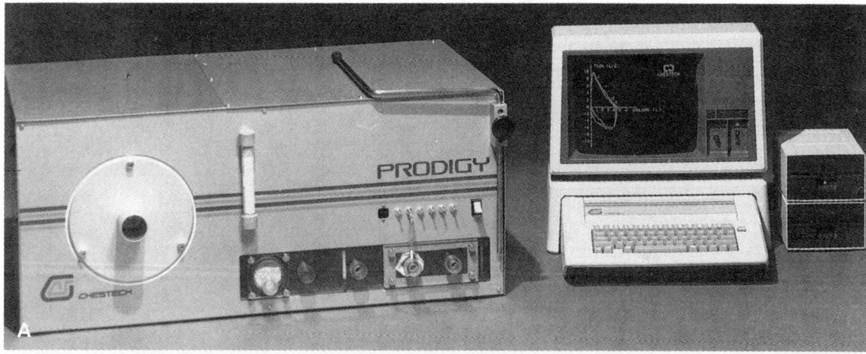

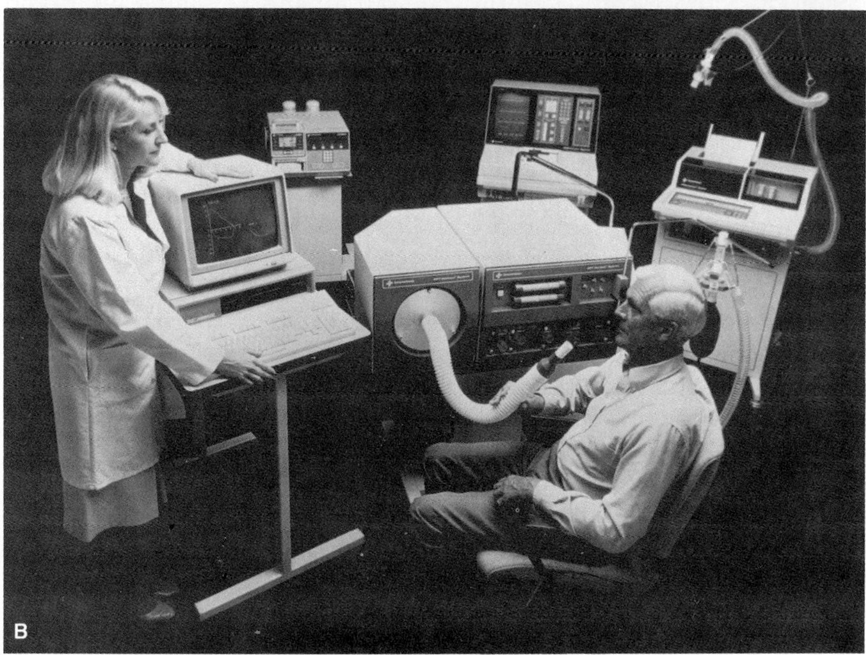

Figure 21-3. A and B. Computer-controlled pulmonary function systems requiring no manual adjustments. (A, courtesy of ChesTech Corporation; B, courtesy of SensorMedics Corporation, Yorba Linda, CA)

Computers in the Blood Gas Laboratory

An interest in the application of computers to the field of blood gases and acid–base balance has long existed. Early work concentrated on the development of interpretation schema to increase the accuracy of acid–base interpretation and subsequent interventions and also served as teaching tools.[1–3] Further efforts were later directed at on-line acquisition of analog data from blood gas analyzers, with subsequent automatic computer interpretation of acid–base status.[4] Martin and Jeffreys[5] described the application of a minicomputer for storing, reporting, and interpreting arterial blood gases in 1983. The advent of the microcomputer, however, has facilitated the more widespread introduction of computer technology into the laboratory itself.

Application of inexpensive microcomputers has significantly increased the efficiency of data management in the blood gas laboratory. Microprocessors built into newer analyzers have further advanced laboratory functions. Microcomputers were first successfully interfaced with manually operated blood gas analyzers in 1979, producing on-line hard copy of results, computer-generated interpretations and selected calculations, and storage of results. Numerous updated commercial applications of this nature exist, either from blood gas analyzer manufacturers, or often from independent software developers. The storage of data on disk has also provided the ability to produce quality control graphics and reports. In some cases, microcomputers have been interfaced with remote printers to transmit results automatically, thus decreasing time required to communicate data while simultaneously eliminating the errors frequently encountered in verbal telephone transmission of blood gas reports.

Newer blood gas analyzing systems are fully automated: microprocessors perform calibration and cleaning functions, control sample size, timing and end-point detection, and provide precision and consistency independent of the operator. Additionally, derived values are rapidly calculated and reported without the need for manual input into another computer system.

Use of computers in the blood gas laboratory improves preparations of quality control reporting and provides a standardized record over time (Fig. 21-4). Application of a simple microcomputer program for in-house computation of a laboratory's mean, standard deviation and coefficient of variation may provide timely feedback and augment a professional data reduction service.[6] Ability to input data into a mainframe system significantly increases the capacity to store, retrieve, and report data and calculations. Highly developed systems, such as the HELP system at LDS Hospital in Salt Lake City, Utah, provide hospital-wide reporting, interpreting, and alerting functions (Fig. 21-5).[7]

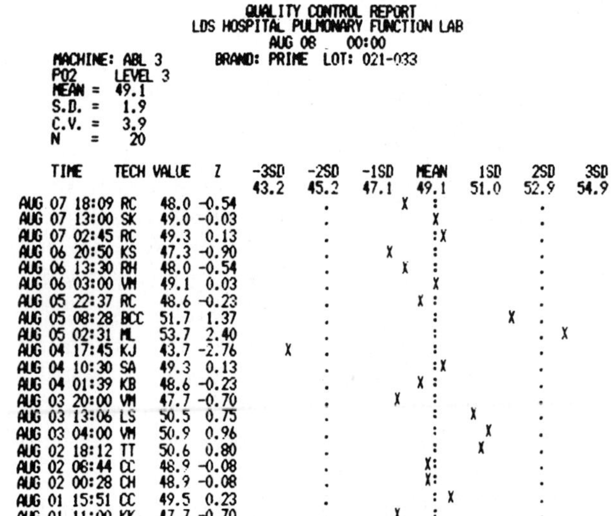
QUALITY CONTROL REPORT
LDS HOSPITAL PULMONARY FUNCTION LAB
AUG 08 00:00
MACHINE: ABL 3 BRAND: PRIME LOT: 021-033
PO2 LEVEL 3
MEAN = 49.1
S.D. = 1.9
C.V. = 3.9
N = 20

-3SD 43.2 | -2SD 45.2 | -1SD 47.1 | MEAN 49.1 | 1SD 51.0 | 2SD 52.9 | 3SD 54.9

TIME	TECH	VALUE	Z
AUG 07 18:09	RC	48.0	-0.54
AUG 07 13:00	SK	49.0	-0.03
AUG 07 02:45	RC	49.3	0.13
AUG 06 20:50	KS	47.3	-0.90
AUG 06 13:30	RH	48.0	-0.54
AUG 06 03:00	VM	49.1	0.03
AUG 05 22:37	RC	48.6	-0.23
AUG 05 08:28	BCC	51.7	1.37
AUG 05 02:31	ML	53.7	2.40
AUG 04 17:45	KJ	43.7	-2.76
AUG 04 10:30	SA	49.3	0.13
AUG 04 01:39	KB	48.6	-0.23
AUG 03 20:00	VM	47.7	-0.70
AUG 03 13:06	LS	50.5	0.75
AUG 03 04:00	VM	50.9	0.96
AUG 02 18:12	TT	50.6	0.80
AUG 02 06:44	CC	48.9	-0.08
AUG 02 00:28	CH	48.9	-0.08
AUG 01 15:51	CC	49.5	0.23
AUG 01 11:00	KK	47.7	-0.70

Figure 21-4. Blood gas quality control data record. (From Gardner RM. Clinical Pulmonary Function Testing, 2nd ed. Intermountain Thoracic Society, Salt Lake City, UT, 1984)

Interpretation of blood gas results by computer has again received considerable attention in recent years. Gardner[7] noted five important steps of computerized blood gas interpretation: (1) determination of acid–base status, (2) determination of oxygenation and oxygen-carrying capacity status, (3) comparison of the most recent results with older values, (4) calculation and reporting of derived values, and (5) alerting of life-threatening conditions.

Hingston and associates[8] evaluated the need for interpretation of blood gases by computer in a physician sample group and concluded that the computer significantly improved the accuracy of interpretation. An interactive diagnostic program offering consultation to health care personnel treating patients with electrolyte and acid–base disorders was described by Moor and Bleich in 1982.[9] Broughton and Kennedy[10] supported computerized interpretations that provide an alerting function, while recommending physician over-reading. Numerous commercial microcomputer software packages for both teaching and reporting purposes have been introduced over the past few years.

Computers in the Intensive Care Unit

Computers in the intensive care unit were first introduced in the early 1960s to track physiologic data. Published reports of such applications proliferated as researchers investigated improved methods of physiologic data collection in an effort to understand shock. Early applications combined sensors of gas concentrations, pressure transducers, electrocardiogram elec-

```
              L D S   H O S P I T A L   B L O O D   G A S   R E P O R T

         ESTHER E          NO.   61534 DR          DANIEL              RM 5N79
FEB 03       PH   PCO2 HCO3   BE   HB  CO/MT PO2 SO2  O2CT %O2  PK/ PL/PP MR/SR
NORMAL HI  7.45  40.0 25.0  2.5 17.0  2/ 1  85  95  22.7
NORMAL LOW 7.35  34.0 19.0 -2.5 13.0  0/ 1  68  93  17.4

03 09:41 V 7.28  52.3 24.0 -3.0 13.4  1/ 0  44  76  14.2 100  32/ 25/ 0 12/ 0
03 09:40 A 7.29  48.2 22.7 -3.9 13.1  1/ 1  70  93  17.2 100  32/ 25/ 0 12/ 0
         SAMPLE #  51, TEMP 35.2, BREATHING STATUS : IMV
         MODERATE ACUTE RESPIRATORY ACIDOSIS
         HYPOVENTILATION (PREVIOUSLY NORMAL)
         CONSIDER DIABETIC KETOACIDOSIS (URINE: GLUCOSE 4+,KETONES 0+)
         O2 CONSUMPTION 176 ML/MIN - CO  5.29 L/MIN
         AV O2 CONTENT DIFF  3.32 (HB 13.25) O2 EXTRACT RATIO  2%
         R-TO-L SHUNT  44%+/-3%
         A-A GRADIENT 482, A/A  13% (EST ALV PO2 552)

03 06:01 V 7.35  45.8 24.9 -0.5 12.7  1/ 0  37  69  12.2  40  26/ 22/ 6 11/ 0
03 06:00 A 7.37  41.3 23.5 -1.1 12.5  1/ 1  49  84  14.8  40  26/ 22/ 6 11/ 0
         SAMPLE #  50, TEMP 35.6, BREATHING STATUS : IMV
         MILD ACID-BASE DISORDER
         O2 CONSUMPTION 163 ML/MIN - CO  5.93 L/MIN
         AV O2 CONTENT DIFF  2.75 (HB 12.60) O2 EXTRACT RATIO  2%
         R-TO-L SHUNT  52%+/-3%
         A-A GRADIENT 144, A/A  25% (EST ALV PO2 193)
         SEVERE HYPOXEMIA  **CONTACT MD OR RN!!!!

03 01:43 V 7.36  48.3 26.9  1.3 13.8  1/ 0  40  69  13.3  41  29/ 23/ 6 11/ 0
03 01:42 A 7.39  42.7 25.5  1.0 13.5  1/ 1  55  86  16.4  41  29/  3/ 6 11/ 0
         SAMPLE #  49, TEMP 36.4, BREATHING STATUS : IMV
         MILD ACID-BASE DISORDER
         O2 CONSUMPTION 209 ML/MIN - CO  6.27 L/MIN
         AV O2 CONTENT DIFF  3.33 (HB 13.65) O2 EXTRACT RATIO  2%
         R-TO-L SHUNT  45%+/-3%
         A-A GRADIENT 142, A/A  28% (EST ALV PO2 197)
         SEVERE HYPOXEMIA BREATHING OXYGEN **CONTACT MD OR RN!!!!

02 22:25 A 7.44  35.3 23.8  0.9 14.1  1/ 0  58  89  17.5  41  32/ 26/ 6 10/ 0
         SAMPLE #  48, TEMP 37.1, BREATHING STATUS : IMV
         NORMAL ARTERIAL ACID-BASE CHEMISTRY
         ESTIMATED R-L SHUNT 73,46,33% (AT AV DIFF OF  0.90, 2.90, 4.90)
         A-A GRADIENT 147, A/A  28% (EST ALV PO2 205)
         SEVERE HYPOXEMIA BREATHING OXYGEN **CONTACT MD OR RN!!!!

02 21:11 V 7.45  37.1 25.6  2.6 14.0  1/ 1  38  70  13.8  41  30/ 23/ 4 10/ 0
02 21:10 A 7.47  35.5 25.7  3.2 13.7  2/ 1  49  85  16.4  41  30/ 23/ 4 10/ 0
         SAMPLE #  47, TEMP 36.9, BREATHING STATUS : IMV
         MILD ACID-BASE DISORDER
         AV O2 CONTENT DIFF  2.90 (HB 13.85) O2 EXTRACT RATIO  2%
         R-TO-L SHUNT  50%+/-3%
         A-A GRADIENT 156, A/A  24% (EST ALV PO2 205)
         SEVERE HYPOXEMIA BREATHING OXYGEN **CONTACT MD OR RN!!!!

   PRELIMINARY INTERPRETATION -- BASED ONLY ON BLOOD GAS DATA.
      ***(FINAL DIAGNOSIS REQUIRES CLINICAL CORRELATION)***
KEY:A=ARTERIAL, V=MIXED VENOUS, C=CAPILLARY, E=EXPIRED CO2, W=WEDGE
    CO=CARBOXY HB, MT=MET HB, O2CT=O2 CONTENT, PK=PEAK, PL=PLATEAU, PP=PEEP
    MR=MACHINE RATE, SR=SPONTANEOUS RATE
          TIME OUT: FEB 03    10:11
```

Figure 21-5. Computerized blood gas report, developed at LDS Hospital, Salt Lake City, Utah. (From Gardner RM, Crapo RO, Morris AH, Beus ML. Computer decision-making in the pulmonary function laboratory. Respir Care 1982;27: 799–808)

trodes, and thermistors to graphically display and trend the condition of the critically ill patient. Manual input of clinical observations and treatments performed usually complemented this on-line acquisition of cardiopulmonary data.

Although there have been many improvements and evolutions, such integrated computer systems remain a fixture of the modern intensive care unit.

Computerized hemodynamic and respiratory monitoring of the critically ill is now considered relatively common throughout the United States.

In 1966, Weil and associates[11] described a four-bed shock research unit at Los Angeles County General Hospital in which a dedicated IBM 1710 computer system was used to collect and process data on a continuous basis. In this experiment, data and programs were stored on magnetic disk. An analog-to-digital converter (ADC) was used to acquire electrical signals. The ADC translates an electrical voltage, which is analogous to a physiologic signal, to a number that can be read and recorded by a computer. Thus, data collected by pressure transducers, biopotential electrodes, thermistors, and manually entered data, are reported by the computer as numerical data. A major research effort of this project was directed toward the development of models to simulate, and thereby predict, selected modes of intensive care treatment. An interest in predictive outcome models persists to this day.

Gardner and coworkers[12] outlined five major tasks of an intensive care unit computer system: (1) acquire physiologic data, (2) communicate data from distant laboratories to the intensive care unit, (3) present and report data in an organized fashion, (4) correlate data, and (5) function as a decision-making tool. Reasons why a computer is useful in monitoring is readily apparent from the list of physiologic variables that are frequently monitored in critically ill patients (Box 21-1).

A further design of a critical care computing system, of special interest to respiratory care practitioners, was described by Nair.[13] In this application, analog data is fed to a computer through an ADC and numerical readings are calibrated and verified by the system.

Box 21-1
Physiologic Variables Frequently Monitored in the Intensive Care Unit

- Arterial blood pressure
- Heart rate
- Temperature
- Hematocrit and hemoglobin concentration
- Urine output rate
- Central venous pressure (CVP)
- Electrocardiogram (ECG)
- Serum electrolytes: Na^+, K^+, Cl^-, HCO_3^-, Ca^{2+}
- Arterial blood gases and pH
- Tidal volume (V_T), respiratory rate (f), minute volume ($\dot{V}_E$)
- Blood volume, plasma volume
- Plasma and urine osmolalities, osmolar and free water clearances
- Electroencephalogram (EEG)
- Intracranial pressure (ICP)
- Pulmonary arterial and precapillary wedge pressures (PAP and PWP)
- Cardiac output and hemodynamic variables
- O_2 transport variables: O_2 delivery, O_2 consumption ($\dot{V}O_2$), and O_2 extraction
- End-tidal CO_2 ($P_{ET}CO_2$), $\dot{V}CO_2$, V_D/V_T
- Mass spectrometry
- Transcutaneous O_2 and CO_2

The computer system can scan selected patient beds and can be programmed to control sampling time and speed. Physiologic data are stored, trended, and displayed in both numerical and graphic form: variables not measured directly are calculated from stored data. This implementation of a computerized respiratory intensive care unit is shown in Figure 21-6.

Computerized Ventilators

Modern electronic ventilators incorporate microprocessors that control and monitor multiple functions and that permit the storage and retrieval of data on demand. Several manufacturers now offer interfaces to personal computers for data management and printing. These newer ventilators are characterized by the use of electromechanical valves, operator-selected ventilation mode, and flow patterns and can provide extensive monitoring. Spearman and Sanders[14] have provided an overview of four representative microprocessor ventilators. All of these ventilators provide data-tending capabilities and can be interfaced with an external computer.

The Puritan-Bennett 7200 ventilator, for example, uses the microprocessor and its associated sensors to monitor and adjust gas flow, monitor airway and system pressure, sample temperature and flow, compensate for gas density, and conduct a Power-On-Self Test (POST) and an Extended Self Test (EST).[15] An independent, preprogrammed electronic circuit provides controlled ventilation in the event of microprocessor failure.

The Puritan-Bennett 7200ae features an expanded microprocessor and memory to permit additional ventilator functions. A digital communications interface (DCI) permits the 7200ae to output formatted information through two RS-232 ports to printers, personal computers, or other remote devices. Other optional, add-on microprocessors include pressure support ventilation, a respiratory mechanics calculator, and waveforms display. Formatted reports include patient data log, chart summary report, ventilator status report (Fig. 21-7), and an Extended Self Test report. The DCI also prints user ID and event ID to give a record of care-related patient procedures.

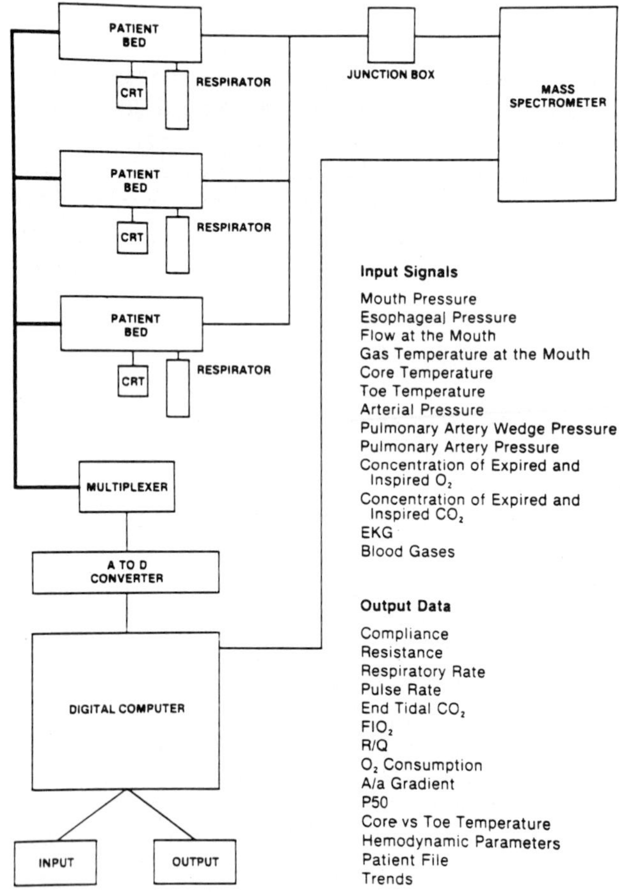

Figure 21-6. Computerized respiratory intensive care unit. (From Nair S. Computers in critical care medicine. In: Shoemaker WC, Thompson WL, Holbrook PR, eds. Textbook of Critical Care Medicine. Philadelphia: WB Saunders, 1984)

```
                         PATIENT DATA LOG
TIME:  10:39  PATIENT ID  1234567890123   ROOM # 9876   DATE: JAN 10
******************************************************************
VENTILATOR SETTINGS
MODE  RR    TV    PF    02    SEN   S PRES  PEEP  WAVE    PLAT  SIGH  NEB
CMV   12.0  0.50  45    21    1.5   0       0.0   SQUARE  0.0   OFF   OFF
******************************************************************
PATIENT DATA                                       1     MINUTE AVERAGE
TIME  RR     MV    MAP    IE                      RR     MV     MAP
        TV    SMV    PAP    PPRES                   TV     SMV    PAP
==================================================================
16:39 ***  ALARM CONDITION - HI PRES LIM        SET POINT - 20        ***
------------------------------------------------------------------
16:39 12.0   6.12   3.8    1.6                    12.0   6.36   3.8
        0.51   0.00   15.1   0.00                   0.53   0.00  15.4

16:40 !!! ALARM SILENCE                  ---------------------------
16:40 !!! ALARM RESET                    ---------------------------
16:40 12.0   6.36   3.9    1.6                    12.0   6.24   3.7
        0.53   0.00   15.3   0.00                   0.52   0.00  15.5

16:41 PRACTITIONER ID 001                ---------------------------
16:41 EVENT ID        254                ---------------------------
16:44 !!! MANUAL INSPIRATION             ---------------------------
16:45 12.0   6.24   3.9    1.6                    12.0   6.24   3.9
        0.52   0.00   15.4   0.00                   0.52   0.00  15.4

16:46 !!! SETTING CHANGE - TIDAL VOLUME   OLD - 0.50   NEW - 0.80   !!!
------------------------------------------------------------------
16:46 ***  ALARM CONDITION - HI PRES LIM      SET POINT - 20          ***
------------------------------------------------------------------
16:46 12.0   9.60   6.4    1.3                    12.0   6.24   6.4
        0.81   0.00   21.4   0.00                   0.52   0.00  16.5
16:46 !!! ALARM SILENCE                  ---------------------------
16:46 !!! ALARM RESET                    ---------------------------

16:47 !!! SETTING CHANGE - HIGH PRES LIM  OLD - 20   NEW - 30       !!!
------------------------------------------------------------------
16:47 12.0   9.72   6.4    1.4                    12.0   9.64   6.4
        0.81   0.00   19.9   0.00                   0.81   0.00  19.9

16:48 !!! SETTING CHANGE - APNEA INTERV   OLD - 20    NEW - 30      !!!
16:48 !!! SETTING CHANGE - APNEA TV       OLD - .50   NEW - .80     !!!
16:48 !!! SETTING CHANGE - APNEA RR       OLD - 12    NEW - 12      !!!
16:48 !!! SETTING CHANGE - APNEA PF       OLD - 45    NEW - 45      !!!
16:48 !!! SETTING CHANGE - APNEA 02       OLD - 21    NEW - 21      !!!
16:48 PRACTITIONER ID 142                ---------------------------

16:50 12.0   9.72   6.4    1.4                    12.0   9.70   6.4
        0.81   0.00   19.9   0.00                   0.81   0.00  19.9

16:55 12.0   9.84   6.3    1.6                    12.0   9.84   6.3
        0.83   0.00   21.3   0.00                   0.83   0.00  21.3

17:00 12.0   9.76   6.5    1.4                    12.0   9.76   6.5
        0.80   0.00   19.7   0.00                   0.80   0.00  19.7

17:05 12.0   9.72   6.4    1.4                    12.0   9.72   6.4
        0.81   0.00   19.9   0.00                   0.81   0.00  19.9
```

Figure 21-7. Computer-generated ventilator data reports, Puritan-Bennett 7200a Ventilator. (Courtesy of Puritan-Bennett Corporation, Lenexa, KS)

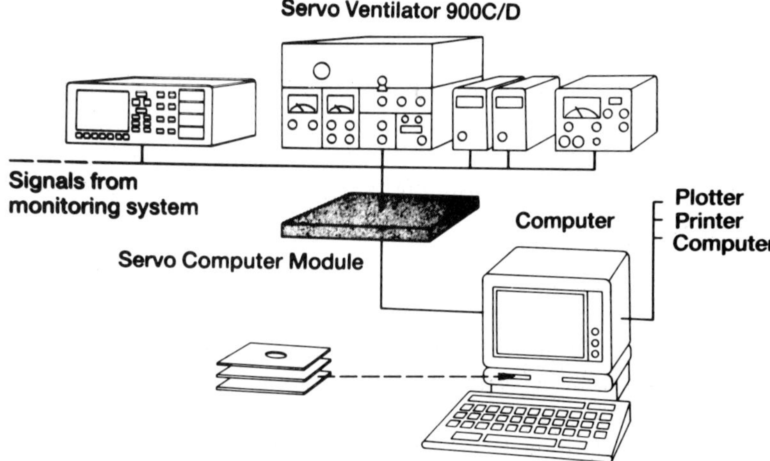

Figure 21-8. The Siemens Servo 900 C/D and Servo Computer Module 990. (Courtesy of Siemens Life Support Systems, Iselin, NJ)

Siemens Corporation has introduced the Computer Aided Ventilation (CAV) system, which includes a personal computer interface (Servo Computer Module 990) and software (Fig. 21-8). The interface module contains 128KB RAM, RS-232 communications ports, and two ports for analog input (eg, pulse oximetry). The module serves as an acquisition, communication, and storing device. The Siemens CO_2 analyzer and Lung Mechanics Calculator can also be connected, as well as any equipment with an analog output. Up to 30 parameters can be monitored by the Servo Computer Module, with 10 stored in a 24-hour trend memory, updated once per minute. Newer software revisions eliminate the need for the Lung Mechanics Calculator, providing this function through the software. Four parameters can be read in real time. The Siemens software is menu driven, to allow access with minimal input. Multiple patient monitoring at a remote site is possible using a data time-sharing or multiplexed device. Graphing and tending capabilities enhance the collection of data (Fig. 21-9).

Advantages of the introduction of computer-aided ventilation include the ability to rapidly modify or update software independent of ventilator hardware. With the addition of alerting functions, interfacing of both analog and digital monitors, the continuing refinement of data storage capacity, and decision-making schema, the interface of the personal computer with the advanced ventilator will be of great interest to the respiratory care practitioner. Spearman and Sanders[14] note, however, that the availability of large volumes of computerized data needs to be approached with some caution, since the accuracy of some monitored data may be questionable, leading to both the accumulation of misleading information and inappropriate alarm functions.

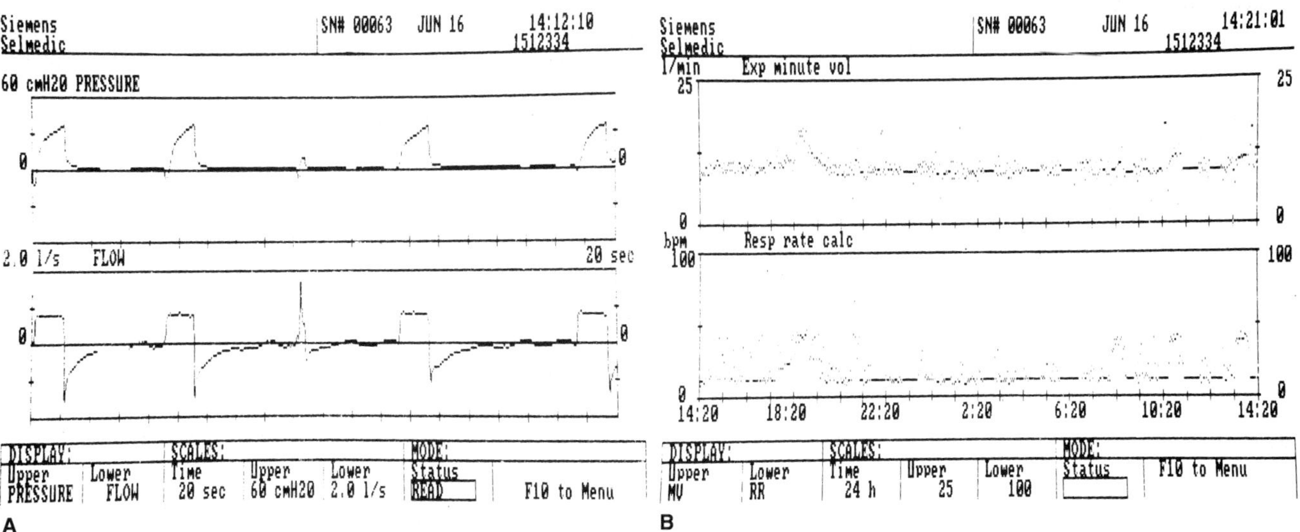

Figure 21-9. (A.) Real-time pressure and flow tracing obtained using Siemens 900C Ventilator and Servo Computer Module 990 with IBM PC. (B.) Twenty-four hour trend report of patient weaning attempt using alternating periods of ventilator support and pressure support. Siemens 900C Ventilator and Servo Computer Module 990 with IBM PC.

Computerized Control of Ventilation

Recent clinical research has involved the experimental investigation of feedback loops with mechanical ventilators, to include the adjustment of minute volume according to measured exhaled CO_2 tension, computer control of positive end-expiratory pressure (PEEP) titration based on changes in lung compliance and functional residual capacity, and computer control of F_{IO_2} based on pulse oximetry saturations.

Thompson[16] notes that interest in closed-loop mechanical ventilation is not new, dating to research performed in 1953.[17] Further studies during the 1960s and 1970s investigated closed-loop control by exhaled CO_2,[18] CO_2 production,[19] and invasive measurement of arterial pH.[20] Research to date indicates that closed-loop ventilation is possible, although the reliability of intra-arterial catheter measurements remains a difficulty. Furthermore, measured exhaled CO_2, used as a signal to control delivered minute volume, may not always approximate arterial CO_2.[16] Thompson notes that the technique of microprocessor-controlled mandatory minute volume, available on several newer ventilators, is the closest approximation to closed-loop control of ventilation currently commercially available.

Computer control of PEEP remains a continuing research interest. East and colleagues[21,22] described the application of a microcomputer to regulate PEEP therapy in dogs using the Siemens Servo 900C ventilator (Fig. 21-10). In their design, three algorithms titrate PEEP: (1) by maximizing static compliance, (2) by maximizing functional residual capacity–based compliance, and (3) by normalizing functional residual capacity. The system adjusts PEEP in 3 cm H_2O steps at 20-minute intervals. The benefits of computer-controlled PEEP may lie in the relatively fast achievement of optimal PEEP levels (within 40 to 60 minutes) using a noninvasive technique and in the potential of automatically tailored PEEP therapy throughout the course of ventilator support. Strickland and Hasson[23] evaluated a computer-controlled ventilator weaning system. The computer-directed system increased or decreased rate and pressure support level based on predetermined limits of respiratory rate and tidal volume. Oxygenation was monitored by pulse oximetry. They found that the computer-based weaning system resulted in fewer blood gases and shorter weaning times. Many questions, however, remain before such applications are widely accepted.

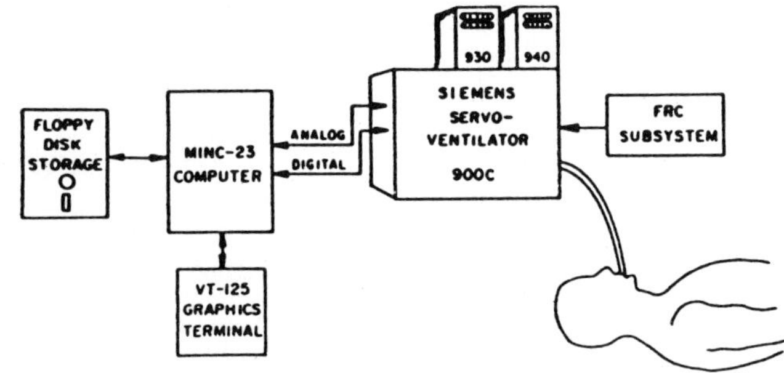

Figure 21-10. Computer-controlled PEEP optimization system. (From East TD, Andriano KP, Pace NL. Computer controlled optimization of positive end-expiratory pressure. Crit Care Med 1986;14:792–797)

Monitoring

Brimm[24] attributes the early use of electronic monitoring to physicians and engineers who adapted monitors of artificial circulation used during heart-lung bypass in the intensive care unit.[24] The early basic interest in physiologic data acquisition and processing, trending, and reporting remains very active today and has been intensified by the rapid changes in technology. Current applications are predominantly in innovative microprocessor uses and the development of advanced software to perform signal analysis. Advances in technology have also led to the development of instruments that can function as noninvasive monitors and also serve as devices to store and trend physiologic data (eg, pulse oximeters and capnographs) (Fig. 21-11).

Computer systems have become inherently smaller, faster, and less expensive, leading to wider application. Modern bedside monitoring systems are often modular and can detect and compensate for artifact and contain decision-making clinical algorithms (eg, dysrhythmia monitoring). Modern systems can also communicate between various instruments and other computers. Many bedside monitors now have keypads or touch-sensitive screens to simplify interactive data entry. In an effort to prevent repetitive transcription of data, with the potential for error, many systems integrate data transmitted directly to the bedside computer system from departments outside the intensive care unit. Brimm[24] notes that this increasing integration of data will result in significant efforts in the future to design a comprehensive computer charting system.[24]

Osborn[25] summarizes three major types of monitoring that are of special interest here. The first type of monitoring, termed *time and limit monitoring,* is relatively simple and is the most widespread: the evaluation of, for example, high or low blood pressure limits. Despite its simplicity, its major deficiency is false alarms. The second type of monitoring is *statistical monitoring,* plotting a patient's data in a multidimensional grid created from a large data bank on critically ill patients. Inferences may be drawn about the patient's probable course by comparing the data with those of similar patients. The limitation here is that such a comparison may not identify the chain of

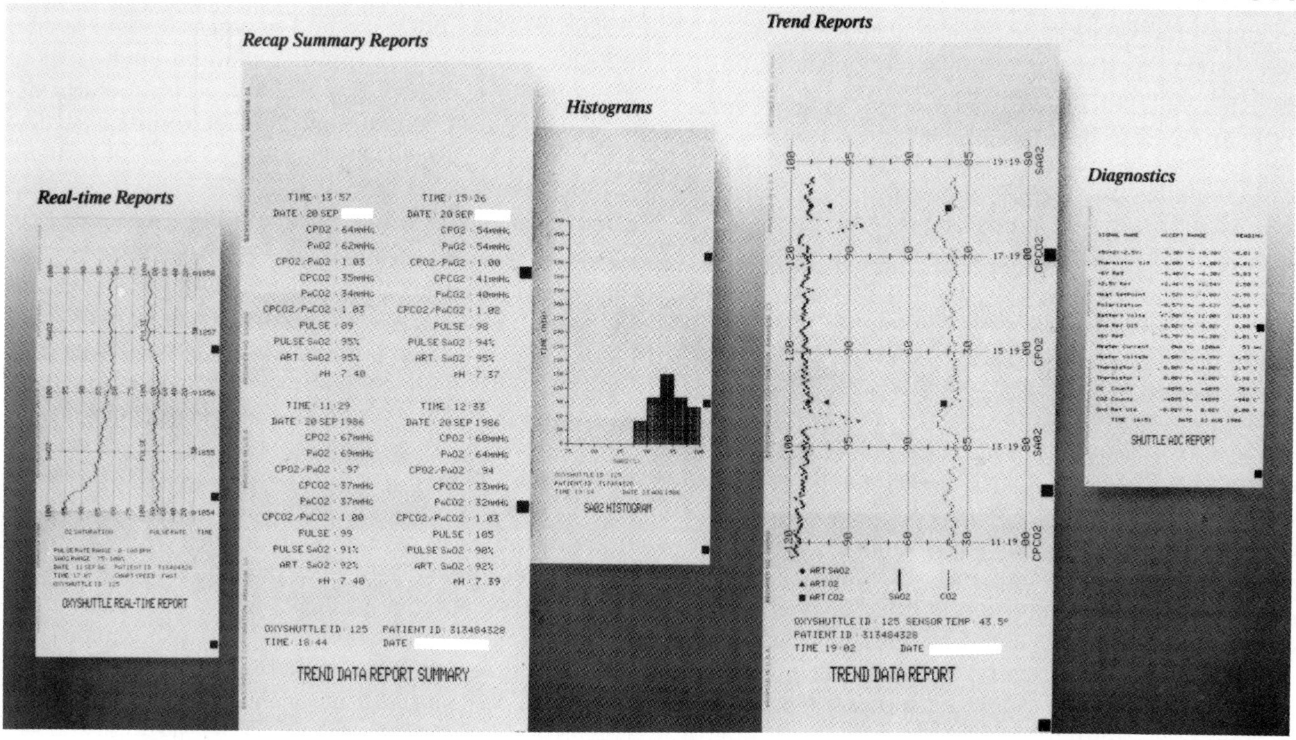

Figure 21-11. Sample reports generated by the OxyShuttle System. (Courtesy of SensorMedics Corporation, Yorba Linda, CA)

causes, nor the specific organ failure. Finally, Osborn describes *integrative monitoring*, based on mathematical modeling and rule-based logic, whose output is diagnostic statements, such as in computer-interpreted electrocardiograms, pulmonary function test results, or arterial blood gas analysis results. Osborn suggests that a successful combination of the three types of monitoring will lead to an ideal intensive care unit computing system. Although it is not yet clear exactly which monitored variable will produce the best monitoring and predictive/prognostic indices, widespread application of computerized monitoring in the intensive care unit will likely lead to a continued refinement of skills and will result in improved care for the critically ill patient.

Clinical Information Systems

The next stage in the evaluation of computers in respiratory care is likely to be in the continuing refinement of applications in clinical information systems. Once restricted to the few institutions that had mainframe systems that could support a detailed reporting and charting subsystem, clinical data management is now also being successfully managed by powerful microcomputers linked to mainframes, or by hand-held computers interfaced with a departmental microcomputer network systems. It is reasonable to speculate that rapid and significant advances will occur in clinical data management in the next few years, as attention begins to turn from capture of physiologic data to the charting and organization of clinical information.[24]

Computer-based information systems can

- Bring order to the clinical chart through standardized computer-generated reports.
- Integrate and increase the general in-house availability of clinical information, especially if the chart is on-line and can be reviewed at the nursing station or bedside terminal.
- Provide trending/graphics capacity to organize and reduce clinical data.
- Improve the readability of the chart.
- Increase the speed and efficiency of charting and laboratory reporting, while reducing labor time.
- Perform automatic performance of many functions (billing, calculations, reporting) from a single input.

Twenty-five to 35% of a health care professional's time is spent doing paperwork.[26–28] Jeromin[29] estimated, in 1982, that only about a dozen respiratory therapy departments in the country had reached a level of substantial computerization and that as many hospitals had failed in the effort. Detailed accounts of two successful, large-scale (mainframe) implementations of clinical information systems for respiratory therapy departments are available elsewhere.[30,31] With the advent of relatively inexpensive, commercial microcomputer-based information systems, however, the successful implementation of respiratory therapy management systems is likely to increase.

Clinical information systems may be developed in-house, developed using input from the hospital to modify a commercial package (eg, IBM Patient Care System), or may include the lease of common-user (unmodified) software (eg, Tenet system). More recently, smaller, microcomputer-based systems have been introduced that are more readily updated or modified. On-line technical assistance is available through telephone line (modem) connections, facilitating corrections and diagnostic evaluations of software or program difficulties.

Both mainframe and microcomputer clinical information systems concentrate on the development of a database that allows storage, retrieval, and reporting capabilities. Data are stored in files containing data fields of alphabetic and numerical data. Given a database arrangement, the computer is able to store and search for data on demand and can construct reports as requested. Common computer functions for a respiratory therapy department can include automatic billing, charting, order entry, treatment records, daily and shift reports, and accounting summaries.

After staff training, a significant component of computerization, and the conversion stage,[32] therapists can input data into the computer from any terminal throughout the hospital (if the system is hospital wide) from dedicated department terminals located in strategic areas, or from within the department itself. If the system is interfaced with the hospital-wide information system, hospital bed census, room changes, discharges, admitting information (sometimes called ADT for admitting, discharge, and transfer functions), and other administrative information is readily available. In most cases, it is desirable and possible to link the department computer system with the hospital information system.

The most common method of access to the hospital information system is through manual keyboards at the nursing stations. The employee is generally assigned an employee number (an electronic signature) and usually a password to permit access to the system. A touch sensitive screen or light pen may be used to select menu items by merely pointing, thus reducing the need for keyboard skills. Most programs are now menu driven, allowing rapid selection of charting or data entry functions. Clinical orders can be entered at the nursing station and automatically sent to the respiratory therapy department (order-entry functions).

Andrews and associates[31] note that up to one half of patient records are in narrative form. Thus, clinical information processing is more difficult than, for example, laboratory numeric reports. A major effort has been to adjust this need to a predefined computer syntax and vocabulary, as well as provide the opportunity for textual comments. To facilitate this process, a questionnaire-entry format provided a logical sequence for data input. Andrews notes that manual clinical charts are organized into chronologically ordered systems. Computers are readily amenable to the logically ordered processes of data entry, organization, storage, and review. An example of a mainframe respiratory care computer charting system is illustrated in Figures 21-12 and 21-13.

More recently, smaller companies have entered the clinical data management market, providing customized, departmental specific systems at a relatively low cost. Such systems are usually microcomputer based. Perhaps the newest innovating in respiratory therapy computer systems is based on the ability of fourth-generation microcomputers, (eg, the IBM PC/AT or Personal System 2) to interface with hand-held computers such as the HP 71 (Fig. 21-14). The combination of the

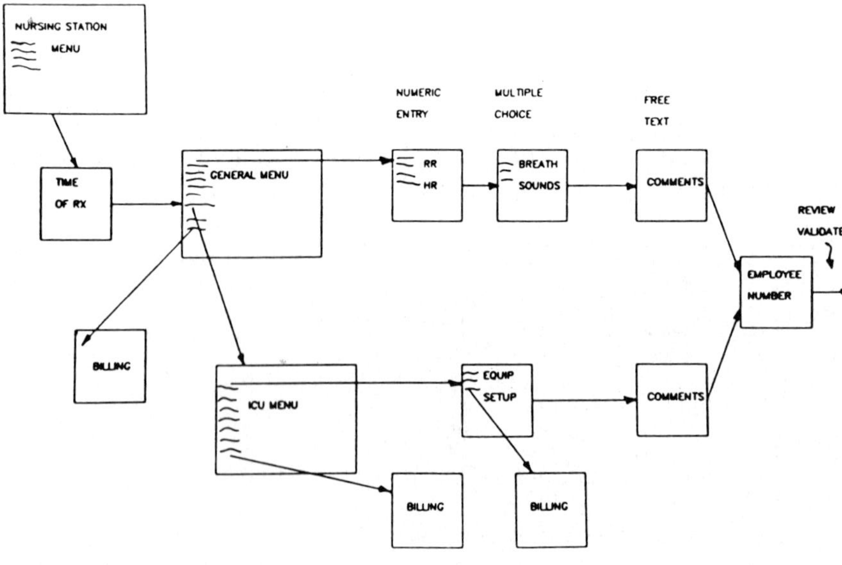

Figure 21-12. Example of main frame computer-based respiratory care charting system. Menu selection facilitates entry of results of respiratory care. (From Andrews RD, Gardner RM, Metcalf SM, Simmons D. Computer charting: An evaluation of a respiratory care computer system. Respir Care 1985;30:695–707)

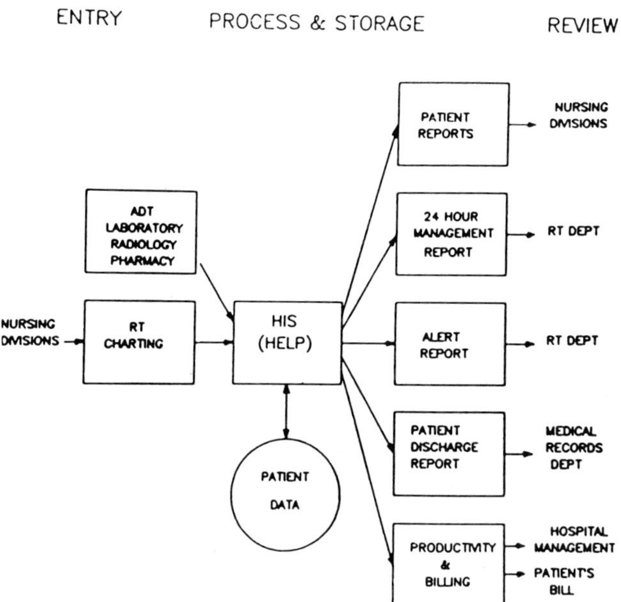

Figure 21-13. Respiratory care charting as processed and distributed by hospital-wide information system (HELP system). (From Andrews RD, Gardner RM, Metcalf SM, Simmons D. Computer chartings: An evaluation of a respiratory care computer system. Respir Care 1985;30:695–707)

two computers, one stationary and the other fully portable, provides the needed mobility for respiratory therapists as they move between units within the hospital. Data captured and entered by the practitioner at the new bedside will thus reflect personal workload, performance, computer charting, new order entries, and other textual comments, during the shift (Fig. 21-15).

As with mainframe systems, background information is first stored by the microcomputer. This is usually done with a large capacity, high acquisition speed, magnetic hard drive, to provide details of employees, floors, computer codes for procedures, physician lists, and standard times for procedures. Significant department organization is necessary before computerization.[29] The hand-held computer system permits the entry of new orders, treatment information, patient file editing or updating, and textual comments entered directly through the hand-held computer keyboard. At the end of the shift, the hand-held computer is connected to the departmental microcomputer, and the information is uploaded to the microcomputer through the interface for filing and sorting recorded data into, for example, patient treatment records, therapist work activity and times, and equipment usage/inventory control and so on. From these data, supervisors can generate work assignments.

Such decentralized systems can be linked to the hospital information system to permit, for example, the sharing of admitting data and facilitate automatic transfer of patient treatment charges to the billing department. Such features are a desirable byproduct of clinical data management programs. Departmental records can be generated daily to document treatments for a patient over a given data range, treatments given by a therapist, time spent in clinical activities compared with standard (expected) times, as well as lists of orders that are due to discontinue within the next 24 hours. Routine backing up of current data files will prevent loss of the data base. Files kept on a hard drive can be archived to magnetic tape at regular intervals.

The interest evident in these smaller systems is based on their flexibility and the decentralized nature of data collection. If data can be successfully gathered at the bedside and entered without the need for access to a nursing station terminal, an increase in clinical productivity and a decrease in manual charting times can reasonably be expected. Managers are especially interested in the capacity of the system to measure and compare productivity and to generate departmental reports for use in performance improvement func-

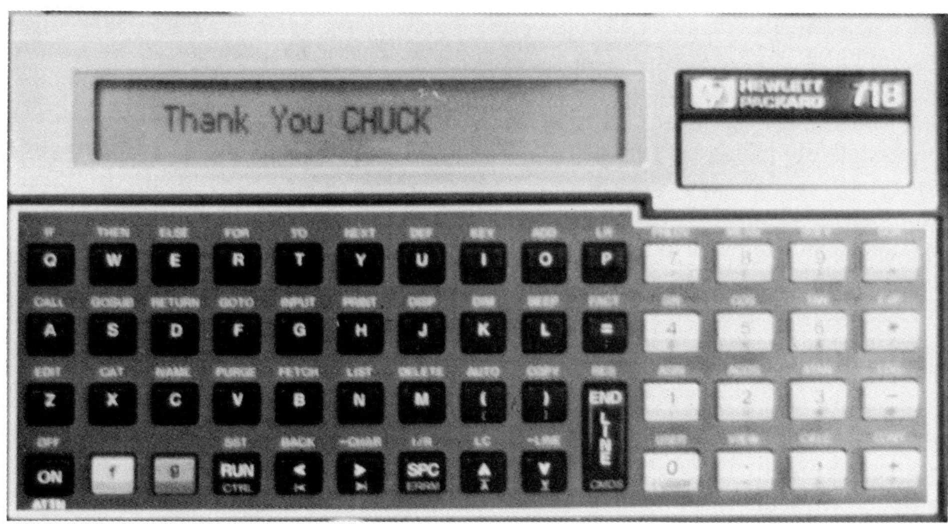

Figure 21-14. Hewlett-Packard 71B hand-held computer; interfaced with IBM-AT.

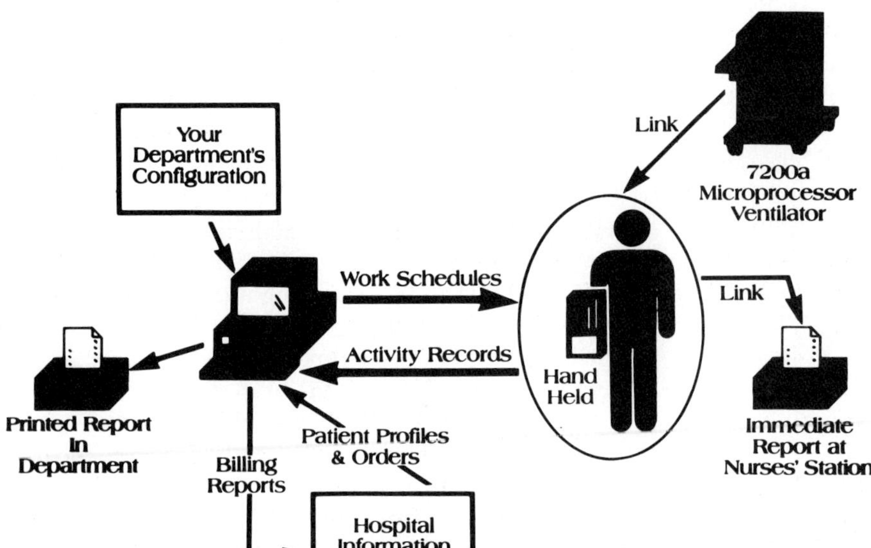

Figure 21-15. Schematic view of respiratory care hand-held computer system. (Courtesy of Puritan-Bennett Corporation, Lenexa, KS)

tions, evaluation of adherence to departmental charting standards, and personnel/staffing functions. A likely development will be the addition of bar code reading capabilities to the hand-held computer to facilitate data entry.

Stand-Alone Applications of Microprocessor-Based Computers

Personal computers were applied in medicine almost as soon as the first machines were commercially available. Progress in application of these devices is even more remarkable considering that the Apple II, the first widely available personal computer, came onto the market in the early 1980s. Major reasons for the popularity of personal computers in medicine are that the hardware is relatively inexpensive, the machine is simple to operate, and, perhaps most significantly, the library of software for medical applications is rapidly increasing.

Shortly before the advent of the personal computer, Cohn and coworkers[33] described the generation of the Automated Physiologic Profile at the bedside of the critically ill, using a powerful desktop calculator and standardized graphic hard-copy output. Because of the success and interest in this early effort, one of the first applications of the personal computer as a stand-alone device was in the intensive care unit.

An early interactive Apple II computer-based program for intensive care unit calculations, intravenous drip rates, and blood gas analysis at the University of Pittsburgh was described in 1982.[34] These programs were subsequently expanded and distributed by the Society of Critical Care Medicine. An advancement of these early programs, adding an interpretive and decision-making function to a computer-generated hemodynamic profile, was described by Marino and Krasner 1984.[35] Numerous commercial applications of these programs are now readily available, with a continuing heavy concentration on hemodynamic and oxygenation profiles.

In a book on the application of microcomputers in the intensive care unit, Dean and Booth[36] provided not only a teaching tool for the health care professional but also included complete listings of software for all programs discussed. These programs are the result of significant effort and development since the late 1970s and include sophisticated versions of emergency drug calculators, hemodynamic profiles, and other routines that can enhance critical care. In fact, the trend toward including public domain software for medical applications has increased in recent years, thus assisting the widespread implementation of such work. An excellent source of noncommercial teaching programs may also be available from the authors of journal articles, who may offer the program on disk upon request. Examples of such sources include arterial blood gas and pulmonary function software,[37] oxygen transport models,[38] and pulmonary and tissue gas exchange models.[39]

Successful commercial applications of educational software have also increased in recent years, despite early charges of simplistic, "page-turner" programs. Although the significance of the personal computer as an education tool has, to date, fallen somewhat short of initial expectations, it holds great promise in professional and in-service education.[40] A full complement of educational, interactive teaching programs for respiratory therapy students is now readily available from several commercial vendors, including problem-solving clinical situations, blood gas and pulmonary function interpretation programs, and more advanced programs for the teaching of trauma care, cardiac care, and other assessment programs. Such programs are widely applied in respiratory therapy, nursing, and medical teaching programs. As instructional programs move from page-turner and drill programs toward simulations, self-paced courses, and instructional dialogues the personal computer will become a significant educational tool.[41]

Literature searches are commonly conducted for research and clinical applications. With a computer-aided search, hundreds of references can be identified in a few minutes. With a modem, the search can be conducted virtually anywhere. In some cases, an entire journal article can be downloaded. Several on-line subscription services are available to assist computerized literature searches. These include Grateful Med, Paper Chase, and BRS Colleague.

Management Applications

Computers are widely applied to management and record-keeping functions owing to the capacity of the microcomputer to store and process large amounts of data. The fact that the hardware is reasonably inexpensive is a major reason for their widespread introduction. Additionally, newer software versions are remarkably easy to learn and require little more than a moderate investment of time to become proficient.

Two major functions of the computer include word processing and spreadsheet applications. Word processing permits the rapid manipulation of large amounts of text and storage on diskette or hard drive. An obvious example of significance for a respiratory therapy department would include the maintenance of the departmental procedure manual on magnetic disk, thus facilitating routine changes and updates without the need for manual correcting and retyping.

Electronic spreadsheets permit the manipulation of large amounts of data, automatic calculation of imbedded formulae, recalculation of all or parts of the data, and graphics capabilities. An example for respiratory therapy applications would be the productivity report, readily calculated based on shift workload reports and paid hours. In the example provided (Fig. 21-16), the individual procedures are assigned a relative value (as in the American Association for Respiratory Care's Uniform Reporting system, or by a system developed in-house) and non–procedure-related tasks are ac-

PAY PERIOD: 6-8 to 6-21

	1	2	3	4	5	6	7	8	9	10	11	12	13	14	SUB	xRVU	TIME
DATE	8	9	10	11	12	13	14	15	16	17	18	19	20	21			
O2 ROUNDS	0.7	1.4	0.3	0.7	1.0	1.2	1.3	1.2	1.2	1.6	1.2	0.8	0.8	0.6	14.0	(.hr)	14.0
EQUIP CHANGE	2.2		1.1	1.0	0.8			1.5		1.5					8.1	(.hr)	8.1
EQUIP CLEAN-UP	1.2	1.5	1.7	1.0	1.2	1.0	1.9	1.1	0.6	1.2	1.1	1.1	0.2	0.4	15.2	(.hr)	15.2
EQUIP REPAIR			0.3			0.2		0.5			0.1				1.1	(.hr)	1.1
EQUIP ASSEMBLY	1.2	0.9	0.5	1.1	1.1	0.9	2.0	1.2	1.0	0.5	1.3	0.9	0.3	0.2	13.1	(.hr)	13.1
EQUIP STOCKING	1.4	1.0	0.7	0.7	0.3	0.8	1.1	0.6	0.6	0.9	0.6	0.5	0.4	0.4	10.0	(.hr)	10.0
EQUIP ORDERING							0.8							0.4	1.2	(.hr)	1.2
SET-UP	48.0	11.0	32.0	27.0	30.0	15.0	17.0	33.0	24.0	29.0	24.0	28.0	26.0	14.0	358.0	.23	82.3
AEROSOL TX	50.0	46.0	48.0	63.0	58.0	47.0	50.0	51.0	43.0	49.0	46.0	52.0	53.0	47.0	703.0	.165	116.0
IPPB															0.0	.33	0.0
USN	2.0	4.0	3.0	4.0	2.0	3.0	5.0	6.0		4.0	3.0		1.0		37.0	.33	12.2
ISB	18.0	31.0	35.0	37.0	31.0	23.0	17.0	15.0	3.0	23.0	37.0	35.0	35.0	22.0	362.0	.165	59.7
CPT	7.0	1.0	5.0	3.0	5.0	7.0	10.0	10.0	19.0	4.0	2.0	2.0	2.0	3.0	80.0	.3	24.0
IND SPUTUM		2.0	1.0	2.0	1.0			7.0							13.0	.4	5.2
MECH VENT/DAY		2.0	3.0	3.0	2.0	2.0	2.0	1.0	3.0	3.0	3.0	3.0	3.0	4.0	34.0	3.6	122.4
VENT MONT/DAY		2.0	3.0	3.0	3.0	3.0	3.0	3.0	3.0	3.0	3.0	3.0	3.0	4.0	39.0	1.0	39.0
CO2 MONT/DAY			1.0		1.0		1.0		1.0		2.0				6.0	1.0	6.0
CPAP/DAY	1.0	1.0	1.0			1.0	1.0	1.0		2.0		1.0	1.0	1.0	11.0	3.6	39.6
PF SCREEN	2.0		1.0		1.0		1.0				1.0	2.0	3.0		11.0	.33	3.6
PFS B & A	1.0	1.0	1.0	1.0	1.0	1.0		1.0	1.0	1.0	1.0				10.0	.58	5.8
SPIROMETRY - B	1.0		1.0			1.0					1.0			1.0	5.0	.57	2.9
SPIROMETRY-B&A		2.0		2.0			2.0		1.0				1.0		8.0	1	8.0
PFT 551						2.0						2.0			4.0	1.25	5.0
PFT 569	1.0	1.0	1.0	1.0		1.0	1.0	1.0	1.0	1.0					9.0	1.5	13.5
O2 TRANS	5.0	11.0	3.0	1.0	3.0	11.0	3.0	5.0	4.0	1.0	1.0	5.0	1.0		54.0	.13	7.0
CPR	1.0	0.5		1.0	1.0	1.0	0.4	2.0	2.0	1.0	1.0		0.5	1.0	12.4	(.hr)	12.4
ABG	9.0	8.0	9.0	7.0	8.0	7.0	8.0	6.0	11.0	10.0	9.0	9.0	8.0	7.0	116.0	.33	38.3
CHARGES	0.6	0.7	0.5	0.4	0.7	0.5	1.0	0.9	1.1	0.8	1.3	0.4	0.8	0.5	10.2	(.hr)	10.2
EAROXI SINGLE	11.0	10.0	7.0	7.0	6.0	6.0	8.0	3.0	11.0	12.0	8.0	8.0	6.0	9.0	112.0	.2	22.4
EAROXI DOUBLE	2.0	2.0	1.0	2.0	2.0	4.0	3.0	2.0	3.0	2.0	2.0	1.0	1.0	2.0	29.0	.2	5.8
EAROXI DAILY	1.0	2.0	2.0	2.0	2.0	2.0	2.0	2.0	2.0	1.0	1.0	1.0	1.0	1.0	22.0	1.0	22.0
STICKERS			0.3			0.6			0.6			0.6			2.1	.2	0.4
NOTES	14.0	12.0	13.0	14.0	13.0	12.0	15.0	13.0	13.0	13.0	12.0	12.0	13.0	12.0	181.0	.2	36.2
OTHER	2.1	1.1	3.0	4.0	4.5	3.0	3.2	2.0	5.1	2.6	7.2	2.6	4.0	3.2	47.6	(.hr)	47.6
															T VAT		810.3
															SEC		79.5
															MAN		90.0
															T PRO		969.8
															ACT HR		1136.7
															PROD		85.3

Figure 21-16. Sample productivity report for 2-week time period, generated by Lotus 1-2-3 electronic spread sheet. (Courtesy of Department of Respiratory Therapy, Community General Osteopathic Hospital, Harrisburg, PA)

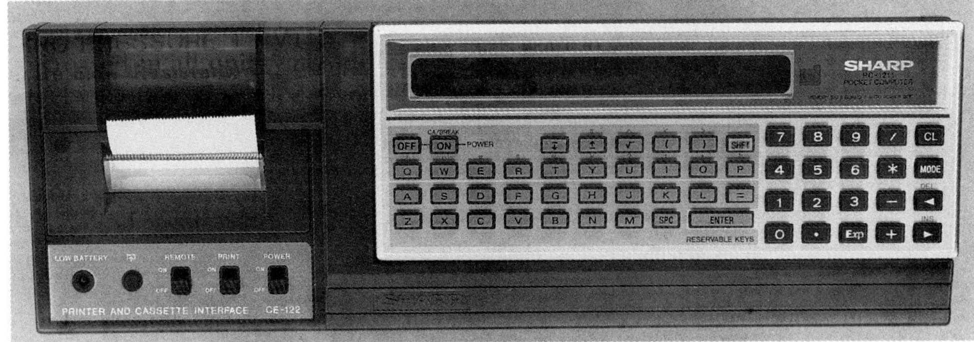

Figure 21-17. First-generation hand-held computer (Sharp PC-1211), with printer interface CE-122.

counted for by accurate time reporting. The data for a 2-week period are multiplied for each category by the relative value unit assigned; then these data are subtotaled, and totals for all procedure and nonprocedure work determined. Finally, hours worked are compared with hours paid and a productivity figure is derived. There are numerous ways to configure productivity reports, with some set by hospital preference or devised by outside consultants. However, the spreadsheet permits the department manager considerable flexibility in the design of his or her own workload and productivity monitoring system.

Significantly, graphs of department procedures and year-to-year comparisons can be used for managerial purposes, to visually demonstrate increasing or decreasing workloads, and to inform staff of department workload on an on-going basis. Graphics can also add a competitive edge to budgeting requests and proposals. An accounting of productivity data over time, in both graphic and tabular form, provides the manager with a useful tool for assessing, and defending, departmental staffing and activity levels.

Hand-Held Computers

During the 1970s, many reports detailed the use of hand-held calculators, programmable in keystroke logic, to facilitate the generation of detailed cardiopulmonary profiles at the bedside.[41–48] These devices, however, were limited by a cryptic numerical output and a lack of decision-making capability.

Hand-held computers (HHCs) first became widely available in 1982 and were quickly applied to computational and interpretive programs for respiratory therapy.[49–52] Among the advantages of the HHC are the extremely low price (from $50 to $250), the memory available (from 2KB to 16KB of RAM, easily upgraded to higher levels with plug-in memory modules), and the fact that the HHC is programmable in the universal computer language BASIC. Experience gained programming and using the HHC is readily transferable to more advanced personal computer applications and may serve as an inexpensive introduction to computers for the novice practitioner.

The HHC is available in three levels of sophistication. The first generation is the least expensive and is not expandable (Fig. 21-17). The second-generation HHC has an expandable memory, by plug-in memory chips, and may be interfaced with peripherals such as line printers and modems (Fig. 21-18). The third generation contains significantly more memory and may be interfaced with printers, modems, and other computers (eg, personal computers) (Fig. 21-19). All HHCs share the common benefits of portability, battery power, decision-making capability, and ease of programming. Despite the limited memory of the first generation HHC, numerous programs useful for both teaching and clinical purposes have been implemented using this device. The first-generation HHC lends itself to simple laboratory calculations and interpretations. Examples include pulmonary calcula-

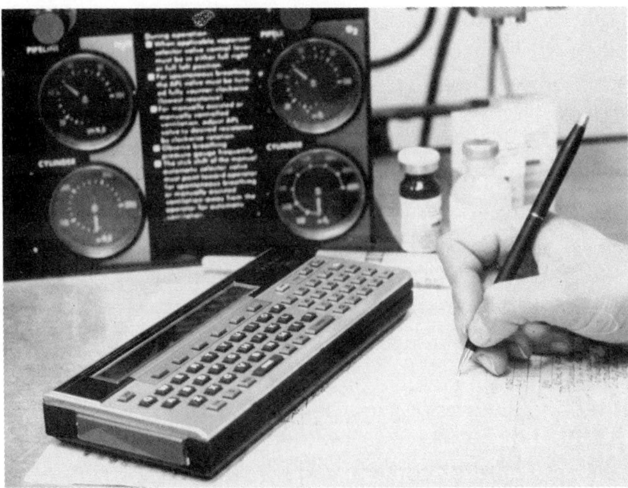

Figure 21-18. Second generation hand-held computer (Sharp PC-1500).

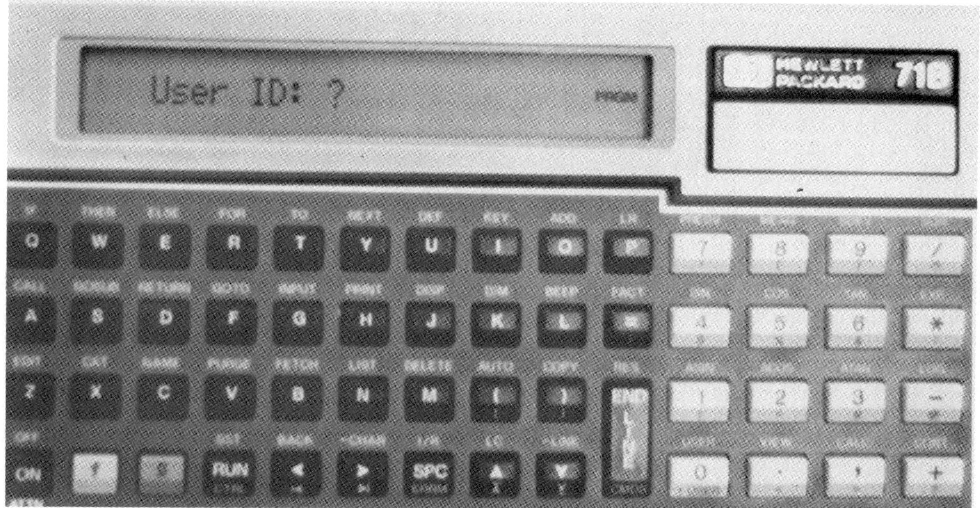

Figure 21-19. Third-generation hand-held computer.

tions[50–52], prediction equations useful in the intensive care unit, cardiopulmonary or hemodynamic profiles,[53–59] and blood gas interpretation.[60] Hess[61] has provided an acid–base teaching program that randomly generates problems for students to test blood gas interpretation skills. Such a program, implemented on an inexpensive HHC, could readily become a part of a library of computer software for education programs in respiratory therapy.

The second-generation HHC, with its expandable memory, is capable of executing advanced decision-making schema, for example, acid–base interpretation by acid–base map.[61–64]

The third-generation HHC is able to store large amounts of data, has expandable memory, and, most importantly, has the ability to interface with personal computers, printers, modems, and video monitors. The third-generation HHC also offers a more extensive set of BASIC functions and statements, user-definable functions, a keyboard that can be customized, and an advanced internal file system. Furthermore, these devices often include built-in software such as word processors, spreadsheets, and communications software. As design of the device is advanced to include rugged construction and a multiscreen, practitioners can expect more manufacturers to offer interfaces to devices such as ventilators and monitors to permit data collection and transfer of information between microprocessors.

Summary

The application of computers in respiratory care and in respiratory care equipment has developed rapidly over the past decade and will continue to expand as computer systems become even less expensive and as the impetus for health care workers to accurately document productivity increases. As microcomputers become more powerful and faster, and as interfaces between other computers multiply, respiratory therapists can expect to have an increasing involvement in computer applications.

It is reasonable to infer that within the next few years rapid and significant advances will occur in both clinical data management hardware and software. This will facilitate the natural progression from the mere acquisition of physiologic data to electronic monitoring, charting, and organization of clinical information. In many cases, portable and personal computers will play an important role in this development.[65]

References

1. Goldberg M, Green SB, Moss ML, Marbach CM, Garfinkel D. Computer-based instruction and diagnosis of acid–base disorders. JAMA 1973;223:269–275.
2. Bleich JL. Computer evaluation of acid–base disorders. J Clin Invest 1969;48:1689–1696.
3. Cohan ML. A computer program for interpretation of blood gas analysis. Comput Biomed Res 1969;2:549–557.
4. Gardner RM, Cannon GH, Morris AH, Olsen KR, Price WG. Computerized blood gas interpretation and reporting system. Computer 1975;January:39–45.
5. Martin L, Jeffreys B. Use of a minicomputers for storing, reporting, and interpreting arterial blood gases, pH, and pleural fluid. Respir Care 1983;28:301–308.
6. DeWitt A. A computer program for quality assurance in the blood gas laboratory. Respir Care 1984;29:371–374.
7. Gardner RM, Crapo RO, Morris AH, Beus ML. Computer decision-making in the pulmonary function laboratory. Respir Care 1982;27:799—808.
8. Hingston DM, Irwin RS, Pratter MR, Dalen JE. A computerized interpretation of arterial pH and blood gas data: Do physicians need it? Respir Care 1982;27:809–815.
9. Moore MJ, Bleich HL. Consulting the computer about acid–base disorders. Respir Care 1982;27:834–838.

10. Broughton JO, Kennedy TC. Interpretation of arterial blood gases by computer (editorial). Chest 1984;85:148–149.
11. Weil MH, Shubin H, Rand W. Experience with a digital computer for study and improved management of the critically ill. JAMA 1966;198:147–152.
12. Gardner RM, Blair JW, Pryor TA, et al. Computer-based ICU data acquisition as an aid to clinical decision-making. Crit Care Med 1982;10:823–830.
13. Nair S. Computers in critical care medicine. In Shoemaker WC, Thompson WL, Holbrook PR, eds. Textbook of Critical Care Medicine. Philadelphia: WB Saunders, 1984.
14. Spearman CB, Sanders HG. The new generation of mechanical ventilators. Respir Care 1987;32:403–414.
15. Dupuis YG. Ventilators: Theory and Clinical Applications. St. Louis: CV Mosby, 1986.
16. Thompson JD. Computerized control of mechanical ventilation: Closing the loop. Respir Care 1987;32:440–444.
17. Frumin JR. Clinical use of a physiological respiratory producing N_2O amnesia-analgesia. Anesthesiology 1957;18:290–299.
18. Kamiyama N, Tachibana N, Yamamura H. Automatic controller for artificial ventilation. Jpn J Anesthesiol 1968;17: 1047–1048.
19. Mitamura Y, Mikami T, Sugara H, Yoshimoto C. An optimally controlled respirator. IEEE Trans Bio-Med 1971;18:330–337.
20. Coon RR, Zyperky EJ, Kampine JP. Systemic arterial blood pH servocontrol of mechanical ventilation. Anesthesiology 1978;49: 201–204.
21. East TD, Andriano KP, Pace NL. Computer controlled PEEP optimization (abstract). Crit Care Med 1985;13:357.
22. East TD, Andriano KP, Pace NL. Computer controlled optimization of positive end-expiratory pressure. Crit Care Med 1986;14: 792–797.
23. Strickland JH, Hasson JH. A computer-controlled ventilator weaning system. Chest 1993;103:1220–1226.
24. Brimm JE. Computers in critical care. Crit Care Nurs Q 1987;9: 53–63.
25. Osborn JJ. Computers in critical care medicine: Promises and pitfalls. Crit Care Med 1982;10:807–810.
26. Jydstrup RA, Gross MJ. Cost of information handling in hospitals. Health Serv Res 1966;1:253–271.
27. Jacobvwitzk K, Strodtman L, Lomas T, Turax T. Micro-computer based data management system for nursing assessment of the diabetic patient. In: Proceedings of the Fifth Annual Symposium on Computers in Medical Care, 1981;755–759.
28. Collen MF, Davis LS, Van Brunt EE, Terdiman JF. Functional goals and problems in large-scale patient record management and automated screening. Fed Proc 1974;33:2376–2379.
29. Jeromin G. Computerization: Are we ready? (editorial) Respir Care 1982;27:846–854.
30. Michelevich DJ, Robinson AL, Rogers C, Dupriest ME, Mize EI. Respiratory therapy as a component of an integrated hospital information system: The Parkland On-Line Information System (POIS). Respir Care 1982;27:846–854.
31. Andrews RD, Gardner RM, Metcalf SM, Simmons D. Computer charting: An evaluation of a respiratory care computer system. Respir Care 1985;30:695–707.
32. Tarrent CAW. Computer conversion: The neglected phase. Comput Health Care 1986;May:26–28.
33. Cohn JD, Engler PE, Del Guercio LRM. The automated physiologic profile. Crit Care Med 1975;3:51–58.
34. Cottrell JJ, Pennock BE, Grenvik A, Rogers RM. Critical care computing. JAMA 1982;248:2289–2291.
35. Marino PL, Kransner J. An interpretive computer program for anlayzing hemodynamic problems in the ICU. Crit Care Med 1984;12:601–602.
36. Dean JM, Booth FV. Microcomputers in Critical Care: A Practical Approach. Baltimore: Williams & Wilkins, 1985.
37. Morris AH, Kanner RE, Crapo DO, Gardner RM. Clinical pulmonary function testing: A manual of uniform laboratory procedures, 2nd ed. Intermountain Thoracic Society, 1984.
38. Morris DA, Granger WM. A block diagram, graphical and microcomputer analysis of the oxygen transport system. Physiologist 1982;25:111–117.
39. Boyle J. A microcomputer program of pulmonary and tissues gas exchange. Ann Biomed Eng 1986;14:425–435.
40. Arons AB. Computer-based instructional dialogs in science courses. Science 1984;224:1051–1056.
41. Ruiz BC, Tucker WK, Kirby RR. A program for calculation of intrapulmonary shunts, blood-gas, and acid–base values with a programmable calculator. Anesthesiology 1975;42:88–95.
42. Shabot MM, Shoemaker WC, State D. Rapid bedside computation of cardiorespiratory variables with a programmable calculator. Crit Care Med 1977;5:105–111.
43. Kenney GNC. Programmable calculator: A program for use in the intensive care unit. Br J Anaesth 1979;51:793–796.
44. Laurent M. Bedside calculation of hemodynamic parameters with a hand-held programmable calculator: I and II. Acta Anesth Belg 1980;31:45–59.
45. Powles ACP, Hershler R, Rigg JRA. A pocket calculator program for non-invasive bedside assessment of cardiopulmonary function. Comput Biol Med 1980;10:143–151.
46. Nahrwold ML. Rapid calculation of derived hemodynamic parameters using a programmable calculator. Anesthesiol Rev 1981;18:15–19.
47. Finlayson DC, Yin A. Calculator assisted cardiorespiratory monitoring. Crit Care Med 1981;9:604–606.
48. Chatburn RL. Computation of cardiorespiratory variables with a programmable calculator. Respir Care 1983;28:447–451.
49. Maxwell C, Silage DA. Hand-held computers in pulmonary medicine (editorial). Respir Care 1983;28:62–66.
50. Silage DA, Maxwell C. A spirometry/interpretation program for hand-held computers. Respir Care 1983;28:35–36.
51. Silage DA, Maxewell C. A lung volume determination/interpretation program for hand-held computers. Respir Care 1983;28: 452–456.
52. Silage DA, Maxwell C. A lung diffusion determination/interpretation program for hand-held computers. Respir Care 1983;28: 452–456.
53. Maxwell C, Hess D, Silage DA. Clinical application of the hand-held computer in respiratory intensive care. Crit Care Q 1983;6: 85–91.
54. Krasner J, Marino PL. The use of a pocket computer for hemodynamic profiles. Crit Care Med 1983;11:826–827.
55. Keller CA, Ruppel G, Hyers T. Bedside computation of cardiopulmonary variables with a hand-held computer (letter). Crit Care Med 1984;12:542.
56. Maxwell C, Hess D, Shefet D. Use of the arterial/alveolar oxygen tension ratio to predict the inspired oxygen concentration needed for a desired arterial oxygen tension. Respir Care 1984;29:1135–1139.
57. Hess D, Maxwell C, Agarwal NN, Silage DA. Hand-held computer applications in critical care medicine: A demonstration. In: Proceedings of the Eighth Annual Symposium on Computer Applications in Medical Care, 1984:1009.
58. Hess D, Maxwell C, Agarwal NN, Silage DA. Hand-held computer applications in critical care medicine. Respir Ther 1985;15: 25–28.
59. Doyle DJ. A simple computer program for obtaining gas exchange indices. Crit Care Med 1985;13:775–776.
60. Hess D, Silage DA, Maxwell C. A blood-gas interpretation program for hand-held computers. Respir Care 1984;29:375–379.
61. Hess D. The hand-held computer as a teaching tool for acid–base interpretation. Respir Care 1984;29:375–379.
62. Silage DA, Maxwell C. An acid–base map/arterial blood gas interpretation program for hand-held computers. Respir Care 1984;29:833–838.
63. Hess D, Eitel D. A portable and inexpensive computer system to interpret arterial blood gases. Respir Care 1986;31:792–795.
64. Doyle DJ. Computer program for bicarbonate dose calculation during cardiac arrest. Crit Care Med 1987;15:283–284.
65. Ash SR, Ulrich DK. Portable and desktop microcomputers for patient care charting. J Med Syst 1986;10:361–373.

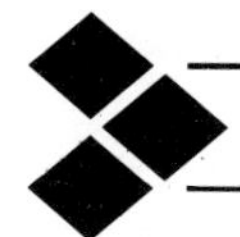

Approval and Surveillance of Medical Devices

Ann Grahm

Richard D. Branson

OBJECTIVES

1. Describe the role of the Food and Drug Administration in regulating medical devices.
2. Compare mandatory and voluntary reporting of device-related problems.
3. Discuss the importance of recognizing and reporting adverse events related to equipment failure and misuse.

KEY TERMS

510(k)
Class III device
investigational device exemption (IDE)
mandatory medical device reporting program (MDR)
medical device
MEDWATCH
premarket application
problem reporting program

Introduction

This chapter is provided as an introduction to the regulatory processes and nonregulatory efforts of the Food and Drug Administration (FDA), including device classification, premarket notification and approval processes, postmarket surveillance, and education programs.

Role of the Food and Drug Administration

The FDA is the only agency mandated to regulate medical devices through the Food, Drug and Cosmetic Act of 1938, with additional authority under the Medical Device Amendments, enacted on May 28, 1976. The Food, Drug, and Cosmetic Act serves to ensure that foods are pure and wholesome, drugs and devices are safe and effective for their intended use, cosmetics are safe and properly labeled, and all packaging and labeling is truthful and informative. In addition, the act regulates biologics and radiation-emitting products such as televisions, microwave ovens, and lasers.

Radiologic products, such as microwave appliances and televisions, regulated separately under the Radiation Control for Health and Safety Act of 1968, are obligated to conform to safety requirements and comply with performance standards separately promulgated under that act.

More recently, the Safe Medical Devices Act of 1990 and Medical Device Amendments of 1992 have expanded FDA controls over user reporting, postmarket surveillance, and device tracking. These acts were signed into law on November 28, 1990, and June 16, 1992.

A medical device is defined as an instrument, apparatus, implement, machine, contrivance, implant, in-vitro reagent, or other similar or related article, including any component, part, or accessory, that does not achieve any of its principal intended purposes through chemical action within or on the body, is not dependent on being metabolized for achievement of any of its principal intended purposes, and which is:

- Recognized in the official National Formulary, or the United States Pharmacopeia (USP)
- Intended for use in the diagnosis of disease or other conditions, or in the cure, mitigation, treatment, or prevention of disease in man or animal
- Intended to affect the structure or function of the body

The FDA regulates all medical devices that are introduced into interstate commerce in the United States, Puerto Rico, and the District of Columbia. The Medical Device Amendments require all medical devices to be placed in one of three increasingly stringent regulatory control categories, as a means to ensure that the device is reasonably safe and effective.

Class I General Controls
Class II Performance Standards
Class III Premarket Approval

Classification is different for pre–Medical Device Amendments devices, post–Medical Device Amendments devices, and transitional devices.

Pre–Medical Device Amendments devices are medical devices in commercial distribution on or before the enactment date of May 28, 1976. The FDA must place all of these devices into Class I, II, or III by issuing regulations. These devices may continue to remain on the market (Table 22-1).

Post–Medical Device Amendments devices are devices that are proposed for commercial distribution after the enactment date of May 28, 1976. To market these devices, it must be determined to be substantially equivalent to a pre–Medical Device Amendments device. Thus, it would be subject to the same requirements as the device to which it is equivalent. If it is not found substantially equivalent, then it is placed in Class III, which requires premarket approval (PMA) before it can be marketed.

Transitional devices are medical devices that were regulated as new devices before the amendments. They are placed, by law, into Class III, requiring PMA approval before marketing.

TABLE 22-1. Breakdown of Devices by Class

Class	Provisions of the MDA
I General Controls	Premarket notification Registration and listing Banning devices Repair, replacement, and refund Adulteration and misbranding Good manufacturing practices (GMP)
II Performance Standards	A performance standard is necessary to ensure safety and effectiveness, ie, design, components, sale restrictions, conformance of performance characteristics.
III Premarket Approval	Necessary to ensure safety and effectiveness; only applies to devices that are life-supporting, life-sustaining, or of substantial importance in preventing impairment to health or present an unreasonable risk of illness or injury.

The classification of devices determines the requirements that manufacturers must meet before distributing their devices into interstate commerce and controls the degree of regulation used to reasonably ensure safety and effectiveness.

The Medical Device Amendments provide the FDA with the authority to regulate devices during all phases of their development, testing, production, distribution, and use. There are approximately 4000 types of medical devices regulated under the legislation, widely ranging in complexity and use.

Premarket Notification

The FDA uses the premarket notification (510k application submission) to determine if a device is, or is not, substantially equivalent to either a pre–Medical Device Amendments device or a reclassified post–Medical Device Amendments device. Refer to Figure 22-1 for the FDA's overview of the substantial equivalence decision-making process. In general, a premarket notification application must be sent to the FDA when introducing a device into distribution for the first time; a product line for the first time, even though the product may have been marketed by another firm previously; or a modification to a device that could alter the safety and effectiveness of a device. A 510k application must contain, among other things:

- Proposed labeling sufficient to describe the devices's intended use, physical composition, method of operation, specifications, and performance claims

510(k) "Substantial Equivalence" Decision-Making Process (Detailed)

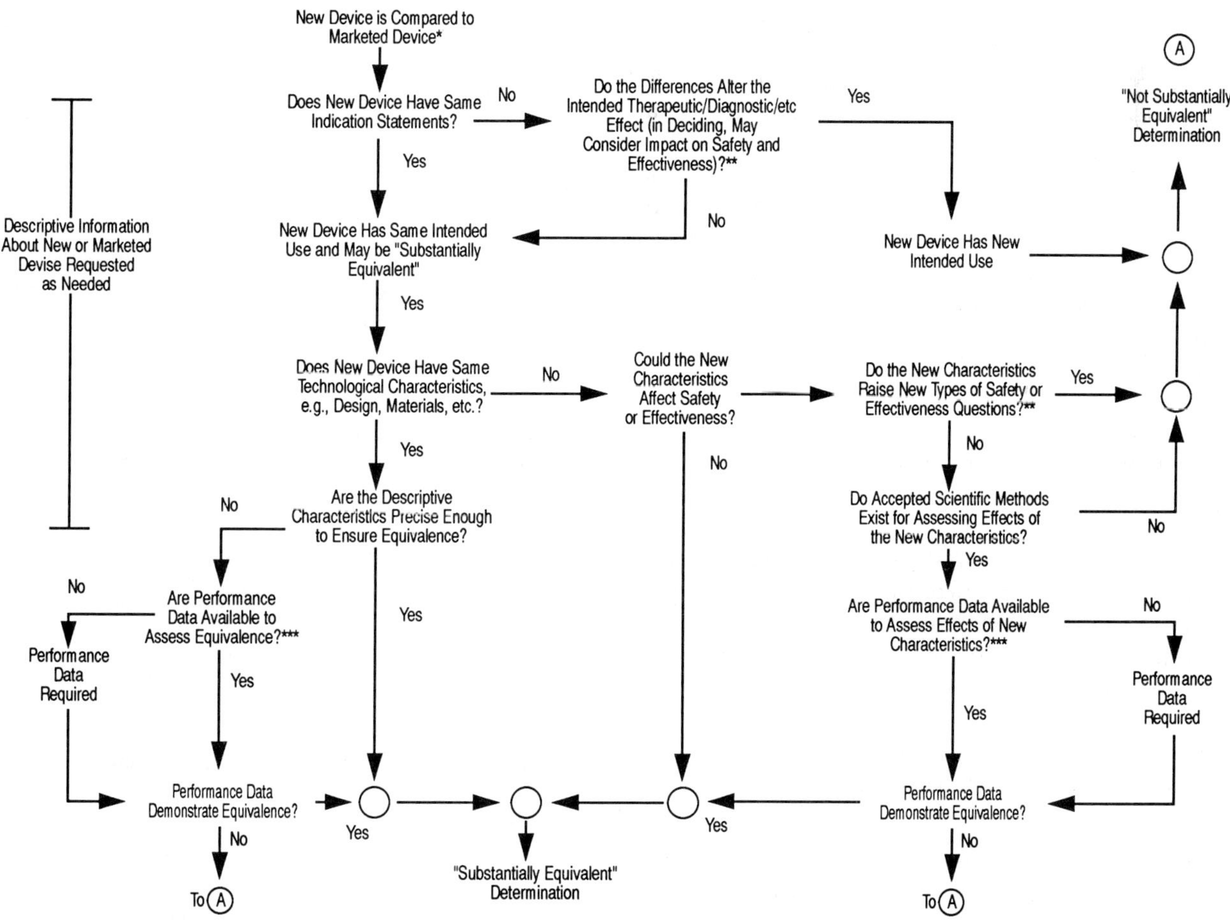

*510(k) Submissions Compare New Devices to Marketed Devices. FDA Requests Additional Information if the Relationship. Between Marketed and "Predicate"(Pre–Amendments or Reclassified Post–Amendments) Devices is Unclear.

**This Decision is Normally Based on Descriptive Information Alone. But Limited Testing Information is Simetimes Required.

***Data May Be in the 510(k), Other 510(k)s, The Center's Classification Files, or the Literature.

Figure 22-1. Flow chart to determine "substantial equivalence" by the Food and Drug Administration.

- A description of how the device is similar to or different from other devices of comparable type or information about what consequences a proposed device modification may have on the device's safety and effectiveness
- Any other information the FDA needs to determine whether the device is substantially equivalent

The amendments require a manufacturer to notify the FDA at least 90 days before it intends to introduce the device, determined to be substantially equivalent, into commercial distribution.

The regulatory provisions for Class I (General Controls) apply to all medical devices. They are the least stringent regulatory controls placed on medical device manufacturers and constitute the minimum required by the FDA for distribution into interstate commerce. These controls require medical device manufacturers to

- Register with the FDA.
- Provide a list of devices they manufacture or distribute.
- Conform to the Good Manufacturing Practices (GMP) regulations.
- Notify health care providers of health risks associated with misbranded, adulterated, or violative products.
- Maintain records and reports that describe the manufacturing methods, facilities, and controls used during manufacturing, packaging, storage, and installation of medical devices.

Examples of anesthesia and respiratory care Class I devices are listed in Box 22-1.

The act provides for the development of performance standards for devices in which general controls are insufficient to ensure safety and effectiveness, when sufficient information exists to develop a performance standard, and when it is necessary to establish a performance standard to provide reasonable assurance of the device's safety and effectiveness. These devices are placed into Class II. Examples of anesthesia and respiratory care Class II devices are listed in Box 22-2.

Box 22-1
Medical Device Classification: Examples of Class I Devices

Esophageal stethoscope
Blow bottle
Nose clip
Ether hook
Nasal oxygen cannula
Breathing mouthpiece
Tracheobronchial suction catheter

Since 1976, the FDA has published its intention to develop mandatory performance standards for several devices, including continuous ventilators and ventilator breathing circuits, cardiac monitors, and central nervous system shunts. Although there are no mandatory medical device performance standards, voluntary standards developed in the medical device area include those of the American Society for Testing and Materials (ASTM), International Standards Organization (ISO), and the USP.

Class III Devices

Premarket Approval Applications

Devices are placed in Class III if insufficient information exists to determine general controls and performance standards may not provide reasonable assurance of safety and effectiveness and if they are life-sustaining, life-supporting, or implantable devices; these devices include those substantially important in preventing impaired health or those that present an unreasonable risk of substantial illness or injury if they do not perform as intended. Devices are also placed in Class III if the FDA has determined the device is not substantially equivalent to a pre–Medical Device Amendments device. In addition, a device the FDA previously regarded as a new drug (transitional devices), such as sutures, were transferred to Class III when the Medical Device Amendments were passed in 1976. To market a Class III device, manufacturers are required to submit a PMA application to the FDA. Examples of Class III anesthesia and respiratory care devices are in Box 22-3.

The manufacturer must submit a PMA application to the FDA that shows the device is safe and effective for its intended use. The application must contain, for example, the indication(s) for use, device descriptions,

Box 22-2
Medical Device Classification: Examples of Class II Devices

Arterial blood sampling kit
Oxygen, nitrous oxide, halothane gas analyzers
Diagnostic spirometers
Nasal, oral airways
Autotransfusion apparatus
Anesthesia breathing circuits
Anesthesia gas machine
Continuous ventilator
All pulmonary function meters
Flowmeters

Box 22-3
Medical Device Classification: Examples of Class III Devices

Indwelling oxyhemoglobin concentration analyzer
Indwelling carbon dioxide analyzer
Lung water monitor
Extracorporeal membrane oxygenators (ECMO)
High-frequency ventilators

marketing history of all countries in which the device has been marketed, summaries of all the significant published and unpublished clinical investigations including summaries of animal and clinical trials, the experimental study design, and data collection and analyses of the results. The summary section of the application contains a methodologic summary of any clinical trials involving human subjects, including the hypothesis of the study, information on the exclusion and selection criteria of subjects, the study population and duration, adverse reactions, patient compliance, device failures, contraindications, and precautions. The FDA is required by law to respond to a PMA application within 180 days. However, applications are frequently put "on hold," pending additional information requested by the FDA to clarify information in the application. In addition, all PMA applications are reviewed by device advisory panels. These 19 panels (see Table 22-3 on page 528) are composed of scientists in the private sector, health care providers, manufacturers, and consumer representatives. Each panel makes recommendations to the FDA for approval, conditional approval, or denial, including review and revision of the labeling that will accompany the device in commercial distribution. The device advisory panel meetings are opened to the public, and meeting dates and times are published in the *Federal Register.*

Investigational Device Exemptions

The scientific data necessary to show safety and effectiveness in humans are often preceded by bench and animal studies to support the claims being made for the device. To undertake clinical human trials to develop these data, a sponsor (eg, the manufacturer of the device) must obtain approval of an investigational device exemption (IDE) application before beginning a clinical trial of an unapproved device. Certain devices are exempt from the requirements of the IDE regulation.

- Devices in commercial distribution when used in accordance with the indications in the labeling in effect at that time
- A device undergoing consumer preference testing, if it does not place persons at risk and is not for safety/effectiveness testing
- A veterinary device
- A laboratory research device
- A custom device, unless it is being used to determine safety and effectiveness for commercial distribution
- A diagnostic device meeting certain criteria

Diagnostic devices may be exempt, if they meet all of the following criteria:

- The diagnostic device is appropriately labeled for research or investigational use only.
- The device is noninvasive.
- The use does not have a significant risk in an invasive sampling procedure.
- The device does not by design or intent introduce energy into the patient.
- The device is not the sole diagnostic procedure.

All other device investigations are subject to the provisions of the IDE regulation and are considered to be either significant or nonsignificant risk. The sponsor of an IDE application must initially determine whether the device presents a significant or nonsignificant risk to the subject. A significant risk device is one that presents a potential for serious risk to the health, welfare, or safety of the subject or is an implant; supports or sustains human life; or is considered substantially important in diagnosing or curing, treating disease, or preventing impairment of human health. Additionally, the institutional review board (IRB) at each institution where the study is to be conducted must make a determination of significant or nonsignificant risk during their review process. Both the sponsor and the IRB should consider the nature of the harm, if any, when considering a study that presents a potential for serious risk. If a device may cause substantial harm to the subjects, the study should be considered a significant risk, especially one in which the potential harm could be life threatening, one that could result in permanent impairment of body functions or permanent damage to a body structure, or one that could necessitate medical or surgical intervention to preclude any permanent impairment.

The sponsor of a significant risk device investigation must obtain both FDA and IRB approval before beginning any investigation. To obtain an IDE approval of a significant risk device investigation a sponsor must

- Develop an investigational plan and assemble reports of prior investigations
- Select qualified investigators, provide them with all the necessary information on the investigational plan and prior investigations, and obtain signed agreements that they will follow the study protocol

- Provide a list of all institutions and IRB chairpersons participating in the study to the FDA
- Provide the amount charged for the device, if sold
- Ensure proper subject monitoring
- Ensure subject (patient) informed consent is obtained
- Submit the above information to the IRB
- Submit all the above information to the FDA and assure the FDA that new significant information will be reported
- Provide to the FDA, IRB, and investigators any adverse device effects reports

In addition, there are several reports that must be submitted to the FDA and/or the IRB over the length of the study for significant risk devices. These reports are listed in Table 22-2.

An IDE application must be approved or disapproved within 30 days of receipt by the FDA; otherwise it is considered deemed approved and the study can begin. Two examples of significant risk devices in anesthesia and respiratory care are extracorporeal membrane oxygenators and high-frequency ventilators (>2.5 Hz). Prior FDA approval is required for certain changes in the investigational plan. However, this approval is not required for deviations in the investigational plan in an emergency use to protect the life or physical well-being of a subject. The sponsor must notify the FDA within 5 working days of any deviations in an emergency.

Sponsors of studies involving nonsignificant risk devices do not have to submit IDE applications to the FDA unless the FDA notifies them otherwise. The FDA considers a nonsignificant risk device investigation to be approved if the device is not a banned device and the sponsor

- Obtains IRB approval after presentation of a nonsignificant risk explanation to the IRB
- Labels the device as investigational
- Maintains IRB approval throughout the investigation
- Ensures that the investigators obtain informed consent for each subject
- Monitors investigations, maintains records, and makes reports
- Complies with prohibitions on promotions, test marketing, and commercialization of the devices
- Does not unduly prolong the investigation

These exemptions can be used to generate clinical data for any class of device, although most IDE applications are granted for Class III devices. Once a device receives final FDA approval, that portion of the IDE application is terminated by the sponsor.

Postmarket Surveillance

Even with increasingly stringent approval processes, devices do fail or malfunction. Surveillance activities are carried out to identify and correct such problems.

Many factors are considered in determining the postmarket risk assessment of a medical device, including whether the use of the devices has caused injury, disease, or death; short- and long-term consequences of a hazard; and a determination of which segments of the population may be at risk. Formal health hazard evaluations (HHE) are conducted when the FDA either becomes aware of a voluntary corrective action by the manufacturer or the field offices request a risk assessment of an incident or device complaint. The Health Hazard Committee, composed of FDA scientists, medical officers, and consumer safety officers meets to determine the risk of adverse health outcomes with the device in question.

To determine the degree of seriousness of a hazard, consideration must be given to inherent risks associated with device use. For example, the patient's diagnosis, natural history of the disease being treated,

TABLE 22-2. Responsibilities for Preparing and Submitting Reports for Significant Risk Devices

	Report Prepared By	
Type of Report	Investigators for	Sponsors for
Unanticipated adverse effect evaluation	Sponsors and IRBs	FDA, investigators and IRBs
Withdrawal of IRB approval	Sponsors	FDA, investigators and IRBs
Progress report	Sponsors, monitors and IRBs	FDA and IRBs
Final report	Sponsors and IRBs	FDA, investigators and IRBs
Emergencies (protocol deviations)	Sponsors and IRBs	FDA
Inability to obtain informed consent	Sponsors and IRBs	FDA
Withdrawal of FDA approval	N/A	IRBs and investigators
Current investigator list	N/A	FDA
Recall and device disposition	N/A	FDA and IRBs
Records maintenance transfer	FDA	FDA
Significant risk determinations	N/A	FDA

risk-to-benefit analysis, and the environment where the device is being used will all be factored into the analysis. Device- or product-related factors, although independent from the previous considerations, are as important and may include issues involving design of the product, performance characteristics, composition of the materials, construction or fabrication, packaging and sterility, instructions for use and labeling, and preventive maintenance. User/patient contributions to the hazard or malfunction involve the "human factors" issues of improper use (unintended by the manufacturer), misuse, abuse, or altered states of vigilance due to fatigue or chemical dependence.

Once the risk has been established, using the information currently available to the field investigators and the committee, the HHE report serves as guidance in classifying the firm's action as a voluntary recall or safety alert and aids in determining any additional regulatory actions, which, depending on the type and severity of the violations, may include seizure, injunction, or criminal prosecution. Manufacturers often conduct their own risk analysis to assess the risk and resolution of the hazard associated with a failed product and usually voluntarily recall products that pose unreasonable risks or substantial harm.

One of the special problems that arises is traceability of products. Length of time on the market, sale of product lines or companies, or wide national or international distributions of products each contributes to difficulties in accounting for all products that may be involved in a recall. In those cases where the FDA finds an unreasonable risk to public health and no more practicable means are available, such as a recall, a notification will be sent by the manufacturer to the appropriate sectors (hospitals, home health care agencies, professional societies) in an effort to eliminate or reduce the risk. Factors the FDA considers in its decision to issue a notification are listed in Box 22-4.

Box 22-4
Factors Determining Notification Orders

Whether a voluntary safety alert has been published
Severity of the harm presented by the risk of using the device
Population and number of individuals at risk
Cause of the risk
Number and traceability of the devices
Assessment of the likelihood that harm will occur
Whether the risk is widespread, nonserious harm to many, or serious harm to a few individuals
Whether notification can eliminate the risk

Device Problem Reporting Program

The Problem Reporting Program is the voluntary reporting system used by health care professionals since its inception in 1974. This nationally established program is endorsed by more than 34 participating professional organizations, including the American Association for Respiratory Care. It is funded by the FDA and administered by the United States Pharmacopeia. Reports can be submitted in writing (Fig. 22-2) or by calling (800-638-6725).

As much detail as possible is encouraged concerning the medical device in question and the circumstances that led to the problem. The U.S. Pharmacopeia forwards the report to the manufacturer and to the FDA for follow-up. Anonymity can be requested, and a special section of the report form addresses these concerns.

Mandatory Medical Device Reporting Program

The FDA has recognized the need for a mandatory reporting system that would yield timely information concerning injuries, death, and malfunctions associated with the use of medical devices. Although merely reporting an event will not reduce the risk of an adverse outcome, it will give the agency information to perform further risk assessments and product development analysis, along with promoting educational programs for users.

The Medical Device Reporting (MDR) regulation requires manufacturers and importers to "notify FDA when they receive information that reasonably suggests that one of their devices has either caused or contributed to a death or serious injury or has malfunctioned in a manner found likely to cause or contribute to a death or serious injury, if it recurred." See Figure 22-3 for a sample MDR report.

A few definitions may be helpful at this point. All manufacturers and importers subject to registration requirements must report events to the FDA. Distributors, other than wholly owned distributors, are not subject to the MDR regulation but are encouraged to report events to the manufacturer, who, then, is required to report events. Information that reasonably suggests, includes, but is not limited to, professional journal articles, medical opinion, or statements made by health care professionals should be reported as events.

Also included are reports or research done by the manufacturers. Serious injury is an injury that is life threatening, causes permanent impairment or damage to body functions, or necessitates medical or surgical intervention to preclude permanent impairment or relieve temporary unanticipated impairment. Unanticipated impairment reflects the manufacturer's assessment of known risks or complications, as stated in the labeling.

(Text continues on page 528)

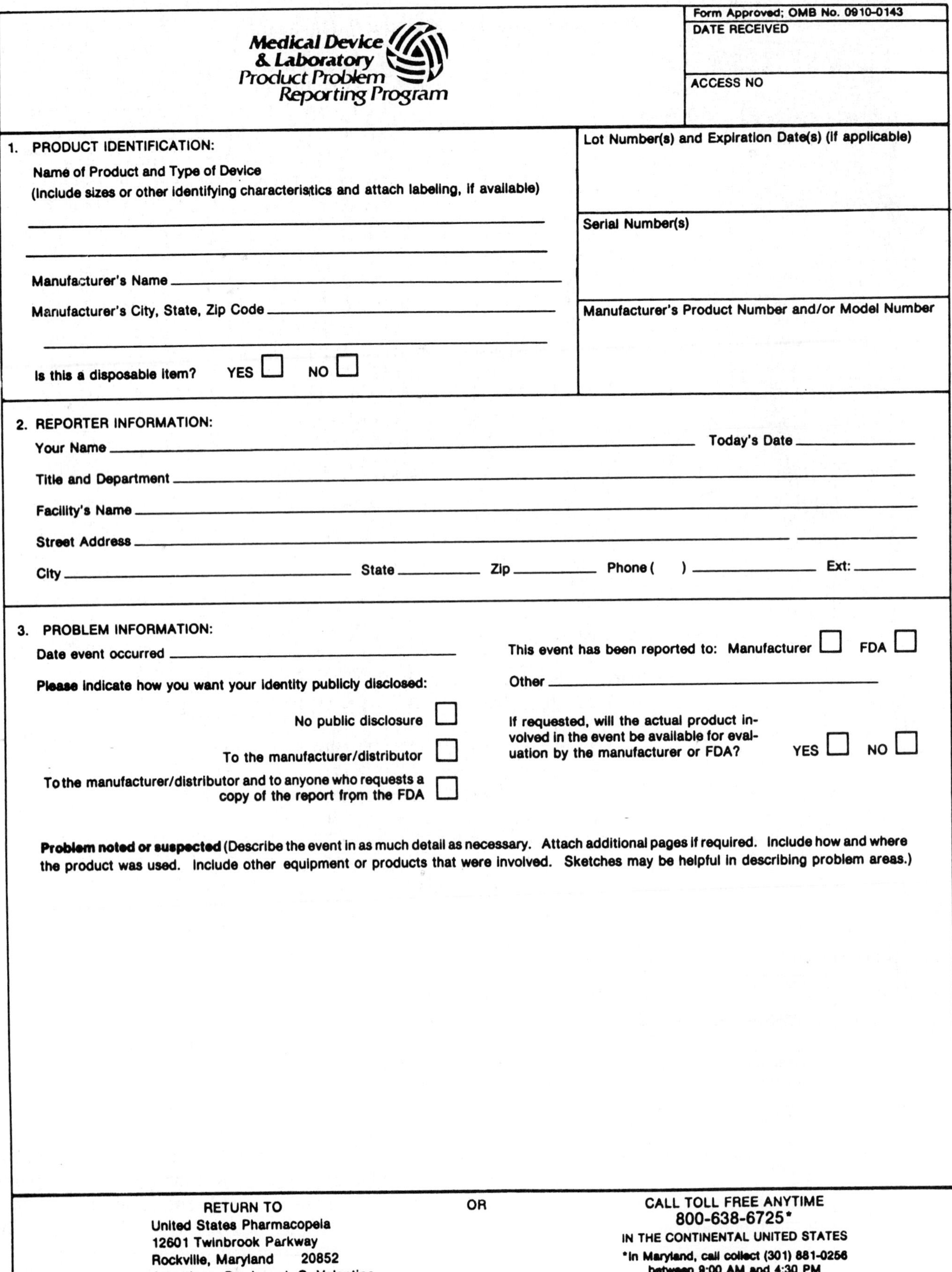

Form Approved; OMB No. 0910-0143

DATE RECEIVED

ACCESS NO

Medical Device & Laboratory Product Problem Reporting Program

1. PRODUCT IDENTIFICATION:

Name of Product and Type of Device
(Include sizes or other identifying characteristics and attach labeling, if available)

____

____

Manufacturer's Name ______________________________

Manufacturer's City, State, Zip Code ______________________________

____

Is this a disposable item? YES ☐ NO ☐

Lot Number(s) and Expiration Date(s) (If applicable)

Serial Number(s)

Manufacturer's Product Number and/or Model Number

2. REPORTER INFORMATION:

Your Name ______________________________ Today's Date ______________

Title and Department ______________________________

Facility's Name ______________________________

Street Address ______________________________ ______________

City ______________ State ______ Zip ______ Phone ( ) ______________ Ext: ______

3. PROBLEM INFORMATION:

Date event occurred ______________________________

Please indicate how you want your identity publicly disclosed:

No public disclosure ☐

To the manufacturer/distributor ☐

To the manufacturer/distributor and to anyone who requests a copy of the report from the FDA ☐

This event has been reported to: Manufacturer ☐ FDA ☐

Other ______________________________

If requested, will the actual product involved in the event be available for evaluation by the manufacturer or FDA? YES ☐ NO ☐

Problem noted or suspected (Describe the event in as much detail as necessary. Attach additional pages if required. Include how and where the product was used. Include other equipment or products that were involved. Sketches may be helpful in describing problem areas.)

RETURN TO
United States Pharmacopeia
12601 Twinbrook Parkway
Rockville, Maryland 20852
Attention: Dr. Joseph G. Valentino

OR

CALL TOLL FREE ANYTIME
800-638-6725*
IN THE CONTINENTAL UNITED STATES
*In Maryland, call collect (301) 881-0256
between 9:00 AM and 4:30 PM

FORM FDA 2516 (3/85)

Figure 22-2. Medical Device and Laboratory Product Problem Reporting Program form.

DEPARTMENT OF HEALTH AND HUMAN SERVICES
PUBLIC HEALTH SERVICE
FOOD AND DRUG ADMINISTRATION

MEDICAL DEVICE REPORT

To:
Center for Devices and Radiological Health
8757 Georgia Avenue (HFZ - 34[illegible])
Silver Spring, MD 20910
(301) 427-7500

FDA USE ONLY

* Optional items

1. DATE RECEIVED BY FDA ______-______-______ (M D Y)
2. ACCESS NO. FDA
3. FDA CODE
4. REPORT RECEIVED BY

DEVICE IDENTIFICATION
5. BRAND NAME
6. COMMON NAME
7. MODEL NO.
8. CATALOG NO.
9. FIRM'S REFERENCE NO.*
10. SERIAL NO.
11. LOT NO.
12. PMA. NO.*

FIRM
13. TYPE
☐ DOMESTIC MFR.
☐ U.S. IMPORTER
14. FIRM NAME
15. CITY
16. ADDRESS
17. STATE
18. ZIP

CONTACT PERSON
19. CONTACT NAME /TITLE
20. PHONE
21. FIRM NAME
22. CITY
23. ADDRESS
24. STATE
25. ZIP

FOREIGN MFR.
26. FIRM NAME
27. ADDRESS *(City, Country, Postal Code)*
28. CONTACT*

INCIDENT INFORMATION
29. DATE OF EVENT ___ ___ ___ (M D Y)
30. TYPE OF REPORT ☐
D - DEATH
I - SERIOUS INJURY
M - MALFUNCTION
31. TYPE OF INJURY *(Enter letter)** ☐
A, B, C, D, E,
F, G, H, Z
32. NUMBER OF PERSONS AFFECTED

33a. DESCRIBE EVENT

33b. ENCLOSURES ☐ YES ☐ NO

SOURCE OF REPORT
34. NAME/TITLE
35. DATE MFR/IMPORTER ALERTED* ______-______-______ (M D Y)
36. FACILITY NAME
37. PHONE*
38. FACILITY ADDRESS *(Include Country)*

ADD. INFO.
39. TO BE SUBMITTED ☐ YES ☐ NO
40. DATE TO BE SUBMITTED ______-______-______ (M D Y)
41. NATURE OF INFORMATION *(Analysis, labeling, etc.)*

EVENT FREQUENCY AND SEVERITY
42. DO YOU HAVE FREQUENCY INFORMATION ☐ OR SEVERITY INFORMATION ☐
ABOUT THIS "TYPE" EVENT AND DOES IT APPEAR IN YOUR PRODUCT LABELING ☐ OR IN FIRM FILES ☐
43. IS THE FREQUENCY OCCURRING MORE THAN USUAL FOR THIS DEVICE ☐
AND IS THIS INFORMATION KNOWN AND AVAILABLE AT THIS TIME ☐
44. IS THE SEVERITY OF THIS EVENT MORE THAN USUAL FOR THIS DEVICE ☐
AND IS THIS INFORMATION KNOWN AND AVAILABLE AT THIS TIME ☐

FORM FDA 3322 (10/87)

Figure 22-3. Health and Human Services Medical Device Report (sample).

TABLE 22-3. Medical Device Reports: January 1985 to February 1988, All Panels: Deaths, Injuries, Malfunctions

Specialty	Deaths	Injuries	Malfunctions	Total
Anesthesiology	263	299	7,333	7895
Cardiovascular	971	19,283	6,312	26,566
Dental	1	122	38	161
ENT	1	35	23	59
Genitourinary	85	1513	1233	2831
Plastic surgery	56	3377	657	4090
General hospital	104	1075	2831	4010
Neurology	15	364	481	860
Ophthalmology	0	1298	423	1721
Orthopedics	22	1133	218	1373
Radiology	15	172	383	570
Clinical chemistry	10	282	1965	2257
Hematology	2	40	476	518
Immunology	0	12	63	75
Microbiology	0	9	18	27
Pathology	2	5	4	11
Clinical toxicology	0	9	86	95
OB-GYN	57	1091	94	1242
Physical medicine	11	148	172	331
Total	1615	30,267	22,810	54,774

Table 22-3 shows all the MDR reports submitted for the first 3 years, according to classification panel. Tables 22-4, 22-5, and 22-6 identify the 10 most frequently reported devices for all panels, according to death, injury, or malfunction. This ranking has been consistent over the 3 years of data collection in MDR. Table 22-7 shows the reporting profile of the anesthesia and respiratory care panel alone, with the 10 most frequently reported devices for deaths, injuries, and malfunctions. Ventilator malfunctions contribute over 56% of all anesthesia and respiratory care products reported. Across all panels, malfunctions account for 55.3% of all reports, with deaths and injuries being reported in 2.9% and 41.8%, respectively. The anesthesia and respiratory care panel differs in that most reports (93%) are malfunctions.

In many events described in the MDR database, manufacturers did not receive or were not able to confirm the patient's condition at the time of the event. The specific procedure or operation being performed or other extenuating circumstances that may have influenced the patient's outcome were not stated in the majority of reports. Interventions, changes in anesthetic management, fluid balance, and length and type of surgery are all important factors in patient outcome. It remains difficult, using MDR data alone, to find a causal relationship between event and outcome under the current reporting regulation. For example, only one device per report is mentioned but, realistically, several devices may in fact be in use for a particular patient at any one time.

MEDWATCH Voluntary Reporting Program

MEDWATCH was introduced by the FDA in 1993 to allow health care professionals to quickly report seri-

TABLE 22-4. Medical Device Reporting: Most Frequently Reported Devices January 1985 to February 1988: Deaths

Device	No. of Deaths
Valve, heart, replacement	255
Defibrillator, low-energy	251
Ventilator, continuous (respirator)	95
Generator, pulse, pacemaker, implantable	91
Electrode, pacemaker, permanent	60
Gas machine for anesthesia or analgesia	55
Catheter, intravascular, diagnostic	54
Pump, infusion	49
Tampon, menstrual, unscented	40
Balloon, intra-aortic and control system	29

TABLE 22-5. Medical Device Reporting: Most Frequently Reported Devices January 1985 to February 1988: Serious Injuries

Device	No. of Injuries
Generator, pulse, pacemaker, implantable	12,364
Electrode, pacemaker, permanent	4629
Prosthesis, implant, breast, saline	1286
Valve, heart, replacement	1074
Prosthesis, breast, noninflatable, silicone	640
Tampon, menstrual, unscented	529
Lens, intraocular	448
Lens, contact (other material)	395
Intrauterine device, contraceptive	346
Pump, infusion	338

TABLE 22-6. Medical Device Reporting: Most Frequently Reported Devices January 1985 to February 1988: Malfunctions

Device	No. of Malfunctions
Ventilator, continuous (respirator)	4122
Generator, pulse, pacemaker, implantable	2216
Gas machine for anesthesia or analgesia	1703
Hexokinase, glucose	1700
Pump, infusion	1027
Electrode, pacemaker, permanent	836
Intravascular administration set	826
Balloon, intra-aortic and control system	520
Humidifier, respiratory gas	370
Set, administration, peritoneal dialysis	360

ous adverse events and product problems occurring with drugs, biologics, medical devices, and special nutritional products. Voluntary reports by health care workers have been essential in identifying postmarket complications. Reporting by respiratory care practitioners concerning dangers associated with heated wire breathing circuits prompted the FDA to issue a safety alert.

MEDWATCH is not intended to record every adverse event that occurs. It is intended to record serious adverse events. A serious adverse event occurs when a device or medication is associated with death, a life-threatening condition, initial or prolonged hospitalization, or congenital anomaly or when medical or surgical intervention was required to prevent permanent disability or damage. A report should be made when suspicion of a serious adverse event is encountered; proving causality is not necessary.

The FDA is also interested in reports concerning improper product labeling, contamination, and product mix-up. Malfunctioning devices that, if used, might result in death or serious injury to patients or caregivers should also be reported.

Reporting through the MEDWATCH program can be accomplished by using the postage-paid MEDWATCH form (Fig. 22-4). A MEDWATCH form may be obtained from the FDA by fax by calling 1-800-FDA-1088.

The importance of serious adverse event (SAE) reporting cannot be overemphasized. Any problems associated with equipment (disposable or reusable) or drugs (over-the-counter or prescription) should be reported to MEDWATCH. MEDWATCH reporting protects reporter confidentiality. However, respiratory care practitioners should realize that reports result in significant scrutiny of the companies in question. Appropriate documentation of the event including date, time, situation of use, patient condition, and equipment serial or lot number should be recorded.

Device Tracking

The 1992 Medical Device Amendments require manufacturers to develop systems to track certain devices. These include devices "the failure of which would be reasonably likely to have serious adverse health consequences, and that are permanently implanted or are a life-sustaining or a life-supporting device used outside a device user facility." These devices include home ventilators and oxygen concentrators.

Nonregulatory Programs

Anesthesia and respiratory therapy equipment has evolved from primitive bellows ventilators and gauze vaporizers to sophisticated microprocessor-controlled devices with integrated alarm systems. Materials research, design changes, and production validation programs have all significantly contributed to overall increases in product safety. However, adverse effects still continue with all equipment. As devices and de-

TABLE 22-7. Medical Device Reporting: January 1985 to February 1988: Most Frequently Reported Anesthesia and Respiratory Care Death, Injury and Malfunction

Device	Death	Injury	Malfunction	Total
Ventilator, continuous	95	56	4122	4273
Anesthesia gas machine	55	61	1703	1819
Humidifier	7	22	370	399
Tracheal tube	14	16	161	191
Apnea monitor	26	7	149	182
Spirometer	3	0	156	159
Blender/mixer	1	3	89	93
Airway pressure monitor	4	0	58	62
Oxygen analyzer	1	0	49	50
Breathing circuit	2	1	41	44

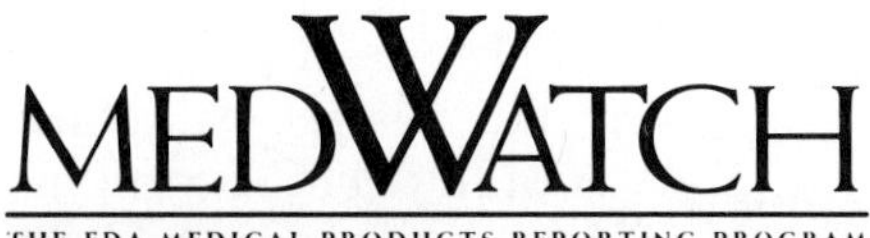

THE FDA MEDICAL PRODUCTS REPORTING PROGRAM

For VOLUNTARY reporting by health professionals of adverse events and product problems

Page ____ of ____

Form Approved: OMB No. 0910-0291 Expires: 12/31/94
See OMB statement on reverse

FDA Use Only (RESP CARE)

Triage unit sequence #

A. Patient information

1. Patient identifier — In confidence
2. Age at time of event: ____ or Date of birth:
3. Sex — ☐ female ☐ male
4. Weight — ____ lbs or ____ kgs

B. Adverse event or product problem

1. ☐ **Adverse event** and/or ☐ **Product problem** (e.g., defects/malfunctions)

2. **Outcomes attributed to adverse event** (check all that apply)
   - ☐ death ____ (mo/day/yr)
   - ☐ life-threatening
   - ☐ hospitalization – initial or prolonged
   - ☐ disability
   - ☐ congenital anomaly
   - ☐ required intervention to prevent permanent impairment/damage
   - ☐ other: ____

3. **Date of event** (mo/day/yr)
4. **Date of this report** (mo/day/yr)
5. **Describe event or problem**
6. **Relevant tests/laboratory data,** including dates
7. **Other relevant history, including preexisting medical conditions** (e.g., allergies, race, pregnancy, smoking and alcohol use, hepatic/renal dysfunction, etc.)

C. Suspect medication(s)

1. **Name** (give labeled strength & mfr/labeler, if known)
   #1
   #2
2. **Dose, frequency & route used** #1 #2
3. **Therapy dates** (if unknown, give duration) from/to (or best estimate) #1 #2
4. **Diagnosis for use** (indication) #1 #2
5. **Event abated after use stopped or dose reduced**
   #1 ☐ yes ☐ no ☐ doesn't apply
   #2 ☐ yes ☐ no ☐ doesn't apply
6. **Lot #** (if known) #1 #2
7. **Exp. date** (if known) #1 #2
8. **Event reappeared after reintroduction**
   #1 ☐ yes ☐ no ☐ doesn't apply
   #2 ☐ yes ☐ no ☐ doesn't apply
9. **NDC #** (for product problems only) – –
10. **Concomitant medical products** and therapy dates (exclude treatment of event)

D. Suspect medical device

1. **Brand name**
2. **Type of device**
3. **Manufacturer name & address**
4. **Operator of device**
   - ☐ health professional
   - ☐ lay user/patient
   - ☐ other: ____
5. **Expiration date** (mo/day/yr)
6. model # ____ catalog # ____ serial # ____ lot # ____ other # ____
7. **If implanted, give date** (mo/day/yr)
8. **If explanted, give date** (mo/day/yr)
9. **Device available for evaluation?** (Do not send to FDA)
   ☐ yes ☐ no ☐ returned to manufacturer on ____ (mo/day/yr)
10. **Concomitant medical products** and therapy dates (exclude treatment of event)

E. Reporter (see confidentiality section on back)

1. **Name, address & phone #**
2. **Health professional?** ☐ yes ☐ no
3. **Occupation**
4. **Also reported to**
   - ☐ manufacturer
   - ☐ user facility
   - ☐ distributor
5. **If you do NOT want your identity disclosed to the manufacturer, place an " X " in this box.** ☐

FDA

Mail to: MEDWATCH
5600 Fishers Lane
Rockville, MD 20852-9787

or **FAX to:** 1-800-FDA-0178

FDA Form 3500 (6/93)

Submission of a report does not constitute an admission that medical personnel or the product caused or contributed to the event.

Figure 22-4. MEDWATCH voluntary reporting form for reporting adverse events and product problems.

livery systems become more complex, user error has become an increasingly large factor in product complaint analysis. In a disconnect study conducted under contract to the FDA, the Arthur D. Little Company found that the incidence of disconnection in breathing circuits is 7% in anesthesia and 9% in critical care units. In documents supporting this study, the Emergency Care Research Institute has recommended three immediate solutions: (1) provision of in-service education through case reviews and risk analysis to aid in anticipation and prevention; (2) the use of oxygen monitors and disconnect alarms in ventilator breathing circuits; and (3) the purchase of equipment that conforms to voluntary standards recommendations. In a majority of practice settings these recommendations are standard.

In a collaborative effort with the American Association of Nurse Anesthetists, American Society of Anesthesiologists, and device manufacturers, the FDA has published a notice of availability in the *Federal Register* on March 28, 1986, of an anesthesia gas machine pre-use checklist.

Several studies on anesthetic mishaps focused on the incidence of pre-use events. The checklist serves as a generic procedure designed to uncover misconnections, some disconnections, high and low pressure leaks, ventilator dysfunction, fail-safe systems, breathing system valve assemblies, and alarms. It is not all inclusive and can easily be modified for use with ventilators.

The FDA has completed, in a joint effort with the American Society of Anesthesiologists, nine videotapes relating to anesthesia practice, including record keeping, mishaps and human errors, adverse outcomes, monitoring, preventive maintenance, disconnections, the pre-use checklist, and an overview of anesthesia practice.

Additionally, cooperative efforts exist between FDA and the National Institutes of Health in the area of home ventilation. A symposium was held in February 1987, sponsored by the National Institutes of Health and supported by the FDA, to bring together government agencies, clinical practitioners, congressional staff, and researchers to help identify issues of health care delivery in the home. This symposium was one of many ongoing efforts in the public and private sector in home health care. The FDA also has representation on the American Society on Testing and Materials F31 Committee on Home Health Care. A survey of durable medical equipment manufacturers was started in late fiscal 1988 to document preventive maintenance practices of durable medical equipment and home health care agencies.

Conclusion

Despite regulatory and nonregulatory efforts, the health care industry cannot have safe and effective device use and FDA-initiated postmarket surveillance programs without the cooperation of health care professionals and manufacturers. It is the responsibility of the end-user, in conjunction with the manufacturer and/or supplier, to understand the use and limitations of particular devices and the consequences of improper use. The FDA understands, despite the importance of assurance of patient safety and proper device function through regulation, that one of the agency's most effective pathways is through patient safety programs and extensive user education programs.

Glossary

AARC abbreviation for the American Association for Respiratory Care, the primary voluntary professional association for respiratory care practitioners.

Absolute humidity the amount of water vapor contained in a gas at a given temperature. Absolute humidity is expressed in milligrams per liter.

Absolute pressure pressure that includes local barometric pressure. At sea level (P_B = 760 mm Hg) a measured pressure of 10 mm Hg yields an absolute pressure of 770 mm Hg.

Accuracy the ability of an instrument to reproduce a known reference value.

Active expiration expiration assisted by the ventilatory muscles or by a ventilator-induced change in transrespiratory pressure causing flow in the expiratory direction.

Adiabatic a process of gas compression or expansion in which no heat energy is added to or taken away from the gas during the process; in adiabatic processes a gas's internal or kinetic energy varies according to changes in its pressure or volume; rapid adiabatic compression can thus result in a dramatic rise in the kinetic energy of a gas, as manifested by a rapid increase in its temperature.

Adsorption the physical adhesion of a thin layer of molecules to the surface of a porous substance.

Aerosol a suspension of solid or liquid particles in a gas.

Aerosol therapy the application of liquid or solid particle suspensions to the airway to achieve specific clinical objectives.

Airway cuff the balloon-like structure at the end of an artificial airway that creates a seal.

Alarm event any condition or occurrence that requires clinician awareness or action.

American symbols standard units for pressure (mm Hg, cm H_2O), volume (mL, L), and flow (L/min, mL/min) and for other variables used in the United States. These are different from Système International (SI) units used throughout the world.

Aneroid barometer a mechanical barometer that employs an evacuated chamber to measure changes in air pressure.

Antiprotozoal a chemical agent effective against protozoa that cause infection.

Antisepsis the destruction of pathogenic microorganisms existing in their vegetative state on living tissue.

Antiseptic a chemical solution capable of antisepsis.

Artificial nose a passive humidification device that works by collecting expired heat and moisture and returning it on the next inspiration.

Asepsis the absence of pathogenic microorganisms; the removal of pathogenic microorganisms or infected material.

Assisted expiration expiratory flow generated by a negative change in transrespiratory pressure due to an external agent (ie, a drop in airway pressure below baseline).

Assisted inspiration inspiratory flow generated by a positive change in transrespiratory pressure due to an external agent (ie, a rise in airway pressure above baseline).

Assisted ventilation the act of continuously assisting inspiration and/or expiration.

Atmosphere absolute (ATA) unit of barometric pressure expressed in atmospheres. 1 ATA = 760 mm Hg.

Atom the smallest form of matter consisting of a nucleus of protons and neutrons and of electrons traveling in orbit around the nucleus.

Atomizer a device used to reduce liquid medication to fine particles in the form of a spray; often used to deliver medication to the nose or throat.

ATPS abbreviation for ambient temperature, ambient pressure, saturated (with water vapor).

ATS American Thoracic Society.

Avogadro's law at a constant temperature and pressure, gases of equal volumes contain equal numbers of molecules.

Babington nebulizer a nebulizer that creates an aerosol by forcing gas through a small hole in a glass sphere that is covered by a thin layer of liquid (usually water).

Bacteria filter a low-resistance, high-efficiency filter capable of removing particles as small as 0.3 μm in diameter.

Bactericidal destructive to bacteria.

Baffle a surface in a nebulizer designed specifically to cause impaction of large aerosol particles, causing either further fragmentation or removal from the suspension through condensation back into the reservoir.

Base excess the difference in the normal buffer base and the actual buffer base in a whole blood sample. Typically expressed in milliequivalents per liter (normal, ± 2 mEq/L).

Beer's law the intensity of a color or of a light ray is inversely proportional to the depth of liquid through which it is transmitted. The absorption is dependent on the number of molecules in the path of the ray.

Bellows spirometer a volume displacement spirometer that expands and contracts like an accordion with one fixed and one movable plate.

Bernoulli's principle a reduction in pressure that occurs near the walls of a tube as gas flow is increased through the tube. This effect only occurs when gas flow is laminar.

Bias flow a continuous flow of gas used during high-frequency oscillation to eliminate carbon dioxide and increase delivered volume.

Bicarbonate HCO_3^-. The ion remaining after the first dissociation of carbonic acid.

Bit the smallest unit of digital information expressed in the binary system of notation (either 0 or 1).

Bland aerosol therapy delivery of aerosolized water or saline to a patient to assist in the removal of secretions.

Blood gas measurement the measurement of blood pH, P_{CO_2}, and P_{O_2} to determine metabolic and respiratory function.

Body humidity the absolute humidity in a volume of gas saturated at a body temperature of 37°C; equivalent to 43.8 mg/L.

Body plethysmography the technique of measuring the residual volume and expiratory reserve volume indirectly using Boyle's law. A device known as a body plethysmograph is used in the determination of these volumes.

Boiling point the temperature at which the vapor pressure of a liquid equals the ambient pressure exerted on the liquid.

Bourdon flowmeter a type of flowmeter that regulates the flow of a gas using a Bourdon tube and a single-stage reducing valve. The Bourdon gauge is recalibrated to read flow, although it measures a change in pressure.

Bourdon gauge a low-pressure flow-metering device always used in conjunction with an adjustable high-pressure reducing valve; the Bourdon gauge employs a fixed-size orifice and operates under variable pressures, as determined by adjustment of the pressure reducing valve.

Boyle's law a gas law that relates a change in volume to a change in pressure at a constant temperature. The law states that if pressure increases, volume will decrease if the temperature remains constant.

Braschi valve a one-way valve placed in the inspiratory limb of a ventilator circuit that facilitates the measurement of auto-PEEP.

Brownian motion the random motion of small particles, such as those in smoke, observed under a microscope. This is caused by the kinetic activity of gas molecules.

Bubble diffuser humidifier a device that produces humidity by routing gas through an underwater diffuser. The diffuser increases the surface area of contact between water and gas.

Bubble humidifier a device that produces humidity by releasing a gas underwater, allowing it to bubble to the surface.

Buffer a chemical substance that, when added to a solution, minimizes fluctuations in pH.

Bulk oxygen system an assembly of equipment and interconnecting piping that has a storage capacity of more than 20,000 cubic feet of oxygen, including unconnected reserves on hand at the site.

Byte a string of binary digits, usually eight, operated on as a basic unit by a digital computer.

Calibration the comparison of an instrument to a known physical standard to assess its accuracy and reproducibility.

Calorimetry measurement of the amount of heat given off by a reaction, group of reactions, or an organism (or organisms).

Canals of Lambert intercommunicating channels between terminal bronchioles and the alveoli that are about 30 μm and appear to remain open even when bronchiolar smooth muscle is contracted.

Capacity the range or limits of measurement by an instrument.

Capnography the process of obtaining a tracing of the amount of carbon dioxide in expired air using a capnograph.

Capnometry the measurement of expired carbon dioxide concentration.

Carboxyhemoglobin a compound produced by the chemical combination of hemoglobin and carbon monoxide.

Carlens tube an endotracheal tube with two lumina that allows separation of gas flow to the left and right lung.

Carrier gas the primary gas flow from a device that contains the aerosol generated from the device.

Cascade humidifier a device that produces humidity by directing gas through a partially submerged tower. The cascade humidifier generally refers to the specific device manufactured by Puritan-Bennett.

Cathode the negative pole or electrode of an electrical source.

Cation an ion that migrates to the cathode (negative electrode) in an electrolytic solution; a positive ion.

Celsius The SI scale for temperature measurement.

Charles' law relates the volume and the temperature of a gas when the pressure remains constant. The law states that as temperature of a gas increases, its volume will increase.

Chest physical therapy (CPT) a collection of therapeutic techniques designed to facilitate clearance of airway secretions, improve the distribution of ventilation, and enhance the efficiency and conditioning of the muscles of respiration; includes positioning techniques, chest percussion and vibration, directed coughing, and various breathing and conditioning exercises.

Clark electrode the Po_2 measuring electrode in a blood gas system, oxygen analyzer, or transcutaneous electrode.

Class III device a device classified by the U.S. Food and Drug Administration as a life support device.

Clinical information systems computerized systems for orders, charting, and billing of procedures.

Closed-circuit calorimetry device that measures oxygen consumption and carbon dioxide production to calculate energy expenditure. Closed circuit refers to the oxygen consumption measurement, which is accomplished by measuring volume loss over time.

Closed-circuit IMV system also called continuous-flow systems; characterized by delivery of gas flow at elevated airway pressure.

Closed-loop control a control scheme in which the actual output of a system is measured and compared with the desired output. If there is a difference caused by external disturbances, the actual output is modified to bring it closer to the desired output.

CO-oximetry the measurement of hemoglobin and oxygen bound to hemoglobin, methemoglobin, and carboxyhemoglobin.

Combined gas law a law that relates temperature, pressure, and volume of a gas under ideal conditions. This is often referred to as the ideal gas law. The law states that $(P_1 \cdot V_1)/T_1 = (P_2 \cdot V_2)/T_2$.

Combustible flammable or apt to catch fire.

Compliance the relative ease at which a body or tissue stretches or deforms. Lung compliance is a measure of volume change per unit pressure change under static conditions.

Compressed gas any material or mixture having in the container an absolute pressure exceeding 40 psi at 70°F, or absolute pressure exceeding 104 psi at 130°F, or any liquid having a vapor pressure exceeding 40 psia at 100°F.

Compressible volume the volume of gas that is not delivered to the patient but is lost in the ventilator circuit due to compression. Compressible volume may be found by multiplying peak inspiratory pressure minus positive end-expiratory pressure by the tubing compliance.

Compressor a device that is designed to compress a gas (usually air). Compressors operate using a diaphragm, piston, or centrifugal impeller to compress the gas entering the device.

Conductivity the power of transmission or conveyance of energy without perceptible motion in the conducting body.

Conjunctival oxygen monitor a device that uses a polarographic oxygen electrode to monitor conjunctival oxygen pressure. Studies have suggested this device may be useful in monitoring the adequacy of cardiopulmonary resuscitation.

Constant airway pressure (CAP) a therapeutic modality that maintains a constant (usually positive) transrespiratory pressure. CAP is not a ventilatory mode because it does not generate a tidal volume, and hypoventilation will occur if the patient becomes apneic.

Continuous positive airway pressure (CPAP) a mode of ventilator operation that allows the patient to breathe spontaneously from a continuous-flow or demand valve at an elevated airway pressure. (same as CAP)

Control circuit the ventilator subsystem responsible for controlling the drive mechanism and/or the output control valves.

Control variable the variable (either pressure, volume, flow, or time) that the ventilator manipulates to cause inspiration. This variable is identified by the fact that its behavior remains consistent despite changes in ventilatory load.

Critical pressure the pressure exerted by a vapor in an evacuated container at its critical temperature.

Critical temperature the highest temperature at which a substance can exist as a liquid, regardless of pressure.

Cryogenic producing extremely low temperatures.

Cuff an inflatable balloon located at the distal tip of some artificial airways (endotracheal tubes, tracheostomy tubes, and esophageal obturator airways). The purpose of the cuff is to seal the airway so that positive pressure may be applied to the lungs and to protect the natural airway from aspiration.

Cuff pressure the pressure exerted by the cuff of an artificial airway on the airway mucosa.

Cycle to end a mechanically supported inspiration.

Cycling mechanism the means by which a ventilator ends the inspiratory phase of mechanical ventilation.

- **Flow cycling** the delivery of gas under positive pressure during inspiration until flow drops to a specified terminal level.
- **Pressure cycling** the delivery of gas under positive pressure during inspiration until an adjustable, preselected pressure has been reached.
- **Time cycling** the delivery of gas under positive pressure during inspiration until an adjustable, preselected time interval has elapsed.
- **Volume cycling** the delivery of gas under positive pressure during inspiration until an adjustable, preselected volume has been delivered.

Dalton's law Dalton's law of partial pressures states that the total pressure of a gas mixture is equal to the sum of the partial pressures of the gases that comprise it. For example, if a gas mixture is composed of gas A, B, and C, the total pressure is equal to the partial pressures of A + B + C.

Database a large collection of data in a computer organized so that it can be expanded, updated, and retrieved.

Decompression illness the development of nitrogen bubbles in joints, tissues, and blood due to inadequate decompression time following hyperbaric treatment. Commonly known as "the bends."

Demand valve a type of mechanical valve that provides gas to a spontaneously breathing patient in response to the pressure or flow gradient developed by the patient's inspiratory effort.

Density a measure of the mass per unit volume of a substance.

Dew point the temperature at which water vapor condenses back to its liquid form.

Differential pressure transducer a type of pressure transducer with two pressure ports separated by a diaphragm. Since two pressures are exerted on the diaphragm, the displacement of it is equal to the pressure difference. These transducers may be strain gauge or variable reluctance transducers.

Diffusion the physical process whereby atoms or molecules tend to move from an area of higher concentration or pressure to an area of lower concentration or pressure.

Diffusion coefficient the rate of diffusion of a gas; in cgs units, the diffusion coefficient is defined as the number of milliliters of a gas at 1 atmosphere of pressure that will diffuse a distance of 1 μm over a square centimeter surface area per minute.

Direct-acting cylinder valve a cylinder valve that operates by a valve stem, opening and closing the valve seat. The stem itself acts directly on the seat to open or close it.

Direct calorimetry measurement of the heat produced by a reaction. Direct calorimetry is distinguished from indirect calorimetry in that direct calorimetry measures the heat production itself.

Disinfectant a chemical agent capable of destroying at least the vegetative phase of pathogenic microorganisms; there are five major categories of disinfectants used in clinical practice: the alcohols, the phenols and their derivatives, the halogens, the aldehydes, and the quaternary ammonium compounds.

Disinfection the process of destroying at least the vegetative phase of pathogenic microorganisms of physical or chemical means.

Distillation the condensation of a vapor obtained by heating a liquid; commonly used to separate out liquids with different boiling points as in the production of oxygen by fractional distillation.

DOT abbreviation for the U.S. Department of Transportation, the department of the federal government responsible for regulating interstate transportation of compressed gases.

Dry powder inhaler a device that allows administration of a dry powdered medication from a capsule by puncturing the capsule and delivering the medication during patient inspiration.

Dry rolling seal spirometer a volume displacement spirometer incorporating a movable piston attached to a cylinder by a soft rolling seal.

Electrode an electrical terminal specialized for a particular electrochemical reaction.

End-expiratory pressure (EEP) the baseline transrespiratory pressure that exists at the end of the expiratory time.

Endotracheal tube an artificial airway that is passed through the mouth or nose and advanced into the trachea. Endotracheal tubes may be cuffed or uncuffed depending on their size.

Esophageal gastric tube airway (EGTA) a modification of the esophageal obturator airway (EOA) that includes a gastric tube that can be extended beyond the distal tip into the stomach to remove air or gastric contents.

Esophageal obturator airway (EOA) the EOA consists of a cuffed hollow tube tipped with a soft plastic obturator at its distal end; the tube passes through a mask and has several holes in its upper portion; once passed into the esophagus, the cuff is inflated, thereby preventing aspiration and allowing ventilation with intermittent positive pressure.

Error the difference between a known reference value and the measured value.

Esophageal pressure pressure measured in the distal third of the esophagus by a balloon catheter. Esophageal pressure approximates pleural pressure.

Evacuate to remove or withdraw from, especially to empty of air and create a vacuum.

Evaporation the change in state of a substance from its liquid to its gaseous form occurring below its boiling point.

Event any condition or occurrence related to mechanical ventilation that requires clinician awareness or action. *Technical events* are those involving inadvertent change in the ventilator's performance. *Patient events* are those involving a change in the patient's clinical status.

Exhalation valve a mushroom- or diaphragm-type valve located on the patient circuit or on a ventilator. During inspiration, the valve is pressurized, closing it so that pressure can build in the patient circuit. Many acute care ventilators incorporate the exhalation valve inside the ventilator, to control flow and positive end-expiratory pressure more accurately.

Expiratory phase (expiration) the part of the ventilatory cycle from the beginning of expiratory flow to the beginning of inspiratory flow.

Expiratory pressure valve a valve that regulates end-expiratory airway pressure during mechanical ventilation or continuous positive airway pressure. Also called PEEP or CPAP valves.

Expiratory time the duration of the expiratory phase.

External compressor a device external to the ventilator used to supply pneumatic source power.

Fahrenheit temperature measurement with a freezing point of water at 32°F and boiling point of water at 212°F.

Feet of sea water (FSW) unit of pressure expressed in feet of seawater (FSW). 33 FSW = 760 mm Hg.

Fenestrated tube a double-cannulated tracheostomy tube that has an opening in the posterior wall of the outer cannula. Removal of the inner cannula allows airflow through the vocal cords, permitting the patient to speak.

Fermentation the oxidative decomposition of substances through enzymes produced by microorganisms.

FDA abbreviation for the U.S. Food and Drug Administration, the federal agency responsible for overseeing the testing and ensuring the purity and effectiveness of drugs (including medical gases).

Fiberoptic laryngoscope a device that uses fiberoptic channels and a light source to allow direct visualization of the vocal cords.

Fick's equation the calculation of cardiac output from measurements of oxygen consumption and arteriovenous oxygen content difference.

Filling density the ratio between the weight of liquid gas put into the cylinder and the weight of water the cylinder could contain if full; for example, the filling density for carbon dioxide is 68%.

Flowmeter a device operated by a needle valve that controls and measures gas flow, according to the principles of viscosity and density.

Flow resistor a type of expiratory pressure valve that maintains pressure by adjusting the size of the orifice (opening) for exhalation. Pressure is constant at a constant flow, but a change in flow causes a change in pressure of the same magnitude.

Flow restrictor a fixed-orifice, constant-pressure, flow-metering device.

Fluid a nonsolid substance that takes the shape of the vessel containing it.

Fluidics a branch of engineering in which hydrodynamic principles are incorporated into flow circuits for such purposes as switching, pressure and flow sensing, and amplification.

Format a specific arrangement in accordance with which computer data are processed, stored, and printed.

French scale a measurement scale used commonly to delineate the diameter of catheters; 1 French unit equals approximately 0.33 mm.

g (also gm) abbreviation for gram.

Galvanic cell a device used to determine the partial pressure of oxygen by measuring the electron current traveling between the anode and cathode.

Gas a thin fluid, like air, capable of indefinite expansion but convertible by compression and cold into a liquid, and eventually a solid.

Gas tension the partial pressure exerted by a gas.

Gastric tonometry the measurement of gastric mucosal pH to determine adequacy of oxygen delivery.

Gauge pressure pressure measured relative to atmospheric pressure.

Graham's law the relative rapidity of diffusion of two gases varies inversely with the square root of their densities.

Graphics the display of pressure, volume, or flow against time in a line or tracing.

Gravity-dependent manometer a pressure measurement device that must remain in an upright position to function.

Hardware the mechanical, magnetic and electronic design, structure, and devices of a computer.

Heat and moisture exchanger an artificial nose that works solely on the physical principles of condensation and evaporation.

Heat and moisture exchanging filter a heat and moisture exchanger that also contains a bacterial/viral filter.

Heat capacity the number of calories required to raise the temperature of 1 g of a substance 1°C (cgs) or 1 pound of a substance 1°F (fps); by definition, the heat capacity of water is 1 cal in the cgs system and 1 BTU in the fps system.

Heated passover humidifier a heated humidifier that relies on transfer of moisture from the surface of the liquid to the gas flowing over it.

Heated wire circuit a ventilator circuit containing a heated wire to prevent condensation.

Henderson-Hasselbalch equation formula relating to pH of a solution to the ratio of bicarbonate ion concentration to free carbon dioxide in solution.

Henry's law the amount of gas dissolved in a given volume of liquid is directly proportional to the partial pressure of that gas in the gas phase.

HEPA abbreviation for high-efficiency particulate air, usually applied to air filtration devices capable of 99.99% efficacy on particulate matter down to 0.3 μm in size.

Hertz (Hz) a unit of frequency equal to 1 cycle per second.

High-flow humidifier a humidification device used to add moisture to high flows of gas (usually > 60 L/min).

High-frequency flow interrupter a device that delivers pulses of gas to the airway by periodically interrupting flow of the gas.

High-frequency jet ventilation a type of high-frequency ventilation characterized by delivery of gas through a small catheter in the endotracheal tube.

High-frequency oscillation a type of high-frequency ventilation characterized by the use of active expiration.

High-frequency percussive ventilation a type of high-frequency ventilation characterized by delivery of pressure limited breaths in short bursts of gas from a venturi.

High-frequency positive-pressure ventilation a type of high-frequency ventilation characterized by a low compressible volume circuit and tidal volume delivery of 3 to 4 mL/kg.

High-frequency ventilation ventilatory support characterized by frequencies greater than 80 breaths per minute and tidal volumes equal to or less than deadspace.

Humidifier a device capable of adding water to a gas as water vapor.

Humidity water in molecular vapor form; *absolute humidity* is a measure of the actual content or weight of water present in a given volume of air; *relative humidity* is the ratio of actual water vapor present in a gas to the capacity of the gas to hold the vapor at a given temperature.

Humidity deficit the difference between the humidity delivered by a device and body humidity (44 mg H_2O/L).

Hyaline membrane disease neonatal respiratory distress syndrome caused by premature birth and surfactant deficiency.

Hygrometer an electronic device used to measure relative humidity.

Hygroscopic having the ability to absorb water and water vapor. Silica gel is a common compound used in medical equipment to absorb water and is sometimes termed a *desiccant.*

Hygroscopic condenser humidifier an artificial nose that has a media treated with a hygroscopic chemical (calcium or lithium chloride) to enhance moisture output.

Hygroscopic condenser humidifier filter a hygroscopic condenser humidifier that contains a filter to prevent transmission of bacteria and viruses.

Hyperbaric pertaining to gases greater than one atmosphere.

Hyperbaric chamber a device capable of exposing a patient to supra-atmospheric pressures.

Hyperbaric oxygenation the therapeutic application of oxygen at pressures greater than 1 atmosphere (760 mm Hg).

Hypobarism of or pertaining to the effects of exposure to pressures less than those normally encountered at sea level; often used to refer to high-altitude sickness.

I:E ratio the ratio of inspiratory to expiratory time during mechanical ventilation; by convention, the ratio is always reduced so that the numerator (inspiratory time) equals 1 (eg, 1:4 or 1:2.5). If inspiration is longer than expiration, the ratio is usually expressed as 2:1 or 4:1.

Imposed work of breathing the additional work of breathing required to overcome devices connected to the patient. These include the endotracheal tube, the breathing circuit, the humidifier, and the ventilator demand valve.

IMV abbreviation for intermittent mandatory ventilation; periodic ventilation with positive pressure, with the patient breathing spontaneously between breaths. These periodic breaths may be controlled (control-mode IMV) or assisted, as with synchronous intermittent mandatory ventilation (SIMV).

Incentive spirometry the application of biofeedback devices (incentive spirometers) to coach and encourage patients to take deeper breaths.

Indirect-acting cylinder valve a type of cylinder valve that employs a diaphragm to open and close the valve seat. Turning the valve stem causes the diaphragm to be displaced through a spring, indirectly opening the valve seat.

Indirect calorimetry determination of heat production of an oxidation reaction by measuring oxygen consumed and carbon dioxide produced and then calculating heat production in calories.

Indwelling located inside the body; commonly refers to invasive diagnostic or therapeutic devices.

Inert not taking part in chemical reactions; not pharmacologically active.

Inertia the tendency of a physical body to oppose any force tending to move it from a position of rest or to change its uniform motion.

Inertial impaction the process of removing large aerosol particles from a carrier gas due to their greater inertia (mass × velocity = inertia). The larger particles (greater mass) travel in a straight path and impact against objects placed in the path (baffles).

Infrared (light) electromagnetic radiation with wavelengths between 10^{-5} and 10^{-4} m; infrared radiation is perceived as heat when it strikes the body.

Infrared absorption spectroscopy a method of detecting gas concentrations based on absorption of infrared light.

Inspiratory phase (inspiration) the part of the ventilatory cycle from the beginning of inspiratory flow to the beginning of expiratory flow. Any inspiratory pause is included in the inspiratory phase.

Inspiratory time inspiratory time (expressed in seconds) is the duration of inspiration during mechanical ventilation. As inspiratory time increases, mean airway pressure increases and the I:E ratio becomes lower.

Inspiratory pause inspiratory pause is a brief pause (0.5 to 2 seconds) at end-inspiration during which pressure is held constant and flow is zero. The purpose of the pause is to improve gas distribution throughout the lungs.

Intermittent mandatory ventilation (IMV) a mode of ventilatory support that allows spontaneous breathing in between mandatory breaths from the ventilator.

Internal compressor a device inside the ventilator used to convert either pneumatic or electric source power into inspiratory pressure.

International symbols the Système International (SI) units for measurement of pressure (kPa), volume (L or mL), temperature (C), and other physiologic variables.

Investigational device exemption (IDE) a designation by the FDA allowing clinical use of a class III device to determine its efficacy.

IPPB abbreviation for intermittent positive-pressure breathing; the application of inspiratory positive pressure, usually with accompanying humidity or aerosol therapy, to a spontaneously breathing patient as a short-term treatment modality, usually for periods not exceeding 15 to 20 minutes.

Isothermic saturation boundary the point in the respiratory tree where inspired gases reach body temperature (37°C) and 100% humidity.

IT abbreviation for implantation tested; as applied to invasive devices, it indicates that the materials used have been shown to be nontoxic to living tissue.

Jargon the special technical language and terms of a particular field or profession.

Kelvin scale the SI temperature scale, with a zero point equivalent to absolute zero. The Kelvin scale has 100 degrees between the measured freezing and boiling points of water and is therefore considered a Centigrade system of temperature measurement. Because 0°K = −273°C, °K = °C + 273.

Keyboard interface between the operator and computer resembling a typewriter keyboard.

kg abbreviation for kilogram.

Kilobyte a unit of capacity equal to 1024 bytes.

Kinetic energy the energy a body possesses through its motion.

Laminar of or pertaining to laminae or layers; specifically refers to a pattern of flow consisting of concentric layers of fluid flowing parallel to the tube wall at linear velocities that increase toward the center.

Laryngoscope an endoscope for examining the larynx.

Latent heat of fusion the additional heat energy needed to effect the changeover of a substance from its solid to its liquid form.

Latent heat of vaporization the heat energy required to vaporize a liquid at its boiling point.

lb abbreviation for pound, the fps system unit of force (and weight at sea level).

Lighted stylet an intubation stylet inserted in the endotracheal tube to aid in tube placement. Visualization of the lighted end near the cricothyroid membrane indicates proper placement.

Limit to set a maximum value for pressure, volume, or flow during mechanically supported inspiration (or expiration); the pre-set maximum value for pressure, volume, or flow during an assisted inspiration (or expiration). Inspiration (or expiration) does not terminate because the limit value has been met.

Linearity the accuracy of an instrument over its entire range of measurement.

Liquefied compressed gas a gas that becomes liquid to a very large extent in containers at ordinary temperatures and at pressures from 25 to 2500 psig. Examples include carbon dioxide and nitrous oxide.

Low-flow humidifier a humidification device used to add moisture to gas flows < 20 L/min.

Low-pass filter a device used to increase resistance to bias flow during high-frequency oscillation for the purpose of increasing mean airway pressure.

Lukens' trap a device placed between the suction catheter and suction tubing that collects a sample of the material suctioned.

Lumen a cavity within any organ or structure of the body or a channel in a tube or catheter.

Magill forceps a device with handles like a hemostat connected to long angled forceps used to assist in placing the endotracheal tube into the trachea.

Mainstream monitor a gas analyzer that monitors the concentration of gases flowing through it.

Mandatory breath an assisted breath that is either initiated or terminated by the ventilator rather than by the patient's physiology or ventilatory drive.

Mandatory medical device reporting program (MDR) FDA program requiring reporting of adverse events related to medical devices.

Manifold a pipe with many connections; in medical gas storage, a collection of gas cylinders linked together for purposes of bulk storage and usually including at least one reserve bank and other safety systems, such as low-pressure alarms.

Mass median aerodynamic diameter that diameter around which the mass of particle diameters is equally distributed.

Mass spectroscopy a device that measures gas concentrations based on their molecular weight.

MDI abbreviation for metered-dose inhaler, a pressurized cartridge used for self-administration of exact dosages of aerosolized drugs.

Mean airway pressure the average pressure that exists at the airway opening over the ventilatory period. It is usually measured as gauge pressure. Mean airway pressure is mathematically equivalent to the area under the time–pressure curve (from the beginning of one breath to the beginning of the next breath) divided by the ventilatory period.

Mechanical aneroid manometers devices that measure gas pressure.

Medical device a device is defined as an instrument, apparatus, implement, machine, contrivance, implant, in vitro reagent, or other similar or related article, including any component, part or accessory, that does not achieve any of its principal intended purposes through chemical action within or on the body and is not dependent on being metabolized for achievement of any of its principal intended purposes.

Medical gas a gas that has been refined and purified according to specifications in the United States Pharmacopeia (USP) intended for human use in the diagnosis or treatment of disease.

Medical gas container a low-pressure, vacuum-insulated vessel containing gas(es) in liquid form.

Medical gas cylinder a tank containing a high-pressure gas or gas mixture at a pressure that may be in excess of 2000 psig.

MEDWATCH voluntary reporting program created by the FDA to allow reporting of medical device failures and adverse events by health care workers.

Megabyte one million bytes.

Mercury barometer a device used to measure air pressure that employs a column of mercury inverted into a mercury reservoir. Gas pressure against the surface of the reservoir causes the mercury column to rise or fall.

Methemoglobin abnormal hemoglobin in which iron has been oxidized that prevents normal oxygen-carrying capacity.

MHz abbreviation for megahertz, a unit of frequency equivalent to 1000 cycles per second (cps).

Milliequivalent (mEq) a quantitative amount of a reacting substance that has a specific chemical combining power; the milligram equivalent weight of a substance is calculated as its gram atomic (or formula) weight divided by its valence ×

0.001; a milliequivalent also represents the number of grams of solute dissolved in 1 mL of a normal solution.

Millimole an SI unit of matter equal to 1/1000 of a mole (a mole is any quantity of matter that contains 6.023×10^{23} atoms, molecules, or ions).

Millisecond (ms) one thousandth of a second.

Millivolt (mV) one thousandth of a volt.

Minute ventilation ($\dot{V}_E$) the total amount of gas moving out of the lungs during 1 minute.

Mixed venous blood blood from the pulmonary artery representing the venous drainage from the whole body.

mL abbreviation for milliliter, or 1/1000 L.

MMV abbreviation for mandatory minute ventilation, a mode of ventilatory support that ensures delivery of a pre-set minimum minute volume, with the patient allowed to breathe spontaneously; should the patient meet the pre-set $\dot{V}_E$ entirely by spontaneous effort, a ventilator in the MMV mode will remain passive, delivering no positive pressure breaths; on the other hand, should the patient's spontaneous $\dot{V}_E$ fall below the pre-set MMV minimum, a ventilator operating in this mode will provide the mechanical support necessary to ensure that the minimum minute ventilation goal is achieved.

Modem a device that converts data to a form that can be transmitted by telephone to data processing equipment where a similar device reconverts it.

Mole the SI unit of matter equal containing 6.023×10^{23} atoms, molecules, or ions.

Molecule the smallest possible quantity of a polyatomic substance that retains the chemical properties of that substance.

Monitor computer display similar to a television screen; also a device that advises, warns, or cautions the caregiver of an event.

Monoplace chamber a hyperbaric chamber capable of treating a single patient.

Mouse a piece of hardware that connects to a computer that replaces the keyboard for accessing documents and features.

msec abbreviation for millisecond.

Multiplace chamber a hyperbaric chamber capable of treating a number of patients and accommodating caregivers.

Nanomole (nM) one-billionth (10^{-9}) mole.

Naris the pair of anterior and posterior openings in the nose that allow the passage of air from the nose to the pharynx.

Nasogastric of or pertaining to the passageway from the nose to the stomach; usually applied to tubes or catheters placed in the stomach through the nose.

Nasopharynx one of the three regions of the throat, situated behind the nose and extending from the posterior nares to the larynx.

Nebulizer a device that produces an aerosol suspension of liquid particles in a gaseous medium using baffling to control particle size.

Needle valve one means of controlling gas flow and pressure. The more the valve is opened, the more flow and pressure are allowed past the valve seat. A common application of a needle valve in plumbing is the faucet on a sink.

NEEP acronym for negative end-expiratory pressure.

NFPA abbreviation for the National Fire Protection Association, a voluntary nongovernmental agency involved in improved methods of fire protection and prevention, including standards for the storage of flammable and oxidizing gases.

NIOSH National Institute of Occupational Safety and Health.

Nonflammable not capable of combustion.

Noninvasive pertaining to a diagnostic or therapeutic technique that does not require the skin to be broken or a cavity or organ of the body to be entered, such as obtaining a blood pressure reading by auscultation with a stethoscope and sphygmomanometer.

Noninvasive respiratory monitor a device that monitors respiratory parameters without crossing the skin barrier.

Nonliquefied compressed gas a gas that does not liquefy at ordinary temperatures and under pressures that range up to 2000 to 2500 psig.

Normocapnia a state characterized by a normal partial pressure of carbon dioxide in the arterial blood (35 to 45 mm Hg).

Nosocomial pertaining to or originating in a hospital, such as a nosocomial infection.

Obturator a device used to block a passage or a canal or to fill in a space, such as the obturator used to insert a tracheostomy tube.

Ohm's law in an electric current passing through a wire, the intensity of the current in amperes equals the electromotive force in volts divided by the resistance.

Open-circuit calorimetry an indirect calorimeter that measures oxygen consumption by determining the difference between inspired and expired oxygen concentrations.

Open-circuit IMV system also called parallel-flow systems; characterized by delivery of gas flow at ambient pressure.

Open-loop control a control scheme in which the output of a system is determined by the initial setting of the controller with no corrections made to accommodate disturbances in the output caused by external factors.

Optode a sensor using light as the signal.

Orifice an entrance or outlet to a body cavity or tube.

Oropharyngeal airways devices placed in the oropharynx to prevent the tongue from falling into the posterior pharynx.

Oropharynx the three anatomic divisions of the pharynx lying behind the oral cavity and midway between the nasopharynx and laryngopharynx.

Orotracheal of or pertaining to the passageway from the mouth to the trachea; usually applied to tubes or catheters placed in the trachea through the mouth, such as an orotracheal tube, or orotracheal suctioning.

Oximeter a photoelectric device (usually noninvasive) used to determine the saturation of blood hemoglobin with oxygen.

Oximetry the process of determining the saturation of hemoglobin with oxygen with an oximeter.

Oxygen analyzer a device that measures the partial pressure on percentage of oxygen in a given gas sample.

Oxygen concentrator (enricher) an electrically powered device capable of physically separating the oxygen in room air from nitrogen, thereby providing an enriched flow of oxygen for therapeutic use.

Oxygen content the quantity of oxygen dissolved in the plasma plus the quantity bound to hemoglobin.

Oxygen delivery system a device used to deliver oxygen concentrations above ambient ($F_{IO_2} > 0.21$) to the lungs through the upper airway.

Fixed-performance oxygen delivery system an oxygen delivery system that can supply all the inspired gas needs of a patient at a given F_{IO_2}; sometimes called high-flow oxygen delivery systems.

Variable-performance oxygen delivery system an oxygen delivery system not capable of meeting all the inspiratory volume or flow needs of the patient, thereby delivering an F_{IO_2} that varies with ventilatory demand; sometimes called low-flow oxygen delivery systems.

Oxygen proportioner a device designed to mix oxygen and air in precise concentrations using proportioning valves. These devices are sometimes referred to as blenders. An oxygen proportioner provides precise concentrations of gas at 50 psi to operate other equipment.

Oxygen saturation the amount of oxygen bound to hemoglobin expressed as a percentage.

Oxygen toxicity the pathologic response of the body and its tissues resulting from long-term exposure to high partial pressure of oxygen; pulmonary manifestations include cellular changes causing congestion, inflammation, and edema.

Oxyhemoglobin the chemical combination resulting from the covalent bonding of oxygen to the ferrous iron pigment in hemoglobin.

Paramagnetic O_2 analyzer a device that measures the partial pressure of oxygen in a gas sample by exploiting the paramagnetic quality of oxygen.

Partial pressure the pressure exerted by a single gas in a gas mixture.

Passive expiration expiration not assisted by the ventilatory muscles or by any ventilator-induced change in transrespiratory pressure causing flow in the expiratory direction.

Peak flowmeter a device that is used to measure a patient's peak expiratory flow rate. This is commonly done to assess the effectiveness of bronchodilator therapy.

PEEP acronym for positive end-expiratory pressure.

Pendelluft movement of gas from "fast" to "slow" filling spaces during breathing; alternatively, the ineffective movement of gas back and forth (accompanied by a mediastinal shifting) between a healthy lung and one with a flail segment caused by a crushing chest injury.

Percuss to strike with short, sharp blows; may be used for diagnosis, as when percussion is used to determine chest resonance, or for therapy, as a component of chest physical therapy.

Percussors mechanical devices (electric or pneumatic) that produce vibrations when applied to the chest wall. Percussors help to improve the effectiveness of chest physiotherapy. They relieve the muscle fatigue experienced by respiratory care practitioners when performing manual percussion.

pH symbol for the logarithm of the reciprocal of the H^+ ion concentration.

Phase one of four significant events that occur during a ventilatory cycle: (1) the change from expiratory time to inspiratory time; (2) inspiratory time; (3) the change from inspiratory time to expiratory time; and (4) expiratory time.

Phase variable a variable (ie, pressure, volume, flow, or time) that is measured and used to initiate some phase of the ventilatory cycle.

Phase variable value the magnitude of a phase variable.

Pharyngeal tracheal lumen airway a device used to allow ventilation in emergency situations when endotracheal intubation is impossible.

pH glass a special type of glass that is permeable to hydrogen ions. This glass is used to develop a potential (voltage) between two solutions of differing pH.

Piezoelectric transducer a transducer capable of converting electrical energy in to physical energy usually in the form of high-frequency vibrations.

Pilot balloon an inflatable chamber near the distal end of the pilot tube that supplies gas pressure and volume to inflate the cuff of an artificial airway. Inflation of the balloon indicates that the cuff contains air. Cuff pressures should be monitored to help prevent pressure necrosis, rather than solely relying on the "feel" of the pilot balloon.

Pilot tube the line that supplies pressure to the cuff of an artificial airway. It is a small-diameter line connected to the artificial airway, and it terminates inside the cuff.

Plethysmography measuring and recording changes in volume of an organ or other part of the body by a plethysmograph.

Pneumotachometer a transducer designed to measure the flow of respiratory gases, usually by measuring pressure differences across a tube of known resistance.

Pneumotachograph an instrument that incorporates a pneumotachometer to record variations in the flow of respiratory gases.

Poiseuille's law describes the relationship between volumetric flow, viscosity, pressure, length, and velocity of a gas flowing through a tube. Poiseuille's law only applies for laminar flow. One important relationship of Poiseuille's law is that as the radius of a tube is decreased by [1/2], the resistance of gas flow increases by 16 times.

Polarity having two poles; in physics, the distinction between a negatively and positively charged pole.

Polarographic of or pertaining to a device or instrument that employs the flow of electrical current between negatively and positively charged poles to measure a physical phenomenon.

Pores of Kohn direct intercommunications between alveoli ranging from 5 to 15 μm in diameter.

Positive end-expiratory pressure (PEEP) the application and maintenance of pressure above atmospheric at the airway throughout the expiratory phase of positive-pressure mechanical ventilation.

Postural drainage the therapeutic use of patient positioning and gravity to facilitate the mobilization of respiratory tract secretions.

Potential energy the energy a body possesses by its position.

Potentiometer a wire-wound variable resistor that operates by changing its effective length, altering its total resistance.

Precision the ability of an instrument to reliably reproduce known reference values over a series of measurements.

Premarket application petition filed by a manufacturer to obtain an investigational device exemption from the FDA.

Pressure force per unit area exerted by a gas or liquid.

Pressure disconnect alarm a device that detects loss of pressure in a ventilation system and warns the operator with an audible and/or visual alarm.

Pressure support ventilation (PSV) pressure-limited assisted ventilation designed to augment a spontaneously generated breath; the patient has primary control over the frequency of breathing, the inspiratory time, and the inspiratory flow.

Preventative maintenance the regularly scheduled testing and service of in-use equipment, designed to prevent failure or malfunction.

Principle of paramagnetism the physical principle that some gases are attracted to the strongest portion of a magnetic field (oxygen is a paramagnetic gas). This principle is employed in the operation of a physical oxygen analyzer.

Printing device output device for a computer that allows hard copies of data to be made.

Programming languages method of communication used to program a computer to run a routine.

Proportioning valve a device that mixes oxygen and air in precise concentrations. These devices operate using a proportioning valve. Sometimes proportioning valves are referred to as blenders.

psi pounds per square inch. Unit of pressure measurement.

psia pounds per square inch absolute; psia is based on a reference point of 0, a perfect vacuum; psia is equal to psig plus atmospheric pressure. At sea level, psig is 0 but psia is 14.7.

psig pounds per square inch gauge.

Psychrometer a wet and dry bulb thermometry device used to measure relative humidity.

Pulmonary artery catheter a catheter inserted into the vena cava and advanced through the right side of the heart until the tip is in the pulmonary arterial tree. Pulmonary artery catheters are used to measure cardiac output and wedge pressure.

Pulse oximeter a monitoring device that measures oxygen saturation noninvasively using red and infrared light.

Quality control the use of statistical analysis in conjunction with known standards to assess an instrument's accuracy, reliability, and reproducibility. Quality control programs also identify technical and random errors that may occur in the operation of the instrument.

Radioaerosol an aerosol with particles that have been labeled with a radioactive isotope and used to assist researchers in analyzing aerosol deposition and clearance in the lung.

Random access memory (RAM) the working space or temporary storage area for the program being used. RAM is erased when the power is turned off.

Read only memory (ROM) the part of the computer's main memory that contains the basic programs that run the computer when it is turned on. ROM cannot be erased.

Reducing valve a device designed to reduce a source gas pressure.

Reference electrode an electrode with a constant potential used with another electrode to complete an electrical circuit through a solution.

Regulator a device designed to control both the pressure and flow of a compressed gas.

Relative humidity the relationship of the actual humidity in a gas sample and the absolute humidity that gas can hold. RH % = actual humidity/absolute humidity.

Resistance impedance to flow in a tube or conduit; quantified as ratio of the difference in pressure between the two points along a tube length divided by the volumetric flow of the fluid per unit time.

Respiratory inductive plethysmography an instrument that indirectly measures tidal volume and respiratory frequency using bands around the chest and abdomen.

Respirometer a device used to measure the volume of respired air or gas.

Response time a measure (usually in milliseconds) of the speed with a mechanical ventilator that can respond to a patient's inspiratory effort and cycle into the inspiratory phase.

Reynold's number the Reynold's number equation is used to predict whether gas flow will be laminar or turbulent. The calculation accounts for the gas's velocity, viscosity density, and diameter of the tube. If the number is less than 2000, flow will be laminar.

Rheostat a variable resistor that controls the flow of electrical current.

Safety system any system designed to prevent or minimize hazards due to human error; in medical gas therapy, a system of connections designed to help prevent accidental interchanging of incorrect equipment or gases during their administration.

- **American Standard Safety System (ASSS)** provides specifications for threaded high-pressure connections between compressed gas cylinders and their attachments.
- **Diameter-indexed safety system (DISS)** provides specifications for threaded low-pressure (less than 200 psig) connections between station outlets, flowmeters, and other therapy devices, such as nebulizers, ventilators, and anesthesia apparatus.
- **Pin-indexed safety system (PISS)** a subsection of the American Standard Safety System applicable only to the valve outlets of small cylinders, up to and including size E, and employing a yoke-and-pin–type connection.

Scissors valve the expiratory valve of the Siemens Servo 900B and 900C ventilators that controls end-expiratory pressure by "pinching" the exhalation with a hinged valve resembling scissors.

Sedimentation the rate at which particles fall out of suspension as related to gravity and the buoyancy provided by the carrier gas.

Sensitivity a measure of the amount of a negative pressure that must be generated by a patient to trigger a mechanical ventilator into the inspiratory phase; alternatively, the mechanism used to set or control this level.

Sensor a device designed to respond to physical stimuli such as temperature, light, magnetism, or movement and transmit resulting impulses for interpretation, recording movement, or operating control.

Servo controlled control of a measured variable by constant input from a signal.

Severinghaus electrode the P_{CO_2} electrode in a blood gas system or transcutaneous electrode.

Sidestream monitor a monitor that samples from the main gas stream through a vacuum pump.

Silica gel crystals crystals used to dry a gas sample; often referred to as desiccant.

SIMV abbreviation for synchronous intermittent mandatory ventilation.

Solenoid valve a type of electromechanical valve that operates using an electromagnet to open the valve. Spring tension usually returns the valve to the closed position.

Solid a firm, compact body that retains its form when not contained.

Solubility coefficient (gas) the volume of gas that can be dissolved in 1 mL of a given liquid at standard pressure and specified temperature.

Solute the substance dissolved in a solution.

Solution a homogeneous and stable mixture of two or more substances, evenly dispersed throughout each other at the molecular level; a saturated solution is one with the maximum amount of solute that can be held by a given volume of a solvent at a constant temperature in the presence of an excess of solute.

Solvent the medium in which a solute is dissolved.

Specific heat the ratio between the amount of heat required to raise the temperature of 1 g of a substance 1°C (cgs) or 1 pound of a substance 1°F at a specific temperature (fps), and the amount of heat required to raise the temperature of 1 g of water 1°C or 1 pound of water 1°F at the specified temperature.

Spectrophotometry the measurement of color in a solution by determining the amount of light absorbed in the ultraviolet, infrared, or visible spectrum; widely used in clinical chemistry to calculate the concentration of substances in solution.

Spinning disk nebulizer a nebulizer that produces an aerosol by drawing water up a siphon tube and using centrifugal force to propel the water droplets.

Spirometer an apparatus designed to measure and record lung volumes and flows.

Spirometry laboratory evaluation of lung function using a spirometer.

Spontaneous breath breath that is both patient initiated and patient terminated; an unassisted breath.

Spontaneous PEEP system a continuous flow system for a spontaneously breathing patient characterized by elevated airway pressure during the expiratory phase. During inspiration, airway pressure is subambient.

Sporicidal destructive to the spore form of bacteria.

Sporicide any agent effective in destroying spores, such as compounds of chlorine and formaldehyde and the glutaraldehydes.

Spreadsheet a grid made up of columns and rows that contain data or formulas often used for financial planning and data collection.

Station outlet the point in a piped medical gas distribution system at which the user normally makes connections and disconnections.

Stepper motor a type of electric motor that moves in discrete positions or steps in response to an input voltage. The voltage applied to the motor determines how far it will move.

Sterile free from any living microorganisms.

Sterilization the complete destruction of all microorganisms, usually by heat or chemical means.

STPD abbreviation for standard temperature, standard pressure, dry.

Stylet a device used to preshape a tube for easier insertion.

Suction catheter a thin tube connected to a vacuum device used for removal of patient secretions.

Sulfhemoglobin sulfur bound to hemoglobin.

Temperature the sensible intensity of heat in any substance; the measure of the average kinetic energy of the molecules making up a substance.

Thermal conductivity the efficiency of heat transfer between objects, measured in (cal/s) × (cm² × C/cm) (cgs).

Thermal equilibrium a condition in which the temperatures of two substances exist at the same temperature; a condition in which heat transfer is in a steady state.

Thermistor an electronic thermometer, the impedance of which varies with temperature; used for measuring minute changes in temperature.

Thermoconductivity measurement the movement or temperature through a body.

Thermophilic growing best under conditions of high temperature.

Thermostat an electrical or mechanical device that regulates and maintains a set temperature in a given system.

Thorpe tube a variable-orifice, constant-pressure, flow-metering device consisting of a tapered transparent tube with a float; the diameter of the tube increases from bottom to top, with the float suspended by flow against the force of gravity at a level determined by the rate of flow.

Threshold resistor a type of expiratory pressure valve that maintains a relatively constant pressure regardless of flow.

Trach button a device used to temporarily obstruct a tracheostomy for the purpose of allowing the patient to breathe normally.

Tracheal tube changer a tube inserted into an endotracheal tube that allows removal of the endotracheal tube and replacement with a new one. The tube changer acts as a guide for placement.

Tracheostomy an opening through the neck into the trachea, through which an indwelling tube may be inserted.

Transcutaneous monitor a device that measures gas tensions across the skin.

Transducer a device capable of converting one form of energy into another and commonly used for measurement of physical events; for example, a pressure transducer may convert the physical phenomenon of force per unit area into an analog electrical signal.

Transfill to fill across; to fill a vessel from another vessel.

Transient expiratory assist pressure (TEAP) a mechanically created, transient baseline pressure that is lower than the end-expiratory pressure of the previous breath. This transient baseline lasts until the volume inspired during the previous breath has been exhaled, at which time the baseline pressure is increased to the previous end-expiratory pressure.

Transpulmonary across the lung; of or pertaining to the difference in a parameter (eg, pressure) between the alveoli and pleural space.

Transrespiratory pressure the pressure difference between airway and body surface (ie, airway pressure − body surface pressure).

Trigger to initiate the inspiratory phase of an assisted breath.

- **Flow trigger** initiation of inspiration following the patient's inspiratory effort exceeding the flow sensitivity setting.
- **Pressure trigger** initiation of inspiration following the patient's inspiratory effort exceeding the pressure sensitivity setting.
- **Time trigger** initiation of inspiration by the ventilator according to the respiratory frequency setting.

Triple point that combination of temperature and pressure that allows the solid, liquid, and vapor forms of a given substance to exist in equilibrium with one another.

Turbinometer an instrument for measuring flow using spinning blades or vanes.

Turbulent flow flow characterized by chaotic molecular movement with formation of irregular eddy currents. Reynold's number > 2000.

Ventilatory period the time from the beginning of inspiratory flow of one breath to the beginning of inspiratory flow for the next breath (total cycle time); the sum of inspiratory time and expiratory time; the reciprocal of ventilatory frequency.

Venturi tube a specially designed tube that includes a dilation of the tube lumen just distal to a constriction; if the angulation of the dilation is not over 15 degrees, the pressure of flowing fluid will be restored nearly to its prerestriction levels.

Venturi's principle a principle which relates a pressure reduction within a diverging duct to the velocity of the gas flowing through it. As velocity increases, the pressure at the tube's restriction decreases. Venturi's principle applies when the gas's flow is noncompressible.

Virucidal destructive to viruses.

Virucide any agent that destroys or inactivates viruses.

Viscosity the internal force that opposes the flow of fluid, either liquids or gases.

Viscous shearing a phenomenon by which gas or a liquid may be entrained into a high-velocity gas stream by shear forces and vortices or eddies.

Volume space occupied by matter measured in milliliters or liters.

Volume-displacement spirometer instrument that measures volume by collecting gas in a leakproof expandable container.

Water column expiratory pressure valve a threshold resistor that uses the weight of a column of water over a diaphragm to maintain expiratory airway pressure.

Water-sealed spirometer a volume displacement spirometer that uses a bell, open at one end, submerged in water.

Water vapor pressure the partial pressure of water in a gas sample. At body temperature and humidity water vapor pressure is 47 mm Hg.

Watt a unit of power equivalent to work done at the rate of 1 joule per second.

WEDGE spirometer a type of bellows spirometer. WEDGE is an acronym for *w*aterless, *e*ffortless, *d*ata-*g*enerating, and *e*lectromechanical.

Weir method equation for calculation of heat production (Kcal) from oxygen consumption and carbon dioxide production.

Wheatstone bridge a sensitive electrical circuit composed of four resisters arranged in a square that allows the measurement of a small change in voltage or current. These are used in conjunction with transducers to measure pressure or flow changes.

Word processor an automated, computerized system, incorporating variously an electronic typewriter, video display terminal, and printer, used to prepare reports, records, and other data.

Yankauer tip a rigid suction tip used to aspirate secretions, blood, or foreign materials from the oropharynx.

Zeolite a commercial name for inorganic sodium-aluminum silicate; due to its ability to absorb both gaseous nitrogen and water vapor from air, zeolite is used extensively in certain oxygen concentrators.

Zone valve a safety valve that is placed in an oxygen piping system such that gas flow may be shut off in the event of a fire or other emergency.

Z-79 an abbreviation for the Z-79 Committee of the American National Standards Institute, a committee that develops standards for anesthesia and ventilatory devices, including anesthesia equipment, reservoir bags, tracheal tubes, humidifiers, nebulizers, and other oxygen-related equipment; when appearing on such equipment, the Z-79 designation signifies that the device meets the design standards established by this voluntary regulatory group.

Index

NOTE: A *t* following a page number indicates tabular material, an *f* following a page number indicates a figure, and a *b* following a page number indicates a box. Drugs are listed under their generic names. When a drug trade name is listed, the reader is referred to the generic name.

A

B

E

N

O

P

Q

R

S

T

W

Y

Z